LIPPINCOTT'S REVIEW FOR
NCLEX•RN

LIPPINCOTT'S REVIEW FOR NCLEX-RN

5th EDITION

Diane M. Billings, RN, EdD, FAAN

Professor of Nursing and Assistant Dean of Learning Resources
Indiana University
School of Nursing
Indianapolis, Indiana

J.B. LIPPINCOTT COMPANY
Philadelphia

Acquisitions Editor: ***Donna L. Hilton, RN, BSN***
Coordinating Editorial Assistant: ***Susan M. Keneally***
Interior Design: ***Ellen Dawson***
Production Manager: ***Janet Greenwood***
Production: ***Tapsco, Inc.***
Compositor: ***Achorn Graphic Services***
Text Printer/Binder: ***The Courier Companies***
Cover Printer: ***Lehigh Press***

Fifth Edition

6 5 4 3

Library of Congress Cataloging-in-Publication Data

Billings, Diane McGovern.
Lippincott's review for NCLEX-RN — 5th ed. / Diane M. Billings.
p. cm.
Rev. ed. of: Lippincott's state board review for NCLEX-RN / Edwina A. McConnell, LuVerne Wolff Lewis. 4th ed. ©1990.
Includes bibliographical references and index.
ISBN 0-397-55058-8 (soft cover)
1. Nursing—Examinations, questions, etc. I. McConnell Edwina A. Lippincott's state board review for NCLEX-RN. II. Title.
III. Title: Review for NCLEX-RN.
[DNLM: 1. Nursing—examination questions. WY 18 B598L 1994]
RT55.M29 1994
610.73'076—dc20
DNLM/DLC
for Library of Congress 93-20781
CIP

Any procedure or practice described in this book should be applied by the health-care practitioner under appropriate supervision in accordance with professional standards of care used with regard to the unique circumstances that apply in each practice situation. Care has been taken to confirm the accuracy of information presented and to describe generally accepted practices. However, the authors, editors and publisher cannot accept any responsibility for errors or omissions or for consequences from application of the information in this book and make no warranty, express or implied, with respect to the contents of the book.

The authors and publisher have exerted every effort to ensure that drug selection and dosage set forth in this text are in accord with current recommendations and practice at the time of publication. However, in view of ongoing research, changes in government regulations, and the constant flow of information relating to drug therapy and drug reactions, the reader is urged to check the package insert of each drug for any change in indications and dosage and for added warnings and precautions. This is particularly important when the recommended agent is a new or infrequently used drug.

Contributors

Susan Bennett, RN, DNS
Assistant Professor of Nursing
Indiana University School of Nursing
Indianapolis, Indiana

Karen Cobb, RN, EdD (Cand.)
Assistant Professor of Nursing
Indiana University School of Nursing
Indianapolis, Indiana

Judith Halstead, RN, DNS
Assistant Professor of Nursing
Indiana University School of Nursing
Indianapolis, Indiana

Patricia Henry, RN, MSN
Lecturer
Indiana University School of Nursing
South Bend, Indiana

Virginia Richardson, RN, DNS (Cand.), CPNP
Assistant Professor of Nursing
Indiana University School of Nursing
Indianapolis, Indiana

Carol Bostrom, RN, MSN
Clinical Assistant Professor
Indiana University School of Nursing
Indianapolis, Indiana

CONTRIBUTORS TO THE PREVIOUS EDITIONS

Janice R. Anderzon, RN, BSN, MS
Clinical Professor, Nursing
University of Wisconsin–Madison
School of Nursing
Madison, Wisconsin

Linda Brown, RN, PhD

Deborah Chyun, RN, BSN, MSN
Lecturer, Cardiovascular Specialty
Medical-Surgical Nursing Program
Yale University
School of Nursing
New Haven, Connecticut

Joanne R. Conger, RN, BSN, MS
Clinical Associate Professor, Emeritus
Adult Medical-Surgical Nursing
University of Wisconsin–Madison
School of Nursing
Madison, Wisconsin

Suzanne Saunders Cooke, RN, CS, MSN
Associate Professor of Clinical Nursing
Texas Tech University Health Sciences Center
School of Nursing
Lubbock, Texas

Richard Creager, RN, BSN
Staff Nurse, Mobile Unit
Meriter Hospital
Madison University
Madison, Wisconsin

Catherine Gray Deering, PhD, RN, CS
Assistant Professor
Clayton State College
Morrow, Georgia

Patricia E. Downing, RN, MN

James A. Fain, PhD, RN
Associate Dean
Nursing
Yale University
School of Nursing
New Haven, Connecticut

Pamela Billings Farley, RN, PhD
Assistant Professor
Department of Nursing
Berea College
Berea, Kentucky

Sarah P. Farrell, RN, MSN, CS

Kathleen A. Furitano, RN, MSN
Pediatric Clinical Nurse Specialist
University of Illinois Hospital
Adjunct Assistant Professor
College of Nursing
University of Illinois
Chicago, Illinois

Collen Gullickson, RN, PhD
Assistant Professor
School of Nursing
University of Wisconsin
Madison, Wisconsin

Diane Hamilton, RN, PhD

Benda Hanson–Smith, RNC, MSN

Marsha L. Heims, RN, EdD
Associate Professor
Department of Family Nursing
Oregon Health Sciences University
Portland, Oregon

Cindy Peterson Helstad, RN, MS
Research Assistant
Center for Health Systems Research and Analysis
University of Wisconsin–Madison
Madison, Wisconsin

Louise M. Juliani, RN, BSN, MS
Charge Nurse
Extended Care Facility
St. Thomas More Benedictine Health Care Center
Canon City, Colorado

Kathryn B. Kolar, RN, MSN
Associate Professor
School of Nursing
University of Mississippi
Jackson, Mississippi

Sara E. Kolb, PhD, RN
Associate Professor
Division of Nursing and the Sciences
Incarnate Word College
San Antonio, Texas

Nancy A. Smyth Markin, RN, PNA, MSN
Professor of Nursing
Oakton Community College
Des Plaines, Illinois

Yondell Masten, RN, C, PhD, OGNP
Professor
Texas Tech University Health Sciences Center
School of Nursing
Lubbock, Texas

Diane M. Matousek, RN, MSN
PhD Candidate
Department of Epidemiology and Public Health
Yale University
School of Medicine
New Haven, Connecticut

Marlene L. McClure, RN, MSN
Professor
Department of Nursing
Pittsburgh State University
Pittsburgh, Kansas

Ellen K. Murphy, MS, JD, FAAN
Associate Professor
School of Nursing
University of Wisconsin–Milwaukee
Milwaukee, Wisconsin

Susan Nitzke, PhD, RD
Associate Professor
Nutritional Sciences
University of Wisconsin–Madison/Extension
Madison, Wisconsin

Linda Denise Oakley, RN, PhD

Joyce M. Olson, RN, MSN
Pediatric Clinical Nurse Specialist
Department of Nursing Services
University of Kansas Medical Center
Kansas City, Kansas

Carol Pederson, PhD, RN
Assistant Professor
School of Nursing
University of Minnesota
Minneapolis, Minnesota

Cherly V. Ratliff, RN, MS, MN

Carol F. Rosenkranz, RN, MN
Education Coordinator
Education Services
Methodist Medical Center
Jackson, Mississippi

Judith K. Sands, RN, EdD
Associate Professor, Director of Undergraduate Studies
University of Virginia
School of Nursing
Charlottesville, Virginia

Lola J. Sasser, RNC, MSN
Associate Professor
University of Mississippi
School of Nursing
Jackson, Mississippi

M. Lisa Sinacore, MSN, RN
Specialty Care/Home Care
Staff Nurse
St. Louis Children's Hospital
St. Louis, Missouri

Suzanne Smith, MSN, RNCS
Associate Professor
College of Nursing and Health Sciences
Winona State University
Winona, Minnesota

Kathryn Lee Sridaromont, RN, MSN
Associate Professor of Clinical Nursing
School of Nursing
Texas Tech University
Health Sciences Center
Lubbock, Texas

Jo Stejskal, RN, EdD
Chairperson, Nursing
Associate Professor
Winona State University
Winona, Minnesota

Barbara Romano Teague, RN, MSN, CPNA
Faculty, University of Kentucky
College of Nursing
Lexington, Kentucky

Bridget Thompson, RN, MSN
Assistant Professor
Family and Community Nursing
University of North Dakota
College of Nursing
Grand Forks, North Dakota

Lynda Zibell, RN, MSN

Preface

Passing the National Council Licensure Examination for Registered Nurses (NCLEX-RN) marks the beginning of a nurse's professional career. *Lippincott's Review for the NCLEX-RN* was developed to help students write this examination successfully, although they have been preparing for it since entering nursing school. The same examination is currently used in all 50 states, the District of Columbia, and United States possessions. Students graduated from baccalaureate, diploma, and associate degree programs in nursing must pass this examination to meet licensure requirements in the United States.

The National Council of State Boards of Nursing, Inc., is an organization with representation from all state boards of nursing. It prepares the test plan used to develop the licensure examination. The test plan is formulated on health care situations that registered nurses commonly encounter and addresses two components: (1) phases of the nursing process and (2) client needs. Representative items test knowledge of these components as they relate to specific health care situations.

This book includes the following major features:

- The introduction explains how the licensure examination is prepared, how to review for it, strategies to help write it successfully, and ways in which to use this book most effectively.
- The test plan developed for the state licensure examination by the National Council of State Boards of Nursing, Inc., was used to prepare this book.
- This book is divided into two sections. The first section represents the four main clinical areas of nursing; the second section is composed of four comprehensive tests. This format enables candidates to review one or more clinical areas and/or to write one or more comprehensive tests, which are designed to resemble NCLEX-RN.
- Each test presents a variety of situations commonly encountered in nursing practice. Just as NCLEX-RN is comprehensive, so are the tests in this book.
- Hundreds of items are new to this edition of the book. Items used from the previous edition have been carefully reviewed and in some instances extensively revised before being included in this edition. Outdated items have been discarded.
- The review tests are grouped according to clinical disciplines so that candidates can review one clinical area at a time.
- The topics tested in all clinical disciplines have been expanded.
- Candidates using this book can evaluate their success on the comprehensive tests. Directions for interpreting self-evaluative results are included.
- Correct answers and rationale are given for all items in this book. The rationales explain why the correct answer is correct, as well as why the distractors are incorrect.
- The study plan "checklist" can be used to systematically develop a study plan.
- Diagnostic grids at the end of each test can be used to identify areas for further study based on content, step of the nursing process, and area of client need.
- The computer disk allows candidates to practice taking computer adaptive tests.
- References are provided at the end of each clinical section. Candidates can verify correct answers, clarify subject matter, or increase knowledge about a specific content area by consulting these references.
- Contributors to the book were selected for their expertise in specific content areas. A national perspective, rather than regional policies and practices, is represented.
- The address and telephone number of the National Council of State Boards of Nursing, Inc., and for each state board of nursing are listed in the Appendix.
- While the target audience of this book is the student preparing to write the licensure examination for registered nurses, other nurses will find it helpful. These nurses include those preparing for challenge examinations, inactive nurses preparing to return to practice, practicing nurses transferring to a different clinical area, and nursing faculty.

I would like to acknowledge the editors and item writers of the previous editions of this book and extend acknowledgment to Edwina A. McConnell for creating a tradition of excellence in NCLEX-RN books. Special thanks to the item writers of this edition—Susan Bennett, Karen Cobb, Judith Halstead, Patricia Henry, and Virginia Richardson; to Bill Collins for designing the answer grids and test item figure; and to Jennifer Morris for the original art work. Thanks also to Donna Hilton, Diana Intenzo, Susan Perry, and Maria Zacierka for their editorial expertise. Finally, thanks to my family for their never-ending support.

Diane M. Billings, EdD, RN, FAAN

Contents

Introduction xv

Section One: Practice Tests

Part I: The Nursing Care of Clients With Psychosocial Health Problems 3

Test 1: Mood Disorders and Crisis Situations 5

The Client With a Major Mood Disorder 5
The Client With Bipolar Disorder, Manic Phase 7
The Client Who Is Depressed 9
The Client With Depressive Disorder and Suicidal Ideation 11
The Client Who Attempts Suicide 13
The Client in Crisis 14

Correct Answers and Rationale *17*

Test 2: Personality Disorders, Organic Disorders, Using a Therapeutic Milieu 29

The Client Who Is Paranoid 29
The Client With Catatonic Schizophrenia 31
The Client With Chronic Mental Illness 32
The Client With an Obsessive-Compulsive Disorder 34
The Client With Organic Mental Syndromes and Disorders 35
Using a Therapeutic Milieu 37

Correct Answers and Rationale *39*

Test 3: Chemical Dependency and Eating Disorders 51

The Client With a Personality Disorder 51
The Client Who Abuses Alcohol 53
The Client With Alcohol Withdrawal 54
The Client Who Is Dependent on Narcotics 56
The Client Who Abuses Barbiturates 57
The Client With an Eating Disorder 58

Correct Answers and Rationale *60*

Test 4: Anxiety, Anger, Abuse, Terminal Illness 71

The Client With Anxiety 71
The Client With Maladaptive Behavior Patterns 72
The Client With Problems Expressing Anger 74
The Client With Family Abuse and Violence 76
The Client With a Psychophysiological Disorder 78
The Client With a Terminal Illness 79

Correct Answers and Rationale *82*

Bibliography 93

Part II: The Nursing Care of the Childbearing Family and Their Neonate 95

Test 1: Antepartum Care 97

The Preconception Client 97
The Pregnant Client Receiving Prenatal Care 99
The Pregnant Client in Childbirth Preparation Classes 103
The Pregnant Client With Risk Factors 105

Correct Answers and Rationale *107*

Test 2: Complications of Pregnancy 119

The Client With Pregnancy-Induced Hypertension 119
The Client With a Hypertensive Disorder 122
The Client With Third Trimester Bleeding 122
The Client With Preterm Labor 123
The Client With Diabetes Mellitus 124
The Client With an Ectopic Pregnancy 125
The Client With a Hydatidiform Mole 126
The Client With Premature Rupture of the Membranes 127

Correct Answers and Rationale *128*

Test 3: The Birth Experience 139

The Primigravida in Labor 139
The Multigravida in Labor 142
The Intrapartal Client With Risk Factors 142

Correct Answers and Rationale *148*

Test 4: Postpartum Care 161

The Postpartal Client With a Vaginal Birth 161
The Postpartal Client Who Breast-Feeds 164
The Postpartal Client Who Bottle Feeds 166
The Postpartal Client With a Cesarean Birth 166
Correct Answers and Rationale *171*

Test 5: The Neonate 183

The Neonatal Client 183
Physical Assessment of the Neonatal Client 184
The Post term Neonate 185
The Neonate With Risk Factors 186
Correct Answers and Rationale *193*

Bibliography 206

Part III: Nursing Care of Children 207

Test 1: Health Promotion 209

Health Promotion for the Infant and Family 209
Health Promotion for the Toddler and Family 210
Health Promotion for the Preschool-Age Child and Family 211
Health Promotion for the School-Age Child and Family 213
Health Promotion for the Adolescent and Family 214
Meetings to Discuss Common Childhood and Adolescent Health Problems 215
Correct Answers and Rationale *218*

Test 2: The Child With Respiratory Health Problems 229

The Client With Tonsillitis 229
The Client With Chronic Otitis Media 230
The Client With Foreign Body Aspiration 231
The Client With Asthma 232
The Client With Cystic Fibrosis and Bronchopneumonia 233
The Client With Sudden Infant Death Syndrome 234
The Client Requiring Cardiopulmonary Resuscitation 235
Correct Answers and Rationale *236*

Test 3: The Child With Cardiovascular Health Problems 247

The Child With a Ventricular Septal Defect 247
The Client With Tetralogy of Fallot 248
The Client With Down Syndrome 249
The Client With Rheumatic Fever 250
The Client With Sickle-Cell Anemia 251
The Client With Iron-Deficiency Anemia 252
The Client With Hemophilia and Acquired Immune Deficiency Syndrome 253
The Client With Leukemia 254
Correct Answers and Rationale *257*

Test 4: The Child With Health Problems of the Upper Gastrointestinal Tract 269

The Client With Cleft Lip and Palate 269
The Client With a Tracheoesophageal Fistula 270
The Client With Imperforate Anus 271
The Client With Pyloric Stenosis 272
The Client With Intussusception 274
The Client With Inguinal Hernia 274
The Client With Hirschsprung's Disease 275
Correct Answers and Rationale *278*

Test 5: The Child With Health Problems of the Lower Gastrointestinal Tract 289

The Client With Diarrhea/Gastroenteritis 289
The Client With Appendicitis 291
The Client With Ingestion of Toxic Substances 292
The Client With Celiac Disease 293
The Client With Phenylketonuria 294
The Client With Colic 295
The Client With Obesity 295
The Client With Cow's Milk Sensitivity 296
Correct Answers and Rationale *298*

Test 6: The Child With Health Problems of the Urinary System 309

The Client With Cryptorchidism 309
The Client With Hydrocele 310
The Client With Hypospadias 311
The Client With Urinary Tract Infection 311
The Client With Glomerulonephritis 312
The Client With Nephrotic Syndrome 314
The Client With Acute/Chronic Renal Failure 315
Correct Answers and Rationale *318*

Test 7: The Child With Neurological Health Problems **329**

The Client With Myelomeningocele 329
The Client With Hydrocephalus 330
The Client With a Seizure Disorder 331
The Client With Meningitis 333
The Client With Infectious Polyneuritis (Guillain-Barré Syndrome) 334
The Client With a Head Injury 335
The Client With a Brain Tumor 336
The Client With a Spinal Cord Injury 337

Correct Answers and Rationale *338*

Test 8: The Child With Musculoskeletal Health Problems **349**

Clients With Musculoskeletal Dysfunction 349
The Client With Cerebral Palsy 350
The Client With Duchenne's Muscular Dystrophy 351
The Client With Congenital Hip Dysplasia 351
The Client With Congenital Clubfoot 352
The Client With Juvenile Rheumatoid Arthritis (JRA) 353
The Client With a Fracture 353
The Client With Osteomyelitis 356

Correct Answers and Rationale *357*

Test 9: The Child With Dermatologic, Endocrine, and Other Health Problems **367**

The Client Who Is Preterm 367
The Infant Who Is Septic 368
The Client With Failure to Thrive 369
The Client With Atopic Dermatitis 369
The Client With Burns 370
The Client With Hypothyroidism 371
The Client With Insulin-Dependent Diabetes Mellitus 372
Clients Who Are Abused 374

Correct Answers and Rationale *375*

Bibliography **386**

Part IV: The Nursing Care of Adults With Medical/Surgical Health Problems **387**

Test 1: The Client With Respiratory Health Problems **389**

The Client With Pneumonia 389
The Client With Tuberculosis 390
The Client With Chronic Obstructive Pulmonary Disease (COPD) 390
The Client With Lung Cancer 391
The Client With Chest Trauma 391
General Questions 392

Correct Answers and Rationale *398*

Test 2: The Client With Cardiovascular Health Problems **409**

The Client With Myocardial Infarction 409
The Client With Congestive Heart Failure (CHF) 410
The Client With Valvular Heart Disease 410
The Client With Hypertension 411
The Client With Angina 411
General Questions 412
The Client With Pernicious Anemia 417
The Client With Hodgkin's Disease 418
The Client Requiring Cardiopulmonary Resuscitation 418
The Client in Shock 419
The Client With Anemia 420
The Clients Who Are Dying 420
General Questions 421

Correct Answers and Rationale *422*

Test 3: The Client With Upper Gastrointestinal Tract Health Problems **439**

The Client With Peptic Ulcer Disease 439
The Client With Cholecystitis 440
The Client With Cancer of the Stomach 441
The Client With Pancreatitis 442
The Client With Hiatal Hernia 444
General Questions 445

Correct Answers and Rationale *447*

Test 4: The Client With Lower Gastrointestinal Tract Health Problems **457**

The Client With Cancer of the Colon 457
The Client With Hepatitis A 458
The Client With Hepatitis B 459
The Client With Hemorrhoids 460
The Client With Inflammatory Bowel Disease 460
The Client With Intestinal Obstruction 462
The Client With Cirrhosis 463
The Client With an Ileostomy 464
General Questions 465

Correct Answers and Rationale *466*

Test 5: The Client With Endocrine Health Problems **477**

The Client With Hyperthyroidism 477
The Client With Diabetes Mellitus 478
The Client With Pituitary Adenoma 478
The Client With Addison's Disease 479
The Client With Cushing's Disease 479
General Questions 480

Correct Answers and Rationale *485*

Test 6: The Client With Urinary Tract Health Problems **495**

The Client With Cancer of the Bladder 495
The Client With Renal Calculi 496
The Client With Acute Renal Failure 498
The Client With Urinary Tract Infection 499
The Client With Pyelonephritis 500
The Client With Chronic Renal Failure 500
General Questions 502

Correct Answers and Rationale *503*

Test 7: The Client With Reproductive Health Problems **513**

The Client With Uterine Fibroids 513
The Client With Breast Cancer 514
The Client With Benign Prostatic Hypertrophy 514
The Client With a Sexually Transmitted Disease 515
The Client With Cancer of the Cervix 516
The Client With Testicular Cancer 516
General Questions 517

Correct Answers and Rationale *522*

Test 8: The Client With Neurological Health Problems **533**

The Client With a Head Injury 533
The Client With Seizures 534
The Client With Cerebrovascular Accident 536
The Client With Parkinson's Disease 537
The Client With Multiple Sclerosis 538
The Unconscious Client 539
The Client in Pain 541

Correct Answers and Rationale *544*

Test 9: The Client With Musculoskeletal Health Problems **557**

The Client With Arthritis 557
The Client With a Hip Fracture 558
The Client With a Herniated Disc 560
The Client With Peripheral Vascular Disease 561
The Client With a Femoral Fracture 562
The Client With a Spinal Cord Injury 563

Correct Answers and Rationale *566*

Test 10: The Client With Sensory Health Problems **577**

The Client With Cataracts 577
The Client With a Retinal Detachment 578
The Client With Glaucoma 580
The Client Undergoing Nasal Surgery 581
The Client With Hearing Disorders 582
The Client With Ménière's Disease 583
The Client With Cancer of the Larynx 583
The Client With Burns 585

Correct Answers and Rationale *587*

Bibliography **599**

Section Two: Postreview Tests

Part V: Comprehensive Tests **603**

Comprehensive Test 1 **605**
Comprehensive Test 2 **627**
Comprehensive Test 3 **649**
Comprehensive Test 4 **671**

Appendix: State Board of Nursing **693**

Introduction

ORGANIZATION AND USE OF THIS BOOK

This book has been developed to help you prepare to write the NCLEX-RN successfully. It is divided into two major sections. The first section contains practice exams representing the four main clinical areas of nursing: psychiatric nursing, obstetrical nursing, pediatric nursing, and medical-surgical nursing. The second section contains four comprehensive exams written to simulate the NCLEX-RN exam. This format enables you to review content in various ways. A computer disk is also included, to help you practice taking computerized adaptive tests (see p. 696 for directions).

You can begin your review by using the practice exams to identify areas of strength and areas needing further study. Each exam contains specific case study situations and miscellaneous questions written in the style of the NCLEX-RN exam. Answers with rationale, coded according to the NCLEX-RN test plan for the step of the nursing process, cognitive level, and client needs, are included at the end of each exam under the heading "Correct Answer and Rationale."

To evaluate your results after completing each exam, divide the number of your correct responses by the total number of questions in the test and multiply by 100. For example, if you answered 72 of 90 items correctly, you would divide 72 by 90 and multiply by 100, for a result of 80%. If you answered more than 75% of the items in an area correctly, you are most likely prepared to answer questions in that area on the NCLEX-RN. But if you answered less than 75% correctly, you need to determine why. Did you answer incorrectly because of lack of content knowledge or because you did not read carefully? Use this information to guide your study.

Use the answer grid at the end of each exam to calculate the percent of items you answered correctly for each area of the test plan (nursing process, cognitive level, and client needs). For example, you can calculate the percentage of correctly answered questions about the nursing diagnosis step of the nursing process; if you missed more than 75% of these questions, you should review information about formulating nursing diagnoses.

After reviewing the specific content areas in the practice exams, take the comprehensive exams. These exams more realistically reflect the NCLEX-RN, which is a comprehensive exam; that is, each test presents a variety of situations commonly encountered in nursing practice and across all clinical disciplines. Underlying knowledge, skills, and abilities related to the basic physiopsychosocial sciences, fundamentals of nursing, pharmacology and other therapeutic measures, communicable diseases, legal and ethical considerations, and nutrition are included in items as needed to plan nursing care for a specific client. The items in the comprehensive exams were also written to test competent nursing practice based on this knowledge and these skills and abilities. After completing each exam, review the answers and rationales to evaluate your results. Use the diagnostic grids to determine the percentage of correct answers in each content area and NCLEX-RN test plan component.

Finally, if you have access to an IBM-compatible personal computer, use the computer disk accompanying this review book to simulate taking computerized adaptive tests. Note how the questions are presented on the computer screen and practice answering questions without using a pencil.

THE TEST PLAN

The National Council Licensure Examination for Registered Nurses (NCLEX-RN) is developed by the National Council of State Boards of Nursing, Inc. The test plan or framework of the examination, which is based on the results of an analysis of the entry-level performance of registered nurses, was used to prepare this book. The test plan is formulated on health care situations that registered nurses commonly encounter and addresses two components: (1) phases of the nursing process and (2) client needs.

NURSING PROCESS

There are five phases of the nursing process: (1) assessment, (2) analysis, (3) planning, (4) implementation, and (5) evaluation.

Assessment. Assessment involves establishing a data base. The nurse gathers objective and subjective information about the client, then verifies the data and communicates information gained from the assessment.

Analysis. Analysis involves identifying actual or potential health care needs/problems based on assessment data. The nurse interprets the data, collects additional data as indicated, and identifies and communicates the client's nursing diagnoses. The nurse also determines the congruency between the client's needs/problems and ability of the health team members to meet these needs.

Planning. Planning involves setting goals for meeting the client's needs and designing strategies to attain these goals. The nurse determines the goals of care, develops and modifies the plan, collaborates with other health team members for delivery of the client's care, and formulates expected outcomes of nursing interventions.

Implementation. Implementation involves initiating and completing actions necessary to accomplish the defined goals. The nurse organizes and manages the client's care; performs or assists the client in performing activities of daily living; counsels and teaches the client, significant others, and health team members; and provides care to attain the established client goals. The nurse also provides care to optimize the achievement of the client's health care goals; supervises, coordinates, and evaluates delivery of the client's care provided by nursing staff; and records and exchanges information.

Evaluation. Evaluation determines goal achievement. The nurse compares actual with expected outcomes of therapy, evaluates compliance with prescribed and/or proscribed therapy, and records and describes the client's response to therapy and/or care. The nurse also modifies the plan, as indicated, and reorders priorities.

The five phases of the nursing process are equally important. Therefore, each is represented by an equal number of items on NCLEX-RN.[1]

CLIENT NEEDS

The health needs of clients are grouped under four broad categories: (1) safe, effective care environment, (2) physiological integrity, (3) psychosocial integrity, and (4) health promotion/maintenance.

Safe, effective care environment. The nurse meets the client's needs for a safe and effective environment by providing and directing nursing care that promotes attainment of client needs. These needs include coordinated care, environmental safety, preparation for treatments and procedures, and safe and effective treatments and procedures.

Physiological integrity. The nurse meets the physiological integrity of clients with potentially life-threatening and/or recurring physiological conditions, and of clients at risk for the development of complications or untoward effects of treatments or management of modalities. The nurse meets the physiological integrity of these clients by providing and directing nursing care that promotes achievement of such needs as physiological adaptation, mobility, comfort, and provision of basic care.

Psychosocial integrity. The nurse meets the client's needs for psychosocial integrity in stress and crisis-related situations throughout the life cycle. The nurse does this by providing and directing nursing care that promotes achievement of the client's needs for psychosocial adaptation and coping/adaptation.

Health promotion/maintenance. The nurse meets the client's needs for health promotion/maintenance throughout the life cycle by providing and directing nursing care that promotes achievement, within the client and significant others, of such needs as continued growth and development, self-care, integrity of support systems, and prevention and early treatment of disease.

Each category of client need is represented on NCLEX-RN, as follows:

1. Safe, effective care environment	25 to 31 percent
2. Physiological integrity	42 to 48 percent
3. Psychosocial integrity	9 to 15 percent[1]
4. Health promotion and maintenance	12 to 18 percent

For further information about NCLEX-RN, write to the National Council of State Boards of Nursing, Inc. For information about the dates, requirements, and specifics of writing the examination in your state, contact your state board of nursing. The addresses and telephone numbers of the National Council of State Boards of Nursing, Inc. and of each state board of nursing are provided in the appendix.

COGNITIVE LEVEL OF QUESTIONS

The cognitive level of questions refers to the type of mental activity required to answer the question as defined in a taxonomy of the cognitive domain.[2] Test questions can be written to test at all levels of the cognitive domain.

The lowest level of the taxonomy is the *knowledge* level, the ability to recall facts about principles, concepts, theories, terms, or procedures. Questions at this level ask you to define, identify, or select. *Comprehension* requires understanding data; questions ask you to interpret, explain, distinguish, or predict. *Application* involves using information in new situations. At this level, you are expected to solve problems, modify plans, manipulate data, and demonstrate appropriate use of information. *Analysis* requires recognizing relationships between parts. Questions at this level ask you to analyze, evaluate, select, differentiate, or interpret data from a variety of sources. The highest level of the cognitive domain is *synthesis.* Here you must put data together in new and meaningful ways.

The test items in the NCLEX-RN are written to test *application* and *analysis* of nursing knowledge. All items in this book have been coded according to the taxonomy of the cognitive domain. As you answer the questions and review your scores, you can determine whether you are able to answer questions at the levels of the cognitive domain tested on the NCLEX-RN exam.

COMPUTER ADAPTIVE TESTING

Beginning in April 1994, NCLEX-RN examinations will be administered in all jurisdictions using computer adaptive testing procedures. Computer adaptive testing (CAT) involves using a computer to randomly generate questions from an item pool to administer individually tailored examinations. CAT has several advantages. For example, an exam can be given in less time, because there are potentially fewer questions for each candidate. CAT exams can also be administered frequently, allowing a graduate of a nursing program to take the exam close to graduation, receive the results quickly, and enter the work force as a registered nurse in less time than is possible with paper and pencil exams. Study results also show that because CAT is self-paced, there is less stress on the candidate.

Here are answers to other questions you may have about CAT.

How is CAT different from paper and pencil tests?

CAT uses the memory and speed of the computer to administer a test for each candidate. The test is generated from a large pool of questions (a test item bank) based on the NCLEX test plan. The examination begins as the computer randomly selects a question of medium difficulty for each candidate. The next question is based on the response to the previous question: If the question is answered correctly, an item of similar or greater difficulty is generated; when it is answered incorrectly, a less-difficult item is selected. Thus, the test is adapted for each individual candidate. Once competence has been determined, the exam is completed at a passing level. CAT for the NCLEX-RN has been field-tested and is psychometrically sound.

Who writes the test questions for the NCLEX-RN?

As with previous examinations, nurse clinicians and nurse educators are nominated by the Council of State Boards of Nursing to serve as item writers. The questions are written to reflect nursing practice in all parts of the country and based on job analysis of the staff nurse conducted every three years by the National Council of State Boards of Nursing, Inc.

Am I getting the same test as my classmates?

The exams for all candidates are derived from the same large pool of test items. They contain comparable questions for each component of the test plan. Although the questions are not exactly the same, they test the same knowledge, skills, and abilities from the test plan.

Will my test be more difficult than my classmate's test?

Each candidate begins the exam with questions of moderate difficulty. After that, each subsequent question is adapted for each candidate, based on the response to the preceding question. The computer constantly recalculates the estimate of competence. If you answer questions of moderate difficulty correctly, the level of difficulty will be increased. On the other hand, if you answer questions of moderate difficulty incorrectly, you will receive easier questions. All of the areas of the test plan are covered, regardless of the number of questions you are asked to answer.

Is CAT fair?

All candidates must meet the requirements of the test plan and achieve the same passing score. Each candidate, therefore, has the same opportunity to demonstrate competence. Although one candidate may answer fewer questions, all candidates have the opportunity to answer a sufficient number of questions to demonstrate competence.

How many questions are on the exam?

Although each exam is individualized, the minimum number of questions is 75. The maximum number of questions is 265. Do not worry if others near you finish early or receive more questions. Focus on doing your best and working at a comfortable speed for you.

How long will it take to finish the exam?

Because each exam is adapted for each candidate, the time will vary. The time will also vary depending on how long it takes to finish each question. Enough time will be allotted for each candidate to demonstrate competence. Most candidates will be able to complete the exam within the maximum 5 hours allotted for the exam.

Can I have a break?

The exam site is designed so that candidates can take breaks. There is a mandatory 10-minute break after 2 hours, and an optional break one and one-half hours after that.

How can I find out where to take the NCLEX-RN?

The Council of State Boards of Nursing contracts with vendors in each state to serve as exam sites. Your school of nursing can inform you of the location nearest you. You can also contact your state board of nursing for information. (See the Appendix for the address.)

What is the physical layout of a typical testing site?

The testing service that administers the NCLEX CAT (Educational Testing Service) has formed a partnership with Sylvan/Kee Systems.[3] The NCLEX is administered at more than 1,200 Sylvan/Kee learning centers nationwide and at various universities and colleges that meet testing site guidelines. Each center has approximately 10 computer stations equipped with adequate lighting and scratch paper for candidates' use. The computers have surge protection devices to prevent data loss. There is also a secured storage area outside of the testing room where you can store personal articles. Each testing center maintains comprehensive security, using audio and video camera monitoring.

How do I schedule an examination?

The first step is to apply to the state board of nursing in the state in which you plan to take the examination. You will receive a ticket of admission from the Educational Testing Service Data Center with information about available testing centers and procedures for making an appointment. Testing centers are open Monday through Saturday, approximately 15 hours each day.

How do I use the computer?

Test questions are presented on the computer screen (monitor); you select your answer and use the keyboard to enter the response (see Fig. 1). The keyboard is simplified to use only two color-coded keys: the "space bar" and the "enter key." You press the "space bar" to highlight the answer, then press the "enter key" once to select your answer and a second time to "enter" your answer into the computer. If you have access to an IBM-compatible personal computer, you can use the practice disk included with this review book to practice selecting and entering answers.

Can I practice entering answers before I take the exam?

At every testing site, written directions are provided at each computer exam station. There also are practice questions on the computer that you can use to be sure you understand how to use the computer before you begin the exam.

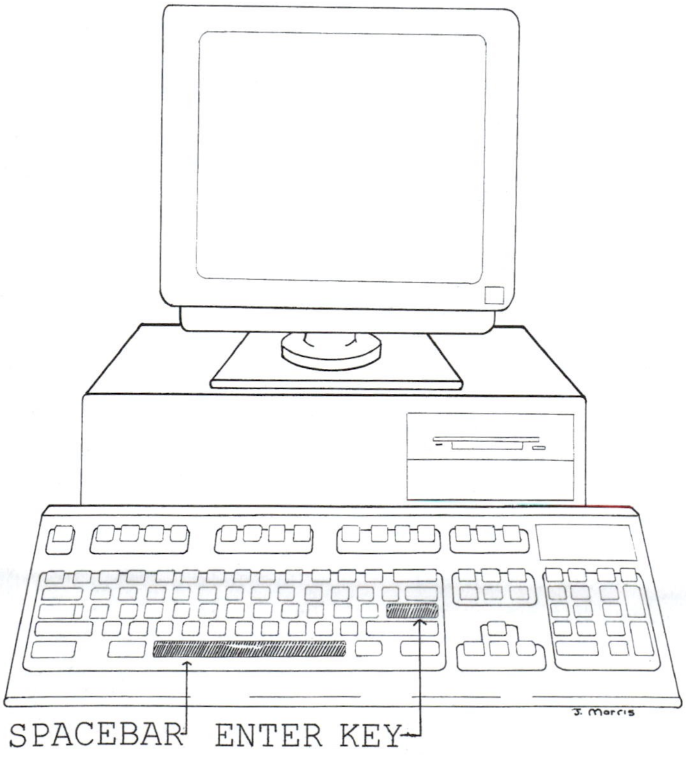

Fig. 1. Computer screen (monitor) and keyboard

Do I need to be experienced with the computer to be able to pass the test?

Field studies conducted by The Council of State Boards of Nursing find that previous computer experience or lack of it has no effect on exam performance. Candidates are able to acquire the necessary computer skills at the testing center.

STUDY PLAN

Studying for the NCLEX-RN exam requires careful planning and preparation. You can make best use of your time and energy by developing a systematic approach to study that includes assessing your study needs, developing a study plan, and using study skills. Use the checklist below to help develop an effective study plan.

CHECKLIST FOR DEVELOPING A STUDY PLAN

1. Review your success in nursing school.
   - ○ I did best in these courses: ________.
   - ○ I needed to study harder in these courses: ________.
   - ○ I had these courses towards the beginning of the curriculum: ________.
   - ○ I scored best on these practice exams in this book: ________.
   - ○ I am not satisfied with my scores on these practice exams in this book: ________.
   - ○ I need further study in these content areas: ________.
   - ○ I need further study in these areas of the nursing process: ________.
   - ○ I need further study in these areas of client needs: ________.
2. Review your test-taking skills.
   - ○ I can identify the components of a test question.
   - ○ I read questions carefully before answering.
   - ○ I can make reasonable "guesses" if I am not certain of the correct answer.
   - ○ I can use the computer to read and answer test questions.
3. Make a study plan.
   - ○ I will study in (location): ________.
   - ○ I will study at these times and dates: ________.
   - ○ I have assembled all of the materials I need to study: ________.
4. Practice managing test anxiety.
   - ○ I can do relaxation and deep breathing exercises.
   - ○ I can visualize success.
   - ○ I can give myself positive feedback.

5. Evaluate your progress.
   - ○ I am on schedule with my study plan.
   - ○ I have reviewed content areas in which I needed to improve my scores.
   - ○ I am building confidence through positive self-feedback.

Assessing Study Needs

The first step in developing a study plan is to determine which content areas you know well and which areas you need to review further. Follow these steps to assess your knowledge, skills, and abilities:

1. Review your success in nursing school. Review your record of achievement in courses in the nursing curriculum. Subjects in which you received high grades, found easy to learn, or in which you have had additional clinical practice or work experience are likely areas of strength. On the other hand, subjects you found difficult to learn or did not achieve high grades in should be areas for concentrated review. Also consider content areas that you have not studied for a while. Recent course work will be most familiar and, therefore, may require the least amount of study.

You can also use the practice exams in this book to identify areas needing further study. Begin with the subjects you find most difficult or in which you have the least confidence. Use the grids at the end of each test to determine areas for further study.

2. Review your test-taking skills. Using effective test-taking skills contributes to exam success. What have you done in the past to make you confident about taking a test? How do you feel when you are in the exam situation? What has worked in the past to help you be successful? Review these strategies, and build on past successes and work on problem areas. Consider additional strategies suggested in the following section, "Test-Taking Strategies." You can practice these skills by simulating the testing situation using the practice tests and comprehensive exams in this review book.

3. Assess your skills for taking computer-administered exams. Although previous computer experience is not necessary to take the NCLEX-RN, you may wish to familiarize yourself with the differences between taking a paper and pencil exam and taking exams administered by the computer. Use the box to the right to review these differences. If you have not used a computer before, find a learning resource center at your college, university, library, or hospital where you can become familiar with basic computer keyboard skills. Use the disk accompanying this review book to simulate the experience of taking questions using a computer. Practice reading questions from the computer screen. If you are used to underlining key words or making notes in the margin of paper and pencil tests, adapt these strategies to reading and answering the questions on the computer screen.

DIFFERENCES BETWEEN PAPER AND PENCIL AND COMPUTER ADMINISTERED EXAMS

Exam Feature	Paper and Pencil Exams	Computer Administered Exams
Question layout	Linear	Blocked, with stem of the question or the case study on the left, options on the right
Question design	Case study with several related questions following the case study	All information related to the question is presented in the stem
Ability to read questions randomly	Yes	No, one question presented at a time
Ability to review or change answer to previous question	Yes	No
Ability to skip question if not sure of answer	Yes	No, must answer each question before receiving the next one
Ability to underline or circle key words; make margin notes	Yes	No
Scratch paper available	Yes	Yes
Proctor	Rotates among tables	Can observe all candidates simultaneously and video monitored
Ergonomics	Sit at desk	Sit at computer
Breaks	Yes	Yes

Developing a Study Plan

Once you have identified areas of strength and areas needing further study, develop a specific plan and begin to study regularly. Students who study a small amount of content over a longer period of time tend to have higher success rates than students who wait until the last few weeks before the exam and then "cram." Consider these suggestions:

1. Identify a place for study. The area should be quiet and have room for your books and papers. This area might be in your home, at your nursing school, or in a library. Be sure your friends and family understand the importance of not interrupting you when you are studying.

2. Establish regular study times. Make "appointments" with yourself to ensure a commitment to study. Frequent, short study periods (1 to 2 hours) are preferable to sporadic, extended study periods. Plan to finish your studying 1 week before the NCLEX-RN exam, last minute "cramming" tends to increase anxiety.

3. Obtain all necessary resources. As you begin to study, it will be helpful to have easy access to textbooks, notes, and study guides. Suggested readings are included at the end of each unit in this book.

4. Make the best use of your time. Make review cards that you can carry with you to study during free moments throughout the day. If possible, you may want to tape record review notes and listen to the tapes on the way to work.

Using Study Skills

Good study skills enable you to acquire, organize, remember, and use the information you need to take the NCLEX-RN examination. These skills include outlining, summarizing, reviewing, and practicing test-taking. Some students prefer studying alone, while others benefit from study groups; know which approach works best for you and develop your study plan accordingly. You can use this book to learn, refine, and practice your study skills. Study skill suggestions include:

1. Use study skills with which you are familiar and that have worked well for you in the past. Recall effective study behaviors you used in nursing school, such as reviewing highlighted text, outlines, or content maps. What are your learning style preferences? Do you study best in a quiet room, or do you prefer music in the background? Are you most alert in the morning or evening? Do you like to eat while you study? Does it help you to concentrate and learn if you make notes as you study? Learn what works best for you and use it to optimize your study plan.

2. Study to learn, not to memorize. NCLEX-RN tests application of knowledge. When reviewing content, continually ask yourself, "How is this information used in client care?"

3. Anticipate questions. As you study, formulate questions around the content. Practice giving rationale for your answer to these questions. If you work in a study group, have each member contribute questions.

4. Study common, not unique, nursing care situations. The NCLEX-RN tests minimum competence for nursing practice; therefore, focus on common health problems and client needs.

5. Simulate test-taking. The comprehensive exams in Part V of this book are designed to simulate the random order in which questions appear in the NCLEX-RN exam. Use these exams to focus on areas of common concern in nursing care, rather than on the traditional content delineations of adult, pediatric, psychiatric, and childbearing clients. Make additional copies of answer sheets, and retake the exams on which you had low scores.

6. Give yourself positive self-feedback. Use positive self-talk strategies to build your confidence. Reward yourself as you study. Engage in a favorite activity after a successful study session.

7. Review your progress. Make a progress checklist identifying content areas. Note as your scores improve. Do not spend time on content you have mastered, on obtaining high scores on the practice exam, or on areas with which you feel confident. Set priorities for study on areas needing additional review.

TEST-TAKING STRATEGIES

Knowing how to take a test is as important as knowing the content being tested. The "how" of test taking, "test-wiseness," can be learned and used to improve test scores. Here are some suggestions for building a repertoire of effective test-taking strategies:

1. Understand the components of the test item. Typically, test items consist of a situation or background information, a question, and four possible answers (see Fig. 2).[4]

The *background (situation)* is a client-based scenario giving information about the client that you need to answer the question. The questions that follow are based on the information given in the situation. As you answer the questions, relate the answer to the background information. Pay particular attention to information about the client's age, family status, health status, ethnicity, or point in the care plan (early admission vs. preparation for discharge).

The *question (stem)* poses the problem to solve. The stem may be written as a direct question such as "What should the nurse do first?", or an incomplete sentence such as "The nurse should. . . .".

Background ⇓ ⇓ Stem

SITUATION:	QUESTION 1:
The parents of children attending an elementary school and a high school invite the school nurse to attend some of their Parent-Teacher Association meetings to discuss common health problems related to their youngsters.	One parent asks about head lice (pediculosis capitis). The nurse discusses the symptoms with the parents. Which of the following symptoms is *most* common when a child has been infected with head lice?
	1. Itching of the scalp. 2. Scaling of the scalp. 3. Serous weeping on the scalp surface. 4. Pinpoint hemorrhagic spots on the scalp surface.

⇑ Answers

Fig. 2. Sample test item, computer adaptive testing format: background (situation), question (stem), and answers (options).

The *answers (options)* are possible responses to the stem. Each stem has one correct option and three incorrect options.

2. Understand which step of the nursing process is being tested. Refer to page xv for an explanation of nursing process questions and review your study grids. For example, as you read the question, determine whether the question is asking you to set priorities (planning) or judge outcomes (evaluation).

3. Understand client needs. As you read the question, consider the question in the context of client needs.

4. Read the question carefully. This is one of the most important aspects of effective test-taking. Do not rush. Ask yourself, "What is this question asking?" and "What is the expected response?". If necessary, rephrase the question in your own words. Do not "read into" a question meaning that is not intended, and do not make a question more difficult than it is. If you do not understand the question, try to figure it out. If, for example, the question is asking about the fluid balance needs of a client with pheochromocytoma and you do not remember what pheochromocytoma is, then try to answer the question based on your knowledge of principles of fluid balance.

5. Look for key words that provide clues to the correct answer. For instance, words such as "except," "not," or "but" can change the meaning of a question; words such as "first", "next", and "most" indicate priority and order of steps.

6. Be sure you understand the meaning of all words in the question. If you see a word you do not know, try to figure out its meaning from a familiar base of the word or from the context of the question.

7. Attempt to answer the question before you see the answers, then look for the answer that is similar to the one you generated.

8. Base answers on nursing knowledge. Remember the NCLEX-RN is used to test for safe practice and that you have learned the information needed to answer the question.

9. If you do not know the answer, make a reasonable guess. "Hunches" and "intuition" are often correct. If you do not know the answer, do not waste time and energy; give yourself permission to not know every question and move on to the next one. In CAT you must answer each question before the next item is administered, and since the level of difficulty will be adjusted as you answer each question, it is likely that you will know the answer to one of the next questions.

TAKING THE NCLEX-RN EXAM

The final step in preparing for the NCLEX-RN exam involves mental and physical preparation. Like an athlete training for competition, you need to be physically and mentally "in shape." Consider these suggestions:

1. Make sure you know the date, time, and place the exam will be given; how to get to the exam site; know how long it takes to drive there; and where you can park. It may be helpful to visit the exam site and see the room where the exam will be given. Visualize yourself in the room, taking the test. Arrive on time for the exam.

2. Make sure you are physically prepared. Get enough rest before the examination; fatigue can impair concentration. If you are working, it may be advisable not to work the day before the exam; if you are working on a shift that is different from the time of the exam, adjust your work schedule several days ahead of time. Avoid planning time-consuming activities (e.g., weddings, vacation trips) immediately before the exam. Do not use any drugs you usually do not use (including caffeine and nicotine), and do not use alcohol for 2 days before the exam. Eat regular meals before the exam. Remember that high-carbohydrate foods provide energy, but excessive sugar and caffeine can cause hyperactivity. Dress comfortably, in layers that can be added or removed according to your comfort level.

3. Manage test anxiety. All test-takers experience some anxiety. A certain amount of anxiety is motivating, but be prepared to control unwanted anxiety. Develop and practice the following anxiety management strategies, and use them during the exam as needed:

- **Mental rehearsal.** Mental rehearsal involves reviewing the events and environment during the examination. Anticipate how you will feel, what the setting will be like, how you will take the exam, what the computer screen will look like, and how you will talk to yourself during the exam. Visualize your success. Rehearse what you will do if you have test anxiety.
- **Relaxation exercises.** Relaxation exercises involve tensing and relaxing various muscle groups to relieve the physical effects of anxiety. Practice systematically contracting and relaxing muscle groups from your toes to your neck to release energy for concentration. You can do these exercises during the exam to promote relaxation.
- **Deep breathing.** Taking deep breaths by inhaling slowly while counting to five and then exhaling slowly while counting to ten increases oxygen flow to the lungs and brain. Deep breathing also decreases tension and helps manage anxiety by focusing you on the breathing and away from troublesome thoughts.
- **Positive self-talk.** Talking to yourself in a positive way serves to correct negative thoughts (e.g., "I can't pass this test"; "I don't know the answers to any of these questions") and reinforces a positive self-concept. Replace negative thoughts with positive ones, telling yourself, "I can do this"; "I studied well and am prepared."
- **Distraction.** Thinking about something else can clear your mind of negative or unwanted thoughts. Think of

something fun, something you enjoy. Plan now what you will think about to distract yourself during the exam.

4. Concentrate. During the exam, be prepared to concentrate. Have tunnel vision. Do not worry if others finish the test before you do. Remember everyone has their own speed for taking tests and that each test is individualized. Do not rush; you will have plenty of time. Focus; do not let noises from the keyboard next to you divert your attention. Do not become overwhelmed by the testing environment. Use positive-self talk as you begin the test.

REFERENCES

1. National Council of State Boards of Nursing, Inc. (1987). NCLEX-RN Test Plan for the National Council Licensure Examination for Registered Nurses. Chicago: The National Council of State Boards of Nursing, Inc.
2. Bloom, B.S. (1956). *Taxonomy of educational objectives, Handbook I: Cognitive domain,* New York: David McKay.
3. Staff (1992). Walk-through of the computerized testing experience: What students will experience when taking NCLEX/CAT. *Issues,* 13(4), 1.
4. Gronlund, N.E. (1988). *How to construct achievement tests.* New York: Prentice-Hall.

LIPPINCOTT'S REVIEW FOR NCLEX•RN

Section ONE

Practice Tests

Part I

The Nursing Care of Clients With Psychosocial Health Problems

Mood Disorders and Crisis Situations

Test 1

The Client With a Major Mood Disorder
The Client With Bipolar Disorder, Manic Phase
The Client Who is Depressed
The Client With Depressive Disorder and Suicidal Ideation
The Client Who Attempts Suicide
The Client in Crisis
Correct Answers and Rationale

Select the one best answer and indicate your choice by filling in the circle in front of the option.

The Client With a Major Mood Disorder

A client is admitted to the hospital's psychiatric unit 1 month after he retired involuntarily. The nurse notes that he keeps his head bowed in a dejected manner and that his facial expression is sad.

1. The nurse visualizes the client's depression from a holistic framework. According to holistic theory, the client's depression should be viewed as a
- ○ 1. reaction to a stressful event.
- ○ 2. symptom of high sugar intake.
- ○ 3. disturbance caused by numerous factors.
- ○ 4. disturbance caused by destructive environmental influences.

2. Using the holistic framework in one-to-one interactions with the client, the nurse should plan to focus primarily on the client's
- ○ 1. dreams and free associations.
- ○ 2. childhood and past life history.
- ○ 3. current feelings and experiences.
- ○ 4. underlying conflicts and defense mechanisms.

3. After a few minutes of conversation, the client wearily asks the nurse, "Why pick me to talk to when there are so many other people here?" Which reply by the nurse would be best?
- ○ 1. "I'm assigned to care for you today, if you'll let me."
- ○ 2. "You have a lot of potential, and I'd like to help you."
- ○ 3. "Why shouldn't I want to talk to you, as well as the others?"
- ○ 4. "You're wondering why I'm interested in you, and not the others?"

4. The nurse meets with the client daily. The client stays mostly in his room and speaks only when addressed, answering briefly and abruptly while keeping his eyes on the floor. At this stage of their relationship, the nurse focuses on the client's ability to
- ○ 1. make decisions.
- ○ 2. relate to other patients.
- ○ 3. function independently.
- ○ 4. express himself verbally.

5. Which of the following client behaviors would best indicate to the nurse that the relationship with the client is in the working phase?
- ○ 1. The client attempts to familiarize himself with the nurse.
- ○ 2. The client makes an effort to describe his problems in detail.
- ○ 3. The client tries to summarize his progress in the relationship.
- ○ 4. The client starts to challenge the boundaries or outer limits of the relationship.

6. The client is concerned that the information he gives to the nurse remains confidential. Which of the following comments would be best for the nurse to make in this situation?
- ○ 1. "If the information you share with me is important in relation to your care, I'll need to share it with the staff."

○ 2. "We can keep the information just between the two of us if you prefer."
○ 3. "I'll share the information with staff members only with your approval."
○ 4. "You can decide whether your physician needs this information for your care."

A client is admitted to the psychiatric unit with complaints of sleep disturbances, fatigue, feelings of uselessness, and inability to concentrate. The client was let go from her place of employment last month due to her inability to keep up with the demands of her position.

7. On the day following an interview during which the client talked at length and tearfully about feeling "useless and old," she failed to keep an appointment with the nurse. Which action would be best for the nurse to take?
○ 1. Assume that the client had a good reason for not coming and let her make the next move.
○ 2. Confront the client with her behavior and ask her to explain the reason for her absence.
○ 3. Seek out the client at the end of the scheduled interview time and tell her she was missed today.
○ 4. Arrange for another session with the client later the same day and say nothing about her absence.

8. The client speaks in a seemingly sincere manner about her former employer who replaced her with a younger person. "He was a wonderful boss. He was the most understanding boss I've ever had. It was a privilege to work for him." Which of the following defense mechanisms is the client most likely using?
○ 1. Sublimation.
○ 2. Suppression.
○ 3. Repression.
○ 4. Reaction formation.

9. The client begins to attend group sessions daily. She explains to the group how she lost her job. Which of the following statements by a group member would be most therapeutic for the client?
○ 1. "Tell us about what you did on your job."
○ 2. "It must have been very upsetting for you."
○ 3. "With your skills, finding another job should be easy."
○ 4. "The company must have had some reason for letting you go."

10. The physician orders a different drug, tranylcypromine sulfate (Parnate), when the client does not respond positively to a tricyclic antidepressant. Which of the following reactions should the client be cautioned about if her diet includes foods containing tyramine?
○ 1. Heart block.
○ 2. Grand mal seizure.
○ 3. Respiratory arrest.
○ 4. Hypertensive crisis.

11. While the client is taking tranylcypromine sulfate (Parnate), the nurse would teach her to especially avoid which food because of its high tyramine content?
○ 1. Nuts.
○ 2. Aged cheeses.
○ 3. Grain cereals.
○ 4. Reconstituted milk.

12. During an interaction with the nurse, the client states "I have nothing to be depressed about. My husband has supported me throughout each of my many hospitalizations. He'll probably leave me this time. I'm an awful person and wife. I'm no good. I can't do anything right." Based on this data, the nurse should consider which of the following as an appropriate nursing diagnosis?
○ 1. Ineffective Individual Coping related to depression, as evidenced by withdrawal.
○ 2. Self-Esteem Disturbance related to numerous hospitalizations, as evidenced by negative self-statements.
○ 3. Dysfunctional Grieving related to imagined loss of husband, as evidenced by negativity.
○ 4. Potential for Self-Directed Violence related to numerous failures, as evidenced by worthlessness.

13. The client has tearfully described her negative feelings about herself to the nurse during their last three interactions. Which of the following goals would be most appropriate for the nurse to include in the care plan at this time? The client will
○ 1. increase her self-esteem.
○ 2. write her negative feelings in a daily journal.
○ 3. verbalize her work-related accomplishments.
○ 4. verbalize three things she likes about herself.

14. The client obtains permission for a 24-hour pass to go home. Which of the following suggestions to the family in preparing for the visit indicates the best understanding of the client's needs?
○ 1. Planning to encourage the client to seek employment outside the home.
○ 2. Limiting friends' visits so that the client can rest during the day.
○ 3. Scheduling a day of interesting activities for the client outside the home.
○ 4. Planning to involve the client in usual at-home pursuits of the immediate family.

15. After a 2-month hospitalization, the client is preparing for discharge. Which of the following subjects would be most helpful to discuss when preparing to terminate the nurse-client relationship?

○ 1. The gains that the client has made during therapy.
○ 2. The plans that the client should make to find a job.
○ 3. The knowledge that the client's daughter is divorcing her husband.
○ 4. The conflicts the client has had with another staff member.

16. The nurse reviews the client counseling sessions with the unit's clinical nurse specialist (CNS). Consulting the CNS serves many purposes, but the overall primary purpose is to
○ 1. increase nurses awareness of client behavior.
○ 2. increase nurses awareness of client thoughts.
○ 3. evaluate nursing practice.
○ 4. evaluate nursing style.

17. Which client reaction in terminating the relationship with the nurse should be considered the most healthy?
○ 1. A lack of response.
○ 2. A display of anger.
○ 3. An attempt at humor.
○ 4. An expression of grief.

The Client With Bipolar Disorder, Manic Phase

A client is admitted to the psychiatric unit accompanied by her husband. She brings six suitcases and three shopping bags. She orders the nurse to carry her bags, to set up a typewriter, and to not touch any of her papers. Her husband states that she has been purchasing items that they cannot afford and has not slept for 4 nights.

18. Which additional information would be a priority for the nurse to seek from the client's husband? The nurse would ask about
○ 1. The client's fluid and food intake.
○ 2. Their current financial status.
○ 3. The client's usual sleeping pattern.
○ 4. Whether the client becomes agitated easily.

19. The husband apologizes to the nurse for his wife's demanding behavior. Which of the following possible replies by the nurse would be best?
○ 1. "I'm sure she's doing the best she can."
○ 2. "It's all right. We have been treated worse."
○ 3. "It must be hard for you to see her like this."
○ 4. "I understand. What happened to set her off like this?"

20. The client puts out her hand and says to the nurse, "Watch out! Here I come." She then puts her hand down and sits in a chair. After determining that the client is not about to harm anyone, the nurse should intervene by
○ 1. giving the client a book of her choice to read.
○ 2. placing the client in isolation to work out her aggression in private.
○ 3. taking the client to a punching bag for exercise to release excess energy.
○ 4. having the client continue to sit while holding her hands to help her gain control of herself.

21. The client is scheduled to go to the radiology department. Before taking the client for her x-ray examination, which of the following actions should the nurse take?
○ 1. Explain the x-ray procedure in simple terms.
○ 2. Provide a detailed explanation of the x-ray procedure.
○ 3. Say nothing before taking her to the x-ray department.
○ 4. Bring another staff member along in case she resists going to the x-ray department.

22. The nurse notes that the client is too busy investigating the unit and overseeing the activities of other clients to eat dinner. To help the client obtain sufficient nourishment, which of the following plans would be best?
○ 1. Serve foods that she can carry with her.
○ 2. Allow her to send out for her favorite foods.
○ 3. Serve food in small, attractively arranged portions.
○ 4. Allow her to enter the unit kitchen for extra food as necessary.

23. Later the same evening, the client appears at the nurses' station with brightly rouged cheeks, ornaments in her hair, and three pairs of false eyelashes, wearing a sheer nightgown, high heels, and bracelets up to her elbows. Which of the following actions should the nurse take in relation to the client's attire?
○ 1. Redirect the client to her room and help her put on proper apparel.
○ 2. Allow the client to wear what she likes and get her involved in a unit activity.
○ 3. Remind the client that she agreed to wear slacks and a shirt when out of her room.
○ 4. Ask the client to put on hospital pajamas, because she has not earned the privilege of wearing her own clothing.

A client with bipolar disorder, manic phase has just sat down to watch television in the lounge.

24. As the nurse approaches the lounge area, the client states, "The sun is shining. Where is my son? I love Lucy. Let's play ball." The client is displaying

○ 1. concreteness.
○ 2. flight of ideas.
○ 3. depersonalization.
○ 4. use of neologisms.

25. The client's speech pattern is related primarily to
○ 1. underlying hostilities.
○ 2. loose ego boundaries.
○ 3. feelings of anxiety.
○ 4. distortions in self-concept.

26. Which of the following responses by the nurse would be the most therapeutic for the client?
○ 1. "Let's talk about what you did today instead."
○ 2. "How does the sun shining relate to your son?"
○ 3. "You're talking nonsense. Why don't you try to stay on one subject?"
○ 4. "I can't follow you. It would help me if you'd speak a little slower."

27. The client is intrusive and disruptive to other clients. He constantly walks about the unit interrupting others. Which plan should the nurse institute first in this situation?
○ 1. Escort the client to his room and explain that he cannot come out until he gets permission.
○ 2. Set limits on the client's behavior. Explain what is expected and what the consequences will be if limits are violated.
○ 3. Ask another staff member to take the client to watch television for the next hour.
○ 4. Bargain with the client. Explain which privileges he can attain if he can control his behavior.

28. Which activity would be most therapeutic for channeling the client's hyperactive behavior? Allowing the client to
○ 1. lead some group activities.
○ 2. clean his room and the dayroom.
○ 3. read to patients who are depressed.
○ 4. exercise and move about as much as possible.

29. Which of the following feeling states does the client's behavior during a manic episode reflect?
○ 1. Guilt, projected onto others.
○ 2. Anger, turned against the self.
○ 3. Distrust, focused on the family.
○ 4. Hostility, directed against the environment.

30. The client sometimes makes inappropriate requests. For example, he calls an office supply store to order many items and charges them to his account. Which of the following nursing interventions would be best in this situation?
○ 1. Tell the client that his request will be filled.
○ 2. Explain to the client that his request is denied.
○ 3. Suggest to the client that part of his request can be met.
○ 4. Call the store to cancel the request without telling the client.

31. The nurse evaluates the client's condition daily. During the client's period of euphoria, the nurse should be especially alert for which conditions?
○ 1. Gastritis and vertigo.
○ 2. Exhaustion and infection.
○ 3. Convulsions and dermatitis.
○ 4. Bradycardia and palpitations.

32. The client has been taking lithium carbonate (Lithane) for hyperactivity, as prescribed by his physician. While the client is taking this drug, the nurse should ensure that he has an adequate intake of
○ 1. sodium.
○ 2. iron.
○ 3. iodine.
○ 4. calcium.

33. Which of the following clinical manifestations would alert the nurse to lithium toxicity?
○ 1. Increasingly agitated behavior.
○ 2. Markedly increased food intake.
○ 3. Sudden increase in blood pressure.
○ 4. Anorexia with nausea and vomiting.

34. After 10 days of lithium therapy, the client's lithium level is 1.0 mEq/L. The nurse knows that this value indicates which of the following?
○ 1. A laboratory error.
○ 2. An anticipated therapeutic blood level of the drug.
○ 3. An atypical client response to the drug.
○ 4. A toxic level.

35. The client expresses the belief that he was born out of wedlock to a famous woman. When dealing with this delusion of grandeur, the nurse should first try to
○ 1. get the client to discuss another topic.
○ 2. involve the client in a simple group project.
○ 3. convince the client that he is wrong in his belief.
○ 4. satisfy the client's implied need to feel important.

A client is irritable and hostile. He becomes agitated and verbally lashes out when his personal needs are not immediately met by the staff.

36. When the client's request for a pass is refused by the physician, he utters a stream of profanities. Which of the following statements best describes the client's behavior? The client's anger is usually
○ 1. not intended personally.
○ 2. a reliable sign of serious pathology.
○ 3. an intended attack on the physician's skills.
○ 4. a sign that his condition is improving.

37. A goal of the client's treatment plan is to reduce his activity and aggression. Which of the following comments by the nurse when the client's anger escalates would best help him move toward his treatment goal?

○ 1. "You must go to your room or into seclusion now."
○ 2. "You're disturbing other clients. If you don't stop, you'll need to go into seclusion."
○ 3. "You have a choice of going to your room voluntarily or being escorted to your room."
○ 4. "Your behavior is disrupting the unit. Let's find a quiet place and talk about what is happening."

38. After two weeks of hospitalization, the client has improved with medication and therapy. Which statement made by the client indicates therapeutic gain and readiness for discharge?

○ 1. "I'm cured now and won't need my medicine when I go home."
○ 2. "I know that I'm getting sick when I get very angry."
○ 3. "My medicine really helps me. I'll be ready to go back to work in a few weeks."
○ 4. "I like feeling high from my illness. It helps me feel great and gives me a lot of energy."

39. The client's wife asks the nurse what she can do to help her husband at home. Which of the following actions by family members on behalf of the client would probably be least helpful?

○ 1. Try to keep the client free from worry and anxiety.
○ 2. Relieve the client of some home responsibilities he had.
○ 3. Develop effective communication techniques with the client at home.
○ 4. Learn to recognize when the client is showing signs of drug toxicity.

40. The client's illness is most likely related to which of the following factors?

○ 1. Having been molested as a preschool-age child.
○ 2. A family history of manic depression.
○ 3. High levels of potassium in the brain.
○ 4. Excessive alcohol intake.

The Client Who Is Depressed

A client is admitted involuntarily by court order to a psychiatric hospital for 90 days. Documents sent with her cite, among other things, that she will not eat because she feels her stomach "is missing" and her bowels have "turned to jelly," and that she views this as "just punishment for my past wickedness and for the evil I've brought on my family."

41. To be evaluated as being legally committable, which of the following criteria did the client most likely have to meet?

○ 1. Psychotic.
○ 2. Tried to harm herself or others.
○ 3. Unable to afford private treatment.
○ 4. Made threatening remarks to friends or relatives.

42. Which of the following rights did the client lose by being admitted involuntarily to a psychiatric hospital? The right to

○ 1. send and receive mail.
○ 2. vote in a national election.
○ 3. make a will or legally binding contract.
○ 4. sign out of the hospital against medical advice.

43. Through which of the following legal methods could the client seek release from the psychiatric hospital if she believed she was being improperly detained?

○ 1. Malpractice suit.
○ 2. Guardianship hearing.
○ 3. Writ of habeas corpus.
○ 4. Lien of property petition.

44. When the client expresses feelings of unworthiness, how would the nurse best respond?

○ 1. "Your family loves you even if you feel unworthy."
○ 2. "Your feeling of being unworthy is just your imagination."
○ 3. "It would be best to try to forget the idea that you are unworthy."
○ 4. "As you begin to feel better, your feelings of unworthiness will begin to disappear."

45. The client has not been eating. After serving the client her tray, which of the following actions by the nurse would be most likely to encourage her to eat?

○ 1. Leave the client's room without comment.
○ 2. Sit beside the client and place the fork in her hand.
○ 3. Tell the client that she will not recover unless she eats.
○ 4. Comment on how good the food looks.

46. The client is to receive tube feedings because she continues to refuse food in any form. Gastric feeding is usually used as a last resort with a suspicious client, because the feedings are very likely to

○ 1. be aspirated.
○ 2. arouse fears of dying.
○ 3. be viewed as an attack.
○ 4. increase irritability.

47. The nurse notes that the client becomes restless and incoherent at night. Besides administering a prescribed medication, which of the following actions by the nurse would be most helpful for the client at this time?

○ 1. Encourage the client to talk about her family.
○ 2. Read to the client with the lights turned down low.
○ 3. Help the client take a cool shower before retiring.
○ 4. Sit quietly with the client until the medication takes effect.

48. The client demands to be left "alone to die." She

states, "If you try to cheat the avenger, you will suffer." Which of the following possible replies by the nurse would be best?

- ○ 1. "I won't let anything harm you."
- ○ 2. "It sounds like you're trying to frighten me."
- ○ 3. "I'm not trying to cheat anyone. What do you mean by that?"
- ○ 4. "I'll leave you alone for 15 minutes. Then I'll be back to see how you're doing."

A client is being admitted to the psychiatric unit. She responds to some of the nurse's questions with one-word answers. Her eyes are downcast, and her movements are very slow. The client's daughter states that her mother has been getting worse for the last 2 months and now is barely eating. She also will not leave her apartment, answer the telephone, or talk to friends.

49. Later that morning, the nurse approaches the client and asks how she feels about being in the hospital. The client does not respond verbally and continues to gaze at the floor. Which of the following actions should the nurse take first?

- ○ 1. Spend time sitting in silence with the client.
- ○ 2. Leave the client alone and tell her that she will be back later to talk.
- ○ 3. Introduce another client to her and ask him to join them.
- ○ 4. Ask another staff member to include the client in an informal group discussion.

50. Which short-term goal should the nurse include in the client's care plan? The client will

- ○ 1. approach the nurse to engage in a one-to-one interaction by the end of the week.
- ○ 2. verbally interact with the nurse for 5 minutes in 1 week.
- ○ 3. problem solve with the nurse in 1 week.
- ○ 4. participate in milieu activities by the end of the week.

51. Which client outcome indicates movement toward reaching the goal stated above? The client

- ○ 1. allows the lab technician to draw her blood.
- ○ 2. begins to mumble inaudibly.
- ○ 3. is not verbally hostile with the nurse.
- ○ 4. begins to occasionally speak to the nurse in short phrases.

52. The nurse observes that the client has bathed, is wearing a clean blouse and slacks, and has combed her hair. Which statement by the nurse would be most helpful for the client?

- ○ 1. "You look good today."
- ○ 2. "I'm glad you're feeling better today."
- ○ 3. "I'm glad you combed your hair today."
- ○ 4. "I like your blouse and slacks."

A client with recurrent, endogenous depression has been hospitalized on the psychiatric unit for 3 days. He exhibits psychomotor retardation, anhedonia, and indecision.

53. Which goal of nursing care should have highest priority if the client demonstrates suicidal tendencies?

- ○ 1. Provide for contact between the client and his wife.
- ○ 2. Use measures to protect the client from harming himself.
- ○ 3. Reassure the client of his worthiness in a gentle manner.
- ○ 4. Maintain a calm environment in which the client can express his feelings and thoughts.

54. The nursing assistant approaches the nurse and states, "The client doesn't know what caused him to be so depressed. He must not want to tell me because he doesn't trust me yet." In responding to this staff member, which of the following statements by the nurse would most accurately describe the client's illness?

- ○ 1. "Endogenous depression is biochemical in nature and isn't caused by an outside stressor or problem. Therefore, the client cannot tell you why he's depressed because he really doesn't know."
- ○ 2. "Endogenous depression can be caused by various stressors. Perhaps the client isn't willing to tell you at this time."
- ○ 3. "Endogenous depression comes from within the person. It's a reaction to a loss. You need to give the client more time to identify the cause or loss."
- ○ 4. "Endogenous depression usually derives from past childhood conflicts. It really isn't important for the client to remember what happened years ago."

55. The client's condition improves, but he still remains alone in his room most of the time. Which of the following statements by the nurse would most likely help the client become involved with a unit activity?

- ○ 1. "Would you like to go to the movie with me today?"
- ○ 2. "I'll be back at 4 o'clock to take you to the movie."
- ○ 3. "I hope you go to the movie this afternoon. It will cheer you up."
- ○ 4. "You might want to go to the movie in the dayroom this afternoon."

56. The physician orders imipramine (Tofranil) for the client. The nurse explains the purpose of the medication to the client. The client asks the nurse, "If I start taking the pills, I'll have to take them the rest of my life, won't I?" Which would be the nurse's most accurate and therapeutic reply?

○ 1. "Your condition determines the need for continued medication."
○ 2. "The medication prescribed is safe and routine."
○ 3. "After your symptoms decrease, the need for medication will be reevaluated."
○ 4. "Are you concerned about taking the medication?"

57. Which of the following health status assessments must be completed before the client starts taking imipramine (Tofranil)?

○ 1. Electrocardiogram (EKG).
○ 2. Urine sample for protein.
○ 3. Thyroid scan.
○ 4. Creatinine clearance test.

58. One nurse strongly believes that all psychiatric medication is a form of "chemical mind control." When the client's wife asks about the efficacy of antidepressant medications, which of the following courses of action would be best for this nurse to take?

○ 1. Give her honest opinion of the treatment.
○ 2. Refer the client's wife to another knowledgeable person for information about the treatment.
○ 3. Explain that there are not enough current statistics about the efficacy of the treatment.
○ 4. Provide a package insert for the wife to read.

59. The nurse develops a medication teaching plan for the client. Which of the following plan components would be least important?

○ 1. A description of possible side effects.
○ 2. An opportunity for the client to express her fears and concerns about the therapy.
○ 3. A description of current research into antidepressant therapy.
○ 4. An explanation of why the first dose of medication is less than a full dose.

60. The client has been taking imipramine (Tofranil) at bedtime for 5 days. The nurse correctly judges that the medication is beginning to produce therapeutic effects when the client

○ 1. asks for a snack of cookies.
○ 2. sleeps 12 to 14 hours a night.
○ 3. states that she can feel her stomach getting better.
○ 4. asks to take the medication in the morning.

61. The client states that imipramine (Tofranil) is helping her feel less depressed but that she is still experiencing dry mouth. Which statement by the client would indicate the need for further teaching?

○ 1. "I've been chewing sugarless gum."
○ 2. "I'm sucking on ice chips."
○ 3. "I'm drinking a lot of water."
○ 4. "I'm sipping water often."

A client has been taking fluoxetine (Prozac) 20 mg qd at 9 a.m. for 7 days.

62. Which of the following would be most important to report to the evening nursing shift?

○ 1. The client received Tylenol at 2 p.m. for a headache. He spent most of the day in his room.
○ 2. The client is still depressed. He refused to participate in group today.
○ 3. The client was weighed this morning; he has lost 4 pounds since admission last week.
○ 4. The client seemed much less depressed today and participated in a card game for the first time since his admission.

The Client With Depressive Disorder and Suicidal Ideation

A nurse who makes weekly rounds of area boarding homes observes a client who was discharged from a psychiatric hospital. The client is irritable and walks about her room slowly and morosely. After 10 minutes the nurse prepares to leave, but the client plucks at her sleeve and quickly asks for help in rearranging her belongings. She also anxiously makes inconsequential remarks to keep the nurse with her.

63. Which of the following statements provides the most likely explanation for the client's behavior? The client

○ 1. is lonely and looking for a way to pass the time.
○ 2. is self-centered and possessive of the nurse's time.
○ 3. needs attention paid to some as yet-unknown concern.
○ 4. desires assistance to improve her room's appearance.

64. The nurse is careful not to act rushed or impatient with the client and gradually learns that the client is very "down" and feels worthless and unloved. In view of the fact that the client had previously made a suicidal gesture, which of the following interventions by the nurse would be a priority at this time?

○ 1. Ask the client frankly if she has thoughts of or plans for committing suicide.
○ 2. Avoid bringing up the subject of suicide to prevent giving the client ideas of self-harm.
○ 3. Outline some alternative measures to suicide for the client to use during periods of sadness.
○ 4. Mention others she has known who have felt like the client and attempted suicide, to draw her out.

65. The nurse would be most concerned about the client's depression when the client states that she

○ 1. feels more tired than usual.
○ 2. has difficulty falling asleep and wakes up early in the morning.
○ 3. no longer watches her favorite television programs.
○ 4. is gaining weight.

66. The client's friend asks the nurse, "What is the best way to act around her when she's so blue?" When considering therapeutic ways to behave with the client, the nurse should recommend that the friend avoid behaving in a way that is
○ 1. firm.
○ 2. serious.
○ 3. cheerful.
○ 4. spontaneous.

During his admission to an impatient psychiatric unit, a client tells the nurse that he has been experiencing headaches that have worsened in the past 2 weeks. He also has difficulty falling asleep and has nightmares when he does sleep. He states, "Nothing matters anymore. Life is nothing and there's nothing left for me. My wife divorced me 3 months ago. No one will want me or love me anymore. I'm not good for anyone."

67. When documenting the admission data, which of the following statements should the nurse include in the client's chart?
○ 1. The client has been depressed since his wife divorced him 3 months ago. He stated, "No one will want or love me anymore." He also complained of headaches and nightmares.
○ 2. The client is suffering from feelings of depression. He complains of headaches and nightmares and exhibits suicidal ideation. He feels unloved and unwanted since his divorce 3 months ago.
○ 3. The client willingly related his recent stressors. Suicidal ideation was also present. His headaches and nightmares have increased during the past 2 weeks.
○ 4. The client verbalized feelings of worthlessness and lack of hope for the future. He exhibited suicidal ideation, stating, "Nothing matters anymore. Life is nothing. No one will want me or love me anymore." The client was divorced 3 months ago. He has difficulty falling asleep and experiences nightmares and headaches, which have increased in the past 2 weeks.

68. From the information provided for this client, which nursing diagnosis would be least accurate?
○ 1. Disturbance in Self-Esteem related to divorce, as evidenced by negative statements about self.
○ 2. Potential for Self-Directed Violence related to lack of hope for the future, as evidenced by suicidal ideation.
○ 3. Sleep Pattern Disturbance related to depressed mood, as evidenced by difficulty falling asleep.
○ 4. Social Isolation related to feelings of worthlessness, as evidenced by withdrawal.

69. Regarding the nursing diagnosis of Potential for Self-Directed Violence, which action should the nurse take first?
○ 1. Instruct the client to seek out staff when he has thoughts of harming himself.
○ 2. Have the client agree to a "no harm" contract.
○ 3. Remove all potentially harmful objects from the client's environment.
○ 4. Assign the client to a double room occupied by another client.

70. The client admits to having thoughts of suicide. He is lethargic, withdrawn, and irritable. In conversations with the nurse, he stresses his faults. When he starts to point out the thing he cannot do, which of the following responses by the nurse would provide the best intervention?
○ 1. "You can do anything you put your mind to."
○ 2. "Try to think more positively about yourself."
○ 3. "Let's talk about your plans for the weekend."
○ 4. "You were able to write a letter to your friend today."

71. At the end of the nurse's shift, the nurse tells the client that she will spend time with him tomorrow and that other staff members are available for him to talk with in the meantime. When the nurse returns to work 3 days later, having been absent due to illness, the client is taciturn and sits staring angrily at her. When dealing with this situation, which of the following actions by the nurse probably would be the least helpful?
○ 1. Commenting that he looks angry.
○ 2. Remaining silent until he decides to talk.
○ 3. Asking him what his thoughts are at the moment.
○ 4. Apologizing for not being able to meet with him as planned.

72. Before the nurse decides which strategy to use with the client, he blurts out, "You hate me, don't you?" Which of the following replies by the nurse would be the most therapeutic?
○ 1. "You're imagining things."
○ 2. "I could never hate anyone."
○ 3. "What did I do or say to give you that impression?"
○ 4. "You're unhappy with me for not being here the last 3 days, aren't you?"

73. Although the client would like comfort, he isolates himself from others because of his anger and pessimism. Which of the following nursing interventions

would be most therapeutic in helping the client deal with his feelings?
- ○ 1. Ignore the angry behavior and focus on his need for comfort.
- ○ 2. Confront the angry behavior and help him learn more positive behaviors.
- ○ 3. Listen to his angry statements and help him plan a schedule to keep occupied.
- ○ 4. Acknowledge the angry behavior and deal with the feeling content of his behavior.

74. The nurse correctly judges that the danger of a suicide attempt is greatest when the client's behavior indicates that he
- ○ 1. has resumed his former life-style.
- ○ 2. has an increased energy level.
- ○ 3. is at a point of deepest despair.
- ○ 4. agrees to visit with an estranged brother.

A 68-year-old client is nearing discharge from the inpatient psychiatric unit to live alone in her apartment. She has improved with medication and treatment and no longer has suicidal ideation. All her family members live out of state.

75. As the nurse helps the client plan an activity program upon her return home, which plan of action would likely be most helpful for the client?
- ○ 1. Finding a volunteer to visit regularly at her apartment.
- ○ 2. Arranging for Meals-on-Wheels.
- ○ 3. Arranging transportation to a senior citizens' social group that meets near her apartment.
- ○ 4. Asking a friend of the client to spend more time with her.

76. In general, it is difficult for a nurse to maintain effective relationships with depressed clients experiencing suicidal ideation because their
- ○ 1. pessimism arouses frustration and anger in others.
- ○ 2. poor personal grooming invites disgust and ridicule from others.
- ○ 3. independence prevents them from asking for assistance.
- ○ 4. laziness keeps them from putting forth the necessary effort to get well.

77. The nurse judges correctly that a client is experiencing an adverse effect from amitriptyline hydrochloride (Elavil) when the client demonstrates
- ○ 1. an elevated blood glucose level.
- ○ 2. insomnia.
- ○ 3. hypertension.
- ○ 4. urinary retention.

78. Which of the following variables should the nurse judge as least likely to indicate high risk when assessing a client's potential for suicide?
- ○ 1. Age.
- ○ 2. Angry behavior.
- ○ 3. Home environment.
- ○ 4. Previous suicidal gesture.

79. A client's goal is: Client will state two alternative actions to take when feeling suicidal in the future. Which of the following client outcomes would indicate the least progress toward meeting this goal?
- ○ 1. The client states that she will volunteer time at a senior day care center.
- ○ 2. The client has written down the telephone number of the suicide help-line and states that she will use it if necessary.
- ○ 3. The client has arranged to join a woman's support group at her church.
- ○ 4. The client is keeping a daily journal of her feelings and problems.

80. Which of the following statements is the best wording of a no-harm, no-suicide contract?
- ○ 1. "I will not think about killing myself."
- ○ 2. "I will not accidentally or on purpose kill myself during the next 24 hours."
- ○ 3. "I will not kill myself until after talking to my doctor."
- ○ 4. "I will not kill myself unless my wife dies."

The Client Who Attempts Suicide

An adolescent female is brought to the hospital emergency room in a state of unconsciousness after having swallowed "a bottle of red pills" 45 minutes earlier. The pills are identified as secobarbital (Seconal). A suicide note is found that asks for forgiveness and states, "I can't live without my boyfriend. He has left me because I'm no good."

81. Which of the following measures should the nurse be prepared to carry out when this client is admitted?
- ○ 1. Forcing fluids.
- ○ 2. Giving a diuretic.
- ○ 3. Inducing vomiting.
- ○ 4. Lavaging the stomach.

82. Which of the following interventions should be of primary concern to the nurse after the client's physical condition is no longer critical?
- ○ 1. Providing the client with a safe environment.
- ○ 2. Ensuring that the client's diet is high in fiber.
- ○ 3. Providing the client with quiet periods for reflection.
- ○ 4. Ensuring that the client's fluid intake is generous.

83. After the client regains consciousness, she says to the nurse, "I can't even kill myself. I can't even do that right." Which of the following responses by the nurse would be most therapeutic at this time?
- ○ 1. "These feelings will pass."
- ○ 2. "Is that how you're feeling?"
- ○ 3. "Why would you feel that way?"
- ○ 4. "You have a great deal to live for."

84. When evaluating the effectiveness of the client's treatment, the nurse can judge that progress is being made when the client's behavior shows an improvement in her
- ○ 1. appetite.
- ○ 2. self-concept.
- ○ 3. activity level.
- ○ 4. gender identity conflict.

85. The client goes to her room and slams the door immediately after the first family therapy session. Later, she tells the nurse, "I'm so mad. The therapist didn't let me tell my side of the story. He just agreed with everything my parents said." Which of the following nursing actions would be most therapeutic in this situation?
- ○ 1. Consider terminating the therapy because it upsets the client.
- ○ 2. Redirect the client to the therapist to tell him how she feels.
- ○ 3. Allow the client to continue to ventilate her feelings to the nurse.
- ○ 4. Suggest to the therapist that he allow the client to tell her side of the story.

86. The adolescent unit where the client is housed uses behavior modification to encourage appropriate client behaviors. Which of the following statements best describes the theory on which behavior modification has been developed?
- ○ 1. Behavior is learned.
- ○ 2. Behavior is related to intrapsychic conflicts.
- ○ 3. Behavioral changes result from stress on the individual and his body systems.
- ○ 4. Behavior is a result of interaction between an individual and the environment.

A client is brought to the inpatient psychiatric unit from the emergency room with a self-inflicted gunshot wound in his arm. He is escorted to the unit by emergency room staff, with his arm bandaged and in a sling.

87. A staff member states to the nurse, "He only hurt his arm, so he probably only wanted to manipulate someone or did it for attention." Which of the following responses by the nurse to the staff member would be most appropriate?
- ○ 1. "All suicide attempts or acts of self-harm are very serious and indicate a cry for help."
- ○ 2. "He really must not have wanted to kill himself, but he certainly injured his arm."
- ○ 3. "He didn't use a lethal method to kill himself, so he must not have been serious about taking his life."
- ○ 4. "It was probably a way to escape a serious problem. The hospital is a safe and secure environment."

88. What client data would be most important for the nurse to consider in deciding to institute suicide precautions because of high-risk behavior? The client
- ○ 1. states that he still has thoughts of harming himself but feels he can control them.
- ○ 2. states that he is worried about his child's reaction.
- ○ 3. expresses guilt and shame about trying to harm himself.
- ○ 4. has recently attempted suicide with a lethal method.

The Client in Crisis

The nurse is employed at a crisis shelter that has several clients each day in a state of severe disorganization. An anxious-looking teenage female is brought to the interviewing room, sobbing and saying that she thinks she is pregnant but does not know what to do.

89. Which of the following nursing interventions would be the most appropriate at this time?
- ○ 1. Ask the client what she had thought of doing.
- ○ 2. Give the client some ideas about what to do next.
- ○ 3. Summarize what the nurse heard and ask the client to confirm the nurse's perceptions.
- ○ 4. Question the client in more detail about her feelings and about what her parents' reactions are likely to be.

90. The client says that she and her boyfriend have engaged in "mostly heavy petting and necking." Which of the following responses by the nurse to the client's comment would be best?
- ○ 1. "You mean you have had sexual intercourse?"
- ○ 2. "Describe what you mean by heavy petting and necking."
- ○ 3. "I think we need to talk about what's involved in sexual intercourse."
- ○ 4. "All you have been doing with your boyfriend is heavy petting and necking?"

91. The client says that she would "rather die than be pregnant." Which of the following responses by the nurse would be most helpful?

○ 1. "Try not to worry until after the pregnancy test."
○ 2. "Pregnancy is normal."
○ 3. "Why are you so upset?"
○ 4. "You're very upset now; it will be easier for you to talk about this if you can relax."

92. The nurse teaches the client about sexual intercourse, contraception, and the like. Which of the following behaviors will the nurse most probably be indirectly responsible for increasing in the client?
○ 1. Promiscuity.
○ 2. Antagonism toward men.
○ 3. Rejection of the female role.
○ 4. Responsibility for sexual encounters.

93. The client states that although she is grateful for the information she has received from the nurse, she does not believe she needs it. "No more fooling around for me!," she states. Which of the following replies by the nurse would be best?
○ 1. "Just in case, why don't you try the pills for a while?"
○ 2. "The last person who said that ended up having a baby."
○ 3. "It's up to you, but if you change your mind, come back and we'll try to help you."
○ 4. "Aren't you being a little bit overconfident about it, as attractive as you must be to the fellows?"

The nurse is responsible for counseling clients who call a crisis shelter hot-line. One night, the nurse talks to two 11-year-old boys on the telephone who think a friend sniffs glue. They say his breath sometimes smells like glue and he acts "drunk." They ask if they should tell their parents about the friend.

94. When formulating a reply, the nurse should be guided by the knowledge that
○ 1. the boys probably fear punishment.
○ 2. sniffing glue is illegal.
○ 3. the boys' observations could be wrong.
○ 4. glue-sniffing is a minor form of substance abuse.

95. The nurse urges the boys to seek help for their friend and warns them that delaying treatment could result in the boy's death. A person who inhales noxious substances is most likely to die from
○ 1. brain lesions.
○ 2. malnutrition.
○ 3. cardiac failure.
○ 4. kidney damage.

The nurse is caring for a client who came to the crisis shelter frightened and behaving aggressively. From the client's friends, the nurse learns that he has been smoking cocaine for the last 3 hours. The client is having a severe reaction to the cocaine and seems to have lost touch with reality. He is very suspicious of his friends who came with him and does not want to talk to the nurse. Suddenly, he yells out, "I'll kill you before I'll let you take me."

96. The nurse should base intervention on knowledge that the client's primary need is
○ 1. physical contact with his friends.
○ 2. isolation from other clients.
○ 3. reassurance from the staff.
○ 4. protection from his own behavior.

97. Which of the following comments by the nurse would be most useful to help the client reestablish his self-control and orientation?
○ 1. "You have no need to be concerned. You're going to be all right."
○ 2. "You have taken a drug you shouldn't have, and it is making you sick."
○ 3. "You're reacting to the cocaine and will soon be past the main drug reaction. You're safe here."
○ 4. "You have a temporary psychosis from taking a psychedelic. Let's watch some television while we wait for it to pass."

98. For this client, using a tranquilizing drug, such as chlorpromazine hydrochloride (Thorazine), to shorten the drug reaction should be avoided because
○ 1. the major tranquilizers can cause a reuptake of the drug in the brain.
○ 2. flashbacks increase in severity when mediating drugs are used to treat the initial reaction.
○ 3. the client's emotions might stem from a source entirely different from the cocaine effects.
○ 4. other incompatible drugs may have been combined with the cocaine that, together with the tranquilizer, might be fatal.

99. As the client describes the effects of cocaine, the nurse should be skeptical if the client says cocaine helps
○ 1. give him energy.
○ 2. him focus on his work.
○ 3. him need less sleep.
○ 4. cope more effectively in social situations.

A client has come to the crisis shelter because she wants to "ask someone a question." Matter-of-factly she asks, "How would you feel if your girlfriend had been raped?" The nurse suspects that the client may have been sexually assaulted.

100. What would be the nurse's best reply to the client's question?

○ 1. "Before I answer, tell me what's really on your mind, okay?"
○ 2. "I haven't thought about it. How would you expect me to feel?"
○ 3. "I'd probably be upset and angry. Do you have a special reason for asking?"
○ 4. "It would bother me. But don't you think there's too much violence these days?"

101. It turns out that the client has been ambivalent about reporting her recent sexual assault. Which of the following beliefs about the rape experience, probably the most widely held in our society, no doubt is contributing to the client's reluctance to speak about being raped? The woman
○ 1. is somehow to blame for the rape.
○ 2. is probably out to "get" the man involved.
○ 3. must show physical injury to prove her innocence.
○ 4. gets more enjoyment than pain from the experience.

102. The client reports that since being raped, she has constantly sought out brightly lit places and the company of friendly people. She also plans to move to another part of the city. When analyzing the client's behavior, the nurse correctly identifies the most likely goal for her maneuvers as
○ 1. self-defense.
○ 2. self-assertion.
○ 3. self-deception.
○ 4. self-gratification.

CORRECT ANSWERS AND RATIONALE

The letters in parentheses following the rationale identify the step of the nursing process (A, D, P, I, E); cognitive level (K, C, T, N); and client need (S, G, L, H). See the Answer Grid for the key.

The Client With a Major Mood Disorder

1. 3. The holistic approach to health care takes into account the whole person and recognizes that many factors can cause health disruptions. Holistic theory believes that all elements of disruption should be examined and eliminated or minimized to allow the person to attain a state of well-being. Reacting to a stressful event, having a high sugar intake, and destructive environmental influences describe specific causes of a disruption in health rather than numerous factors influencing the client as a whole. (A, C, L)

2. 3. A holistic approach is used when a nurse focuses on current life experiences to help a client identify disruptions in his life that are causing ill health. Focusing on dreams and free associations, childhood and past life history, and underlying conflicts and defense mechanisms describe psychoanalytically based therapy. (P, C, L)

3. 4. The nurse is using a therapeutic technique of restatement when she reiterates the client's comment in the form of a question. This technique best helps the client continue the conversation with an expression of his feelings. Telling the client that the nurse is assigned to care for him and that is why she is there is impersonal and implies that the client is being uncooperative. Telling the client that the nurse is there because the client has potential for improvement implies that other clients perhaps do not have this potential. Asking the client a question with the word "why" challenges him and demands an explanation. None of these approaches is as effective as using the technique of restatement. (I, N, L)

4. 4. When working with a client who speaks little, answers briefly, and looks at the floor, the nurse should focus on the simplest type of behavior (that is, behavior requiring the least effort for the client). The relationship described in this item is the orientation phase, when self-expression and verbalization are more appropriate goals than decision making, relating to others, and functioning independently. (P, N, L)

5. 2. This nurse–client relationship is most probably in the working phase. The client's effort to describe his problems to the nurse illustrates that the client has gone beyond testing and acquainting himself with a new relationship and is now working on his problems. The relationship is in an orientation phase when the client attempts to familiarize himself with the nurse and challenges boundaries of the relationship. The relationship is in a termination phase when the client summarizes and evaluates his progress. (A, T, L)

6. 1. The nurse should make sure that the client understands she will need to discuss information given by the client when, in her judgment, the information is necessary in relation to his therapy. This is a judgment the client is unable to make with safety. Telling a client that she can keep information confidential and will not share it with anyone places the nurse in a difficult position. If the client tells her something that she considers vital information for others on the health team, she would need to break a promise to the client if she feels that she must share the information. (I, N, S)

7. 3. The responsibility for maintaining a relationship with a client rests with the nurse. If a client misses a scheduled interview, the nurse is assuming responsibility for the relationship by seeking her out at the end of the scheduled interview time and telling her she was missed. To confront the client with her absence and ask her to explain it is nontherapeutic and threatening. To arrange another session with the client and to say nothing about the missed appointment does not keep to the terms of the nurse–client contract and offers little help to the client. The nurse makes an assumption without knowing the facts if she believes the patient has good reason for not keeping her appointment. She is not assuming responsibility when she waits for the client to make the next move in this situation. (P, N, L)

8. 4. Reaction formation is a defense mechanism that occurs when a person expresses an attitude or feeling opposite from his unconscious feelings or attitudes. The client compliments her employer when, unconsciously, she most likely does not like him because he fired her. Sublimation involves directing unacceptable impulses into constructive channels. Suppression is a conscious effort to overcome unacceptable thoughts or desires. Repression is a defense mechanism that occurs when a person excludes or bars painful experiences and thoughts from her state of consciousness. (A, T, L)

9. 2. It is most therapeutic when clients in group sessions help each other explore feelings further and when they demonstrate understanding of each other. In this situation asking the client to describe her work and indicating that the company must have had a reason for firing her avoid discussing the client's feelings. Suggesting to the client that she will have no trouble finding another job offers false hope without full knowledge of the situation. (E, N, L)

10. 4. Tranylcypromine sulfate (Parnate) is a monoamine oxidase (MAO) inhibitor. A client taking this drug in combination with foods or beverages rich in tyramine is likely to have a hypertensive crisis. The medication should be discontinued and the physician notified if the client exhibits symptoms related to an impending hypertensive crisis, such as headaches, diaphoresis, palpitations, pallor, nausea and vomiting, and chest pain. (D, K, L)

11. 2. Aged and strong cheeses are tyramine-rich foods and, when ingested in combination with MAO inhibitors, can cause a severe hypertensive crisis. Other foods and beverages rich in tyramine include aged meat and other nonfresh meat, liver, dried fish, any fermented high-protein food (e.g., yeast extracts and concentrates), Italian broad beans (pods), green bean pods, wine, beer, and ale. In many instances, the following caffeine-containing foods and beverages are also restricted: coffee, tea, cocoa, chocolate, and caffeine-containing soft drinks. (I, T, L)

12. 2. Negative self-statements are directly related to how the client views and feels about herself. The comments reflect a feeling of low self-esteem because of the psychopathology of the illness necessitating or related to her many hospitalizations. The negative view of self is a prominent theme underlying her verbalizations. Information concerning whether the client is withdrawn or is going to hurt herself is absent. The client only imagines that her husband will leave her because of her view of herself. (D, T, L)

13. 4. Describing and verbalizing feelings are necessary and normal because the client has usually repressed or blocked feelings which is partly responsible for the client's pain. Expressing feelings are a prerequisite before the nurse can intervene in how the client thinks or behaves. Stating a goal like increasing self-esteem is too global and non-specific. Writing feelings in a journal will not benefit the client since she has verbalized them to the nurse. Verbalizing work-related accomplishments is too specific and focuses on only one client aspect. Focusing on what the client likes about herself is too broad for what the client thinks is important to her. Asking the client to identify only three qualities does not overwhelm the client. (P, N, L)

14. 4. Planning to involve the client in usual at home pursuits of the immediate family is best when the client is to go home for a 24-hour pass. There are no indications that this client requires extra rest or unusual activities. It is too early for the client to start looking for employment and may not even be appropriate for this client. (P, N, L)

15. 1. Terminating a nurse–client relationship is a weaning process. Subjects such as plans for finding employment, divorce plans of a family member, and conflicts during hospitalization do not aid this weaning. Discussing the gains that the client has made during hospitalization does. The content focuses on gains made in treatment, feelings about termination, and saying goodbye. Introducing new material at termination may be a distraction and stall termination. (P, T, L)

16. 3. The overall purpose of reviewing the client's counseling sessions with the clinical nurse specialist is to evaluate nursing practice. Awareness of client behavior and client thoughts and evaluation of nursing style are parts of nursing practice. (I, C, L)

17. 4. Grief is a direct and appropriate response to termination of a positive relationship and indicates acceptance of termination. Anger is healthy when openly expressed but is a less healthy reaction than grief. A lack of response may be interpreted as indifference, but it represents a profound emotional reaction that the patient is unable to express. Humor may be a defense against feelings of loss. (E, C, L)

The Client With a Bipolar Disorder, Manic Phase

18. 1. Assessing nutritional status is a priority in this situation. A client with bipolar disorder, manic phase commonly does not have time to eat or drink because of their state of constant activity and easy distractability. Altered nutritional status and constant physical activity can lead to malnutrition, weight loss, and physical exhaustion. These states can lead to death if appropriate intervention is not instituted. Financial status is neither important nor something that the nurse can intervene with. Clients with bipolar disorder, manic phase typically go on spending sprees, have disturbed sleep patterns, and exhibit hostility when their personal desires are limited. (A, N, L)

19. 3. When the client's husband apologizes for her behavior, it is best to focus on the husband's feelings and be supportive of him. To say that the client is doing the best she can and that the nurse is used to being treated worse by clients ignores the husband's feelings. To ask what caused the client's behavior suggests criticism of the client and asks the husband for a judgment that he may not be able to make accurately. (I, T, L)

20. 3. If a client with overactive behavior acts aggressively, the nurse must first take measures to protect herself and others from harm. However, when the aggression subsides, efforts should be made to provide activity that is most likely to decrease tension and energy, such as using a punching bag. Reading a book, holding the client's hands, or placing her in isolation to work out aggression in private will not meet her needs to reduce energy and tension. However, when selecting an activity for a hyperactive client, care should be taken so that the activity does not overstimulate an already overactive client. (I, T, L)

21. 1. It is best to explain the x-ray procedure to the client in simple terms. Saying nothing or giving overly detailed explanations is inappropriate; the client needs some explanation, but details are unnecessary. There is no indication that additional help is needed for this client. (I, T, L)

22. 1. Because the client is very active, it would be best to give her food she can carry with her and eat as she moves. Allowing the client in the unit kitchen is impractical, and she most likely would be too busy to eat anyway. Allowing the client to send out for her favorite foods and serving food in small, attractively arranged portions do not meet the problem of ensuring that the active client has proper nourishment. (I, T, L)

23. 1. Explanations are unlikely to be of value for this client. It is best to assist the client into proper attire in a matter-of-fact way. At this point, the nurse needs to assist the client in setting limits on her behavior. (I, T, L)

24. 2. The client is demonstrating flight of ideas. Concreteness involves interpreting another person's words literally. Depersonalization refers to feelings of strangeness concerning the environment or the self. A neologism is a word coined by a client. (A, C, L)

25. 3. The anxiety the client feels gives rise to the distorted thinking displayed in such speech patterns as flight of ideas. Loose ego boundaries, underlying hostilities, and distortions in self-concept have little, if any, relation to the thought disorder described here. (D, T, L)

26. 4. The nurse takes responsibility for not being able to understand the client when she asks the client to speak more slowly so she can follow her train of thought. This is least likely to arouse anxiety in the client. Although helping the client make adequate connections between events is desirable, the manner in which it is done (when the nurse asks how the sun shining relates to her son) offers a threat by requiring that the client analyze thoughts and describe why they occur. Changing the subject by suggesting that the client talk about what she did yesterday is not helpful and does not focus on the client's needs. Reprimanding the client by indicating that she is talking nonsensically also is not helpful for the client in this situation. (I, T, L)

27. 2. Setting limits on behavior and explaining consequences if the limits are violated will inform the client about which behaviors are unacceptable and will set limits on manipulative behavior. The client becomes aware of what is expected and what will happen if he is not responsible for his own behavior. Taking the client to his room and telling him that he can come out when permitted does not teach him what behavior is acceptable, give him the opportunity to accept responsibility for himself, or clearly define consequences from the inability to control himself. Asking a staff member to take the client to watch television is not appropriate because, in addition to the above, the client most likely cannot sit for an hour and the television may be too stimulating. The nurse should never bargain, argue, or reason with this type of client. Rather, the nurse states what the limits are, what is expected, and what will occur if limits are not adhered to. (P, N, L)

28. 2. Channeling activities through constructive tasks, such as cleaning, allows the client to express aggressive behavior. During periods of client hyperactivity, it is generally advisable not to involve the client in activities with other clients because the technique tends to be nontherapeutic. Allowing the hyperactive client to exercise and move about as much as possible is likely to lead to exhaustion. (P, N, L)

29. 4. During a manic phase, the client is unlikely to show evidence of feelings of guilt, anger, or distrust. Hostility is a more characteristic feeling. (D, C, L)

30. 2. Here, the nurse has a responsibility to deny the client's request because it is inappropriate and financially irresponsible. Limit-setting is also an important part of working with clients, especially those in a very hyperactive phase of their illness. (I, T, L)

31. 2. The client should be observed for physical exhaustion, which predisposes to infections when a hyperactive client experiences euphoria and becomes overactive. (D, N, L)

32. 1. Sodium is necessary for renal excretion of lithium carbonate (Lithane). A low sodium intake results in retention of lithium and eventual lithium toxicity. (I, T, L)

33. 4. Clinical manifestations of lithium toxicity include anorexia, nausea and vomiting, diarrhea, coarse hand tremors, twitching, lethargy, decreased urine output, decreased blood pressure, and impaired consciousness. (D, T, L)

34. 2. The therapeutic blood level range for lithium is between 0.6 and 1.4 mEq/L for adults. A level of 1.0 can be anticipated after 10 days of treatment. (D, T, L)

35. 4. When a client has delusions of grandeur, it is not helpful to change the topic of discussion, involve him in a group project, or try to convince him that his thoughts are erroneous. It is far better to try to satisfy his implied need to feel important, because this recognizes the cause of the behavior and helps make him feel important. (I, N, L)

36. 1. Staff members sometimes are the recipients of a client's angry behavior because they are "safe targets" and are available for attack. The display of anger is rarely intended to be personal. Nor is such behavior necessarily a sign of serious pathology, an attack on a physician's skills, or a sign that the client's condition is improving. (E, N, L)

37. 3. Whenever possible, the client should first be given choices when action must be taken because of behavior. In this situation, this is best accomplished by telling the client that he has a choice of going to his room voluntarily or being escorted to his room. The client's room should be used first; if this does not help, then seclusion may be indicated. Because the client's anger is increasing, the situation is beyond discussion. (I, T, L)

38. 3. The client's statements reflecting cure and not needing medication are unrealistic and inaccurate. The presence of anger does not indicate illness. The feeling of anger is normal. Enjoyment of the state that mania produces implies that the client may not take his medication. It also implies that he does not understand the personal, family, medical, and social problems that the manic phase entails. (E, N, L)

39. 1. For the client going home, it is best to suggest that, if possible, he be relieved of some home responsibilities, that better communication be developed, and that family members learn to recognize signs of toxicity while the client is on drug therapy. It is unrealistic and impractical to attempt to eliminate worry and anxiety from a client's environment. (I, N, L)

40. 2. A family history of bipolar disorder is commonly present. A history of child molestation, high potassium levels in the brain, and drinking alcohol have not been found to be of etiologic significance for this illness. (D, T, L)

The Client Who is Depressed

41. 2. A client is legally committable when she tries to harm herself or others. (D, T, S)

42. 4. A person who has been involuntarily committed to a hospital for the mentally ill loses the right to leave the hospital of his own accord. He does not necessarily lose rights to vote, make a will or contract, or send and receive mail. (D, T, S)

43. 3. A writ of habeas corpus is defined as an order requiring that a prisoner (in this case, the client) be brought before a judge or into court to decide whether he is being held lawfully. Its purpose is to obtain liberation of a person held without just cause. (D, T, S)

44. 4. When the client feels unworthiness, she reflects low self-esteem. Presenting another set of facts in a manner that is accepting of the client but avoids a power struggle is necessary. Telling the client that her feelings are imaginary, that her family still loves her, and that she should try to forget ideas of unworthiness disregard her feelings and may be perceived as rejection. (I, T, L)

45. 2. Sitting beside the client and placing the fork in her hand are likely to stimulate the depressed client to eat. Sitting with the client also conveys a message of having time for her and of caring. Leaving the client alone, telling her that she must eat to recover, and trying to encourage her by saying the food looks good are techniques that are less likely to interest the client in eating. (I, T, L)

46. 3. The suspicious person characteristically views others as wishing to attack him. Attempting to feed the client through a gastrostomy tube is likely to be interpreted as an attack. A gastrostomy feeding is no more likely to be aspirated by this client than by any other client. Gastrostomy feeding is safe when proper technique is used. A client is unlikely to view gastrostomy feeding as a sign of approaching death or to become increasingly irritable toward others. (D, N, L)

47. 4. Doing something with or to this client is unlikely to help restlessness and incoherence. It is best to sit quietly with the client until the medication takes effect. A warm bath might be helpful, but not a cool shower. (I, T, L)

48. 4. When this client wants to be "left alone to die," it is best to leave the client for a few minutes, then return to see how the client is getting along. This response acknowledges the client's request and also lets the client know that the nurse will be back shortly. It responds to reality. Telling the client that the nurse will not allow anything to hurt the client, that the nurse is not trying to cheat the client, and that the client may be trying to frighten the nurse all are responding to delusional material. (I, T, L)

49. 1. The nurse's sitting in silence with the client shows that the nurse accepts the client and cares about her. It also will help the client get to know the nurse, initiate a feeling of comfort with the nurse, and lead to development of trust. The nurse would not persist in asking the client questions or attempt to engage her in conversation, because these measures would only overwhelm the client at this time. Leaving the client alone does not promote comfort or trust with the nurse. Telling the client that the nurse will be back to talk later will only burden the client with the nurse's expectation to talk, which the client may not be likely to meet. Including the client in group discussion will increase her discomfort and anxiety and will not be therapeutic at this time. (I, T, L)

50. 2. The goal of client-nurse interaction for 5 minutes is a realistic one to work toward based on the severity of the client's illness. This implies that the client will have gained some measure of trust in the nurse. Expecting the client to take the initiative to approach the nurse to interact in 1 week is probably unrealistic. Participating in milieu activities and problem solving are unrealistic goals at this time. The client must first start talking with the nurse before she can tolerate groups or participate in group activities. The client would feel too anxious and overwhelmed if urged too soon to participate in groups. (P, T, L)

51. 4. Speaking in short phrases with the nurse directly indicates the client's feeling of beginning comfort and trust in the nurse. Allowing the lab technician to draw blood is passive behavior. Verbalizing hostility to the nurse and displacing anger onto the nurse could be therapeutic for this client in that she would be venting feelings instead of avoiding them. Mumbling inaudibly is not helpful to the client or the nurse. (E, T, L)

52. 3. Relating to the client that she combed her hair points out a visible accomplishment to the client and reinforces positive self-care behavior. Telling the client that she looks good implies that the client did not look good yesterday. Telling the client that she is glad she is feeling better today may be an erroneous interpretation. The client may feel just as depressed as before. Stating that she likes the client's blouse and slacks implies that the nurse did not like the client's clothing before this time. (I, T, L)

53. 2. Whenever a client is suicidal, steps must be taken to prevent the client from harming herself. Other goals of care are less important than being sure the client does not carry out the threat of suicide. All threats of suicide should be taken seriously and proper precautions should be taken to protect the client from self-harm. (P, T, L)

54. 1. The cause of endogenous depression is believed to be biochemical and not a reaction to a loss. It is caused by an imbalance or decreased availability of norepinephrine, serotonin, and possibly dopamine, so the client cannot identify a specific outside cause or a loss. Reactive depression is a reaction to a loss or a stressor. It is wrong to consider that lack of trust or slow thinking are reasons why the client will not identify the cause of his depression. However, problems and stressors in the client's life are usually present, and he can discuss them with the staff when he is willing or able to. (I, N, L)

55. 2. A depressed client is often ambivalent; that is, he both wants to and does not want to carry out an activity. This client should not be given choices that allow him to say no. His disinterest may not really indicate a wish to be left alone. Making an appointment to take a client to a unit activity is more helpful than allowing the client to say he does not wish to go or leaving it up to the client to decide on his own. (I, T, L)

56. 3. This response provides the most complete information about both the current and future treatment plan and answers the question asked by the client. (I, T, L)

57. 1. Because tricyclic antidepressants such as imipramine (tofranil) cause tachycardias and EKG changes, an EKG should be done before the client takes the medication. Other side effects include urinary retention, constipation, and drowsiness. Imipramine is administered cautiously to clients receiving thyroid medication. (A, C, L)

58. 2. When strongly opposed to a type of therapy, the nurse should refer people who ask about the therapy to another knowledgeable person for information. If the nurse gives the client and family an honest opinion, it may cause the client and family to lose confidence in prescribed therapy. It would be dishonest to tell the client and family that the nurse does not know enough about the treatment to be of help. Just providing a copy of the package insert is impersonal and likely to be of little help. (P, T, L)

59. 3. A medication teaching plan includes information relevant to the client's care. A description of current research about antidepressant therapy is not essential unless the client is participating in a research protocol. (P, T, L)

60. 1. Improved appetite and improved sleep patterns indicate that the medication is having a therapeutic effect. Oversleeping could indicate oversedation. (E, T, L)

61. 3. Dry mouth is a common side effect of tricyclic antidepressants. Drinking copious amounts of water does not eliminate this side effect and can be physiologically detrimental, possibly leading to electrolyte imbalance. (E, N, L)

62. 4. A sudden lift in mood could indicate that the client has decided to commit suicide. Headache and loss of appetite are side effects of the medication and not life threatening. A full therapeutic effect could take up to 4 weeks, so a continuance of the depressive state would not be a cause for concern at this time. (E, N, L)

The Client With Depressive Disorder and Suicidal Ideation

63. 3. This client most likely needs attention paid to some unknown concern. Her behavior should be considered meaningful but not as yet fully understood. The client is also showing signs of agitated depression. Judging that the client is lonely and looking for a way to pass time, that she is self-centered and possessive of the nurse's time, or that she desires assistance to improve her room's appearance are conclusions or value judgments based on insufficient data in this situation. (D, N, L)

64. 1. Investigating the presence of suicidal thoughts and plans by overtly asking the client if she is thinking of or planning to commit suicide is a priority nursing action in this situation. Direct questioning about thoughts or plans related to self-harm does not give a person the idea to harm himself. Self-harm is an individual decision. To avoid the subject when a client appears suicidal is unwise; the safest procedure is to investigate. It would be premature in this situation to outline alternative measures to suicide or to describe other clients who have attempted suicide. (I, N, L)

65. 2. Sleep disturbances are markers of the biologic changes associated with depression and indicate increased severity. Feelings of fatigue, decreased interest in usual activities, and changes in appetite are common symptoms of depressed mood. (E, T, L)

66. 3. Cheerfulness and gaiety have a tendency to make a depressed person feel more guilty and unworthy. It is helpful to be firm and businesslike or serious with a depressed client and to behave naturally and spontaneously. (I, T, L)

67. 4. The nurse documents specific behavioral, emotional, and somatic clues, including objective and subjective data, as succinctly as possible to relate accurate and complete information about the client. This documentation is important not only when the client is admitted but also throughout the hospitalization. Charting information in vague terms leaves room for varied interpretations. (E, N, L)

68. 4. All four client problems and nursing diagnoses could apply to a client with depression and suicidal ideation. Social isolation is a typical problem of depressed clients; however, information is lacking regarding whether the client is withdrawn, and further assessment would be needed to consider it as a problem. (D, T, L)

69. 3. Client safety is the nursing priority. The nurse would remove potentially harmful objects from the environment to minimize the occurrence of self harm. Instructing the client to seek out staff when he has thoughts of harming himself gives the staff an opportunity to intervene and provide relief in discussing his feelings. Having the client agree to a no harm contract is important because the client is participating in being responsible for his own behavior. The nurse assigns the client to a double room so he is not alone. (I, T, L)

70. 4. Pointing out the client's progress by describing what he can now do is therapeutic. Telling the client that he can do anything he puts his mind to, encouraging him to think more positively about himself, and talking about weekend plans may prove more frustrating than helpful for a client who is already finding fault with himself. Also, by suggesting that the client and nurse make plans for the client's weekend changes the subject that the client introduced in the conversation. (I, T, L)

71. 2. When the nurse is unable to keep an appointment and the client appears angry about it when the nurse returns to work, the nurse should comment that the client looks angry, ask the client what her thoughts are at the moment, and apologize for not being able to meet as planned. In this situation, it would be least helpful to remain silent until the client chooses to speak. The nurse should take the initiative and give the client every opportunity to ventilate anger and express other feelings and thoughts. (I, T, L)

72. 3. A good rule of thumb is to let the client bring up his own topics for discussion and to explore clues more fully, especially if they relate to the client's feelings about the nurse. A nurse who states that the client is unhappy because she was absent is reading the client's mind. It would be impersonal for the nurse to say that she could not hate anyone. Telling the client that she is imagining things is not therapeutic and belittles the client. (I, T, L)

73. 4. Helping a depressed client learn to express feelings instead of turning the negative ones inward is an important goal of therapy. Confronting the angry behavior and helping the client learn more positive behaviors are more likely to be useful for a client who is more active than depressed. Ignoring the client's behavior and planning a schedule while the client expresses anger avoids the client's feelings. (I, T, L)

74. 2. Suicide attempts are more likely soon after depression lifts, when the client has more energy to act on her thoughts and impulses. A client may not have the energy to commit suicide during times of greatest depression. The client's energy level, rather than her status, is related to the danger involved. (E, N, L)

75. 3. Arranging for a volunteer visitor, a friend to visit, and Meals-on-Wheels all increase the client's activity but do not get her out of the house and increase her social resources as transportation to the senior group does. (P, T, H)

76. 1. Depressed clients are difficult to relate to because of their hopelessness and general apathy. The concomitant feelings of hopelessness and lack of success experienced by the nurse may lead her to withdraw or to feel angry with the client. Poor personal grooming is typical of clients with depression and suicidal ideation but can be managed by the nurse. Depressed clients are typically dependent on others. They are not motivated by laziness and are usually conscientious and dependable. (D, C, L)

77. 4. Depressed clients have sleep disturbances, and hence the property of sedation in a drug is valuable. Often, these clients are treated with antipsychotic, antidepressant, and antiparkinsonism agents simultaneously. An additive effect may cause urinary retention and paralytic ileus, serious problems that should be reported promptly. Insomnia, elevated blood glucose level, and hypertension are not associated with amitriptyline hydrochloride (Elavil) therapy. (E, N, L)

78. 2. Anger is a low risk factor for suicide, certainly less significant than such factors as age, home environment, and previous suicidal gestures. Anger turned outward is usually more positive than anger turned inward. (D, T, L)

79. 4. Recording feelings and problems daily would not be an adaptive action helpful to the client who feels suicidal. In fact, it probably would increase the client's focusing on negative thoughts and occurrences. Volunteering at a senior day care center will enhance the client's self-esteem as well as provide a measure of socialization outside of the home and structure to her day. Joining a woman's support group will provide the client with a support system. Expressing a willingness to call the suicide help line if necessary will provide the client with support and appropriate intervention. Concrete plans when thinking about suicide provide adaptive coping methods. (E, N, L)

80. 2. Agreeing to not kill oneself until after talking to a physician or unless one's spouse wife dies implies that the possibility of self-harm is still possible. Not thinking about killing oneself does not eliminate the possible impulsive behavior or action of self-harm. Agreeing to not kill oneself purposely or accidentally for 24 hours implies agreement to be partly responsible for one's own behavior and safety. In this situation, the nurse would renew the contract each day, if necessary, after assessing the client. (E, T, L)

The Client Who Attempts Suicide

81. 4. Stomach contents should be removed to prevent further absorption of the secobarbital. Lavage is preferred to induced vomiting in an unconscious client to prevent aspiration of stomach contents. Forcing fluids and giving a diuretic are inappropriate measures in this situation. (P, N, G)

82. 1. The primary nursing responsibility for a suicidal client is to provide a safe environment and to protect the patient from harming himself or herself. (P, T, G)

83. 2. When the client criticizes herself for not being able to commit suicide successfully, it is most therapeutic when the nurse makes a comment that encourages the client to elaborate and ventilate her feelings, such as, "Is that how you feel?" To tell the client that her feelings will pass or that she has a great deal to live for discounts her feelings. A comment that includes the word "why" asks the client to defend her feelings and tends to be nontherapeutic. (I, T, L)

84. 2. An improved self-concept indicates that the clients therapy is effective. A poor self-concept is a very common sign of depression and almost always occurs in the suicidal client. Appetite and activity level are not necessarily decreased in depression. Gender identity conflict is common in adolescence, but is not a sign of depression. (E, T, L)

85. 2. Because self-responsibility is part of the focus of family therapy, direct communication between the persons involved in the situation is encouraged. Learning to express oneself clearly and to give direct feedback is part of healthy communication. Here, terminating therapy because it upsets the client and suggesting to the therapist that the client be allowed to speak do not allow the client to deal directly with the person she is angry with and discourages the client from taking responsibility for her own feelings. It is satisfactory to allow a client to ventilate to a nurse, but in this situation it would be best for the client to open communication with her therapist. (I, T, L)

86. 1. Behavior modification originates from learning theories stating that behavior is learned or determined by its consequences and can be reinforced or extinguished. The psychodynamic model of behavior is reflected in the theory that behavior is related to intrapsychic conflicts. The interpersonal model of behavior is reflected in the theory that behavioral changes result from stress on the individual and his body systems. The systems model is reflected in the theory that behavior results from interaction between an individual and the environment. (E, C, L)

87. 1. The nurse must always consider all suicide attempts as very serious. Even though the attempt may result in minimal injury, it is still a cry for help and an extremely dysfunctional method of coping. To think of a suicide attempt as a form of manipulation or means to gain attention is irresponsible and leads to unsafe nursing practice. It also minimizes the client's pain and disregards his intent. Even if a client is ambivalent about suicide, accidental suicide results in loss of life. Using a gun is a high risk and lethal method of suicide. Other high risk methods include jumping, hanging, carbon monoxide poisoning, and staging a car crash. (I, N, L)

88. 4. Suicide precautions are instituted for a client who has made a recent suicide attempt using a lethal method. The client is at high risk for suicide, and his life must be protected and safety maintained.

Feelings of being in control of suicidal thoughts, expressing guilt and shame about the suicide attempt, and worrying about a child's reaction indicate a lower risk for suicide. Recent suicide attempts using a lethal method always indicates the need for suicide precautions. (E, N, L)

The Client in Crisis

89. 3. For the client who believes she is pregnant and comes to a crisis center for help, it would be best for the nurse first to summarize the client's comments and ask the client to confirm her perceptions. The first step in the nursing process is assessment, which includes obtaining accurate information about the client. Other interventions can then follow. (I, T, L)

90. 2. When the client describes what she has been doing in sexual encounters with her boyfriend, the nurse's best and initial response is to gather data that will help her determine meanings of terms the clients uses. Other comments at this time are less effective because they assume an understanding of what the client has said. (I, T, L)

91. 4. Because persons in the midst of emotional crises find it difficult to focus their thinking, the goal of the nursing intervention is to return the client to noncrisis functioning and to reduce anxiety. Pointing out the level of distress that the client is actually experiencing is the first step in attaining this goal. (I, T, L)

92. 4. Sex education has the goal of increasing one's knowledge about sex, which ordinarily leads to taking more responsibility for his or her sexual behavior. (E, N, L)

93. 3. When the client says she needs no more help because she is going to stop "fooling around," the nurse should make a comment that lets the client know the door is open for her to return. The nurse leaves the decision to the client, but does not threaten or push her own point of view. Nor does the nurse put the client down or ridicule her. (I, T, L)

94. 1. Telephoning the crisis shelter indicates that the boys are alarmed but are reluctant to talk with their parents. The nurse should focus on helping the boys talk with their parents. Because of their ages and the problem, the boys may fear that their parents will assume that they have been sniffing glue. (D, N, L)

95. 3. Persons who inhale noxious substances, such as glues, risk cardiac failure because of overexertion when under the influence of the substance. Respiratory failure is another cause of death from inhalant use. Liver and kidney damage may occur with prolonged use, but are not the most common cause of death. (D, T, L)

96. 4. The client may be experiencing delusions secondary to cocaine intoxication, which diminish reality testing and make the client fearful. Because the client is a potential danger to himself and to others, he should be protected from his own behavior. (P, N, L)

97. 3. To help the client reestablish self-control and orientation, it would be best for the nurse to make a truthful statement about what is happening and explain what to expect. Telling the client that he has no need for concern offers false assurance. It is not helpful to "moralize" by berating the client for what he did. A statement with technical terms that the client may not understand is futile. Television is generally contraindicated for a client suffering ill effects after using cocaine. (I, T, L)

98. 4. Major tranquilizers should not be given to shorten the drug reaction because of the danger (possibly fatal) of drug incompatibility. Street drugs are often combined with other substances. (D, N, L)

99. 2. Cocaine is a stimulant that increases activity and causes sleeplessness. Cocaine use may make the user feel more comfortable in social situations. It does not improve concentration or work performance. (D, T, L)

100. 3. When the client asks how the nurse would feel if his girlfriend had been raped, and the nurse believes that the question is most probably personal, the nurse should give a straightforward response while focusing on the client. It is better not to respond to the client's question with a probing question. A nurse who asks for the client's opinion on how the nurse should feel is asking the client to analyze the nurse's feelings rather than her own. The client's problem is ignored if the nurse changes the subject of the conversation. (I, T, L)

101. 1. Many people still believe that a woman who has been raped is somehow responsible for the rape. Less often do people assume that a raped woman was out to "get" the man involved or that the woman enjoyed the experience. A woman does not have to show physical injury to prove that she has been raped. (D, N, L)

102. 1. A client who has been raped who seeks out brightly lit places and the company of friends and plans to move to another part of the city is exhibiting self-defense to help avoid being raped again. (D, N, L)

NURSING CARE OF CLIENTS WITH PSYCHOSOCIAL HEALTH PROBLEMS

TEST 1: Mood Disorder and Crisis Situations

Directions: Use this answer grid to determine areas of strength or need for further study.

NURSING PROCESS

A = Assessment
D = Analysis, nursing diagnosis
P = Planning
I = Implementation
E = Evaluation

COGNITIVE LEVEL

K = Knowledge
C = Comprehension
T = Application
N = Analysis

CLIENT NEEDS

S = Safe, effective care environment
G = Physiological integrity
L = Psychosocial integrity
H = Health promotion/maintenance

		Nursing Process					Cognitive Level				Client Needs			
Question #	Answer #	A	D	P	I	E	K	C	T	N	S	G	L	H
1	3	A						C					L	
2	3			P				C					L	
3	4				I					N			L	
4	4			P						N			L	
5	2	A							T				L	
6	1				I					N	S			
7	3			P						N			L	
8	4	A							T				L	
9	2					E				N			L	
10	4		D				K						L	
11	2				I				T				L	
12	2		D						T				L	
13	4			P						N			L	
14	4			P						N			L	
15	1			P					T				L	
16	3				I			C					L	
17	4					E		C					L	
18	1	A								N			L	
19	3				I				T				L	
20	3				I				T				L	
21	1				I				T				L	
22	1				I				T				L	
23	1				I				T				L	

ANSWER GRID: 1

Nursing Process

A = Assessment
D = Analysis, nursing diagnosis
P = Planning
I = Implementation
E = Evaluation

Cognitive Level

K = Knowledge
C = Comprehension
T = Application
N = Analysis

Client Needs

S = Safe, effective care environment
G = Physiological integrity
L = Psychosocial integrity
H = Health promotion/maintenance

		Nursing Process					Cognitive Level				Client Needs			
Question #	Answer #	A	D	P	I	E	K	C	T	N	S	G	L	H
24	2	A						C					L	
25	3		D						T				L	
26	4				I				T				L	
27	2			P						N			L	
28	2			P						N			L	
29	4		D					C					L	
30	2				I				T				L	
31	2		D							N			L	
32	1				I				T				L	
33	4		D						T				L	
34	2		D						T				L	
35	4				I					N			L	
36	1					E				N			L	
37	3				I				T				L	
38	3					E				N			L	
39	1				I					N			L	
40	2		D						T				L	
41	2		D						T		S			
42	4		D						T		S			
43	3		D						T		S			
44	4				I				T				L	
45	2				I				T				L	
46	3		D							N			L	
47	4				I				T				L	
48	4				I				T				L	
49	1				I				T				L	
50	2			P					T				L	
51	4					E			T				L	
52	3				I					N			L	

Nursing Process

A = Assessment
D = Analysis, nursing diagnosis
P = Planning
I = Implementation
E = Evaluation

Cognitive Level

K = Knowledge
C = Comprehension
T = Application
N = Analysis

Client Needs

S = Safe, effective care environment
G = Physiological integrity
L = Psychosocial integrity
H = Health promotion/maintenance

		Nursing Process					Cognitive Level				Client Needs			
Question #	Answer #	A	D	P	I	E	K	C	T	N	S	G	L	H
53	2			P					T				L	
54	1				I					N			L	
55	2				I				T				L	
56	3				I				T				L	
57	1	A						C					L	
58	2			P					T				L	
59	3			P					T				L	
60	1					E			T				L	
61	3					E				N			L	
62	4					E				N			L	
63	3		D							N			L	
64	1				I					N			L	
65	2					E			T				L	
66	3				I				T				L	
67	4					E				N			L	
68	4		D						T				L	
69	3				I				T				L	
70	4				I				T				L	
71	2				I				T				L	
72	3				I				T				L	
73	4				I				T				L	
74	2					E				N			L	
75	3			P					T					H
76	1		D					C					L	
77	4					E				N			L	
78	2		D						T				L	
79	4					E				N			L	
80	2					E			T				L	
81	4			P						N		G		

ANSWER GRID: 3

NURSING PROCESS

A = Assessment
D = Analysis, nursing diagnosis
P = Planning
I = Implementation
E = Evaluation

COGNITIVE LEVEL

K = Knowledge
C = Comprehension
T = Application
N = Analysis

CLIENT NEEDS

S = Safe, effective care environment
G = Physiological integrity
L = Psychosocial integrity
H = Health promotion/maintenance

		Nursing Process					Cognitive Level				Client Needs			
Question #	Answer #	A	D	P	I	E	K	C	T	N	S	G	L	H
82	1			P					T			G		
83	2				I				T				L	
84	2					E			T				L	
85	2				I				T				L	
86	1					E		C					L	
87	1				I					N			L	
88	4					E				N			L	
89	3				I				T				L	
90	2				I				T				L	
91	4				I				T				L	
92	4					E				N			L	
93	3				I				T				L	
94	1		D							N			L	
95	3		D						T				L	
96	4			P						N			L	
97	3				I				T				L	
98	4		D							N			L	
99	2		D						T				L	
100	3				I				T				L	
101	1		D							N			L	
102	1		D							N			L	
Number Correct														
Number Possible	102	6	22	16	40	18	1	9	57	35	4	2	95	1
Percentage Correct														

Score Calculation:
To determine your **Percentage Correct**, divide the **Number Correct** by the **Number Possible**.

ANSWER GRID: 4

Personality Disorders, Organic Disorders, Using a Therapeutic Milieu

Test 2

The Client Who is Paranoid
The Client With Catatonic Schizophrenia
The Client With Chronic Mental Illness
The Client With an Obsessive-Compulsive Disorder
The Client With Organic Mental Syndromes and Disorders
Using a Therapeutic Milieu
Correct Answers and Rationale

Select the one best answer and indicate your choice by filling in the circle in front of the option.

The Client Who is Paranoid

A client glances disdainfully around the adult inpatient unit on his arrival at the hospital. He is neatly and attractively dressed and clutches a leather briefcase tightly in his arms.

1. The client refuses to let the nurse touch his briefcase or check it for valuables or contraband. How would the nurse best learn of the briefcase's contents?

○ 1. Obtaining help to take the briefcase away from the client.
○ 2. Asking the client to open the briefcase while he describes its contents.
○ 3. Inspecting the briefcase when the client is temporarily out of the room.
○ 4. Telling the client that he must follow hospital policy if he wishes to stay.

2. As the nurse stands near the window in the client's room, the client shouts, "Come away from the window! They'll see you!" Which of the following responses by the nurse would be best?

○ 1. "Who are 'they?' "
○ 2. "No one will see me."
○ 3. "You have no reason to be afraid."
○ 4. "What will happen if they do see me?"

3. The nurse should recognize that moving away from the window quickly as the client requested is contraindicated, because it would

○ 1. reveal a lack of poise in the nurse.
○ 2. make the client feel the nurse is only humoring him.
○ 3. indicate nonverbal agreement with the client's false ideas.
○ 4. let the client think he will have his way when he wishes.

4. The client thinks he is being followed by "foreign agents" who are after "secret papers" in his briefcase. What thought disorder does this indicate?

○ 1. Idea of reference.
○ 2. Idea of influence.
○ 3. Delusion of grandeur.
○ 4. Delusion of persecution.

5. The client's thoughts of being followed by foreign agents after secret papers indicates which nursing diagnosis?

○ 1. Sensory-Perceptual Alteration: Visual related to increased anxiety, as evidenced by inappropriate responses.
○ 2. Alteration in Thought Processes related to increased anxiety, as evidenced by delusional thinking.
○ 3. Impaired Verbal Communication related to disordered thinking, as evidenced by loose associations.
○ 4. Social Isolation related to mistrust, as evidenced by withdrawal.

6. The client is suspicious of the staff members and

other clients and has paranoid delusions. To help establish a therapeutic relationship with the client, which of the following plans would be best?
- ○ 1. Initiate conversations with the client whenever he becomes agitated.
- ○ 2. Set aside specific times each day for conversations with the client.
- ○ 3. Allow the client to initiate conversations when he feels ready for them.
- ○ 4. Plan conversations with the client at frequent but unspecified times during the day.

7. During a conversation with the nurse, the client suddenly jumps up, begins pacing, and wrings his hands. In this situation, what would be the nurse's best course of action?
- ○ 1. Take the client for a walk to help reduce his restlessness.
- ○ 2. Change the subject of conversation.
- ○ 3. Share the nurse's observations with the client and comment that he appears anxious.
- ○ 4. Suggest that the nurse leave and point out to him that he does not appear to want to talk now.

8. The client is to receive haloperidol (Haldol). To prevent the client from possibly "cheeking" the medication, the drug should be given in?
- ○ 1. Liquid form.
- ○ 2. Capsule form.
- ○ 3. Suppository form.
- ○ 4. As an intramuscular injection.

9. After 3 days of taking haloperidol, the client shows an inability to sit still, is restless and fidgety, and paces around the unit. Of the following extrapyramidal adverse reactions, the client is showing signs of
- ○ 1. dystonia.
- ○ 2. akathisia.
- ○ 3. parkinsonism.
- ○ 4. tardive dyskinesia.

10. Which of the following medications can the nurse anticipate administering to treat the client's extrapyramidal side effects?
- ○ 1. Chlordiazepoxide (Librium).
- ○ 2. Benztropine mesylate (Cogentin).
- ○ 3. Imipramine hydrochloride (Tofranil).
- ○ 4. Thioridazine hydrochloride (Mellaril).

11. Which of the following observations about the client would warrant the most prompt reporting and the use of safety precautions? The client
- ○ 1. cries when he talks about his divorce.
- ○ 2. starts a petition to end the curfew hour.
- ○ 3. declines to attend a daily group therapy session.
- ○ 4. names another client as his adversary.

12. The client exhibits ideas of reference, concrete thinking, and withdrawn behavior. The nursing assistant assigned to care for the client comments to the nurse, "That client! He surely gets on my nerves. Just who does he think he is?" Which of the following replies by the nurse would be best?
- ○ 1. "It sounds as though you are angry with him."
- ○ 2. "You shouldn't talk about a client that way."
- ○ 3. "I wonder if you might try to consider his feelings."
- ○ 4. "We can consider changing your client assignment."

13. The secure atmosphere of the hospital eventually helps effect a decrease in the client's paranoid ideation. All of the following activities of the nurse very likely contributed to the client's recovery *except*
- ○ 1. encouraging the client to take responsibility for his actions.
- ○ 2. acting as a role model for the client in everyday social situations.
- ○ 3. minimizing promises to the client but keeping those that are made.
- ○ 4. letting the client see the nurse talking with other clients outside of his hearing range.

14. When making plans for the client's discharge from the hospital, the nurse should use remaining interactions with the client primarily to
- ○ 1. explain possible causes of his illness.
- ○ 2. discuss the termination of the nurse-client relationship.
- ○ 3. teach about the medications he will use at home.
- ○ 4. give advice on how to handle possible future problems.

15. The client's refusal to eat because he fears something has been placed in his food is delusional thinking that most clearly demonstrates that he is
- ○ 1. aware of his dependency on others.
- ○ 2. sensitive to others' thoughts and feelings.
- ○ 3. making excuses for refusing to cooperate with staff.
- ○ 4. unable to differentiate between thoughts and external reality.

16. The team leader overhears a nursing assistant respond to the client's statement that he is the only person alive who has the answer to the world food shortage with, "How can that be? Tell me more." When discussing the effects of questioning a client closely about his false ideas, the team leader should tell the nursing assistant that this helps the client to
- ○ 1. reverse his thinking.
- ○ 2. explain his thinking.
- ○ 3. share more of his thinking.
- ○ 4. clarify some of his thinking.

17. Which of the following characteristics of a suspicious client makes it especially difficult for the nurse to establish and maintain a therapeutic relationship with him?

○ 1. Tendency to question others' motives.
○ 2. Tendency to ridicule and belittle others.
○ 3. Tendency to believe he is right and others are wrong.
○ 4. Tendency to see others as part of the conspiracy against him.

18. The nurse should avoid using touch with a paranoid client because touch may
○ 1. be misinterpreted by the client.
○ 2. arouse transference feelings in the client.
○ 3. lead to dependency on the part of the client.
○ 4. inhibit development of trust in the relationship.

19. The client spends most of the day alone in his room. He sits in the milieu momentarily but then retreats to his room, interacting only minimally with the nurse and others. Considering these behaviors, the nurse should first take which approach with this client?
○ 1. Initiate brief, frequent contacts with the client.
○ 2. Allow the client to isolate himself in his room.
○ 3. Invite the client to work on a puzzle.
○ 4. Invite the client to attend community meeting.

20. Which short-term goal would be most therapeutic for a schizophrenic client with a nursing diagnosis of Self-Care Deficit related to apathy, as evidenced by unwillingness to shower and dress self? The client will
○ 1. verbalize the need to shower and dress himself by the end of 1 week.
○ 2. recognize the need to shower and dress self by the end of 1 week.
○ 3. explain reasons why he should shower and dress himself by the end of 1 week.
○ 4. shower and dress himself by the end of 1 week.

The Client With Catatonic Schizophrenia

A client brought to the hospital by her husband is wearing sandals, revealing dirty and swollen feet, and a wrinkled dress with a stain on the front. She moves slowly and looks confused.

21. The initial goal of the nurse who admits the client should be focused on
○ 1. making the client feel safe and accepted.
○ 2. helping the client get acquainted with others.
○ 3. giving the client information about the program.
○ 4. providing the client with clean and comfortable clothes.

22. When asked about herself during the admission interview, the client stares blankly at the nurse and mutters unintelligibly. The nurse would best chart this behavior as
○ 1. "not able to answer questions at this time."
○ 2. "uncooperative during admission procedure."
○ 3. "responded to questions with a blank look and incomprehensible mumble."
○ 4. "stared when asked questions and was disoriented and incoherent."

23. The client begins to express herself verbally on occasion. Which of the following nursing actions should be credited with helping a mute client express herself verbally?
○ 1. Asking questions that draw the client out.
○ 2. Using hand signals to entice the client to communicate.
○ 3. Making open-ended statements followed with silence.
○ 4. Expressing perceptions about what the client is experiencing.

24. The client often does the opposite of what she is requested to do. For example, if asked to stand up, she sits down; if asked to dress, she undresses. In view of the client's negativism, which of the following actions would be best for the nurse to take to get the client to the dining room for meals?
○ 1. Ask her to eat in her room away from the other clients.
○ 2. Wait for her to get hungry enough to come to the dining room by herself.
○ 3. Tell her it is time for lunch and lead her firmly by the arm to the dining room.
○ 4. Promise her a reward if she eats in the dining room and get help to take her there if she refuses.

25. When upset, the client curls into a fetal position in bed. Which of the following defense mechanisms is she using when she displays behavior reminiscent of an earlier level of emotional development?
○ 1. Fixation.
○ 2. Regression.
○ 3. Substitution.
○ 4. Symbolization.

26. To help the client's progress, the nurse pays close attention to nonverbal communication whenever conversing with the client. Which of the following statements best describes why this is important? Nonverbal communication
○ 1. conveys feelings more accurately than does verbal communication.
○ 2. reveals inner defects in a person better than does verbal communication.
○ 3. allows for a healthier expression of negative emotions than do verbal communication.
○ 4. provides better concealment for true feelings than does verbal communication.

27. The client has been hospitalized for 2 weeks and is showing signs of progress daily. After visiting the

client one evening, the client's husband complains to the nurse, "Why isn't she well yet? Aren't you people doing your job?" Which of the following replies by the nurse would be the most therapeutic?
- ○ 1. "You're anxious for your wife to get better. Shall we talk about it for a while?"
- ○ 2. "She's really doing a lot better than you think. It won't be long before she'll be home again."
- ○ 3. "We're doing the best we can. She has deep-seated conflicts that cannot be cured overnight."
- ○ 4. "I know it's difficult for you. But you wouldn't want to rush her and have her get worse again, would you?"

28. The client's children are being cared for by her mother-in-law. One day after a visit with her children, the client becomes agitated and shaky and whispers to the nurse, "That woman has turned my children against me." Which of the following interventions would be best for the nurse to make first?
- ○ 1. Arrange for a social service consultation.
- ○ 2. Ask family members to limit their visiting with the client.
- ○ 3. Determine who the client is referring to.
- ○ 4. Assign a staff member to watch the client carefully for the rest of the day.

29. The physician prescribes fluphenazine decanoate (Prolixin Decanoate) for the client. What is this drug's outstanding characteristic?
- ○ 1. It is inexpensive and can be self-administered.
- ○ 2. It relieves symptoms quickly.
- ○ 3. It needs to be administered only once every 2 to 4 weeks.
- ○ 4. It has fewer side effects than the other major tranquilizers.

30. To evaluate the effects of fluphenazine on the client, it is *least* important for the nurse to regularly monitor the client's
- ○ 1. weight.
- ○ 2. white blood cell count.
- ○ 3. blood pressure.
- ○ 4. pulmonary function.

31. Psychotic clients may suddenly behave in an impulsive, hyperactive, unpredictable manner. Which of the following approaches would be best for the nurse to use first if the client would become violent?
- ○ 1. Provide a physical outlet for the client's energies.
- ○ 2. Let the client know that her behavior is not acceptable.
- ○ 3. Get help to handle the situation safely.
- ○ 4. Use heavy sedation to keep the client calm.

32. The client will be discharged with a 1-week supply of clozapine (Clozaril). Which client statement indicates an accurate understanding of the nurse's teaching about his medication?
- ○ 1. "I need to call my doctor in 2 weeks for a checkup."
- ○ 2. "I need to keep my appointment here at the hospital next week for a blood test."
- ○ 3. "I can drink alcohol, can't I?"
- ○ 4. "I can take over-the-counter sleeping medication if I have trouble sleeping, can't I?"

The Client With Chronic Mental Illness

33. The nurse interested in working with the chronically mentally ill knows the needs of this large client population include all of the following except
- ○ 1. community-based treatment programs.
- ○ 2. psychosocial rehabilitation.
- ○ 3. employment opportunities.
- ○ 4. better custodial care in long-term hospitals.

34. The nurse is offered a position as a psychiatric nurse in a psychosocial rehabilitation program. The nurse knows that the role will include all the following functions except
- ○ 1. teaching independent living skills.
- ○ 2. assisting clients with living arrangements.
- ○ 3. assisting clients in insight-oriented therapy.
- ○ 4. linking clients with community resources.

A client in the program has worked as a hotel maid for the last 3 years. She tells the nurse she is thinking of quitting her job because "voices on television are talking about me."

35. What would be the most important thing for the nurse to do first?
- ○ 1. Get information about the client's medication compliance.
- ○ 2. Remind the client that hearing voices is a symptom of her illness with which she can cope.
- ○ 3. Check with the client's employer about her work performance.
- ○ 4. Arrange for the client to be admitted to a psychiatric hospital for a short stay.

36. The client tells the nurse she stopped taking chlorpromazine hydrochloride (Thorazine) 2 weeks ago because she is better and wants "to make it on my own without this damned medicine." Which of the following would be the nurse's most therapeutic response?
- ○ 1. "You've told me about other times like this when you stopped taking your medication and got sick again. Please don't do it again this time."

○ 2. "You're a smart girl. You know what will happen if you don't take your medication. Why do you want to be so bad to yourself?"
○ 3. "I know you get tired of taking the medication, especially when you're doing well. Is there any special reason you decided to stop right now?"
○ 4. "Maybe you're ready for a short holiday from the thorazine. I'll talk it over with the physician. But you need to keep taking it until I talk with him."

A nurse working at an outpatient mental health center primarily with the chronically mentally ill receives a telephone call from the mother of a client who lives at home. The client's mother reports that the client refuses to go to the sheltered workshop where she has worked for the last year, and that she has been taking her medication.

37. What should the nurse do first?
○ 1. Call the director of the sheltered workshop for information about the client.
○ 2. Reserve an inpatient bed in the hospital.
○ 3. Ask to speak to the client.
○ 4. Make an appointment to see the client.

38. The director of the sheltered workshop tells the nurse that the client had done well until last week when a new person started at the workshop. This new person worked faster than the client and took her place as leader of the group. Based on this information, which of the following would be the most appropriate nursing intervention?
○ 1. Make a home visit and tell the client that if she does not return to the workshop, she will lose her place there.
○ 2. Ask the director to assign the client to another work group when she returns to the workshop.
○ 3. Make an appointment to meet the client at the mental health center and ask her about the situation.
○ 4. Arrange placement for the client in a skill training program.

39. The client tells the nurse that she quit going to the workshop because "the job doesn't pay enough." She reports that her sister just finished school and bought a car, and says that she plans to look for an office job like her sister. Which of the following characteristics of a chronically mentally ill young adult best explains the client's behavior?
○ 1. Difficulty accepting the role of client.
○ 2. Low self-esteem.
○ 3. Lack of coping resources.
○ 4. High expectations of self in achieving social goals.

40. The mental health center has a psychoeducational program for families of the chronically mentally ill. The nurse invites the client's parents to attend the program. The nurse's actions are based on the knowledge that the desired outcomes of these psychoeducational programs include all of the following except helping the families
○ 1. feel less guilty about the client's illness.
○ 2. develop a support network with other families.
○ 3. improve their conflicted relationship.
○ 4. recognize the client's strengths more accurately.

A client who has not left the bus station for 3 days is brought to the mental health center by a police officer because she had been "bothering people." She denies this, will not give her name, and holds tightly to her purse. She refuses to talk to anyone except to say, "You have no right to keep me here. I have money and I can take care of myself." The police can hold her for disturbing the peace but think she needs psychiatric evaluation.

41. Which of the following factors would be most relevant to a decision about this client's disposition?
○ 1. She seems able to care for herself.
○ 2. She has no known family.
○ 3. She is not known to the mental health center.
○ 4. She has $500 in cash and says she will go to a hotel.

42. The decision is made to admit the client involuntarily on an emergency basis. The nurse on the inpatient unit explains the involuntary hospitalization process to the client, who listens quietly. Which of the following statements made by the nurse would be inaccurate?
○ 1. "You're in the hospital because the psychiatrist who saw you earlier thinks that you are unable to care for yourself right now."
○ 2. "You're free to talk to a lawyer if you'd like to do so."
○ 3. "You cannot leave the hospital until the doctor or a judge thinks you can take care of yourself."
○ 4. "You cannot have any visitors while you're here involuntarily."

43. The nurse informs the staff members that the physician is discharging the client because involuntary commitment is not indicated. The nursing assistant states, "How can her physician be so cruel? She should stay in the hospital instead of the bus station." Which of the following responses would be best for the nurse to make to the nursing assistant?
○ 1. "I agree with you. She does have symptoms of mental illness."

○ 2. "Even though the client may have a mental illness, she is not gravely disabled or dangerous to herself or others."
○ 3. "The client wants to leave, so the physician is not going to put her through the commitment process."
○ 4. "The client has a home to go to and family to support her. She doesn't need to be here."

44. As the nurse helps the client prepare for discharge, the client says, "You know, I've been in lots of hospitals and I know when I'm sick enough to be there. I'm not that sick now. You don't need to worry about me." Which of the following would be the most therapeutic response by the nurse?
○ 1. "We're worried about you. Is there any way we can help you now?"
○ 2. "We could have helped you more if you had told us more."
○ 3. "You told us you were a visitor here. Is there any information you need before you leave the hospital?"
○ 4. "How do you know when you need to be in the hospital?"

45. The nurse has been asked to develop a medication education program for clients in the rehabilitation program. When developing the course outline, the nurse should plan to include all of the following topics except
○ 1. a categorization of a wide variety of psychotropic drugs.
○ 2. interventions for common side effects of psychotropic drugs.
○ 3. the role of medication in treating chronic illness.
○ 4. the effect of combining common street drugs with psychotropic medication.

46. The nurse has been asked to orient a new nurse to the psychosocial rehabilitation program. To ensure that the new nurse understands the concept of chronic mental illness, the nurse would include all of the following information in the orientation program except that
○ 1. the chronically mentally ill have been labeled deviant by society, and much of their behavior is related to this role identity.
○ 2. although care of the chronically mentally ill is an important goal, the ultimate goal of long-term treatment is cure of the psychiatric disorder.
○ 3. the chronically mentally ill have both primary and secondary symptoms of psychiatric illness.
○ 4. the development of chronic mental illness follows a common, predictable pattern.

47. The nurse at the mental health center has been asked to develop an in-service program for the staff about young adult chronically mentally ill clients. Which of the following characteristics would the nurse most likely find common to this group of clients?
○ 1. They have minimal experience with lengthy periods of hospitalization.
○ 2. They accept the client role easily.
○ 3. They have a low incidence of substance abuse.
○ 4. They have lower expectations of achieving social goals of employment and relationships than do older chronically mentally ill clients.

The Client With an Obsessive-Compulsive Disorder

A client released from a psychiatric hospital 1 year ago has been seeing a nurse for outpatient follow-up care. The client arrives late for an appointment. During the interview, he fidgets restlessly, has trouble remembering what topic is being discussed, and says he thinks he is "going crazy."

48. Which of the following statements by the nurse would best deal with the client's feeling about "going crazy"?
○ 1. "I see that this concerns you, but what does 'crazy' mean to you?"
○ 2. "Most people feel that way occasionally. You're no different from anyone else."
○ 3. "I don't know enough about you to judge. Why don't you tell me more about yourself?"
○ 4. "You sound perfectly sane to me. Maybe your perception of the word "crazy" is different from mine."

49. The client reveals that he was late for his appointment because of "my dumb habit. I have to take off my socks and put them back on 41 times! I can't stop until I do it just right." The nurse judges correctly that the client's behavior most likely represents an effort to
○ 1. relieve his anxiety.
○ 2. control his thoughts.
○ 3. gain attention from others.
○ 4. express hostility toward his mother.

50. A decision is made not to hospitalize the client. Of the following abilities the client has demonstrated, the one that probably most influenced the decision not to hospitalize him is his ability to
○ 1. hold a job.
○ 2. relate to his peers.
○ 3. perform activities of daily living.
○ 4. behave in an outwardly normal manner.

51. The staff considers it important to decrease the client's dependence on others. To meet this goal, when the client says, "What time is it?" which of the following replies would be the most effective for a staff member to make?

○ 1. "My watch says 10 o'clock."
○ 2. "What time do you think it is?"
○ 3. "Has anyone else got the time?"
○ 4. "There's a clock behind you on the wall."

52. The client eats slowly and is always the last to finish lunch, which makes it difficult for the group to start its 1 p.m. outing. Which of the following approaches would be the best plan of action for this problem?
○ 1. Change the time of the outing to accommodate the client.
○ 2. Arrange for the client to start eating earlier than the others.
○ 3. Plan to go without the client so that he will have ample time for his lunch.
○ 4. Inform the client that he will have to eat faster so that the group can leave on time.

53. The client wants to take up a hobby and asks the day-care nurse for some suggestions. From a therapeutic standpoint, which of the following activities would be the most desirable for the client?
○ 1. Swimming.
○ 2. Solo flying.
○ 3. Drama club.
○ 4. Photography.

A client tells the nurse that he checks all lights to be sure they are off 26 times before he can leave his house. He knows his behavior is senseless but he can't stop. He rarely sees his friends anymore, because they "are fed up with his being late everytime they plan to get together." Besides, he "really is too busy to see them" because of "all the things going on at work."

54. Which of the following nursing diagnoses would be least appropriate for this client?
○ 1. Fear.
○ 2. Diversional Activity Deficit.
○ 3. Social Isolation.
○ 4. Powerlessness.

55. In considering the client's immediate needs, the nurse would include all of the following client outcomes except, the client will
○ 1. increase expression of feelings.
○ 2. connect feelings with behavior.
○ 3. use two adaptive coping behaviors to deal with anxiety.
○ 4. make a decision about one of his problems.

56. The client reports that before he leaves home to go anywhere, he counts the money in his wallet as many as 12 times. The best explanation for the client's motives when performing this particular ritual is that he is attempting to
○ 1. channel excessive sexual energy into an appropriate habit.
○ 2. compensate for not having enough money to spend as a child.
○ 3. avoid the embarrassment of having a shortage of funds on hand.
○ 4. substitute emotions unacceptable to him with a relatively acceptable activity.

57. Which of the following actions would be best for the nurse to take when the nurse observes the client in a ritualistic pattern of behavior?
○ 1. Isolate the client so that he will not disturb others.
○ 2. Observe the client closely for marked changes in behavior.
○ 3. Remind the client that he can control his behavior if he wishes.
○ 4. Enable the client to continue so that he will not become more agitated.

58. Which of the following qualities is most important for the nurse interacting with obsessive-compulsive clients?
○ 1. Patience.
○ 2. Compassion.
○ 3. Friendliness.
○ 4. Self-confidence.

59. The client has been taking clomipramine (Anafranil) for his obsessive-compulsive disorder. He tells the nurse, "I'm not really better and I've been taking the medication faithfully for the past week just like it says on this prescription bottle." Which of the following actions would the nurse do first?
○ 1. Tell the client to stop taking the medication and call the physician.
○ 2. Tell the client to continue taking the medication as prescribed, because it takes 5–10 weeks for a full therapeutic effect.
○ 3. Encourage the client to call his physician in 1 week and to continue taking his medication.
○ 4. Ask the client if he has resumed smoking cigarettes.

60. The nurse could initially recommend all of the following methods of treatment to a client with obsessive-compulsive disorder except
○ 1. relaxation exercises.
○ 2. thought stopping.
○ 3. meditation.
○ 4. exposure therapy.

The Client With Organic Mental Syndromes and Disorders

A 72-year-old female client is brought by ambulance to the hospital's psychiatric unit from a nursing home where she has been a client for 3 months. Transfer data indicate that she has become increasingly confused and disoriented and has become a "management problem."

61. In which of the following ways should the hospital admission routine be modified for an older, confused person like the client? The client should be
- ○ 1. left alone to promote recovery of her faculties and composure.
- ○ 2. medicated to ensure her calm cooperation during the admission procedure.
- ○ 3. allowed sufficient extra time in which to gain an understanding of what is happening to her.
- ○ 4. given a tour of the unit to acquaint her with the new environment in which she will live.

62. The client is to undergo a series of diagnostic tests to determine whether or not her dementia is treatable. Treatable forms of dementia (those with symptoms that can be arrested or reversed) include those caused by all of the following disorders except
- ○ 1. cerebral abscess.
- ○ 2. multiple sclerosis.
- ○ 3. syphilitic meningitis.
- ○ 4. electrolyte imbalance.

63. An electroencephalogram (EEG) is ordered for the client. The procedure is most accurately described as one that
- ○ 1. is somewhat painful but short.
- ○ 2. does not involve the use of electrical shock.
- ○ 3. tests the client's intelligence but not her sanity.
- ○ 4. enables the examiner to know what the client is thinking.

64. The night before her EEG, which of the following preparations will most probably be required for the client?
- ○ 1. Washing her hair.
- ○ 2. Taking a laxative.
- ○ 3. Going to bed early.
- ○ 4. Providing a sample of her handwriting.

65. After the diagnostic tests are completed, the client's mental condition is found to be due to cerebral arteriosclerosis. Because no known cure exists for this disorder, which of the following attitudes should the nursing staff try to influence the client (and each other) to adopt?
- ○ 1. A hopeful attitude.
- ○ 2. A resigned attitude.
- ○ 3. A concerned attitude.
- ○ 4. A nonchalant attitude.

66. In addition to disturbances in her mental awareness and in her orientation to reality, the client is also likely to show loss of ability in
- ○ 1. speech.
- ○ 2. judgment.
- ○ 3. endurance.
- ○ 4. balance.

67. The client exhibits memory loss, confusion, and wandering behavior. Of the following comments by the nurse, which would provide the best reality orientation for the client when she first awakens in the morning?
- ○ 1. "Do you remember who I am or what day it is today?"
- ○ 2. "Hello, did you sleep well? Which dress would you like to wear today, the yellow or the green one?"
- ○ 3. "Here I am again, your favorite nurse. Today is Tuesday, so there will be pancakes for breakfast this morning."
- ○ 4. "Good morning. This is your second day in Memorial Hospital and I'm your nurse for today. My name is Ms. Daly."

68. Because of the client's age and organic impairment, which of the following courses of action should most certainly be included in the plan of care?
- ○ 1. Have two people accompany the client when she is up and about.
- ○ 2. Make sure all objects that the client could trip over are removed from her path.
- ○ 3. Put the client's favorite belongings in a safe place so that she will not lose them.
- ○ 4. Give the client her medications in liquid form to make certain that she swallows them.

69. The client roams about the hospital unit at night, disturbing the sleep of other clients. When asked why she walks about, she complains of being lost and unable to sleep. A large sign is posted on the door of her room to help her locate it. Which of the following programs would be best for dealing with the client's insomnia?
- ○ 1. A daily afternoon nap to prevent overtiredness at night.
- ○ 2. Administration of a hypnotic drug at bedtime.
- ○ 3. Enough active exercise daily so she will be comfortably tired at night.
- ○ 4. A cup of hot tea with lemon before bed to promote a feeling of well-being.

70. Phenothiazines rather than barbiturates may occasionally be prescribed to treat severe insomnia for the client primarily because barbiturates tend to cause
- ○ 1. eventual kidney damage.
- ○ 2. respiratory and cardiac depression.
- ○ 3. delirium and paradoxical excitement.
- ○ 4. loss of rapid-eye-movement stages during sleep.

71. The client's daughter says that her mother wore the same dirty, worn out undergarments for weeks at home. Of the following techniques, which would be best for the nurse to follow with the client during

hospitalization to prevent further regression in her personal hygiene habits?
- ○ 1. Accept her need to go without bathing if she so desires.
- ○ 2. Make her assume responsibility for her own physical care.
- ○ 3. Encourage her to do as much self-care as she can.
- ○ 4. Do most of her physical care while letting her think she did it herself.

72. A nurse on the unit often avoids the client's company, preferring to associate with clients of her own age group or younger. Which of the following factors is most likely responsible for this nurse's extreme discomfort with older clients and her unconscious avoidance of them?
- ○ 1. Fears and conflicts about aging.
- ○ 2. Dislike of physical contact with older people.
- ○ 3. A desire to be surrounded by beauty and youth.
- ○ 4. Recent experiences with her mother's elderly friends.

73. One day when she is more alert than usual, the client asks the nurse to help her make out her will. Which of the following possible responses by the nurse would be best in this situation?
- ○ 1. "I'm not a lawyer, but I'll do what I can for you."
- ○ 2. "You have a long way to go before you'll need to do that. Let's wait on it a while, shall we?"
- ○ 3. "I don't believe in getting involved in legal matters, but maybe I can find another nurse who'll help you."
- ○ 4. "You need to consult an attorney because I'm not trained in such matters. Is there a family lawyer I can call for you?"

74. The client is allowed to reminisce about her past life. What effect can reminiscing by an elderly client be expected to have on her functioning in the hospital?
- ○ 1. Increase the client's confusion and disorientation.
- ○ 2. Subject the client to the others' impatient responses.
- ○ 3. Decrease the client's feelings of isolation and loneliness.
- ○ 4. Keep the client from participating in therapeutic activities.

75. The client's daughter brings an article about Alzheimer's disease to the nurse and says, "This sounds just like Mother. Are you sure she doesn't have Alzheimer's? Maybe she should be in a special treatment program." Which of the following responses by the nurse would be *inaccurate?*
- ○ 1. "Your mother's symptoms are common to a number of brain disorders."
- ○ 2. "You may be right. I'll talk with the physician about doing more tests so we can know for sure."
- ○ 3. "Even if we were certain that she has Alzheimer's, the treatment that will help her is the same as what she is getting."
- ○ 4. "As we learn more about how the brain ages, it is possible to diagnose these problems more accurately."

76. What clinical manifestation is uncommon to clients with organic mental disorders including Alzheimer's disease?
- ○ 1. Agnosia.
- ○ 2. Sleep disturbances.
- ○ 3. Problems with long-term memory retrieval.
- ○ 4. Elevated mood.

77. The client's daughter is convinced that her mother has Alzheimer's disease. She asks the nurse, "Does this disease run in families? Will this happen to me when I get old?" The nurse should base the response on the knowledge that which of the following factors is not associated with increased incidence of Alzheimer's disease?
- ○ 1. Excessive alcohol consumption.
- ○ 2. Head trauma.
- ○ 3. Family history of Alzheimer's disease.
- ○ 4. Old age.

A client exhibits confusion and severe memory loss. At 11:30 a.m., he tells the nurse that he is going to work and proceeds to walk toward the door.

78. The nurse should take which of the following actions?
- ○ 1. Remind him that he retired from his job 10 years ago.
- ○ 2. Tell him that she'll accompany him for a short walk outdoors.
- ○ 3. Divert his attention toward the dining room where lunch is being served.
- ○ 4. Tell him that he does not have to go to work today.

79. With a client experiencing delirium, the nurse prioritizes interventions to first maintain
- ○ 1. orientation.
- ○ 2. life.
- ○ 3. optimal level of functioning.
- ○ 4. consistency in routine.

Using a Therapeutic Milieu

The nurse is employed in a psychiatric hospital, working toward providing a therapeutic milieu for clients.

80. The primary purpose of managing the milieu on a psychiatric unit is to ensure that the environment will

○ 1. help clients meet treatment goals.
○ 2. meet the comfort needs of clients and staff.
○ 3. allow the staff to observe and evaluate clients.
○ 4. facilitate implementation of physicians' orders.

81. For a closed or locked unit, the nurse judges the milieu as therapeutic, because priorities are given to
○ 1. socialization and self-understanding.
○ 2. education and vocation counseling.
○ 3. safety, structure, and support.
○ 4. developing communication, social, and leisure skills.

82. A client asks the nurse for a medication because he is "feeling nervous." In terms of a therapeutic milieu, what would be the nurse's best response to the client's request?
○ 1. "Let's sit down and talk about your feelings of nervousness."
○ 2. "Why don't you play ping-pong with another client?"
○ 3. "Try lying down awhile and thinking about something else."
○ 4. "I'll call your doctor and get an order for some medication."

83. It is least important that the nurse take steps to set limits for which of the following clients?
○ 1. The client who uses the telephone most of the day.
○ 2. The client whose behavior is disturbing other clients.
○ 3. The client whose attire is offensive to the nursing staff.
○ 4. The client whose behavior indicates that she may harm herself.

84. Several adolescents are playing the stereo loudly in a common recreation area, and the adult clients are complaining about the loud music. As a first step in setting limits in this situation, the nurse should set limits
○ 1. on permissible volume while the stereo is being used.
○ 2. by prohibiting the use of the stereo in the recreation area.
○ 3. by turning down the volume while the stereo is on.
○ 4. by explaining to the adults that the adolescents need recreational activity.

85. An elderly client diagnosed with organic mental disorder is showing signs of confusion, short attention span, and mood swings. Which of the following activities would be best suited for this client? Having the client
○ 1. join others going on a field trip.
○ 2. become a member in group therapy.
○ 3. meet with an assertiveness training group.
○ 4. participate in a reality-orientation group.

86. A hyperkinetic 5-year-old child exhibits signs of extreme restlessness, short attention span, and impulsiveness. Which of the following ways that the nurse could alter the child's milieu would likely be most therapeutic for him?
○ 1. Increase the child's sensory stimulation and activity.
○ 2. Limit the child's opportunities to display anger and frustration.
○ 3. Define behaviors of the child that will be acceptable and those that will be unacceptable.
○ 4. Allow the child freedom to choose activities in which to participate and other children with whom to associate.

87. A 15-year-old male client shows signs of mild intoxication. When questioned, he states that another client, whom he refuses to name, gave him beer. The best course of action to initiate at this time would be to
○ 1. search the client's room for beer.
○ 2. call a community meeting to deal with the problem.
○ 3. try to persuade the client to tell who gave him the beer.
○ 4. call the physician to obtain additional orders.

CORRECT ANSWERS AND RATIONALE

The letters in parentheses following the rationale identify the step of the nursing process (A, D, P, I, E); cognitive level (K, C, T, N); and client need (S, G, L, H). See the Answer Grid for the key.

The Client Who Is Paranoid

1. 2. When a client refuses to have his belongings checked for valuables or contraband according to hospital policy, the least threatening course of action is to ask him to open his briefcase while he describes its contents. Getting help to take the briefcase away from the client is a threatening maneuver. Inspecting the briefcase while the client is out of his room involves secrecy and is less desirable than an open discussion with the client. Telling the client that he must observe hospital policy to stay is threatening and probably inaccurate as well. (P, T, L)

2. 1. Asking the client who "they" are when he is fearful helps the nurse understand his behavior and is least demanding of the client. The client is very unlikely to accept statements that indicate no one will see the nurse and that there is no reason to be afraid. Asking the client what will happen if someone sees the nurse is also unlikely to be acceptable and validates the client's delusion. (I, T, L)

3. 3. The client's behavior is likely to be reinforced when the nurse takes steps to agree with the false ideas he holds. The nurse's action of moving away from the window as the client requests is less likely to be interpreted as a lack of poise, an effort to humor the client, or an admission of giving in to the client's wishes. (E, N, L)

4. 4. The client's thought process is best defined as a delusion of persecution. A delusion of grandeur involves an exaggerated idea of one's importance or identity. An idea of reference assumes that the remarks and behavior of others apply to oneself. An idea of influence refers to the belief that persons or objects have control over one's behavior. (D, C, L)

5. 2. The nursing diagnosis Alteration in Thought Processes related to increased anxiety, as evidenced by delusional thinking, most accurately reflects this client's problem given the data. Sensory-Perceptual Alteration, Impaired Verbal Communication, and Social Isolation are nursing diagnoses typically present in clients with thought disorders and paranoia. Additional data would be needed to support these diagnoses. (D, N, L)

6. 2. To promote a therapeutic relationship with a suspicious client, it is best to set aside periods for conversation at the same time each day. During each phase of a therapeutic relationship, the nurse should be as consistent as possible. It is less satisfactory to use unspecified times or to allow the client to initiate meetings. It is difficult to have meaningful conversations that promote a therapeutic relationship when meetings occur only when the client is agitated, although the nurse may need to intervene at those times as well. (P, T, L)

7. 3. When the client becomes restless during a conversation with the nurse, the best course of action is to help him recognize and acknowledge his feelings and share observations with him. Other courses of action, such as changing the subject, taking him for a walk, and leaving him, do not encourage him to express anxiety. (I, T, L)

8. 1. It is generally best to try giving a medication in its liquid form if the patient "fights" taking it. If he refuses to swallow or expectorates the medication, the intramuscular route then can be used, although it too will probably meet with resistance. (P, T, L)

9. 2. The client's behavior is best defined as akathisia. Dyskinesia is characterized by twitching or involuntary muscular movement. Dystonia is characterized by uncoordinated spasmodic movements. (D, N, L)

10. 2. The drug of choice for a client experiencing extrapyramidal side effects to haloperidol (Haldol) is benztropine mesylate (Cogentin) because of its anticholinergic properties. Chlordiazepoxide (Librium) is a minor tranquilizer, or antianxiety agent. Imipramine hydrochloride (Tofranil) is an antidepressant. Thioridazine hydrochloride (Mellaril) is a major tranquilizer, or antipsychotic agent. (D, N, L)

11. 4. The client exhibits aggression against his perceived adversary when he names another client as his adversary. The staff will need to watch him carefully for signs of impending violent behavior that may injure others. Crying about a divorce would be appropriate, not pathologic, behavior. A petition to end the curfew hour would be a positive, direct action aimed at a bothersome situation. Declining to attend group therapy needs follow-up but may be due to any number of unknown reasons. (E, N, L)

12. 1. Like clients, health personnel have feelings and rights. Here, the nurse recognizes the assistant's angry feelings without scolding her or dismissing her feelings. (I, T, L)

13. 4. The suspicious client is likely to experience an increase in paranoid ideation when he sees his nurse talking with other clients outside of his hearing range. Taking actions that encourage the client to take responsibility for his own actions, having nurses as role models, and minimizing promises while keeping those that are made are unlikely to arouse feelings of suspicion and conspiracy. (E, N, L)

14. 2. When preparing to discharge the client from the hospital, the nurse should work toward ending the relationship and exploring reactions to the separation. Giving advice is not recommended. Health teaching is important, but during final interactions with the client it is of primary importance to work toward ending the nurse-client relationship. Furthermore, the health teaching should not be left until the last minute. (P, T, L)

15. 4. Delusional thinking refers to a belief that is not validated by reality and is maintained even when proof is given to the contrary. Here, the client is unable to differentiate between his thoughts and external reality. Some suspicious clients demonstrate sensitivity to the thoughts and feelings of others, but this is not evidence of delusional thinking. (D, T, L)

16. 2. Questioning a client closely about his false ideas places him on the defensive, and he will most likely continue to defend his unrealistic point of view even more vigorously. Close questioning is unlikely to lead the client to reverse, share, or clarify his thinking. (P, T, L)

17. 4. The suspicious client characteristically considers others to be part of a conspiracy against him. Behaviors such as questioning the motives of others, ridiculing and belittling others, and believing that he is right and others are wrong are more easily managed and are not central to the core problem of suspicion. (D, C, L)

18. 1. Touch should be used cautiously with clients, especially paranoid clients who have poor reality testing and who project their own feelings and impulses. The clients may easily misinterpret the use of touch. (P, C, L)

19. 1. Brief, frequent contacts with the client would be the first approach used by the nurse to convey caring and acceptance to the client to facilitate trust and promote a feeling of self-worth. Allowing the client to isolate himself in his room increases his isolative behavior and allows withdrawal into self and from others. Inviting the client to community meeting and to work on a puzzle would be appropriate interventions later, after the client feels some comfort with and trust in the nurse. (I, T, L)

20. 4. Showering and dressing himself by the end of 1 week is most therapeutic to the client. A client with schizophrenia often appears to be apathetic and lack initiative. These effects are typically related to the ambivalence associated with schizophrenia. The client may tell the nurse that he will shower and dress and be able to explain why he should shower and dress but be unable to do so because of the ambivalence that impedes his ability to initiate and complete self-care. (E, N, L)

The Client With Catatonic Schizophrenia

21. 1. It is important to help make the client feel safe and accepted. Helping the client get acquainted with others and giving her information about the program are important but are of lower priority at admission. Providing the client with clean clothes is desirable but less important than conveying feelings of safety and trust. (P, T, L)

22. 3. The best charting describes exactly what the client did and said in a particular situation. Noting that the client was unable to answer questions, was uncooperative, and was disoriented and incoherent do not follow this basic principle of documenting and also are not objective descriptions. (E, N, L)

23. 3. The best approach for a client who has difficulty expressing herself verbally is to use a nondemanding, open-ended statement. When the client is ready to talk, the silences following the statement will give him the opportunity to do so. Asking the client questions, using hand signals, and assuming what the client is experiencing are ineffective for this client. (I, T, L)

24. 3. Punishment and reward are likely to be of little value when a client does the opposite of what she is asked to do. The client simply may not eat if allowed to decide when to go to the dining room. The best course of action is to firmly lead the client to the dining room. This type of positive and firm approach is also needed to help increase the client's socialization. (I, T, L)

25. 2. A client's behavior is best described as regression when it is typical of an earlier stage of development. Fixation means not progressing beyond a given level of development. Substitution means replacing unacceptable ideas with more acceptable ones. Symbolization occurs when one idea or object comes to stand for another. (D, T, L)

26. 1. It has been shown that nonverbal communication usually conveys feelings more accurately than does verbal communication. Words often are used to cover feelings, whereas nonverbal communication offers less opportunity to hide true feelings. (D, C, L)

27. 1. The nurse demonstrates her interest in the feelings the husband expresses about his wife and provides an opportunity to discuss them by acknowledging his anxiety and offering to converse with him. Statements to the husband that indicate the staff is doing the best it can, that the client is better than the husband thinks, and that rushing through treatment may make matters worse give the husband no reassurance and disregard his feelings. (I, T, L)

28. 3. The nurse needs to know who the client is referring to and should try to obtain this information from the client. Arranging for a social service consultation and assigning someone to watch the client are premature, although they may be indicated later. Asking the family to limit visits would not be helpful in gaining an understanding of the situation. (I, T, L)

29. 3. An outstanding characteristic of fluphenazine decanoate (Prolixin Decanoate) is that it can be effective even when administered relatively infrequently. (D, C, L)

30. 4. It is least important to check the results of pulmonary function tests for the client receiving fluphenazine decanoate (Prolixin Decanoate). Weight checks are indicated because a side effect of this drug is edema with weight changes. The client should be monitored for blood dyscrasias. Blood pressure may fluctuate while the drug is being used and should be monitored. (I, C, L)

31. 3. The recommended first course of action is to prevent accidents and injuries when a client becomes violent. In this situation, it would be best to call for help to handle the situation safely. Other actions may be taken later, after safety is ensured. (I, T, L)

32. 2. Mandatory weekly white blood cell counts are used to detect developing agranulocytosis, which can be fatal and occurs in 1–2% of clients taking clozaril. This medication is also associated with risk of seizures; this risk is dose dependent, meaning that it increases in moderate to high doses (600–900 mg/day). Use of alcohol and over-the-counter medications is contraindicated. Patients should be taught to report lethargy, weakness, fever, sore throat, malaise, mucus membrane ulceration, or other possible signs of infection or flu-like complaints. (E, N, L)

The Client With Chronic Mental Illness

33. 4. Among the needs of the chronically mentally ill are community-based treatment programs, psychosocial rehabilitation programs, and appropriate employment opportunities. During necessary periods of hospitalization active treatment, rather than custodial care, is needed. (D, C, L)

34. 3. The nurse's role in a psychosocial rehabilitation program involves teaching the client to live independently by using interpersonal skills and community resources. Insight-oriented psychotherapy is not beneficial for this client population. (P, C, L)

35. 1. Symptom exacerbation is most often related to noncompliance with the prescribed medication regimen. Therefore, obtaining information about the client's compliance is the first priority. Helping the client recognize the symptoms and her ability to manage them and checking with her employer are appropriate, but not the first priority. Hospitalization is not indicated, because the client is still working and can talk about the symptoms. (I, T, L)

36. 3. Recognizing the client's feeling and her progress while obtaining more information is the most therapeutic response. Reminding the client of her previous related experience is also appropriate but could be done more therapeutically. To suggest the possibility of a drug holiday when symptoms are recurring is clinically unsound. (I, T, L)

37. 3. The nurse will speak with the client to question her about perceptions or reasons interfering with going to the sheltered workshop. This conveys that the nurse is interested and willing to help the client. Calling the director of the workshop can only be done if the nurse receives the client's permission. If the nurse needs additional information about the client's progress, making an appointment would be a method to assess further problems. Reserving an empty bed is not appropriate until the nurse has assessed the client's needs. (I, T, L)

38. 3. Making an appointment with the client at the mental health center to explore her feelings and behavior acknowledges the client's importance and makes her a partner in resolving the problem. Threatening the client with loss of a position at the workshop, asking for a new assignment for her at the workshop, or changing her program are premature actions. (I, T, L)

39. 4. Because chronically mentally ill young adults have not been hospitalized for long periods, they have not learned or accepted lower role expectations and continue to expect to achieve the same social goals as non-mentally ill peers. While low self-esteem and lack of coping resources are common in this client group, the client's behavior does not demonstrate these characteristics. (D, T, L)

40. 3. Psychoeducational groups for families aim to provide education about the biochemical etiology of psychiatric disease to reduce family guilt, about symptoms and symptom management, about medication, about family networking, and about ways of coping with a mentally ill family member. (D, C, L)

41. 1. This client's ability to care for herself is most relevant to a decision about her disposition. If she is gravely disabled or needs treatment to care for herself, involuntary hospitalization is indicated whether or not she is known to the mental health center. Having monetary resources does not necessarily mean that she will be able to use them to care for herself. (P, N, L)

42. 4. Clients have a right to see visitors regardless of admission status. Involuntary hospitalization requires a psychiatrist state-of-need. Release requires medical and/or legal approval. Any client admitted involuntarily has the right to legal counsel. (I, T, L)

43. 2. To be committed involuntarily, a client must not only be suffering from a mental illness but must be gravely disabled (unable to care for self or come to harm if discharged) or dangerous to self or others. Having a mental illness alone is not grounds for commitment. Having a supportive family or home and not wanting treatment are not reasons to not pursue involuntary commitment if indicated or necessary to ensure the well-being of the client or another individual. (I, T, L)

44. 1. It is most therapeutic to let the client know of the staff's continued concern and ask her what might be useful to her. Making the point that she did not use the hospital well is not therapeutic on discharge. Offering information and reviewing the client's knowledge of symptoms are both therapeutic responses. (I, T, L)

45. 1. The psychotropic drugs used to treat chronic mental illness are more appropriate for the teaching plan than are a variety of psychotropic drug categories. Teaching should be focused on the needs and interests of the target audience. Such topics as interventions for common side effects of psychotropic drugs, the role of medication in treating chronic mental illness, and the effects of using common street drugs with psychotropic medication should be included in the teaching program. (P, T, L)

46. 2. Care rather than cure is the treatment focus with the chronically mentally ill. This group has been labeled deviant, and many of the secondary symptoms develop in response to the deviant role they are assigned. Primary symptoms are those associated with the psychiatric illness, such as hallucinations and delusion. While individual variation exists, the development of chronic mental illness follows a predictable pattern. (P, T, L)

47. 1. Chronically mentally ill young adults are between ages 18 and 35. Due to deinstitutionalization they did not experience long periods of hospitalization in which to learn the chronic client role and accompanying decreased self-expectations so commonly seen in older chronically mentally ill clients. Substance abuse is very common in this client population. (D, C, L)

The Client With an Obsessive-Compulsive Disorder

48. 1. When the client says he thinks he is "going crazy," it is best for the nurse to ask him what "crazy" means to him. Before moving toward consensual validation, the nurse must have a clear idea of what the client means by his words and actions. (I, T, L)

49. 1. The client exhibiting obsessive-compulsive behavior is attempting to control his anxiety. The compulsive component of the behavior is performed to relieve or avoid anxiety. Obsessive-compulsive disorder is an anxiety-related disorder. (D, C, L)

50. 3. A client able to take care of his basic nutritional needs is probably not sufficiently incapacitated by his illness to require hospitalization. The ability to behave normally is of lesser importance in this decision, depending on the client's family's or significant others' tolerance of the behavior. The client's abilities to hold a job and relate to his peers may be considered in making the decision but are not valid criteria for hospitalization. (D, N, L)

51. 4. To decrease the client's dependence on others, when he asks what time it is, the staff member should point out the clock for him. Telling the client the time or asking someone else the time increases his dependence. It is belittling to ask the client what time he thinks it is. (I, T, L)

52. 2. Letting the client eat earlier meets his needs for more time and also the group's need to depart for the outing on time. It also protects the client from being resented by others and lets him be included in group activity. Changing the time of an activity to meet the needs of one client is undesirable and may be impractical as well. (P, T, L)

53. 3. Drama clubs are good for their social and self-expressive qualities. This client needs outlets that are creative and oriented toward others. Swimming, solo flying, and photography are hobbies with few social and other-oriented qualities. (P, N, L)

54. 1. Diversional Activity Deficit, Social Isolation, and Powerlessness are appropriate nursing diagnoses for this client. There is no data to support the problem of fear for the client in this situation. Data supporting Powerlessness includes statements of "I know it's senseless. I can't stop." Being too busy at work to see friends and rarely seeing friends anymore support Diversional Activity Deficit and Social Isolation. (D, N, L)

55. 4. Clients with an obsessive-compulsive disorder are typically rigid and controlled in their thinking and behavior. They find it difficult to be introspective and to express or even recognize their feelings. Increasing identification and expression of feelings and connecting feelings with behaviors may prove helpful. Learning and using adaptive coping behaviors when anxious would be appropriate for the client, because anxiety underlies the need for the disorder. The primary gain experienced by the client with obsessive-compulsive disorder is relief of anxiety. Learning how to manage anxiety decreases the need for obsessions and compulsions. Problem identification and decision making would not be helpful to the client at this time nor realistically possible for the client to engage in. (P, N, L)

56. 4. The dynamics of compulsive activity involve a

defense against anxiety by persistently doing something else (that is, a substitution activity). This behavior occurs each time threatening thoughts or impulses appear. Channeling excessive sexual energy into an appropriate habit describes a defense mechanism that is almost always healthy (sublimation). Judgment that the client counts money repeatedly to compensate for not having enough money to spend as a child or to avoid the embarrassment of running short of money is based on insufficient data and represents an oversimplification of the client's problem. (D, N, L)

57. 4. It is best to accept compulsive behavior in a comparatively permissive manner. The client may become restless and anxious if the ritualistic activity is denied him. Isolating the client, observing him for marked changes in behavior, and reminding him that he can control his behavior if he wishes are unwarranted or inappropriate measures in this situation. (I, T, L)

58. 1. Although compassion, friendliness, and self-confidence may be desirable to some degree in caring for a client with an obsessive-compulsive disorder, it is considered most important that the nurse demonstrate patience. It takes the client a long time to complete necessary tasks. Unless nurses are patient, they can easily become frustrated, upset, or angry. The obsessive-compulsive client cannot be hurried. (D, C, L)

59. 2. It takes 5–10 weeks of clomipramine (Anafranil) therapy to derive full therapeutic effect for clients with obsessive-compulsive disorder. Clomipramine (Anafranil) is related to the tricyclic antidepressants. When taken for depression, 2–4 weeks of therapy is needed for therapeutic effect. Asking the client if he has resumed smoking is appropriate, because smoking increases the metabolism of clomipramine, necessitating a dosage adjustment to achieve therapeutic effect—but it would not be the first statement to make to this client. (I, T, L)

60. 3. Relaxation exercises, thought stopping, and exposure therapy are potentially therapeutic and beneficial for a client with obsessive-compulsive disorder. Meditation would not be helpful for the client because of increased anxiety, which interferes with concentration, thinking, and focusing. After obsessions and/or compulsions decrease, the client may find meditation helpful and calming. (P, N, L)

The Client With Organic Mental Syndromes and Disorders

61. 3. When admitting an elderly client, especially one who is confused and disoriented, it is best to give the client extra time in which to gain an understanding of what is happening to her. This will help her get her bearings and adjust to a new environment. In this situation, it would be less desirable to leave the client alone, medicate her, or try to orient her to the new environment. (I, T, L)

62. 2. Multiple sclerosis is a progressive chronic disease; its course cannot be reversed, although clients may experience periodic remissions. Cerebral abscess, syphilitic meningitis, and electrolyte imbalance are treatable, and cure is possible. (D, C, L)

63. 2. Electroencephalography records the electrical activity in the brain. It does not involve the use of electrical shock, is not painful, does not test the client's intelligence, and does not let others know what the client is thinking. (D, C, L)

64. 1. The client's hair should be free of oils, sprays, and lotion before an EEG; hence, client preparation includes a shampoo. Taking a laxative, going to bed early, and providing a handwriting sample are not indicated for an EEG. (P, T, L)

65. 1. People of all ages need to sense future well-being. They must have hope for things to come and believe in growth and change to live life to its fullest. Health personnel need to foster this feeling of hopefulness and subscribe to it to help clients attain well-being, even when the prognosis appears poor. (P, T, L)

66. 2. Basic symptomatology demonstrates that clients with chronic organic mental disorders experience defects in memory, orientation, and intellectual functions, such as judgment and discrimination. Loss of other abilities is less typical. (D, N, L)

67. 4. To promote reality orientation, the nurse should be as specific as possible when addressing a confused and disoriented client. Such comments as indicating what day it is, where the client is, and the nurse's name can help. Asking the client questions about her environment is likely to be challenging and may decrease the client's self-esteem. Stereotyped comments give the client no basic information; nor is it helpful when the nurse provides mostly irrelevant information. (I, T, L)

68. 2. When caring for a client with organic mental impairment, it may be necessary to have two people accompany her when she ambulates, place her favorite things in safekeeping, and give medications in a liquid form to be sure she swallows them. However, it is most essential to remove objects in the client's path of ambulation to help prevent falls. (P, T, L)

69. 3. A client with insomnia is more likely to sleep well if she feels tired at bedtime, which is likely if she had enough daily exercise so that she is comfortably tired at night. Having the client take a daily afternoon nap is likely to interfere with night-time sleep. Offering the client tea at bedtime is unlikely to promote sleep, especially if the tea contains caffeine, which may lead to further wakefulness. Sedatives should be used only as a last resort, because they are likely to be habit-forming. (P, T, L)

70. 3. Delirium, confusion, and excitement are signs of barbiturate toxicity. Barbiturates are less preferable than other sedatives for a client who is often confused and disoriented. (D, N, L)

71. 3. The best procedure for helping the client remain independent and observe good hygiene habits is to encourage her to do as much self-care as she is capable of doing. For this client, it would be inappropriate to accept her poor personal hygiene habits. It would be impractical and unrealistic to expect the client to start taking care of all her hygiene needs. To do all of the client's hygienic care would cause further dependence, and it would be dishonest to care for the client while letting her think she did it herself. (I, T, L)

72. 1. The most likely reason for a nurse's discomfort with elderly clients is that she has not examined her own fears and conflicts about aging. Until she does, it is unlikely that she will feel comfortable with elderly clients. (E, N, L)

73. 4. A will is an important legal document, and it is best to have one prepared with the help of an attorney. It would be unwise to help the client, because a nurse is not a lawyer. Asking the client to delay preparing the will just avoids the problem. It is also not helpful to seek out another nurse to help the client prepare a will. (I, T, L)

74. 3. Reminiscing can help reduce depression in an elderly client and lessens feelings of isolation and loneliness. It gives the client permission to be old. (D, C, L)

75. 2. The cluster of symptoms, including increased confusion and disorientation, that led to the client's admission are common to a number of organic mental disorders for which the treatment is similar. Although medical science is rapidly learning more about the aging brain, no definitive test for Alzheimer's exists. Changes found at autopsy are the most definitive known markers at this time. (I, T, L)

76. 4. Elevated mood states are uncommon in clients with organic mental disorders. Irritability, anxiety, and depression are more common mood states. Agnosia (decreased ability to recognize both people and objects), sleep disturbances, and problems with long-term memory are common. (D, C, L)

77. 1. Alcohol consumption in persons with Alzheimer's disease has not been found to be greater than that in persons without Alzheimer's disease. A family history of the disease, a history of head trauma, and advanced age have all been linked to increased incidence. (I, T, L)

78. 3. The client who is a fantasy or reminiscent wanderer can be helped most by diverting his attention toward an activity to relieve boredom or tension. Reminding the client with severe memory loss that he retired from his job 10 years ago will not help him and may increase his frustration. Telling the client that the nurse will accompany him for a short walk outdoors reflects poor judgment by the nurse and may compromise the client's safety. Telling the client that he does not have to work today can further confuse the client and reinforce his fantasy and disorientation. (I, T, L)

79. 2. Nursing interventions that maintain life are a priority for the client with delirium. Facilitating orientation, optimal functioning, and consistency in daily routine are of less importance whether caring for a client with delirium or a client with dementia. Maintaining an optimal level of functioning is the primary goal for a client with dementia. (P, T, L)

Using a Therapeutic Milieu

80. 1. A therapeutic milieu is an environment that helps clients meet treatment goals. Meeting the comfort needs of clients and staff, allowing staff to observe and evaluate clients, and facilitating the implementation of physicians' orders are significant but are not the primary purpose of managing the milieu. (D, C, L)

81. 3. Clients on a closed or locked inpatient psychiatric unit are typically acutely ill. Providing safety, structure, and support are immediate priorities in the therapeutic milieu for clients with cognitive impairment and inability to handle stress. Socialization, self-understanding, education, vocational counseling, and leisure, social, and communication skills are important for clients in the therapeutic milieu who are less acutely ill. As clients improve, they become better organized in their thinking and more capable of tolerating stress. They would then be more apt to benefit from additional groups and therapies. (E, N, L)

82. 1. The nurse should take the time to listen to the client to discover more about his feelings before making an assessment or intervening. Calling the physician is an intervention made without complete data. Giving advice by suggesting that the client rest or play a game with another client is not therapeutic in this situation. (I, T, L)

83. 3. The nurse should judge the client's behavior in relation to the milieu and clarify the behavior's effect on the milieu, not on personal values held by staff members. Overusing the telephone, behavior that disturbs other clients, and behavior that may harm the client are situations requiring a degree of limit setting. (E, N, L)

84. 1. The nurse should state the limits clearly to a client who is disturbing others. The limits should be objective and fair and should reflect the situation at hand. The client should be included in decision making when possible, but the nurse is ultimately responsible. (P, T, L)

85. 4. Because the client has impaired memory, attention, and concentration, a reality orientation group is recommended to help her maintain an optimal level of functioning. Entering group therapy, going on a field trip, and meeting with an assertiveness training group are likely to be too stressful or stimulating to the client and may increase her frustration and decrease her sense of accomplishment. (P, T, L)

86. 3. Children need to know what behaviors are acceptable and what behaviors are unacceptable. They feel more secure when boundaries are clear and when policies concerning their behavior are consistently enforced. Increasing sensory stimulation and activity, limiting opportunities to display anger and frustration, and allowing freedom to choose activities would tend to increase stress and frustration for the hyperkinetic child. (P, T, L)

87. 2. The milieu should be used to increase peer support and handle confrontation when necessary. For adolescents, peer pressure is generally more effective in changing behavior than the staff's influence. Searching the client's room and trying to persuade a client who was involved to tell on his friends are authoritarian actions and may increase mistrust of the staff. Calling a physician is not necessary at this time. (I, T, L)

NURSING CARE OF CLIENTS WITH PSYCHOSOCIAL HEALTH PROBLEMS

TEST 2: Personality Disorders and Organic Disorders, Using a Therapeutic Milieu

Directions: Use this answer grid to determine areas of strength or need for further study.

NURSING PROCESS

A = Assessment
D = Analysis, nursing diagnosis
P = Planning
I = Implementation
E = Evaluation

COGNITIVE LEVEL

K = Knowledge
C = Comprehension
T = Application
N = Analysis

CLIENT NEEDS

S = Safe, effective care environment
G = Physiological integrity
L = Psychosocial integrity
H = Health promotion/maintenance

		Nursing Process					Cognitive Level				Client Needs			
Question #	Answer #	A	D	P	I	E	K	C	T	N	S	G	L	H
1	2			P					T				L	
2	1				I				T				L	
3	3					E				N			L	
4	4		D					C					L	
5	2		D							N			L	
6	2			P					T				L	
7	3				I				T				L	
8	1			P					T				L	
9	2		D							N			L	
10	2		D							N			L	
11	4					E				N			L	
12	1				I				T				L	
13	4					E				N			L	
14	2			P					T				L	
15	4		D						T				L	
16	2			P					T				L	
17	4		D					C					L	
18	1			P				C					L	
19	1				I				T				L	
20	4					E				N			L	
21	1			P					T				L	
22	3					E				N			L	
23	3				I				T				L	

ANSWER GRID: 1

Nursing Process

A = Assessment
D = Analysis, nursing diagnosis
P = Planning
I = Implementation
E = Evaluation

Cognitive Level

K = Knowledge
C = Comprehension
T = Application
N = Analysis

Client Needs

S = Safe, effective care environment
G = Physiological integrity
L = Psychosocial integrity
H = Health promotion/maintenance

		Nursing Process					Cognitive Level				Client Needs			
Question #	Answer #	A	D	P	I	E	K	C	T	N	S	G	L	H
24	3				I				T				L	
25	2		D						T				L	
26	1		D					C					L	
27	1				I				T				L	
28	3				I				T				L	
29	3		D					C					L	
30	4				I			C					L	
31	3				I				T				L	
32	2					E				N			L	
33	4		D					C					L	
34	3			P				C					L	
35	1				I				T				L	
36	3				I				T				L	
37	3				I				T				L	
38	3				I				T				L	
39	4		D						T				L	
40	3		D					C					L	
41	1			P						N			L	
42	4				I				T				L	
43	2				I				T				L	
44	1				I				T				L	
45	1			P					T				L	
46	2			P					T				L	
47	1		D					C					L	
48	1				I				T				L	
49	1		D					C					L	
50	3		D							N			L	
51	4				I				T				L	
52	2			P					T				L	

Answer Grid: 2

Nursing Process

A = Assessment
D = Analysis, nursing diagnosis
P = Planning
I = Implementation
E = Evaluation

Cognitive Level

K = Knowledge
C = Comprehension
T = Application
N = Analysis

Client Needs

S = Safe, effective care environment
G = Physiological integrity
L = Psychosocial integrity
H = Health promotion/maintenance

		Nursing Process					Cognitive Level				Client Needs			
Question #	Answer #	A	D	P	I	E	K	C	T	N	S	G	L	H
53	3			P						N			L	
54	1		D							N			L	
55	4			P						N			L	
56	4		D							N			L	
57	4				I				T				L	
58	1		D					C					L	
59	2				I				T				L	
60	3			P						N			L	
61	3				I				T				L	
62	2		D					C					L	
63	2		D					C					L	
64	1			P					T				L	
65	1			P					T				L	
66	2		D							N			L	
67	4				I				T				L	
68	2			P					T				L	
69	3			P					T				L	
70	3		D							N			L	
71	3				I				T				L	
72	1					E				N			L	
73	4				I				T				L	
74	3		D					C					L	
75	2				I				T				L	
76	4		D					C					L	
77	1				I				T				L	
78	3				I				T				L	
79	2			P					T				L	
80	1		D					C					L	
81	3					E				N			L	

Answer Grid: 3

Nursing Process

A = Assessment
D = Analysis, nursing diagnosis
P = Planning
I = Implementation
E = Evaluation

Cognitive Level

K = Knowledge
C = Comprehension
T = Application
N = Analysis

Client Needs

S = Safe, effective care environment
G = Physiological integrity
L = Psychosocial integrity
H = Health promotion/maintenance

		Nursing Process					Cognitive Level				Client Needs			
Question #	Answer #	A	D	P	I	E	K	C	T	N	S	G	L	H
82	1				I				T				L	
83	3					E				N			L	
84	1			P					T				L	
85	4			P					T				L	
86	3			P					T				L	
87	2				I				T				L	
Number Correct														
Number Possible	87	0	25	23	30	9	0	17	49	21	0	0	87	0
Percentage Correct														

Score Calculation:

To determine your **Percentage Correct**, divide the **Number Correct** by the **Number Possible**.

Chemical Dependency and Eating Disorders

Test 3

The Client With a Personality Disorder
The Client Who Abuses Alcohol
The Client With Alcohol Withdrawal
The Client Who Is Dependent on Narcotics
The Client Who Abuses Barbiturates
The Client With an Eating Disorder
Correct Answers and Rationale

Select the one best answer and indicate your choice by filling in the circle in front of the option.

The Client With a Personality Disorder

A client is readmitted to the hospital psychiatric unit. His history of impulsive acts and aggressive behavior toward others, including his wife, has resulted in problems with the police. He has been unable to hold a job for longer than 2 months and feels no remorse about using others for personal gain.

1. The client is called a "manipulator" by a nurse because in the past, he played staff members against each other for favors and made them angry with each other. When the staff analyzes the nurse's comment, they correctly judge that labeling the client as a manipulator is most likely to

- ○ 1. prevent staff from expecting too much of the client.
- ○ 2. prevent staff from seeing the client as he really is.
- ○ 3. help staff find ways to prevent the client from mocking them.
- ○ 4. help staff identify approaches for appropriate therapy for the client.

2. An attitude by the nurse that would most likely foster a therapeutic relationship between the nurse and the client who tries to manipulate people is

- ○ 1. sympathy.
- ○ 2. aloofness.
- ○ 3. strictness.
- ○ 4. consistency.

3. The client makes derogatory comments toward the nurse when the nurse does not allow him to eat breakfast in his room. He states, "You're inadequate and don't know what you're doing. The evening nurse always lets me eat in my room. In fact, the nurse brings me my supper tray and gets me what I want." Based on this information, which nursing diagnosis would be most appropriate for this client?

- ○ 1. Self-Esteem Disturbance related to dependency needs, as evidenced by attempts to manipulate staff.
- ○ 2. Potential for Violence related to antisocial character, as evidenced by verbal threats to the nurse.
- ○ 3. Ineffective Individual Coping related to lack of ego strength, as evidenced by impulsiveness.
- ○ 4. Impaired Social Interaction related to low self-esteem, as evidenced by dysfunctional interactions with wife.

4. To decrease the client's manipulation of staff, the nurse would include which of the following measures in the plan?

- ○ 1. Convey an accepting attitude toward the client regardless of his behavior.
- ○ 2. Ignore the client's derogatory comments and use diversional activities.
- ○ 3. Explain the consequences of manipulative behavior and maintain staff consistency.
- ○ 4. Consistently give the client negative feedback about his behavior and tell him what he should do.

5. Because the client has a potential for violence and aggressive behavior, which short-term goal would be most appropriate for the nurse to include in the plan of care? The client will

- ○ 1. not harm others while on the unit.

○ 2. discuss feelings of anger with the nurse in 1 week.
○ 3. ask the nurse for medication when upset.
○ 4. verbalize reasons for his anger to the nurse in 1 week.

A 16-year-old client is readmitted to the psychiatric hospital's adolescent unit. She recently ran away from home for the fifth time this year and while hitchhiking in a state of drug-induced euphoria on a freeway was picked up by the police. She is accompanied to the unit by her juvenile worker.

6. The nurse recognizes that it is difficult to maintain control in the relationship with this client. Which of the following actions would be best for the nurse to take when feeling outmaneuvered by this client?
○ 1. Seek help from the other staff members.
○ 2. Request to be assigned to a different client.
○ 3. Discuss feelings of frustration with the client.
○ 4. Focus attention on the client's nonadaptive behavior.

7. In the course of their conversation, the client tells the nurse bitterly, "My parents are mean. They don't care about me at all." Which of the following responses by the nurse would be the least therapeutic?
○ 1. "You feel that your parents don't care about you."
○ 2. "What would be a sign to you that your parents cared?"
○ 3. "I'm sure your parents have your best interests at heart."
○ 4. "Tell me more about your parents being mean and not caring."

8. The client is quick to learn about the problems of other people and to use this knowledge for her own amusement. She makes a target of a 15-year-old withdrawn girl and has the other clients tease and play tricks on her. Of the following people, who would probably have the most influence in helping the client change her behavior?
○ 1. Physician.
○ 2. Peer group.
○ 3. Juvenile worker.
○ 4. Religious counselor.

9. When planning the client's nursing care, the nurse should take into account which of the following traits that the client also would be likely to display?
○ 1. Poor judgment.
○ 2. Faulty memory.
○ 3. Low intelligence.
○ 4. Disordered thinking.

A client is in treatment at the day hospital. This is her seventh admission. She has been unable to hold even part-time jobs and has had four abortions in the last 4 years. She is now living with her family after being evicted from her apartment. She complains of feeling "empty and lonely," and her arms are scarred from frequent self-mutilation.

10. Which of the following personality disorders does this client exhibit?
○ 1. Antisocial personality disorder.
○ 2. Avoidant personality disorder.
○ 3. Borderline personality disorder.
○ 4. Compulsive personality disorder.

11. Which nursing diagnosis would be least appropriate for this client?
○ 1. High Risk for Self-Mutilation.
○ 2. Personality Identity Disturbance.
○ 3. Self-Esteem Disturbance.
○ 4. Sensory-Perceptual Alteration.

12. The client has become attached to a part-time nurse and frequently refuses to share her history with any other staff member. She tells this nurse that other staff members mistreat her, that she can trust only her, and that she fears for her safety during the nurse's absence. This common defense mechanism is known as
○ 1. reaction formation.
○ 2. splitting.
○ 3. projection.
○ 4. denial.

13. The client repeatedly states that she is not like the other clients and asks the staff for special privileges. She does not follow the rules about using the telephone or watching television. An immediate and major focus of this client's nursing care plan would be to
○ 1. enforce the unit rules consistently.
○ 2. limit the client's contact with others.
○ 3. obtain vocational training for the client.
○ 4. ignore the client's behavior.

14. The client describes her personal history with sadness. Her mother died when she was 2 years old, and her life was chaotic and disorganized. She lived with a number of relatives and in foster homes. In planning the client's care, the nurse attempts to promote completion of the developmental task on which the client would most likely have been working when her mother died. According to Erikson, this basic task is the achievement of
○ 1. trust.
○ 2. independence.
○ 3. safety.
○ 4. autonomy.

15. As the client's discharge date approaches, she asks to stay in the program and makes threats to "do

something" to herself if discharged. The staff remains firm on the discharge date. Which of the following interventions would be most important to ensure the client's safety?
○ 1. Request an immediate extension for the client.
○ 2. Ask the client to leave early.
○ 3. Transfer the client to another hospital.
○ 4. Assess the seriousness of the client's threats.

The Client Who Abuses Alcohol

A friend accompanies the client to the hospital's substance abuse unit, where he is to be admitted for detoxification from alcohol.

16. The client consumed about 6 ounces of alcohol just before coming to the hospital. Which of the following methods would be best for the nursing staff to use to promote alcohol destruction in the client's body?
○ 1. Give the client black coffee to drink.
○ 2. Walk the client around the unit following a cold shower.
○ 3. Have the client breathe pure oxygen through a face mask.
○ 4. Provide the client with a restful room so that he can sleep off the effects of alcohol.

17. Hospital policy requires that the client's belongings be searched for contraband on admission. In view of the client's drinking problem, which of his possessions is most likely to be confiscated by the nursing staff?
○ 1. Hair dressing.
○ 2. Electric razor.
○ 3. Shaving cream.
○ 4. Antiseptic mouthwash.

18. While obtaining a nursing history, the nurse questions the client about the amount of alcohol he consumes daily. The nurse can expect the client to likely answer the question by
○ 1. exaggerating the amount.
○ 2. underestimating the amount.
○ 3. indicating that he does not know the amount.
○ 4. expressing uncertainty about the amount.

19. The most important reason for investigating the amount of alcohol the client has consumed during the 24 to 48 hours before admission is to help determine
○ 1. how far the disease has progressed.
○ 2. the severity of withdrawal.
○ 3. whether the client will experience delirium tremens.
○ 4. whether the client should be considered an alcoholic.

20. Of the following nursing diagnoses, which would the nurse correctly judge to be most important during the early detoxification period?
○ 1. Sleep Pattern Disturbance.
○ 2. Self-Esteem Disturbance.
○ 3. Ineffective Individual Coping.
○ 4. Knowledge Deficit.

21. Which of the following medications is most likely to be prescribed for the client during withdrawal from alcohol to provide sedation and to ease some of the anxiety and discomfort of the withdrawal process?
○ 1. Paraldehyde (Paral).
○ 2. Lorazepam (Ativan).
○ 3. Phenytoin sodium (Dilantin).
○ 4. Temazepam (Restoril).

22. To assess the client's physiological response and the effectiveness of the medication prescribed specifically for alcohol withdrawal, the nurse would first
○ 1. assess the client's nutritional status.
○ 2. assess the client for tremors in the extremities.
○ 3. monitor the client's vital signs.
○ 4. monitor the client's sleep pattern.

23. The client could not remember the events of the past weekend, although he had receipts in his pockets from several shops where he made purchases on Saturday. This problem illustrates what condition?
○ 1. Blackout.
○ 2. Hangover.
○ 3. Dry drunk syndrome.
○ 4. Alcoholic hallucinosis.

24. After a day of abstinence, the client has coarse tremors of the hands, making it hard for him to feed himself. He asks the nurse low long it will be before his "shakes" go away. On which of the following statements should the nurse base the response? The tremors
○ 1. can only be relieved by alcohol intake.
○ 2. usually disappear after about 2 days of abstinence.
○ 3. may persist for several days or even longer after alcohol intake has stopped.
○ 4. are a permanent condition due to irreversible central nervous system damage.

25. The client craves a drink while withdrawing from the alcohol. Which of the following measures is the best way to help him resist the urge to drink?
○ 1. A locked-door policy.
○ 2. A routine search of visitors.
○ 3. One-to-one supervision by the staff.
○ 4. Support from other alcoholic clients.

26. The client ashamedly tells the nurse that he hit his wife during a recent argument and asks the nurse if she thinks his wife will ever forgive him. Which of the following replies by the nurse would be best in this situation?

○ 1. "Perhaps you could call her up and find out."
○ 2. "That's something you can explore in family therapy."
○ 3. "It would depend on how much she really cares for you."
○ 4. "You seem to have some feelings about hitting your wife."

27. The client's wife agrees to meet with her husband's therapist but says she has "about had it" with her husband's "foolishness and bad temper." Which of the following organizations would probably be the most helpful to her in obtaining additional assistance and support in coping with her alcoholic spouse?
○ 1. Alateen.
○ 2. Al-Anon.
○ 3. Narcotics Anonymous.
○ 4. Alcoholics Anonymous.

28. The client is beginning to participate in the alcohol treatment program. Which nursing approach would be most effective in decreasing his denial about his alcoholism?
○ 1. Give him reading materials about the disease of alcoholism.
○ 2. Point out concrete problems that are a direct consequence of his alcoholism.
○ 3. Explain the physiological effects of alcohol on the body.
○ 4. Teach him assertiveness techniques.

29. The nurse is teaching members of the client's group how to give each other constructive feedback. Which of the following statements by the nurse best illustrates constructive feedback?
○ 1. "I think you're a real con artist."
○ 2. "You're dominating the conversation."
○ 3. "You interrupted John twice in 4 minutes."
○ 4. "You don't give anyone a chance to finish talking."

30. The client is started on a regimen of disulfiram (Antabuse). A valuable and expected result of successful disulfiram therapy is that it
○ 1. decreases the need for alcohol.
○ 2. acts to deter alcohol consumption.
○ 3. improves the alcoholic's ability to drink limited amounts of alcohol.
○ 4. creates a nerve block so that the effects of alcohol are not felt.

31. Which client statement would indicate to the nurse that further teaching about disulfiram (Antabuse) is necessary?
○ 1. "I can drink one or two beers and not get sick while on Antabuse."
○ 2. "I need to stop taking Antabuse for at least 2 weeks before I can drink alcohol without experiencing an alcohol-Antabuse reaction."
○ 3. "A metallic or garlic taste in my mouth is normal when starting on Antabuse."
○ 4. "Reading labels on cough syrup, after-shave lotion, and mouthwash is important because they might contain alcohol."

32. While on disulfiram therapy, the client becomes nauseated and vomits severely. The nurse is justified in judging that the client has most probably
○ 1. developed an allergy to disulfiram.
○ 2. been given an overdose of disulfiram accidentally.
○ 3. been drinking alcohol while on disulfiram therapy.
○ 4. developed gastritis as a result of disulfiram therapy.

33. A daily lecture series on alcoholism is conducted by the counselors on the substance abuse unit where the client is housed. The counselors should explain that the client will most likely experience which of the following symptoms of alcoholism during the chronic stage of the disease?
○ 1. Increased alcohol tolerance.
○ 2. Vague feelings of apprehension and doom.
○ 3. Feelings of grandiosity and increasing combativeness.
○ 4. The desire to switch to a different form of alcoholic beverage.

34. Which of the following suggestions would be most appropriate for the nurse to make to members of the client's family concerning how they can best help promote a supportive environment for him at home? Suggest that the family members
○ 1. follow a program offered by Al-Anon.
○ 2. obtain counseling in a mental health clinic.
○ 3. refrain from discussing alcoholism in their home.
○ 4. make sure that no alcoholic beverages are served in the home.

35. Which of the following remarks that the client might make before his discharge would show the most realistic analysis of his situation in relation to avoiding future drinking problems?
○ 1. "I promise I'll never get drunk again."
○ 2. "I'm going to try hard to stay away from that first drink."
○ 3. "I'll just have one or two drinks at the most, now and then."
○ 4. "I can whip this drinking business if my wife keeps off my back."

The Client With Alcohol Withdrawal

A client enters the hospital for treatment of cirrhosis of the liver. She is accompanied by her husband.

36. The nurse who admitted the client comments to another nurse, "Cirrhosis. She must be an alcoholic."

The practice of automatically attributing an overindulgence in alcohol to people with cirrhosis is an example of
- ○ 1. an ideology.
- ○ 2. a stereotype.
- ○ 3. a mental set.
- ○ 4. a halo effect.

37. Nurses can best avoid developing premature, biased views of a client by
- ○ 1. reading about the client's illness.
- ○ 2. asking others for their opinions of the client.
- ○ 3. acquainting oneself with others of the client's kind.
- ○ 4. personally getting to know what the client is really like.

38. The physician notes on the medical record that the client has a 7-year history of drinking a six pack of beer and some wine every day. The unit secretary reads the physician's notes and exclaims, "I have a friend who drinks more than that! Would he be considered an alcoholic?" Which of the following possible replies by the nurse shows the best understanding of alcoholism as a social disease?
- ○ 1. "Not if he drinks with others and not alone."
- ○ 2. "Not if he sticks to beer and avoids the hard liquor."
- ○ 3. "Not if he drinks only in the evening or on weekends."
- ○ 4. "Not if he is able to get along well at work and at home."

39. The client sees no connection between her liver disorder and her alcohol intake. She believes that she drinks "very little" and that her family is "making something out of nothing." Which of the following defense mechanisms is the client using?
- ○ 1. Denial.
- ○ 2. Displacement.
- ○ 3. Rationalization.
- ○ 4. Reaction formation.

40. Attempts by health team members to force the client to face the fact that she is an alcoholic and to break her defenses would most likely lead to
- ○ 1. insight and rehabilitation.
- ○ 2. hallucinations and psychosis.
- ○ 3. restlessness and psychosis.
- ○ 4. disorganization and depression.

41. Medications for the client include a B-complex vitamin. The client wants to know why she must take this vitamin. What would be the nurse's best response?
- ○ 1. "The beer you have been drinking has caused you to become vitamin depleted."
- ○ 2. "Your daily alcohol consumption causes malnutrition."
- ○ 3. "The B vitamins help reduce the long-term effects of alcohol withdrawal."
- ○ 4. "The amount of vitamins in the wine you drink is very low."

42. The nurse teaches the client about the value of good nutrition and the B vitamins. Which of the following statements would the client most likely make in response to the teaching?
- ○ 1. "This is all so complicated. Maybe I'll feel better after a good night's sleep."
- ○ 2. "I've been wondering why I felt so bad. I just need vitamins."
- ○ 3. "I don't know why you're telling me all of this. I don't drink enough to cause these problems."
- ○ 4. "I don't see what this has to do with me."

43. Besides cirrhosis, the client suffers from numbness, itching, and pain in her extremities and is prone to footdrop. This disorder of the nervous system is termed
- ○ 1. neuralgia.
- ○ 2. Bell's palsy.
- ○ 3. neurasthenia.
- ○ 4. peripheral neuritis.

44. Numbness, itching, and pain in the extremities indicates which of the following nursing diagnoses?
- ○ 1. Alteration in Comfort.
- ○ 2. Impaired Skin Integrity.
- ○ 3. Anxiety.
- ○ 4. Self-Care Deficit.

45. The client has neurologic damage. As a precautionary measure, the nurse must be especially careful when
- ○ 1. cleansing the client's skin.
- ○ 2. massaging the client's feet.
- ○ 3. turning the client from side to side.
- ○ 4. applying heat to the client's lower legs.

46. A noncaffeinated beverage is substituted for the client's usual morning coffee. This measure is taken because
- ○ 1. clients transfer their oral dependency needs symbolically to coffee.
- ○ 2. regular coffee aggravates tremors and interferes with sleep.
- ○ 3. clients tend to abuse coffee in the same way they once abused alcohol.
- ○ 4. regular coffee has a diuretic effect that interferes with hydration.

47. The client receives the appropriate medical and nursing treatment for her liver disorder and neurologic ailments, and her condition improves slightly. However, after 5 days in the hospital, she begins to thrash about in bed, pulling the sheets and yelling, "Go away, bugs, go away!" Which of the following nursing notes best sums up the client's behavior?
- ○ 1. Restless, disoriented, and hallucinating.
- ○ 2. Agitated and experiencing visual hallucinations.
- ○ 3. Fidgety and out of contact with reality.

○ 4. Seeing "bugs" in her bedclothes and slapping at them.

48. When the client thrashes in bed and yells, "Go away, bugs, go away," this behavior indicates which of the following nursing diagnoses?
○ 1. Sensory-Perceptual Alteration.
○ 2. Sleep Pattern Disturbance.
○ 3. Altered Thought Processes.
○ 4. Ineffective Individual Coping.

49. Which of the following measures should be included in the nursing care plan when the client has delirium tremens?
○ 1. Restrain her and keep the room quiet.
○ 2. Touch her before saying anything and tell her where she is.
○ 3. Have someone stay with her and keep a light on in the room.
○ 4. Tell her she is having nightmares and that she will be better soon.

50. For the client experiencing delirium tremens, which of the following physician orders should the nurse question?
○ 1. Chlordiazepoxide 25 mg po qid.
○ 2. Chlordiazepoxide 100 mg q 4h prn for agitation.
○ 3. Chlorpromazine 100 mg q 4h prn for agitation.
○ 4. Thiamine 100 mg IM qd for 3 days.

51. When developing a one-to-one relationship with the client after she is physiologically stable, the nurse should use the first meeting to determine the client's
○ 1. healthy coping mechanisms.
○ 2. most probable reasons for alcohol abuse.
○ 3. knowledge about Alcoholics Anonymous.
○ 4. childhood experiences that predispose to alcoholism.

52. The client's husband tells the nurse that he also drinks heavily in the evenings and would like to stop. The nurse suggests that he attend Alcoholics Anonymous, but he says, "I went to one men's meeting and all they did was swear and brag about how drunk they got." Which of the following responses would be best for the nurse to make?
○ 1. "That's too bad. I can see how you might have been turned off by the experience."
○ 2. "Not everyone finds Alcoholics Anonymous helpful. There are other therapies available."
○ 3. "The Alcoholics Anonymous meetings vary from group to group. Have you thought about giving it another try?"
○ 4. "If you really want to stop your drinking, you would go back to Alcoholics Anonymous whether you liked it or not."

53. The client's husband asks the nurse about requirements to become a member of Alcoholics Anonymous. Which reply by the nurse is accurate?
○ 1. "Resolve to abstain from alcohol and to help others to do so."
○ 2. "Admit that you are powerless over alcohol and that you need help."
○ 3. "Analyze the wrongs you have done while drinking and try to make amends for them."
○ 4. "Turn your life over to a higher power and seek to improve contact with that power through meditation."

54. The client is to be discharged from the hospital. What information is likely to be most helpful in her efforts to stop drinking?
○ 1. Dependency on her husband to help her stop drinking.
○ 2. The disease concept of alcoholism.
○ 3. The stages of alcoholism.
○ 4. The importance of perseverance in her efforts to change her behavior.

The Client Who Is Dependent on Narcotics

A client is brought to the hospital's emergency room by a friend, who states, "I guess he had some bad junk (heroin) today."

55. In assessing the client, the nurse would likely find which of the following symptoms?
○ 1. Increased heart rate, dilated pupils, and fever.
○ 2. Tremulousness, impaired coordination, increased blood pressure, and ruddy complexion.
○ 3. Decreased respirations, constricted pupils, and pallor.
○ 4. Eye irritation, tinnitus, and irritation of nasal and oral mucosa.

56. The client is in a light coma. Which nursing diagnosis would receive the highest priority?
○ 1. Ineffective Individual Coping.
○ 2. Ineffective Breathing Pattern.
○ 3. Alteration in Nutrition.
○ 4. Self-Care Deficit.

57. Which nursing intervention would receive the lowest priority for the client with a heroin overdose?
○ 1. Prepare for CPR.
○ 2. Monitor vital signs.
○ 3. Monitor breathing pattern.
○ 4. Discuss treatment options.

58. After administering naloxone (Narcan), a narcotic antagonist, the nurse should monitor the client carefully for signs of
○ 1. cerebral edema.
○ 2. kidney failure.
○ 3. seizure activity.
○ 4. respiratory depression.

59. The client has a history of occasional cocaine use. Which of the following telltale signs would tell the nurse that the client has recently abused this drug?
○ 1. Red, excoriated nostrils.

○ 2. Clear, constricted pupils.
○ 3. White patchy areas on the tongue.
○ 4. Lumpy abscesses in intramuscular areas.

60. The client is admitted to the chemical dependency unit with heroin dependency. After about 12 hours, he develops signs of heroin withdrawal. Of the following signs and symptoms of opiate withdrawal, which occur late, rather than early, in the course of withdrawal?
○ 1. Vomiting and diarrhea.
○ 2. Yawning and diaphoresis.
○ 3. Lacrimation and rhinorrhea.
○ 4. Restlessness and nervousness.

61. The client has numerous complaints of discomfort while abstaining from heroin. Which of the following nursing orders on the client's care plan would be the least advisable and effective?
○ 1. Be empathetic but firm with the client's complaints.
○ 2. Promise to reevaluate the client's withdrawal plan to ease his discomfort.
○ 3. Prepare the client in advance for minor discomforts that might occur.
○ 4. Inform the client of alternative methods, such as warm baths, for dealing with aches and pains.

62. Knowing the client's history, the nursing staff suggest that he be tested for the human immunodeficiency virus (HIV). But he refuses, saying, "No way! I never share needles. None of my friends have it. And anyway, I'm straight." When teaching the client about AIDS, the nurse should include all of the following information except that
○ 1. people can be infected with the virus without having symptoms of the disease.
○ 2. the virus can be transmitted through heterosexual intercourse.
○ 3. asymptomatic people cannot transmit the infection.
○ 4. due to the client's high-risk life-style, testing is especially important.

63. The nursing staff is concerned about possible HIV exposure among other clients on the unit and themselves. Which of the following precautionary measures is the least important?
○ 1. Strict handwashing procedures.
○ 2. A private room for the client.
○ 3. Wearing gloves when handling body fluids.
○ 4. Increased caution in disposing of needles and syringes.

64. The client starts methadone therapy. Which of the following signs would alert the nurse to acute methadone toxicity?
○ 1. Fever.
○ 2. Colitis.
○ 3. Renal shutdown.
○ 4. Respiratory depression.

65. Which of the following characteristics of methadone contributes most greatly to the drug's potential for abuse?
○ 1. It blunts the craving for heroin.
○ 2. It blocks the pleasurable effects of heroin.
○ 3. It is equally effective at low or high doses.
○ 4. It lessens the severity of withdrawal symptoms.

66. Which of the following measures would be the most feasible to ensure the therapeutic use of methadone and to prevent its abuse?
○ 1. Monitor the client's urine drug levels.
○ 2. Administer the methadone in injection form.
○ 3. Supervise the client when administering liquid methadone.
○ 4. Use methadone only for a hospitalized client.

67. While the client is in chemical dependency rehabilitation, which nursing intervention would be least appropriate?
○ 1. Call Narcotics Anonymous to tell them to expect the client after discharge.
○ 2. Enforce unit policies.
○ 3. Confront the client's inappropriate behaviors.
○ 4. Help the client to express feelings.

68. When discussing Narcotics Anonymous, the nurse should explain that the client needs to
○ 1. stay drug-free one day at a time.
○ 2. be "clean" of drugs at the meetings.
○ 3. abstain from drugs for the rest of his life.
○ 4. commit a certain amount of time to the organization.

69. The client's eventual success or progress when out of the hospital can probably best be measured by what factor?
○ 1. the kinds of friends he makes.
○ 2. the number of drug-free days he has.
○ 3. the way he gets along with parents.
○ 4. the amount of responsibility his job entails.

70. Which of the following physical disorders is the heroin addict least likely to develop as a result of the addiction?
○ 1. Hepatitis.
○ 2. Pneumonia.
○ 3. Tuberculosis.
○ 4. Cholelithiasis.

The Client Who Abuses Barbiturates

A client is brought by ambulance to the hospital emergency room after taking an overdose of barbiturates. A male friend arrives a short time later, carrying some of the client's personal belongings.

71. The client went into shock at home and is semicomatose on admission. If death occurs shortly, the cause of death would most likely be

○ 1. kidney failure.
○ 2. cardiac standstill.
○ 3. internal hemorrhaging.
○ 4. respiratory depression.

72. The client's friend reports that the client has been taking about eight "reds" (800 mg of secobarbital [Seconal]) daily, besides drinking more alcohol than usual. Which of the following terms best describes the interaction of barbiturates and alcohol?
○ 1. Additive.
○ 2. Suppressive.
○ 3. Potentiating.
○ 4. Antagonistic.

73. The client's friend asks anxiously, "Do you think she will live?" Which of the following replies would be best for the nurse to make?
○ 1. "We can only wait and see."
○ 2. "Do you know her well?"
○ 3. "She is very ill and may not live."
○ 4. "Her condition is serious. You sound very worried about her."

74. The nurse talks further with the client's friend and tries to determine the nature of their relationship. Which of the following motivations provides the best justification for the nurse's inquiries?
○ 1. To ascertain the friend's capabilities as a source of support for the client.
○ 2. To encourage the friend to realize the seriousness of the client's condition.
○ 3. To determine whether the friend can be trusted with confidential information about the client.
○ 4. To learn whether the client's relationship with the friend may have caused the suicide attempt.

75. Before her hospitalization, the client needed increasingly larger doses of barbiturates to achieve the same euphoric effect she initially realized from their use. From this information, the nurse should plan care taking into account that the client is likely suffering from drug
○ 1. tolerance.
○ 2. addiction.
○ 3. habituation.
○ 4. dependence.

76. By which of the following symptoms could the client probably have been identified as a chronic user of barbiturates in the days before her hospitalization?
○ 1. Drooling, fainting, and illusions.
○ 2. Sluggishness, ataxia, and irritability.
○ 3. Diaphoresis, twitching, and sneezing.
○ 4. Suspiciousness, tachycardia, and edema.

77. The client's vital signs stabilize, and she later awakens in a confused state. Which of the following nursing measures would be least appropriate while the client is recovering from sedative overdose?
○ 1. Maintain seizure precautions for the client.
○ 2. Close the windows in the vicinity of the client.
○ 3. Use a p.r.n. order for a medication for anxiety and agitation.
○ 4. Use short, complete sentences when speaking to the client.

78. Following a dose–response test, the client receives pentobarbital sodium (Nembutal) at a nonintoxicating maintenance level for 2 days and at decreasing doses thereafter. This regimen is prescribed primarily to help prevent possibly fatal
○ 1. psychosis.
○ 2. convulsions.
○ 3. hypotension.
○ 4. hypothermia.

79. During an interaction with the nurse, the client states that her "life has gone down the tubes" since her divorce 6 months ago. After she lost her job and apartment, she "took those pills to sleep and not wake up." From these data, the nurse would give the highest priority to which of the following nursing diagnoses?
○ 1. Self-Esteem Disturbance.
○ 2. Potential for Self-Directed Violence.
○ 3. Ineffective Individual Coping.
○ 4. Sleep Pattern Disturbance.

80. Based on the client's loss of her husband through divorce, the loss of her job and apartment, and her drug dependency, the nurse includes the nursing diagnosis Self-Esteem Disturbance on the client's care plan. Based on this information, which of the following short-term goals is appropriate? The client will discuss with the nurse
○ 1. feelings related to her losses.
○ 2. two actions to improve her life.
○ 3. effects of drugs on her life.
○ 4. three strengths that she has.

81. The staff notices that the client spends most of her time with the young adult clients, most of whom have also misused drugs. This group of clients is a dominant force on the unit, keeping the non-drug users entertained with stories of their "highs." In which of the following ways would staff best deal with this problem?
○ 1. Providing additional recreation.
○ 2. Breaking up drug-oriented discussions.
○ 3. Speaking with the clients individually about their behavior.
○ 4. Bringing up for discussion staff observations of the clients' drug-oriented conversations at the weekly client group meetings.

The Client With an Eating Disorder

A client has been referred to a nurse-led group for compulsive overeaters at the mental health clinic by her physician.

82. During the initial interview with the nurse, the client states, "I can't stand myself and the way I look." Which of the following statements by the nurse would be most therapeutic?

- ○ 1. "All the group members feel the same as you do."
- ○ 2. "I don't think you look bad at all."
- ○ 3. "Don't worry. You'll be back in shape soon."
- ○ 4. "Tell me more about your feelings."

83. It is desirable for group members to use functional roles in the group to obtain the most benefit from the group. In which of the following instances is a group role (versus an individual role) being used by one of the members? The member

- ○ 1. shows the group the latest pictures of her child.
- ○ 2. insists that everyone try her favorite reducing diet.
- ○ 3. makes quiet comments to the person sitting next to her.
- ○ 4. proposes an alternative task to keep from thinking about food.

84. The group members learn that many people in the American culture have difficulty with weight control because they unconsciously equate food with

- ○ 1. love and affection.
- ○ 2. power and control.
- ○ 3. status and prestige.
- ○ 4. survival and growth.

85. The client states that her sister has been using amphetamines for weight control for a long time. If the sister is described as having the following symptoms, which one is least likely to be related to prolonged use of amphetamines

- ○ 1. Gastritis.
- ○ 2. Drug dependency.
- ○ 3. Emotional lability.
- ○ 4. Depression between doses.

86. The client has gained 35 pounds in 7 weeks. Before her admission to the psychiatric unit, she refused to see her friends or to leave her house. Which of the following nursing diagnoses would be most appropriate for this client?

- ○ 1. Ineffective Individual Coping.
- ○ 2. Self-Esteem Disturbance.
- ○ 3. Diversional Activity Deficit.
- ○ 4. Anxiety.

87. Which of the following nursing interventions would be least appropriate for this client?

- ○ 1. Invite her to participate in an informal craft activity.
- ○ 2. Ask the dietician to meet with her.
- ○ 3. Tell her to record what she eats throughout the day.
- ○ 4. Explain to her that obesity can be the result of maladaptive coping with stress.

An adolescent client is admitted to the psychiatric unit for rapid weight loss associated with anorexia nervosa. She is 5 feet, 2 inches tall and weighs 70 pounds.

88. Physical manifestations most likely to be found during nursing assessment include

- ○ 1. tachycardia, hypertension, and hyperthyroidism.
- ○ 2. tachycardia, hypertension, and iron deficiency anemia.
- ○ 3. hypotension, elevated serum potassium level, and vitamin C deficiency.
- ○ 4. bradycardia, hypotension, and cold sensitivity.

89. The nurse establishes which of the following nursing diagnoses as being of highest priority for this client?

- ○ 1. Self-Esteem Disturbance.
- ○ 2. Ineffective Individual Coping.
- ○ 3. Altered Nutrition: Less than Body Requirements.
- ○ 4. Body Image Disturbance.

90. A behavioral program for weight gain is instituted as part of the nursing care plan. Which of the following nursing interventions would be most specific to attainment of the program goal?

- ○ 1. Provide emotional support and active listening.
- ○ 2. Give positive rewards for gradual weight gain.
- ○ 3. Help the client identify her problematic eating behaviors.
- ○ 4. Initiate intravenous hyperalimentation.

91. The nurse enters the client's room and finds her doing sit-ups. What would be the nurse's best approach?

- ○ 1. Wait until she finishes and ask her why she feels the need to exercise.
- ○ 2. Remind her that if she loses weight, she will lose privileges.
- ○ 3. Ask her to stop doing the sit-ups and direct her to a quiet activity.
- ○ 4. Leave the room and allow her to exercise in private.

92. What would be the most appropriate and realistic outcome for the client for this hospitalization?

- ○ 1. Her weight is stable and she is willing to begin outpatient group therapy.
- ○ 2. Her weight is within the normal range and she no longer feels the need to diet.
- ○ 3. Her discharge weight is 15% more than her admission weight.
- ○ 4. Her eating behaviors have changed, and she reports feeling better.

CORRECT ANSWERS AND RATIONALE

The letters in parentheses following the rationale identify the step of the nursing process (A, D, P, I, E); cognitive level (K, C, T, N); and client need (S, G, L, H). See the Answer Grid for the key.

The Client With a Personality Disorder

1. 2. Labels may cause staff to make assumptions about the client, discount the client's point of view, and cause the client to live up to the label in a self-fulfilling prophecy. (E, N, L)

2. 4. It is most important that the nurse maintain a consistency approach when dealing with the client who manipulates others. The nurse should set limits on the client's behavior and then consistently enforce these limits to help prevent manipulation. Strictness for its own sake is not appropriate with this client, nor is sympathy or aloofness. (P, N, L)

3. 1. The client's statements to the nurse reflect an attempt to manipulate the nurse to fulfill his desires and are related to his dependency needs. This behavior reflects the client's low self-esteem and is an attempt to assert his superiority and deny his true feelings about himself. The client is not verbally threatening the nurse or acting impulsively. There is no evidence of dysfunctional interactions with his wife, although this may be a problem. (D, N, L)

4. 3. The client must be aware of the outcomes or consequences of his behavior. Explanations must be clear and concise and conveyed in a matter-of-fact manner. Consistency of approach from the entire staff in following through will help decrease manipulation. Accepting all behaviors or ignoring them is not helpful or safe for the client and others on the unit. Accepting the client but not his behaviors guards against the client feeling rejected and increases his sense of worth. Giving negative feedback and telling him what he should do can be threatening to the client with low self-esteem and may only increase his manipulative behavior. (P, T, L)

5. 2. Discussing angry feelings with the nurse will help the client identify his feelings, express them appropriately, and decrease his anxiety. Not harming others is desirable but is more of a long-term goal and does not help the client to learn how to appropriately handle his feelings. Asking the nurse for medication is not helpful and just helps the client avoid dealing with his feelings. Medication may be needed when the client cannot control his behavior or calm down. Antianxiety agents are not usually prescribed for clients with antisocial personality disorder, because these clients often have problems with alcohol or drugs. Verbalizing reasons for his anger implies that the client needs to justify his feelings and helps him displace his feelings onto others without looking at himself and his role in a situation. (P, N, L)

6. 1. When a nurse is having problems dealing with a client, it is best to admit to the need for help and seek the assistance of other staff who can help. (I, T, L)

7. 3. When the client makes a derogatory comment about her parents, a good technique is to help the client discuss her feelings in more detail and to be more specific about her sweeping conclusion. It would be least therapeutic to state that her parents have her best interests at heart, because this accuses the client of being unfeeling or wrong about her parents. (I, T, L)

8. 2. Most teenagers respond best to their peers and less well to persons of authority, such as physicians, juvenile workers, and religious counselors. (E, N, L)

9. 1. The person with antisocial attitudes frequently uses extremely poor judgment. The person is typically of above-average intelligence, has an intact memory, and is a clever rather than a disordered thinker. (D, N, L)

10. 3. This client's primary diagnosis is borderline personality disorder, characterized by impulsive, often self-mutilating behavior and unstable, intense personal relationships. Antisocial personality disorder is characterized by failure to accept social norms, which often results in unlawful behavior. The avoidant personality demonstrates social withdrawal and hypersensitivity to criticism. The compulsive personality is preoccupied with details and rules, to the exclusion of other life activities. (E, N, L)

11. 4. Sensory-perceptual alteration is the least appropriate nursing diagnosis for this client. There is no evidence to support disordered thinking, hallucinations, or delusions. During periods of extreme stress, the client with a borderline personality disorder may experience transient psychotic symptoms. (D, N, L)

12. 2. Splitting refers to a primitive defense mechanism, as well as learned behavior, in which manipulation becomes an adaptive style. Reaction formation is a defense in which negative feelings are replaced with positive ones. Projection involves attributing one's own negative traits to someone else. Denial is a defense mechanism used to resolve emotional conflict and allay anxiety by disavowing thoughts or external realities that are consciously intolerable. (D, C, L)

13. 1. Consistent enforcement of unit rules will help the borderline client control her behavior. Ignoring the behavior leads to an increase in the behavior to evoke a response from the staff. If the client assumes control of the behavior, the client has little opportunity to learn increased responsibility for the behavior. Although vocational plans will be important for discharge planning, they are not an immediate priority. (P, T, L)

14. 4. The achievement of autonomy is the basic task of 2-year-olds. Developing a sense of trust is a task for infants; becoming independent more appropriately describes adolescent tasks. Safety is not a developmental task. (D, N, L)

15. 4. Assessment is an ongoing process throughout treatment. Any suicidal statement must be assessed. Extending the hospital stay would encourage dependency and manipulation. Early discharge is not indicated and may be seen as a punitive staff response to a client threat. Transfer without careful assessment of need would also encourage dependency. (I, T, L)

The Client Who Abuses Alcohol

16. 4. The rate of alcohol destruction is not influenced by drinking black coffee, walking after a cold shower, or breathing pure oxygen. Alcohol is destroyed and oxidized in the body at a slow, steady rate. Therefore, it would be best to have the client sleep off the effects of the alcohol. (I, T, L)

17. 4. Antiseptic mouthwashes often contain alcohol and should be taken from clients entering a substance abuse unit, unless labeling clearly indicates that the product does not contain alcohol. Such personal care items as hair dressing and shaving cream do not contain alcohol. An electric razor should present no problem for a client being admitted for the treatment of alcoholism as long as it is in good working order. (E, N, L)

18. 2. The alcoholic usually underestimates the amount of alcohol consumed. He may be unaware of how much he really drinks or may fail to admit, even to himself, how much he really consumes. (D, T, L)

19. 2. The amount of alcohol consumed in the last 24 to 48 hours helps determine how much medication the client needs to relieve withdrawal symptoms when a client is admitted for the treatment of alcoholism. It will not help determine how far the disease has progressed or whether the client should be considered an alcoholic. It is difficult to predict delirium tremens during withdrawal, but if the client has had them previously, he may likely have them again. (E, N, L)

20. 1. Alcoholism disrupts sleeping and eating habits. Most alcoholics are undernourished and in need of extra nourishment and rest. Self-esteem Disturbance, Ineffective Individual Coping, and Knowledge Deficit reflect potential client problems which the nurse would include in the plan of care when the client's physiological status has stabilized and alcohol detoxification nears completion. (E, N, L)

21. 2. Antianxiety agents such as lorazepam (Ativan) and chlordiazepoxide (Librium) are commonly used to ease symptoms during alcohol withdrawal. The anticonvulsant phenytoin sodium (Dilantin) does not relieve anxiety, nor does paraldehyde (Paral), which is used primarily for its hypnotic and sedative effects. Temazapam (Restoril) is a sedative-hypnotic not used for alcohol withdrawal. (E, N, L)

22. 3. Monitoring vital signs provides information regarding the client's physiological status during alcohol withdrawal and his physiological response to the antianxiety agent used during detoxification. Vital signs will reflect the degree of central nervous system irritability, indicating the effectiveness of the medication in easing withdrawal symptoms. Assessing the client's nutritional status, sleep pattern, and presence of tremors are less immediate and indirect means of assessing physiological status during alcohol detoxification. (I, N, L)

23. 1. A client is said to be suffering from a blackout when he cannot recall what he has been doing while under the influence of alcohol. Common symptoms of a hangover, including headaches and gastrointestinal distress, typically follow heavy alcohol consumption. In dry drunk syndrome, a person has not been drinking but acts grandiose, impatient, and uses many defense mechanisms. Alcohol hallucinosis occurs after ending or reducing heavy drinking and is marked by auditory hallucinations. (D, C, L)

24. 3. The client suffering with alcoholism may experience tremors for several days or even longer after alcohol intake has stopped. (I, T, L)

25. 4. Group support has proven more successful than individual attention from the staff in influencing positive behavior in alcoholics. Locked doors do not help clients change behavior or develop their own controls. Searching visitors is impractical and externally oriented. (I, T, L)

26. 4. The client is feeling remorse about hitting his wife. Here, it is best to make a comment that will help him focus on his feelings and ventilate them. Reflecting what the client has said is a good technique to accomplish these goals. Comments that give advice to the client or hedge the issue are less satisfactory. (I, T, L)

27. 2. Al-Anon is for the mates of alcoholics. Alateen is for the children of alcoholics. Alcoholics Anonymous is for the alcoholic. Narcotics Anonymous is for the abuser of narcotic substances. (P, C, L)

28. 2. The nurse would discuss concrete problems that are directly due to the client's alcoholism to confront the client and increase his awareness of how alcohol has gotten him into trouble. Providing the client with reading material about the disease of alcoholism, explaining the physiological effects of alcohol, and teaching assertiveness techniques are all important interventions for the client in alcohol rehabilitation but less effective in decreasing denial. (I, T, L)

29. 3. A nurse using group therapy with clients is giving constructive feedback to the group by describing specifically what was seen and heard in an objective rather than judgmental, manner. The nurse is following this principle in telling a client how often he has interrupted the group within a set period of time. (I, T, L)

30. 2. Disulfiram (Antabuse) helps curb the impulsiveness of the problem drinker. Any disulfiram in the body reacts with the alcohol to produce marked discomfort. (D, C, L)

31. 1. Any amount of alcohol consumed while taking disulfiram can cause an alcohol-disulfiram reaction. The reaction experienced is in proportion to the amount of alcohol ingested. The alcohol–disulfiram reaction can begin in 5–10 minutes after alcohol is ingested. Symptoms can be mild, as in flushing, throbbing in head and neck, nausea, and diaphoresis. Other symptoms include vomiting, respiratory difficulty, hypotension, vertigo, syncope, and confusion. Severe reactions involve respiratory depression, convulsions, coma, and even death. (E, N, L)

32. 3. Nausea with severe vomiting is common when the client drinks alcohol. Other typical signs and symptoms of an alcohol disulfiram reaction include vasodilation in the upper body, palpitations, hyperventilation, headache, and dyspnea. Severe reaction can be life-threatening. (D, N, L)

33. 2. Vague feelings of apprehension and doom appear during the chronic phase of alcohol addiction. Such symptoms as an increased alcohol tolerance, feelings of grandiosity and combativeness, and a desire to switch to a different form of alcoholic beverage usually appear at an earlier stage of the disease. (P, C, L)

34. 1. Alcoholism involves the entire family. The organization Al-Anon can help family members understand and live more comfortably with an alcoholic person and learn to deal with his behavior. Counseling in a mental health program is not ordinarily recommended. Behavior in the home such as avoiding the subject of alcoholism in the client's presence and making sure that alcohol is not served in the home puts the onus of responsibility for helping the alcoholic on family members, whereas in reality it is the client who must take responsibility for maintaining sobriety after a course of treatment. (P, T, L)

35. 2. The most realistic analysis in relation to avoiding future drinking problems in the alcoholic client who has completed a course of therapy occurs when the client says he is going to try hard to stay away from his first drink. The alcoholic must understand that he cannot take even one drink without returning to his old drinking habits. It is unwise for the alcoholic to promise he will never drink again; this almost tempts the alcoholic to return to drinking. The alcoholic who believes he will do fine if his "wife keeps off my back" has a doubtful future in terms of abstinence; he is placing the responsibility for his behavior on his wife rather than on himself. (E, N, L)

The Client with Alcohol Withdrawal

36. 2. Stereotype refers to the concept of labeling that categorize persons into groups. To say that a client is an alcoholic because he has cirrhosis of the liver is an example of stereotyping. Ideology is a manner of thinking characteristic of an individual. Mental set refers to a readiness to organize an individual's perceptions in a particular way. The halo effect is a tendency to be influenced by a general impression of a person (favorable or unfavorable) when rating one of his specific traits. (D, C, L)

37. 4. The best way to learn to know a client is to get to know him personally. Depending on others and books are poor substitutes. (P, C, L)

38. 4. The alcoholic is usually differentiated from the person who consumes greater-than-average quantities of alcohol by his inability to get along in his social relationships at work and at home. Behaviors such as drinking alone, drinking only beer and wine, and drinking only in the evenings and on weekends do not differentiate alcoholics from nonalcoholics. (I, T, L)

39. 1. The person using denial as a defense mechanism refuses to acknowledge an aspect of reality. This client is using denial when she refuses to acknowledge that she has a problem with alcohol. Displacement involves transferring a feeling to a more acceptable substitute object. Rationalization involves substituting one reason for a behavior for the real reason motivating the behavior. Reaction formation is when an opposite attitude takes the place of the real attitudes or impulses that the individual harbors. (D, C, L)

40. 4. When health team members attempt to break down a client's defense mechanism, the client is likely to become disorganized and depressed. The defense should not be attacked directly, for it may lead to complete disorganization in the face of a crisis or may give way to depression. (E, N, L)

41. 3. Denial is a major symptom of alcohol dependence. It is helpful if confrontation can be avoided during the first few days of withdrawal. This response gives accurate information with minimal confrontation. (I, T, L)

42. 3. Denial is a major factor in the client's response to treatment at this time. This response best demonstrates her denial. (E, T, L)

43. 4. Typical symptoms of peripheral neuritis include numbness, itching, and pain in the extremities and a predisposition to footdrop. Neurasthenia is neurotic behavior in which the main pattern is motor and mental fatigue. Neuralgia refers to severe pain along the course of a nerve. Bell's palsy is a type of facial paralysis involving the seventh cranial nerve. (D, C, L)

44. 1. The client with peripheral neuritis experiences pain, itching, and numbness of the extremities. Impaired Skin Integrity, Anxiety, and Self-Care Deficit are problems that could result if appropriate nursing and medical interventions are not instituted. (D, N, S)

45. 4. Clients often require help to keep their skin clean. Massaging the feet may be important in some instances, and turning from side to side is an essential nursing measure for many clients. However, a client with neurologic disorders is likely to have sensory changes. Therefore, it is particularly important to guard against burns, because the client may not feel heat on the skin. (I, T, G)

46. 2. Regular coffee contains caffeine, which acts as a psychomotor stimulant. Hence, serving coffee to the alcoholic client may add to her tremors and wakefulness. (E, N, L)

47. 4. Nursing notes most helpful to others are those that describe exactly what the client did and said. Technical terms used to describe behavior may be misinterpreted by others. (E, N, L)

48. 1. The client is experiencing sensory-perceptual alteration related to alcohol withdrawal, as evidenced by stating, "Go away, bugs." The client's thrashing reflects her agitation. Visual hallucinations, disorientation, and agitation are symptoms of delirium tremens. (D, N, L)

49. 3. The client with delirium tremens should not be left unattended. Unintentional suicide is a possibility when the client attempts to get away from hallucinations. Shadows created by dim lights are likely to cause illusions. Such measures as restraining the client, touching her before saying anything, and telling her where she would likely add to her agitation. Explaining that she is having a nightmare and that she will soon be better are untruthful statements that offer false assurance. (P, T, L)

50. 3. The nurse should question the order for chlorpromazine (Thorazine) 100 mg q 4h prn for agitation. Chlorpromazine is a major tranquilizer and antipsychotic that decreases the seizure threshold. During alcohol withdrawal, central nervous system irritability is present, and seizures can occur at this time. The nurse would question this drug order because of the increased risk of seizure. (D, N, L)

51. 1. In early one-to-one helping relationships with this client, focusing on the positive aspects and on healthy coping mechanisms likely would help increase the client's self-esteem. Seeking out reasons for alcohol abuse and delving into childhood experiences that predispose to alcoholism describe more traditional mental health therapies that have not proven very successful. An alcoholic should have a good understanding of Alcoholics Anonymous, but this should not be the focus in early meetings with this client. (P, T, L)

52. 3. It would be best for the nurse to support Alcoholics Anonymous without threatening the client's husband and encourage him not to judge the group on the basis of one meeting. Offering sympathy and making judgments about the meeting are not recommended. Because this is the first meeting with the man, it would be inappropriate to suggest that he give up on Alcoholics Anonymous and look at other therapies. (I, T, L)

53. 2. Alcoholics Anonymous requires that the alcoholic admit that he is powerless over alcohol and that he needs help. Eligibility for membership in Alcoholics Anonymous does not require that the applicant resolve to abstain from drinking, help others to do so, analyze the wrongs he has done, make amends for wrongs committed, or turn his life over to a higher power. (I, T, L)

54. 4. Information about the importance of continued efforts to change her behavior takes into account the fact that alcohol dependence is a difficult problem but that the client can conquer it. This approach is nonjudgmental and places the responsibility to not drink on the client. (E, N, L)

The Client Who is Dependent on Narcotics

55. 3. Common signs of heroin overdose are respiratory depression, pale or cyanotic skin and lips, pinpoint pupils, shock, cardiac arrhythmias, and convulsions. Death may occur from respiratory depression and pulmonary edema. Increased heart rate, dilated pupils, and increased temperature may indicate stimulant abuse. Tremulousness, impaired coordination, increased blood pressure, and a ruddy complexion may indicate alcohol intoxication. Eye irritation, double vision, tinnitus, and irritated mucous membranes could indicate inhalant intoxication. (A, N, L)

56. 2. The client's ineffective breathing pattern should receive the highest priority. Respiratory depression occurs with heroin overdose due to central nervous system depression. (D, N, L)

57. 4. The nurse monitors vital signs and breathing pattern, and prepares for emergency intervention like cardiopulmonary resuscitation. Discussing treatment modalities for chemical dependency while the client is physically unstable would be an inappropriate action. (I, T, L)

58. 4. After administering naloxone (Narcan), the nurse should monitor the client's respiratory status carefully. The drug is short-acting, and the client may fall back into a coma with respiratory depression again after its effects wear off. (I, T, L)

59. 1. Cocaine is usually sniffed through the nostrils. This may cause red excoriated nostrils due to local irritation. (A, T, L)

60. 1. Vomiting and diarrhea are usually late, rather than early, signs of heroin withdrawal. (A, C, L)

61. 2. When a client complains of discomfort while abstaining from heroin, it would be least desirable for the nurse to tell him that she will reevaluate the client's withdrawal plan for easing the client's discomforts. Better courses of action for this client include being empathetic but firm and explaining alternative methods, such as warm baths, to deal with discomfort. Also, it would be important to prepare the client in advance for the discomfort that likely will occur as heroin is withdrawn. (I, T, L)

62. 3. Clients who test positive for human immunodeficiency virus (HIV) can transmit the infection when they experience no symptoms or only mild nonspecific symptoms. Given this client's life-style, the probability of exposure to the virus is high. Thus, testing is important. The virus's long incubation period means that individuals can be infected without exhibiting disease symptoms. The virus can be transmitted through heterosexual intercourse if one partner is infected. (I, N, L)

63. 2. A private room is not indicated unless necessitated by the presence of another infection. Protection from HIV infection includes wearing gloves before touching mucous membranes and blood or other body fluids. Needles should not be broken or recapped; rather, the syringe and needle should be placed in a puncture-resistant container. Handwashing is the foundation of infection control. (I, T, L)

64. 4. A common sign of methadone toxicity is respiratory depression. Fever, colitis, and renal shutdown are not associated with methadone toxicity. (A, T, L)

65. 3. Methadone is equally effective at low or high doses. The danger is that clients may take small doses and sell the excess to drug abusers. (E, N, L)

66. 3. The best way to keep methadone out of the illicit drug market is to administer the liquid form under direct supervision. (I, T, L)

67. 1. Calling Narcotics Anonymous to tell them to expect the client is inappropriate and unnecessary, as it increases the client's dependency on the nurse. It is the client's responsibility to make arrangements for attending meetings. Enforcing unit policies and confronting inappropriate behaviors like manipulation and use of defense mechanisms such as projection are part of the nurse's role in drug rehabilitation. Helping the client to express feelings appropriately through the use of assertiveness techniques teaches the client appropriate interpersonal skills. (I, T, L)

68. 1. Narcotics Anonymous suggests that a person plan only one day at a time. It is too frightening and unrealistic for the client to agree to be "clean" of drugs at Narcotics Anonymous meetings and abstain from drugs the rest of his life. Members do not have to commit a certain amount of time to the organization, although members free of drug use for a certain period often voluntarily work with the organization. (I, T, L)

69. 2. The best judgment concerning progress is based on the number of drug-free days the client has. The longer one is free of drugs, the better the prognosis. The kinds of friends the client has, the way he gets along with parents, and the degree of responsibility his job requires could possibly influence his success, but judgments concerning success are best based on the number of days that he is drug free. (D, N, L)

70. 4. The heroin addict is least likely to develop cholelithiasis as a result of drug abuse. Drug addicts are prone to such disorders as hepatitis, pneumonia, and tuberculosis, primarily due to poor sanitation and an unhealthful life-style. (D, C, L)

The Client Who Abuses Barbiturates

71. 4. The most likely cause of death from barbiturate overdose is respiratory failure. Cardiac arrest is not common. Circulatory depression may occur. (D, N, L)

72. 1. Combining barbiturates and alcohol is dangerous because the two are depressants, and an additive effect results. The agents do not enhance the effects of each other, nor do they suppress each other or act as antagonists. (D, C, L)

73. 4. When a friend asks if a seriously ill client will live, it is best for the nurse to respond by explaining the seriousness of the client's condition and acknowledging the friend's concern. This type of comment does not offer false hope. It is stereotypical to say that one can only "wait and see" if the client dies while offering no support. By asking the friend to describe his relationship with the client, the nurse is not focusing on the problem. Simply to say that the client is very ill and may not live is harsh and nonsupportive. (I, T, L)

74. 1. In this situation, the nurse should focus on the client and her needs for support. The nurse inquires about the relationship between the friend and the client to learn whether the friend is a source of support for the client. The focus of attention at this time is not centered on the seriousness of the client's condition. It is irrelevant to attempt to learn whether the relationship may be a factor in the client's suicide attempt and whether the friend can be trusted with confidential information at this time. (A, N, L)

75. 1. Tolerance for a drug occurs when a client requires increasingly large doses to obtain the desired effect. Addiction is the highest degree of physical and psychological dependence, and withdrawal is accompanied by severe physical symptoms. The drug-dependent person cannot keep drug intake under control and finds it hard to function without its effects. Habituation is defined as a mild degree of dependence. (D, T, L)

76. 2. Typical signs and symptoms of barbiturate abuse include sluggishness, difficulty walking, and irritability. Judgment and understanding are impaired, and speech is slurred and confused. The client acts drunk as from alcohol but does not have the odor of alcohol on his breath. (A, C, L)

77. 3. For the client who is confused when she begins to awaken after taking a large dose of barbiturates, the nurse should plan to maintain seizure precautions, close windows, and speak to her in short, complete sentences. Giving a medication for anxiety and agitation would be inappropriate, because it could add to the depressant effects of the barbiturates that the client took. (I, N, L)

78. 2. Generalized convulsions may occur on the second or third day of withdrawal from barbiturates. Without treatment, as described in this item, the convulsions may be fatal. Postural hypotension and psychoses are possibilities but are unlikely to be fatal; they are unrelated to the pentobarbital sodium regimen. Hyperthermia, rather than hypothermia, occurs during withdrawal. (D, C, L)

79. 2. The nurse would give the highest priority to the nursing diagnosis Potential for Self-Directed Violence. Self-Esteem Disturbance, Ineffective Individual Coping, and Sleep Pattern Disturbance are all possible nursing diagnoses but not as important as the client's suicide attempt. (D, N, L)

80. 1. The most appropriate short-term goal is for the client to discuss feelings related to her losses. The nurse would help the client identify and describe her feelings to help her become aware of her feelings and to help her verbalize these feelings instead of turning them inward or internalizing them. (P, N, L)

81. 4. This situation points out how a group of clients can have an undesirable influence on another client. It would probably be best for a nurse who becomes aware of such a situation to discuss her observations with the group at one of their regular therapy sessions. The problem involves all of the clients in the group, and discussing it with them gives all members an opportunity to offer suggestions. It will likely be futile to try to break up the group's drug-oriented discussions. Providing additional recreation and speaking to clients on an individual basis do not approach the problem in a direct manner. (I, T, L)

The Client With an Eating Disorder

82. 4. The nurse would want to hear more about the client's feelings to assess for potential underlying causes of the eating disorder and to assess the overeating as a maladaptive response. Telling the client that all the group members feel the same, to not worry because she'll be back in shape soon, or that she doesn't look so bad minimizes and ignores the client's feelings and focuses on the weight problem itself. (I, T, L)

83. 4. A member of the group is assuming a functional role when she proposes an alternate task to keep from thinking about food. She acts in the role of a contributor to the group. Showing pictures of children, insisting that everyone try a favorite reducing diet, and making comments to another group member are examples of individual role behavior that are irrelevant to the group task. Showing pictures of one's child in a group is an example of a "blocker." The person who insists that everyone try her recipe is a special-interest pleader. The person making comments to another group member is withdrawing from the group. (A, N, L)

84. 1. Through the ages, communication has occurred around food. Honor is extended through food, and punishment is given by withholding food. Food is commonly recognized as giving comfort, because it often serves this purpose during childhood. Hence, in our culture food is often equated with love and affection. (D, C, L)

85. 1. Adverse effects associated with amphetamine use include drug dependency, emotional lability, and depression between doses. Gastritis is not associated with amphetamine use. (A, C, L)

86. 2. Based on the data, the most appropriate nursing

diagnosis is Self-Esteem Disturbance related to weight gain, as evidenced by withdrawal. (D, T, L)

87. 3. Telling the client who is withdrawn and an overeater to record what she eats throughout the day focuses her attention on her eating problem and will probably decrease her self-esteem and increase her withdrawal. It is more beneficial to invite the client to an informal craft activity where socialization can occur, which may have a positive effect on the client's self-esteem. Asking the dietician to meet with the client and discussing overeating as a maladaptive response to stress are therapeutic in that the client can learn important information about nutrition and stress and coping. (I, T, L)

88. 4. Bradycardia, hypotension, and cold sensitivity reflect the slowed metabolism that occurs with severe weight loss. Tachycardia and hypertension reflect increased metabolic rate, which is inconsistent with anorexia nervosa. Hyperthyroidism and elevated serum potassium are atypical with anorexia. Vitamin C deficiency and anemia may occur, but they are not hallmark symptoms of the disorder. (A, C, L)

89. 3. The nursing diagnosis Altered Nutrition: Less than Body Requirements receives the highest priority at this time. Self-starvation is life threatening, and gradual weight gain is a priority. Self-Esteem Disturbance, Ineffective Individual Coping, and Body Image Disturbance may be applicable to the client with anorexia nervosa but are of less importance than self-starvation. (D, N, L)

90. 2. Behavioral programs involve rewards and punishments to elicit specific behavioral responses. Emotional support and listening are general interventions not specific to the program goal. Identifying problematic eating behaviors is a general intervention related to behavioral programs, but is not specific to a behavioral program for weight gain. Hyperalimentation may be used as a last resort but is a physiologic, not a behavioral, intervention. Rapid weight gain is psychologically intolerable and physically dangerous for the client. (I, T, L)

91. 3. The primary goal with severe anorexia is to promote weight gain through behavior modification. This involves actively monitoring and interrupting undesirable behaviors, even against the client's protests. Waiting for the client to finish exercising may be polite but exacerbates weight loss as more calories are burned. Threatening future loss of privileges does not motivate a client who is in the middle of a compulsion. Active intervention is required to prevent continued weight loss. (I, T, L)

92. 1. The goal of hospitalization for anorexia is to stabilize the client's weight and facilitate entry into outpatient care. Weight gain in the hospital may not be sustained unless the client receives follow-up help for the underlying problem. Most clients do not achieve a normal weight in the hospital and require continued follow-up. The urge to diet can continue for years following hospitalization. A change in eating behaviors does not address the central issue of dangerous weight loss and psychiatric disturbance. (E, N, L)

NURSING CARE OF CLIENTS WITH PSYCHOSOCIAL HEALTH PROBLEMS

TEST 3: Chemical Dependency and Eating Disorders

Directions: Use this answer grid to determine areas of strength or need for further study.

NURSING PROCESS

A = Assessment
D = Analysis, nursing diagnosis
P = Planning
I = Implementation
E = Evaluation

COGNITIVE LEVEL

K = Knowledge
C = Comprehension
T = Application
N = Analysis

CLIENT NEEDS

S = Safe, effective care environment
G = Physiological integrity
L = Psychosocial integrity
H = Health promotion/maintenance

		Nursing Process					Cognitive Level				Client Needs			
Question #	**Answer #**	A	D	P	I	E	K	C	T	N	S	G	L	H
1	2					E				N			L	
2	4			P						N			L	
3	1		D							N			L	
4	3			P					T				L	
5	2			P						N			L	
6	1				I				T				L	
7	3				I				T				L	
8	2					E				N			L	
9	1		D							N			L	
10	3					E				N			L	
11	4		D							N			L	
12	2		D					C					L	
13	1			P					T				L	
14	4		D							N			L	
15	4				I				T				L	
16	4				I				T				L	
17	4					E				N			L	
18	2		D						T				L	
19	2					E				N			L	
20	1					E				N			L	
21	2					E				N			L	
22	3				I					N			L	
23	1		D					C					L	

ANSWER GRID: 1

Nursing Process

A = Assessment
D = Analysis, nursing diagnosis
P = Planning
I = Implementation
E = Evaluation

Cognitive Level

K = Knowledge
C = Comprehension
T = Application
N = Analysis

Client Needs

S = Safe, effective care environment
G = Physiological integrity
L = Psychosocial integrity
H = Health promotion/maintenance

		Nursing Process					Cognitive Level				Client Needs			
Question #	Answer #	A	D	P	I	E	K	C	T	N	S	G	L	H
24	3				I				T				L	
25	4				I				T				L	
26	4				I				T				L	
27	2			P				C					L	
28	2				I				T				L	
29	3				I				T				L	
30	2		D					C					L	
31	1					E				N			L	
32	3		D							N			L	
33	2			P				C					L	
34	1			P					T				L	
35	2					E				N			L	
36	2		D					C					L	
37	4			P				C					L	
38	4				I				T				L	
39	1		D					C					L	
40	4					E				N			L	
41	3				I				T				L	
42	3					E			T				L	
43	4		D					C					L	
44	1		D							N	S			
45	4				I				T			G		
46	2					E				N			L	
47	4					E				N			L	
48	1		D							N			L	
49	3			P					T				L	
50	3		D							N			L	
51	1			P					T				L	
52	3				I				T				L	

ANSWER GRID: 2

NURSING PROCESS

A = Assessment
D = Analysis, nursing diagnosis
P = Planning
I = Implementation
E = Evaluation

COGNITIVE LEVEL

K = Knowledge
C = Comprehension
T = Application
N = Analysis

CLIENT NEEDS

S = Safe, effective care environment
G = Physiological integrity
L = Psychosocial integrity
H = Health promotion/maintenance

		Nursing Process					Cognitive Level				Client Needs			
Question #	Answer #	A	D	P	I	E	K	C	T	N	S	G	L	H
53	2				I				T				L	
54	4					E				N			L	
55	3	A								N			L	
56	2		D							N			L	
57	4				I				T				L	
58	4				I				T				L	
59	1	A							T				L	
60	1	A						C					L	
61	2				I				T				L	
62	3				I					N			L	
63	2				I					N			L	
64	4	A							T				L	
65	3					E				N			L	
66	3				I				T				L	
67	1				I				T				L	
68	1				I				T				L	
69	2		D							N			L	
70	4		D					C					L	
71	4		D							N			L	
72	1		D					C					L	
73	4				I				T				L	
74	1	A								N			L	
75	1		D						T				L	
76	2	A						C					L	
77	3				I					N			L	
78	2		D					C					L	
79	2		D							N			L	
80	1			P						N			L	
81	4				I				T				L	

ANSWER GRID: 3

NURSING PROCESS

A = Assessment
D = Analysis, nursing diagnosis
P = Planning
I = Implementation
E = Evaluation

COGNITIVE LEVEL

K = Knowledge
C = Comprehension
T = Application
N = Analysis

CLIENT NEEDS

S = Safe, effective care environment
G = Physiological integrity
L = Psychosocial integrity
H = Health promotion/maintenance

		Nursing Process					Cognitive Level				Client Needs			
Question #	**Answer #**	A	D	P	I	E	K	C	T	N	S	G	L	H
82	4				I				T				L	
83	4	A								N			L	
84	1		D					C					L	
85	1	A						C					L	
86	2		D						T				L	
87	3				I				T				L	
88	4	A						C					L	
89	3		D							N			L	
90	2				I				T				L	
91	3				I				T				L	
92	1					E				N			L	
Number Correct														
Number Possible	92	9	26	11	30	16	0	17	37	38	1	1	90	0
Percentage Correct														

Score Calculation:

To determine your **Percentage Correct**, divide the **Number Correct** by the **Number Possible.**

Anxiety, Anger, Abuse, Terminal Illness

Test 4

The Client With Anxiety
The Client With Maladaptive Behavior Patterns
The Client With Problems With Expression of Anger
The Client With Family Abuse and Violence
The Client With a Psychophysiological Disorder
The Client With a Terminal Illness
Correct Answers and Rationale

Select the one best answer and indicate your choice by filling in the circle in front of the option.

The Client With Anxiety

A client is brought to the hospital emergency room by his brother. On admission, the client is perspiring profusely, breathing rapidly, and complaining of dizziness and palpitations. Problems of a cardiovascular nature are ruled out. The client's diagnosis is tentatively listed as acute anxiety reaction.

1. The emergency room nurse observes that the client is hyperventilating. Which of the following measures would be best to try first to ease the symptoms caused by hyperventilation?
- ○ 1. Have the client breathe into a paper bag.
- ○ 2. Instruct the client to put his head between his knees.
- ○ 3. Give the client a low concentration of oxygen via nasal cannula.
- ○ 4. Tell the client to take several deep, slow breaths and exhale normally.

2. The client was later admitted to the inpatient psychiatric unit for further evaluation and treatment, based on his urgent plea for help. The client is aware that his anxiety is of neurotic origin. Neurotic anxiety differs from normal anxiety in that it is
- ○ 1. out of proportion to the cause.
- ○ 2. lessened with the passage of time.
- ○ 3. a rational response to an objective danger.
- ○ 4. easily traceable to a consciously recognized stimulus.

3. Which of the following nursing actions would be *inappropriate* on the client's admission to the unit?
- ○ 1. Support the client's attempts to discuss feelings.
- ○ 2. Respect the client's personal space.
- ○ 3. Reassure the client of his safety.
- ○ 4. Confront the client's dysfunctional coping behaviors.

4. In caring for the client with a nursing diagnosis of Anxiety (panic), the nurse would consider which of the following goals to be primary? Reduce the client's
- ○ 1. secondary gains.
- ○ 2. physical activities.
- ○ 3. level of anxiety.
- ○ 4. need for security.

5. The client often jumps when spoken to and complains of feeling uneasy. He says, "It's as though something bad is going to happen." All of the following nursing measures are likely to reassure the client except
- ○ 1. being physically present.
- ○ 2. being technically competent.
- ○ 3. conveying optimistic verbalizations.
- ○ 4. communicating a respectful attitude.

6. During a conversation with the client, the nurse observes the client shaking his leg and tapping his fingers on the table next to him. Which statement by the nurse would be most helpful to the client at this time?
- ○ 1. "I see that you're anxious. I'll be back later when you're calmer."
- ○ 2. "I noticed that your leg is shaking and you're tapping your fingers on the table. How are you feeling now?"
- ○ 3. "I'll get you something to help you feel less anxious."

○ 4. "I know that you feel anxious. Let's discuss something more pleasant."

7. The nursing diagnosis for this client is Social Isolation related to severe anxiety, as evidenced by withdrawal into his room. An appropriate long-term goal related to this nursing diagnosis is that the client will
○ 1. attend group meetings with a staff member by discharge.
○ 2. initiate interactions with the nurse when feeling anxious.
○ 3. express two adaptive methods of coping with anxiety.
○ 4. participate in milieu activities by discharge.

8. What is the main reason that the activities planned for the client are directed toward increasing his contact with other people?
○ 1. to relieve his boredom.
○ 2. to reduce his egocentricity.
○ 3. to keep him safely occupied.
○ 4. to prevent him from regressing.

9. In working with the client with an anxiety-related disorder, the ultimate nursing goal is to
○ 1. reduce the client's anxiety to a manageable level.
○ 2. help the client decrease denial and avoidance about his feelings and link feelings with behaviors.
○ 3. assist the client with problem solving and developing adaptive coping behaviors.
○ 4. use supportive confrontation when the client avoids painful issues.

10. The client seldom experiences feelings of panic and has been participating in groups on the inpatient unit. He tells the nurse, "I still have problems falling asleep without tossing and turning." Of the following nursing actions, which would be most helpful to the client?
○ 1. Teach him relaxation exercises.
○ 2. Tell him to ask his doctor for medication.
○ 3. Recommend that he watch television until he gets sleepy.
○ 4. Advise him to ride the exercise bicycle for 10 minutes before retiring for the night.

11. Alprazolam (Xanax) is prescribed to treat moderate to severe anxiety. The client will derive all of the following benefits from this anxiolytic except
○ 1. decreasing focus on somatic symptoms of anxiety.
○ 2. decreasing psychological symptoms of anxiety.
○ 3. increasing the likelihood that the client will participate in group.
○ 4. decreasing the potential of physical and psychological dependence.

12. While the client is taking chlordiazepoxide (Librium), he should be taught to avoid ingesting
○ 1. coffee.
○ 2. cheese.
○ 3. alcohol.
○ 4. shellfish.

13. The client has been taking buspirone (Buspar) for 2 days as prescribed. Which statement made by the client indicates a need for further teaching?
○ 1. "I can take Buspar as I need it when I'm anxious."
○ 2. "I may not feel better for 7 to 10 days."
○ 3. "I can't become physically dependent on Buspar."
○ 4. "I need to take Buspar with food."

14. Upon discharge, the client is referred to the outpatient clinic for follow-up. Which of the following hospital-learned abilities is probably most important for the continued alleviation of anxiety symptoms?
○ 1. He recognizes when he is feeling anxious.
○ 2. He understands the reasons for his anxiety.
○ 3. He can alter his methods of handling anxiety.
○ 4. He can describe the situations preceding his feelings of anxiety.

15. The physician in the outpatient clinic tells the nurse that he is prescribing an antianxiety agent for the client. The nurse would question an order for
○ 1. biperiden hydrochloride (Akineton).
○ 2. oxazepam (Serax).
○ 3. hydroxyzine pamoate (Vistaril).
○ 4. propanolol (Inderal).

16. The client complains of muscular tension and is wringing his hands. He tells the nurse, "Help me. I don't know what to do to feel better. I feel jumpy inside." The nurse would assess the client's anxiety level to be
○ 1. mild (+1).
○ 2. moderate (+2).
○ 3. severe (+3).
○ 4. panic (+4).

17. Which behavior would the nurse least expect from the client with an anxiety-related disorder prior to discharge from an inpatient unit? The client
○ 1. uses adaptive strategies to reduce anxiety.
○ 2. uses avoidance when uncomfortable.
○ 3. recognizes mild anxiety as helpful for personal changes.
○ 4. describes the side effects of his medication.

The Client With Maladaptive Behavior Patterns

A 19-year-old client is admitted to a psychiatric unit with a nonspecific diagnosis of personality disorder. He is accompanied by his mother and a lawyer who tells the nurse that he hopes his client will "stay out of mischief until we get the messes straightened out."

18. According to the client's mother, the client "always was a mean little boy, forever playing pranks on people and teasing the small animals in the neighborhood. Now he's just a bigger prankster and less easy to control." In view of the client's history, which of the following courses of action would likely be the most effective for the nursing staff to follow initially?

- ○ 1. Let the client know the staff has the authority to subdue him if he gets unruly.
- ○ 2. Keep the client isolated from the other clients until he is better known by the staff.
- ○ 3. Provide the client with a list of rules while emphasizing that he will have to pay for any damage he causes.
- ○ 4. Closely observe the client's behavior on the unit to establish a baseline pattern of physical and social functioning.

19. After the client has been on the unit for a few days, the nurses notice that he uses his shortness and unattractiveness as an excuse for not attending various social functions, such as the weekly dance. Which of the following interventions would be best to take first to deal with the client's avoidance of social functions?

- ○ 1. Tell the client he will need a better excuse than his appearance for not participating.
- ○ 2. Explain to the client that everyone's cooperation is necessary to make the program a success.
- ○ 3. Confront the client with the fact that he is using his appearance as an excuse to avoid socializing.
- ○ 4. Insist that the client come up with some alternative ways to spend the time when he should be socializing.

20. A staff member asks the client after one of his loud belches, "Do you wonder why people find you repulsive?" This comment most likely will make the client feel

- ○ 1. defensive and defiant.
- ○ 2. insulted and indignant.
- ○ 3. ashamed and remorseful.
- ○ 4. embarrassed and unhappy.

21. The client's past history of cruelty and current crass behavior arouse feelings of anxiety and antagonism in staff and other clients. What is the most likely reason for these responses? The client's behavior is

- ○ 1. beyond comprehension.
- ○ 2. viewed as alien to their value system.
- ○ 3. easily misinterpreted as to its meaning.
- ○ 4. seen as only too understandable by others.

22. The client attempts to provoke the male nurse by yelling, "Hey nursie, where's your hat and purse?" In relation to being baited by the client, which of the following actions is best for the nurse to take?

- ○ 1. Ignore the client's kidding to avoid reinforcing it.
- ○ 2. Smilingly shake his head no at the client to stop his teasing.
- ○ 3. Use feminine gestures to indicate acceptance of the client's ribbing.
- ○ 4. Challenge the client to an arm-wrestling match to prove his masculinity.

23. The client on the inpatient unit tells the nurse that he likes to call places and make bomb threats. He says that he enjoys watching the people being evacuated and the police running in and out of the buildings. Which of the following replies by the nurse would be least helpful in encouraging the client to examine the meaning and effects of such messages?

- ○ 1. "What does it do for you to tell me that?"
- ○ 2. "You could be sent to jail for that, you know."
- ○ 3. "You make bomb threats and everybody hops, is that right?"
- ○ 4. "You expect me to be shocked by what you're saying?"

24. Which nursing diagnosis specifically relates to the client who likes to call places and make bomb threats?

- ○ 1. Potential for Violence directed at others.
- ○ 2. Ineffective Individual Coping.
- ○ 3. Self-Esteem Disturbance.
- ○ 4. Social Isolation.

25. One evening the client takes the nurse aside and whispers, "Don't tell anybody, but I'm going to call in a bomb threat to this hospital tonight." Of the following actions by the nurse, which would best preserve the client's trust in the nurse and provide the best protection for all concerned parties?

- ○ 1. Warn the client that his phone privileges will be taken away if he abuses them.
- ○ 2. Offer to disregard the client's plan if he does not go through with it.
- ○ 3. Say nothing to anyone until the client has actually completed the call, then notify the proper authorities.
- ○ 4. Explain to the client that this information will have to be shared immediately with the staff and the physician.

26. Constructive discipline is applied each time the client behaves in a cruel manner. At those times, which of the following ideas is the most basic and most important for the staff to convey to the client?

- ○ 1. The client is accepted although his behavior may not be.
- ○ 2. Everyone must cope with some restrictions on his actions.
- ○ 3. No one would bother with the client if the staff did not care about him.
- ○ 4. If the client cannot control his behavior, then others will have to control it for him.

A client on the inpatient psychiatric unit has a history of impulsive antisocial tendencies. He feels no remorse for any of his actions and is egocentric.

27. In planning care for the client, the nurse considers all of the following aspects as important *except*

○ 1. short-term goals should be realistic.
○ 2. long-lasting maladaptive patterns of behavior are impossible to change during one short-term hospital stay.
○ 3. behavior modification should not be used.
○ 4. explaining to the client the effects of his behavior on others will be helpful.

28. The client-nurse relationship develops so that they are able to delineate and concentrate on a goal to help the client increase his social skills. The nurse is talking with the client about being able to socialize at mealtime without being disruptive. While discussing this topic, it would be best for the nurse to focus the discussion on the client's
○ 1. strengths and responsibilities in the situation.
○ 2. manipulation and disruption in similar situations.
○ 3. explanations concerning his behavior at mealtimes in the past.
○ 4. rationalizations of his behavior.

29. The nurse judges that the client's problematic behavior stems from feelings of resentment toward his mother. The client's resentment seems to represent an attempt to punish his mother for what he perceives as her lack of concern for him. The best thing for the nurse to do with this information is to
○ 1. explain it to the client but in an indirect manner.
○ 2. assist the client to discover it gradually for himself.
○ 3. record it on the client's chart so that the psychiatrist can deal with it.
○ 4. include the client's mother in therapy sessions so that she can discover it for herself.

30. If the client and his mother improve their relationship and the client accomplishes the normal developmental task of identity, which of the following age-related developmental tasks should he be expected to master next?
○ 1. Intimacy.
○ 2. Integrity.
○ 3. Autonomy.
○ 4. Productivity.

31. Which of the following terms best describes the client's sense of self-awareness of his attitudes, defense mechanisms, and behaviors?
○ 1. Insight.
○ 2. Rapport.
○ 3. Lucidity.
○ 4. Cathexis.

32. During the latter part of the client's hospitalization, his progress slows and he seems to be making more enemies than friends. Which of the following evaluations of this situation is probably most accurate?
○ 1. He has too many problems to overcome.
○ 2. He has been unable to develop trust in the nurse.
○ 3. He is reacting to the termination of hospitalization.
○ 4. He is experiencing only a temporary setback in his overall progress.

33. In treating the client with antisocial behavior patterns, the nurse would help the client achieve all of the following outcomes in relation to impulsive behavior except
○ 1. identify feelings before acting impulsively.
○ 2. express sorrow and remorse for his impulsive actions.
○ 3. describe how his actions affect others.
○ 4. identify impulsive acts that have resulted in problems with others.

The Client With Problems Expressing Anger

A client is admitted to the psychiatric hospital for evaluation after numerous incidents of threatening, angry outbursts and two episodes of hitting a coworker at the grocery store where he works. The client is very anxious and tells the nurse who admits him, "I didn't mean to hit him. He made me so mad that I just couldn't help it. I hope I don't hit anyone here."

34. Which of the following responses is the nurse's most therapeutic response?
○ 1. "You'd better not hit anyone here, even if you do get mad."
○ 2. "Tell me more about what happened."
○ 3. "It sounds like you were quite angry. When you feel angry here, you'll need to tell us about it instead of hitting."
○ 4. "I'm sure you didn't mean to hit him and that it won't happen here."

35. The nurse knows that providing a safe environment for the client and the other clients is a nursing care priority. Which of the following is the most important initial action the nurse should take to ensure a safe environment?
○ 1. Let other clients know that he has a history of hitting others so that they will not provoke him.
○ 2. Put him in a private room and limit his time out of the room to when staff can be with him.
○ 3. Tell him that hitting others is not acceptable behavior and ask him to let a staff member know when he begins feeling angry so they can talk.
○ 4. Obtain an order for a medication to decrease his anxiety.

36. The client rushes out of the day room, where he has been watching TV with other clients. He is hyperventilating, flushed, and his fists are clenched. He states to the nurse, "That bastard! He's just like Tom. I almost hit him." Which of the following would be the nurse's best response?
○ 1. "You're angry and you did well to leave the situa-

tion. Let's walk up and down the hall while you tell me about it."

○ 2. "Even if you're angry, you can't use that language here."

○ 3. "I'm glad you left the situation. Why don't you go to your room and calm down. I'll come in soon to talk."

○ 4. "I can see you're angry. Let me get you some Ativan to help you calm down. Then we'll talk about what happened."

37. Based on the client's potential for violence toward others and inability to cope with anger, which short-term goal would be most helpful? The client will

○ 1. acknowledge his angry feelings.

○ 2. describe situations that provoke angry feelings.

○ 3. list how he's handled his anger in the past.

○ 4. verbalize his feelings in an appropriate manner.

38. In developing a nursing care plan for the client, the staff decides to take an educational approach. All of the following would be appropriate steps in the plan except

○ 1. assisting the client to recognize anger.

○ 2. identifying all the important people in the client's life with whom he is angry.

○ 3. identifying alternative ways to express anger.

○ 4. practicing expressing anger.

39. Which of the following factors in the client's history is least likely to contribute to his difficulty in coping with anger?

○ 1. A history of abuse as a child.

○ 2. Frequent drinking episodes.

○ 3. A family history of bipolar disorder.

○ 4. A learning disability.

40. In the first group meeting after the client is admitted, another client sits near the nurse and says loudly, "I'm sitting here because I'm afraid of Ted. He's so big and I heard him talk about hitting people." Which of the following responses by the nurse would be the most therapeutic?

○ 1. "Everyone is here for different problems. You know you don't have to worry. We'll keep you safe."

○ 2. "Ted is new to the group. Since he doesn't know anyone here, let's go around and introduce ourselves."

○ 3. "You don't know Ted yet. Once you get to know him, I'm sure you won't be afraid."

○ 4. "It can be frightening to have new people on the unit. The purpose of this group is for people to get to know each other so we can talk together about things like being afraid."

41. A female client in the group states, "My doctor tells me I need to get mad more and not let people tell me what to do. Maybe she thinks I should be more like Ted." To respond appropriately to this client, it is most important that the nurse understand that

○ 1. denial of anger and the inability to be assertive can be as serious a problem as the aggressive expression of anger.

○ 2. it is appropriate for a woman to deny her anger, because assertive behavior in women is not culturally acceptable.

○ 3. because clients frequently distort what they are told by physicians, it is unlikely that the client has been told what she reports.

○ 4. because both clients are about the same age, the female client is trying to help Ted feel accepted by the group.

42. In talking about discharge with his nurse, the client says, "It's been easy not to get mad and hit people here because the staff won't let me. It's not the same at work." What would be the nurse's most effective response?

○ 1. "We have helped, but you're the one who decided not to hit when you were angry. You can do that at work, too."

○ 2. "Lots of people feel this way. You're just worried about leaving the hospital. You've learned so much that you won't have any problems at work."

○ 3. "You sound worried about going back to work. The things you've learned here can help at work, too. Let's talk about what you learned and how you can use it."

○ 4. "It's hard to leave the hospital, I know. But you're better and need to get back to work. You'll be OK, I know."

43. The client states to the nurse, "My doctor says I'm really mad inside and I'm passive-aggressive. I don't know what she means. You know I don't get angry. Do you think I'm passive-aggressive?" Which of the following responses by the nurse would be most inappropriate?

○ 1. "Most people get mad sometimes. Can you remember any times when you've felt angry about something?"

○ 2. "Since this is something you've discussed with your doctor, I think you need to keep talking to her about it."

○ 3. "Do you have any thoughts about what your doctor meant?"

○ 4. "I think it's hard for you to recognize when you feel angry, and that means you can't express it very well."

44. The treatment team recommends that the client take an assertiveness training course offered in the hospital. Which of the following behaviors indicates that the client is becoming more assertive?

○ 1. He begins to arrive late for unit activities.

○ 2. He asks the nurse to call his employer about his insurance.

○ 3. He tells his roommate that smoke bothers him and asks him not to smoke.

○ 4. He follows the nurse's advice and asks his doctor about being passive-aggressive.

45. Which of the following physiological responses does *not* occur when a client is angry?
○ 1. Increased respiratory rate.
○ 2. Decreased blood pressure.
○ 3. Increased muscle tension.
○ 4. Decreased peristalsis.

46. Which of the following psychological responses to anger is least common in psychiatric clients?
○ 1. Decreased self-esteem.
○ 2. Feelings of invulnerability.
○ 3. Fear of retaliation.
○ 4. Feelings of guilt.

47. Anger is a common human emotion that nurses commonly encounter when caring for clients with psychosocial alterations. Which of the following statements is *least* accurate and *least* useful to the nurse caring for clients who express anger?
○ 1. Anger can be an adaptive response and should be discussed with the client.
○ 2. Feeling angry may frighten the client and cause anxiety.
○ 3. When a client is angry, it is usually because the nurse has done something wrong.
○ 4. Anger is frequently used by a client to keep the nurse from getting too close.

48. Which of the following factors is most important for the nurse to consider when assessing the angry client's potential for violence?
○ 1. The time of day and level of activity on the unit.
○ 2. The attitude of the staff toward the angry client.
○ 3. The staff–client ratio.
○ 4. The client's past history of violent behavior.

49. Indirect expression of anger is more common than direct expression. Which of the following client behaviors is most likely to be an indirect expression of anger?
○ 1. Responding sarcastically to an invitation to join a unit activity.
○ 2. Refusing to take medication.
○ 3. Organizing a card game with other clients.
○ 4. Shouting at another client.

The Client With Family Abuse and Violence

The client, a married homemaker, has been referred to the mental health center because she is depressed.

50. Seeing the client for the first time, the nurse notices bruises on her upper arms and asks about them. After denying any problems, the client starts to cry and says, "He didn't really mean to hurt me, but I hate the kids to see. I'm so worried about them." During the interview, it would be most important for the nurse to determine
○ 1. the type and extent of abuse in the family.
○ 2. the potential of immediate danger to the client and her children.
○ 3. the resources available to the client.
○ 4. whether the client wants to be separated from her husband.

51. The client describes her husband as a "good man" who works hard and provides well for his family. She does not work outside the home and states that she is proud to be a wife and mother just like her own mother. The family pattern that the client describes best illustrates which characteristic of abusive families?
○ 1. Tight, impermeable boundaries.
○ 2. Imbalanced power ratio.
○ 3. Role stereotyping.
○ 4. Dysfunctional feeling tone.

52. The client agrees to meet with the nurse the following week. Before the nurse terminates the meeting with the client, which nursing action is most important?
○ 1. Give the client the telephone numbers of a shelter or a safe house and the crisis line.
○ 2. Advise the client to leave her husband.
○ 3. Tell the client not to do anything that could upset her husband.
○ 4. Ask the client what she could do to deescalate the situation at home.

53. As the nurse learns more about the client and her family, which of the following characteristics is the nurse *least* likely to find to be true about the abuser?
○ 1. Between episodes of abuse, he has a warm, empathetic relationship with his wife.
○ 2. He grew up in an abusive family.
○ 3. He is a college graduate and has a stable work history.
○ 4. He abuses alcohol.

54. In planning care for the client, the nurse should include all of the following measures *except*
○ 1. being compassionate and empathetic.
○ 2. teaching the client about abuse and the cycle of violence.
○ 3. explaining to the client her personal and legal rights.
○ 4. sharing feelings of frustration with the client.

55. The nurse discusses the client and her family in a staff meeting. Which of the following statements made by other staff members is likely to be most helpful to the nurse in developing a treatment plan?
○ 1. "This client sounds like a lot of women I know who don't want to change. You can try family therapy, if the husband will come."

○ 2. "Have you thought about suggesting that she attend the group for women in abusive families?"
○ 3. "I think the police should be notified in case he hits her again and she wants to call them."
○ 4. "Have you thought about calling the client's mother to find out what she knows about the family?"

56. In assessing the client's methods of coping, which method would the nurse least expect to find her using?
○ 1. Assertiveness.
○ 2. Self-blame.
○ 3. Alcohol abuse.
○ 4. Suicidal thoughts.

57. During the third session with the nurse, the client states, "I don't know what to do anymore. He doesn't want me to go anywhere while he's at work, not even to visit my friends." Which of the following nursing diagnoses would the nurse formulate in respect to this data?
○ 1. Violence related to abusive husband, as evidenced by victim's statement of being battered.
○ 2. Self-Esteem Disturbance related to victimization, as evidenced by not being able to leave the house.
○ 3. Powerlessness related to abusive husband, as evidenced by inability to make decisions.
○ 4. Ineffective Individual Coping related to victimization, as evidenced by crying.

58. As the nurse develops a treatment plan for the client, which of the following factors would be *least* important to consider?
○ 1. The abuser's refusal to be involved in treatment.
○ 2. The client's coping skills.
○ 3. The recent promotion of the client's husband.
○ 4. The birthday party for the client's child next week.

59. The client tells the nurse that her 8-year-old daughter refuses to go to school because she is afraid her mother will not be home when she returns. Which of the following is the most therapeutic response for the nurse to make?
○ 1. "She must be feeling insecure right now. Let her stay home with you for a few days to reassure her."
○ 2. "Children often feel responsible for trouble in the family. Have you talked with her about what she's afraid might happen?"
○ 3. "You know she's too young to be home alone after school. If you can't be there, you should find someone else to meet her so she won't be afraid."
○ 4. "She's aware of the trouble in the family and is worried about what might happen. Would you like to have her talk to the child therapist here? I think it would be helpful."

60. After months of treatment, the client tells the nurse that she has decided to stop treatment. There has been no abuse during this time and she feels better able to cope with the needs of her husband and children. In discussing this decision with the client, it would be most important for the nurse to
○ 1. tell the client that this is a bad decision that she will regret.
○ 2. find out more about the client's decision.
○ 3. warn the client that abuse often stops when one partner is in treatment, only to begin again later.
○ 4. remind the client of her duty to protect the children by continuing treatment.

A third-grade child is referred to the mental health clinic by the school nurse because he is fearful, anxious, and socially isolated.

61. After meeting with the client, the nurse talks with his mother, who says, "It's that school nurse again. She's done nothing but try to make trouble for our family since my son started school. And now you're in on it." Which of the following responses by the nurse is least likely to help her develop a relationship with this family?
○ 1. "The school nurse is concerned about your son and is only doing her job. Does this bother you?"
○ 2. "We see a number of children who go to your son's school. He isn't the only one, if you're worried about that."
○ 3. "You sound pretty angry with the school nurse. Can you tell me what has happened?"
○ 4. "It sounds like you've had some bad experiences with the school. Let me tell you why your son was referred, and then you can tell me about your concerns."

62. The client's mother tells the nurse that last year was a very bad time for the family. Her husband was unemployed, and she worked a second job to help. Twice during the year, she slapped her son repeatedly when he refused to obey. She says it has not happened again and that the family is "back to normal." After assessing the family, the nurse decides that the child is not at risk for abuse. Which of the following observations would *least* support this decision?
○ 1. The parents have a caring and supportive relationship.
○ 2. The client has not talked about violence during his visits.
○ 3. The infrequent episodes were limited to a time of intense family stress.
○ 4. The parents have a defensive attitude toward the school nurse.

The Client With a Psychophysiological Disorder

A client is admitted to the hospital with a diagnosis of chronic ulcerative colitis. He reports frequent bouts of diarrhea that have caused him to lose 10 pounds in the last month.

63. Because this is the client's fourth admission to the hospital in the last 9 months, he is familiar to the nurse caring for him. Which of the following remarks by the nurse on admission would be most beneficial to the client?

○ 1. "It's nice to see you again. Did you get lonesome for us on the outside?"
○ 2. "I thought we had seen the last of you for a while. What are you doing back?"
○ 3. "It's been 2 months since you were last here. What do you think about being back in the hospital?"
○ 4. "I see you have your old room again. No need to explain things to you, since you're such an old pro."

64. The client becomes tense and nauseated when he hears the cart containing meal trays approaching. Which of the following practices would be best to prevent the premeal buildup of tension that the client experiences?

○ 1. Reroute the meal cart so that the client will not be disturbed by it.
○ 2. Order a special early tray for the client to let him finish eating before the meal cart comes.
○ 3. Turn on the client's television or radio before meals to mask the noise of the approaching meal cart.
○ 4. Arrange for someone to keep the client engaged in a relaxing activity or conversation before mealtimes.

65. The client should be involved in suitable activities in his room while his illness is being treated. These activities should be chosen based on which of the following attributes?

○ 1. Conducive to rest and relaxation.
○ 2. Enhance improvement of social skills.
○ 3. Include insight and self-awareness experiences.
○ 4. Involve manual dexterity rather than intellectual processes.

66. The physician recommends that the client have a partial bowel resection and an ileostomy. Later, the client says to the nurse, "That doctor of mine surely likes to play big. I'll bet the more he can cut, the better he likes it." Which of the following replies by the nurse would be most therapeutic?

○ 1. "You sound upset. We can talk about it if you'd like."
○ 2. "What do you mean by that?"
○ 3. "Aren't you being a bit hard on him? He's trying to help you."
○ 4. "Does that remark have something to do with the operation he wants you to have, by any chance?"

67. The client becomes increasingly morose and irritable after thinking more about his physician's recommendations. He is rude to his visitors and pushes nurses away when they attempt to give him medications and treatments. Which of the following nursing interventions would be best when the client has a hostile outburst?

○ 1. Offer the client positive reinforcement each time he cooperates.
○ 2. Encourage the client to discuss his immediate concerns and feelings.
○ 3. Continue with the assigned tasks and duties as though nothing has happened.
○ 4. Encourage the client to direct his anger at staff members who can handle his angry outbursts.

68. Arrangements are made for a member of the ileostomy club to meet with the client. Which of the following aims illustrates the chief purpose for having a representative from the club visit the client preoperatively?

○ 1. To let the client know that he has resources in the community to help him.
○ 2. To provide support for the physician's plan of therapy for the client.
○ 3. To show the client support and provide realistic information on the ileostomy.
○ 4. To convince the client that he will not be disfigured and can lead a full life.

A client is transferred to the medical unit from intensive care after suffering a myocardial infarction 5 days ago.

69. The client states to the nurse, "My secretary should be here by now. I don't have time to lie around here and do nothing. I've never had time to relax and I don't plan on starting now." Based on this initial data, the nurse would consider all of the following nursing diagnoses *except*

○ 1. Ineffective Individual Coping.
○ 2. Knowledge Deficit.
○ 3. Powerlessness.
○ 4. Anxiety.

70. The client further states to the nurse, "Please hand me the telephone. I need to check on what's keeping my secretary. She should have been here 30 minutes ago." Which of the following responses by the nurse would be most therapeutic?

○ 1. "Perhaps she's delayed by traffic. Give her 15 more minutes."
○ 2. "You've just had a myocardial infarction. Let's talk about what that means."
○ 3. "You really don't care about the fact that you're sick, do you?"
○ 4. "Do you realize you've just had a myocardial infarction?"

71. Which action by the client would be least indicative of his understanding of his illness and ability to make changes in his life-style?
○ 1. "I told my secretary to bring my airline ticket to me before I'm discharged tomorrow so I don't miss my meeting."
○ 2. "These relaxation tapes sound okay; I'll see if they help me."
○ 3. "No more working 10 hours a day for me unless it's an emergency situation."
○ 4. "I talked with my wife yesterday about working on a new budget together."

72. The client refuses to eat lunch and rudely tells the nurse to get out of his room. What would be the nurse's best response?
○ 1. "I'll leave, but you need to eat."
○ 2. "I'll get you something for your pain."
○ 3. "Your anger doesn't bother me. I'll be back later."
○ 4. "You sound angry. What is upsetting you?"

73. As the client tells the nurse about his painful headaches, the nurse feels sympathy for the client instead of empathy. Which of the following descriptions best defines empathy?
○ 1. To identify with another person's feelings.
○ 2. To have parallel feelings with another person.
○ 3. To feel condolence and agreement with another person.
○ 4. To experience and perceive the feelings of another person.

74. The nurse correctly recognizes that an obstacle to the client's therapy is present when the client is
○ 1. closed off emotionally from others.
○ 2. highly intelligent and manipulative.
○ 3. prone to become dependent on the therapist.
○ 4. unable to tolerate the therapist's suggestions and guidance.

75. The most important distinction for the nurse to make between a psychophysiological disorder, such as ulcerative colitis, and a somatoform disorder, such as conversion reaction, is that a psychophysiological disorder may be
○ 1. consciously selected by the person.
○ 2. fatal to the person if left untreated.
○ 3. relieved when the mental conflict is arrested.
○ 4. handled by the person with a characteristic attitude of indifference.

76. Certain personality characteristics are often attributed to persons with ulcerative colitis. Based on this theory, which of the following traits should the nurse expect to see in a client with this disorder?
○ 1. Self-reliance.
○ 2. Decisiveness.
○ 3. Perfectionism.
○ 4. Ambitiousness.

77. One evening the client directs a stream of profanities at the nurse, then abruptly hangs his head and pleads, "Please forgive me. Something just came over me. Why do I say those things?" The nurse should judge that the client is exhibiting what behavior?
○ 1. Punning.
○ 2. Confabulation.
○ 3. Flight of ideas.
○ 4. Emotional lability.

A client with peptic ulcers takes little responsibility for her self-care.

78. To minimize secondary gains, the nurse includes all of the following measures in this client's care plan except
○ 1. giving the client simple choices.
○ 2. having consistent expectations of what the client can do.
○ 3. spending additional time with the client when she complains of body aches.
○ 4. recognizing the client when she does something for herself.

79. The nurse correctly judges that the dynamics underlying the client's passivity regarding self-care center around
○ 1. the need to be perfect.
○ 2. identity problems.
○ 3. dependency needs.
○ 4. mistrust of the nurse's abilities.

80. Of the following possible effects of chronic invalidism on the client's family, the most detrimental to their interrelationships would most probably be that the illness may make family members feel
○ 1. guilty and dominated.
○ 2. put upon and overworked.
○ 3. superior and self-sufficient.
○ 4. sympathetic and concerned.

The Client With a Terminal Illness

This client, who is dying of AIDS, is admitted to the inpatient psychiatric unit because he attempted suicide. His close friend recently died from AIDS.

81. The client states to the nurse, "What's the use of living? My time is running out." What is the nurse's best response?
- ○ 1. "Let's talk about making some good use of that time."
- ○ 2. "Don't give up. There could be a cure for AIDS tomorrow."
- ○ 3. "You're in a lot of pain. What are you feeling?"
- ○ 4. "Life is precious and worth living."

82. One of the staff members says to the nurse, "Why are we carrying out suicide precautions? It's pointless and a waste of time." The nurse should
- ○ 1. assign the staff member to other clients.
- ○ 2. ask the psychiatric clinical nurse specialist to meet with the staff member.
- ○ 3. agree with the staff member and discontinue suicide precautions.
- ○ 4. call for a multidisciplinary staff meeting.

83. The client begins to talk about his feelings related to his illness and the loss of his friend. He begins to cry. What would be the nurse's best response?
- ○ 1. Give the client some Kleenex and tell him it is okay for him to cry.
- ○ 2. Tell the client to stop crying and that everything will be okay.
- ○ 3. Busy herself with sorting the client's mail.
- ○ 4. Change the subject.

84. One of the client's visitors tells the nurse, "I wish we would have taken that trip to Europe last year. We just kept putting it off and now I'm furious that we didn't go." Which of the following stages of adaptation to dying is the client's friend most likely experiencing?
- ○ 1. Anger.
- ○ 2. Denial.
- ○ 3. Bargaining.
- ○ 4. Depression.

85. The nurse who usually is most effective when caring for the client and helping his friend deal with death is one who
- ○ 1. has contemplated her own death and mortality.
- ○ 2. attends continuing education classes on death and dying.
- ○ 3. can provide caring and physical care while remaining distant emotionally.
- ○ 4. views dying persons as distinct populations of people in need of comfort.

86. Which of the following philosophies would most likely help the client and his family best cope during the final stages of the client's illness?
- ○ 1. Live each day as it comes as fully as possible.
- ○ 2. Relive the pleasant memories of days gone by.
- ○ 3. Expect the worst and be grateful when it does not happen.
- ○ 4. Plan ahead for the remaining good times that will be spent together.

A 13-year-old male client is admitted to the hospital for the third time. His illness is diagnosed as acute lymphatic leukemia. The liaison psychiatric nurse is asked by the team leader to help the nursing staff work more effectively with this terminally ill child and his family.

87. One of the nurses says to the liaison nurse, "Whenever I go to the client's room, I feel that I have to smile and act happy even though I want to cry when I see him." Which of the following responses by the liaison nurse would be best in this situation?
- ○ 1. "Call me when you feel that way. We can talk it over at the time."
- ○ 2. "Try not to show emotion, such as crying. You'll likely upset the client."
- ○ 3. "Keep smiling. The client and his parents need all the support they can get."
- ○ 4. "Tell the client that you feel bad that he is ill. If it seems appropriate, you can cry too."

88. Because the client is increasingly prone to outbursts concerning his treatments, which of the following approaches by the nurse would likely be most helpful in gaining his cooperation?
- ○ 1. Tell him how the treatment can be expected to help him each time.
- ○ 2. Describe the probable effect on his body that missing a treatment would have.
- ○ 3. Ask him to be a good boy and to not make the treatment any harder for himself or the staff.
- ○ 4. Promise to give him a backrub every 2 hours if he does not make a fuss about the treatment.

89. The client suspects that he will not live. However, others talk about only pleasant matters with him and maintain a persistently cheerful facade around him. What will the client most likely feel as a result of such behavior?
- ○ 1. Relief.
- ○ 2. Isolation.
- ○ 3. Hopefulness.
- ○ 4. Independence.

90. Most authorities would agree that the client's parents should be told as much about the client's disease and prognosis as
- ○ 1. they wish to know.
- ○ 2. the nurse believes they can understand.
- ○ 3. the physician can tell them.
- ○ 4. their clergyman thinks is advisable for them to know.

91. The liaison nurse suggests that some recreational diversion be planned for the client. In particular, these recreational activities should
- ○ 1. be of a nonviolent nature.
- ○ 2. stimulate the imagination.
- ○ 3. require some physical effort.
- ○ 4. be geared to early adolescent interests.

92. The client's sister asks the nurse, "Can you check my blood? When my brother got the measles so did I. And I think I have this, too." Appropriate actions by the nurse would include all of the following *except*
- ○ 1. asking the client's doctor to take a sample of the sister's blood.
- ○ 2. explaining that leukemia is not a communicable disease.
- ○ 3. discussing the sister's concern with her parents.
- ○ 4. telling the sister's parents about a group for siblings of clients with terminal illness.

93. When talking with the nurse, the client's 15-year-old brother says, "We used to play pretty rough games together. Maybe some of the bruises he got when I tackled him caused this." What would be the nurse's most helpful response?
- ○ 1. "Don't feel guilty. You didn't cause your brother's illness."
- ○ 2. "I can see you're worried about this. Let's talk about how people get leukemia."
- ○ 3. "Here is some information about leukemia for you to read. You'll see you didn't cause it."
- ○ 4. "Lot's of people worry about things like this. It isn't your fault."

94. During the nursing shift report, the team leader lists tasks and routines completed for the terminally ill client. Which of the following kinds of behavior is the nurse most likely demonstrating when she emphasizes the technical aspects of caring for a dying client?
- ○ 1. Tactful behavior.
- ○ 2. Efficient behavior.
- ○ 3. Objective behavior.
- ○ 4. Defensive behavior.

CORRECT ANSWERS AND RATIONALE

The letters in parentheses following the rationale identify the step of the nursing process (A, D, P, I, E); cognitive level (K, C, T, N); and client need (S, G, L, H). See the Answer Grid for the key.

The Client With Anxiety

1. 1. The best way to ease symptoms caused by hyperventilation is to have the client breathe into a paper bag. Having the client put his head between his knees, giving him low concentrations of oxygen, and having him take deep, slow breaths and exhale normally will not alleviate symptoms of hyperventilation. (I, T, G)

2. 1. Neurotic anxiety is out of proportion to its cause. Normal anxiety decreases lessening with time, is a rational response to an objective danger, and is easily traceable to a consciously recognized stimulus. (D, C, L)

3. 4. Supporting the client in his attempts to discuss feelings, respecting personal space, and reassuring him about his safety promote a therapeutic nurse-client relationship and prevent escalation of anxiety. Confronting dysfunctional coping behaviors or defense mechanisms will most likely be viewed as a threat and increase anxiety. (I, T, L)

4. 3. Reducing anxiety is a primary goal for the client with the nursing diagnosis Anxiety (panic). Problem solving and developing adaptive measures to cope with anxiety are goals to work toward after anxiety is reduced. Reducing secondary gain or benefits, support, and attention that the client receives from others because he is sick is important, but not as immediate as helping the client reduce anxiety. Physical activities such as walking help relieve nervous energy. The client's need to feel secure is also important in maintaining a lower anxiety level or minimizing anxiety. (P, T, L)

5. 3. Making optimistic statements avoids the client's feelings and offers little help when he feels uneasy. Being present, demonstrating competence, and respecting how the client feels are helpful for an anxious client. (I, T, L)

6. 2. The nurse helps the client to recognize that he is feeling anxious by pointing out his behaviors to him. The nurse then attempts to help the client recognize his anxiety and describes his feelings to help him connect behaviors with feelings. Telling the client that she will be back later, will get something to help him feel less anxious, and changing the subject are not helpful to the client. The client wants to avoid or ignore his anxiety, which will not help him to deal with his feelings. (I, T, L)

7. 4. An appropriate long-term goal for the client who withdraws into his room because of severe anxiety is the client who will participate in milieu activities by discharge. Attending group with a staff member is a short-term goal related to the problem of social isolation. Initiating interactions with the nurse when anxious does not relate to social isolation and would be an appropriate outcome to be expected earlier during the client's hospitalization. Expressing two adaptive methods of coping with anxiety does not relate to the problem of social isolation but would be an appropriate outcome related to the nursing diagnosis Ineffective Individual Coping. (P, T, L)

8. 2. The client who is withdrawn due to severe anxiety tends to be self-focused and needs a range of outside interests to help divert attention from himself. (P, N, L)

9. 3. Problem solving and building adaptive coping behaviors to deal with anxiety is the nurse's ultimate goal when working with the client who has an anxiety-related disorder or an unmanageable anxiety level (severe or panic level). Reducing a client's anxiety to a manageable level, helping the client decrease denial and avoidance about feelings, and linking behaviors with feelings are important goals that are more immediate and short-term and assist the client in reaching the ultimate goal of managing his anxiety adaptively. Supportive confrontation is used when the client avoids painful issues that he needs to deal with during his recovery. Supportive confrontation is used by the nurse for a client experiencing mild to moderate anxiety, not during severe and panic levels. (P, T, L)

10. 1. Relaxation exercises would be most helpful because they provide the client with an adaptive mechanism to manage stress and produce a physiological response opposite that of anxiety. The relaxation response decreases pulse rate, blood pressure, and respiration rate. Telling the client to ask his doctor for medication avoids the problem and implies that the client is incapable of managing his behavior adaptively. Recommending the client watch television avoids the client's needs and may not be helpful in dealing with his anxiety. Advising the client to ride the exercise bicycle at bedtime will produce a physiological response opposite to that of relaxation by increasing pulse, respirations, and blood pressure. (I, T, L)

11. 4. Alprazolam (Xanax) is a benzodiazepene used on

a short-term or temporary basis because physical and psychological dependence can occur as well as tolerance. It is used to treat psychological and somatic symptoms of anxiety and as an adjunct to other treatments. (D, C, L)

12. 3. Using alcohol or any central nervous system depressant when taking chlordiazepoxide (Librium) is contraindicated because of additive effects. (P, C, L)

13. 1. Buspirone (Buspar), an anxiolytic, is not administered on an as-needed basis because it has a delayed onset of therapeutic action. Therapeutic effects may be experienced in 7–10 days, with full effects not occurring for 3–4 weeks. This drug is not known to cause physical or psychological dependence. (E, N, L)

14. 3. The client with anxiety may be able to learn to recognize when he is feeling anxious, understand the reasons for his anxiety, and be able to describe situations that preceded his feelings of anxiety. However, he is likely to continue to experience symptoms unless he has also learned to alter his behavior so as to handle his anxiety successfully. (E, N, L)

15. 1. Biperiden hydrochloride (Akineton) is used to treat Parkinson's disease. Propanolol (Inderal) is a beta-adrenergic blocker used to relieve physical symptoms of anxiety. Oxazepam (Serax) and hydroxyzine pamoate (Vistaril) are anti-anxiety agents. (E, N, L)

16. 3. This client is manifesting a severe (+3) level of anxiety. Physically, his muscles are tense and he is wringing his hands. Intellectually, his perceptual capacity is restricted and he is internally focused. Problem solving is difficult. Emotionally, he is using somatization and wants to feel better. (A, N, L)

17. 2. Before the client is discharged from the inpatient unit, he would not be expected to use avoidance when uncomfortable. During the course of hospitalization, the client would have learned to identify uncomfortable feelings, use effective problem-solving methods, and learn adaptive coping behaviors to deal with uncomfortable and anxious feelings. (E, N, L)

The Client With Maladaptive Behavior Patterns

18. 4. The best initial course of action when admitting a client is to observe him to get to know him and to establish baseline information. This is part of the assessment phase of the nursing process. Isolating a client is not recommended unless there is a very good reason for it. An example would be the very active, combative client who is dangerous to himself and others. Interventions such as telling the client that the staff has authority to subdue him or providing the client with rules he must follow threaten the client and likely will promote trouble. (A, T, L)

19. 3. The antisocial client needs to be confronted by his behavior to learn what is expected of him and how to achieve what is expected. An intervention that indicates the client needs a better excuse than he is using to avoid a social function encourages the use of excuses and belittles the client. The client is unlikely to cooperate when he is told that he should try to make a social event successful. Having the client use an activity other than the one he has planned avoids dealing with a problem and is not a good first action. (I, T, L)

20. 1. When the nurse asks the client if he understands why others find him repulsive, the client is likely to feel defensive and defiant. The question is belittling, and a natural tendency is to counterattack the threat to the self-image. Because the person with an antisocial personality is egocentric and unconcerned about his effect on others, he is unlikely to feel ashamed, remorseful, or embarrassed. (E, N, L)

21. 2. Society tends to stigmatize those who deviate from the dominant value system. Therefore, the client's behavior is a source of anxiety because it is alien to the staffs' and other clients' value systems. (E, N, L)

22. 1. This client is trying to provoke the nurse into a reaction when he taunts him. Behavior that is reinforced will continue. Behavior that is not reinforced tends to become extinguished. Hence, ignoring the client's comment is the best course of action. The other responses would tend to reinforce the client's behavior. (I, T, L)

23. 2. In this situation it is least helpful to respond to the client's comment by moralizing, such as by saying that he could go to jail for making these threats. It is better to validate and clarify the meaning of the client's message. Such comments give feedback to the client and promote self-evaluation. (I, T, L)

24. 1. Potential for violence directed at others is evidenced by the client who threatens others, acts on impulse, and is aggressive toward others. (D, T, L)

25. 4. When this client says that he plans to make a bomb threat to the hospital, the possible results are too serious to risk bargaining with the client. The best course of action, and the one most likely to promote trust, is to tell the client honestly what must be done about the bomb threat. It is possible that the client is also asking to be stopped and that he is indirectly pleading for help. (I, T, L)

26. 1. The most basic and important idea to convey to the client is that, as a person, he is accepted although his behavior may not be. (P, T, L)

27. 3. Behavior modification can be helpful to the client when positive reinforcements are used to reinforce desired behaviors. Realistic short term goals are important as first steps to changing long lasting maladaptive patterns of behavior. (P, T, L)

28. 1. The best approach here is to capitalize on the client's strengths and his responsibilities in a given situation. Clients such as this one are skillful at placing the blame or focus on others. The interaction should be present-oriented and have a positive focus. (I, T, L)

29. 2. Therapy is usually most effective when the client is helped to understand why he behaves as he does. The client is not likely to accept the therapist's insight until he understands himself. Explaining the client's behavior to him is usually not beneficial. Documenting the client's behavior so that the physician can deal with a problem delegates a nursing responsibility to someone else. Bringing the client's mother into therapy sessions at this time is likely to focus on someone other than the client. (I, T, L)

30. 1. Intimacy is a developmental task of early adulthood. It is mastered after a sense of identity is established, normally during adolescence. A sense of integrity is a developmental task of the elderly. A sense of autonomy is a developmental task of early childhood. A sense of productivity, or generativity, is a developmental task of middle adulthood. (D, C, L)

31. 1. The term "insight" best describes the client's self-awareness and self-understanding. Rapport is the manner in which the client and nurse perceive each other and relate to each other; it is a positive feeling. Lucidity is the state of being intelligible or clearly understood by others. Cathexis refers to an emotional investment in a person, object, or idea. (D, C, L)

32. 3. Various behaviors, including a slowing of progress, may surface during the final phases of the relationship between the client and nurse. The nurse needs to redirect the client to the issues of termination and help him deal with the feelings associated with termination. (E, N, L)

33. 2. The client with an antisocial personality disorder does not feel guilt, sorrow, or remorse for his actions. Immediate gratification without regard for the rights of others and hasty decisions often result because of his inability to tolerate frustration. (E, N, L)

The Client With Problems Expressing Anger

34. 3. Describing acceptable behavior to the client focuses on the immediate problem. Asking the client to explain what happened is a therapeutic statement likely to elicit assessment data; however, it is less focused on the client's immediate problem. Threatening statements do not elicit further information and are not therapeutic. (I, T, L)

35. 3. The nurse clearly addresses behavioral expectations and provides alternatives for the client. Isolating the client and making others responsible for the client's behavior are inappropriate, because they do not include the client in managing his behavior. Medication may be helpful but does not involve the client in responsibility for his behavior. (I, T, L)

36. 1. The nurse acknowledges and labels the client's emotion and acknowledges his appropriate behavior. Recognizing the client's physiological arousal, the nurse suggests an activity and stays with him. Setting limits on the client's language does not acknowledge his control. Offering the client medication suggests that he cannot control his behavior. (I, T, L)

37. 4. Verbalizing feelings, especially feelings of anger, in an appropriate manner is an adaptive method of coping and reduces the chance of the client acting out his feelings toward others. Acknowledging feelings of anger and describing situations that precipitate angry feelings are important outcomes in helping the client reach his goal of appropriately verbalizing his feelings but are not ends in themselves. Asking the client to list how he has handled anger in the past is helpful if the nurse discusses coping methods with the client. Based on this client's history, this would not be helpful, because the nurse and client are aware of the client's aggression toward others. (P, T, L)

38. 2. Identifying individuals with whom the client is angry is not important to the overall plan. Helping the client recognize anger, identifying alternative ways to express anger, and practicing the expression of anger are all steps in the process of teaching the client to recognize and respond appropriately to anger. (P, T, L)

39. 3. Childhood abuse, alcohol abuse, and learning disabilities are all associated with angry, impulsive behavior. A family history of bipolar disorder predisposes the client to that illness but is not specifically associated with difficulty in coping with anger. (A, C, L)

40. 4. This response acknowledges the client's feelings and helps the group accept a new member. The nurse's response should acknowledge the client's fear and address the purpose of the group but should not provide false reassurance. (I, T, L)

41. 1. Both denial of anger with passive, unassertive behavior and the aggressive expression of anger are maladaptive behavior patterns. Gender-based stereotypes of assertive behavior are not conducive to mental health. Options 3 and 4 are unwarranted assumptions based on inadequate data. (E, N, L)

42. 3. The nurse acknowledges the client's concern and provides an opportunity to review his progress and to prepare for the work situation. Option 1 is therapeutic but does not review the client's progress or prepare him for the work situation. Options 2 and 4 provide false reassurance. (I, T, L)

43. 2. Refusing to discuss the client's concerns is inappropriate. It is important to help the client recognize that anger is a normal emotion and to invite the client to talk about her concern about the label passive-aggressive. (I, T, L)

44. 3. By requesting that her roommate respect her rights, the client is asserting herself. Arriving late is often passive resistance; asking the nurse to call is dependent behavior. Asking the doctor is more assertive, but the client relies on the nurse's direction to do so. (E, N, L)

45. 2. Blood pressure, as well as respiratory rate and muscle tension, increase in anger due to the autonomic nervous system response to epinephrine secretion. Peristalsis decreases. (A, C, L)

46. 2. Fear of retaliation, guilt, and decreased self-esteem are common psychological responses to feelings of anger. Although anger may provide an initial feeling of strength and invulnerability, this is rarely a sustained response. (E, N, L)

47. 3. Anger has many sources and functions. The nurse who personalizes the anger misses an opportunity to understand its meaning to the client. Anger is an adaptive response in many situations and serves to energize the client. To understand the use of anger, the nurse must discuss it with the client. Anger also causes anxiety and can serve to protect the client from closeness. (D, C, L)

48. 4. Violent behavior is more likely when there is a demand for high activity, when there is inadequate staffing, and when the staff feels hopeless about a client. However, the client's past history of violent behavior is the most accurate predictive factor. (A, T, L)

49. 1. Sarcasm is frequently used to express anger indirectly. Refusing medication and shouting are both more direct expressions of angry, negative feelings. Assuming responsibility for a unit activity is a positive, assertive action. (E, N, L)

The Client With Family Abuse and Violence

50. 2. The safety of the client and her children is the immediate concern. If there is immediate danger, action must be taken to protect them. The level of abuse in the family, the client's plans, and the available resources are also important considerations in developing a treatment plan but are not the most important concerns. (A, N, L)

51. 3. Impermeable boundaries, imbalanced power ratio, and dysfunctional feeling tone are all common in abusive families. However, the traditional and rigid gender roles described by the client are examples of role stereotyping. (D, N, L)

52. 1. The nurse would provide the client with resources or support systems to turn to when the next battering incident occurs. It is inappropriate to advise the client to leave her husband. The client should not be pushed or coerced into leaving her husband until she is ready. Telling the client not to do anything to upset her husband and asking her what she could do to deescalate the situation at home places blame for the violence on the client. (I, T, L)

53. 1. Lack of empathy characterizes relationships in abusive families. It is more likely that the relationship is built around the abuser's need for power and control. A history of family violence and low self-esteem are common among abusers. The idea that only poorly educated, poorly employed men are abusive is a myth. Most alcohol abusers batter their partners whether or not they are drinking at the time. (D, N, L)

54. 4. Sharing feelings of frustration with the client is inappropriate. The nurse's feelings of frustration are not unusual, and she needs to discuss these feelings with a clinical supervisor to better understand and deal with them. (P, T, L)

55. 2. Group therapy with women with similar problems may help the client reduce her isolation and sense of shame. The idea that abuse victims do not want to change is inaccurate and leads to feelings of hopelessness among professionals. Contacting other people about the client and family without the client's consent violates confidentiality. (I, T, L)

56. 1. Self-blame, substance abuse, and suicidal thoughts and attempts are possible dysfunctional coping methods used by abuse victims. The nurse would least likely find assertiveness in the victim. The victim is usually compliant with the spouse and feels guilt, shame, and some responsibility for the battering. (A, C, L)

57. 3. The data here best support the nursing diagnosis of powerlessness related to abusive husband, as evidenced by inability to make decisions. (D, T, L)

58. 4. While any event in a family can contribute to an abusive episode, the birthday party is less important to treatment planning than the husband's promotion, a potential major stressor. His refusal of treatment and the client's coping skills are both very important in treatment planning. (P, N, L)

59. 4. It is important that the nurse address the family problem and include the client in making decisions about her daughter. Allowing the child to remain at home and having someone else at home to meet her ignores the basic family problem. Asking the client to talk to her daughter is appropriate but is not a sufficient intervention in this situation. (I, T, L)

60. 2. The nurse needs more information about the client's decision before deciding what intervention is most appropriate. Judgmental responses could make it difficult for the client to return for treatment should she want to do so. (I, T, L)

61. 1. Defending the school nurse puts the client's mother on the defensive and stifles communication. All the other responses address, either directly or indirectly, the mother's concerns and ask for her view of the situation. This approach is important in building a relationship with the family. (I, T, L)

62. 4. A strong defensive reaction by parents to an appropriate concern by a teacher or other professional may indicate family problems. A caring, supportive relationship among family members and infrequent episodes of abuse during a time of intense family stress are not characteristic of abusive families. (E, N, L)

The Client With a Psychophysiological Disorder

63. 3. When this client returns to the hospital for the fourth time in 9 months, it is best for the nurse to acknowledge his readmission and give him an opportunity to express his feelings. Telling the client it is nice to see him and asking him if he had become lonesome serve little purpose except as social comments. Telling the client that she thought she had seen the last of him and asking him what he is doing back in the hospital could be interpreted as being rude and challenging. The nurse is making an assumption when she states that the client will not need to be oriented to the hospital because of previous admissions. (I, T, L)

64. 4. Using people for therapeutic interventions is usually more helpful than manipulating the environment, as is the case when a client becomes upset when he hears meal trays approaching. Tension is less likely to develop when a client is interpersonally involved than when the time element in relation to eating has been altered. (P, T, L)

65. 1. Activity within physical limits is desirable. However, the emphasis of treatment lies in providing rest and freedom from emotional stress to the greatest extent possible for a client suffering with a psychophysiological disorder. This goal is best met when activities that promote rest and relaxation are chosen for the client. The goal is less well met by activities that promote improvement of social skills, insight and self-awareness, and manual rather than intellectual dexterity. (D, T, L)

66. 2. Here, when the client seems to be questioning his physician's goals, it is best for the nurse to present an open statement by repeating part of what the client said and asking him what he means by what he said. This technique helps the client express his feelings. It is less therapeutic to tell the client that he sounds upset, that he is being hard on his physician, or that his remark apparently has something to do with the surgery he is about to undergo. (I, T, L)

67. 2. When this client has hostile outbursts, it is best for the nurse to help him express his feelings. This serves as a release valve for the client. Other actions by the nurse are less therapeutic than helping the client express himself. (I, T, L)

68. 3. Preoperative visits and talks with clients who have made successful adjustments to ileostomies are helpful and may tend to make the client less fearful of the operation and its consequences. (D, C, L)

69. 3. The nurse would consider the diagnoses Ineffective Individual Coping, Knowledge Deficit, and Anxiety when working with a client with a psychophysiological disorder. Powerlessness would not be appropriate, because the client projects an image of a person who works hard, does not take time to relax, and is usually in charge and productive. (A, N, L)

70. 2. The nurse presents reality to the client about his condition to help decrease his denial about his physical status. The nurse conveys that she is concerned about him and willing to help him understand his illness. Stating that the secretary could be delayed by traffic is not appropriate and shows poor judgment. Options 3 and 4 are responses that are belittling to the client, may cause the client to become defensive, and convey the nurse's frustration. (I, T, L)

71. 1. Leaving the hospital and immediately flying to a meeting indicates poor judgment by the client and little understanding of what he needs to change regarding his life-style. Expressing a willingness to try relaxation tapes, not working 10 hours a day, and working on a new budget with his wife shows that the client understands some of the changes he needs to make to decrease his stress and lead a more healthy life-style. (E, N, L)

72. 4. The best response is one that directly expresses the nurse's observations to the client and offers the client the opportunity to openly vent and talk about her feelings or concerns to decrease somatization or the need to express feelings through physical symptoms. Leaving, offering to provide pain medication, and stating that anger does not bother the nurse ignores the client's needs and does not help the client. (I, T, L)

73. 4. Empathy refers to the ability to feel as another

person feels and to be able to understand and respond to the feelings. Having parallel feelings with another person and feeling condolence and agreement with another person describe sympathy more accurately than empathy. Identifying with another person's feelings is only part of the process of empathizing with another person. (D, C, L)

74. 1. Clients with psychophysiological disorders tend to close themselves off emotionally from others and do not reveal their feelings easily. These characteristics are often an obstacle in therapy. These clients may expect the therapist to help them without having to disclose feelings. (E, T, L)

75. 2. Psychophysiological disorders, if untreated, may prove fatal. Persons with psychophysiological disorders do not select the physical ailment they suffer from, find relief from physical symptoms when a mental conflict is arrested, or handle the symptoms with an attitude of indifference. (D, C, L)

76. 3. Persons with ulcerative colitis commonly have a personality described as obsessive-compulsive. Behaviors such as perfectionism, conformity, rigidity, being emotionally on guard, and obstinacy are typical. (A, C, L)

77. 4. This client directs profanities at the nurse and then is sorry for his behavior. This type of behavior illustrates emotional lability, which is a readily changeable or unstable emotional affect. Punning is using a word when it can have two or more meanings, or a play on words. Confabulation involves replacing memory loss by fantasy to hide confusion; it is unconscious behavior. Flight of ideas refers to a rapid succession of verbal expressions that jump from one topic to another and are only superficially related. (D, T, L)

78. 3. The nurse would minimize the time she spends with the client when she engages in complaining behavior to decrease somatization and the secondary gain of getting attention. Giving the client simple choices encourages independent decision-making and responsibility for herself. Being consistent in expectations of the client decreases manipulation of the nurse. Giving recognition when the client does something for herself rewards the client for appropriate, responsible behavior. (I, T, L)

79. 3. Clients with peptic ulcers are thought to be dependent or overly independent and ambitious, depending on factors in the client's life. Perfectionism, identity problems, and mistrust of staff's abilities are not specific to clients with peptic ulcers. (D, N, L)

80. 1. When a family member has been chronically ill, feelings of guilt and domination tend to cause the greatest amount of intrapsychic conflict in the family's interrelationships. These feelings are not easy to express and communicate openly. Hence, feelings of guilt and domination tend to have the most negative and destructive effect on interrelationships in terms of behavioral symptoms. (D, C, L)

The Client With a Terminal Illness

81. 3. The nurse recognizes the client's pain, hopelessness, and sense of loss related to his condition and the loss of his friend and encourages him to express his feelings. Giving the client permission to talk about his feelings of sadness, loss, and hopelessness and listening to him is an important nursing intervention for the dying client. "Let's talk about making good use of the time you have left," "Don't give up," and "Life is worth living" are statements that ignore the client's needs and inhibit his expression of feelings. (I, T, L)

82. 4. The nurse would call for a multidisciplinary staff meeting because she recognizes the need for staff members to share their feelings of anger, frustration, and grief. Because nurses focus on saving human lives, any feelings of hopelessness regarding a dying client can interfere with the client's care and management. Assigning the staff member to other clients and calling the clinical nurse specialist to deal with the staff member ignores the entire staff's needs and does nothing to immediately help the situation. The psychiatric clinical nurse specialist would be included in the staff meeting to help the entire staff deal with their feelings. Agreeing with the staff member and discontinuing suicide precautions is highly inappropriate. (I, T, L)

83. 1. The nurse would give the client a facial tissue and tell him it's okay to cry to convey her acceptance and empathy. The client needs understanding and encouragement to talk about his feelings. He needs to know that it is natural and normal to have tremendous feelings of loss and sadness and needs the nurse to help him cope with intense feelings. Telling the client to stop crying, busying oneself in the client's room, and changing the subject are not helpful to the client because they ignore his needs and inhibit the expression of emotion. (I, T, L)

84. 1. The client's friend appears to be experiencing anger in this situation, much of which stems from feelings of guilt. During the stage of denial, the friend is more likely to deny the client's diagnosis and prognosis. During the stage of bargaining, the friend tends to offer to do certain things in exchange for more time before the client dies. In the stage of depression, the friend is likely to make few or no comments and act dejected. (D, T, L)

85. 1. It is best to examine one's own feelings about

death and dying before caring for the terminally ill client. Many authorities consider self-examination of one's own finiteness essential before one can successfully meet the needs of a dying client. (E, N, L)

86. 1. It is best when supporting the friend or family of a terminally ill client to focus on the present, the "here and now." This can be accomplished by living each day at a time to its fullest. Friends and families also want to know what to expect and want someone to listen to them as they express grief over death. (D, C, L)

87. 4. Clients very often sense a nurse's feelings. Therefore, when the nurse becomes emotionally upset while caring for the terminally ill child, it is best for her to share her emotions with the child when it seems appropriate. It is also acceptable to cry. Trying not to show emotion and trying to smile regardless of how one feels are inappropriate responses. It is of little help to the client or the nurse who is upset if the nurse waits until a later time when she can speak to someone about the situation. (I, T, L)

88. 1. Here, the best course of action when the client has outbursts concerning his treatments is to tell him how the treatment can be expected to help him. Describing the effect on his body if he misses a treatment is a negative approach and may be threatening to the client. The client is likely to feel angry if told to be a "good boy" during treatments. Offering to give the client a backrub if he does not fuss does not give him the information to which he is entitled. (I, T, L)

89. 2. Children are aware of and show anxieties about death at an earlier age than was once thought, and they recognize false cheerfulness. They tend to experience isolation and loneliness when those around them are trying to hide or mask the truth. They are then left to face the realities of death alone. (D, N, L)

90. 1. Most authorities recommend that the parents of an ill child, including a child who is terminally ill, should be told as much as they wish to know. The nurse can determine this by talking with the parents and child. (P, C, L)

91. 4. Recreational activities selected for this 13-year-old client should be geared to the client's interests. Activities that are physical in nature are likely to be too strenuous for a terminally ill child. Activities of a nonviolent nature and those that stimulate the child's imagination are satisfactory, but the first criterion should be that the activity be appropriate for the client's age level. (P, C, L)

92. 1. Taking a blood sample is an unnecessary, invasive procedure that would not directly address the child's fear. Providing an age-appropriate explanation and alerting the parents to the sibling's concern and the resources available to assist siblings with the terminal illness are all appropriate interventions. (I, T, L)

93. 2. A response that acknowledges the brother's concern and provides him with information is most helpful. Providing reassurance without addressing the expressed concern and providing information without acknowledging the expressed concern are not as helpful as acknowledgment plus information. (I, T, L)

94. 4. The nurse caring for a terminally ill client who reports only tasks and routines completed for the client is probably behaving defensively. It is very likely that this nurse has not come to grips with death and dying. (A, T, L)

NURSING CARE OF CLIENTS WITH PSYCHOSOCIAL HEALTH PROBLEMS

TEST 4: Anxiety, Anger, Abuse, Terminal Illness

Directions: Use this answer grid to determine areas of strength or need for further study.

NURSING PROCESS

A = Assessment
D = Analysis, nursing diagnosis
P = Planning
I = Implementation
E = Evaluation

COGNITIVE LEVEL

K = Knowledge
C = Comprehension
T = Application
N = Analysis

CLIENT NEEDS

S = Safe, effective care environment
G = Physiological integrity
L = Psychosocial integrity
H = Health promotion/maintenance

		Nursing Process					Cognitive Level				Client Needs			
Question #	Answer #	A	D	P	I	E	K	C	T	N	S	G	L	H
1	1				I				T			G		
2	1		D					C					L	
3	4				I				T				L	
4	3			P					T				L	
5	3				I				T				L	
6	2				I				T				L	
7	4			P					T				L	
8	2			P						N			L	
9	3			P					T				L	
10	1				I				T				L	
11	4		D					C					L	
12	3			P				C					L	
13	1					E				N			L	
14	3					E				N			L	
15	1					E				N			L	
16	3	A								N			L	
17	2					E				N			L	
18	4	A							T				L	
19	3				I				T				L	
20	1					E				N			L	
21	2					E				N			L	
22	1				I				T				L	
23	2				I				T				L	

ANSWER GRID: 1

NURSING PROCESS

A = Assessment
D = Analysis, nursing diagnosis
P = Planning
I = Implementation
E = Evaluation

COGNITIVE LEVEL

K = Knowledge
C = Comprehension
T = Application
N = Analysis

CLIENT NEEDS

S = Safe, effective care environment
G = Physiological integrity
L = Psychosocial integrity
H = Health promotion/maintenance

		Nursing Process					Cognitive Level				Client Needs			
Question #	Answer #	A	D	P	I	E	K	C	T	N	S	G	L	H
24	1		D						T				L	
25	4				I				T				L	
26	1			P					T				L	
27	3			P					T				L	
28	1				I				T				L	
29	2				I				T				L	
30	1		D					C					L	
31	1		D					C					L	
32	3					E				N			L	
33	2					E				N			L	
34	3				I				T				L	
35	3				I				T				L	
36	1				I				T				L	
37	4			P					T				L	
38	2			P					T				L	
39	3	A						C					L	
40	4				I				T				L	
41	1					E				N			L	
42	3				I				T				L	
43	2				I				T				L	
44	3					E				N			L	
45	2	A						C					L	
46	2					E				N			L	
47	3		D					C					L	
48	4	A							T				L	
49	1					E				N			L	
50	2	A								N			L	
51	3		D							N			L	
52	1				I				T				L	

ANSWER GRID: 2

Nursing Process	**Cognitive Level**	**Client Needs**
A = Assessment	K = Knowledge	S = Safe, effective care environment
D = Analysis, nursing diagnosis	C = Comprehension	G = Physiological integrity
P = Planning	T = Application	L = Psychosocial integrity
I = Implementation	N = Analysis	H = Health promotion/maintenance
E = Evaluation		

		Nursing Process					Cognitive Level				Client Needs			
Question #	Answer #	A	D	P	I	E	K	C	T	N	S	G	L	H
53	1		D							N			L	
54	4			P					T				L	
55	2				I				T				L	
56	1	A						C					L	
57	3		D						T				L	
58	4			P						N			L	
59	4				I				T				L	
60	2				I				T				L	
61	1				I				T				L	
62	4					E				N			L	
63	3				I				T				L	
64	4			P					T				L	
65	1		D						T				L	
66	2				I				T				L	
67	2				I				T				L	
68	3		D					C					L	
69	3	A								N			L	
70	2				I				T				L	
71	1					E				N			L	
72	4				I				T				L	
73	4		D					C					L	
74	1					E			T				L	
75	2		D					C					L	
76	3	A						C					L	
77	4		D						T				L	
78	3				I				T				L	
79	3		D							N			L	
80	1		D					C					L	
81	3				I				T				L	

ANSWER GRID: 3

NURSING PROCESS

A = Assessment
D = Analysis, nursing diagnosis
P = Planning
I = Implementation
E = Evaluation

COGNITIVE LEVEL

K = Knowledge
C = Comprehension
T = Application
N = Analysis

CLIENT NEEDS

S = Safe, effective care environment
G = Physiological integrity
L = Psychosocial integrity
H = Health promotion/maintenance

		Nursing Process					Cognitive Level				Client Needs			
Question #	Answer #	A	D	P	I	E	K	C	T	N	S	G	L	H
82	4				I				T				L	
83	1				I				T				L	
84	1		D						T				L	
85	1					E				N			L	
86	1		D					C					L	
87	4				I				T				L	
88	1				I				T				L	
89	2		D							N			L	
90	1			P				C					L	
91	4			P				C					L	
92	1				I				T				L	
93	2				I				T				L	
94	4	A							T				L	
Number Correct														
Number Possible	94	10	19	14	35	16	0	17	53	24	0	1	93	0
Percentage Correct														

Score Calculation:

To determine your **Percentage Correct**, divide the **Number Correct** by the **Number Possible.**

BIBLIOGRAPHY

American Psychiatric Association (1987). *Diagnostic and statistical manual of mental disorders* (3rd ed.). Washington, DC: Author.

Arnold, E., & Boggs, K. (1989). *Interpersonal relationships: professional communication skills for nurses.* Philadelphia: WB Saunders.

Baumann, A., Johnston, N., & Antai-Ontong, D. (1990). *Decision making in psychiatric and psychological nursing.* St. Louis: Mosby Yearbook.

Beck, C., Rawlins, R., & Williams, S. (1988). *Mental health-psychiatric nursing: A holistic life-cycle approach.* St. Louis: Mosby-Times Mirror.

Burgess, A.W. (1990). *Psychiatric nursing in the hospital and the community* (5th ed.). Norwalk, CT: Appleton and Lange.

Doenges, M., Townsend, M., & Moorhouse, M.F. (1989). *Psychiatric care plans: Guidelines for client care.* Philadelphia: F.A. Davis.

Fawcett, C. (1993). *Family psychiatric nursing.* St. Louis: Mosby Yearbook.

Gary, F., & Kavanagh, C.K. (1991). *Psychiatric mental health nursing.* Philadelphia: J.B. Lippincott.

Gordon, M. (1991). *Manual of nursing diagnosis: 1991–1992.* St. Louis: Mosby Yearbook.

Haber, J., Hoskins, P.P., Leach, A.M., & Sideleau, B.V. (1987). *Comprehensive psychiatric nursing.* New York: McGraw-Hill.

Haber, J., McMahon, A.L., Price-Hoskins, P., & Sideleau, B.F. (1992). *Comprehensive psychiatric nursing.* (4th ed.) St. Louis: Mosby Yearbook.

Hamdy, R.C., Turnbull, J., Lancaster, M., & Norman, L. (1990). *Alzheimer's Disease: A handbook for caregivers.* St. Louis: Mosby Yearbook.

Janosik, E., & Davies, J. (1989). *Psychiatric mental health nursing* (2nd ed.). Boston: Jones & Bartlett.

Johnson, B. (1993). *Psychiatric-mental health nursing: Adaptation and growth* (3rd ed.). Philadelphia: J.B. Lippincott.

Keltner, N., Schweke, L., & Bostrom, C. (1991). *Psychiatric nursing: A psychotherapeutic management approach.* St. Louis: C.V. Mosby.

Kinney, J. (1991). *Clinical manual of substance abuse.* St. Louis: Mosby Yearbook.

Lewis, S., Grainger, R.D., McDowell, W.A., Gregory, R.J., & Messner, R.L. (1989). *Manual of Psychosocial Nursing Interventions: Promoting Mental Health in Medical-Surgical Settings.* Philadelphia: W.B. Saunders.

McFarland, G.K., & Thomas, M.D. (1991). *Psychiatric-mental health nursing: Application of the nursing process.* Philadelphia: J.B. Lippincott.

McFarland, G.K., Wasli, E., & Genety, E. (1992). *Nursing diagnosis and process in psychiatric-mental health nursing* (2nd ed.). Philadelphia: J.B. Lippincott.

Servonsky, J., & Opas, S.R. (1987). *Nursing management of children.* Boston: Jones & Bartlett.

Shives, L.R. (1990). *Basic concepts of psychiatric-mental health nursing, 2/e.* Philadelphia: J.B. Lippincott.

Stuart, G., & Sundeen, S. (1991). *Principles and practice of psychiatric nursing* (4th ed.). St. Louis: C.V. Mosby.

Townsend, M.C. (1990). *Drug guide for psychiatric nursing.* Philadelphia: F.A. Davis.

Townsend, M.C. (1991). *Nursing diagnoses in psychiatric nursing: A pocket guide for care plan construction* (2nd ed.). Philadelphia: F.A. Davis.

Varcarolis, E. (1990). *Foundations of Psychiatric-mental health nursing.* Philadelphia: W.B. Saunders.

West, P., & Evans, C.L. (1992). *Psychiatric and mental health nursing with children and adolescents.* Gaithersburg: Aspen Publishers.

Wilson, H., & Kneisl, C. (1989). *Psychiatric nursing.* Menlo Park, CA: Addison-Wesley.

Part II

The Nursing Care of the Childbearing Family and Their Neonate

Antepartum Care

Test 1

The Preconception Client
The Pregnant Client Receiving Prenatal Care
The Pregnant Client in Childbirth Preparation Classes
The Pregnant Client With Risk Factors
Correct Answers and Rationale

Select the one best answer and indicate your choice by filling in the circle in front of the option.

The Preconception Client

A 20-year-old nulligravida visits a family planning clinic. She states that she and her boyfriend are planning their wedding and want to plan the spacing of their children.

1. Before beginning to counsel the client about sexuality, the nurse should first
- ○ 1. obtain a sexual history from the client in a private setting.
- ○ 2. have the client undergo a complete physical examination.
- ○ 3. suggest that the client's sexual partner attend the counseling sessions.
- ○ 4. discuss reproductive system anatomy and physiology with the client.

2. Most authorities recommend that the nurse can best prepare to counsel clients concerning sexuality when the nurse first has
- ○ 1. personal experience in a sexual relationship.
- ○ 2. reviewed the extensive literature on human sexuality.
- ○ 3. developed an awareness of his or her own feelings, values, and attitudes related to sexuality.
- ○ 4. completed a formal educational program for preparation as a clinical specialist in sexual counseling.

3. The nurse formulates a nursing diagnosis of Knowledge Deficit related to ovulation and fertility management due to misinformation. Which of the following statements related to ovulation should be included in the client's teaching plan?
- ○ 1. Ovulation only occurs during the menstrual period, so precautions need to be taken only during this period.
- ○ 2. Women who practice natural methods of family planning usually do not know when they have ovulated.
- ○ 3. Most women can tell they have ovulated by the severe pain that accompanies ovulation.
- ○ 4. Most women ovulate about 2 weeks before the beginning of the next menstrual period.

4. Following a discussion about conception and fertilization, the client asks the nurse, "How long does it take for sperm to reach an ovum?" What is the nurse's best response?
- ○ 1. "Under ideal conditions, sperm can reach the ovum in 1 to 5 minutes."
- ○ 2. "Millions of sperm reach the ovum within an hour."
- ○ 3. "Thousands of sperm enter the fallopian tube within 30 minutes."
- ○ 4. "Only one sperm will actually fertilize the ovum, and this usually takes 48 hours."

5. The client asks the nurse, "Why do people who use natural methods to prevent pregnancy have a high failure rate?" The nurse's best response is based on the knowledge that natural methods
- ○ 1. are very frustrating for both partners.
- ○ 2. require extensive record keeping.
- ○ 3. can be 100% effective if done correctly.
- ○ 4. depend on knowing when ovulation occurs.

6. The nurse instructs the client about oral contraceptive agents. Following instruction, the nurse knows that the client has understood the instructions from what client statement?
- ○ 1. "Oral contraceptives need to be used with spermacides during the first year of use."
- ○ 2. "Only a few minor side effects are associated with oral contraceptives."
- ○ 3. "Oral contraceptives work by inhibiting ovulation and changing the consistency of cervical mucous."
- ○ 4. "Persons with a history of thromboembolic disease can use oral contraceptives if they are carefully monitored."

A 34-year-old multigravida is seen in the family planning clinic following the delivery of her fourth child 6 months ago.

7. The client says that her husband objects to using "rubbers" (condoms) for contraception. What is the nurse's best response?
- ○ 1. "Most men think that it's the female who doesn't like condoms."
- ○ 2. "Why do you think he objects?"
- ○ 3. "A lot of men don't like to use condoms."
- ○ 4. "Skin condoms, rather than latex, can prevent sexually transmitted diseases."

8. The client inquires about using a diaphragm for contraception. In planning the teaching for this client, the nurse should include which of the following?
- ○ 1. The diaphragm should be removed once every 48 hours.
- ○ 2. Most women who use diaphragms develop symptoms of toxic shock syndrome.
- ○ 3. A diaphragm can be obtained without a prescription.
- ○ 4. The diaphragm should be left in for 6–8 hours after intercourse.

9. The client asks the nurse "What do men do if they want to be sterilized?" The nurse should respond that a commonly used procedure involves clamping or cutting the
- ○ 1. epididymis.
- ○ 2. seminal vesicles.
- ○ 3. ejaculatory duct.
- ○ 4. ductus deferens.

10. Following a discussion about various sexual myths with the client, the nurse realizes that the client needs further instruction when she says
- ○ 1. "Alcohol acts as a depressant for sex."
- ○ 2. "Sexual intercourse should be avoided during menstruation."
- ○ 3. "Masturbation can be used to achieve orgasm."
- ○ 4. "Having an orgasm is not a necessary part of a satisfactory sexual experience."

11. The nurse discusses sexual arousal and orgasm with the client. The nurse asks the client which *primary* anatomic structure in the female is involved in sexual arousal and orgasm. The nurse's teaching will be considered effective if the client's answer is the
- ○ 1. vagina.
- ○ 2. clitoris.
- ○ 3. mons pubis.
- ○ 4. labia minora.

The nurse is conducting a 2-hour class for a group of married couples on the topic of human sexuality.

12. In preparing for the presentation, the nurse plans to include a discussion of why foreplay during intercourse is important. Which of the following should be included in the teaching plan? In addition to arousing the sexual urge, foreplay helps to
- ○ 1. relax the vaginal orifice.
- ○ 2. increase vaginal secretions.
- ○ 3. delay premature clitoral orgasm.
- ○ 4. prevent early ejaculation in the male.

13. One of the class participants asks several questions about becoming pregnant. She says "How do sperm ever manage to reach the ovum?" The nurse's best response is that "Sperm are propelled in the female primarily by
- ○ 1. cilia in the female reproductive tract."
- ○ 2. movement of the sperm's tail-like portion."
- ○ 3. peristalsis-like contractions in the cervix and uterus."
- ○ 4. gravity and the force generated by ejaculation."

14. One of the participants says that her sister-in-law is unable to become pregnant. The nurse explains that one reason for the diagnosis of infertility in a female is
- ○ 1. absence of an ovary.
- ○ 2. dilated hymenal ring.
- ○ 3. blocked fallopian tubes.
- ○ 4. obstructed Bartholin's gland duct.

15. After learning about fertilization, one of the participants asks where it occurs in the body. The nurse responds correctly that fertilization of the ovum normally occurs in the
- ○ 1. ovary.
- ○ 2. uterus.
- ○ 3. corpus luteum.
- ○ 4. fallopian tube.

A 21-year-old client visits the obstetrician's office because she "thinks I might be pregnant." She has missed one menstrual period.

16. The client tells the nurse that she wants to find out if she is pregnant. A radioimmunoassay test is performed. The nurse instructs the client that this pregnancy test is
- ○ 1. highly accurate within 7 days after conception.
- ○ 2. identical to a home pregnancy test.
- ○ 3. a positive sign of pregnancy.
- ○ 4. based on an antigen-antibody reaction.

17. After instructing the client about the radioimmunoassay test, the nurse knows that the client understands the instructions when she says which hormone is used for this test?

○ 1. Estrogen.
○ 2. Luteinizing hormone.
○ 3. Follicle-stimulating hormone.
○ 4. Human chorionic gonadotrophin.

18. The client reports that she has had urinary frequency, breast tenderness, and occasional nausea. The nurse determines that the client may be experiencing signs of pregnancy considered
○ 1. presumptive.
○ 2. probable.
○ 3. positive.
○ 4. pervasive.

19. While waiting for the results of the pregnancy test, the client says that she has heard that women still die during childbirth from hemorrhage. What is the nurse's best response?
○ 1. Tell the client not to worry about that right now.
○ 2. Instruct the client that maternal deaths do not occur as a result of modern technology.
○ 3. Ask the client why she would ask about death when she isn't certain she is pregnant.
○ 4. Gather additional data related to the client's concerns about pregnancy and delivery.

20. The client tells the nurse that she is a junior in college and plans to marry her boyfriend in a year. She says, "A baby right now will sure affect us financially. Neither one of us wants to quit college." What is a priority nursing diagnosis for this client at this time?
○ 1. Knowledge Deficit related to lack of understanding about first trimester changes.
○ 2. Fear related to lack of desire to be pregnant.
○ 3. High Risk for Altered Nutrition related to the desire to conceal pregnancy.
○ 4. Anxiety related to initial encounter with the health care system.

21. The client's pregnancy test is negative. She tells the nurse that she would like to learn more about the natural family planning method of taking the basal body temperature. After instruction, the nurse knows that the client understands the instructions from what statement?
○ 1. "I should take my temperature every evening before going to bed."
○ 2. "It doesn't matter when I take my temperature, as long as I take it once a day."
○ 3. "It's important that I take my temperature every morning before I get out of bed."
○ 4. "Since this method is so ineffective, I should use another form of family planning."

A client and her husband are seen in the fertility clinic because she has been unable to conceive. The couple have been married for 5 years. The couple have had a complete physical examination, and the husband has been found to have a mildly low sperm count.

22. Based on these assessment data, what is the priority nursing diagnosis for this couple?
○ 1. Grief related to inability to conceive.
○ 2. Knowledge Deficit related to anatomy and physiology of male fertility.
○ 3. Ineffective Family Coping related to infertility.
○ 4. Fatigue related to extensive diagnostic testing.

23. The client states "We're not sure how the treatments for infertility work." What is the nurse's best response?
○ 1. "For artificial insemination, sperm is inseminated at the time of ovulation through the cervix."
○ 2. "In vitro fertilization involves the direct transfer of ova and washed sperm into the fallopian tubes."
○ 3. "Gamete intrafallopian transfer (GIFT) requires the use of another man's sperm."
○ 4. "Clomid is a fertility drug derived from certain hormones."

24. An appropriate goal for this couple would be that by the end of the first visit, the couple will
○ 1. choose an appropriate method of treatment.
○ 2. discuss alternatives to infertility, such as adoption.
○ 3. describe each of the potential treatment modalities.
○ 4. discuss reasons for low sperm production.

The Pregnant Client Receiving Prenatal Care

A 24-year-old nulligravida schedules an appointment at the prenatal clinic because she has "missed two menstrual periods."

25. From the initial interview the nurse learns that the first day of the client's last menstrual period was March 13. According to Naegele's rule, the nurse determines that the client's estimated due date is
○ 1. June 20.
○ 2. October 6.
○ 3. November 6.
○ 4. December 20.

26. While the nurse is preparing the client for a pelvic examination, the client says "I'm afraid of this examination." What is the nurse's best response?
○ 1. "I'll be with you to explain everything the nurse practitioner is doing."
○ 2. "Nearly all new mothers have some fears about this type of examination."

○ 3. "Please tell me more about what you mean when you say you're afraid."
○ 4. "The examination won't take too long. You'll be draped to ensure privacy."

27. The nurse practitioner determines that the client is at approximately 10 weeks gestation. At this time it is possible to assess
○ 1. a softening of the lower uterine segment.
○ 2. approximate weight of the infant at term.
○ 3. cholasma on the face and forehead.
○ 4. whether quickening has occurred.

28. The client states, "I just can't believe that I'm going to have a baby!" What is the nurse's best response?
○ 1. "Would you like some pamphlets on the childbirth experience?"
○ 2. "These feelings are normal for first-time mothers."
○ 3. "You shouldn't have doubts now. Your pregnancy has been confirmed."
○ 4. "Would you like me to make an appointment for you at the mental health clinic for counseling on pregnancy?"

29. The nurse evaluates the client's expression of surprise at the confirmation of pregnancy as an indication of
○ 1. normal ambivalence.
○ 2. rejection of the pregnancy.
○ 3. acceptance of the pregnancy.
○ 4. need for further developmental assessment.

30. The nurse formulates a nursing diagnosis for the client. What is the priority diagnosis at this time?
○ 1. Impaired Social Interaction related to pregnancy confirmation.
○ 2. Decreased Cardiac Output related to pregnancy.
○ 3. Ineffective Family Coping: Compromised related to pregnancy.
○ 4. Altered Nutrition related to increased demands of pregnancy.

A client and her husband are seen in the antepartal clinic. The client had a positive pregnancy test and is now approximately 11 weeks pregnant.

31. The client's husband tells the nurse that he has been experiencing nausea and vomiting and fatigue along with his wife. The nurse determines that the client's husband is experiencing
○ 1. couvade syndrome.
○ 2. mittelschmerz.
○ 3. stress.
○ 4. jealousy.

32. The client tells the nurse that she has been vomiting after breakfast nearly every morning. Which of the following measures should the nurse suggest to help the client cope with early morning nausea and vomiting?
○ 1. Sip whole milk at breakfast.
○ 2. Drink only warm liquids for breakfast.
○ 3. Eat dry, unsalted crackers before arising in the morning.
○ 4. Drink a carbonated beverage before arising in the morning.

33. The client asks the nurse if sexual activity should change during pregnancy if no complications exist. The nurse should instruct the client that
○ 1. the couple should practice coitus interruptus during pregnancy.
○ 2. it is generally agreed that sexual activity need not be altered during pregnancy.
○ 3. it is best to avoid sexual intercourse until the client is at least 16 weeks gestation.
○ 4. ideally, the couple should have sexual intercourse not more often than once a week during pregnancy.

34. When instructing the client about drinking alcoholic beverages during pregnancy, the nurse should include which of the following?
○ 1. Limit drinking to beer and wine.
○ 2. Abstain from drinking alcoholic beverages.
○ 3. Drink no more than 1 ounce of liquor per day.
○ 4. Dilute liquor with water or soda before drinking it.

35. The nurse has instructed the client about desired weight gain during pregnancy. The nurse's teaching is considered effective when the client makes what statement?
○ 1. "A maximum weight gain of about 20 pounds (9kg) is recommended."
○ 2. "Weight gain has little significance as long as I don't feel hungry."
○ 3. "A weight gain of approximately 12 pounds (5.5 kg) each trimester is recommended."
○ 4. "Weight gain varies, but a range of 25 to 35 pounds (11.4 to 16 kg) is usually considered normal."

A 24-year-old primipara is seen in the prenatal clinic for her first visit. She is at approximately 8 weeks gestation.

36. The nurse explains to the client that she will need to take vitamins with iron during her pregnancy. The nurse suggests that the absorption of supplemental iron can be increased by taking it
○ 1. at bedtime.

○ 2. between meals.
○ 3. at the same time every day.
○ 4. with a good source of vitamin C.

37. The nurse also instructs the client to increase her dietary intake of iron. Which of the following foods should the nurse instruct the client to include in her diet?
○ 1. Beef and pork.
○ 2. Bananas and figs.
○ 3. Carrots and tomatoes.
○ 4. Cottage cheese and yogurt.

38. The nurse instructs the client about the importance of sufficient protein in her diet. The nurse knows that the instructions have been effective if the client indicates that she includes which of the following foods in her daily diet?
○ 1. Beans and nuts.
○ 2. Mushrooms and melons.
○ 3. Spinach and turnip greens.
○ 4. Citrus fruits and tomatoes.

39. The nurse plans to instruct the client to include foods rich in folic acid (folacin) in her meal planning. An appropriate goal for the client is that every day she will eat two servings of
○ 1. fresh fruit.
○ 2. dairy products.
○ 3. whole wheat bread.
○ 4. green leafy vegetables.

40. The client asks the nurse why vitamin C intake is so important during pregnancy. What is the nurse's best response?
○ 1. "Vitamin C is required to promote blood clot and collagen formation."
○ 2. "Supplemental vitamin C in large doses can prevent the fetus from becoming infected."
○ 3. "Eating moderate amounts of foods high in vitamin C can help metabolize carbohydrates."
○ 4. "Studies have shown that vitamin C helps the placenta grow."

41. The nurse plans to instruct the client to increase her intake of magnesium, which aids the synthesis of proteins, nucleic acids, and fats. Which of the following foods should the nurse encourage the client to include in her daily diet?
○ 1. Olives.
○ 2. Pears.
○ 3. Oranges.
○ 4. Spinach.

A 30-year-old multipara has been receiving regular prenatal care. She visits the obstetrician's office with her husband at 13 weeks gestation for a routine visit.

42. The client tells the nurse that she has not felt the baby move. The nurse interprets this as
○ 1. normal, because quickening is not usually felt until 24 weeks gestation for multiparous clients.
○ 2. unusual, because most multiparous clients experience quickening by 10 weeks gestation.
○ 3. evidence that the client's estimated date of delivery is not correct.
○ 4. normal, because most multiparous clients experience quickening at 17 weeks.

43. The physician schedules the client for a diagnostic ultrasound to assess fetal growth. After instructing the client about the ultrasound procedure, the nurse considers the teaching effective when the client makes what statement?
○ 1. "The procedure requires the use of a needle which will be inserted into the uterus."
○ 2. "I can't have anything to eat or drink after midnight on the day of the procedure."
○ 3. "I may feel some pain and discomfort after the procedure."
○ 4. "I need to drink 32 to 40 ounces of fluid 1 hour before the procedure."

44. An important assessment for the nurse to make for the pregnant client in the second trimester is whether or not the client has
○ 1. experienced quickening.
○ 2. bought a cradle for the infant.
○ 3. been wearing maternity clothes.
○ 4. experienced nausea and vomiting.

45. What is an appropriate nursing measure to facilitate the client's husband's involvement in the pregnancy during the second trimester?
○ 1. Suggest that the client's husband develop a new hobby.
○ 2. Help the husband identify new acquaintances at work.
○ 3. Encourage the husband to listen to the fetal heart beat.
○ 4. Refer the husband to an expectant fathers' bowling team.

46. The nurse plans to perform Leopold's maneuvers to examine the client's abdomen. To help make the client feel more comfortable and make the results more accurate, the nurse should have the client
○ 1. empty her bladder.
○ 2. lie on her left side.
○ 3. hyperventilate for 2 minutes.
○ 4. avoid eating immediately before the procedure.

47. The nurse observes that the client has a brown discoloration across her nose and cheeks. The nurse determines that this facial discoloration is
○ 1. an indication that the fetus is male.
○ 2. potentially serious and may require laser treatment.

○ 3. will fade if an antihistamine is prescribed.
○ 4. without clinical significance and usually disappears after delivery.

A primipara is seen in the nurse midwive's office at 22 weeks gestation.

48. The nurse midwife performs Leopold's maneuvers on the client to
○ 1. turn the fetus in the uterus.
○ 2. ease the fetus into the pelvis.
○ 3. assess the location of the placenta.
○ 4. determine the fetal position.

49. While the client is lying supine on the examination table, she tells the nurse midwife that she is feeling dizzy. After observing that the client is pale and perspiring freely, the nurse midwife should
○ 1. turn the client onto her left side.
○ 2. obtain the client's blood pressure.
○ 3. assess the client for vaginal bleeding.
○ 4. lower the client's head between her knees.

50. The client tells the nurse midwife, "I hope I don't get varicose veins. What causes them?" The nurse midwife explains that varicose veins are usually due to
○ 1. decrease in normal cardiac output.
○ 2. increase in maternal blood volume.
○ 3. interference with venous return from extremities.
○ 4. constriction in the blood vessel walls in the extremities.

51. The client tells the nurse midwife that she and her husband wish to drive to visit relatives who live several hundred miles away. The nurse should make which of the following recommendations concerning automobile travel? Automobile travel during pregnancy *should*
○ 1. be avoided during the first half of pregnancy.
○ 2. be limited to 1- to 2-hour trips.
○ 3. include intermittent rest periods.
○ 4. be safe, but the pregnant woman should avoid driving.

52. When the client complains of leg cramps, the nurse midwife suggests which exercise to relieve the cramps?
○ 1. Sit until the leg cramps disappear.
○ 2. Alternately flex and extend the legs.
○ 3. Push upward on the toes and downward on the knees.
○ 4. Lie flat in bed with the legs extended.

53. The client tells the nurse midwife that she has been experiencing heartburn. Which preventive measure should the nurse midwife suggest?
○ 1. Eat smaller and more frequent meals.
○ 2. Take Alka-Seltzer with water after meals.
○ 3. Decrease fluid intake to three glasses daily.
○ 4. Take 1/2 teaspoon of baking soda with water.

A 15-year-old client is seen in the prenatal clinic with her boyfriend. The client is at approximately 16 weeks gestation with her first pregnancy.

54. The client tells the nurse that she has been experiencing ankle edema. After instructing the client about ankle edema during pregnancy, the nurse knows that the client understands the instructions when she says that she will
○ 1. wear knee-high hose instead of pantyhose.
○ 2. complete all tasks that require standing at one time.
○ 3. reduce her fluid and vitamin C intake.
○ 4. dorsiflex her feet frequently.

55. The physician orders alpha-fetoprotein (AFP) screening for the client. In planning instruction for the client about the test, the nurse should stress that alpha-fetoprotein studies
○ 1. are not usually very accurate until 18 weeks gestation.
○ 2. require a freshly voided maternal urine specimen.
○ 3. with elevated levels are associated with trisomy 13.
○ 4. with elevated levels are associated with neural tube defects.

56. The client tells the nurse that she is "exhausted" because she has been unable to sleep at night. Following instruction about strategies to promote sleep, the nurse realizes that the client needs further instruction when she says she should
○ 1. drink hot chocolate before going to bed.
○ 2. ask her boyfriend to give her a soothing backrub.
○ 3. place pillows at her back and between her legs.
○ 4. practice deep-breathing exercises before she goes to sleep.

57. The nurse reinforces the client's need for continued prenatal care throughout the pregnancy. Why is this especially important for adolescent clients?
○ 1. Pregnancy-induced hypertension is the most prevalent medical complication in adolescents.
○ 2. These clients usually place their infants for adoption, and psychologic support is necessary.
○ 3. Adolescents prefer individual counseling related to nutrition.
○ 4. The baby's father usually deserts the mother in the second trimester.

58. The client weighs 100 pounds and has only gained

1 pound since becoming pregnant. She states, "I haven't had any appetite." What is the most appropriate nursing diagnosis for this client?

○ 1. Knowledge Deficit related to nutrition.
○ 2. Noncompliance with diet related to body image.
○ 3. Altered Nutrition, Less than Body Requirements related to lack of appetite.
○ 4. Altered Growth and Development related to poor appetite.

59. At her prenatal visit at 38 weeks gestation, the client tells the nurse that she is voiding frequently. While assessing the client, the nurse questions her concerning symptoms of pyuria, hematuria, and dysuria. When the client reports no symptoms, the nurse should

○ 1. weigh the client.
○ 2. assess the client for lightening.
○ 3. obtain a urine specimen.
○ 4. ask the client if she's felt the baby move.

The Pregnant Client in Childbirth Preparation Classes

A primipara and her husband voice an interest in the childbirth preparation classes offered in the community. They have their physician's support for delivery in a birthing center. The client is at approximately 6 weeks gestation.

60. The couple asks the nurse when they will first be able to hear the baby's heart beat. What is the nurse's best response?

○ 1. "The baby's heart beat can be heard with a doppler early in the third trimester."
○ 2. "Using a stethoscope, the heart beat can be heard as early as 6 weeks."
○ 3. "I think you should be worrying about other things right now."
○ 4. "The heart beat can be heard as early as 8 to 10 weeks with a doppler."

61. The couple asks when they should begin the preparation for childbirth classes that discuss nutrition during pregnancy and infant feeding. The best response by the nurse would be to suggest that the couple start attending

○ 1. as soon as the client experiences quickening.
○ 2. after the client has read pamphlets on the anatomy and physiology of reproduction.
○ 3. during the first trimester of pregnancy.
○ 4. in the late second or early third trimester.

62. The client reports a history of varicose veins. The nurse instructs the client to lie down with her feet elevated and a pillow under her left hip to avoid vena cava syndrome. The nurse knows the client has understood the instructions when the client states that the purpose of this is to

○ 1. strengthen the valves in the legs.
○ 2. increase the muscle tone of the legs.
○ 3. facilitate drainage of the extremities.
○ 4. decrease the supply of blood through the arteries.

63. The client asks the nurse how to prepare her breasts for breast-feeding. The nurse's best response is to instruct her to

○ 1. wear a supportive but loose-fitting bra.
○ 2. tug and roll the nipples between the thumb and forefinger.
○ 3. rub the nipples with a terrycloth towel when drying them after bathing.
○ 4. pat the nipples once a day with a gauze sponge moistened with alcohol.

64. The nurse plans to teach the client to alternately contract and relax the pubococcygeal muscle (Kegel exercises) several times a day. The nurse explains that the primary purpose of these exercises is to

○ 1. prevent vulvar varicosities.
○ 2. relieve lower back discomfort.
○ 3. strengthen the perineal muscles.
○ 4. strengthen the abdominal muscles.

Ten couples are enrolled in an early preparation for childbirth class, which will be taught over a 6-week period by a registered nurse.

65. The nurse plans instruction on anatomy and physiology of pregnancy and fetal development. Which of the following would be appropriate to include in the teaching plan? The umbilical cord contains

○ 1. one vein and one artery.
○ 2. two veins and one artery.
○ 3. one vein and two arteries.
○ 4. two veins and two arteries.

66. The nurse is planning a 2-hour childbirth preparation class focused on labor and delivery. Included in the plan will be the normal sequence of maneuvers the fetus goes through during labor and delivery if the head is the presenting part. Which of the following should the nurse plan to include in the instructions?

○ 1. Engagement, external rotation, flexion, and expulsion.
○ 2. Descent, flexion, external rotation, internal rotation, extension, and expulsion.
○ 3. Descent, flexion, internal rotation, extension, external rotation, and expulsion.
○ 4. Internal rotation, descent, engagement, expulsion, and external rotation.

67. A woman in the class asks how much blood will be

lost during delivery. What is the nurse's best response?

○ 1. "The maximum blood loss considered within normal limits is 500 ml."
○ 2. "The minimum blood loss considered within normal limits is 700 ml."
○ 3. "Most women lose very little blood during delivery."
○ 4. "It would be very unusual if you lost more than 100 ml during delivery."

68. Following instruction about the amnionic fluid and sac during the preparation for childbirth class, the nurse knows that a client needs further instructions by which statement?

○ 1. "The amnionic fluid helps to dilate the cervix."
○ 2. "The fetus is protected from injury by the amnionic fluid."
○ 3. "Immune bodies are provided to the fetus by the amnionic fluid."
○ 4. "One function of the amnionic fluid and sac is to keep the fetus at an even temperature."

Six couples all having their first child are enrolled in a childbirth preparation class during the third trimester. The classes last 6 weeks and are taught by a registered nurse.

69. One of the clients asks the nurse what to do about backaches. The best exercise for the nurse to suggest to relieve backache is

○ 1. sit-ups.
○ 2. leg lifts.
○ 3. knee bends.
○ 4. pelvic rock.

70. As the nurse evaluates all causes of pain during labor, she decides to teach the class participants that the primary cause of pain in the first stage of labor is

○ 1. hypoxia of the abdominal muscles.
○ 2. cultural responses in our society.
○ 3. pressure on the bladder.
○ 4. dilatation and effacement of the cervix.

71. Which of the following questions asked by a pregnant client's husband would require the nurse to gather additional assessment data?

○ 1. "Should I look for a new job?"
○ 2. "Can we afford to have a baby?"
○ 3. "What kind of parents will we be?"
○ 4. "Will I be able to help my wife during labor?"

72. The nurse has instructed the class participants about methods to cope with discomforts of labor. The nurse realizes that one of the pregnant clients needs further instruction when she says that she has been practicing

○ 1. effleurage.
○ 2. progressive relaxation.
○ 3. various chest breathing patterns.
○ 4. rapid, deep breathing techniques.

73. After the first class session, a pregnant client tells the nurse that she has had some vaginal discharge and local itching. The nurse's best action is to advise the client

○ 1. to schedule an appointment at the clinic for an examination.
○ 2. to take a vinegar douche under low pressure.
○ 3. that her symptoms are normal.
○ 4. to avoid sexual intercourse, because labor may be beginning.

The nurse is responsible for teaching preparation for parenthood classes to a group of pregnant teenagers. The 2-hour classes meet once a week for 6 weeks.

74. One client asks the nurse, "How is the baby's sex determined? I want to have a boy." The nurse explains that the chromosome combination that must exist to produce a male infant is

○ 1. XX.
○ 2. XY.
○ 3. XYY.
○ 4. XXY.

75. The nurse has instructed the group about the functions of the placenta. Following the instruction, the nurse knows that a client needs further instructions when she says that the hormones produced by the placenta include

○ 1. aldosterone.
○ 2. progesterone.
○ 3. human placental lactogen.
○ 4. human chorionic gonadotrophin.

76. The nurse plans to instruct the group about the placenta and that the fetus obtains oxygen through the umbilical cord. Which of the following should be included in the teaching plan?

○ 1. The fetal blood vessel with the highest oxygen content is the umbilical vein.
○ 2. About 20% of umbilical cords have only two vessels.
○ 3. A velamentous insertion exists when the cord inserts centrally at the placenta.
○ 4. A nuchal cord has no protective covering of Wharton's jelly.

77. The nurse plans to emphasize the need for continued prenatal care and well-baby care following delivery. Which of the following should be included in the teaching plan?

○ 1. The infant mortality rate is defined as the number of infant deaths under age 1 year per 1,000 live births.

○ 2. The perinatal mortality rate is defined as the number of fetal deaths per 1,000 live births.
○ 3. The neonatal mortality rate is defined as the number of infant deaths under age 6 months per 1,000 live births.
○ 4. More than 50% of women in the United States do not receive prenatal care, and this contributes to the high infant mortality rate.

A 25-year-old primigravida visits the prenatal clinic during her second trimester. The client began receiving prenatal care at 7 weeks gestation.

78. The client asks the nurse, "How early can the sex be determined. I'm scheduled for an ultrasound next week." The nurse's response is "The sex of the fetus can be determined as early as
○ 1. 8 weeks gestation."
○ 2. 10 weeks gestation."
○ 3. 12 weeks gestation."
○ 4. 16 weeks gestation."

79. The client reports frequent constipation. To help relieve constipation, the nurse should instruct the client to
○ 1. use glycerine suppositories as needed.
○ 2. drink a glass of hot water in the morning.
○ 3. avoid highly seasoned foods.
○ 4. use a mild laxative, such as milk of magnesia, as needed.

80. The client complains of discomfort from hemorrhoids. The nurse realizes that the client needs further instruction from which statement?
○ 1. "I can reinsert the hemorrhoid with my finger."
○ 2. "Avoiding constipation is important to relieve hemorrhoids."
○ 3. "Ice packs, warm soaks, and topical ointments can provide temporary relief."
○ 4. "Daily doses of aluminum hydroxide gel can help prevent hemorrhoids."

81. The client tells the nurse that she experiences leg cramps frequently. The nurse explains that this is most likely due to
○ 1. low potassium intake.
○ 2. too much exercise.
○ 3. imbalanced calcium/phosphorus ratio.
○ 4. overuse of laxatives.

The nurse is responsible for a 2-hour presentation on the anatomy and physiology of pregnancy for 25 nursing students.

82. The nurse plans to instruct the group about the development of the placenta. Which of the following should be included in the teaching plan?
○ 1. The placenta is formed by the fusion of chorionic villi and the decidua basalis.
○ 2. The weight of a term placenta is 1,000 to 1,500 grams.
○ 3. Most substances with a molecular weight greater than 500 grams readily cross the placenta by diffusion.
○ 4. Due to the placenta's complex structure, viruses are not able to cross it.

83. A student asks what the placenta does during pregnancy. The nurse's best response is that the placenta performs functions similar to the
○ 1. brain.
○ 2. lungs.
○ 3. muscles.
○ 4. spleen.

84. During the presentation, a student asks, "How many days after conception does the fertilized ovum implant in the uterine wall?" The nurse's best response is that this process normally takes
○ 1. 3 days.
○ 2. 7 days.
○ 3. 11 days.
○ 4. 15 days.

85. After describing the pelvic changes that occur during pregnancy, the nurse determines that the group understands the instructions when a student states that the uterus receives its blood supply directly from the uterine artery and the
○ 1. iliac artery.
○ 2. ovarian artery.
○ 3. hypogastric artery.
○ 4. uterosacral artery.

86. The nurse plans to discuss various diagnostic tests to determine fetal well-being. Which of the following should be included in the teaching plan?
○ 1. Fetal biophysical profile involves assessing breathing movements, body movements, tone, amnionic fluid volume, and fetal heart rate reactivity.
○ 2. A reactive nonstress test is an ominous sign and requires further evaluation with fetal echocardiography.
○ 3. Contraction stress testing is performed on most pregnant women and can be initiated as early as 20 weeks gestation.
○ 4. Amniocentesis for lung maturity studies requires admission to the hospital and a full bladder.

The Pregnant Client With Risk Factors

A primigravida is admitted to the hospital at 12 weeks gestation. She has abdominal cramping and bright red vaginal spotting. Her cervix is not dilated.

87. Based on the client's symptoms, the nurse determines that the client is most likely experiencing a
- ○ 1. missed abortion.
- ○ 2. threatened abortion.
- ○ 3. inevitable abortion.
- ○ 4. incomplete abortion.

88. The client is discharged when her symptoms subside, although she is still having slight vaginal spotting occasionally. Before discharge, the nurse should instruct the client to
- ○ 1. weigh herself daily.
- ○ 2. follow a salt-free diet temporarily.
- ○ 3. save her perineal pads for inspection.
- ○ 4. have intercourse no more often than once a week.

89. After the client passes some of the products of conception, she returns to the hospital for a dilatation and curettage (D & C). The nurse determines that the client is most likely experiencing which type of abortion?
- ○ 1. Missed.
- ○ 2. Induced.
- ○ 3. Threatened.
- ○ 4. Incomplete.

90. The nurse administers butorphanol tartrate (Stadol) as ordered, primarily to
- ○ 1. prevent nausea.
- ○ 2. reduce discomfort.
- ○ 3. control hemorrhage.
- ○ 4. promote uterine contractility.

91. Postoperatively, the nurse finds the client crying. Which of the following comments by the nurse would be best in this situation?
- ○ 1. "Why are you crying?"
- ○ 2. "Will a pill help your pain?"
- ○ 3. "I'm sorry you lost your baby."
- ○ 4. "You can always try again to get pregnant."

A 30-year-old multipara is admitted to the hospital's surgical unit following a spontaneous abortion and a dilatation and curettage (D & C).

92. After assessing the client, the nurse suggests that she receive pentazocine hydrochloride (Talwin), primarily to
- ○ 1. inhibit lactation.
- ○ 2. aid uterine involution.
- ○ 3. relieve abdominal discomfort.
- ○ 4. prevent conception for about 6 weeks.

93. The nurse finds the client crying and overtly upset. Which of the following nursing diagnoses is best for the client at this time?
- ○ 1. Knowledge Deficit related to the loss.
- ○ 2. Powerlessness related to loss and grief.
- ○ 3. Spiritual Distress related to anxiety.
- ○ 4. Anxiety related to low self-esteem.

94. The nurse determines that the client is Rh negative and her husband is Rh positive. Analysis of the client's blood indicates that she is unsensitized. The nurse administers human anti-D globulin (Rhogam) before the client is discharged from the hospital, to prevent the client from
- ○ 1. becoming Rh positive.
- ○ 2. developing Rh sensitivity.
- ○ 3. developing AB antigens in the blood.
- ○ 4. becoming pregnant with an Rh-positive fetus.

CORRECT ANSWERS AND RATIONALE

The letters in parentheses following the rationale identify the step of the nursing process (A, D, P, I, E); cognitive level (K, C, T, N); and client need (S, G, L, H). See the Answer Grid for the key.

The Preconception Client

1. 1. When acting as a sexuality counselor, the nurse should begin by obtaining a sexual history from the client. Obtaining a history is part of the assessment phase of the nursing process. Only after the nurse has collected necessary information can the data be analyzed and plans formulated, implemented, and evaluated. While a complete physical examination, including a Pap smear, is often warranted, this can be done later. There is no need to include the client's sexual partner at this time, nor any need to discuss anatomy and physiology until after the sexual history has been obtained. (I, T, H)

2. 3. A nurse must develop an awareness of his or her own feelings, values, and attitudes about human sexuality to be effective as sexual counselors. A nurse who recognizes his or her own beliefs can be more sensitive and objective when confronted with others' beliefs. Having sexual experience, reviewing the literature, and completing a formal educational program may help, but these activities do not replace good self-understanding. (I, N, H)

3. 4. Ovulation occurs approximately 2 weeks before menstruation begins. Stated another way, the menstrual period begins approximately 2 weeks after ovulation. Ovulation does not usually occur during the menstrual period when the endometrium is being shed. Clients can be taught to determine when ovulation occurs (e.g., cervical mucous changes, basal body temperature changes). Although some women consistently experience some pelvic discomfort during ovulation (mittelschmerz), severe pain is rare. (P, N, H)

4. 1. Sperm can reach the ovum in only 1 to 5 minutes under ideal conditions. This is a very important point to make with a client seeking information related to contraception. Many people believe that the time interval is much longer and that they can wait to take steps to prevent conception until after intercourse, which is usually too late. (I, N, H)

5. 4. Natural methods of fertility management depend on knowing when ovulation occurs. Regular menstrual cycles can vary by 1 or 2 days in either direction. The calendar method, basal body temperature method, cervical mucous method, and the symptothermal method are all natural methods of fertility management. Although some recordkeeping is necessary, it is not extensive. Although sexual spontaneity may be restricted for several days, this is not necessarily frustrating for both partners. Even if the selected method is done correctly, first year failure rates range from 2–10%. (D, N, H)

6. 3. Oral contraceptive agents inhibit ovulation by suppressing follicle-stimulating hormone (FSH) and luteinizing hormone. Among the many side effects of oral contraceptives include nausea, vomiting, fluid retention, increased vaginal discharge, cholasma, headaches, weight gain, thromboembolic disorders, hepatic adenoma, and possible hypertension. A history of thromboembolic disease is an absolute contraindication to using oral contraceptive agents. (E, N, H)

7. 2. The nurse is trying to assess the client and her husband further. If one partner has objections to using a condom, the nurse should explore the basis of the objections. The nurse may need to provide the client with accurate information and dispel myths related to fertility management. Open-ended questions often elicit more information. Telling the client that most men believe it is the female that does not like condoms, or that a lot of men do not like to use condoms, is not helpful. Both latex and skin condoms prevent sexually transmitted disease. (A, T, H)

8. 4. A diaphragm should be left in place for 6 to 8 hours after intercourse. More spermicidal cream or jelly should be used if intercourse is repeated during this period. The client should be instructed to remove the diaphragm at least once every 24 hours. Cases of toxic shock syndrome are infrequent, but clients should be instructed in the danger signs: fever, diarrhea, rash, vomiting, and muscle aches. A client cannot obtain a diaphragm without a prescription. Each woman must be fitted individually by a skilled practitioner. (P, N, H)

9. 4. In vasectomy, a common procedure for male sterilization, the ductus deferens (vas deferens) is cut and tied. Coagulation may also be used to create an obstruction in the vas deferens. (I, N, H)

10. 2. Intercourse during menstruation is not harmful. Alcohol acts as a central nervous system depressant and acts accordingly on the libido (sexual drive). Masturbation can be used to achieve orgasm. An orgasm is not always necessary for a satisfactory sexual experience. (E, N, H)

11. 2. Composed of erectile tissue, the clitoris is especially sensitive to foreplay and movements of the shaft of the penis against its surface. (E, N, H)

12. 2. Sexual arousal helps increase vaginal secretions, which help prepare the vagina for penile penetration and increase comfort during sexual intercourse by lubricating the vagina. Foreplay does not necessarily relax the vaginal orifice. Foreplay does not delay clitoral orgasm or premature ejaculation; in fact, it can trigger these. (P, N, H)

13. 2. The sperm's tail propels it along the female reproductive tract. Muscle action in the uterus may help move sperm toward the fallopian tube, but no peristalsis-like contractions occur in the cervix and uterus. (I, N, H)

14. 3. Occluded or obstructed fallopian tubes make conception impossible, because the sperm cannot reach the ovum. Such conditions as absent ovary, dilated hymenal ring, or obstructed Bartholin's duct do not result in infertility. (I, N, H)

15. 4. Fertilization normally occurs in the fallopian tubes. If the fertilized ovum does not move into the uterus, the condition is known as a tubal pregnancy. A tubal pregnancy is one type of ectopic pregnancy. (I, N, H)

16. 1. The radioimmunoassay pregnancy test is highly accurate within 7 days after conception. It uses an antiserum with specificity for the beta subunit of human chorionic gonadotrophin (hCG) in blood plasma. Over-the-counter or home pregnancy tests are performed on urine and use the hemagglutination-inhibition method. A positive pregnancy test is a probable sign of pregnancy. Certain conditions other than pregnancy, such as choriocarcinoma, can cause elevated hCG levels. The radioimmunoassay pregnancy test is not based on an antigen-antibody reaction. (I, N, H)

17. 4. Human chorionic gonadotrophin is the hormone used in most pregnancy tests. Estrogen stimulates uterine development during pregnancy. Luteinizing hormone stimulates ovulation. Follicle stimulating hormone is involved in follicle maturation during the menstrual cycle. (E, N, H)

18. 1. Amenorrhea, urinary frequency, breast tenderness, nausea, vomiting, and fatigue are considered presumptive or subjective changes of pregnancy. Probable or objective signs of pregnancy include Goodell's sign (softening of the cervix), Chadwick's sign (discoloration of the mucous membranes of the cervix, vagina, and vulva), and Hegar's sign (softening of the isthmus of the uterus). Other probable signs include enlargement of the abdomen, uterine souffle, and Braxton-Hicks contractions. Positive or diagnostic signs of pregnancy include detection of the fetal heartbeat, detection of fetal movements by a trained examiner, and ultrasound identification of a fetus. (D, N, H)

19. 4. The client's concerns about death during childbirth provided the nurse with an opportunity to gather additional data. Telling the client not to worry is not helpful. Maternal death does occur, even with modern technology. Leading causes of maternal mortality in the United States include embolism, pregnancy-induced hypertension, hemorrhage, ectopic pregnancy, and infection. Asking the client why she would ask about death when she isn't certain she is pregnant may not provide data that would be helpful in planning care. (A, N, H)

20. 2. The most appropriate priority diagnosis from the data available is Fear related to lack of desire to be pregnant. The client has stated that pregnancy would be a financial burden. The nurse does not know whether the client is pregnant, so Knowledge Deficit is not appropriate. From the available data, it is not clear whether the client is at high risk for altered nutrition, nor has the client expressed anxiety. (D, N, H)

21. 3. The client using the basal body temperature method should take her temperature for 5 minutes every morning on awakening and before arising or starting any activity. At this time, temperature is least likely to be influenced by other factors. A slight drop in body temperature before ovulation occurs in some but not all women. A woman cannot determine exactly when ovulation occurs until it has actually happened. Depending on the client's motivation and the ability to perform the procedure correctly, this can be an effective fertility management method. (E, N, H)

22. 1. A common reaction for infertile couples is Grief. There are no data to suggest Knowledge Deficit, Ineffective Family Coping, or Fatigue. (D, N, L)

23. 1. For artificial insemination, sperm is introduced through the cervix at the time of ovulation. In vitro fertilization involves removal of a mature ovum from a woman's ovary, fertilization with sperm in a petri dish, and reimplantation of the embryo into the woman's uterine cavity. Gamete intrafallopian transfer (GIFT) does *not* require the use of another male's sperm. Clomid is a nonhormonal fertility drug. (I, N, H)

24. 3. By the end of the first visit, the couple should be able to identify potential treatment modalities. They should consider all the various treatments before selecting one. The first visit is not the appropriate time to decide on treatment. The couple may desire information about alternatives, but there are not enough data to suggest that a specific treatment modality may not be successful. The husband is already aware of his low sperm count. Although it might be helpful for the couple to review reasons for low sperm production, this is not a priority goal at this time. (P, N, H)

The Pregnant Client Receiving Prenatal Care

25. 4. When using Naegele's rule to determine the estimated due date, count back 3 calendar months from the first day of the last menstrual period and add 7 days. This means the client's due date is December 20. Measurement of fundal height and ultrasonography are also used to determine gestational age. (I, N, H)

26. 3. When the client expresses fear of the examination, it is best for the nurse to say something that allows the client to describe her feelings. The nurse can then gather additional data to aid planning and implementation of nursing care. It is of no help to a fearful client when the nurse describes his or her own role or says that nearly all new mothers have similar fears. Telling the client that the examination will not take long or that she will be draped for privacy ignores her fears. (I, N, S)

27. 1. By 10 weeks gestation, the uterus has enlarged to about twice its normal size. Chadwick's sign (bluish coloring of the vaginal mucosa) is noted as early as the 6th week. Hegar's sign (softening of the lower uterine segment) may be noted at 6 to 8 weeks. Fetal movements (quickening) cannot be palpated until about 18 to 20 weeks. (A, N, H)

28. 2. This client is expressing a feeling about having a baby. The nurse responds to the client's feeling by explaining that such feelings are normal and experienced by many women early in pregnancy. Studies have shown that a common reaction to pregnancy is summarized as "someday, but not now." Fathers must also come to terms with the pregnancy. The nurse practitioner's confirmation of the pregnancy is something the client already knows. Offering a pamphlet on pregnancy does not respond to the couple's feelings. There is no indication that the client is in need of psychological counseling. (I, N, H)

29. 1. When a pregnancy is confirmed, the initial reaction is surprise at the reality of conception, regardless of whether the pregnancy was planned or unplanned. Expressions of surprise and wrong timing reflect the predominant feeling of ambivalence common during the first trimester. Acceptance of the pregnancy is a developmental task of pregnancy. Rejection of the pregnancy, especially in the first trimester, may result in a decision to terminate it. (D, N, L)

30. 4. The priority nursing diagnosis at this time relates to nutrition and the necessary health teaching. Pregnancy places additional demands on the body, and adequate nutrition is important for fetal well-being. No data are presented to suggest impaired social interaction or ineffective family coping. Cardiac output is increased, not decreased, during pregnancy. (D, N, H)

31. 1. Couvade syndrome is one in which the expectant father experiences some of the discomforts of pregnancy along with the pregnant woman as a means of identifying with the pregnancy. The expectant father is not experiencing mittelschmerz, which is the term for the lower abdominal discomfort felt by some women during ovulation. There are no data to suggest that the symptoms are related to stress or jealousy. (D, N, H)

32. 3. Eating a dry high carbohydrate food, such as crackers or dry toast, before arising in the morning often relieves the early morning nausea and vomiting that many pregnant women experience. Eating high-fat foods or drinking fluids tend to exacerbate the condition for many women. (I, N, H)

33. 2. It is generally agreed that couples need not change their pattern of sexual activity during pregnancy unless complications arise. Some women find intercourse uncomfortable during the first and third trimesters due to the common discomforts of pregnancy. During the third trimester, the couple should consider coital positions other than male superior, such as side-by-side, female superior, and vaginal rear entry. Intercourse is contraindicated when bleeding or ruptured membrane occurs. After 32 weeks gestation, women with a history of preterm labor should be advised of the possible risks of coitus. (I, T, H)

34. 2. There is no definitive answer as to how much alcohol can be safely consumed by a pregnant woman. Therefore, it is recommended that pregnant clients be taught to abstain from drinking alcohol during pregnancy. Maternal alcohol use may result in fetal alcohol syndrome, marked by mild to moderate mental retardation, physical growth retardation, central nervous system disorders, and feeding difficulties. (P, N, H)

35. 4. The National Academy of Sciences Institute of Medicine recommends that women gain between 25 and 35 pounds (11.4 to 16 kg) during pregnancy. These guidelines were developed to decrease the risk of intrauterine growth retardation. (I, N, H)

36. 4. Absorption of supplemental iron and nonmeat sources of iron is enhanced by combining them with meat or a good source of vitamin C. Gastrointestinal upset is more likely when iron is taken on an empty stomach. The pregnant woman who experiences gastrointestinal upset should be taught to take iron tablets with meals to decrease adverse gastrointestinal symptoms. However, iron absorption is reduced 40–50% if tablets are taken with meals. (I, N, G)

37. 1. Foods high in iron include almost all seafoods and meats, including shellfish, as well as green vegetables. Eggs, while high in cholesterol, are also rich in iron. Poor sources of iron include carrots, tomatoes, bananas, figs, cottage cheese, and yogurt. Milk and milk products are valuable sources of calcium but poor sources of iron. (I, N, G)

38. 1. Rich sources of protein include meat, fish, poultry, beans, nuts, milk, eggs, cheese, and wheat germ. Such foods as mushrooms, melons, spinach, turnip greens, citrus fruits, and tomatoes are poor sources of protein but good sources of other nutrients. (E, N, G)

39. 4. Green leafy vegetables, such as asparagus, spinach, brussels sprouts, and broccoli are rich sources of folic acid. A well-balanced diet must include whole grains, dairy products, and fresh fruits; however, these foods are not rich in folic acid. (P, N, G)

40. 1. Vitamin C is required to promote blood clot and collagen formation. Vitamin C deficiency has been associated with premature rupture of the membranes and pregnancy induced hypertension. High doses of vitamin C are not recommended. Neonates exposed to excessive doses of vitamin C have developed symptoms of scurvy after birth. High doses of vitamin C do not prevent the fetus from becoming infected. Vitamin C does not help to metabolize carbohydrates, although thiamine is a coenzyme in carbohydrate metabolism. Vitamin C does not affect placental growth. Folacin needs are increased during pregnancy to assist with fetal and placental growth. (I, N, G)

41. 4. Spinach and other dark leafy green vegetables are excellent sources of magnesium. Other good sources include dried beans, nuts, soybeans, whole-grain cereals, milk, meat, and seafood. Olives are high in sodium but not magnesium. Pears are good sources of niacin but not magnesium. Oranges provide vitamin C but are not high in magnesium. (P, N, G)

42. 4. Although some women may perceive quickening between 14 and 20 weeks gestation, most multiparous women experience it at approximately 17.5 weeks gestation. It is not unusual or abnormal for a client at 13 weeks gestation not to experience quickening. (D, N, G)

43. 4. A full bladder helps in the visualization of the fetus. A client does not need to restrict food or fluid intake on the day of the procedure. The diagnostic ultrasound is a procedure that uses high-frequency sound waves, not needles. It is a painless procedure, although the client may experience discomfort from a full bladder. The client should not experience pain following the procedure. (E, N, H)

44. 1. Assessment during the second trimester requires the nurses to determine whether the client has felt fetal movement. Quickening provides evidence that the fetus is a real person. Perceiving the baby as a person usually increases excitement about the pregnancy, as evidenced by wearing maternity clothes and making purchases for the nursery. The client should experience decreased nausea and vomiting in the second trimester. (A, N, G)

45. 3. The father's involvement in the pregnancy can be facilitated during the second trimester by watching and feeling fetal movements and by hearing the fetal heartbeat. Developing new time-consuming interests outside the home may indicate that the father is not coping positively with the changes precipitated by the pregnancy. (A, N, G)

46. 1. The client should empty her bladder before the nurse palpates the abdomen to perform Leopold's maneuvers. This increases the client's comfort and makes palpation more accurate. The client should be lying in a supine position with the head slightly elevated for greater comfort and the knees drawn up slightly. The client does not need to hyperventilate or avoid eating before the procedure. (P, N, H)

47. 4. Discoloration on the face that commonly appears during pregnancy, chloasma usually disappears after delivery and is of no clinical significance. The client bothered by her appearance may be able to decrease its prominence with makeup. No treatment is necessary for this condition. It is not related to the sex of the fetus. (D, N, G)

48. 4. Leopold's maneuvers are used to determine the position of the fetus in the uterus. Locating the back of the fetus makes it easier to assess the fetal heart rate, which can best be heard through the fetal back. Leopold's maneuvers are not used to turn the fetus in the uterus, to ease the fetus into the pelvis, or to assess the location of the placenta. (D, N, G)

49. 1. The most common reason a pregnant client may feel dizzy, become pale, and perspire freely when lying supine is pressure on the vena cava from the enlarging uterus. The condition is often referred to as vena cava syndrome, or supine hypotensive syndrome. It can be alleviated by turning the client onto her left side. Measuring the client's blood pressure or lowering her head between her knees is not helpful. The symptoms are not related to vaginal bleeding. (I, N, G)

50. 3. The enlarging uterus exerts pressure on blood vessels carrying blood to and from the lower part of the body, especially the extremities, and predisposes to varicosities. Prevention and management of varicosities includes avoiding anything that places constriction on the legs or thighs, such as round garters or knee-high hose. Supportive hose or elastic stockings may be helpful. Lying down with feet elevated several times a day can also promote venous return. Cardiac output is increased during pregnancy, not decreased. Increased maternal blood volume and constricted blood vessel walls in the extremities do not cause leg varicosities. (I, N, G)

51. 3. Automobile travel is not contraindicated during pregnancy unless the client develops complications. The client traveling by automobile should be advised to take intermittent rest periods of 10 to 15 minutes every 2 hours. This stimulates the circulation, which becomes sluggish during long periods of sitting. There is no reason why the client cannot drive, if no complications exist. (I, N, H)

52. 3. Leg cramps are thought to result from excessive amounts of phosphorus absorbed from milk products. Pushing up on the toes and down on the knees is an effective measure to relieve leg cramps. Keeping the legs warm and elevating them are good preventive measures. Sitting will not relieve cramps, nor will lying with the legs extended. Flexing and extending the legs is not helpful. (I, N, G)

53. 1. Heartburn can occur at any time during pregnancy. Contributing factors include stress, tension, worry, fatigue, caffeine, and smoking. Eating smaller and more frequent meals may help prevent heartburn. The client should be advised to avoid fatty foods, Alka-Seltzer, baking soda, and Fizrin, which are high in sodium. Increasing fluid intake may help, by diluting gastric juices. (I, N, G)

54. 4. Frequent foot dorsiflexion facilitates circulatory fluid return in the lower extremities by stimulating muscle contraction. Other strategies to decrease ankle edema include avoiding standing or sitting for long periods, and resting with the legs and hips elevated several times a day. Restrictive bands on knee-high hose should be avoided to aid circulation. Reducing fluid vitamin C intake is not helpful. (E, N, G)

55. 4. Alpha-fetoprotein is found in the fetal circulation, maternal serum, and amnionic fluid. Elevated levels are associated with neural tube defects such as anencephaly and spina bifida. Elevated levels also have been associated with multiple gestation, fetal death, abdominal wall defects, teratomas, fetal distress, and normal fetuses. Maternal serum is assessed between 15 and 20 weeks gestation. Decreased levels are associated with genetic defects such as trisomy 13, trisomy 18, and trisomy 21. (P, N, H)

56. 1. Chocolate contains caffeine, which should be avoided. A warm caffeine-free beverage such as herbal tea, a soothing backrub, extra pillows to support a side-lying position, and relaxation techniques can all be helpful to induce sleep. (E, N, H)

57. 1. The most significant medical complication in pregnant adolescents is pregnancy-induced hypertension. Prenatal care is often the most critical factor influencing pregnancy outcome. Other risks for adolescents include low-birth-weight infants, preterm labor, iron deficiency anemia, and cephalopelvic disproportion. Infants of adolescent mothers are usually not placed for adoption. Adolescent mothers have better nutrition when they attend group classes and are subject to peer pressure. Adolescent fathers may abandon the mothers at any time during the pregnancy; however, some adolescent fathers are supportive throughout the pregnancy. (D, N, H)

58. 3. The most appropriate nursing diagnosis for this client is Altered Nutrition, Less than Body Requirements related to lack of appetite. She has gained only 1 pound and states that she has no appetite. It is important that the nurse gather additional data to determine the reason for the client's poor appetite. There are no data to support Knowledge Deficit or Noncompliance. Although the pregnant adolescent may be experiencing Altered Growth and Development related to the pregnancy, this is not the priority diagnosis. (D, N, H)

59. 2. Most primigravid clients and many multigravid clients experience lightening 1 or 2 weeks before delivery. This indicates that the fetus has descended into the pelvis. Lightening helps the mother breathe easier, because there is less pressure on the chest cavity. However, she may experience frequency of urination, because the fetal presenting part compresses the bladder. If the client has no symptoms of pyuria, hematuria, or dysuria, frequency is most probably caused by lightening; the nurse should assess for this. Leopold's maneuvers can help determine whether the fetus has descended into the pelvis. There is no reason to weigh the client, obtain a urine specimen, or ask about fetal movement based on the data presented. (I, N, H)

The Pregnant Client In Childbirth Preparation Classes

60. 4. With doppler ultrasound, the fetal heartbeat can be heard as early as 8 to 10 weeks gestation. With a stethoscope, the heartbeat cannot be heard until 17 to 20 weeks gestation. Telling the client to worry about other things right now is not helpful. (I, N, H)

61. 3. Early pregnancy classes are appropriate for clients seeking early obstetric care. These classes focus on maternal nutrition, minor discomforts of pregnancy, and newborn nutrition. Most clients make the decision to breast-feed or bottle feed by the sixth month of pregnancy. Toward the end of the second trimester or the beginning of the third trimester, couples are usually psychologically ready for termination of the pregnancy and are ready for classes dealing with labor and delivery, newborn care, and postpartum care. The clients do not need to read pamphlets before attending childbirth classes. Quickening occurs between 17 and 20 weeks gestation; there is no reason that the couple should wait until this occurs to attend childbirth classes. (I, N, H)

62. 3. Elevating the legs enhances venous return and decreases venous stasis, helping relieve varicosities. It does not strengthen vessel valves, increase muscle tone, or decrease the blood supply to the arteries. (E, N, H)

63. 2. Tugging and rolling the nipples between the thumb and forefinger is thought to be beneficial in distributing natural lubrication from Montgomery's tubercles, stimulating blood flow to the breast, and developing a protective layer of skin over the nipples. These are all goals of nipple preparation. Rubbing the nipples with a terrycloth towel removes protective lubrication and should be avoided. Alcohol may remove normal oils and may predispose the client to cracked nipples. Some authorities recommend massaging the nipples with a cream. (I, N, H)

64. 3. Kegel exercises help strengthen the perineal muscles, tone the vagina, prevent hemorrhoids, and control stress incontinence. (P, N, H)

65. 3. The umbilical cord normally consists of two arteries and one vein. Oxygen and other nutrients are carried to the fetal circulation by the umbilical vein. The oxygen-poor blood is pumped back to the placenta by the fetal heart through two umbilical arteries. A single umbilical artery is sometimes associated with congenital anomalies. (P, N, H)

66. 3. If the head is the presenting part, the normal maneuvers during labor and delivery are descent, flexion, internal rotation, extension, external rotation, and expulsion. These maneuvers occur as the fetal head passes through the maternal pelvis. (P, N, H)

67. 1. In a normal delivery and for the first 24 hours after delivery, a total blood loss not exceeding 500 ml is considered normal. (I, N, H)

68. 3. Amnionic fluid does not provide the fetus with immune bodies, but it does help dilate the cervix, protect the fetus from injury, and keep the fetus at an even temperature. (E, N, H)

69. 4. The pelvic rock or pelvic tilt seems to help strengthen back muscles, which helps alleviate backaches during pregnancy. The exercise is done as follows: With hands on hips, alternately "tuck" the buttocks under, then relax. The exercise may be done while standing, sitting, lying, or on hands and knees. (I, N, H)

70. 4. Pain during the first stage of labor is primarily due to dilatation of the cervix, hypoxia of the uterine muscle cells during contraction, stretching of the lower uterine segment, and pressure on adjacent structures. A client's perceptions of pain and cultural background can influence pain. During the second stage of labor, pain is thought to be due to hypoxia of the contracting uterine muscle cells, distention of the perineum and vagina, and pressure on the adjacent structures. (I, N, H)

71. 1. Concerns about financial capabilities commonly intensify during the third trimester, and it is not unusual for the expectant father to ask about the affordability of an infant. However, it is not common for the father to ask if he should look for a new job. Further assessment is required in this situation. Other common concerns of expectant couples are what kind of parents will they be and if the father can help during labor. (A, N, L)

72. 4. Hyperventilation causes maternal respiratory alkalosis, resulting in reduced placental oxygen exchange for the fetus. For this reason, rapid breathing in labor is no longer advocated. Techniques that decrease discomfort during labor are progressive relaxation, effluerage (except during the transition phase of labor), and various chest-breathing patterns. (E, N, G)

73. 1. Increased vaginal discharge is normal during pregnancy, but local itching is associated with infections, such as those due to *Trichomonas vaginalis* or *Candida albicans.* The client's symptoms must be further assessed by a health professional as the client may need treatment. Douches are not commonly prescribed during pregnancy. These symptoms are not associated with onset of labor. (I, N, G)

74. 2. Female sex cells normally contain two X chromosomes; male cells, one X chromosome and one Y chromosome. The mature ovum always has the X type, but the spermatozoon may be either X or Y. The male partner determines the sex of the fetus. If a male X chromosome combines with the ovum, the infant will be a female (XX). If a male Y chromosome combines with the ovum, the infant will be a male (XY). (I, N, H)

75. 1. Produced by the adrenal cortex, aldosterone stimulates the maternal kidney tubules to reabsorb sodium and water. Human placental lactogen (HPL), human chorionic gonadotrophin (HCG), and progesterone are three of the hormones produced by the placenta during pregnancy. (P, N, H)

76. 1. Oxygenated blood flows through the umbilical vein to the fetus. Blood leaving the fetus to return to the placenta flows through the two umbilical arteries. About 1% of umbilical cords have only one artery.

A velamentous cord does not insert centrally into the placenta. A nuchal cord exists when the cord is wrapped around the fetus' neck. (P, N, H)

77. 1. Infant mortality rate is defined as the number of deaths of infants under age 1 year per 1,000 live births. The perinatal mortality rate is defined as the number of deaths per 100,000 live births plus stillbirths. The neonatal mortality rate is the number of deaths of infants under age 28 days per 100,000 live births. An estimated one-third of pregnant clients do not receive prenatal care. (P, N, H)

78. 4. Fetal sex can be determined as early as 16 weeks gestation. (I, N, H)

79. 2. Measures to relieve constipation include drinking a glass of hot water in the morning, increasing bulk and roughage in the diet, increasing fluid intake, and exercising regularly. It is best not to suggest laxatives or suppositories, because a client may become dependent on them. Laxatives should be used only when diet, fluid intake, and exercise do not relieve the problem and after consultation with the nurse or physician. (I, N, G)

80. 4. Aluminum hydroxide gel can be helpful in relieving leg cramps but is not helpful to relieve the discomfort of hemorrhoids. Effective measures include reinserting the hemorrhoid while in a side-lying position, avoiding constipation, applying ice packs, taking warm soaks, and applying topical creams and ointments. (E, N, G)

81. 3. The exact cause of leg cramps is unknown, but contributing factors may include inadequate calcium intake, imbalanced calcium/phosphorus ratio, and pressure of the enlarged uterus on the pelvic nerves. Fatigue and poor circulation can also contribute to the problem. Lack of potassium intake, too much exercise, and frequent laxative use do not contribute to leg cramps. (D, N, G)

82. 1. The placenta is formed by fusion of the chorionic villi and the decidual basalis. The weight of a term placenta is 400 to 600 grams, or about one-sixth the weight of the newborn. Most substances with a molecular weight of less than 500 grams diffuse readily through the placenta. Larger molecules have more difficulty, with the exception of immune Y-globulin G (IgG). Many viruses, such as rubella, chickenpox, mumps, measles, cytomegalic inclusion disease, and *Treponema pallidum,* may cross the placenta and infect the fetus. (P, N, H)

83. 2. During pregnancy, the placenta performs the same functions in the embryo/fetus as the lungs, kidney, and stomach (respiration, elimination, nutrition). It does not perform functions normally performed by the brain, muscles, or spleen. (I, N, H)

84. 2. The fertilized ovum remains in the fallopian tube for about 3 days and in the uterus for about 4 days before it implants in the uterine wall. (I, N, H)

85. 2. The uterus receives its blood supply from the uterine and ovarian arteries. The ovarian artery is a branch of the aorta. It enters the broad ligament and supplies the ovary with blood, while its main stem makes its way to the upper margin of the uterus. (E, N, H)

86. 1. The fetal biophysical profile includes fetal breathing movements, fetal body movements, tone, amniotic fluid volume, and fetal heart rate reactivity. A reactive nonstress test is a sign of fetal well-being and does not require further evaluation. Contraction stress testing or oxytocin challenge testing should be performed only on women at risk. The contraction stress test is rarely performed before 28 weeks gestation, because of the possibility of initiating labor. Amniocentesis can be performed on an outpatient basis, and the client should empty the bladder before the procedure. (P, N, G)

The Pregnant Client With Risk Factors

87. 2. In a threatened abortion, there is vaginal bleeding or spotting. The cervix is not dilated, and abdominal cramping may occur. An inevitable abortion is characterized by more bleeding and cramping than a threatened abortion; the cervix is dilating, and termination of the pregnancy cannot be prevented. In an incomplete abortion, some but not all of the products of conception have been expelled; usually, the placenta remains. In a missed abortion, the fetus is dead but has not been expelled from the uterus. (D, N, G)

88. 3. The client threatening to abort may be sent home if she has only slight bleeding or spotting and is free of abdominal pain. However, she should be taught to save her perineal pads and tissue or clots passed for inspection to determine whether she is expelling any products of conception. She should refrain from having sexual intercourse, because coitus is likely to increase bleeding and cramping. A light or regular diet is satisfactory. She does not need to weigh herself daily. (I, N, G)

89. 4. In an incomplete abortion, part of the products of conception are retained—most commonly, the placenta. The internal cervical os has begun to dilate. In a missed abortion, the fetus dies in utero but is not expelled. If the fetus remains in utero beyond six weeks, fetal autolysis results in the release of thromboplastin, and disseminated intravascular coagulation (DIC) can develop. A threatened abortion results when bleeding and cramping occur but the cervix remains closed and no products of conception have been expelled. An induced abortion is an elective termination of the pregnancy. (D, N, G)

90. 2. Butorphanol tartrate (Stadol) exerts an analgesic effect. It does not prevent nausea, cause uterine contraction, or control hemorrhage. (D, N, G)

91. 3. After a spontaneous abortion, the client and family members can be expected to suffer from grief for several months or longer. The acute phase of grieving lasts approximately 6 weeks. When offering support, a simple statement such as, "I'm sorry you lost your baby" is appropriate. Therapeutic communication techniques help the client and family understand the meaning of the loss, move less stressfully through the grief process, and share feelings. Asking why the client is crying suggests that the nurse sees no need for the client's sorrow. Offering the client an analgesic is not appropriate. Telling the client that she can get pregnant again is not therapeutic. (I, N, L)

92. 3. Pentazocine hydrochloride (Talwin) is an analgesic; it does not provide contraceptive protection, inhibit lactation, or promote uterine involution. (D, N, G)

93. 2. Crying and being overtly upset is related to the client's feeling of powerlessness over the loss. There is no information to support the nursing diagnoses of Knowledge Deficit, Spiritual Distress, or Anxiety. (D, N, L)

94. 2. Rh sensitization can be prevented by human anti-D globulin, which clears the maternal circulation of Rh-positive cells before sensitization can occur, thereby blocking maternal antibody production. (D, N, G)

NURSING CARE OF THE CHILDBEARING FAMILY AND THEIR NEONATE

TEST 1: Antepartum Care

Directions: Use this answer grid to determine areas of strength or need for further study.

NURSING PROCESS

A = Assessment
D = Analysis, nursing diagnosis
P = Planning
I = Implementation
E = Evaluation

COGNITIVE LEVEL

K = Knowledge
C = Comprehension
T = Application
N = Analysis

CLIENT NEEDS

S = Safe, effective care environment
G = Physiological integrity
L = Psychosocial integrity
H = Health promotion/maintenance

		Nursing Process					Cognitive Level				Client Needs			
Question #	Answer #	A	D	P	I	E	K	C	T	N	S	G	L	H
1	1				I				T					H
2	3				I					N				H
3	4			P						N				H
4	1				I					N				H
5	4		D							N				H
6	3					E				N				H
7	2	A							T					H
8	4			P						N				H
9	4				I					N				H
10	2					E				N				H
11	2					E				N				H
12	2			P						N				H
13	2				I					N				H
14	3				I					N				H
15	4				I					N				H
16	1				I					N				H
17	4					E				N				H
18	1		D							N				H
19	4	A								N				H
20	2		D							N				H
21	3					E				N				H
22	1		D							N			L	
23	1				I					N				H

ANSWER GRID: 1

NURSING PROCESS

A = Assessment
D = Analysis, nursing diagnosis
P = Planning
I = Implementation
E = Evaluation

COGNITIVE LEVEL

K = Knowledge
C = Comprehension
T = Application
N = Analysis

CLIENT NEEDS

S = Safe, effective care environment
G = Physiological integrity
L = Psychosocial integrity
H = Health promotion/maintenance

		Nursing Process					Cognitive Level				Client Needs			
Question #	Answer #	A	D	P	I	E	K	C	T	N	S	G	L	H
24	3			P						N				H
25	4				I					N				H
26	3				I					N	S			
27	1	A								N				H
28	2				I					N				H
29	1		D							N			L	
30	4		D							N				H
31	1		D							N				H
32	3				I					N				H
33	2				I				T					H
34	2			P						N				H
35	4				I					N				H
36	4				I					N		G		
37	1				I					N		G		
38	1					E				N		G		
39	4			P						N		G		
40	1				I					N		G		
41	4			P						N		G		
42	4		D							N		G		
43	4					E				N				H
44	1	A								N		G		
45	3	A								N		G		
46	1			P						N				H
47	4		D							N		G		
48	4		D							N		G		
49	1				I					N		G		
50	3				I					N		G		
51	3				I					N				H
52	3				I					N		G		

ANSWER GRID: 2

Nursing Process

A = Assessment
D = Analysis, nursing diagnosis
P = Planning
I = Implementation
E = Evaluation

Cognitive Level

K = Knowledge
C = Comprehension
T = Application
N = Analysis

Client Needs

S = Safe, effective care environment
G = Physiological integrity
L = Psychosocial integrity
H = Health promotion/maintenance

		Nursing Process					Cognitive Level				Client Needs			
Question #	Answer #	A	D	P	I	E	K	C	T	N	S	G	L	H
53	1				I					N		G		
54	4					E				N		G		
55	4			P						N				H
56	1					E				N				H
57	1		D							N				H
58	3		D							N				H
59	2				I					N				H
60	4				I					N				H
61	3				I					N				H
62	3					E				N				H
63	2				I					N				H
64	3			P						N				H
65	3			P						N				H
66	3			P						N				H
67	1				I					N				H
68	3					E				N				H
69	4				I					N				H
70	4				I					N				H
71	1	A								N			L	
72	4					E				N		G		
73	1				I					N		G		
74	2				I					N				H
75	1			P						N				H
76	1			P						N				H
77	1			P						N				H
78	4				I					N				H
79	2				I					N		G		
80	4					E				N		G		
81	3		D							N		G		

Answer Grid: 3

Nursing Process

A = Assessment
D = Analysis, nursing diagnosis
P = Planning
I = Implementation
E = Evaluation

Cognitive Level

K = Knowledge
C = Comprehension
T = Application
N = Analysis

Client Needs

S = Safe, effective care environment
G = Physiological integrity
L = Psychosocial integrity
H = Health promotion/maintenance

		Nursing Process					Cognitive Level				Client Needs			
Question #	Answer #	A	D	P	I	E	K	C	T	N	S	G	L	H
82	1			P						N				H
83	2				I					N				H
84	2				I					N				H
85	2					E				N				H
86	1			P						N		G		
87	2		D							N		G		
88	3				I					N		G		
89	4		D							N		G		
90	2		D							N		G		
91	3				I					N			L	
92	3		D							N		G		
93	2		D							N			L	
94	2		D							N		G		
Number Correct														
Number Possible	94	6	19	17	38	14	0	0	3	91	1	28	5	60
Percentage Correct														

Score Calculation:

To determine your **Percentage Correct**, divide the **Number Correct** by the **Number Possible**.

Complications of Pregnancy

Test 2

The Client With Pregnancy-Induced Hypertension
Pregnant Clients With Hypertensive Disorders
The Pregnant Client With Third Trimester Bleeding
The Pregnant Client With Preterm Labor
The Pregnant Client With Diabetes Mellitus
The Client With an Ectopic Pregnancy
The Pregnant Client With a Hydatidiform Mole
The Pregnant Client With Premature Rupture of the Membranes
Correct Answers and Rationale

Select the one best answer and indicate your choice by filling in the circle in front of the option.

The Client With Pregnancy-Induced Hypertension

A 17-year-old unmarried client visits the prenatal clinic at 32 weeks gestation. She has been receiving care at the clinic and has early signs of pregnancy-induced hypertension.

1. The nurse assesses the client for possible risk factors for pregnancy-induced hypertension. Which of the following would be most important for the nurse to assess?
- ○ 1. Primigravid status.
- ○ 2. Unmarried status.
- ○ 3. ABO incompatibility.
- ○ 4. Upper socioeconomic level.

2. The nurse assesses the client for symptoms typical of mild pregnancy-induced hypertension. Which of the following data indicate mild pregnancy-induced hypertension?
- ○ 1. Blood pressure of 160/110 mm Hg on two separate occasions.
- ○ 2. Proteinuria, >5 grams/24 hours.
- ○ 3. Urine output <400 ml/24 hours.
- ○ 4. Swelling of fingers, hands, face, and ankles.

3. The nurse formulates a nursing diagnosis for the client. Which of the following would be most appropriate?
- ○ 1. Knowledge Deficit related to diet and exercise during pregnancy.
- ○ 2. Fluid Volume Deficit related to fluid shift from intravascular to extravascular space.
- ○ 3. High Risk for Injury related to cerebral vasospasm.
- ○ 4. High Risk for Injury to fetus related to inadequate placental perfusion.

4. The nurse assesses the client's blood pressure. Which of the following data would confirm the client's diagnosis of mild pregnancy-induced hypertension?
- ○ 1. Systolic blood pressure of at least 140 mm Hg.
- ○ 2. Diastolic blood pressure above 90 mm Hg.
- ○ 3. An increase in systolic and diastolic pressures of at least 20 mm Hg above baseline pressures.
- ○ 4. An increase above baseline pressure of at least 30 mm Hg systolic and 15 mm Hg diastolic.

5. The nurse plans to instruct the client in care while the client is at home. Which of the following is an appropriate goal for the client? The client will
- ○ 1. return to the prenatal clinic in 1 month.
- ○ 2. exhibit decreased edema following 1 week of a low-protein, low-salt diet.
- ○ 3. rest on the left side during the day, with bathroom privileges.
- ○ 4. immediately report adverse reactions from oral magnesium sulfate medication.

6. The nurse teaches the client about how pregnancy-induced hypertension affects the growing fetus. The nurse realizes that the client needs further instruc-

tions when she says that pregnancy-induced hypertension can lead to
○ 1. stillbirth.
○ 2. prematurity.
○ 3. congenital anomalies.
○ 4. intrauterine growth retardation.

A 21-year-old primigravida is diagnosed with mild pregnancy-induced hypertension at 36 weeks gestation. She is being treated at home and visits the prenatal clinic twice weekly.

7. The nurse instructs the client to keep a record of fetal movement patterns at home. The nurse determines that the instructions are effective when the client says that she will count the number of times the baby moves
○ 1. during a 10-minute period three times a day.
○ 2. for 20 minutes after lunch each day.
○ 3. for 30 minutes every morning before arising.
○ 4. during a 12-hour period.

8. The nurse plans to instruct the client about nutrition during pregnancy. The teaching plan includes instructing the client to avoid overcooking vegetables, because this practice destroys vitamin
○ 1. A.
○ 2. C.
○ 3. E.
○ 4. K.

9. The client reports that she has been taking a supplemental mineral and vitamin preparation daily. In addition to the mineral and vitamin supplement, the nurse instructs the client to increase her dietary intake of
○ 1. iron.
○ 2. vitamin D.
○ 3. magnesium.
○ 4. riboflavin.

10. The client states that she frequently ingests clay. The nurse assesses the client for symptoms of
○ 1. obesity.
○ 2. lactose intolerance.
○ 3. hypocalcemia.
○ 4. anemia.

11. At the nurse's request, the client records her typical daily menu as follows:

Breakfast: 4 oz. orange juice, two pieces of toast, two strips of bacon, and coffee with sugar
Lunch: bean burrito and cola drink
Dinner: beef and bean taco salad in a flour tortilla shell and iced tea.
Snack: two cookies

Which of the following food supplements to this menu would best provide the necessary nutrients for the client for one day?
○ 1. One glass of milk with each meal, one egg, one serving of green beans, one serving of broccoli, one pear, and one apple.
○ 2. One vanilla milkshake, one serving of meat, one banana, and two slices of bread with two pats of margarine.
○ 3. One glass of milk with each meal and one at bedtime, one dish of custard, one serving of meat, one apple, and one banana.
○ 4. One glass of milk with each meal, two eggs, two slices of whole wheat bread, two pats of margarine, one apple, and one serving of sliced carrots.

A 26-year-old primipara visits the prenatal clinic for her regular visit at 34 weeks gestation. She is diagnosed with mild pregnancy-induced hypertension.

12. The client tells the nurse she takes mineral oil for occasional constipation. The nurse instructs the client to
○ 1. take the mineral oil with juice to increase the action of the mineral oil.
○ 2. avoid mineral oil because it interferes with the absorption of fat soluble vitamins.
○ 3. avoid mineral oil because it causes nausea and vomiting in pregnant clients.
○ 4. use the mineral oil at least every other day or as needed to prevent constipation.

13. When the client complains of flatulence, the nurse instructs her to
○ 1. decrease the number of meals eaten each day.
○ 2. avoid eating gas producing foods.
○ 3. drink carbonated beverages several times a day.
○ 4. drink a teaspoon of bicarbonate of soda in water as necessary.

14. The client asks the nurse what causes heartburn. The nurse explains that heartburn during pregnancy is due to
○ 1. increased peristaltic action.
○ 2. displacement of the stomach by the uterus.
○ 3. increased secretion of hydrochloric acid.
○ 4. backflow of stomach contents into the esophagus.

15. The nurse asks the client how often the baby has moved today. She replies that she hasn't counted the baby's movements today, but that yesterday the baby moved six times over a 12-hour period. The nurse determines that the fetus
○ 1. requires follow-up evaluation by a physician.

○ 2. is showing signs of central nervous system maturation.
○ 3. could be experiencing an increase in deep sleep periods.
○ 4. is moving an adequate number of times.

16. One week following her prenatal visit, the client calls the nurse and says she has had a continuous headache for two days. She says she is nauseated and does not want to take aspirin. Which of the following responses by the nurse is most appropriate?
○ 1. "Take two Tylenol tablets. They aren't as likely to upset your stomach."
○ 2. "I think the doctor should see you today. Can you come to the clinic this morning?"
○ 3. "I can't prescribe on the telephone. I will make an appointment for you for next week."
○ 4. "I'll talk to the doctor and have a prescription for some medication phoned in to your pharmacy."

A 17-year-old primipara at 38 weeks gestation is scheduled for admission to the hospital with a diagnosis of severe pregnancy-induced hypertension.

17. In reviewing the client's prenatal records, which of the following data would be most indicative of the client's diagnosis of severe pregnancy-induced hypertension?
○ 1. Polyuria.
○ 2. Urine specific gravity of 1.04.
○ 3. Proteinuria below 3 grams in 24 hours.
○ 4. Weight gain of less than 1 pound in 1 week.

18. In planning for the client's admission, the nurse selects the most appropriate room for the client from the following available choices?
○ 1. A brightly lit room close to the nurse's station.
○ 2. A room in the intensive care unit where the client can be monitored.
○ 3. A quiet room where staff can observe the client frequently.
○ 4. A room on a surgical unit where the client can be transferred quickly to the operating room if necessary.

19. When preparing the room before the client's admission, the nurse should make sure that which of the following equipment is readily available in the room?
○ 1. Ultrasonography machine.
○ 2. Padded siderails.
○ 3. In-and-out catheterization kit.
○ 4. Flashlight.

20. Soon after admission, the physician orders 5% dextrose in Ringer's solution and magnesium sulfate intravenously. Before administering the magnesium sulfate, the nurse should first assess
○ 1. fetal heart rate.
○ 2. maternal pulse rate.
○ 3. maternal temperature.
○ 4. maternal respiratory rate.

21. The nurse monitors the client during magnesium sulfate administration. If the client develops magnesium toxicity, the nurse obtains the antidote drug
○ 1. calcium gluconate.
○ 2. diazepam (Valium).
○ 3. levallorphan (Lorfan).
○ 4. nalorphine hydrochloride (Nalline).

22. The nurse assesses the client receiving magnesium sulfate for symptoms of hypermagnesemia. An important sign for the nurse to note first is
○ 1. hyperactivity.
○ 2. rapid pulse rate.
○ 3. tingling in the fingers.
○ 4. decreased deep tendon reflexes.

A 15-year-old primigravida at 34 weeks gestation is admitted to the hospital via ambulance. She is taken to the labor area with a diagnosis of severe pregnancy-induced hypertension. On admission, her blood pressure is 150/100 mm Hg and her reflexes are +3 with no clonus.

23. In planning for the client's care, the nurse formulates which of the following priority goals?
○ 1. The client will not develop seizures during the first 48 hours.
○ 2. The client will exhibit decreased generalized edema within 12 hours.
○ 3. The client will have increased urinary output within 4 hours.
○ 4. The client will be sedated and have decreased reflex excitability within 12 hours.

24. A continuous intravenous infusion of 5% dextrose in Ringer's solution is administered. Which of the following signs should the nurse report immediately?
○ 1. Proteinuria.
○ 2. Facial flushing.
○ 3. Moist rales in lung fields.
○ 4. Urinary output exceeding intake.

25. The client's blood pressure climbs to 164/110 mm Hg. Which of the following symptoms would suggest to the nurse that the client may be about to convulse?
○ 1. Fetal movements.
○ 2. Severe headache.
○ 3. Feeling of warmth.
○ 4. Inability to void.

26. If the client begins to convulse due to eclampsia, the nurse's first action is to
○ 1. pad the siderails.

○ 2. apply wrist and ankle restraints.
○ 3. increase the flow rate of the intravenous infusion.
○ 4. suction the mouth and nasopharynx to keep the airway open.

27. The nurse should suggest that the client assume which position while on bedrest?
○ 1. Supine.
○ 2. Semi-Fowler's.
○ 3. Left lateral.
○ 4. Trendelenburg.

28. The nurse formulates a nursing diagnosis for the client. The most appropriate diagnosis at this time is
○ 1. High Risk for Injury related to possibility of convulsions.
○ 2. Knowledge Deficit related to signs and symptoms of pregnancy-induced hypertension.
○ 3. Fluid Volume Deficit related to inadequate fluid intake.
○ 4. Noncompliance related to inability to cope with the situation.

A 16-year-old unmarried primigravida at approximately 35 weeks gestation is admitted to the hospital's labor unit in early active labor, accompanied by her mother. The client has been seen in the prenatal clinic twice weekly for the last 2 weeks for mild pregnancy-induced hypertension.

29. After admission, the client tells the nurse about the baby's father. While assessing the client's support systems, the nurse gathers additional data. If the relationship between the client and the baby's father is typical, the father is most likely
○ 1. an older man who has taken advantage of the client.
○ 2. a younger male with whom the client has engaged in sexual experimentation.
○ 3. one of many males with whom the client has had a series of casual sexual relationships.
○ 4. a member of the client's peer group with whom the client has had a long-term sexual relationship.

30. The client asks the nurse, "What is the cure for my high blood pressure?" The nurse's best response is
○ 1. strict bedrest.
○ 2. delivery of the infant.
○ 3. sedation with magnesium sulfate.
○ 4. administration of hydralazine (Apresoline).

31. The nurse assesses the client for symptoms of HELLP syndrome. Which of the following data would require the nurse to notify the physician immediately?
○ 1. Platelet count >100,000.
○ 2. Hemoglobin 12.5.
○ 3. Epistaxis.
○ 4. Facial flushing.

The Client With a Hypertensive Disorder

A 36-year-old multigravida visits the prenatal clinic for the first time at 8 weeks gestation. She has been diagnosed with chronic hypertension and is taking methyldopa (Aldomet) daily.

32. When counseling the client about diet during pregnancy, the nurse realizes that the client needs further instruction when she says
○ 1. "I should eliminate all salt from my diet."
○ 2. "A high-protein diet is recommended."
○ 3. "Moderate salt intake is okay."
○ 4. "I need to eat more meat and beans each day."

33. The client's blood pressure is 160/110 mm Hg. The client asks the nurse if she will need to continue taking medication for hypertension. The nurse's best response is that the antihypertensive drug of choice during pregnancy is
○ 1. phenobarbital.
○ 2. diazepam.
○ 3. methyldopa.
○ 4. morphine.

34. After instructing the client about the need for frequent prenatal visits, the nurse determines that the instructions have been effective when the client says
○ 1. "I may develop rheumatic heart disease because of my high blood pressure."
○ 2. "I need to be monitored closely because I may develop preeclampsia."
○ 3. "I may have a very large infant and will probably need a cesarean section."
○ 4. "I may develop placenta previa, so I need to be monitored carefully."

The Client With Third Trimester Bleeding

A 28-year-old gravida 2, para 1 at 32 weeks gestation is admitted to the hospital because of vaginal bleeding.

35. In planning the client's care, one of the first actions the nurse lists in the nursing care plan is to
○ 1. perform a vaginal examination.
○ 2. provide a cleansing enema.
○ 3. shave the abdomen and perineal area.
○ 4. check the fetal heart rate and maternal blood pressure.

36. The nurse assesses the client for symptoms of abruptio placenta, noting especially
○ 1. uterine contractions.
○ 2. abdominal rigidity.
○ 3. lack of pain.
○ 4. early membrane rupture.

37. While collecting data about the client's life-style, which of the following factors might lead the nurse to suspect a medical diagnosis of abruptio placenta?
○ 1. Cigarette smoking.
○ 2. History of placenta accreta.
○ 3. Previous low transverse cesarean delivery.
○ 4. Malnutrition.

38. The nurse assesses the client for symptoms of placenta previa, noting especially
○ 1. painless vaginal bleeding.
○ 2. a boardlike fundus.
○ 3. intermittent pain with spotting.
○ 4. dull lower abdominal pain.

39. The client asks, "What's the difference between abruptio placenta and placenta previa?" The nurse's best response is to explain that implantation of abruptio placenta is
○ 1. normal.
○ 2. abnormal.
○ 3. outside the uterus.
○ 4. in the lower uterine segment.

40. If the client develops symptoms of disseminated intravascular coagulation and hypofibrinogenemia as a sequelae to abruptio placenta, the nurse would plan to
○ 1. assist with a cesarean section.
○ 2. administer whole blood.
○ 3. administer fresh frozen plasma.
○ 4. assist with a double setup.

A 34-year-old multigravida at 36 weeks gestation is admitted to the hospital with a diagnosis of partial placenta previa.

41. In explaining the diagnosis, the nurse tells the client that the partial placenta previa implantation site
○ 1. is near the internal cervical os.
○ 2. covers the entire internal cervical os.
○ 3. covers a portion of the internal cervical os.
○ 4. lies within 5 cm of the internal cervical os.

42. After giving instructions about the cause of the vaginal bleeding, the nurse determines that the teaching has been effective when the client says that the bleeding results from
○ 1. premature labor.
○ 2. a heavy bloody show.
○ 3. a large-for-gestational age fetus.
○ 4. exposure of maternal blood sinuses.

43. The nurse formulates a nursing diagnosis for the client soon after admission. Which of the following nursing diagnoses is most appropriate at this time?
○ 1. Fluid Volume Deficit related to vaginal bleeding.
○ 2. Fear related to unknown outcome of fetus.
○ 3. Pain related to uterine contractions.
○ 4. Ineffective Family Coping related to hospitalization.

44. The client begins to have excessive vaginal bleeding soon after admission, and an emergency cesarean section is planned. In planning care for the client, the first nursing measure should be to
○ 1. shave the abdomen and perineal area.
○ 2. ask family members to wait in the waiting room.
○ 3. check the status of the fetus.
○ 4. start intravenous fluid infusion.

45. Following the cesarean delivery, the nurse assesses the client for possible uterine atony by
○ 1. checking the skin sutures every 15 minutes for 1 hour.
○ 2. supporting the incision and palpating the fundus every 15 minutes for 1 hour.
○ 3. observing the amount of lochia immediately after delivery.
○ 4. noting the amount of bleeding on the abdominal dressings.

The Client With Preterm Labor

A multigravida at 28 weeks gestation is admitted to a perinatal center with contractions of moderate intensity occurring every 3 to 4 minutes. The client, who has previously delivered two nonviable fetuses, is crying on admission. She is accompanied by her husband.

46. The client is a candidate for therapy with ritodrine (Yutopar). Which of the following would be most important for the nurse to assess before beginning ritodrine therapy?
○ 1. Level of consciousness.
○ 2. Fatigue level.
○ 3. Estimated fetal size.
○ 4. Cervical dilatation.

47. After gathering initial assessment data, the nurse formulates a nursing diagnosis for the client. The most appropriate nursing diagnosis at this time is
○ 1. Pain related to intense uterine ischemia.
○ 2. Ineffective Family Coping related to constant attention to pregnancy.
○ 3. Noncompliance related to treatment of preterm labor.

○ 4. Fear related to unknown outcome of labor and possible preterm delivery.

48. While administering intravenous ritodrine the nurse assesses the client for which common side effect?
- ○ 1. Obesity.
- ○ 2. Seizure activity.
- ○ 3. Itching.
- ○ 4. Tachycardia.

49. The nurse monitors the client's laboratory studies during ritodrine therapy. The nurse explains to the client that an increase in blood plasma volume is confirmed by
- ○ 1. decreased hemoglobin level.
- ○ 2. protein in the urine.
- ○ 3. decreased blood glucose levels.
- ○ 4. increased serum calcium levels.

50. The client's contractions are monitored with an external electronic monitor. The nurse places the tokodynamometer disc
- ○ 1. over the top of the fundus.
- ○ 2. over the body of the fetus.
- ○ 3. on the left side of the abdomen.
- ○ 4. at the site of discomfort during a contraction.

51. The external electronic monitor is used to monitor the fetal heart rate. If the fetus is in left occipitoanterior position, the nurse should place the transducer
- ○ 1. near the client's umbilicus.
- ○ 2. 2 inches above the symphysis pubis.
- ○ 3. over the fetal back.
- ○ 4. midway between the client's umbilicus and symphysis pubis.

A 34-year-old multigravida at 36 weeks gestation is admitted to the hospital. The client has experienced two stillbirths.

52. On admission to the antenatal unit, the nurse determines that the fetal heart rate is 140 beats per minute. The nurse should
- ○ 1. document this as an abnormal reading.
- ○ 2. notify the attending physician.
- ○ 3. continue to monitor the client and fetus.
- ○ 4. check the fetal heart rate again in 5 minutes.

53. An ultrasound is scheduled for the client before an amniocentesis. After teaching the client about the purpose of the ultrasound, the nurse determines that the client needs further instruction when she says that ultrasound is done to
- ○ 1. locate the placenta.
- ○ 2. measure the biparietal diameter.
- ○ 3. determine where to insert the needle.
- ○ 4. identify a pool of amnionic fluid.

54. The client asks, "Why is the L/S ratio so important?" The nurse's best response is that a lecithin/sphingomyelin (L/S) ratio of 2:1 indicates fetal
- ○ 1. lung maturity.
- ○ 2. congenital anomalies.
- ○ 3. coagulation defects.
- ○ 4. kidney maturity.

55. The nurse formulates a nursing diagnosis for the client. The most appropriate diagnosis for a client undergoing antenatal testing is
- ○ 1. Pain related to the diagnostic testing.
- ○ 2. Anxiety related to diagnostic tests for fetal well-being.
- ○ 3. Ineffective Family Coping related to hospitalization.
- ○ 4. Fear related to impending labor and delivery.

56. To instruct the client about the "shake test" to be performed on the amnionic fluid, the nurse should plan to explain that the "shake test" evaluates the stability of the foam after amnionic fluid, normal saline, and ethyl alcohol are combined and helps determine the maturity of the fetal
- ○ 1. biliary system.
- ○ 2. urinary system.
- ○ 3. vascular system.
- ○ 4. pulmonary system.

57. After teaching the client about potential complications following amniocentesis that must be reported immediately, the nurse determines that the client understands the instructions when she says that she should immediately report
- ○ 1. nausea.
- ○ 2. vaginal bleeding.
- ○ 3. urinary frequency.
- ○ 4. irregular, painless uterine tightness.

The Client With Diabetes Mellitus

A 27-year-old primigravida at 20 weeks gestation is seen in the high-risk prenatal clinic. She is an insulin-dependent diabetic.

58. A nonstress test is performed, and the results are documented as reactive. The nurse tells the client that the test results indicate
- ○ 1. fetal heart rate accelerations and well-being.
- ○ 2. the need for a contraction stress test.
- ○ 3. the need for continuous monitoring.
- ○ 4. no evidence of fetal anomalies.

59. A contraction stress test is scheduled after explaining the purpose of the test, the nurse determines that the client understands the instructions when she states that the test is done to detect fetal

○ 1. cardiac anomalies.
○ 2. compromise during contractions.
○ 3. breathing movements.
○ 4. amnionic fluid volume.

60. The client states that the contraction stress test performed 1 week ago was negative. The nurse determines that the fetal heart rate pattern showed
○ 1. no late decelerations.
○ 2. frequent accelerations.
○ 3. inconsistent late decelerations.
○ 4. no accelerations.

61. The client is scheduled for a fetal biophysical profile. To instruct the client about this test, the nurse plans to explain that it
○ 1. provides results in approximately 2 weeks.
○ 2. is an uncomfortable invasive procedure.
○ 3. requires the client to be NPO for 8 hours before the test.
○ 4. is noninvasive and yields rapid results.

A 30-year-old multigravida at 10 weeks gestation is receiving prenatal care in a high-risk clinic. She is an insulin-dependent diabetic.

62. The nurse discusses the importance of keeping blood glucose levels near normal throughout the pregnancy. The nurse explains to the client that as pregnancy progresses, her insulin needs will
○ 1. increase.
○ 2. decrease.
○ 3. remain constant.
○ 4. cannot be predicted.

63. After explaining the complications of pregnancy that occur with diabetes, the nurse determines that the client needs further instruction when she says that one complication is
○ 1. infection.
○ 2. ketoacidosis.
○ 3. oligohydramnios.
○ 4. pregnancy-induced hypertension.

64. When planning to teach the client how to monitor glucose control and insulin dosage at home, the nurse should explain that the most accurate method for glucose assessment is
○ 1. urine testing.
○ 2. blood glucose testing.
○ 3. 50 g 1-hour screen.
○ 4. 3-hour glucose tolerance testing.

65. The client reports that she participated in strenuous aerobic exercise before becoming pregnant. She asks the nurse if she can continue exercising. What is the nurse's best response?
○ 1. "You probably should discontinue exercising while pregnant."
○ 2. "You need to ask your doctor if this type of exercise will affect the fetus."
○ 3. "You can continue exercising as before, but you should eat a carbohydrate or protein snack before exercising."
○ 4. "It's probably not a good idea, this type of exercise could injure the developing fetus."

66. After teaching about symptoms of hypoglycemia and hyperglycemia, the nurse determines that the client understands the instructions when she says that hypoglycemia may be manifested by
○ 1. polyuria.
○ 2. fatigue.
○ 3. drowsiness.
○ 4. nervousness.

67. At 39 weeks gestation, the client is admitted to the hospital for induction of labor. The client receives intravenous infusions of 5% glucose solution and of insulin. If at 10 a.m. the client's blood glucose level is 80 mg/100 ml of blood and at 11 a.m. it is 90 mg/100 ml, the nurse should
○ 1. increase the insulin dosage immediately.
○ 2. decrease the insulin dosage promptly.
○ 3. keep the insulin dosage unchanged.
○ 4. obtain another bloood glucose reading.

68. The client asks the nurse about insulin needs during the postpartum period. The nurse should instruct the client that during the postpartum period, insulin requirements
○ 1. fall significantly.
○ 2. usually increase.
○ 3. depend on the length of labor.
○ 4. increase if the client breast-feeds.

The Client With an Ectopic Pregnancy

A 24-year-old client is admitted to the hospital. It is suspected that she is pregnant, with gestation occurring outside the uterus.

69. Because the client is suspected of having an ectopic pregnancy, on admission it is particularly important for the nurse to assess whether or not she
○ 1. has recently had intercourse.
○ 2. has been pregnant before.
○ 3. is currently taking birth control pills.
○ 4. knows when her last menstrual period began.

70. Sonography confirms that the client has an ectopic pregnancy. The nurse explains that in an ectopic pregnancy, implantation of the fertilized ovum most commonly occurs in the

○ 1. ovary.
○ 2. cervix.
○ 3. fallopian tube.
○ 4. peritoneal cavity.

71. The nurse formulates a nursing diagnosis for the client soon after admission. The most appropriate diagnosis for the client is
○ 1. Anticipatory Grieving related to the loss of the pregnancy.
○ 2. Fear related to the outcome of the pregnancy.
○ 3. Ineffective Family Coping related to hospitalization.
○ 4. High Risk for Infection related to probable urinary stasis.

72. The nurse assesses the client for symptoms of a tubal rupture, noting especially
○ 1. uncontrollable vomiting.
○ 2. sharp abdominal pain.
○ 3. excessive vaginal bleeding.
○ 4. marked abdominal distention.

73. The client is scheduled for emergency surgery. Before surgery, the nurse assesses the client's blood pressure and
○ 1. uterine cramping.
○ 2. pupillary reflexes.
○ 3. vaginal discharge.
○ 4. pulse rate.

A 36-year-old client is admitted to the hospital with possible ruptured ectopic pregnancy.

74. For which of the following procedures should the nurse plan to prepare the client soon after admission?
○ 1. Dilatation and curettage.
○ 2. Culdocentesis.
○ 3. Evacuation of the uterus.
○ 4. Shirodkar-Barter cerclage.

75. After admission, it is most important for the nurse to assess the client's health history for
○ 1. infectious hepatitis.
○ 2. incompetent cervix.
○ 3. late onset of menarche.
○ 4. pelvic inflammatory disease.

76. Following surgery, the nurse instructs the client about potential complications. The nurse determines that the client needs further instructions when she states that a potential complication is
○ 1. pain.
○ 2. edema.
○ 3. fever.
○ 4. bleeding.

The Client With a Hydatidiform Mole

A multiparous client thought to be at 16 weeks gestation (based on uterine size) calls the prenatal clinic and reports that she is experiencing such severe morning sickness that she has not "been able to keep anything down for 3 days."

77. On receiving the call, the nurse should recommend that the client
○ 1. take sips of carbonated beverages.
○ 2. come to the prenatal clinic that day.
○ 3. consider obtaining psychological counseling.
○ 4. eat saltine crackers before arising in the morning.

78. The client visits the clinic. Due to the client's excessive vomiting, the nurse assesses her urine for
○ 1. protein.
○ 2. albumin.
○ 3. glucose.
○ 4. acetone.

79. If the client's excessive vomiting continues, the nurse should assess for symptoms of
○ 1. hypocalcemia.
○ 2. hyponatremia.
○ 3. hypokalemia.
○ 4. hypoglycemia.

80. The nurse explains to the client that hyperemesis gravidarum is thought to be related to high levels of the hormone
○ 1. progesterone.
○ 2. estrogen.
○ 3. somatotropin.
○ 4. gonadotropin.

81. The client is admitted to the hospital for further evaluation. Based on the client's history, it is particularly important that the nurse further assess for
○ 1. abdominal pain.
○ 2. bright red bleeding.
○ 3. yellowish vaginal discharge.
○ 4. dehydration.

82. The client is to receive intravenous therapy and asks the nurse when she will be able to eat again. The nurse explains that oral intake of food and fluids will be
○ 1. withheld indefinitely until acidosis is corrected.
○ 2. given in small quantities when desired.
○ 3. given as clear liquids after 24 hours if vomiting stops.
○ 4. withheld until hyperalimentation and intravenous therapy successfully replace lost electrolytes.

A 38-year-old client at approximately 14 weeks gestation is admitted to the hospital with a diagnosis of complete hydatidiform mole.

83. Soon after admission, the nurse assesses the client for symptoms of
- ○ 1. pregnancy-induced hypertension.
- ○ 2. gestational diabetes.
- ○ 3. hypothyroidism.
- ○ 4. polycythemia.

84. Following a dilatation and curettage to evacuate the molar pregnancy, it is especially important that the nurse assess for
- ○ 1. hypertension.
- ○ 2. hemorrhage.
- ○ 3. abdominal distention.
- ○ 4. chorioamnionitis.

85. After explaining the need for follow-up care after evacuation of the mole, the nurse determines that the client understands the instructions when she says that she is at risk for developing
- ○ 1. severe anemia.
- ○ 2. choriocarcinoma.
- ○ 3. invasion of the mole into the ovaries.
- ○ 4. polyps in the fallopian tubes.

The Client With Premature Rupture of the Membranes

A 26-year-old client at 28 weeks gestation is admitted to the hospital with premature rupture of the membranes.

86. Following admission, it is particularly important for the nurse to assess for symptoms of
- ○ 1. urinary tract infection.
- ○ 2. uterine rupture.
- ○ 3. small-for-gestational age fetus.
- ○ 4. anemia.

87. The client begins to have contractions every 10 minutes. The physician orders intravenous magnesium sulfate. The nurse explains to the client that the primary purpose of magnesium sulfate is to
- ○ 1. provide sedation.
- ○ 2. combat hypomagnesia.
- ○ 3. improve fetal pulmonary function.
- ○ 4. inhibit contractions.

88. After 24 hours, the client's contractions stop. She is to be discharged with home monitoring. After teaching the client about preterm labor symptoms, the nurse determines that she needs further instructions when she says.
- ○ 1. "I should call the doctor if my contractions occur every hour for 4 hours."
- ○ 2. "If I start having contractions, I should empty my bladder."
- ○ 3. "I should report contractions occurring every 10 minutes for an hour."
- ○ 4. "I should lie on my left side if contractions begin."

89. The client is readmitted at 34 weeks gestation in active labor. The physician orders intramuscular administration of betamethazone. Following administration, the nurse plans to assess the client for symptoms of
- ○ 1. hypoglycemia.
- ○ 2. infection.
- ○ 3. urinary retention.
- ○ 4. hypertension.

90. The client delivers a viable male infant weighing 1,701 grams (3 lb, 12 oz), who is transferred to the neonatal intensive care unit. Following delivery, the nurse plans to assess the client for feelings of
- ○ 1. relief.
- ○ 2. euphoria.
- ○ 3. guilt.
- ○ 4. empathy.

CORRECT ANSWERS AND RATIONALE

The letters in parentheses following the rationale identify the step of the nursing process (A, D, P, I, E); cognitive level (K, C, T, N); and client need (S, G, L, H). See the Answer Grid for the key.

The Client With Pregnancy-Induced Hypertension

1. 1. Pregnancy-induced hypertension occurs more often in primigravidas, adolescents, women of lower socioeconomic status, primigravidas over age 35, women with family history of pregnancy-induced hypertension and women with additional complications such as multiple gestation, diabetes mellitus, Rh incompatibility, and hydatidiform mole. ABO incompatibility, upper socioeconomic status, and unmarried status are not risk factors. (A, N, G)

2. 4. Generalized edema, with swelling of the face, hands, fingers, and ankles, often occurs with mild pregnancy-induced hypertension. Blood pressure readings of 160 mm Hg systolic and 100 mm Hg diastolic, proteinuria, and oliguria (urine output <400 ml/24 hr) are signs of severe pregnancy-induced hypertension. (D, N, G)

3. 2. Based on the information provided, the most appropriate nursing diagnosis is Fluid Volume Deficit related to fluid shift from intravascular to extravascular space. There are no data to suggest knowledge Deficit or High Risk for Injury, either to the client or the fetus. The potential for these diagnoses exist, particularly if the client indicates a knowledge deficit or her condition deteriorates. (D, N, G)

4. 4. The diagnosis of mild pregnancy-induced hypertension is based on an increase of 30 mm Hg or greater in systolic pressure and 15 mm Hg or greater in diastolic pressure. From 120/80 mm Hg to 140/90 mm Hg is usually considered the general range of blood pressure in mild pregnancy-induced hypertension. Both systolic and diastolic pressures increase in pregnancy-induced hypertension (D, N, G)

5. 3. The client with mild-pregnancy induced hypertension is often treated at home. Restricting activities is of prime importance, and bed rest for most of the day is recommended. The left lateral recumbent position is recommended to decrease pressure on the vena cava, which increases venous return, circulatory volume, and renal and placental perfusion. A decrease in angiotensin II improves renal blood flow, lowers blood pressure, and increases diuresis. The client should be monitored twice weekly. Her diet needs to be well balanced, with ample protein. If magnesium sulfate is necessary, as in severe pregnancy-induced hypertension, the drug is usually administered intravenously. (P, N, G)

6. 3. Congenital anomalies are not associated with hypertensive disease. Such conditions as stillbirth, prematurity, and intrauterine growth retardation are associated with pregnancy-induced hypertension. (E, N, G)

7. 4. Numerous methods have been proposed to record the maternal perceptions of fetal movement. A commonly used method is the Cardiff "count to 10" method. The client begins counting fetal movements at a specified time (e.g., 8 A.M.), and notes the time when the tenth movement is felt. If 10 movements are not felt in a 12-hour period, the client should notify the health care provider. Another method involves monitoring the fetal movements over 1 hour. The client should report if fewer than three movements are felt. (E, N, G)

8. 2. Heat destroys certain nutrients in food, particularly water-soluble vitamins such as vitamin C, thiamine, and folacin. Therefore, it is best to cook vegetables in the shortest time and with the least amount of water possible. It is preferable to eat raw fruits and vegetables when possible. (P, N, G)

9. 1. A healthy, well-balanced diet can provide adequate amounts of all vitamins and minerals except iron and folic acid. Supplemental vitamins are often prescribed to ensure adequate mineral and vitamin intake. (I, N, G)

10. 4. All pregnant clients should be screened for pica, or the ingestion of nonfood substances such as clay, dirt, or starch. Screening the client for anemia is important, because clients who practice pica commonly are anemic. Obesity, lactose intolerance, and hypocalcemia are not usually associated with pica. (A, N, G)

11. 1. According to the newest ADA guidelines, the recommended daily diet during pregnancy includes:

Dairy products: four servings
Meat: four servings
Breads and cereals: four or more servings
Vegetables: one serving of dark green or orange/yellow, two servings of others.
Fruits and fruit juices: one serving of citrus, two or more servings of others.

The client's diet includes no milk or dairy products. It does include four servings of meat/protein, one serving of vegetables (salad), and four servings of bread products. Therefore, the client needs four servings of dairy products (three glasses of milk, one egg), two servings of vegetables (e.g., green beans, broccoli), and two servings of fruit or fruit juices (e.g., pear, apple). (D, N, G)

12. 2. The client should be advised to avoid taking mineral oil because it interferes with absorption of fat-soluble vitamins from the intestinal tract. Harsh laxatives are contraindicated. If dietary measures and increased fluid intake do not prevent constipation and a mild laxative is indicated, the client should contact the physician or other health care provider. A stool softener or a mild laxative may be prescribed. Mineral oil does not cause nausea and vomiting. (I, N, G)

13. 2. Flatulence is an annoying and fairly common discomfort of pregnancy. Suggestions to help overcome it include avoiding large meals, chewing food well, and avoiding gas-producing foods, such as carbonated beverages. Bicarbonate of soda should be avoided during pregnancy because of the potential for electrolyte imbalance. (I, N, H)

14. 4. Heartburn is caused by stomach contents entering the distal end of the esophagus, producing a burning sensation. (I, N, H)

15. 1. Fewer than 10 fetal movements in a 12-hour period is not reassuring and should be reported to the physician. (D, N, G)

16. 2. A client with pregnancy-induced hypertension complaining of a continuous headache for 2 days should be seen by a health care provider immediately. Continuous headache is a symptom of severe pregnancy-induced hypertension, and immediate care is recommended. (I, N, G)

17. 2. Signs of severe pregnancy-induced hypertension include blood pressure of 160/110 mm Hg or greater measured at two different times at least 6 hours apart, oliguria, proteinuria of 5 g or greater in 24 hours and a urine specific gravity of 1.04 or greater. (D, N, H)

18. 3. The client with severe pregnancy-induced hypertension may develop eclampsia, characterized by convulsions. To decrease the likelihood of convulsions, it would be best to place this client in a quiet room. This helps decrease unnecessary stimuli that could trigger a convulsion. The room should be conveniently located for frequent observations by nursing personnel. In many hospitals, the client is admitted to the labor area, where she and the fetus can be closely monitored. (P, N, G)

19. 2. Because the client with severe pregnancy-induced hypertension may develop eclampsia and convulsions, certain equipment must be readily available should seizure activity start. Of the choices available, the padded side rails are the most appropriate choice. Other equipment should be available to aspirate mucus, to administer oxygen, to insert an indwelling catheter, and to administer emergency drugs. An indwelling catheter may be necessary to most accurately determine urine output. (P, N, G)

20. 4. A central nervous system depressant used as an anticonvulsant for severe pregnancy-induced hypertension, magnesium sulfate may depress respirations to a dangerously low and even life-threatening level. This drug should not be administered without first consulting the physician if the client's respiratory rate is below 12 to 14 breaths per minute. Although fetal heart rate and maternal temperature and pulse are important, respiratory rate is the most important vital sign to assess before administering magnesium sulfate. (I, N, G)

21. 1. The antidote for magnesium sulfate is calcium, commonly administered as calcium gluconate. It should be readily available when magnesium sulfate is being administered. Diazepam (Valium), levallorphan (Lorfan), and nalorphine hydrochloride (Nalline) are not antidotes for magnesium sulfate. (I, N, G)

22. 4. Typical signs of hypermagnesemia include decreased deep tendon reflexes, lethargy progressing to coma with increasing toxicity, and impaired respiration. The nurse should check the client's patellar, biceps, and radial reflexes regularly during magnesium sulfate therapy. Hyperactivity and tingling in the fingers are common symptoms of hypocalcemia. A rapid pulse rate commonly occurs in hypomagnesemia. (A, N, G)

23. 1. The highest priority for a client with severe pregnancy-induced hypertension is to prevent seizures and deliver the infant safely. Efforts to decrease edema, reduce blood pressure, increase urine output, limit kidney damage, and maintain sedation are desirable, but are not as important as preventing convulsions. (P, N, G)

24. 3. When assessing a client receiving an intravenous infusion, the nurse should promptly report moist rales in the lung fields, which indicate fluid overload and pulmonary edema. Proteinuria can be expected in the client with pregnancy-induced hypertension. Urine output greater than intake is desirable, because the client typically retains excess fluids. Flushed skin is probably unrelated to pregnancy-induced hypertension. (I, N, G)

25. 2. A common symptom of an impending convulsion is severe headache. Such symptoms as fetal movements, warmth, or inability to void are not precursors of an eclamptic convulsion. (D, N, G)

26. 4. The client showing signs of impending convulsion should be protected from injury. Suctioning mucus from the client's mouth and nasopharynx and administering oxygen can be done during the clonic phase, when thrashing has subsided. The side rails should have been padded before the client was placed in the bed, to prevent injury. Gentle restraint, best done with the nurse's hands, may be necessary during a convulsion, but restraining the client's arms and ankles is not advised. Increasing intravenous fluid infusion will not prevent a convulsion. (I, N, G)

27. 3. To prevent potential fetal injury from decreased placental perfusion, the best maternal position is the left lateral position. Supine, semi-Fowler's, and Trendelenburg positions are not advised for clients with severe pregnancy-induced hypertension. (I, N, G)

28. 1. The best nursing diagnosis at this time is High Risk for Injury related to possibility of convulsions. The client has severe pregnancy-induced hypertension with elevated blood pressure. There are no data to suggest Fluid Volume Deficit, Knowledge Deficit, or Noncompliance. (D, N, G)

29. 4. The partner of an unmarried pregnant adolescent is usually a member of her peer group. Usually, they have had a long-term relationship. (A, N, L)

30. 2. The only known cure for pregnancy-induced hypertension is delivery of the fetus. Early diagnosis and careful management are used to control the disorder. Medical treatment for severe pregnancy-induced hypertension includes bedrest, a high-protein, moderate-sodium diet, restoration of fluid and electrolyte balance, sedation, and antihypertensive medications. Medical treatment for eclampsia includes steps to control convulsions, correct hypoxia and acidosis, lower blood pressure, and stabilize the client for delivery. (I, N, G)

31. 3. HELLP syndrome involves hemolysis, elevated liver enzymes, and low platelet count (below 100,000). This syndrome is sometimes associated with severe pregnancy-induced hypertension. Women with HELLP syndrome and their offspring have high morbidity and mortality rates and should be cared for in a tertiary care center. Symptoms include anemia, pallor, fatigue, anorexia, and dyspnea. Signs of liver dysfunction include nausea and vomiting, right upper quadrant pain, jaundice, and malaise. Signs of disseminated intravascular coagulation (DIC)—epistaxis, hematuria, petechiae, bleeding gums, and GI tract bleeding—should be reported immediately. Platelet count greater than 100,000, hemoglobin of 12.5, and facial flushing are not symptomatic of HELLP syndrome or DIC. (D, N, G)

The Client With a Hypertensive Disorder

32. 1. Moderate salt intake is acceptable. Clients with chronic hypertension should have adequate protein intake. Protein intake of 1.5 g/kg of body weight is recommended for a client with proteinuria. Meat and beans are good sources of protein. (E, N, H)

33. 3. Methyldopa (Aldomet) is the antihypertensive drug of choice for pregnant clients with chronic hypertension. There is a risk of fetal depression with phenobarbital and diazepam (Valium). Morphine is usually administered intramuscularly or intravenously for sedation during labor. (I, N, G)

34. 2. Women with chronic hypertension during pregnancy are at risk for such complications as preeclampsia (about 25%), abruptio placenta, and intrauterine growth retardation. These clients do not have a greater risk for large fetuses, heart disease, or placenta previa. However, factors associated with placenta previa include multiparity and advanced maternal age. (E, N, G)

The Client With Third Trimester Bleeding

35. 4. When a client is admitted with bleeding in the third trimester of pregnancy, the nurse should first assess fetal heart rate and maternal blood pressure. Vaginal examination and an enema are contraindicated for this client, as excessive vaginal bleeding may occur if placenta previa is present. The client is not in labor and delivery is not imminent, so shaving the abdomen and perineal area is not necessary (I, N, G)

36. 2. The most typical symptom of abruptio placenta is a rigid or boardlike uterus. Pain is common. The amnion does not ordinarily rupture, nor do uterine contractions occur. (A, N, G)

37. 1. The true cause of abruptio placenta is unknown. Possible contributing factors include excessive intrauterine pressure caused by hydramnios or multiple pregnancy, cigarette smoking, alcohol ingestion, trauma, increased maternal age and parity, cocaine abuse, and amniotomy. A previous low transverse cesarean section delivery is associated with increased risk of placenta previa. History of placenta accreta or malnutrition is not associated with abruptio placenta. (D, N, G)

38. 1. The most characteristic sign of placenta previa is painless vaginal bleeding during the third trimester of pregnancy. Placenta previa occurs when the placenta attaches in the lower segment of the uterus or over the cervical os. Bleeding depends on the number of sinuses exposed. (A, N, G)

39. 1. Abruptio placenta is defined as the premature separation of a normally implanted placenta. (I, N, H)

40. 3. Treatment of hypofibrinogenemia includes administration of fresh frozen plasma. Anemia is treated by administering packed red cells. Vaginal birth without an episiotomy is the preferred method of delivery. A double setup is the procedure used to detect placenta previa. (P, N, G)

41. 3. Implantation of the partial placenta previa occurs over a portion of the internal cervical os, but it is not completely covered as in a complete placenta previa. A low placental implantation site is near the internal cervical os. (I, N, G)

42. 4. Bleeding precipitated by placenta previa results from exposure of the maternal sinuses when placental villi are torn from the uterine wall as the lower uterine segment contracts and dilates in the later weeks of pregnancy. Bleeding is not initiated because of premature labor, a heavy bloody show, or a large-for-gestational age fetus. (E, N, G)

43. 2. The most appropriate diagnosis at this time is Fear related to concern for own personal status and the outcome of the fetus. The client is only at 36 weeks gestation, and delivery would produce a preterm infant. There are no data to suggest Fluid Volume Deficit, Pain, or Ineffective Family Coping, although these are possible diagnoses for future care. (D, N, G)

44. 4. The client experiencing excessive blood loss prior to delivery needs fluid and/or blood replacement. The first priority is to begin intravenous infusion. Fetal heart rate should be monitored with continuous electronic monitoring equipment, and oxygen may be administered to alleviate hypoxia of the client and fetus. There is no need to ask the family members to leave, as the client may be fearful and family members can be supportive. An indwelling catheter is often required and the client may need an abdominal shave, but the priority is to start the intravenous infusion. (P, N, G)

45. 2. Every postpartum client, regardless of the type of delivery, is at risk for uterine atony and hemorrhage. Even though an abdominal incision and abdominal dressing are present, the nurse should palpate the fundus gently while supporting the incision every 15 minutes for at least 1 hour. This should be done more frequently if bleeding is moderate or severe. The nurse should also observe and note any bleeding on the abdominal incision dressings, but this is not an accurate measure of uterine atony. The sutures do not need to be inspected every 15 minutes. The nurse should note the amount of lochia immediately after delivery and during the recovery period, usually about 2 hours. (I, N, G)

The Client With Preterm Labor

46. 4. Pharmaceutical agents to suppress labor are ordinarily contraindicated for a client with cervical dilatation of 5 cm or greater. Level of consciousness, fatigue level, and estimated size of the fetus should be investigated but do not contraindicate the use of ritodrine. (A, N, G)

47. 4. For this client, who is crying on admission and has lost two fetuses in the past, the most appropriate diagnosis is Fear related to outcome of labor and possible preterm birth. No evidence in this situation suggests Pain related to uterine ischemia, Ineffective Family Coping, or Noncompliance. (D, N, L)

48. 4. Maternal side effects of ritodrine therapy include tachycardia, occasionally premature ventricular contractions, increased stroke volume, increased blood pressure, palpitations, tremors, nausea and vomiting, and shortness of breath. The physician should be notified before increasing the ritodrine dosage if maternal pulse is 120 beats per minute or greater. Other adverse effects include hyperglycemia, metabolic acidosis, pulmonary edema, increased plasma volume, and anemia. Obesity does not preclude using ritodrine. Itching and seizure activity are not associated with ritodrine therapy. (A, N, G)

49. 1. Increased blood plasma volume cause a type of blood dilution that causes a decrease in hemoglobin and hematocrit levels. Hyperglycemia, not hypoglycemia, is associated with ritodrine therapy. Proteinuria is not associated with ritodrine therapy and blood plasma volume. Increased serum calcium levels are not associated with ritodrine therapy. (I, N, S)

50. 1. As the uterus contracts, the abdominal wall rises and, when external monitoring is used, presses against the transducer. This movement is transmitted into an electrical current, which is then recorded. For best results, the tokodynamometer should be placed at the top of the fundus, where uterine displacement during contractions is greatest. (I, N, G)

51. 3. To monitor fetal heart rate, the best placement of the doppler is over the fetal back. (I, N, G)

52. 3. Fetal heart rate is normally between 120 and 160 beats per minute. The nurse should continue to monitor the client and fetus. This is not an abnormal reading, so there is no need to notify the physician. There is no indication that fetal heart rate needs to be checked again in 5 minutes. (I, N, G)

53. 2. Before amniocentesis, an ultrasound is valuable in locating the placenta, locating a pool of amnionic fluid, and showing the physician where to insert the needle. Assessing gestational age by measuring the biparietal diameter of the fetus is not a prerequisite to performing amniocentesis. Late in pregnancy, biparietal diameter may be difficult to measure because of fetal position or engagement. (E, N, S)

54. 1. A lecithin/sphingomyelin (L/S) ratio of 2:1 indicates fetal lung maturity. Lecithin is a major component of pulmonary surfactant in the fetus. Surfactant is necessary for lung expansion in the newborn. The L/S ratio does not detect congenital anomalies, coagulation defects, or kidney maturity. (I, N, S)

55. 2. For this client, who has experienced two stillbirths, the most appropriate diagnosis is Anxiety related to diagnostic tests for fetal well-being. There is minimal pain with most antepartal diagnostic tests. There is no indication that the client is demonstrating Ineffective Family Coping or Fear related to impending labor and delivery at this time. (D, N, L)

56. 4. The "shake test" helps determine the maturity of the fetal pulmonary system. The test is based on the fact that surfactant will foam when mixed with ethanol. The more stable the foam, the more mature the fetal pulmonary system. Although the "shake test" is inexpensive and provides rapid results, problems have been noted with its reliability. Fast-negative results can occur. For this reason, the L/S ratio is usually performed in conjunction with the "shake test." (P, N, S)

57. 2. Following amniocentesis, the client should promptly report vaginal discharge or bleeding or a decrease in fetal movement. Nausea, urinary frequency, and irregular painless uterine tightness (Braxton-Hicks contractions) are not complications of amniocentesis. (E, N, G)

The Client With Diabetes Mellitus

58. 1. A nonstress test that is reactive indicates fetal heart rate accelerations and well-being. The nonstress test is considered reactive when two or more fetal heart rate accelerations occur, along with fetal movement, during a 10- to 20-minute period. The baseline fetal heart rate should be in the normal range of 120–160 beats per minute. Each acceleration should have a duration of 15 seconds, and the acceleration should have an amplitude greater than 15 beats per minute. Based on a reactive nonstress test, there is no indication for a contraction stress test; however, contraction stress tests are often scheduled for insulin-dependent diabetic clients in the latter part of pregnancy. The client does not need continuous monitoring. The nonstress test does not detect fetal anomalies; however, cardiac abnormalities may be suspected if the fetal heart rate is abnormal. (I, N, G)

59. 2. The contraction stress test is performed on high-risk clients, such as insulin-dependent diabetic clients. The test subjects the fetus to uterine contractions, during which fetal heart rate is monitored. Contractions compress the arteries to the placenta. A fetus with adequate oxygen reserve will tolerate transient oxygen reductions, and the fetal heart rate will remain normal. The test is performed either by nipple stimulation, which releases oxytocin from the maternal posterior pituitary gland, or by intravenous oxytocin administration. The test is not performed to detect cardiac anomalies, breathing movements, or amnionic fluid volume. (E, N, G)

60. 1. A negative contraction stress test, indicating no fetal heart rate decelerations, is considered normal. A positive contraction stress test indicates fetal compromise. A suspicious contraction stress test would demonstrate inconsistent late decelerations. An absence of fetal heart rate accelerations is considered a nonreactive positive contraction stress test. (D, N, G)

61. 4. The fetal biophysical profile assesses five parameters: fetal heart rate reactivity, fetal breathing movements, gross fetal body movements, fetal tone, and amnionic fluid volume. Fetal heart rate reactivity is determined by a nonstress test, the other four parameters are by ultrasound scanning. The test is noninvasive, and results are available as soon as it is completed and interpreted. The procedure is not uncomfortable and does not require that the client be NPO for 8 hours before the test. (P, N, S)

62. 1. Progressive insulin resistance is characteristic of pregnancy. It is not unusual for insulin needs to increase by as much as four times the nonpregnant dose. This resistance is due to the production of human placental lactogen, also called human chorionic somatotropin (HCS), by the placenta. This hormone, and to a lesser degree, estrogen and progesterone, are insulin antagonists. (I, N, G)

63. 3. The pregnant diabetic client is at higher risk for complications, such as infection, polyhydramnios, and ketoacidosis, than the pregnant nondiabetic client. Infants of diabetic mothers may be larger than average and have a greater incidence of congenital anomalies. (E, N, G)

64. 2. The most accurate method for home glucose monitoring is blood testing. Various devices are available for blood glucose testing. Urine testing is not as accurate as blood testing. In pregnancy, the renal threshold for glucose is lower, resulting in lower urine glucose levels than usually seen in nonpregnant adults. The 50 g 1-hour test is used to screen pregnant women with risk factors for diabetes. The 3-hour glucose tolerance test is used to diagnose diabetes. (P, N, G)

65. 3. While pregnancy is not an optimum time to begin vigorous exercise, a well-controlled diabetic client who has regularly engaged in exercise may continue to do so. She should be reminded to eat a carbohydrate or protein snack before exercising to prevent hypoglycemia. The fetus is well protected in the amnionic sac, and exercise is not harmful. (I, N, G)

66. 4. Nervousness is an early sign of hypoglycemia. Polyuria, fatigue, and drowsiness are manifestations of hyperglycemia. Hypoglycemia is the most common cause of coma in clients with diabetes. (E, N, G)

67. 3. In general, it is desirable to maintain a blood glucose level between 60 mg/100 ml and 110 mg/100 ml. Because this client's blood glucose level is in the normal range, no action is required. Diabetic clients should have their blood glucose monitored hourly while labor is being induced. (I, N, G)

68. 1. During the postpartum period, insulin needs fall significantly. If the client breast-feeds, lower blood glucose levels decreases the insulin requirements. The length of the client's labor does not influence insulin needs. (I, N, H)

The Client With an Ectopic Pregnancy

69. 4. It may be important to obtain information from a client with suspected ectopic pregnancy concerning when she last had intercourse, whether she is taking birth control pills, and whether she has been pregnant previously. However, it is of particular importance to determine when she started her last normal menstrual period. Such information helps establish an accurate diagnosis. Usually the client with an ectopic pregnancy will have missed a menstrual period or two and often suspects or knows she is pregnant. If the client's menstrual cycle is irregular, she may be unaware she is pregnant. (A, N, G)

70. 3. An ectopic pregnancy is defined as any gestation located outside the uterus. Approximately 95% of ectopic pregnancies occur in the fallopian tube. (I, N, G)

71. 1. The most appropriate nursing diagnosis for this client is Anticipatory Grieving related to the loss of the pregnancy. This is a crisis for the client, and she needs emotional support. There are no data to suggest the diagnoses Fear, Ineffective Family Coping, or Infection related to urinary stasis. (D, N, L)

72. 2. The most common symptom of tubal rupture is severe abdominal pain and referred shoulder pain. The pain is knifelike in quality and in a lower abdominal quadrant. Slight vaginal bleeding, often described as spotting, also is common. Vomiting and abdominal distention are not associated with tubal rupture in ectopic pregnancy. (A, N, G)

73. 4. Fallopian tube rupture is an emergency situation because of extensive bleeding into the peritoneal cavity. Shock will soon develop if precautionary measures are not taken. The nurse readying a client for surgery should be especially careful to monitor blood pressure and pulse rate for signs of impending shock. The nurse should be prepared to administer fluids, blood, or plasma expanders as necessary through an intravenous line that should already be in place. (A, N, G)

74. 2. Symptoms of ruptured ectopic pregnancy are not always obvious. If bleeding into the pelvic cavity is extensive, then vaginal examination causes intense pain and blood is detected in the cul-de-sac of Douglas. Culdocentesis will validate the diagnosis. Aspiration of nonclotting blood is indicative of ectopic pregnancy. Laparoscopy, ultrasound, and laparotomy will also confirm the diagnosis. Dilatation and curettage is not indicated for ruptured ectopic pregnancy. The uterus is not evacuated, because the pregnancy is located outside the uterus. A Shirodkar-Barter cerclage is used for an incompetent cervix, not ectopic pregnancy. (P, N, S)

75. 4. Anything that causes a narrowing or constriction in the fallopian tubes so that a fertilized ovum cannot be properly transported to the uterus for implantation predisposes to an ectopic pregnancy. Pelvic inflammatory disease is the most common cause of constricted or narrow tubes. Developmental defects are other possible causes. The incidence of ectopic pregnancy has increased dramatically over the past several years. (A, N, G)

76. 2. The client should not experience edema. Symptoms that the client should report include pain, bleeding, and temperature elevation. (E, N, G)

The Client With a Hydatidiform Mole

77. 2. A client at 16 weeks gestation who has had "morning sickness" but now has been vomiting for 3 days should visit the clinic that day, if possible. Although early morning nausea often occurs in the first trimester, pernicious vomiting or hyperemesis gravidarum in the second trimester may indicate complications. The client's symptoms should be investigated further. (I, N, G)

78. 4. Combustion cannot be completed when fat is burned in the body in the absence of carbohydrates. Improper fat metabolism results in acetone and diacetic acid in the urine from the starvation this client is experiencing. All pregnant clients have their urine tested for protein and glucose; based on this client's symptoms, her urine should also be screened for acetone. (I, N, G)

79. 3. Gastrointestinal secretion losses from excessive vomiting, as well as from diarrhea and excessive perspiration, can result in hypokalemia, as well as acidosis, if precautionary measures are not taken. (A, N, G)

80. 2. Although the cause of hyperemesis is still unclear, it is thought to be related to high estrogen levels or to trophoblastic activity or gonadotrophin production. Hyperemesis is also associated with infectious conditions, such as hepatitis or encephalitis, intestinal obstruction, peptic ulcer, and hydatidiform mole. (I, N, H)

81. 4. Based on this client's history of hyperemesis gravidarum, it is particularly important for the nurse to assess for additional signs and symptoms of dehydration. Common signs and symptoms of dehydration include scanty urine output, lassitude, and fever. The client should not experience abdominal pain or bright red bleeding. With hydatidiform mole, any vaginal bleeding is usually brownish or "prune-colored." The client should not have any yellowish vaginal discharge. (A, N, G)

82. 3. Usually the client remains NPO for at least 24 hours with intravenous therapy. If the client is not vomiting after 24 hours, she may be offered clear liquids. If she tolerates liquids, dry toast, crackers, or cereal may be given every 2 to 3 hours. Hyperalimentation is started only if other measures fail. (I, N, G)

83. 1. Hydatidiform mole is suspected when the following symptoms are present: brownish or "prune-colored" vaginal bleeding, anemia, absence of fetal heart rate, passage of hydropic vessels, uterine enlargement greater than expected for gestational age, elevated hCG levels, and pregnancy-induced hypertension. (A, N, G)

84. 2. Following dilatation and curettage for evacuation of the mole, the nurse should assess the client's vital signs and monitor for signs of hemorrhage. The client should not experience abdominal distention, and the pregnancy-induced hypertension is usually resolved following evacuation. Symptoms of infection are important to assess, but chorioamnionitis is an inflammation of the amnionic fluid membranes. With complete mole, no embryonic/fetal tissue or membranes are present. (A, N, G)

85. 2. A client who has had a hydatidiform mole removed should have regular checkups to rule out the presence of choriocarcinoma, which may complicate the client's clinical picture. The client's hCG levels are monitored for 1 to 2 years. During this time, she should be advised not to become pregnant, as this will be reflected in rising hCG levels. Severe anemia, invasion of the mole, and polyps in the fallopian tubes are not associated with hydatidiform mole. (E, N, G)

The Client With Premature Rupture of the Membranes

86. 1. It is particularly important that the nurse assess for symptoms of infection, particularly urinary tract infection. Although the cause of premature rupture of the membranes is unknown, it has been associated with incompetent cervix, infection, trauma, and multiple pregnancies. The client should be assessed for a small-for-gestational age fetus and anemia, but these are not related to premature rupture of membranes. Uterine rupture is not associated with premature rupture of the membranes. (A, N, G)

87. 4. The primary purpose of the magnesium sulfate is to inhibit uterine contractions. Compared to intravenous ritodrine, magnesium sulfate causes fewer side effects. In some institutions, prostaglandin synthesis inhibitors such as indomethacin (Indocin) are being investigated. The client may experience a sedative effect from magnesium sulfate. This drug is not given to combat hypomagnesia, and it does not improve the fetal pulmonary system. (I, N, G)

88. 1. The client should report contractions occurring every 10 minutes or less for 1 hour, or if fluid leakage occurs. If the client experiences preterm labor symptoms for more than 15 minutes, she should empty her bladder, rest on the left side, palpate for uterine contractions, and call the health care provider. It is not necessary for the client to call the health care provider if she experiences contractions every hour for 4 hours, but she should monitor the contraction pattern to determine increasing frequency. (E, N, H)

89. 2. Maternal side effects of betamethazone (Celestone, Solupan) include increased risk of infection, initiation of lactation, gastrointestinal bleeding, weight gain, edema, and pulmonary edema when used concurrently with tokolytics. Hypoglycemia may occur in the neonate, but not the mother. Urinary retention and hypertension are not considered side effects of betamethazone. (P, N, G)

90. 3. Following a preterm delivery, a client often feels guilty. With therapeutic communication skills, the nurse can help her express these feelings and to identify and implement appropriate coping mechanisms. The client should be taken to the neonatal intensive care unit as soon as possible after the delivery, to promote the bonding process. (P, N, L)

NURSING CARE OF THE CHILDBEARING FAMILY AND THEIR NEONATE

TEST 2: Complications of Pregnancy

Directions: Use this answer grid to determine areas of strength or need for further study.

NURSING PROCESS

A = Assessment
D = Analysis, nursing diagnosis
P = Planning
I = Implementation
E = Evaluation

COGNITIVE LEVEL

K = Knowledge
C = Comprehension
T = Application
N = Analysis

CLIENT NEEDS

S = Safe, effective care environment
G = Physiological integrity
L = Psychosocial integrity
H = Health promotion/maintenance

		Nursing Process					Cognitive Level				Client Needs			
Question #	Answer #	A	D	P	I	E	K	C	T	N	S	G	L	H
1	1	A								N		G		
2	4		D							N		G		
3	2		D							N		G		
4	4		D							N		G		
5	3			P						N		G		
6	3					E				N		G		
7	4					E				N		G		
8	2			P						N		G		
9	1				I					N		G		
10	4	A								N		G		
11	1		D							N		G		
12	2				I					N		G		
13	2				I					N				H
14	4				I					N				H
15	1		D							N		G		
16	2				I					N		G		
17	2		D							N				H
18	3			P						N		G		
19	2			P						N		G		
20	4				I					N		G		
21	1				I					N		G		
22	4	A								N		G		
23	1			P						N		G		

ANSWER GRID: 1

NURSING PROCESS

A = Assessment
D = Analysis, nursing diagnosis
P = Planning
I = Implementation
E = Evaluation

COGNITIVE LEVEL

K = Knowledge
C = Comprehension
T = Application
N = Analysis

CLIENT NEEDS

S = Safe, effective care environment
G = Physiological integrity
L = Psychosocial integrity
H = Health promotion/maintenance

		Nursing Process					Cognitive Level				Client Needs			
Question #	Answer #	A	D	P	I	E	K	C	T	N	S	G	L	H
24	3				I					N		G		
25	2		D							N		G		
26	4				I					N		G		
27	3				I					N		G		
28	1		D							N		G		
29	4	A								N			L	
30	2				I					N		G		
31	3		D							N		G		
32	1					E				N				H
33	3				I					N		G		
34	2					E				N		G		
35	4				I					N		G		
36	2	A								N		G		
37	1		D							N		G		
38	1	A								N		G		
39	1				I					N				H
40	3			P						N		G		
41	3				I					N		G		
42	4					E				N		G		
43	2		D							N		G		
44	4			P						N		G		
45	2				I					N		G		
46	4	A								N		G		
47	4		D							N			L	
48	4	A								N		G		
49	1				I					N	S			
50	1				I					N		G		
51	3				I					N		G		
52	3				I					N		G		

ANSWER GRID: 2

Nursing Process

A = Assessment
D = Analysis, nursing diagnosis
P = Planning
I = Implementation
E = Evaluation

Cognitive Level

K = Knowledge
C = Comprehension
T = Application
N = Analysis

Client Needs

S = Safe, effective care environment
G = Physiological integrity
L = Psychosocial integrity
H = Health promotion/maintenance

		Nursing Process					Cognitive Level				Client Needs			
Question #	Answer #	A	D	P	I	E	K	C	T	N	S	G	L	H
53	2					E				N	S			
54	1				I					N	S			
55	2		D							N			L	
56	4			P						N	S			
57	2					E				N		G		
58	1				I					N		G		
59	2					E				N		G		
60	1		D							N		G		
61	4			P						N	S			
62	1				I					N		G		
63	3					E				N		G		
64	2			P						N		G		
65	3				I					N		G		
66	4					E				N		G		
67	3				I					N		G		
68	1				I					N				H
69	4	A								N		G		
70	3				I					N		G		
71	1		D							N			L	
72	2	A								N		G		
73	4	A								N		G		
74	2			P						N	S			
75	4	A								N		G		
76	2					E				N		G		
77	2				I					N		G		
78	4				I					N		G		
79	3	A								N		G		
80	2				I					N				H
81	4	A								N		G		

ANSWER GRID: 3

Nursing Process

A = Assessment
D = Analysis, nursing diagnosis
P = Planning
I = Implementation
E = Evaluation

Cognitive Level

K = Knowledge
C = Comprehension
T = Application
N = Analysis

Client Needs

S = Safe, effective care environment
G = Physiological integrity
L = Psychosocial integrity
H = Health promotion/maintenance

		Nursing Process					Cognitive Level				Client Needs			
Question #	Answer #	A	D	P	I	E	K	C	T	N	S	G	L	H
82	3				I					N		G		
83	1	A								N		G		
84	2	A								N		G		
85	2					E				N		G		
86	1	A								N		G		
87	4				I					N		G		
88	1					E				N				H
89	2			P						N		G		
90	3			P						N			L	
Number Correct														
Number Possible	90	17	15	13	32	13	0	0	0	90	6	70	5	9
Percentage Correct														

Score Calculation:

To determine your **Percentage Correct**, divide the **Number Correct** by the **Number Possible**.

The Birth Experience

Test 3

The Primigravida in Labor
The Multigravida in Labor
The Intrapartal Client With Risk Factors
Correct Answers and Rationale

Select the one best answer and indicate your choice by filling in the circle in front of the option.

The Primigravida in Labor

A 22-year-old primigravid client at 40 weeks gestation is admitted to the hospital in the first stage of labor.

1. The client is admitted to the labor area in the latent phase of the first stage of labor with contractions lasting 20 seconds. In assessing the client's emotional status, the nurse anticipates that she will be
- ○ 1. serious.
- ○ 2. irritable.
- ○ 3. happy.
- ○ 4. panicky.

2. The client asks how long she will be in labor. The nurse's best response is to explain that for primigravidas, labor usually lasts
- ○ 1. 10 hours.
- ○ 2. 14 hours.
- ○ 3. 18 hours.
- ○ 4. 22 hours.

3. The nurse performs a nitrazine test to determine whether the client's membranes have ruptured. The nurse notifies the physician of probable membrane rupture if the nitrazine paper is
- ○ 1. blue.
- ○ 2. olive.
- ○ 3. orange.
- ○ 4. yellow.

4. The client says, "The doctor said the baby is at 'minus one.' What does that mean?" After providing instruction, the nurse determines that teaching has been effective when the client states that the fetal presenting part is located
- ○ 1. 1 cm above the ischial spines.
- ○ 2. 1 cm below the ischial spines.
- ○ 3. 1 fingerbreadth above the ischial spines.
- ○ 4. 1 fingerbreadth below the ischial spines.

5. At 6 cm dilatation, the client receives a continuous lumbar epidural block. Following administration of this anesthesia, it is most important for the nurse to assess the client's
- ○ 1. blood pressure.
- ○ 2. urine output.
- ○ 3. level of anesthesia.
- ○ 4. level of consciousness.

6. The client delivers a viable male neonate who is given a score of 8 on the Apgar rating system. The nurse determines that the neonate's physical condition is
- ○ 1. good.
- ○ 2. fair.
- ○ 3. poor.
- ○ 4. critical.

A 32-year-old primigravida at 39 weeks gestation is admitted to the hospital in active labor. The client's husband accompanies her to the labor area.

7. The nurse performs Leopold's maneuvers. When the client asks what these maneuvers are for, the nurse's best response is to explain that they help determine
- ○ 1. fetal presentation.
- ○ 2. fetal heart rate.
- ○ 3. intensity of contractions.
- ○ 4. frequency of contractions.

8. The client's husband coaches her with breathing and relaxation techniques as they were taught in childbirth preparation classes. When the client reaches the transition phase of labor, she screams out, "I can't do this anymore!" The nurse should suggest to the client's husband that he
- ○ 1. leave the room, until his wife gains control.
- ○ 2. ask his wife if she wants analgesia.
- ○ 3. tell his wife that she is doing well and it will be over soon.

○ 4. talk to his wife while maintaining direct eye contact and breathe with her.

9. The nurse formulates a nursing diagnosis for the client in the transitional phase of labor. The most appropriate diagnosis is
- ○ 1. Altered Urinary Elimination Patterns related to pressure on the bladder.
- ○ 2. Impaired Gas Exchange related to hyperventilation.
- ○ 3. Ineffective Family Coping related to fear and anxiety.
- ○ 4. Pain related to increasing frequency and intensity of uterine contractions.

10. The client delivers a viable neonate. The physician orders oxytocin intravenously following delivery of the placenta. Which of the following data would indicate that the placenta is about to be delivered?
- ○ 1. The abdominal wall relaxes noticeably.
- ○ 2. The cord lengthens outside the vagina.
- ○ 3. The client complains of back pain.
- ○ 4. The uterus falls below the level of the symphysis pubis.

11. While the client holds and looks at her neonate, she begins to cry. The nurse correctly interprets this behavior as indicating that the client is
- ○ 1. disappointed in the baby's sex.
- ○ 2. grieving over the loss of the pregnancy.
- ○ 3. experiencing a normal response to the birth.
- ○ 4. likely to have trouble with bonding.

12. The client asks when she can start breast-feeding her baby. The nurse's best response is to instruct the client that breast-feeding can begin
- ○ 1. immediately after birth.
- ○ 2. in about 2 hours, after the baby is bathed.
- ○ 3. in about 8 hours, after the baby has had some rest.
- ○ 4. after determining the patency of the baby's esophagus with formula feeding.

A 24-year-old primigravida is admitted to the hospital in early labor. On admission, she is 2 cm dilated.

13. Following admission, the client asks if she must remain in bed. What is the nurse's best response?
- ○ 1. "It's best to stay in bed to help prevent the cord from prolapsing."
- ○ 2. "You may walk around, but let me know immediately if your membranes rupture."
- ○ 3. "It's best to stay in bed and lie on your left side so the baby can receive a good supply of oxygen."
- ○ 4. "You may get up to the bathroom, but the rest of the time you should stay in bed."

14. The nurse instructs the client in active relaxation techniques to help her cope with the pain of contractions. The nurse determines that the client understands the instructions when she says that active relaxation includes
- ○ 1. relaxing uninvolved body muscles during uterine contractions.
- ○ 2. accepting a supreme power that can help relieve the discomfort of uterine contractions.
- ○ 3. considering the discomfort of uterine contractions to be more psychological than physical.
- ○ 4. assuming a state of mind that is open to suggestion from a coach during uncomfortable uterine contractions.

15. The client asks the nurse what effleurage means. The nurse's best response is to explain that effleurage is a type of massage involving
- ○ 1. deep kneading of muscular tissues.
- ○ 2. secure grasping of muscular tissues.
- ○ 3. light stroking of the skin surface.
- ○ 4. punctuated tapping on the skin surface.

16. At the beginning of labor, the nurse observes moderately increased bloody vaginal discharge (show). The nurse's best action is to
- ○ 1. check fetal descent by performing Leopold's maneuvers.
- ○ 2. perform a vaginal examination to determine cervical dilatation.
- ○ 3. check for rupture of the membranes with nitrazine paper.
- ○ 4. notify the physician of premature separation of the placenta.

17. The client asks the nurse why she can have only fluids while in labor. After providing an explanation, the nurse determines that the teaching has been effective from which client statement?
- ○ 1. "Solid foods tend to cause nausea and vomiting."
- ○ 2. "The digestive process is normally slow."
- ○ 3. "Most clients aren't hungry during labor."
- ○ 4. "My body has a sufficient store of nutrients, so eating is unnecessary."

18. On assessment, the nurse determines that her cervix is 6 cm dilated, with contractions occurring every 3–4 minutes. While assessing the client's mental status, the nurse anticipates that her mental attitude will now reflect feelings of
- ○ 1. depression.
- ○ 2. excitement.
- ○ 3. seriousness.
- ○ 4. irritability.

A 19-year-old primigravida at 38 weeks gestation is admitted to the hospital in active labor. Her mother accompanies her to the labor unit.

19. On admission, the client is breathing rapidly and complains of feeling dizzy and light-headed. She is 7 cm dilated. The nurse determines that she is most likely experiencing effects of
- ○ 1. normal active labor.
- ○ 2. elevated blood pressure.
- ○ 3. hyperventilation.
- ○ 4. shortness of breath.

20. The client is not completely dilated, but has a strong urge to push. The nurse's best course of action at this time is to
- ○ 1. position the client for pushing.
- ○ 2. administer a prescribed sedative.
- ○ 3. suggest that the client use a pant-blow pattern of breathing.
- ○ 4. let the client push, but tell her to push as gently as possible.

21. For the client in the transition phase of labor, the nurse's primary action is to provide
- ○ 1. extra fluids.
- ○ 2. extra blankets.
- ○ 3. distraction from the pain.
- ○ 4. encouragement and support.

22. The physician tells the client that she is beginning the second stage of labor. The nurse realizes that the client understands the second stage of labor from which of the following statements about it?
- ○ 1. "I'm having bloody show."
- ○ 2. "My membranes have ruptured."
- ○ 3. "My contractions are very strong."
- ○ 4. "My cervix is completely dilated."

23. Following delivery of a viable female neonate, the client makes comments to her mother about the baby. Which of the following comments should the nurse interpret as a possible sign of potential maternal-infant bonding problems?
- ○ 1. "She's so cute."
- ○ 2. "I wish she were a boy."
- ○ 3. "She looks just like me."
- ○ 4. "I want to nickname her 'Sugar Bear.'"

A 23-year-old primigravida at 40 weeks gestation is admitted to the hospital in the latent phase of labor. She is accompanied by her husband.

24. The nurse instructs the client about skin massage and the gate control theory of pain. Which of the following statements would be appropriate for the nurse to include in this instruction?
- ○ 1. The gating mechanism is located at the pain site.
- ○ 2. Pain perception is decreased if anxiety is present.
- ○ 3. A technique to assist the gating mechanism involves shallow chest breathing.
- ○ 4. The gating mechanism is in the spinal cord.

25. The nurse explains that according to the gate control theory of pain, a closed gate means that the client should experience
- ○ 1. no pain.
- ○ 2. dull pain.
- ○ 3. light pain.
- ○ 4. reduced pain.

26. The nurse teaches the client how to use personalized concentration points or ideas to promote muscular relaxation during labor. The nurse determines that this teaching has been effective when the client says that the points or ideas serve as a
- ○ 1. projection for pain.
- ○ 2. distraction from pain.
- ○ 3. rationalization for pain.
- ○ 4. counterirritant for pain.

27. The nurse formulates a plan for assessing the client's blood pressure during labor. The client's nursing care plan should specify that her blood pressure will be monitored
- ○ 1. every 4 hours until delivery.
- ○ 2. every hour between contractions during the active phase of labor.
- ○ 3. every hour during a contraction during the active phase of labor.
- ○ 4. every 2 hours until the transition phase of labor.

28. The client is progressing, but is still in the latent phase of labor. She is happy and appears relaxed, although she is aware of labor contractions. At this time, the nurse suggests to the client's husband that he can be of most assistance by
- ○ 1. keeping a record of her urinary output.
- ○ 2. playing a game of cards that he and she enjoy.
- ○ 3. suggest that she receive an epidural block.
- ○ 4. suggest that she practice rapid, shallow breathing.

29. The client has progressed to 5 cm dilatation and is starting to feel considerable discomfort during contractions. The nurse suggests that the client change from slow chest breathing to
- ○ 1. shallow abdominal breathing.
- ○ 2. deep chest breathing.
- ○ 3. rapid panting breathing.
- ○ 4. pursed-lip breathing.

A 15-year-old primigravida is admitted to the hospital in active labor. She is at 36 weeks gestation and is 8 cm dilated. She has had only one prenatal visit.

30. Soon after admission, the nurse determines that the client is hyperventilating. The nurse's most appropriate action is to have the client breathe

○ 1. several whiffs of oxygen.
○ 2. into a paper bag.
○ 3. rapidly and shallowly.
○ 4. with forceful expiration.

31. Due to the hyperventilation, the nurse assesses the client for symptoms of
○ 1. metabolic acidosis.
○ 2. metabolic alkalosis.
○ 3. respiratory acidosis.
○ 4. respiratory alkalosis.

32. The client complains of severe back pain during labor. The nurse assesses fetal position through vaginal examination and tells the client that her severe back pain is most likely due to the fetus being in what position?
○ 1. Occipitodiagonal.
○ 2. Occipitoanterior.
○ 3. Occipitoposterior.
○ 4. Occipitotransverse.

33. In planning for delivery, the nurse anticipates that due to the fetal position and severe back labor, the client will
○ 1. require a cesarean section.
○ 2. need an extensive episiotomy.
○ 3. have a precipitate delivery.
○ 4. experience marked discomfort.

34. Based on the client's symptoms, the most appropriate nursing diagnosis is
○ 1. Anxiety related to lack of support.
○ 2. Noncompliance related to lack of prenatal care.
○ 3. Pain related to unexpected and intense back discomfort.
○ 4. High Risk for Injury related to lack of control during transition.

The Multigravida in Labor

A 31-year-old multigravida at 39 weeks gestation is admitted to the hospital in active labor.

35. Soon after admission, the client's membranes rupture spontaneously. The client is 6 cm dilated at +1 station. The nurse's first action is to
○ 1. assess the contraction pattern.
○ 2. note the color, amount, and odor of the amniotic fluid.
○ 3. prepare the client for imminent delivery.
○ 4. change the client's position.

36. An intravenous solution of 5% dextrose in Ringer's solution is started, and an epidural anesthetic is administered. The client's contractions and fetal heart rate are being monitored with external electronic equipment. The nurse determines that there is a variable deceleration pattern on the fetal heart rate. The nurse's most appropriate action is to
○ 1. change the client's position.
○ 2. increase the intravenous fluid infusion rate.
○ 3. prepare the client for a cesarean section.
○ 4. shave the client's perineum in preparation for delivery.

37. The client is 10 cm dilated and begins to push. The nurse notes early decelerations of the fetal heart rate and instructs the client about the most likely cause of the early decelerations. Following the instructions, the nurse determines that the teaching has been effective when the client says that the early deceleration pattern is due to
○ 1. cord compression.
○ 2. fetal malpresentation.
○ 3. fetal head compression.
○ 4. inadequate placental perfusion.

38. The physician determines that low forceps are needed to assist in delivery. The nurse explains to the client that low forceps are used when the fetal skull
○ 1. has reached the perineum with the scalp visible between contractions.
○ 2. is at a station of +2 or more.
○ 3. is engaged but above +2 station.
○ 4. has reached the level of the ischial spines.

39. The client delivers a viable neonate. Approximately 10 minutes after delivery, she complains of a chill. The nurse assesses her further by gathering data related to her
○ 1. temperature, pulse, and respirations.
○ 2. need for analgesic medication.
○ 3. desire for a warm blanket.
○ 4. volume of blood loss.

40. Following delivery, the nurse formulates a nursing diagnosis. The most appropriate diagnosis at this time is
○ 1. Pain related to exhaustive pushing efforts.
○ 2. Knowledge Deficit related to self-care during the postpartum period.
○ 3. High Risk for Injury related to effects of epidural anesthesia.
○ 4. Fluid Volume Excess related to intravenous fluid administration.

The Intrapartal Client With Risk Factors

A 39-year-old multiparous client at 40 weeks gestation is admitted to the hospital in active labor. She has been diagnosed with Class II heart disease.

41. When assessing the client after admission to the labor unit, the nurse should obtain which of the following data first?

○ 1. Fetal movement and activity.
○ 2. The client's last food and fluid intake.
○ 3. Frequency of contractions.
○ 4. The client's desire to breast-feed or bottle-feed her infant.

42. To ensure cardiac emptying and adequate oxygen during labor, the nurse encourages the client to
○ 1. breathe rapidly during a contraction.
○ 2. limit the number of visitors.
○ 3. remain in a side-lying position.
○ 4. refuse analgesia and anesthesia.

43. The nurse prepares the client for lumbar epidural anesthesia. Before anesthesia administration, the nurse instructs the client to assume which of the following positions?
○ 1. Sitting.
○ 2. Side-lying.
○ 3. Knee-chest.
○ 4. Supine.

44. Based on the client's medical diagnosis of Class II heart disease, during labor the nurse will frequently assess her for
○ 1. reactions to ergot products.
○ 2. excessive discomfort from contractions.
○ 3. symptoms of infection.
○ 4. moist rales in the lower lungs.

45. The nurse plans to instruct the client about pushing during the second stage of labor. Which of the following should be included in the teaching plan? The client should push when
○ 1. she feels the urge.
○ 2. she feels a contraction.
○ 3. the nurse observes bulging of the perineum.
○ 4. the nurse palpates the onset of a contraction.

A 22-year-old primigravida at 39 weeks gestation is admitted to the hospital for induction of labor. The client is a Class B, insulin-dependent diabetic.

46. Before starting the induction with intravenous oxytocin, the nurse should
○ 1. position the client on her right side.
○ 2. evaluate the contraction pattern.
○ 3. monitor fetal heart rate by continuous electronic monitoring for 15 minutes.
○ 4. test the client's urine for glucose.

47. The nurse plans care for the client in labor. Which of the following is essential to include in the plan for a pregnant diabetic client?
○ 1. Measure urine output every hour.
○ 2. Administer insulin subcutaneously every 4 hours.
○ 3. Check urine for protein every 2 hours.
○ 4. Monitor blood glucose levels every hour.

48. The nurse begins induction of labor with an intravenous oxytocic agent. The infusion rate is increased every 20 minutes as indicated. During the induction, the nurse should
○ 1. remain with the client continuously.
○ 2. keep the client awake during induction.
○ 3. change the client's position every ½ hour.
○ 4. discontinue infusion when the contractions are 5 to 6 minutes apart.

49. The nurse formulates a nursing diagnosis for the client. The most appropriate nursing diagnosis at this time is
○ 1. Knowledge Deficit related to glucose metabolism and management.
○ 2. Pain related to prolonged labor and uterine ischemia.
○ 3. Fear related to probable need for cesarean section.
○ 4. Potential for High Risk for Injury to mother and fetus related to dysfunctional carbohydrate metabolism.

50. The fetus is in a cephalic presentation. After the physician performs an amniotomy, the nurse determines that the amnionic fluid is meconium stained. As a result, the nurse gathers additional data related to the
○ 1. fetal heart rate.
○ 2. amniocentesis findings.
○ 3. fetal position.
○ 4. estimated fetal size.

51. The client is at −2 station when the membranes are ruptured. Immediately after the membranes are ruptured, the nurse should
○ 1. position the client on her left side.
○ 2. prepare for a precipitous delivery.
○ 3. determine the client's blood pressure.
○ 4. check for prolapsed umbilical cord.

A 26-year-old primigravida at 40 weeks gestation is admitted to the hospital's labor unit for induction of labor. The client's membranes rupture spontaneously, and there is evidence of meconium staining.

52. The nurse plans the client's care for the labor period. Which of the following would be important to include in the care plan if there is evidence of late fetal heart rate decelerations during induction of labor?
○ 1. Inform the client about the status of the fetus.
○ 2. Prepare the client for an immediate cesarean section.
○ 3. Evaluate the contraction pattern.

○ 4. Discontinue the oxytocin infusion.

53. The nurse instructs the client about the procedures that will be performed on the neonate immediately after delivery to prevent meconium aspiration. The nurse determines that the instructions have been effective when the client states that the neonate will be
- ○ 1. suctioned as soon as the head is delivered.
- ○ 2. intubated after delivery.
- ○ 3. given oxygen by mask after delivery.
- ○ 4. given a drug to dilate the bronchi after delivery.

54. The client has a history of smoking one to two packs of cigarettes daily. In response to a question, the nurse tells the client that due to her smoking, the neonate is likely to have a
- ○ 1. higher-than-average pulse rate.
- ○ 2. below-average hemoglobin.
- ○ 3. below-average birth weight.
- ○ 4. above-average respiratory rate.

55. The nurse instructs the client about the purpose of the episiotomy. The nurse determines that the client has understood the instructions when she says that an episiotomy
- ○ 1. shortens the second stage of labor.
- ○ 2. relieves pressure on the rectum.
- ○ 3. prevents perineal lacerations.
- ○ 4. facilitates the third stage of labor.

A multigravida is admitted to the hospital in active labor. The client's and the fetus's conditions have been good since admission.

56. The client calls out to the nurse, "The baby is coming!" The nurse's first action is to
- ○ 1. inspect the perineum.
- ○ 2. time the contractions.
- ○ 3. auscultate the fetal heart rate.
- ○ 4. contact the physician.

57. It appears that delivery is imminent and the nurse has no help immediately available. The nurse's first action is to
- ○ 1. have the client push with a contraction.
- ○ 2. administer a prescribed analgesic to the client.
- ○ 3. prepare a clean area on which to deliver the neonate.
- ○ 4. lower the head of the bed to a flat position.

58. To help the client remain calm and cooperative during the delivery, what is the nurse's best response?
- ○ 1. "The baby is coming. Relax and everything will be fine."
- ○ 2. "Do you want me to call your husband?"
- ○ 3. "Even though the baby is coming, the doctor will be here soon."
- ○ 4. "The baby is coming. I'll explain what's happening and guide you as we go along."

59. The nurse plans to deliver the neonate's head
- ○ 1. between contractions.
- ○ 2. at the end of a contraction.
- ○ 3. at the peak of a contraction.
- ○ 4. at the beginning of a contraction.

60. As the head is being delivered, the nurse should
- ○ 1. tell the client to push forcefully.
- ○ 2. check for an umbilical cord around the neonate's neck.
- ○ 3. apply gentle traction on the neonate's anterior shoulder.
- ○ 4. place gentle pressure on the client's fundus with one hand.

61. Following delivery of the neonate, the nurse delivers the placenta by
- ○ 1. asking the client to bear down forcefully.
- ○ 2. massaging the fundus for a few minutes.
- ○ 3. observing for signs of placental separation before taking any action.
- ○ 4. pulling gently on the cord until the placenta appears.

A 30-year-old multigravida at 37 weeks gestation is admitted to the hospital in early labor. She is pregnant with twins.

62. The twins are continually monitored with electronic fetal monitoring. Following instructions about the purpose of the electronic monitoring, the nurse determines that the client understands the instructions when she says that an electronic monitor
- ○ 1. takes much less time to use.
- ○ 2. causes less discomfort.
- ○ 3. provides a continuous recording of fetal heart rate.
- ○ 4. allows greater mobility.

63. In addition to electronic monitoring, the nurse plans to assess the client during labor more frequently for symptoms of
- ○ 1. urinary frequency.
- ○ 2. oligohydramnios.
- ○ 3. pregnancy-induced hypertension.
- ○ 4. polycythemia.

64. While the client is in active labor at 5 cm dilatation, the nurse observes contractions occurring at a rate of two to three in a 10-minute period. The nurse's most appropriate action is to
- ○ 1. note the fetal heart rate patterns.
- ○ 2. notify the physician.
- ○ 3. administer a prescribed sedative.

○ 4. have the client flex her thighs up against her abdomen.

65. The client delivers a male neonate and a female neonate. The twins are considered dizygotic twins. The nurse instructs the client that dizygotic twins result from the fertilization of
○ 1. one ovum with one sperm.
○ 2. one ovum with two sperm.
○ 3. two ova with one sperm.
○ 4. two ova with two sperm.

66. During the immediate postpartum period, the client experiences uterine atony. The nurse assesses her further for symptoms of
○ 1. thrombophlebitis.
○ 2. puerperal infection.
○ 3. uterine rupture.
○ 4. postpartum hemorrhage.

67. The twin neonates require additional hospitalization after the client is discharged. In planning the family's care, an appropriate goal for the nurse to formulate is: The parents will
○ 1. discuss the jealousy that will occur later in life between the twins.
○ 2. touch, hold, and participate in care of the twins on a daily basis.
○ 3. visit the twins twice weekly while they are hospitalized.
○ 4. identify complications that may occur as the twins develop.

A primigravida is admitted to the hospital's labor and delivery unit in active labor. She is almost 2 weeks postterm.

68. The nurse instructs the client in techniques of pushing to use during the second stage of labor. The nurse determines that the client needs further instructions when she says she will need to
○ 1. be in a semi-Fowler's position or a position of comfort.
○ 2. flex her thighs onto her abdomen before bearing down.
○ 3. exert downward pressure as though she were having a bowel movement.
○ 4. hold her breath for several bearing-down efforts during each contraction.

69. The client desires a bilateral pudendal block anesthetic before delivery. The nurse explains that this type of anesthesia will relieve discomfort primarily in her
○ 1. back.
○ 2. uterus.
○ 3. cervix.
○ 4. perineum.

70. Following the bilateral pudendal block anesthesia and delivery, the nurse assesses the neonate for potential side effects of the anesthetic, especially noting
○ 1. heart rate.
○ 2. respiratory rate.
○ 3. color.
○ 4. blood pressure.

71. The nurse explains to the client that deep suctioning of the neonate's nasopharynx can lead to
○ 1. injury to the tender mucous membranes.
○ 2. inhibition of the normal effort to clear mucus.
○ 3. stimulation of the vagus nerve.
○ 4. excessive removal of carbon dioxide.

72. The neonate is in good condition. After suctioning to clear the airway following delivery, the nurse should next
○ 1. administer oxygen therapy.
○ 2. ensuring adequate warmth.
○ 3. assist with intubation.
○ 4. perform cardiac massage.

A 30-year-old primigravida delivers a viable male infant more than 2 weeks postterm.

73. At 5 minutes after birth, the nurse evaluates the neonate using the Apgar scoring chart. After assessing heart rate, respiratory effort, muscle tone, and reflex irritability, the nurse should next assess the neonate's
○ 1. eyes.
○ 2. color.
○ 3. suck reflex.
○ 4. urethral patency.

74. Because the neonate is postmature, the nurse assesses carefully for symptoms of
○ 1. hyperglycemia.
○ 2. hypoglycemia.
○ 3. anemia.
○ 4. elevated temperature.

A primigravida at 39 weeks gestation is admitted to the hospital in early active labor. There is question about whether her pelvis is adequate for vaginal delivery.

75. After 5 hours of active labor, the client's cervical dilatation is 5 cm, with 80% effacement—the same as 2 hours before. Contractions are 8 to 10 minutes apart, lasting 45 seconds. The nurse determines that the client is most likely experiencing

- ○ 1. cephalopelvic disproportion.
- ○ 2. prolonged latent phase.
- ○ 3. effects of sedative medication.
- ○ 4. hypertonic contraction pattern.

76. An ultrasound is scheduled to obtain pelvic measurements. After teaching the client about the purpose of the ultrasound, the nurse determines that she understands the instructions when she says that the most important pelvic measurement is the

- ○ 1. true conjugate.
- ○ 2. bi-ischial diameter.
- ○ 3. diagonal conjugate.
- ○ 4. transverse diameter.

77. The physician elects to perform a cesarean section. When the nurse takes the consent form to the client for signing, the client's husband says, "I'll sign it. I always take care of our business affairs." The nurse's most appropriate response is to

- ○ 1. ask the client if this is satisfactory to her.
- ○ 2. have the client's husband sign the consent form.
- ○ 3. ask the client to sign the consent form.
- ○ 4. ask the doctor if this is satisfactory.

78. The nurse plans to instruct the client about preparation for the cesarean section. Which of the following should the nurse include in the teaching plan?

- ○ 1. Insertion of an indwelling catheter.
- ○ 2. Administration of a narcotic medication.
- ○ 3. Sterilization of the abdomen.
- ○ 4. Requirement that the client's husband remain in the waiting room.

A multigravida is admitted to the hospital for a trial labor and possible vaginal birth. She has a history of previous cesarean delivery because of fetal distress.

79. After several hours of active labor, the physician orders nalbuphine (Nubain). The nurse evaluates the drug as effective when the client says

- ○ 1. "At least now I'll be able to get some sleep."
- ○ 2. "The contractions don't seem as intense as before."
- ○ 3. "I'm numb from my waist down."
- ○ 4. "I feel less nauseous now."

80. While monitoring fetal heart rate, the nurse observes minimal variability and a rate of 130 beats per minute. The nurse explains to the client that the decreased variability is most likely due to

- ○ 1. maternal hypoventilation.
- ○ 2. fetal distress.
- ○ 3. cephalopelvic disproportion.
- ○ 4. affects of analgesic medication.

81. The fetus develops severe bradycardia and fetal distress, and an emergency cesarean section is performed under general anesthesia. When the nurse plans care for the client during the postoperative period, which of the following measures would be most important to include?

- ○ 1. Observe for delayed breast milk production.
- ○ 2. Monitor for symptoms of hypertension.
- ○ 3. Carefully assess uterine tone.
- ○ 4. Evaluate for symptoms of postpartal infection.

82. A neonatologist is present in the operating room following delivery. The nurse explains to the client's husband that the neonatologist is present because neonates born by cesarean delivery tend to have increased incidence of

- ○ 1. cold stress.
- ○ 2. convulsions.
- ○ 3. umbilical cord infections.
- ○ 4. respiratory distress syndrome.

83. The nurse assesses the client's emotional status following the cesarean delivery. Which of the following expressions of emotion would warrant further assessment by the nurse?

- ○ 1. Relief.
- ○ 2. Frustration.
- ○ 3. Indifference.
- ○ 4. Disappointment.

A 34-year-old multigravida at 36 weeks gestation is admitted to the hospital in active labor. She is diagnosed with Rh sensitization.

84. The client's contractions and the fetal heart rate are monitored electronically. The nurse detects a sinusoidal pattern of fetal heart rate. The nurse explains to the client that this is usually due to

- ○ 1. severe fetal anemia.
- ○ 2. maternal anesthesia.
- ○ 3. fetal hyperactivity.
- ○ 4. prematurity.

85. The fetus is in a frank breech presentation. The client's membranes rupture spontaneously, and the nurse documents the color of the fluid as yellowish. The nurse explains to the client that this is usually due to

- ○ 1. Rh sensitization.
- ○ 2. breech presentation.
- ○ 3. amniotic fluid embolism.
- ○ 4. polyhydramnios.

86. Following spontaneous rupture of the membranes, if the cord prolapses, the nurse should plan to immediately

○ 1. relieve pressure on the cord.
○ 2. expedite delivery.
○ 3. turn the client to a supine position.
○ 4. replace the cord into the vagina.

87. The client delivers a viable male neonate via cesarean section. The neonate is scheduled for an immediate exchange transfusion. In planning the neonate's care during the exchange transfusion, the nurse would include which of the following measures?

○ 1. Administer calcium gluconate intravenously before the procedure.
○ 2. Monitor the neonate's status before and during the procedure.
○ 3. Maintain a cool environment.
○ 4. Administer 1 ounce of formula by mouth just before the procedure.

A 28-year-old multigravida with suspected acute pyelonephritis is admitted to the hospital at 32 weeks gestation.

88. In planning care for the client, the nurse would include which of the following measures in the nursing care plan?

○ 1. Assess the client for chills, high fever, and flank pain.
○ 2. Prepare the client for intravenous penicillin therapy.
○ 3. Instruct the client about the need for a probable cesarean delivery.
○ 4. Observe the client for possible uterine hemorrhage.

89. The client's health history reveals herpes simplex virus type 2. The client is currently asymptomatic and without lesions. The nurse explains that because of the viral infection, she should plan to

○ 1. have a cesarean delivery.
○ 2. take the medication acyclovir (Zovirax), as prescribed, throughout the remainder of her pregnancy.
○ 3. have a vaginal delivery if no lesions are present.
○ 4. bottle-feed rather than breast-feed after delivery.

90. At 37 weeks gestation, the client is admitted to the hospital in active labor. She has a precipitous labor and spontaneously delivers a viable neonate. During the immediate postpartum period, the nurse should monitor the client closely for symptoms of

○ 1. ineffective bonding.
○ 2. excessive bleeding.
○ 3. intrauterine infection.
○ 4. urinary stasis.

CORRECT ANSWERS AND RATIONALE

The letters in parentheses following the rationale identify the step of the nursing process (A, D, P, I, E); cognitive level (K, C, T, N); and client need (S, G, L, H). See the Answer Grid for the key.

The Primigravida in Labor

1. 3. In the first stage of labor when complications are absent and contractions are still not strong, the client is usually not very uncomfortable. She is usually excited that the "big day" has finally arrived, and she can expect to be happy and eager. As labor progresses, she becomes serious and ready to "get down to work." As transition approaches, she is likely to become irritable, tired, and, sometimes, panicky. (A, C, L)

2. 2. The average length of labor for a primigravida is approximately 12 to 14 hours; for a multigravida, 8 to 10 hours. (I, C, H)

3. 1. The nitrazine test helps determine the pH of fluid. The membranes have likely ruptured if the pH of the fluid is above 6.5 and the nitrazine paper turns blue-green, blue-grey, or deep blue. If the pH of the fluid is below 6.0, the fluid is most likely vaginal secretions and the paper will turn olive or olive-yellow. (A, C, G)

4. 1. The ischial spines are used as landmarks to determine the descent of the fetal presenting part. The station −1, means that the presenting part is 1 centimeter above the level of the ischial spines. The station +1 means that the presenting part is 1 centimeter below the level of the ischial spines. Fingerbreadths are not used as measurements in determining station. (E, N, H)

5. 1. One complication of regional anesthesia is hypotension. It may develop because the anesthetic acts as a sympathetic blocker. The nurse should monitor maternal blood pressure, pulse, and respiration and fetal heart rate every 5 minutes until delivery and should report any drop in blood pressure immediately. To overcome hypotension, administration of intravenous fluids is usually increased. Ephedrine can also be administered. The person responsible for administering the anesthesia is also responsible for determining the level of anesthesia. The client will normally remain conscious while under the influence of regional anesthesia, such as an epidural block. (A, N, G)

6. 1. The Apgar rating system rates a neonate on the basis of heart rate, respiratory effort, muscle tone, reflex irritability, and color at 1 minute and again at 5 minutes after birth. The neonate receives a score between 0 and 10. The higher the score, the better the neonate's condition. A score between 4 and 6 indicates fair condition. A score between 0 and 3 indicates critical condition. (D, N, G)

7. 1. Leopold's maneuvers assist in identifying fetal presentation and position. The procedure should be performed between contractions and after the client empties her bladder. There are four maneuvers. For the first maneuver, the nurse palpates the upper abdomen with both hands to determine whether the head or the buttocks fills the fundus. For the second maneuver, the nurse places one palm on each side of the abdomen and locates the fetal back. In the third maneuver, the nurse determines what fetal part is located at the inlet by gently grasping the lower portion of the abdomen, just above the symphysis pubis. In the fourth maneuver, the nurse faces the client's feet and attempts to locate the fetal brow, moving the hands down the sides of the uterus toward the pubis. Leopold's maneuvers are often performed before initial auscultation of the fetal heart rate. (D, N, G)

8. 4. The transition stage of labor requires reinforcement of techniques learned during preparation for childbirth classes. It is best when the husband speaks to his wife using direct eye contact and breathes with her when she loses control during the transition stage. This often helps her regain control. The client should be encouraged to focus on one contraction at a time at this point in labor. Telling the husband to leave the room is not appropriate. When the client reaches transition, or 8–10 cm dilatation, it is usually too late for analgesia. Telling the client that it will soon be over does not help her gain control. (I, N, H)

9. 4. During transition, contractions are increasing in frequency, duration, and intensity. The most appropriate nursing diagnosis is Pain related to strength and duration of the contractions. There are no data to suggest Altered Urinary Elimination, Impaired Gas Exchange, or Ineffective Family Coping. (D, N, G)

10. 2. The most reliable sign that the placenta has detached from the uterine wall is the cord lengthening outside the vagina. Oxytocin is administered to promote uterine contractions and thereby control postpartum bleeding. (D, N, G)

11. 3. Childbirth is a very emotional experience. An expression of happiness with tears is a very normal reaction. (D, N, G)

12. 1. A neonate is active and alert very soon after birth, if no complications exist. The American Academy of Pediatrics recommends beginning breast-feeding as soon as possible after delivery. A neonate that will be breast-fed should not be given formula by bottle at this time. Many institutions provide sterile water for the initial feeding to assess for esophageal atresia. Because colostrum is not irritating if aspirated and is readily absorbed by the neonate's respiratory system, breast-feeding can be done immediately after birth. (I, N, G)

13. 2. Most authorities suggest that a woman in an early stage of labor be allowed to walk if she wishes, as long as no complications are present. Birthing centers or single-room maternity units allow women considerable latitude without much supervision at this stage of labor. However, if the client's membranes rupture, it would be wise for the nurse to check for potential prolapsed cord. (I, N, G)

14. 1. Childbirth educators use various techniques and methods to prepare parents for labor and delivery. Active relaxation involves relaxing uninvolved muscle groups while contracting a specific group and using chest breathing techniques to lift the diaphragm off the contracting uterus. Hypnosis is a technique in which the client assumes a state of mind that makes her open to suggestions from an attendant or coach. (E, N, H)

15. 3. Light stroking of the skin, effleurage is often used with the Lamaze method of childbirth preparation. (I, N, G)

16. 2. Increased bloody show normally occurs when cervical dilatation increases. Fetal descent is unrelated to show. Rupture of the fetal membranes will result in the escape of amnionic fluid, not bloody show. Premature separation of the placenta is usually accompanied by bleeding, frequently concealed. (I, N, G)

17. 2. Recommendations for food and fluid intake during labor varies widely in the literature and in clinical practice. Gastric emptying is slower in pregnancy, and the potential for nausea and vomiting poses a risk for aspiration of stomach contents. Clients are often limited to clear fluids or ice chips, and many institutions have a policy of administering intravenous fluids. Even without food in the stomach, nausea and vomiting are common late in the first stage of labor. (I, N, G)

18. 3. As the client progresses into the first stage of labor and the contractions become stronger and closer together, she typically becomes less talkative and more serious. She tends to turn her thoughts inward as she begins to concentrate on the work at hand. (D, N, L)

19. 3. When a client is hyperventilating during labor, she is eliminating more carbon dioxide than usual. As a result, she becomes lightheaded or dizzy. Being lightheaded or dizzy is not correlated with normal active labor, elevated blood pressure, or shortness of breath. (D, N, G)

20. 3. Pushing during the first stage of labor when the urge is felt but the cervix is not completely dilated may produce swelling and make labor more difficult. The client should be encouraged to use a pant blow (blow-blow) pattern of breathing to help overcome the urge to push. Administering a sedative or instructing the client to push lightly is not recommended. (I, N, G)

21. 4. During the transition phase of the first stage of labor, the client needs encouragement and support. This is a difficult and painful time, when contractions are especially strong. During this phase, the client usually finds it very difficult to maintain self-control. Everything else seems secondary to her as she progresses into the second stage of labor and delivery. (I, N, G)

22. 4. The second stage of labor begins with complete cervical dilatation and ends with delivery. Show normally is bloody during the first stage of labor, especially when in the transition phase. The membranes often rupture in the second stage of labor, but they may also rupture earlier—in some instances, even before labor begins. Contractions can be strong in the first stage of labor as well as in the second stage. (E, N, H)

23. 2. Expressions of disappointment with the baby's sex may signal problems with maternal-infant bonding. Hostile or very low key (passive) behavior toward the baby may also be a cue to potential bonding problems. (D, N, L)

24. 4. According to the gate control theory of pain perception, when the endings of small peripheral nerve fibers detect a stimulus, they transmit it to cells in the dorsal horn of the spinal cord. These impulses pass through a network of cells in the spinal cord called the substantia gelatinosa, and a synapse occurs that returns the transmission to the peripheral site through a motor nerve. The impulse is then transmitted via the spinal cord to the brain, where the impulse is perceived as pain. Gate control mechanisms in the spinal cord are capable of halting these impulses (closing the gate), so pain is not perceived. (I, N, G)

25. 1. According to the gate control theory of pain, a closed gate means that the client should feel no pain. (I, N, G)

26. 2. Personalized concentration points or ideas serve as a distraction from pain. They do not act as a projection, rationalization, or counterirritant for pain. (E, N, G)

27. 2. During active labor, the client's blood pressure should be monitored every hour between contractions. If the client exhibits hypotension or hypertension, blood pressure should be monitored more frequently. Blood pressure normally increases during a contraction, which is why it is best to measure blood pressure between contractions. (P, N, G)

28. 2. While the client is fairly comfortable and in early labor, distraction activities (e.g., reading, television, cards, or games) are recommended. In addition, the client should be encouraged to use appropriate breathing techniques, particularly slow chest breathing. No information given in this situation indicates that it is necessary to keep an accurate record of this client's urine output, although she should be encouraged to void every 2 to 3 hours to prevent bladder distention. (I, N, G)

29. 1. The psychoprophylaxis method of childbirth suggests using slow chest breathing until it becomes ineffective during labor contractions, then to switch to shallow abdominal breathing during the peak of a contraction. When transition nears, a pant-blow pattern of breathing is used. (I, T, G)

30. 2. The symptoms of hyperventilation result from excess carbon dioxide elimination from the body. Hence, rebreathing into a paper bag or cupping the hands is beneficial. This increases the carbon dioxide intake during respiration. Taking whiffs of oxygen, breathing rapidly and shallowly, and breathing with forceful expirations will likely aggravate the condition. (I, N, G)

31. 4. The carbon dioxide insufficiency that occurs during hyperventilation will lead to respiratory alkalosis. (A, N, G)

32. 3. When a client complains of severe back pain during labor, the fetus is most likely in an occipitoposterior position. This means that the fetal head presses against the client's sacrum, which causes marked discomfort during contractions. Repositioning the client and providing sacral backrubs may help alleviate the discomfort. Transverse and anterior occiput positions do not cause pressure on the sacrum. Occipitodiagonal is not a fetal position. (I, N, G)

33. 4. The client with back pain during labor experiences marked discomfort, more so than when the fetus is in the anterior position. Severe back pain during labor does not necessarily require a cesarean delivery or an extensive episiotomy. The physician may elect to do an episiotomy, but it is not necessarily required. It is unlikely that a primigravida with a fetus in an occipitoposterior position will have a precipitous delivery. (P, N, S)

34. 3. The most appropriate nursing diagnosis at this time is Pain related to unexpected and intense back discomfort. There is no information to indicate the diagnoses Anxiety, Noncompliance, and High Risk for Injury. (D, N, S)

The Multigravida in Labor

35. 2. The nurse's first action when membranes rupture spontaneously is to check the odor, consistency, and volume of the amniotic fluid. For this client the fetal head is engaged and at +1 station, so there is little likelihood of cord prolapse. However, when the fetal head is not engaged, checking for cord prolapse is the first priority when the membranes spontaneously rupture. Amniotic fluid is usually straw-colored. Greenish-brown fluid (meconium) indicates that the fetus has suffered a hypoxic event. Yellowish fluid may indicate fetal anemia, hypoxia, or intrauterine infection. All clients have their contractions monitored while in labor. Delivery is not imminent if the client is 6 cm dilated, but multigravidas may progress quickly, especially after rupture of the membranes. Changing the client's position is not necessary simply because the membranes have ruptured. (I, T, G)

36. 1. Variable decelerations usually indicate cord compression. After the membranes rupture, variable decelerations are common. This decreases protection to the cord, particularly as the fetus descends the birth canal. Repositioning the client often helps to correct this fetal heart rate pattern. If repositioning is not successful, the clinician may choose to perform amnioinfusion—infusion of sterile saline solution into the uterus via sterile catheter. This procedure helps take the pressure off the cord. Increasing the intravenous fluid rate is not helpful. There is no need to prepare the client for a cesarean delivery at this time. Delivery is not imminent, so shaving the perineum is not necessary. (In fact, there is controversy as to whether shaving should be performed at all.) (I, N, G)

37. 3. Early decelerations are usually due to pressure on the fetal head as the fetus progresses through the birth canal. These decelerations mirror the contraction pattern and are usually benign, unless the pattern occurs in early labor. If this pattern is demonstrated in early labor, it may indicate cephalopelvic disproportion. Variable decelerations are associated with cord compression. Malpresentations are not usually associated with early decelerations. Inadequate placental perfusion is associated with late fetal heart rate decelerations. (E, N, G)

38. 2. The American College of Obstetricians and Gynecologists has classified forceps applications into three categories: outlet, low, and midforceps. When the fetal skull is at +2 or higher station, this is considered low forceps. Forceps applied when the fetal skull is seen on the perineum and the scalp is visible between contractions are called outlet forceps. Midforceps application occurs when the head is engaged but above +2 station. Forceps application is not indicated if the fetal skull is at the level of the ischial spines. (I, N, G)

39. 3. A chill shortly after delivery is not uncommon. Warm blankets can help provide comfort for the client. The nurse should also explain that the reaction is normal. It has been suggested that the shivering response is caused by a difference in internal and external body temperatures. A different theory proposes that the women is reacting to fetal cells that have entered the maternal bloodstream via the placental site. It takes time to produce a temperature change following a chill. An analgesic is not indicated. The volume of blood loss is not necessarily related to a chill. (A, N, G)

40. 3. The most appropriate diagnosis at this time is High Risk for Injury related to the effects of the epidural anesthesia. The client may have no sensation in her lower abdomen and legs for several hours following delivery. Care should be taken to avoid injury, and ambulation should be delayed until sensation has returned. There are no data to suggest Pain due to exhaustive pushing or Fluid Volume Excess. Knowledge Deficit related to self-care during the postpartum period is not a priority. The client is a multigravida and should have some knowledge related to postpartum self-care. (D, N, G)

The Intrapartal Client With Risk Factors

41. 3. When admitting a client to the hospital's labor unit, the nurse needs to obtain certain information about the client promptly to plan care. Particularly with a multigravida, the information should most certainly include the frequency, intensity, and duration of labor contractions. In addition, the nurse should determine when the labor began, whether the membranes have ruptured, and the client's estimated delivery date. From this information, the nurse gets a quick overview of the client's status and can then proceed to plan effective care. Whether the client has felt fetal movement, when she last had food or fluids, and whether she wishes to breastfeed are important, but less influential in initial plans for care. (A, N, G)

42. 3. A side-lying or semi-Fowler's position helps to ensure cardiac emptying and adequate oxygenation. In addition, oxygen by mask, analgesics and sedatives, diuretics, prophylactic antibiotics, and digitalis may be warranted. Breathing rapidly during a contraction, limiting the number of visitors, and refusing analgesia or anesthesia do not help the load on the cardiac system. (I, N, G)

43. 2. Lumbar epidural anesthesia is usually administered with the client in a left side-lying position with shoulders parallel and legs slightly flexed. (I, N, G)

44. 4. The nurse should auscultate the client's lungs frequently for evidence of rales, which may indicate cardiac decompensation. Vital signs and fetal status also must be monitored. Pulse rate above 100 beats per minute or respiratory rate above 25 breaths per minute may indicate cardiac decompensation. Clients with cardiac disease are not given ergot products. The client should not experience excessive discomfort with contractions, as sedation and anesthesia are advised. Symptoms of infection are important to note, but cardiac status is more important for the laboring client who may suffer cardiac decompensation. (A, N, G)

45. 4. A client who has received lumbar epidural anesthesia usually does not feel the urge to push. The nurse is responsible for informing the client when the contraction begins by palpating the fundus for a contraction. Bulging of the perineum results from pushing. (P, N, G)

46. 3. Before beginning intravenous oxytocin infusion, the nurse should obtain a baseline measurement of fetal heart rate. If the fetal heart rate pattern shows fetal distress, the client is not a candidate for induction. The client should be positioned on her left side for optimal placental perfusion and to avoid vena cava syndrome. The client is not in labor, so there are no contractions to monitor. There is no indication that the client's urine should be tested before intravenous oxytocin infusion. (I, N, S)

47. 4. Metabolic changes occurring during labor and delivery require close monitoring of the diabetic client's blood glucose level—every hour, during labor. There is no indication that the client's urine output needs to be measured every hour. Insulin, if needed, is usually given intravenously and will depend on the client's blood sugar levels. There is no indication that the client's urine should be checked for protein every 2 hours. However, because pregnant diabetic clients are more prone to pregnancy-induced hypertension, any evidence of protein in the urine should be reported. (P, N, G)

48. 1. Induction of labor with an oxytocic agent carries risks. It is essential that a nurse remain with the client at all times to monitor uterine contractions and fetal heart rate. Even if the client is being monitored with electronic monitoring equipment, a nurse needs to remain at the bedside. Oxytocin administration carries a risk of water intoxication and uterine rupture. There is no need to keep the client awake during the procedure, nor does the client need to change position every 1/2 hour. The usual protocol is to increase the dosage of the oxytocin in accordance with institutional policy, until a regular contraction pattern is established, at which time the infusion should be maintained at that rate or decreased. The infusion should be discontinued and the physician notified if fetal distress is noted or if contractions occur less than 2 minutes apart or last longer than 60 seconds. (I, N, G)

49. 4. The most appropriate diagnosis at this time is Potential for Injury to mother and fetus related to dysfunctional carbohydrate metabolism. The normal changes of carbohydrate metabolism that occur during pregnancy make control of diabetes more difficult. Diabetic mothers have a higher incidence of pregnancy-induced hypertension, polyhydramnios, preterm birth, and larger-than-usual fetus and often have decreased placental perfusion. Infants of diabetic mothers may have polycythemia, congenital anomalies, and respiratory distress. There is no information to support the diagnoses Knowledge Deficit and Pain related to prolonged labor. There is no indication that the client will require cesarean delivery at this time. (D, N, S)

50. 1. A common sign of fetal distress due to an inadequate transfer of oxygen to the fetus is meconium-stained fluid. Because the fetus has suffered hypoxia, close fetal heart rate monitoring is necessary. Amniocentesis findings, fetal position, and estimated fetal size are not related to meconium staining. In a breech presentation, some meconium-stained fluid may be present. (A, N, G)

51. 4. With the fetus at −2 station, the cord may prolapse as amniotic fluid rushes out. The nurse should inspect the perineal area to detect cord prolapse immediately after the amniotomy. The color, amount, and odor of the amniotic fluid should be noted. Fetal heart rate should be monitored. The client's optimal position is on the left side, but this is not a priority at this time. The client is not having a precipitous delivery with the fetal skull at −2 station. Maternal blood pressure should be monitored throughout labor, but this is not a priority at this time. (I, N, G)

52. 4. Late decelerations of fetal heart rate signals poor placental perfusion. The nurse should stop the oxytocin infusion and report the pattern to the attending clinician. The client should be turned to her left side, and oxygen may be administered. If the pattern persists or if decreased variability occurs, then delivery may be indicated. The nurse should provide information about fetal well-being throughout the labor process. Immediate cesarean delivery is not indicated unless the pattern persists. The contraction pattern is monitored throughout the induction of labor, but the priority here is to discontinue the oxytocin infusion. (I, N, G)

53. 1. Aspiration of meconium is best prevented by suctioning the neonate's nasopharynx immediately after the head is delivered and before the shoulders and chest are delivered. As long as the chest is compressed in the vagina, the infant will not inhale and aspirate meconium in the upper respiratory tract. Meconium aspiration blocks the air flow to the alveoli, leading to potentially life-threatening respiratory complications. Based on the information provided, there is no need for intubation, oxygen, or medication at this time. (E, N, S)

54. 3. Neonates born to mothers who smoke tend to have lower-than-average birth weights. Maternal smoking is not related to higher pulse rate, below-average hemoglobin, or increased respiratory rate unless complications arise, such as pre-term birth or respiratory distress. (I, N, G)

55. 1. An episiotomy serves several purposes. It shortens the second stage of labor, substitutes a clean surgical incision for a tear, and decreases undue stretching of perineal muscles. An episiotomy helps prevent tearing of the rectum but does not necessarily relieve pressure on the rectum. Although an episiotomy usually helps prevent tearing, this may still occur. An episiotomy does not facilitate the third stage of labor, which extends from delivery of the neonate to delivery of the placenta. (E, N, S)

56. 1. When the client says the baby is coming, the nurse should first inspect the perineum and observe for crowning. It is vital in this situation that the nurse validate the client's statement. If the client is not delivering precipitously, the nurse can calm her and use appropriate breathing techniques. Timing contractions is not the priority action. Fetal heart rate is monitored throughout the labor process. The nurse should try to obtain assistance if delivery is imminent, but should never leave the client. Delivery may occur before the physician arrives. (I, N, S)

57. 3. The nurse should immediately prepare a clean area for delivery when birth is imminent and no additional help is available. Most hospital labor units have emergency delivery packs with sterile towels, a bulb syringe, and a cord clamp. The nurse should remember to use universal precautions and don a pair of sterile gloves for the delivery. Trying to delay the birth is contraindicated. The nurse should instruct the client to pant or pant-blow to decrease the urge to push. Pushing the head out quickly can cause tearing of the perineum. An analgesic is not warranted. The head of the bed should be elevated to about 45 degrees, not lowered. The client should assume a position of comfort. (I, N, G)

58. 4. The nurse should remain calm during a precipitous delivery. Explaining to the client what is happening as the birth progresses and how she can assist is likely to help her remain calm and cooperative. Maintaining eye contact is also beneficial. The cliche "everything is fine" is not appropriate. Asking the client if her husband should be called is not appropriate when birth is imminent and no help is available. Saying that the physician will be there soon may not be an accurate statement and is not very reassuring if the client is concerned about the delivery. (I, N, L)

59. 1. It is best to deliver the neonate's head between contractions to prevent the head from emerging suddenly, with subsequent tearing of the perineum and possible cerebral damage to the neonate. The nurse should support the perineum with one hand while controlling delivery of the head with the other hand. (P, N, S)

60. 2. As soon as the neonate's head is delivered, the nurse should check the neck for the umbilical cord. A cord encircling the neck should be pulled down gently and slipped over the head. This is done to avoid cutting off the infant's oxygen supply, which may occur if the infant's shoulder presses on the cord during delivery, interrupting the blood supply through the cord. If the cord is too tight around the neck to be removed, it should be double-clamped and cut before the rest of the body is delivered, to prevent asphyxiation. The neonate should then be delivered quickly. Having the client push forcefully may cause tearing of the perineum. The nurse will not apply gentle traction on the infant's anterior shoulder until the cord has been checked and the head delivered. Placing pressure on the client's fundus is not helpful. (I, N, G)

61. 3. The best course of action is to wait for a sign of placental separation. Pulling on the cord before the placenta is delivered may cause inversion of the uterus. Signs of placental separation include lengthening of the umbilical cord, a slight gush of dark blood, and a change in the contour of the fundus from discoid to globula. After separation occurs, the client can be asked to bear down. Massaging the fundus is not helpful. (I, N, G)

62. 3. A major advantage of monitoring fetal heart rate electronically is that it provides for a continuous recording of the heart rate during and between contractions. A fetoscope allows only a sampling of readings and is not as accurate in determining variables in fetal heart rate. Electronic monitoring may require less nursing time, but this is not a major advantage for using it. The client may have some discomfort from wearing the belts continuously, but these can be removed now and then. The client is less mobile with the monitoring belts in place. Newer electronic monitoring devices do not use belts and are more comfortable. (E, N, H)

63. 3. The client should be carefully assessed for symptoms of pregnancy-induced hypertension, which is more common in clients expecting twins. Urinary frequency may occur as the uterus impinges on the bladder, but this is not unusual. Oligohydramnios and polycythemia are not typically associated with twin gestations. Anemia is more common than polycythemia. (P, N, G)

64. 2. The nurse should contact the physician because the client is most likely experiencing hypotonic uterine contractions. These contractions tend to be painful but ineffective. The usual treatment is oxytocin augmentation, unless cephalopelvic disproportion exists. The heart rates of both fetuses will be continuously monitored. There is no indication that a sedative is necessary. Having the client flex her thighs up against her abdomen may be done in the second stage of labor when she is pushing. (I, N, H)

65. 4. Dizygotic, or fraternal, twins develop from two ova and two sperm. They may be of the same sex, but their chances of resembling each other are no greater than that of any siblings. Identical, or monozygotic, twins develop from a single ovum and single sperm. (I, N, H)

66. 4. Uterine atony means that the uterus is not firm or boggy because it is not contracting. This can lead to postpartum hemorrhage. Clients with multiple gestation, polyhydramnios, prolonged labor, or large-for-gestational age fetus are more prone to uterine atony. Thrombophlebitis, puerperal infection, and uterine rupture are not associated with uterine atony. (I, N, G)

67. 2. It is important that the parents be allowed to touch, hold, and participate in care of the twins whenever they desire. Ideally, this will be on a daily basis, to promote parent-infant bonding. It is not appropriate to discuss jealousy between the twins, as this may not occur. Having the couple visit the twins twice weekly is not appropriate; they should visit and provide care whenever they desire. Identifying complications that may occur is not appropriate. (P, N, H)

68. 4. The client should use exhale breathing while pushing to avoid the adverse physiologic effects of the Valsalva maneuver, which occurs with prolonged breath-holding during pushing. The technique for exhale breathing includes inhaling several deep breaths, holding the breath for 5 to 6 seconds, and exhaling slowly every 5 to 6 seconds through pursed lips while continuing to hold the breath. The Valsalva maneuver can also be avoided by exhaling continuously while pushing. Semi-Fowler's position enhances the effectiveness of the abdominal muscle efforts during pushing, but the client can assume a squatting or side-lying position if desired. The client should flex her thighs and exert downward pressure while pushing. (E, N, H)

69. 4. A bilateral pudendal block is used for vaginal deliveries to relieve pain primarily in the perineum and vagina. It does not relieve discomfort in the uterus, cervix, or back. Pudendal block anesthesia is adequate for episiotomy and its repair. (I, N, G)

70. 1. Adverse effects on the neonate following pudendal block include bradycardia, hypotonia, reduced responsiveness, and seizures. These complications are thought to be related to accidental injection of the fetal scalp. The neonate's respiratory rate and color are monitored closely after birth, but deviations are not related to the pudendal anesthesia. The neonate's blood pressure is not routinely monitored unless complications exist. (I, N, G)

71. 3. Deep suctioning of the nasopharynx immediately after birth carries the danger of stimulating the vagus nerve, which causes a slow heartbeat. Careless suctioning can injure the neonate's mucous membranes. Routine suctioning does not decrease the neonate's normal efforts to clear mucus. Oversuctioning may remove too much oxygen (not carbon dioxide), which can cause respiratory distress. (I, N, G)

72. 2. A neonate in good condition needs to be kept warm. This reduces cold stress and potential respiratory problems. The infant can be evaluated under a radiant warmer or wrapped in dry, warm blankets on the mother's abdomen. A neonate in good condition does not need oxygen therapy, intubation, or cardiac massage. (I, N, G)

73. 2. The Apgar scoring system evaluates the neonate at 1 minute and again at 5 minutes after birth, assessing color, heart rate, respiratory effort, muscle tone, and reflex irritability. (I, N, G)

74. 2. Postmature neonates frequently have difficulty maintaining adequate glucose reserves. Other common problems include meconium aspiration syndrome, polycythemia, congenital anomalies, seizure activity, and cold stress. These complications are primarily due to a combination of advanced gestational age, placental insufficiency, and continued exposure to amniotic fluid. (I, N, G)

75. 1. If a client has been in active labor and there is no change in effacement or cervical dilatation after 2 hours, the nurse should suspect cephalopelvic disproportion. The client is not experiencing a prolonged latent phase (dilatation 0–3 cm), effects of sedation, or a hypertonic contraction pattern. (D, N, G)

76. 1. The true conjugate, or obstetric conjugate, is the most important measurement when judging the adequacy of a client's pelvis for a normal vaginal delivery. (E, N, G)

77. 3. Preparation for cesarean delivery is similar to preparation for any abdominal surgery. The client must give informed consent. Another person may not sign for the client, unless the client is unable to sign the form. If this is the case, only certain designated persons may do so legally. The husband does not need to sign the form unless his wife is unable to do so. (I, N, S)

78. 1. An indwelling catheter ensures that the urinary bladder will remain empty during surgery and so is common before cesarean delivery. A narcotic medication will depress the neonate, so it usually is not prescribed. The client's skin cannot be sterilized. The husband may join his wife in the operating room if he desires; he is not required to remain in the waiting room. (P, N, G)

79. 2. Nalbuphine (Nubain), a synthetic agonist-antagonist similar to butorphanol and pentzocine, is used for analgesia during labor. Although the client may rest or fall asleep after administration, it is not a sedative. The client should not experience numbness from this drug. The drug is not given to counteract nausea. (E, N, G)

80. 4. Decreased variability may be seen in various conditions; however, it is most commonly due to analgesic administration. Other factors that can cause decreased variability include anesthesia, deep fetal sleep, anencephaly, prematurity, hypoxia, tachycardia, brain damage, and arrhythmias. Maternal hypoventilation and cephalopelvic disproportion are not commonly associated with decreased variability. The fetal heart rate is 130 beats per minute, so the fetus is not in distress. (I, N, G)

81. 3. The postoperative care of a client who has received general anesthesia for a cesarean delivery should include frequent assessment of uterine tone, as uterine atony is more common after general anesthesia. General anesthesia also carries a greater risk for maternal vomiting and aspiration. The client may experience hypotension. General anesthesia is not related to delayed breast milk production or postpartal infection; however, clients with surgical incisions are more prone to infection during the postpartum period. (P, N, G)

82. 4. Respiratory distress syndrome is more common in neonates delivered by cesarean section than in those delivered vaginally. Such conditions as convulsions, cold stress, and umbilical cord infections are not more common in cesarean delivery. (I, N, G)

83. 3. Further assessment is warranted if the client expresses indifference. This may indicate a potential problem with maternal-infant bonding. It is not unusual for a client who experiences an emergency cesarean section to feel relief, frustration, and disappointment. With therapeutic communication skills, the nurse can help the client express these feelings and adjust to the postoperative period. (A, N, L)

84. 1. An ominous sign, the sinusoidal pattern is usually associated with Rh isoimmunization, severe anemia, and asphyxiation. It can also be attributed to the administration of nalbuphine hydrochloride (Nubain) and intravenous butorphanol tartrate (Stadol). Because no medication has been given to this client, the pattern suggests fetal anemia. Internal fetal monitoring should be instituted and cesarean delivery considered. (I, N, G)

85. 1. Amniotic fluid is normally clear. Yellowish fluid indicates Rh sensitization. The yellowish color is related to fetal anemia and bilirubin. In a breech presentation, it is not uncommon for the amniotic fluid to be greenish due to meconium expelled by the fetus. Amniotic fluid embolism is not related to the fluid color. This dangerous situation may occur naturally after a difficult labor or from hyperstimulation of the uterus. Amniotic fluid may leak into the maternal circulation. Symptoms include respiratory distress, circulatory collapse, acute hemorrhage, tachycardia, hypotension, chest pain, and cyanosis. Amniotic fluid embolism is a medical emergency, and maternal mortality is high. Polyhydramnios refers to an excessive volume of amniotic fluid. (I, N, G)

86. 1. The first step in cord prolapse is to relieve pressure on the cord. Immediate measures include lowering the client's head by using the Trendelenburg position or knee-chest position so that the fetal presenting part will move away from the pelvis, and moving the fetal presenting part off the cord by applying pressure through the vagina with a sterile gloved hand. Oxygen may be administered. Immediate cesarean delivery is usually performed. The nurse should not attempt to replace the cord into the vagina. (P, N, G)

87. 2. Nursing responsibilities during exchange transfusion include assembling the equipment, preparing the neonate and parents, assisting the physician during the procedure, monitoring the neonate's status before and during the procedure, and maintaining careful records. Calcium gluconate is not given before the procedure, but may be administered intravenously after each 100 ml of blood infusion, if indicated. The neonate should be in a warm environment, preferably under a radiant warmer, and should be NPO for at least 4 hours before the procedure to prevent possible aspiration. The parents should be kept informed of the neonate's condition. (P, N, G)

88. 1. A client with possible acute pyelonephritis should be closely assessed for chills, high fever, and flank pain. In addition, the client is at risk for preterm labor and intrauterine growth retardation. Pyelonephritis is not treated with penicillin. The client will not be required to have a cesarean delivery, unless severe fetal complications develop. The client is not at risk for uterine hemorrhage. (P, N, G)

89. 3. The Infectious Disease Society for Obstetrics and Gynecology has issued guidelines for the management of clients with herpes simplex virus type 2. If no lesions are present, vaginal delivery should be attempted. For a client with visible lesions, cesarean delivery should be planned. Acyclovir (Zovirax) is not recommended during pregnancy. There is no contraindication to breast-feeding if the client desires. (I, N, H)

90. 2. A client who experiences a precipitous labor and delivery is at increased risk for excessive uterine bleeding, lacerations of the soft tissues, and potential uterine rupture. Ineffective bonding, intrauterine infection, and urinary stasis are not associated with precipitous labor and delivery. (I, N, G)

NURSING CARE OF THE CHILDBEARING FAMILY AND THEIR NEONATE

TEST 3: The Birth Experience

Directions: Use this answer grid to determine areas of strength or need for further study.

NURSING PROCESS

A = Assessment
D = Analysis, nursing diagnosis
P = Planning
I = Implementation
E = Evaluation

COGNITIVE LEVEL

K = Knowledge
C = Comprehension
T = Application
N = Analysis

CLIENT NEEDS

S = Safe, effective care environment
G = Physiological integrity
L = Psychosocial integrity
H = Health promotion/maintenance

		Nursing Process					Cognitive Level				Client Needs			
Question #	Answer #	A	D	P	I	E	K	C	T	N	S	G	L	H
1	3	A						C					L	
2	2				I			C						H
3	1	A						C				G		
4	1					E				N				H
5	1	A								N		G		
6	1		D							N		G		
7	1		D							N		G		
8	4				I					N				H
9	4		D							N		G		
10	2		D							N		G		
11	3		D							N		G		
12	1				I					N		G		
13	2				I					N		G		
14	1					E				N				H
15	3				I					N		G		
16	2				I					N		G		
17	2				I					N		G		
18	3		D							N			L	
19	3		D							N		G		
20	3				I					N		G		
21	4				I					N		G		
22	4					E				N				H
23	2		D							N			L	

ANSWER GRID: 1

NURSING PROCESS

A = Assessment
D = Nursing diagnosis
P = Planning
I = Implementation
E = Evaluation

COGNITIVE LEVEL

K = Knowledge
C = Comprehension
T = Application
N = Analysis

CLIENT NEEDS

S = Safe, effective environment
G = Physiological integrity
L = Psychosocial integrity
H = Health promotion/maintenance

		Nursing Process					Cognitive Level				Client Needs			
Question #	Answer #	A	D	P	I	E	K	C	T	N	S	G	L	H
24	4				I					N		G		
25	1				I					N		G		
26	2					E				N		G		
27	2			P						N		G		
28	2				I					N		G		
29	1				I				T			G		
30	2				I					N		G		
31	4	A								N		G		
32	3				I					N		G		
33	4			P						N	S			
34	3		D							N	S			
35	2				I				T			G		
36	1				I					N		G		
37	3					E				N		G		
38	2				I					N		G		
39	3	A								N		G		
40	3		D							N		G		
41	3	A								N		G		
42	3				I					N		G		
43	2				I					N		G		
44	4	A								N		G		
45	4			P						N		G		
46	3				I					N	S			
47	4			P						N		G		
48	1				I					N		G		
49	4		D							N	S			
50	1	A								N		G		
51	4				I					N		G		
52	4				I					N		G		

ANSWER GRID: 2

Nursing Process

A = Assessment
D = Nursing diagnosis
P = Planning
I = Implementation
E = Evaluation

Cognitive Level

K = Knowledge
C = Comprehension
T = Application
N = Analysis

Client Needs

S = Safe, effective environment
G = Physiological integrity
L = Psychosocial integrity
H = Health promotion/maintenance

		Nursing Process					Cognitive Level				Client Needs			
Question #	Answer #	A	D	P	I	E	K	C	T	N	S	G	L	H
53	1					E				N	S			
54	3				I					N		G		
55	1					E				N	S			
56	1				I					N	S			
57	3				I					N		G		
58	4				I					N			L	
59	1			P						N	S			
60	2				I					N		G		
61	3				I					N		G		
62	3					E				N				H
63	3			P						N		G		
64	2				I					N				H
65	4				I					N				H
66	4				I					N		G		
67	2			P						N				H
68	4					E				N				H
69	4				I					N		G		
70	1				I					N		G		
71	3				I					N		G		
72	2				I					N		G		
73	2				I					N		G		
74	2				I					N		G		
75	1		D							N		G		
76	1					E				N		G		
77	3				I					N	S			
78	1			P						N		G		
79	2					E				N		G		
80	4				I					N		G		
81	3			P						N		G		

Answer Grid: 3

NURSING PROCESS

A = Assessment
D = Nursing diagnosis
P = Planning
I = Implementation
E = Evaluation

COGNITIVE LEVEL

K = Knowledge
C = Comprehension
T = Application
N = Analysis

CLIENT NEEDS

S = Safe, effective environment
G = Physiological integrity
L = Psychosocial integrity
H = Health promotion/maintenance

		Nursing Process					Cognitive Level				Client Needs			
Question #	Answer #	A	D	P	I	E	K	C	T	N	S	G	L	H
82	4				I					N		G		
83	3	A								N			L	
84	1				I					N		G		
85	1				I					N		G		
86	1			P						N		G		
87	2			P						N		G		
88	1			P						N		G		
89	3				I					N				H
90	2				I					N		G		
Number Correct														
Number Possible	90	9	12	12	46	11	0	3	2	85	9	65	5	11
Percentage Correct														

Score Calculation:

To determine your **Percentage Correct**, divide the **Number Correct** by the **Number Possible.**

Postpartum Care

Test 4

The Postpartal Client With a Vaginal Birth
The Postpartal Client Who Breast Feeds
The Postpartal Client Who Bottle Feeds
The Postpartal Client With a Cesarean Birth
Correct Answers and Rationale

Select the one best answer and indicate your choice by filling in the circle in front of the option.

The Postpartal Client With a Vaginal Birth

A primigravida has delivered her first baby, with labor, delivery, recovery, and the postpartum period in the same hospital room.

1. When instilling erythromycin ointment into the neonate's eyes, the nurse should place the medication
- ○ 1. on the cornea.
- ○ 2. at the inner canthus.
- ○ 3. at the outer canthus.
- ○ 4. in the lower conjunctival sac.

2. The physician orders an intramuscular injection of phytonadione (AquaMephyton) for the neonate. The nurse explains to the client that this medication will be injected in which of the neonate's muscles?
- ○ 1. Deltoid.
- ○ 2. Gluteus medius.
- ○ 3. Gluteus maximus.
- ○ 4. Vastus lateralis.

3. When the nurse accidentally bumps the bassinet, the neonate throws out its arms, hands opened, and begins to cry. Following instructions, the nurse determines that the mother understands this reflex when she states that it is the
- ○ 1. Moro reflex.
- ○ 2. rooting reflex.
- ○ 3. grasping reflex.
- ○ 4. tonic neck reflex.

4. In response to the nurse's question about how she is feeling, the client replies that she is "tired, sore, and hungry." She then begins to relate her birth experience. Based on the assessment data, the nurse determines that the client is in which phase of the postpartal psychological adaptation process?
- ○ 1. Giving up.
- ○ 2. Taking in.
- ○ 3. Letting go.
- ○ 4. Taking hold.

5. In planning care for the client for the first 24 hours, the nurse should plan for her primary concerns, which will most likely focus on her
- ○ 1. baby.
- ○ 2. husband.
- ○ 3. own comfort.
- ○ 4. mothering skills.

6. The nurse plans to teach the client about infant care when the client is in which phase of postpartal psychological adaptation?
- ○ 1. Taking in.
- ○ 2. Letting go.
- ○ 3. Taking hold.
- ○ 4. Letting down.

The nurse is caring for a 24-year-old primipara following a spontaneous vaginal delivery under local anesthesia.

7. About 4 hours after delivery, the client says she needs to urinate. The nurse should
- ○ 1. catheterize the client.
- ○ 2. offer her a bedpan.
- ○ 3. check her bladder for distention.
- ○ 4. assist her in ambulating to the bathroom.

8. While the client is taking her first shower after delivery, the nurse remains nearby to assess her for
- ○ 1. chilling.
- ○ 2. fainting.
- ○ 3. vomiting.
- ○ 4. hemorrhaging.

9. Twelve hours after delivery, the nurse documents that involution is progressing normally after palpating the client's fundus
- ○ 1. slightly above the level of the umbilicus.
- ○ 2. midway between the umbilicus and the symphysis pubis.

○ 3. barely above the upper margin of the symphysis pubis.
○ 4. at the level of the umbilicus, deviated to the left.

10. Assessing the client on the second postpartum day, the nurse notes an ecchymotic area to the right of the perineum. The nurse should
○ 1. apply an ice bag to the perineum.
○ 2. continue with the client's usual care.
○ 3. increase the number of sitz baths from three to six each day.
○ 4. contact the physician for further orders.

The nurse is caring for a multipara who has just delivered a viable male neonate vaginally under epidural block anesthesia. The client has a midline episiotomy.

11. The nurse notes that the client's bladder is distended. The nurse explains that this is most likely due to
○ 1. having delivered a term neonate.
○ 2. a bladder infection.
○ 3. pressure of the uterus on the bladder.
○ 4. edema in the lower urinary tract area.

12. The nurse formulates a nursing diagnosis for the client. An appropriate diagnosis is
○ 1. High Risk for Infection related to labor process and episiotomy.
○ 2. Fatigue related to lengthy labor process.
○ 3. Fluid Volume Excess related to intravenous fluid therapy.
○ 4. Urinary Retention related to trauma of delivery.

13. The client asks the nurse about postpartum exercises. The nurse instructs the client that the most appropriate exercise to start with on the first postpartum day is to assume a
○ 1. sitting position, lie back, and then return to a sitting position.
○ 2. prone position, then do push-ups by using the arms to lift the upper body.
○ 3. supine position with the knees flexed, then inhale deeply while allowing the abdomen to expand and exhale while contracting the abdominal muscles.
○ 4. supine position with the knees flexed, then bring the chin onto the chest wall while inhaling and reach for the knees by lifting the head and shoulders while exhaling.

14. The client seems embarrassed when the nurse observes her talking to her baby. The nurse explains that most neonates
○ 1. prefer high-pitched speech with tonal variations.
○ 2. respond to low-pitched speech with a sameness of tone.
○ 3. like cooing sounds rather than words.
○ 4. cannot hear well enough to be aware of speech until about age 4 weeks.

15. Eight hours after delivery, the client is unable to urinate; the nurse prepares to catheterize her. When inserting the catheter, the nurse feels resistance. The nurse's most appropriate action is to
○ 1. remove the catheter and wait about an hour before trying to reinsert it.
○ 2. pull the catheter back about ½ inch before trying to move it inward again.
○ 3. allow the labia to fall into place and then gently advance the catheter again.
○ 4. ask the client to bear down gently as if to void and slowly advance the catheter 2 to 3 inches.

The nurse is caring for a primipara who delivered a viable neonate by spontaneous vaginal delivery under local anesthesia.

16. After teaching the client about lochia, the nurse determines that she understands the instructions when she says that on the second postpartum day, the lochia should be
○ 1. pink.
○ 2. white.
○ 3. dark red.
○ 4. dark yellow.

17. The client asks the nurse, "Why does my baby spit up the formula after feeding?" The nurse's best response is to explain that the regurgitation is thought to result from
○ 1. an immature cardiac sphincter.
○ 2. a small stomach in relation to total body size.
○ 3. slow peristaltic action.
○ 4. inappropriate feeding methods.

18. The nurse teaches the client to provide visual stimulation to the neonate, explaining that this is best accomplished by
○ 1. maintaining eye contact with him.
○ 2. holding him so he can look outdoors.
○ 3. wiggling her fingers in front of his eyes.
○ 4. moving a brightly colored rattle in front of his eyes.

19. The client asks the nurse how often she should hold her baby without "spoiling him." The nurse's best response is to instruct her to hold him
○ 1. only when he is fussy.
○ 2. as much as she desires.
○ 3. only when feeding him.
○ 4. occasionally, but use an infant seat.

20. The nurse on the night shift finds the client drenched

in perspiration. The nurse formulates which of the following nursing diagnoses for the client?
- ○ 1. Altered Urinary Elimination related to infection.
- ○ 2. Impaired Thermoregulation related to room temperature.
- ○ 3. Altered Protection related to effects of anesthesia.
- ○ 4. Fluid Volume Excess related to normal postpartal elimination process.

The nurse is caring for a 25-year-old primipara who delivered a viable neonate vaginally under spinal block anesthesia.

21. After teaching the client about spinal anesthesia during the immediate postpartum period, the nurse determines that she understands the instructions when she says
- ○ 1. "A possible side effect is a spinal headache."
- ○ 2. "After 20 to 30 minutes, I'll be able to walk to the bathroom."
- ○ 3. "After 1 hour, I can walk if I drink lots of fluids."
- ○ 4. "I won't be able to care for my baby during the first day after delivery."

22. When assessing the client 24 hours after delivery, the nurse determines that the fundus is firm but to the right of midline. Based on this finding, the nurse further assesses for
- ○ 1. constipation.
- ○ 2. uterine atony.
- ○ 3. urine retention.
- ○ 4. retention of blood clots.

23. The client asks the nurse, "Can my baby see?" The nurse's best response is that neonates
- ○ 1. can see only moving objects.
- ○ 2. can see within a limited range.
- ○ 3. cannot see but can distinguish light from dark.
- ○ 4. cannot see until 1 week after birth.

24. The client asks the nurse, "How can I tell whether my baby is spitting up or vomiting?" The nurse explains that in contrast to regurgitated material, vomited material is characterized by
- ○ 1. variable amounts.
- ○ 2. a curdled appearance.
- ○ 3. a brownish color.
- ○ 4. usually occurring before a feeding.

25. On the evening before the client is to be discharged, she begins to cry and says that she is worried about being able to care for her baby adequately. The nurse determines that she is experiencing the
- ○ 1. taking in phase of childbearing and exhibiting typical signs of depression.
- ○ 2. postpartal blues phase of childbearing and needs psychological counseling.
- ○ 3. letting down phase of childbearing and needs help to assume responsibility for neonatal care.
- ○ 4. taking hold phase of childbearing and reacting to her feelings of inadequacy in relation to neonatal care.

26. The client asks the nurse what contraception method she and her husband should use until she has her 6-week postpartum examination. The nurse explains that the most appropriate contraception method is
- ○ 1. condom with spermicide.
- ○ 2. diaphragm with K-Y jelly.
- ○ 3. vinegar douche.
- ○ 4. rhythm method.

The nurse is caring for a 17-year-old unmarried primipara. The client's family is very supportive, and the client intends to keep the baby.

27. The client is to receive a rubella vaccine during the postpartum period. In planning instructions for the client before the injection, the nurse should include which of the following in the teaching plan?
- ○ 1. The vaccine prevents a future fetus from becoming infected.
- ○ 2. Pregnancy should be avoided for 3 months after the immunization.
- ○ 3. The vaccine is being given during the postpartum period because the client didn't receive immunization in the antepartal period.
- ○ 4. The injection will immunize the client against the 7-day measles.

28. The client changes her baby's diaper for the first time, and the nurse evaluates her mothering skills. While caring for the adolescent primipara, the nurse should focus on her need for
- ○ 1. praise and encouragement.
- ○ 2. prolonged verbal instructions.
- ○ 3. her mother to assist her.
- ○ 4. special psychological counseling.

29. After teaching the client how to care for the umbilical cord, the nurse determines that the instructions have been effective when the client states that care of the cord area should be done with
- ○ 1. soap and water.
- ○ 2. petroleum jelly.
- ○ 3. hydrogen peroxide.
- ○ 4. alcohol pledgets.

30. The client tells the nurse that she gained 25 pounds during pregnancy and asks how long it will take to return to her normal prepregnant weight. The

nurse's best response is to explain that this will most likely occur in
- ○ 1. 2 weeks.
- ○ 2. 6 weeks.
- ○ 3. 8 weeks.
- ○ 4. 10 weeks.

31. The client tells the nurse that she and her baby will be living with her parents so that she can finish high school. The nurse formulates which of the following nursing diagnoses for the client?
- ○ 1. Anxiety related to return to high school.
- ○ 2. Ineffective Individual Coping related to unrealistic expectations.
- ○ 3. Family Coping, Potential for Growth, related to addition of new family member.
- ○ 4. High Risk for Infection related to lack of information about self-care.

The Postpartal Client Who Breast-Feeds

At 26 weeks gestation, a 24-year-old primigravida decides to breast-feed her baby. She discusses this with a nurse in the prenatal clinic and with the nurse after delivery.

32. The client says, "I'm worried that I won't be able to nurse my baby because my breasts are so small." The nurse's best response is to explain that
- ○ 1. breast size does not influence the ability to nurse.
- ○ 2. women with small breasts tend to produce less milk than women with large breasts.
- ○ 3. the woman's belief in her ability to nurse is less important than breast size.
- ○ 4. the baby can grasp the nipples more easily on small breasts than on large breasts.

33. The prenatal clinic nurse plans to instruct the client about inverted nipples. Which of the following measures should be included in the teaching plan?
- ○ 1. Wear a supportive brassiere cut open at the nipples.
- ○ 2. Brush the nipples lightly with a terrycloth towel daily.
- ○ 3. Do nothing until late in the pregnancy, as the nipples usually correct themselves.
- ○ 4. Push the areolar tissues away from the nipples, then grasp the nipples to tease them out of the tissues.

34. During the 30th week of gestation, the client calls the prenatal clinic nurse and states that fluid is leaking from her nipples. The nurse explains that she
- ○ 1. is producing colostrum, which indicates that her breasts are being readied for nursing.
- ○ 2. has milk coming in early and should pump her breasts until delivery.
- ○ 3. should visit the prenatal clinic as soon as possible, because the physician will most likely prescribe medication.
- ○ 4. should limit sodium intake because the client is retaining fluids, which results in the discharge.

35. The client delivers a viable neonate at term. The nurse instructs the client to avoid taking any medications unless prescribed by the physician, because many drugs have been found to
- ○ 1. suppress milk production.
- ○ 2. depress the neonate's appetite.
- ○ 3. be excreted in breast milk to the nursing neonate.
- ○ 4. interfere with the milk ejection reflex.

36. If a medication is prescribed, the nurse should instruct the client to take the medication
- ○ 1. during a feeding.
- ○ 2. midway between feedings.
- ○ 3. immediately after a feeding.
- ○ 4. immediately before a feeding.

37. After the delivery, the client asks the nurse, "How often should I try to breast-feed?" The nurse's best response is
- ○ 1. every 2 to 3 hours.
- ○ 2. every 4 to 5 hours.
- ○ 3. whenever she desires.
- ○ 4. when the baby is hungry or crying.

A multipara delivered a viable male neonate 12 hours ago. The client plans to breast-feed her baby, although she bottle-fed her first two children.

38. The client tells the nurse that she has "cramps" every time she breast-feeds. The nurse should
- ○ 1. offer the client a prescribed analgesic.
- ○ 2. advise the client to breast-feed less often.
- ○ 3. suggest that the client ambulate more often.
- ○ 4. recommend that the client take a prescribed laxative.

39. When a multipara complains of "cramps" or afterpains, the nurse explains that these are caused by
- ○ 1. blood loss during delivery.
- ○ 2. retention of small placental tags.
- ○ 3. excessive stretching of the uterus.
- ○ 4. release of oxytocin during nursing.

40. When counseling the client about diet and nutrition during lactation, the nurse stresses that it is especially important to increase intake of
- ○ 1. fats.
- ○ 2. protein.
- ○ 3. calories.
- ○ 4. vitamin K.

41. The client asks if she needs to adjust her fluid intake while breast-feeding. The nurse explains that

○ 1. satisfying a normal appetite for fluids is appropriate.
○ 2. increased fluid intake is recommended to foster milk production.
○ 3. decreased fluid intake is recommended to avoid diluting the quality of the milk.
○ 4. definite recommendations have not been established for fluid intake during lactation.

42. The nurse explains to the client that the primary action that stimulates the neonate to open the mouth and grasp the nipple is to
○ 1. pull down on his chin.
○ 2. squeeze his cheek gently.
○ 3. place the nipple into his mouth.
○ 4. brush his lips lightly with the nipple.

43. Following instructions about burping the neonate, the nurse determines that the client understands when she says that babies
○ 1. eat more if they are burped frequently.
○ 2. who are fed on demand rarely need to be burped.
○ 3. who nurse properly do not need to be burped.
○ 4. who are breast-fed usually do not swallow as much air as bottle-fed infants.

A primipara delivered a viable neonate 4 hours ago. The client plans to breast-feed.

44. The nurse plans to teach the client how to prevent nipple soreness. Which of the following should be included in the teaching plan?
○ 1. Perform breast-feeding every 4 hours to promote emptying of the breasts.
○ 2. Place as much of the areola of the breast as possible into the baby's mouth.
○ 3. Pull the nipple out of the baby's mouth quickly when breast-feeding is completed.
○ 4. Encourage the baby to grasp only the nipple and not the areola during breast-feeding.

45. The nurse teaches the client how to express milk manually, instructing her to use her thumb and forefinger to
○ 1. alternately compress and release the nipple.
○ 2. compress and release the breast at the edge of the areola.
○ 3. slide forward from the edge of the areola toward the end of the nipple.
○ 4. roll the nipple while exerting a gentle pull on the nipple.

46. After teaching the client how to store breast milk, the nurse determines that she needs further instructions when she says that breast milk
○ 1. should be stored in clean glass containers.
○ 2. should be labeled with the date, time, and amount.
○ 3. can be safely stored for 48 hours in the refrigerator.
○ 4. that is frozen should be thawed in the refrigerator for a few hours.

47. The nurse plans to instruct the client in methods to prevent breast engorgement. Which of the following measures should be included in the teaching plan?
○ 1. Increase her activities slowly.
○ 2. Wear a supportive brassiere.
○ 3. Empty both breasts regularly.
○ 4. Decrease fluid intake for 24 to 48 hours.

48. The client tells the nurse that she plans to return to work in 6 months and will probably wean her baby then. The client asks the nurse, "How will I stop producing milk when I want to wean the baby?" The nurse's best response is that
○ 1. the milk supply will diminish as the baby nurses less.
○ 2. the physician will order a medication to stop lactation when the client decides to stop breast-feeding.
○ 3. wearing a tight breast binder usually effectively suppresses lactation.
○ 4. the milk supply normally diminishes at approximately 6 months after delivery.

49. On the third postpartum day, the client tells the nurse that she is aware of a "letdown sensation" in her breasts and asks what causes it. The nurse explains that the letdown sensation is stimulated by which hormone?
○ 1. Estrogen.
○ 2. Oxytocin.
○ 3. Prolactin.
○ 4. Progesterone.

An 18-year-old primipara delivered a viable male neonate 2 hours ago. She has decided to breast-feed, and her 19-year-old husband supports her decision. The neonate has a strong sucking reflex.

50. The client tells the postpartum nurse, "I'm going to need lots of help with breast-feeding since I've never done this before." When assessing the client, the nurse should
○ 1. determine her level of motivation to breast-feed.
○ 2. evaluate the literature on breast-feeding that she has read.
○ 3. perform a physical examination of her breasts.
○ 4. assess her nutritional status.

51. The nurse formulates which priority nursing diagnosis for the client?

○ 1. Potential for Breast Engorgement related to lack of knowledge about breast-feeding.
○ 2. High Risk for Sore Nipples related to infant's strong suck.
○ 3. Knowledge deficit related to inexperience with breast-feeding.
○ 4. Fear related to lack of confidence about being able to breast-feed.

52. The client asks the nurse if she should supplement breast-feeding with formula feeding. The nurse's best response is that
○ 1. bottle supplements tend to confuse the baby and should be avoided.
○ 2. to prevent jaundice, bottle supplements are appropriate.
○ 3. the husband may feel left out if bottle supplements are not used.
○ 4. the baby must suck more vigorously on a bottle than a breast, so supplements should be avoided.

53. On the third postpartum day, the client experiences breast engorgement. To relieve engorgement, the nurse plans to teach the client that before nursing her baby, she should
○ 1. take a cool shower.
○ 2. rub her nipples gently with lanolin.
○ 3. express a little milk.
○ 4. massage her breasts vigorously.

The Postpartal Client Who Bottle Feeds

The nurse discusses formula preparation with a group of postpartal clients on the hospital's maternity unit.

54. The nurse explains that commercial, premodified formulas are diluted to have approximately the same number of calories per ounce as human milk, normally about
○ 1. 10.
○ 2. 20.
○ 3. 30.
○ 4. 40.

55. The nurse plans to instruct the clients about the number of calories each day per pound of body weight that a neonate requires for normal growth and development. Which of the following should be included in the teaching plan? The nurse should explain that the number of calories required per pound of body weight is
○ 1. 20 to 25.
○ 2. 30 to 35.
○ 3. 40 to 45.
○ 4. 50 to 55.

A 24-year-old primigravida is admitted to the hospital's maternal-newborn unit following a vaginal delivery of a viable female neonate at term. The client plans to bottle-feed the infant.

56. After teaching the client about bottle-feeding, the nurse determines that she needs further instructions when she says
○ 1. "Bottle-fed babies up to 6 months of age may gain as much as 1 ounce per day."
○ 2. "Iron-fortified formulas are usually recommended."
○ 3. "Bottle-fed babies will usually regain their birth weight by 10 days of age."
○ 4. "Cow's milk is an acceptable alternative to formula once the baby is 5 months old."

57. The nurse plans to teach the client how to prepare the bottles and formula using the aseptic method of sterilization. Which of the following measures should be included in the teaching plan?
○ 1. Place all equipment in a large kettle of water and boil for 5 minutes.
○ 2. Cover the sterilizer and boil all equipment for 25 minutes.
○ 3. Clean nipples separately to avoid contamination.
○ 4. Enough formula for 48 hours may be prepared and stored in the refrigerator.

58. The nurse teaches the client to position the neonate in what position following a feeding?
○ 1. On the right side.
○ 2. On the left side.
○ 3. Prone with the head elevated.
○ 4. Supine with the head elevated.

59. The client asks, "How do I care for the nipples after bottle-feeding my baby?" The nurse's best response is to instruct the client to
○ 1. scrub the nipples in warm soapy water.
○ 2. wash the nipples under hot running water.
○ 3. boil the nipples for a short time before handling them.
○ 4. soak the nipples in mild disinfectant before washing them.

The Postpartal Client With a Cesarean Birth

A 22-year-old primigravida has delivered a term female neonate by cesarean section due to cephalopelvic disproportion.

60. The client is on a full liquid diet as tolerated following the cesarean delivery. Before providing a full liquid lunch, the nurse should assess the client's

○ 1. breath sounds.
○ 2. ability to ambulate.
○ 3. bowel sounds.
○ 4. degree of pain.

61. During the postoperative period, the client com plains of "gas pains." The nurse instructs her to
○ 1. eat ice chips.
○ 2. maintain bedrest.
○ 3. drink orange juice.
○ 4. increase activity.

62. After determining that the client's fundus is firm and at midline, the nurse has the client ambulate for the first time after delivery. A moderate amount of lochia rubra gushes from the client's vagina. The nurse should
○ 1. return the client to bed and notify the physician.
○ 2. return the client to bed in the Trendelenburg position.
○ 3. help the client to return to bed and administer oral ergotrate.
○ 4. continue to ambulate the client and explain that the gush is normal.

63. While changing the neonate's diaper, the client asks the nurse about some red-tinged drainage from the neonate's vagina. The nurse determines that her teaching has been effective when the client says
○ 1. "It's of no concern because it is such a small amount."
○ 2. "The cause of vaginal bleeding in neonates is unknown."
○ 3. "Sometimes baby girls have a small amount of vaginal bleeding from hormones received from the mother."
○ 4. "Vaginal bleeding in neonates is caused by a temporary bleeding problem. The neonate needs medication."

64. A week after the client is discharged, she calls the maternity unit and says that she is afraid she is "losing her breast milk. The baby had been nursing every 4 hours, but now she's crying to be fed every 2 hours." The nurse explains to the client that the neonate's behavior is due to
○ 1. being unable to digest the breast milk properly.
○ 2. the mother having a temporary decrease in the milk supply.
○ 3. the mother not allowing the neonate to suck long enough with each feeding.
○ 4. the neonate is having a temporary growth spurt and requires more feedings.

A multiparous client delivered her third child prematurely, and the neonate died shortly after birth. The client is Rh negative and the neonate was Rh positive.

65. The client asks to see her baby soon after its death. In responding to her request, the nurse should
○ 1. allow her to view the neonate only if it is physically normal.
○ 2. allow her to view the neonate as desired to help facilitate in the grief process.
○ 3. not allow her to view the neonate, because this may precipitate postpartum depression.
○ 4. not allow her to view the neonate, because it is the nurse's responsibility to protect the client from unnecessary trauma.

66. The client is a candidate for RhoGam. The nurse plans to administer the medication
○ 1. within 1 hour after delivery.
○ 2. before delivery of the placenta.
○ 3. within 72 hours after delivery.
○ 4. before discharge from the hospital.

67. The physician orders a Betke-Kleihauer test on the client prior to administration of RhoGam. The nurse instructs the client that this is to determine whether the client has
○ 1. developed an ABO incompatibility.
○ 2. experienced prior Rh sensitization.
○ 3. had a transfusion reaction sometime in the past.
○ 4. had a larger fetomaternal bleed than usual and requires additional RhoGam.

68. The client asks how she should tell her 4-year-old son about the baby's death. The nurse should instruct the client
○ 1. "Tell your son that God took the baby to heaven."
○ 2. "Explain to him that death is a long sleep."
○ 3. "I think your son is too young to understand what happened."
○ 4. "Your son may be lonely at first. Tell me how you think he will feel."

A 34-year-old multiparous client is admitted to the hospital in active labor. The client delivers a 7 pound, 15 ounce (3,600 g) neonate vaginally under local anesthesia and has a midline episiotomy.

69. This is the client's seventh pregnancy. The client has one set of twins, and all the children are living. The neonates were all term and the client has no history of abortion. Using the TPAL method, the nurse documents the client as
○ 1. 6,007.
○ 2. 7,006.
○ 3. 8,017.
○ 4. 8,008.

70. In developing a plan of care for the client, the nurse reviews her prenatal, labor, and delivery records.

Of the following data in the client's record, which requires further assessment by the nurse?
- ○ 1. Vaginal laceration.
- ○ 2. Leukocytosis of 15,000/mm.
- ○ 3. Blood loss of 500 ml at delivery.
- ○ 4. Temperature of 100°F 2 hours after delivery.

71. Before assessing the client's perineum, the nurse places her in which of the following positions?
- ○ 1. Sim's.
- ○ 2. Fowler's.
- ○ 3. Prone.
- ○ 4. Supine.

72. The client is diagnosed with a puerperal infection. The nurse explains to the client that the most likely contributor to the infection is
- ○ 1. maternal age over 30.
- ○ 2. vaginal manipulation and trauma.
- ○ 3. use of low forceps for delivery.
- ○ 4. antepartal infection before labor.

73. The physician orders intravenous antibiotic therapy with ampicillin sodium (Polycillin). Before administering this drug, the nurse should
- ○ 1. ask the client if she has any drug allergies.
- ○ 2. assess the amount of lochia.
- ○ 3. place the client in a supine position.
- ○ 4. check the client's blood pressure.

74. During intravenous antibiotic therapy for puerperal infection, the nurse encourages the client to maintain which position?
- ○ 1. Trendelenburg.
- ○ 2. Sim's.
- ○ 3. Semi-Fowler's.
- ○ 4. Prone.

A 39-year-old grand multipara is admitted to the postpartum unit following a cesarean delivery because of fetal distress. The client weighed 305 pounds at her last prenatal visit.

75. The nurse plans to assess the client for signs and symptoms of thromboembolic disease. Which of the following assessments should be included in the nursing care plan?
- ○ 1. Homan's sign.
- ○ 2. Chandler's sign.
- ○ 3. Deep tendon reflexes.
- ○ 4. Costovertebral angle tenderness.

76. The physician orders prophylactic heparin (Panheparin) therapy. After instructing the client about the purpose of the medication, the nurse determines that she understands when she says that the drug will
- ○ 1. make her blood thinner.
- ○ 2. hasten discharge of lochia.
- ○ 3. promote uterine involution.
- ○ 4. prevent blood clot formation.

77. While the client is receiving heparin (Panheparin), the nurse plans to keep which of the following drugs available to counteract bleeding complications due to heparin overdose?
- ○ 1. Calcium carbonate.
- ○ 2. Protamine sulfate.
- ○ 3. Magnesium sulfate.
- ○ 4. Methergine.

78. The nurse instructs the client to report any symptoms of pulmonary embolism immediately, including
- ○ 1. dry skin.
- ○ 2. chest pain.
- ○ 3. edema.
- ○ 4. slow pulse.

79. The client is to be discharged while on heparin therapy. After teaching her about signs of hemorrhage during heparin therapy, the nurse determines that she needs further instructions when she states that which symptoms must be reported?
- ○ 1. Epitaxis.
- ○ 2. Bleeding gums.
- ○ 3. Ankle edema.
- ○ 4. Petechiae.

A 28-year-old multipara is admitted to the postpartum unit following a vaginal delivery. On the second postpartum day, the client is diagnosed with cystitis and the physician orders antibiotic therapy.

80. The nurse plans to instruct the client about self-care during treatment. Which of the following measures should be included in the teaching plan?
- ○ 1. Limit fluid intake to 1 quart daily.
- ○ 2. Empty the bladder every 2 to 4 hours.
- ○ 3. Wear nylon underwear every day.
- ○ 4. Avoid breast feeding until the treatment is completed.

81. The nurse formulates which priority nursing diagnosis for the client?
- ○ 1. Fear related to effects of therapy.
- ○ 2. Ineffective Family Coping related to prolonged hospitalization.
- ○ 3. Dysuria related to lengthy labor.
- ○ 4. Pain related to dysuria and frequency.

82. The client asks, "Can I still continue to breast-feed my baby?" The nurse's best response is that breast-feeding
- ○ 1. can continue as long as she desires.

○ 2. should be alternated with bottle-feeding to allow her to rest.
○ 3. can continue when the antibiotic therapy is stopped.
○ 4. is contraindicated, and she should switch to bottle-feeding.

A 30-year-old multipara is admitted to the postpartum unit following cesarean delivery for abruptio placenta. She plans to breast-feed. Her neonate weighs 10 pounds, 2 ounces (4,593 g). The client is receiving intravenous Ringer's lactate solution in her left arm.

83. While assessing the client 4 hours after delivery, the nurse determines that her fundus is "boggy." The nurse's first action is to
○ 1. continue massaging the fundus.
○ 2. contact the physician.
○ 3. increase intravenous fluid infusion.
○ 4. check the patency of the indwelling catheter.

84. The client develops symptoms of early postpartum hemorrhage. In planning care for the client, the nurse should include which of the following measures in the care plan?
○ 1. Administration of Prostin 15M intramuscularly.
○ 2. Administration of undiluted oxytocin.
○ 3. Fundal massage every 30 minutes.
○ 4. Preparation for emergency laparoscopy.

85. The client asks, "Why am I bleeding so much?" The nurse's best response is that the most likely cause of uterine atony is
○ 1. trauma during delivery.
○ 2. oxytocin use during labor.
○ 3. lengthy and prolonged labor.
○ 4. overdistention of the uterus.

86. The nurse formulates which priority nursing diagnosis for the client?
○ 1. Altered Tissue Perfusion related to excessive uterine bleeding.
○ 2. Knowledge Deficit related to lack of information on postpartum care.
○ 3. Fluid Volume Excess related to excessive intravenous fluids.
○ 4. Potential for Hypertension related to use of oxytocin.

87. The client asks, "If I get pregnant again, will I need to have a cesarean section?" The nurse's best response is that vaginal delivery after a cesarean delivery is
○ 1. possible if the client has not had a classic uterine incision.
○ 2. possible if the client has a history of short labors.
○ 3. not possible, because it may rupture the uterus during labor.
○ 4. not possible unless the client has a small-for-gestational age fetus.

A 26-year-old primipara is seen in the postpartum clinic 2 weeks after she delivered a viable female neonate. The client has been breast-feeding and is diagnosed with infectious mastitis.

88. The client asks, "Can I continue breast-feeding?" The nurse's best response is that breast-feeding should be
○ 1. continued and the neonate fed frequently.
○ 2. continued only if symptoms decreased.
○ 3. discontinued for 48 hours until antibiotic therapy is completed.
○ 4. discontinued because the infant may become infected.

89. After teaching the client about treatment of infectious mastitis, the nurse determines that she needs further instructions when she says
○ 1. "I can apply heat to the infected area."
○ 2. "I should increase my fluid intake."
○ 3. "I'll need to take antibiotics for 10 days."
○ 4. "I need to avoid analgesics while I'm taking antibiotics."

90. The client develops an abscess, which is surgically incised. In planning care for this client, which of the following measures would be important to include in the nursing care plan?
○ 1. Change the sterile dressings every 4 hours.
○ 2. Instruct her in bottle-feeding and formula preparation.
○ 3. Remove the sterile packing after 4 hours.
○ 4. Teach her how to pump her breasts.

A 16-year-old unmarried primipara is admitted to the postpartum unit following low forceps delivery of a viable male neonate. The client has a fourth-degree laceration and a midline episiotomy. The neonate is being placed for adoption.

91. After providing instruction about episiotomy care, the nurse determines that the client understands the teaching when she says
○ 1. "I should use plain, cool water to clean the episiotomy area."
○ 2. "I wipe the area from front to back using a blotting motion."

○ 3. "Sitz baths with cool water should be taken once a day."
○ 4. "Ice packs can help decrease swelling and should be used for 48 hours."

92. Four hours after delivery, the client asks if she can feed her baby. The nurse's best response is
○ 1. "I'll bring the baby to you for feeding."
○ 2. "We should ask your physician if this is a good idea."
○ 3. "It's not a good idea for you to hold and feed the baby."
○ 4. "I'll check with the social worker to see if the adopting parents will permit this."

93. One week after delivery, the client visits the postpartum clinic complaining of excessive lochia rubra with clots. The physician orders methylergonovine maleate (Melthergine) 0.2 mg intramuscularly. Before administering this drug, the nurse should monitor the client's
○ 1. blood pressure.
○ 2. pulse.
○ 3. respirations.
○ 4. temperature.

94. The client says, "I've been crying a lot the last few days. I just feel so depressed sometimes. Why is this?" What is the nurse's best response?
○ 1. "These feelings are symptoms of postpartum blues and are normal. Do you want to talk about it?"
○ 2. "I think you're probably overreacting to being a new mother. You'll be fine."
○ 3. "It's unusual for mothers to feel depressed. Talk to your doctor; he may want to prescribe medication."
○ 4. "This may be a symptom of a serious mental illness. Do you want me to make an appointment for you at the mental health clinic?"

A client who has just delivered expresses anxiety to the postpartum nurse over the fact that her brother has Down syndrome.

95. After teaching the client about Down syndrome, the nurse determines that the client needs further instructions when she says
○ 1. "Down syndrome is an abnormality that can result from an extra chromosome."
○ 2. "Down syndrome is a form of mental retardation."
○ 3. "There is no method available to determine if my baby has Down syndrome."
○ 4. "Babies born to older mothers are more likely to have Down syndrome."

CORRECT ANSWERS AND RATIONALE

The letters in parentheses following the rationale identify the step of the nursing process (A, D, P, I, E); cognitive level (K, C, T, N); and client need (S, G, L, H). See the Answer Grid for the key.

The Postpartal Client With a Vaginal Birth

1. 4. An eye medication is best instilled into the lower conjunctival sac, starting at the inner canthus. Much of the medication is likely to be lost if it is placed in the inner or outer canthus. The medication may irritate and damage the cornea if placed on it. Erythromycin eye ointment (Ilotycin) is an effective prophylactic treatment against *Neisseria gonorrhea* and *Chlamydia trachomatis.* (I, N, G)
2. 4. The vastus lateralis muscle is most commonly recommended for intramuscular injections in the neonate. The muscle affords the best tissue and the least likelihood of injuring other structures. The gluteus muscles are not recommended because of the danger of injuring the sciatic nerve. The deltoid muscle is too small in a neonate for intramuscular administration. (I, N, S)
3. 1. The Moro, or startle, reflex occurs when the neonate responds to stimuli by extending the arms, hands open, and then moving the arms in an embracing motion. The Moro reflex should be present at birth but disappears at about age 3 months. The grasping reflex is present when the neonate grasps an object placed in the hand. The rooting reflex is present when the neonate turns the head and opens the mouth after being stimulated on the cheek. This reflex is also called the sucking reflex. The tonic neck reflex is demonstrated when the neonate while lying supine, turns the head to one side. (E, N, H)
4. 2. The client is in the taking in phase up to 3 days following birth. During this time food and sleep are a major focus for the client. In addition, she works through the birth experience to sort out reality from fantasy and clarify any misunderstandings. The taking hold phase is the second phase of postpartal psychological adaptation; the letting go phase is the final phase. (D, N, L)
5. 3. During the taking in phase of maternal postpartum adjustment, the client's primary concern is with her own needs. This phase usually lasts 1 to 3 days after birth. (P, N, L)
6. 3. Beginning after completion of the taking in phase, the talking hold phase lasts about 10 days. During this phase, the client is concerned with her need to resume control of all facets of her life in a competent manner. At this time, she is ready to learn self-care and infant care skills. The letting go phase is the final phase of postpartal psychological adaptation. (P, N, L)
7. 4. Because the client delivered under local anesthesia, she should have full mobility in her legs. Usually she can begin ambulating well enough to walk to the bathroom, with the nurse's assistance, at 4 hours after delivery. It is usually unnecessary to use a bedpan. Catheterization should be used only as a last resort if a client is unable to void following delivery. (I, N, G)
8. 2. Clients sometimes feel faint when ambulating for the first time after delivery. This results from the sudden change in blood circulation in the body. Primarily for this reason, the nurse remains nearby while the client takes her first shower after delivery. (I, N, H)
9. 1. The height of the uterus felt slightly above the umbilicus is normal approximately 12 hours after delivery. Unless complications occur, this client could expect normal progress of involution. Immediately after delivery, however, the top of the fundus will normally be midway between the umbilicus and the symphysis pubis. It descends at a rate of approximately one fingerbreadth each day. It will be barely palpable above the upper margin of the symphysis pubis 7 to 10 days after delivery. Although there is individual variation, these are the common normal ranges. (I, N, G)
10. 2. No special treatment is indicated when an ecchymotic area is observed on the second postpartum day. Applying ice is effective immediately to reduce bleeding or swelling but should not be done on the second postpartum day. Heat is appropriate, but three sitz baths a day is adequate. (I, N, G)
11. 4. Edema is commonly present in the area of the lower urinary tract following delivery. This condition often makes it difficult to start voiding. Hyperemia of the bladder mucosa also commonly occurs. The combination of hyperemia and edema predisposes to decreased sensation to void, overdistention of the bladder, and incomplete bladder emptying. Nursing care of the postpartum client should include careful monitoring of the bladder to help prevent urine retention and its associated problems. (I, N, G)
12. 4. The most appropriate nursing diagnosis is Urinary Retention related to the trauma of delivery. The client is not at a high risk for infection, although some risk is present. With adequate cleanliness and hygiene, infection can be prevented. There is no indication that the client is experiencing fatigue from a

lengthy labor. Typically, during the immediate postpartum period the client experiences a fluid volume deficit from lack of fluid intake and blood/fluid loss during delivery. (D, N, G)

13. 3. After an uncomplicated delivery, postpartum exercises may begin on the first postpartum day with exercises to strengthen the abdominal muscles. This is done by inhaling deeply while allowing the abdomen to expand and then exhaling while contracting the abdominal muscles. Such exercises as reaching for the knees, push-ups, and sit-ups are ordinarily too strenuous for the first postpartum day but may be done later in the postpartum period. Kegel exercises should be done often in the postpartal period to restore perineal and vaginal muscle tone. Increased lochia or pain indicates overactivity; the client should be instructed to decrease activity if this occurs. (I, N, H)

14. 1. Providing stimulation and speaking to neonates is very important, and the nurse should encourage the client to do so. Some authorities believe that speech is the most important type of sensory stimulation for a neonate. Neonates respond best to speech with tonal variations and a high-pitched voice. While cooing can be used, a neonate does respond to words, and these should be used as a stimulus to language development. A neonate can hear all sounds louder than about 55 decibels. (I, N, H)

15. 4. The catheter may have caused a temporary spasm at the internal sphincter, resulting in resistance. The nurse should ask the client to bear down gently as if to void, to promote sphincter relaxation. This technique usually helps overcome a temporary spasm. If the catheter is removed entirely, a new sterile catheter must be obtained and a second attempt made to introduce it. Pulling the catheter out a bit and allowing the labia to fall into place are contraindicated because of the danger of introducing organisms that could cause a urinary tract infection. (I, N, G)

16. 3. The vaginal discharge that normally occurs for 2 to 3 days after delivery, lochia rubra, contains mostly blood and is dark red in color. The discharge then becomes more serous and watery, at which time it is called lochia serosa. About the 10th day after delivery, the discharge becomes thinner, scanty, and almost without color and is called lochia alba. (E, N, G)

17. 1. Initial regurgitation in the neonate may be due to excessive mucous and gastric irritation from foreign substances in the stomach from birth. Later regurgitation is thought to be due to the neonate's immature cardiac sphincter. It represents an overflow of stomach contents and is probably due to feeding the neonate too fast or too much. Regurgitation is normal, but vomiting or forceful fluid expulsion is not. (I, N, G)

18. 1. Neonates like to look at eyes, and eye-to-eye contact is a good way to provide visual stimulation. The parent's eyes are circular, move from side to side, and become larger and smaller; neonates have been observed to fix on them. In general, neonates prefer circular objects of darkness against a white background. (I, N, H)

19. 2. Holding and patting neonates helps them develop trust in caregivers. Tactile stimulation is important and should be encouraged. Holding neonates often is unlikely to "spoil" them. (I, N, H)

20. 4. Excessive perspiration is common during the puerperium. The most appropriate nursing diagnosis is Fluid Volume Excess related to normal postpartal elimination. There are no data to suggest urinary tract infection, impaired thermoregulation, or altered protection related to effects of anesthesia. (D, N, G)

21. 1. A potential side effect of spinal (subarachnoid) block anesthesia is a spinal headache. This anesthesia also may produce hypotension, bladder dysfunction, and, in some cases, total spinal blockade with respiratory paralysis. Controversy exists as to the treatment of spinal headaches. Keeping the client flat in bed and providing overhydration are usually of little value. Providing abdominal support with a tight binder may provide some relief. Effects of the anesthetic usually last 1 to 3 hours, and the injection is given just before delivery. So it is unlikely that the anesthetic will have worn off in 20 to 30 minutes or even 1 hour. The client can care for the neonate as soon as she desires to do so. (E, N, G)

22. 3. A full bladder is likely to push the uterus to the right of midline, so the nurse should further assess for symptoms of urine retention. When the bladder is empty, it normally is nonpalpable and lies approximately in the midline. A full bladder can prevent the uterus from contracting properly (uterine atony); hemorrhage can occur. Here, the client's uterus is firm. Deviation of the fundus is not related to constipation or retention of blood clots. (A, N, G)

23. 2. The neonate has immature oculomotor coordination, an inability to accommodate for distance, and poorly developed eyes, visual nerves, and brain. However, the normal neonate can see clearly within about 9 to 12 inches. (I, N, G)

24. 2. Vomited material has been digested and looks very much like curdled milk, with a sour odor. Vomiting usually occurs between feedings and empties the stomach of its contents. In contrast, regurgitation is undigested material; it does not have a sour odor and occurs during or immediately after feeding. The amount of material is not a reliable guide in distinguishing vomiting from regurgitation. (I, N, H)

25. 4. A primipara often has concerns about her ability to care for her infant properly during the taking hold phase. She is working toward independence and autonomy and wants to be able to perform well. She needs emotional support, advice on how to manage, reassurance, and reinforcement of appropriate behavior. The let down phase, sometimes called the postpartum blues, is characterized by irritability and generally occur later in the postpartum period. Psychological counseling is rarely necessary. (D, N, G)

26. 1. A condom with spermicide is often recommended for contraception after delivery until the client's 6-week postpartal examination. The diaphragm must be refitted, which is usually done at the 6-week examination. A vinegar douche is not an effective method of contraception. The rhythm method is not effective, because the client is unlikely to be able to determine when ovulation has occurred until her menstrual cycle returns. Women who are not breast-feeding can use oral contraceptive agents. (I, N, G)

27. 2. Following administration of rubella vaccine, the client should be instructed to avoid pregnancy for at least 3 months to prevent toxic effects of the vaccine to the fetus. The vaccine does not protect a future fetus from infection. The vaccine is not given to pregnant clients, even though they are not immune. The injection immunizes the client against the 3-day or German measles, not the 7-day measles. (P, N, G)

28. 1. The adolescent client may have special needs during the postpartum period. Praise and encouragement of her mothering skills are important for confidence and self-esteem. She does not need prolonged verbal instructions, lengthy explanations may overwhelm the first-time mother. It is not essential that the client's mother assist her; however, the nurse can instruct the client while her mother is present. Special psychological counseling is not necessary. (I, N, H)

29. 4. It is best to care for the neonate's umbilical cord area by cleaning it with pledgets moistened with alcohol. The alcohol promotes drying and helps decrease the risk of infection. Sometimes, an antibiotic ointment may be used instead of alcohol. Such agents as hydrogen peroxide, petroleum jelly, and soap and water are not as effective as alcohol or an antibiotic ointment. At home, the client can use cotton balls moistened with alcohol. (E, N, H)

30. 2. In most cases, unless complications develop or the client has gained excessive weight during the antepartal period, she can expect to return to prepregnant weight by 6 weeks. Many clients lose 14–20 pounds by 2 weeks postpartum. (I, N, H)

31. 3. The most appropriate nursing diagnosis based on the information provided is Family Coping, Potential for Growth, related to addition of new family member. There is no information to support the diagnoses Anxiety, Ineffective Individual Coping to unrealistic expectations, and High Risk for Infection. (D, N, L)

The Postpartal Client Who Breast-Feeds

32. 1. Various hormones have a role in lactation. The pituitary hormone prolactin has a central role. Breast size is not important as long as there is glandular tissue to secrete the milk. Various factors can influence milk supply, such as suckling, emptying of the breasts, diet, exercise, rest, level of contentment, and stress. The fat in breast tissue plays no role in milk production. Women with small breasts do not produce less milk. The client's belief in her ability to breast-feed is important. The size of the breast does not influence the neonate's ability to grasp the nipple. The neonate may have difficulty grasping inverted nipples. (I, N, H)

33. 4. The areolar tissues can be pushed in and away from the nipples, then the nipples grasped and pulled out gently. Using a Woolrich breast shield, which pushes the nipples through openings in the shield, also can help overcome inverted nipples. A cut-open brassiere is not effective. Brushing the nipples with a terrycloth towel is not advised. Inverted nipples usually do not correct themselves. (P, N, H)

34. 1. During the last trimester of pregnancy, a client may experience fluid leakage from the nipples. This is colostrum, a precursor of milk. The client should keep her nipples clean so that colostrum does not dry and cause sore and cracked nipples. (I, N, H)

35. 3. Various medications can be excreted in the breast milk and affect the nursing neonate. The client should avoid all nonprescribed medications. Some medications can suppress milk production; these may be prescribed for clients who bottle-feed. Medications usually do not affect the neonate's appetite or interfere with the milk ejection reflex. (I, N, G)

36. 3. Taking a prescribed drug after breast-feeding will help minimize the neonate's exposure to the drug, because drugs are most highly concentrated in the body soon after they are taken. (I, N, G)

37. 1. Soon after delivery, the client should breast-feed her baby every 2 to 3 hours unless her milk supply is established. Feeding every 4 to 5 hours is not often enough. The client may only feel like feeding less often, so this is not appropriate. The neonate may be sleepy during the first 24 hours after birth, so his state of hunger or crying is not reliable. (I, N, G)

38. 1. Multiparas tend to experience cramps when breast-feeding more frequently than primiparas. This is because breast-feeding releases oxytocin, which causes uterine muscles to contract. The uterine muscles tend to be more tonically contracted after delivery in primiparas. An analgesic is most commonly offered to provide relief from discomfort.

Breast-feeding less often is not advised. Ambulation or laxative use is not helpful. (I, N, G)

39. 4. Breast-feeding stimulates the oxytocin secretion, which causes the uterine muscles to contract. These contractions account for the discomfort associated with "afterpains." The cramps are not related to blood loss. "Afterpains" tend to be more common when small placental tags have been retained, when the uterus has been excessively stretched (twins), and with increasing parity. (I, N, H)

40. 3. One of the most important factors for the lactating mother to include in the diet is calories. An inadequate calorie intake can reduce milk volume, but should not affect milk quality. (I, N, H)

41. 2. Increased fluid intake is recommended during lactation to foster milk production and to replace the fluids that the baby consumes with nursing. Inadequate fluid intake may decrease milk volume. The daily recommendation is eight to ten glasses of fluids, including water, juice, milk, and soup. (I, N, H)

42. 4. Lightly brushing the neonate's lips with the nipple causes the neonate to open the mouth the begin sucking. Such techniques as pulling down on the chin, squeezing the cheek, or placing the nipple directly in the mouth force the mouth open or force the neonate to take the nipple. The neonate should be taught to open the mouth and grasp the nipple on his or her own. The neonate should not be forced to nurse. (I, N, H)

43. 4. Breast-fed neonates do not swallow as much air as bottle-fed neonates, but they still should be burped. Neonates do not eat more if they are burped frequently. Neonates fed on demand need to be burped. (E, N, H)

44. 2. Several methods can be used to prevent nipple soreness. Placing as much of the areola as possible into the neonate's mouth is one method. Other methods include changing position with each nursing so that different areas of the nipples receive the greatest stress from nursing and avoiding breast engorgement, which makes it difficult for the neonate to grasp the nipple. In addition, nursing more frequently, so that a ravenous neonate is not sucking vigorously at the beginning of feedings, and feeding on demand to prevent overhunger are helpful. Air-drying the nipples and exposing them to light have also been recommended. Some authorities have suggested using warm tea bags, which contain tannic acid, as compresses to help healing. (P, N, H)

45. 2. The best technique for expressing milk from the breast is alternately compressing and releasing the breast at the edge of the areola. With the thumb on top and two fingers on the bottom of the breast at the edge of the areola, the client pushes in toward her chest and then squeezes her thumb and fingers together while pulling forward on the areola, without sliding her fingers or thumb on her skin. Manipulating the nipples may injure them. (I, N, H)

46. 1. Breast milk should not be stored in clean glass containers, because immunoglobin tends to stick to glass bottles and the containers should be sterile. The client should use sterile plastic containers labeled with date, time, and amount. Stored breast milk can be safely kept in the refrigerator for 48 hours or in a freezer for 2 months. Frozen breast milk should be thawed in the refrigerator for a few hours, placed under warm tap water, then shaken. (E, N, H)

47. 3. If at all possible, it is better to prevent breast engorgement. The best technique is to empty the breasts regularly and frequently with feedings. Engorgement is less likely when the mother and neonate are together, as in single room maternity care or continuous rooming-in, because nursing can be done conveniently to meet the neonate's and mother's needs. Increasing activity and wearing a supportive brassiere will not prevent engorgement. Decreasing fluid intake is not advised. (P, N, H)

48. 1. The milk supply diminishes normally as the infant nurses less. Gradual weaning by eliminating one feeding at a time over several weeks is the best recommendation. Medication to suppress lactation is most effective when started as soon after delivery as possible. Mechanical methods of suppressing lactation (a breast binder) are most effective when used as soon after delivery as possible. The milk supply persists beyond 4 to 6 months after delivery if the breasts are emptied regularly. (I, N, H)

49. 2. Oxytocin brings on the letdown reflex when milk is carried to the nipples. Prolactin stimulates milk production. Estrogen influences development of female secondary sex characteristics and controls menstruation. Progesterone increases the lobes, lobules, and alveoli of the breasts prenatally. A lactating mother can experience the letdown reflex suddenly when she hears her baby cry or when she anticipates a feeding. (I, N, G)

50. 1. Successful breast-feeding depends on the client's willingness and motivation to breast-feed. Women who have a strong desire to breast-feed tend to continue breast-feeding longer. They are often more tolerant of the discomforts of breast-feeding and more accepting of the need for frequent feedings. The type of literature is not a significant factor in successful breast-feeding. Physical examination of the client's breasts is not necessary. Although adequate nutrition during lactation is important, even clients who have had poor nutrition can be taught how to improve their diets. (A, N, H)

51. 3. The most appropriate initial nursing diagnosis for this client is Knowledge Deficit related to inexperience with breast-feeding. The client is not at any higher of a risk for engorgement than other clients who may have breast-fed before. The client may have a risk for sore nipples, but the nursing diagnosis should involve pain or discomfort, not just simply high risk for sore nipples. There is no evidence that the client is fearful. (D, N, H)

52. 1. Bottle supplements tend to cause nipple confusion in the neonate and should be avoided. Once in a while, if the client is tired, a bottle supplement may be given to the neonate by another caregiver. The husband can become involved in other aspects of the neonate's care besides feeding. Bottle supplements are not appropriate to prevent jaundice, although if neonatal bilirubin level is excessive, some pediatricians recommend temporary discontinuation of breast-feeding. Neonates suck less vigorously on a bottle than on the breast. (I, N, G)

53. 3. Various measures may be tried to relieve breast engorgement. Expressing a little milk before nursing, massaging the breasts gently, or taking a warm shower before feeding may all be helpful to improve milk flow. Applying lanolin to the nipples or taking a cool shower does not relieve breast engorgement. (I, N, H)

The Postpartal Client Who Bottle-Feeds

54. 2. Human milk normally contains about 20 calories per ounce. (I, N, H)

55. 4. As a general rule, most neonates require 50 to 55 calories per pound of body weight, or about 117 calories per kilogram of weight, each day. (P, N, H)

56. 4. Neither unmodified cow's milk nor skim milk is an acceptable alternative for newborn nutrition. The American Academy of Pediatrics recommends that infants be given breast milk or formula until age 1 year. However, the American Academy of Pediatrics Committee on Nutrition has decreed that cow's milk could be substituted in the second 6 months of life, but *only if* the amount of milk calories does not exceed 65% of total calories and iron is replaced by solid foods. The protein content in cow's milk is too high, is poorly digested, and may cause gastrointestinal tract bleeding. Bottle-fed infants may gain as much as 1 ounce per day up to age 6 months. Iron-fortified formulas are recommended. Bottle-fed neonates may regain their birth weight by 10 days of age. (E, N, H)

57. 1. With the aseptic method of bottle/nipple sterilization, all equipment is placed in a large kettle of water and boiled for 5 minutes. Another pan is used to boil the water for making the formula. The terminal sterilization method requires placing the prepared bottles in a large kettle or bottle sterilizer and then boiling for 25 minutes. In the aseptic method, nipples do not need to be cleaned separately. Only enough formula for 24 hours should be prepared ahead of time and stored in the refrigerator. (P, N, H)

58. 1. To aid digestion, the neonate should be placed on the right side after a feeding. (I, N, H)

59. 1. Nipples should be washed in warm soapy water. They may be weakened by the temperature of dishwashers. The nipples do not need to be boiled. A mild disinfectant is not appropriate. (I, N, H)

The Postpartal Client With a Cesarean Birth

60. 3. Before providing the client with a full liquid lunch, the nurse should first assess for the presence of bowel sounds. Breath sounds, the ability to ambulate, and degree of pain are all important to assess, but not in relation to the client's diet. (I, N, G)

61. 4. During the first few days postpartum, the accumulation of gas in the intestines may cause discomfort. Measures to decrease gas pain discomfort include increasing activity, leg exercises, avoiding carbonated or very hot or cold beverages, avoiding using ice or straws, and maintaining a high-protein liquid diet for the first 24 to 48 hours. A rectal tube may also be used. A gastric or intestinal tube is sometimes used when other measures fail. Eating ice chips, maintaining bedrest, or drinking cold orange juice will not help relieve the discomfort from gas pains. (I, N, H)

62. 4. Lochia can be expected to increase when the client is first ambulated. Lochia tends to pool in the uterus and vagina when the client is recumbent and flows out when the client arises. If bright red bleeding continues, the client should be put to bed. Massaging the fundus is not indicated, because the lochia is normal. (I, N, G)

63. 3. Estrogen is believed to cause slight vaginal bleeding in the female neonate. The condition disappears spontaneously, so there is no need for concern. No treatment is necessary. (E, N, H)

64. 4. Neonates normally increase breast-feeding during periods of rapid growth (growth spurts). These can be expected at age 10 to 14 days, 5 to 6 weeks, $2\frac{1}{2}$ to 3 months, and $4\frac{1}{2}$ to 6 months. Each growth spurt is usually followed by a regular pattern. (I, N, H)

65. 2. If the client wishes to view her baby's body, she has the right to do so. Viewing the body has been found to help the grieving process. (I, N, L)

66. 3. For maximum effectiveness, RhoGam should be administered within 72 hours after delivery. Most Rh negative clients also receive RhoGam during the prenatal period at 28 weeks gestation. (I, N, G)

67. 4. The Betke-Kleihauer test can detect greater-than-usual fetomaternal bleeding and requires additional RhoGam. The test does not determine whether the client has an ABO incompatibility or has experienced a transfusion reaction in the past. The indirect Coomb's test can determine if excess antibodies are present from a prior Rh sensitization. (I, N, G)

68. 4. In this situation, it is best for the nurse to first learn something about the child and then allow the client to express how she thinks he may feel. Offering opinions and giving advice are not recommended. It is better for the nurse to explore various courses of action and leave the final decision to the mother. A youngster who is told that God took a loved one or that the loved one is asleep may become afraid of God or afraid to go to sleep. (I, N, L)

69. 4. The TPAL acronym (T = number of term infants, P = number of preterm infants, A = abortions, and L = number of currently living children) is useful for recording a client's obstetric history. This client has had eight term infants, no preterm infants, and no abortions and has eight living children. (I, N, G)

70. 1. Localized infection may occur in the puerperium at laceration, episiotomy, or abdominal incision sites. During pregnancy and the puerperium, the white blood cell count may be slightly elevated. Blood loss of 500 ml is within normal limits. Temperature of 100°F 2 hours after delivery is usually due to dehydration. (A, N, G)

71. 1. The best position for assessing an episiotomy is Sim's position, with the top leg over the bottom leg. The nurse lifts the top buttock and exposes the perineum and anus for assessment. (I, N, G)

72. 2. Vaginal examination during labor results in deposits of pathogens in the cervix and later invasion of the decidua by the pathogens. Vaginal trauma, such as laceration, increases the risk of infection. Maternal age over 30, use of low forceps, or antepartal infection before labor do not contribute to puerperal infection. (I, N, G)

73. 1. Before administering ampicillin sodium (Polycillin) intravenously, the nurse should ask the client if she has any drug allergies. Antibiotic therapy can cause adverse side effects such as rash or even anaphylaxis. Assessing the amount of lochia is important for all postpartum clients, but not necessary before antibiotic therapy. Placing the client in a supine position and checking her blood pressure are not necessary. (I, N, G)

74. 3. The nurse should encourage the client to maintain a semi-Fowler's position, which promotes comfort and facilitates drainage. (I, N, H)

75. 1. Homan's sign (tenderness or pain due to calf pressure as the foot is dorsiflexed) commonly signals deep leg vein thromboembolic disease. Costovertebral angle tenderness (Chandelier's sign) indicates potential urinary tract infection. Deep tendon reflexes are assessed for central nervous system irritability in pregnancy-induced hypertension. (P, N, G)

76. 4. Heparin (Panheparin) therapy is ordered to prevent clot formation. A side effect of heparin therapy during the puerperium is increased lochia flow. (E, N, G)

77. 2. Protamine sulfate is a heparin antagonist given intravenously to counteract bleeding complications caused by heparin overdose. Calcium carbonate is not used as a heparin antagonist. Magnesium sulfate is used to treat preterm labor and pregnancy-induced hypertension. Methergine is used to treat late postpartum hemorrhage. (P, N, G)

78. 2. A major complication of deep vein thrombosis is pulmonary embolism. Signs and symptoms, which may occur suddenly and require immediate treatment, include severe chest pain, apprehension, cough (possibly accompanied by hemoptysis), tachycardia, fever, hypotension, diaphoresis, pallor, shortness of breath, and friction rub. Dry skin, edema, and slow pulse are not symptoms of pulmonary edema. (P, N, G)

79. 3. Signs of hemorrhage include hematuria, epistaxis, ecchymosis, and bleeding gums. Ankle edema is not symptomatic of hemorrhage. (E, N, G)

80. 2. The client diagnosed with cystitis needs to void every 2 to 4 hours while awake to keep her bladder empty. In addition, she should maintain adequate fluid intake and wear cotton-crotch underwear. Breast-feeding is not contraindicated during treatment. (P, N, H)

81. 4. The priority nursing diagnosis is Pain related to dysuria and frequency. There are no data to suggest Fear or Ineffective Coping. Dysuria related to lengthy labor is not a nursing diagnosis. (D, N, G)

82. 1. The client can continue to breast-feed as often as she desires. Continuation of breast-feeding is limited only by the client's discomfort or malaise. The antibiotic should be chosen carefully to avoid affecting the neonate through the breast milk. (I, N, G)

83. 1. The most frequent cause of a "boggy" fundus shortly after delivery is relaxation of the uterine muscles, or uterine atony. The nurse's first action would be to massage the fundus. If the fundus does not become firm with this action, the nurse may need to call the physician. Adding oxytocin to the intravenous solution and increasing the flow rate may be necessary, if fundal massage is not effective. Checking indwelling catheter patency may be necessary if the catheter is plugged or dislodged and the bladder is not being emptied. (I, N, G)

84. 1. Early postpartal hemorrhage occurs in the first 24 hours postpartum. Postpartal hemorrhage is defined as blood loss greater than 500 ml. Rapid intravenous oxytocin infusion, oxygen therapy, and fundal massage to contract the uterus are usually effective. If bleeding persists, the nurse inspects the cervix and vagina for lacerations. If atony does not respond, then 250 mcg of 15-methyl prostaglandin F2 (Prostin 15M) may be administered intramuscularly. Repeat doses can be given every 15 to 30 minutes, if necessary. Undiluted oxytocin should not be administered, because it can cause severe hypotension. Severe uncontrolled hemorrhage may necessitate hysterectomy. (P, N, G)

85. 4. The most likely cause of this client's uterine atony is overdistention of the uterus from the 10 pound, 2 ounce (4,593 g) neonate. Trauma during delivery is not a likely cause. Although excessive oxytocin use and lengthy or prolonged labor can contribute to uterine atony, this client had a cesarean section for abruptio placenta; it is not likely that she had a long labor or received excessive oxytocin. Besides a large infant, polyhydramnios and bleeding from abruptio placenta or placenta previa can also contribute to uterine atony during the postpartum period. (I, N, H)

86. 1. The priority nursing diagnosis is Altered Tissue Perfusion related to excessive uterine bleeding. There are no data to suggest Knowledge Deficit related to postpartum care or Fluid Volume Excess. The client is at risk for shock and hypotension, not hypertension, because of the excessive uterine bleeding. (D, N, G)

87. 1. Vaginal birth after a previous cesarean delivery can be attempted if the client has not had a classic uterine incision. This type of incision carries a danger of uterine rupture. A physician must be available, and a cesarean delivery must be possible within 30 minutes. A history of short labors or a small-for-gestational age neonate is not a criterion for vaginal birth after cesarean delivery. (I, N, G)

88. 1. The client being treated for infectious mastitis should continue to breast-feed often. Treatment also includes bedrest, increased fluid intake, local heat application, analgesics, and antibiotic therapy. Continually emptying the breasts decreases the risk of breast abscess. (I, N, G)

89. 4. There is no reason why this client cannot take mild analgesic medications while on antibiotic therapy. The client should apply heat to the infected area, increase fluid intake, and continue taking the antibiotics for 10 days. (E, N, G)

90. 4. Breast-feeding should continue during therapy for infectious mastitis, so the client should be taught how to pump her breasts. Dressings do not need to be charged every 4 hours, nor does the packing need to be removed every 4 hours. The client does not need instruction in formula preparation or bottle-feeding. (P, N, H)

91. 2. The nurse should instruct the client to cleanse the perineal area with warm, soapy water and wipe from front to back with a blotting motion. Plain cool water is not helpful. Sitz baths taken three or four times a day can help increase circulation to the area. Ice packs are helpful for the first 24 hours. (E, N, H)

92. 1. After birth, the client should decide whether she wants to see her baby and/or participate in care. Seeing and caring for the neonate often facilitates the grief process. Asking the physician is not necessary. Telling the client that it is not a good idea to hold and feed the neonate is inappropriate. There is no need to check with the client's social worker. The client has the right to make decisions regarding care of her baby. (I, N, H)

93. 1. Methylergonovine maleate (Methergine) can cause hypertension; so the nurse should monitor the client's blood pressure before and after administration. Assessing pulse, respiration, and temperature is important for all postpartum clients, but not specific to Methergine administration. (I, N, G)

94. 1. The client is most likely experiencing postpartum depression or the postpartum "blues." An estimated 50 to 70% of women experience some degree of postpartum depression. Explaining that these feelings are normal and asking if she would like to talk about them can be very helpful. Telling her that she is overreacting and will be fine is not helpful. She does not need medication and does not exhibit symptoms of serious mental illness. (I, N, L)

95. 3. Various methods can determine whether a neonate has Down syndrome. The simian crease and genetic studies can be indicative of this disorder. The degree of mental retardation is difficult to predict in a neonate. Down syndrome is an abnormality that can result in an extra chromosome, and it is one form of mental retardation. Older mothers (over age 35) have a higher incidence of Down syndrome children, but this disorder can occur regardless of the mother's age. (E, N, H)

NURSING CARE OF THE CHILDBEARING FAMILY AND THEIR NEONATE

TEST 4: Postpartum Care

Directions: Use this answer grid to determine areas of strength or need for further study.

NURSING PROCESS

A = Assessment
D = Analysis, nursing diagnosis
P = Planning
I = Implementation
E = Evaluation

COGNITIVE LEVEL

K = Knowledge
C = Comprehension
T = Application
N = Analysis

CLIENT NEEDS

S = Safe, effective care environment
G = Physiological integrity
L = Psychosocial integrity
H = Health promotion/maintenance

		Nursing Process					Cognitive Level				Client Needs			
Question #	Answer #	A	D	P	I	E	K	C	T	N	S	G	L	H
1	4				I					N		G		
2	4				I					N	S			
3	1					E				N				H
4	2		D							N			L	
5	3			P						N			L	
6	3			P						N			L	
7	4				I					N		G		
8	2				I					N				H
9	1				I					N		G		
10	2				I					N		G		
11	4				I					N		G		
12	4		D							N		G		
13	3				I					N				H
14	1				I					N				H
15	4				I					N		G		
16	3					E				N		G		
17	1				I					N		G		
18	1				I					N				H
19	2				I					N				H
20	4		D							N		G		
21	1					E				N		G		
22	3	A								N		G		
23	2				I					N		G		

ANSWER GRID: 1

NURSING PROCESS

A = Assessment
D = Analysis, nursing diagnosis
P = Planning
I = Implementation
E = Evaluation

COGNITIVE LEVEL

K = Knowledge
C = Comprehension
T = Application
N = Analysis

CLIENT NEEDS

S = Safe, effective care environment
G = Physiological integrity
L = Psychosocial integrity
H = Health promotion/maintenance

		Nursing Process					Cognitive Level				Client Needs			
Question #	Answer #	A	D	P	I	E	K	C	T	N	S	G	L	H
24	2				I					N				H
25	4		D							N		G		
26	1				I					N		G		
27	2			P						N		G		
28	1				I					N				H
29	4					E				N				H
30	2				I					N				H
31	3		D							N			L	
32	1				I					N				H
33	4			P						N				H
34	1				I					N				H
35	3				I					N		G		
36	3				I					N		G		
37	1				I					N		G		
38	1				I					N		G		
39	4				I					N				H
40	3				I					N				H
41	2				I					N				H
42	4				I					N				H
43	4					E				N				H
44	2			P						N				H
45	2				I					N				H
46	1					E				N				H
47	3			P						N				H
48	1				I					N				H
49	2				I					N		G		
50	1	A								N				H
51	3		D							N				H
52	1				I					N		G		

ANSWER GRID: 2

NURSING PROCESS

A = Assessment
D = Analysis, nursing diagnosis
P = Planning
I = Implementation
E = Evaluation

COGNITIVE LEVEL

K = Knowledge
C = Comprehension
T = Application
N = Analysis

CLIENT NEEDS

S = Safe, effective care environment
G = Physiological integrity
L = Psychosocial integrity
H = Health promotion/maintenance

		Nursing Process					Cognitive Level				Client Needs			
Question #	Answer #	A	D	P	I	E	K	C	T	N	S	G	L	H
53	3				I					N				H
54	2				I					N				H
55	4			P						N				H
56	4					E				N				H
57	1			P						N				H
58	1				I					N				H
59	1				I					N				H
60	3				I					N		G		
61	4				I					N				H
62	4				I					N		G		
63	3					E				N				H
64	4				I					N				H
65	2				I					N			L	
66	3				I					N		G		
67	4				I					N		G		
68	4				I					N			L	
69	4				I					N		G		
70	1	A								N		G		
71	1				I					N		G		
72	2				I					N		G		
73	1				I					N		G		
74	3				I					N				H
75	1			P						N		G		
76	4					E				N		G		
77	2			P						N		G		
78	2			P						N		G		
79	3					E				N		G		
80	2			P						N				H
81	4		D							N		G		

ANSWER GRID: 3

NURSING PROCESS

A = Assessment
D = Analysis, nursing diagnosis
P = Planning
I = Implementation
E = Evaluation

COGNITIVE LEVEL

K = Knowledge
C = Comprehension
T = Application
N = Analysis

CLIENT NEEDS

S = Safe, effective care environment
G = Physiological integrity
L = Psychosocial integrity
H = Health promotion/maintenance

		Nursing Process					Cognitive Level				Client Needs			
Question #	Answer #	A	D	P	I	E	K	C	T	N	S	G	L	H
82	1				I					N		G		
83	1				I					N		G		
84	1			P						N		G		
85	4				I					N				H
86	1		D							N		G		
87	1				I					N		G		
88	1				I					N		G		
89	4					E				N		G		
90	4			P						N				H
91	2					E				N				H
92	1				I					N				H
93	1				I					N		G		
94	1				I					N			L	
95	3					E				N				H
Number Correct														
Number Possible	95	3	8	14	57	13	0	0	0	95	1	45	7	42
Percentage Correct														

Score Calculation:

To determine your **Percentage Correct**, divide the **Number Correct** by the **Number Possible**.

ANSWER GRID: 4

The Neonate

Test 5

The Neonatal Client
Physical Assessment of the Neonatal Client
The Postterm Neonate
The Neonate With Risk Factors
Correct Answers and Rationale

Select the one best answer and indicate your choice by filling in the circle in front of the option.

The Neonatal Client

The nurse notes that for almost an hour after birth, the neonate was awake, alert, and startled and cried easily. Respirations rose to 70 per minute, and heart rate on two occasions was 160 beats per minute.

1. After sleeping quietly for about 2 hours, the neonate then awoke with a start, cried, extended and flexed all four extremities, and then choked, gagged, and regurgitated some mucus. The nurse should
- ○ 1. call the physician, as the neonate appears to have hypoglycemia.
- ○ 2. change the neonate's position and aspirate mucus as necessary.
- ○ 3. place the neonate in an incubator, as these signs suggest a need for additional oxygen and humidity.
- ○ 4. wrap the neonate in a blanket and offer formula.

2. During the first feeding, the nurse observes the neonate gagging on mucus and becoming cyanotic. The nurse should first
- ○ 1. start mouth-to-mouth resuscitation.
- ○ 2. administer 100% oxygen by mask.
- ○ 3. raise the neonate's head and pat the back gently.
- ○ 4. clear the neonate's airway with suction or gravity.

3. The nurse is able to retract the neonate's foreskin only slightly beyond the urethral opening without using force. Before cleansing the penis, the nurse should
- ○ 1. retract the foreskin as far as it will move back easily.
- ○ 2. use gentle but steady force to retract the foreskin gradually farther each day.
- ○ 3. leave the foreskin in place and prepare to use a bulb syringe to help with cleansing.
- ○ 4. leave the foreskin in place and report the condition to the physician for possible corrective measures.

4. The neonate weighed 8 pounds, 1 ounce (3,700 g) at birth. At age 3 days he weighs 7 pounds, 12 ounces. The nurse instructs the mother to
- ○ 1. continue feeding on demand, as the weight loss is within normal limits.
- ○ 2. increase the amount of formula to prevent further dehydration.
- ○ 3. switch to a different formula, as the current one appears inadequate.
- ○ 4. give additional feedings, because the weight loss indicates inadequate intake.

5. To assess the neonate for jaundice, the nurse
- ○ 1. blanches the skin on the forehead.
- ○ 2. blanches the skin on the buttocks.
- ○ 3. observes the skin in natural daylight.
- ○ 4. observes the skin when the neonate cries.

6. The nurse instructs the mother that the neonate's posterior fontanel will normally close by age
- ○ 1. 2 to 3 months.
- ○ 2. 6 to 8 months.
- ○ 3. 12 to 18 months.
- ○ 4. 20 to 24 months.

A viable female neonate is delivered vaginally at 40 weeks gestation. The neonate has Apgar scores of 9 at 1 minute and 10 at 5 minutes after birth.

7. Soon after delivery the neonate receives an injection of vitamin K. After explaining the purpose of vitamin K, the nurse determines that the mother understands when she says that it is given to the neonate because
- ○ 1. neonates have no intestinal bacteria.
- ○ 2. neonates are susceptible to avitaminosis.
- ○ 3. hemolysis of the fetal red blood cells destroys vitamin K.

○ 4. the neonate's liver does not produce vitamin K.

8. After delivery, the mother asks the nurse, "Why is my baby under the warmer?" After explaining why, the nurse determines that the mother needs further instructions when she states that the neonate is under the warmer to prevent
○ 1. hypothermia.
○ 2. hypoglycemia.
○ 3. hyperglycemia.
○ 4. acidosis.

9. When instructing the mother about the neonate's need for sensory and visual stimulation, the nurse should plan to explain that the most highly developed sense in the neonate is
○ 1. taste.
○ 2. smell.
○ 3. touch.
○ 4. hearing.

10. The nurse assesses the neonate's cry as infrequent and very high-pitched. The nurse should
○ 1. tell the mother that this is normal.
○ 2. notify the physician, as this may indicate a neurological problem.
○ 3. stimulate the neonate to cry more often.
○ 4. assess the neonate for tachypnea.

11. The nurse notes small, shiny white specks on the neonate's gums and hard palate. The nurse should
○ 1. place the neonate in isolation.
○ 2. notify the physician promptly.
○ 3. send a sterile specimen on a swab to the laboratory.
○ 4. continue to monitor the neonate, as these spots are normal.

12. During the initial assessment, the nurse notes that the neonate's hands and feet are bluish-colored. The nurse should
○ 1. wrap the neonate warmly.
○ 2. massage the neonate's extremities.
○ 3. administer oxygen to the neonate promptly.
○ 4. report the cyanosis to the physician promptly.

Physical Assessment of the Neonatal Client

The nurse is responsible for assessing a male neonate approximately 24 hours old. The neonate was delivered vaginally.

13. The nurse should plan to assess the neonate's physical condition
○ 1. midway between feedings.
○ 2. immediately after a feeding.
○ 3. after the neonate has been NPO for 8 hours.
○ 4. immediately before a feeding.

14. The nurse notes a swelling on the neonate's scalp that crosses the suture line. The nurse documents this condition as
○ 1. cephalhematoma.
○ 2. caput succedaneum.
○ 3. hemorrhagic edema.
○ 4. perinatal caput.

15. The neonate was born at term and weighed 7 pounds, 8 ounces (3,400 g) at birth. After teaching the mother about the neonate's weight, the nurse determines that the mother understands the instructions when she says that the neonate is
○ 1. large for gestational age.
○ 2. small for gestational age.
○ 3. average for gestational age.
○ 4. slightly above normal for gestational age.

16. The nurse measures the circumference of the neonate's head and chest, then explains to the mother that when the two measurements are compared, the head is normally about
○ 1. the same size as the chest.
○ 2. 2 cm larger than the chest.
○ 3. 2 cm smaller than the chest.
○ 4. 4 cm larger than the chest.

17. After explaining the neonate's cranial molding, the nurse determines that the mother needs further instructions from which statement?
○ 1. "The molding is caused by an overriding of the cranial bones."
○ 2. "The degree of molding is related to the amount and length of pressure on the head."
○ 3. "The molding will disappear in a few days."
○ 4. "The fontanels may be damaged if the molding doesn't resolve quickly."

The nurse is responsible for the initial assessment of a term female neonate, approximately 4 hours old.

18. The nurse documents the neonate's anterior fontanel as normal, since it is shaped like a
○ 1. circle.
○ 2. square.
○ 3. diamond.
○ 4. triangle.

19. To evaluate the patency of the neonate's nostrils, the nurse
○ 1. inserts a catheter through each nostril.
○ 2. covers the mouth and ausculates the chest on each side.
○ 3. observes for ciliary movements within each nostril.
○ 4. occludes one nostril at a time and observes for respiratory effort.

20. The nurse assesses the neonate's chest. Which of the following findings warrants further investigation?
- ○ 1. Heart murmur.
- ○ 2. Expiratory grunt.
- ○ 3. Bronchial breath sounds.
- ○ 4. Fine crackles at the end of deep inspiration.

21. The nurse instructs the mother about normal reflexes. The nurse determines that she understands the instructions when she describes the tonic neck reflex as when the neonate
- ○ 1. touches the chin on the acromial process of either shoulder.
- ○ 2. pulls both arms and does not move the chin beyond the point of the elbows.
- ○ 3. turns the head to the left side, extends the left extremities, and flexes the right extremities.
- ○ 4. turns the head to the left side, extends all extremities and flexes, then promptly relaxes them.

22. The mother expresses concern when it is discovered that the neonate's eyes are crossed. The nurse explains to the mother that strabismus in a neonate is considered
- ○ 1. normal, because the eyes drift until the neonate can see.
- ○ 2. normal, because there is lack of eye muscle coordination in neonates.
- ○ 3. abnormal, because this indicates that eye movements are of unequal strength and need surgical intervention.
- ○ 4. abnormal, because most neonates can focus the eyes well.

23. After noting a white cheeselike substance on the neonate's body creases, the nurse should
- ○ 1. remove it with oil.
- ○ 2. notify the physician.
- ○ 3. allow it to remain on the skin.
- ○ 4. brush it off with a dry cotton ball.

A term neonate is to be released from the hospital at 2 days of age. The nurse performs a physical examination before discharge.

24. The nurse examines the neonate's hands and palms. Which of the following findings requires further assessment?
- ○ 1. Many creases across the palm.
- ○ 2. Absence of creases on the palm.
- ○ 3. A single crease on the palm.
- ○ 4. Two large creases across the palm.

25. The mother asks when the "soft spots" close. The nurse explains that the neonate's anterior fontanel will normally close by age
- ○ 1. 2 to 3 months.
- ○ 2. 6 to 8 months.
- ○ 3. 12 to 18 months.
- ○ 4. 20 to 24 months.

26. While performing the physical assessment, the nurse explains to the mother that in a term neonate, sole creases are
- ○ 1. absent near the heels.
- ○ 2. evident under the heels only.
- ○ 3. spread over the entire foot.
- ○ 4. evident only forward of the transverse arch.

27. Laboratory findings indicate that the neonate's hemoglobin is 16g/100 ml of blood. The nurse should
- ○ 1. document this as a normal finding.
- ○ 2. assess for symptoms of polycythemia.
- ○ 3. notify the physician promptly.
- ○ 4. explain to the mother that the neonate may need a transfusion.

28. While assessing the neonate's eyes, the nurse notes the following: absence of tears, corneas of unequal size, constriction of the pupils in response to bright light, and presence of a red circle on the pupils on ophthalmoscopic examination. Which of these findings warrant further assessment?
- ○ 1. Absence of tears.
- ○ 2. Corneas of unequal size.
- ○ 3. Constriction of pupils.
- ○ 4. Presence of red circle on pupils.

29. After teaching the mother about the neonate's positive Babinski reflex, the nurse determines that the mother understands the instructions when she says that a positive Babinski reflex indicates
- ○ 1. immature muscle coordination.
- ○ 2. immature central nervous system.
- ○ 3. possible lower spinal cord defect.
- ○ 4. possible injury to nerves that innervate the feet.

The Postterm Neonate

The nurse is caring for a neonate delivered by cesarean section at 42 weeks gestation. The neonate weighed 9 pounds, 1 ounce (4.1 kg) and had Apgar scores of 7 at 1 minute and 9 at 5 minutes after birth.

30. While assessing the neonate, the nurse explains to the mother that postterm neonates typically have
- ○ 1. oily skin.
- ○ 2. a long, thin body.
- ○ 3. very little scalp hair.
- ○ 4. abundant lanugo.

31. When the neonate is 2 hours old, the nurse notes increased respiratory rate and tremors of the hands and feet. A priority nursing diagnosis is

○ 1. Ineffective Airway Clearance related to excessive mucous.
○ 2. Hyperthermia related to heat from radiant warmer.
○ 3. Decreased Cardiac Output related to excessive size.
○ 4. Altered Nutrition, Less than Body Requirements related to depleted glycogen stores.

32. Because of postmaturity, an appropriate goal to accomplish is: Before discharge, the neonate will
○ 1. establish parental bonding.
○ 2. gain 5 ounces.
○ 3. maintain normal temperature.
○ 4. maintain a normal hemoglobin level.

33. Following circumcision, the nurse observes a small amount of bright red bleeding from the circumcision site. The nurse's first action is to
○ 1. notify the physician immediately.
○ 2. continue to monitor the circumcision site.
○ 3. secure the diaper tightly to apply pressure on the site.
○ 4. apply gentle pressure to the site with a sterile gauze pad.

34. When the neonate is age 5 days, the nurse notes the following: frequent hiccups, gray-blue eyes, red rash on face, and white patches in the mouth. Which of these findings warrant further assessment?
○ 1. Frequent hiccups.
○ 2. Gray-blue eyes.
○ 3. Red rash on face.
○ 4. White patches in mouth.

A male neonate is admitted to the nursery following a vaginal delivery with low forceps. He is postterm and weighs 9 pounds (4,000 g).

35. During initial assessment, the nurse detects Ortolani's sign. The nurse should
○ 1. document this as a normal finding.
○ 2. notify the physician promptly.
○ 3. wrap the neonate securely in a warm blanket.
○ 4. obtain an order for phototherapy.

36. Following circumcision via a Plastibell, the nurse instructs the neonate's mother to cleanse the circumcision site with
○ 1. mild soap.
○ 2. warm water.
○ 3. betadine solution.
○ 4. antibiotic ointment.

37. The mother asks the nurse if anything can be done about the neonate's feet, which appear flat. The nurse's best response is that the neonate
○ 1. can be expected to have flat-appearing feet for several years.
○ 2. should be seen by a pediatrician for further evaluation.
○ 3. is likely to injure his feet if encouraged to walk at an early age.
○ 4. will need to wear corrective shoes when beginning to walk.

The Neonate With Risk Factors

A female neonate is being delivered by cesarean section due to placenta previa. She is classified as preterm and appropriate for gestational age.

38. As the neonate is removed from the uterus, which of the following should the nurse plan to do first?
○ 1. Stimulate her to cry.
○ 2. Administer oxygen.
○ 3. Place her in a resuscitator.
○ 4. Aspirate mucus from her mouth.

39. The neonate is to be given oxygen via a mask attached to a hand-operated bag. While administering the oxygen, the nurse positions the neonate on her
○ 1. left side, with the neck slightly flexed.
○ 2. back, with the head turned slightly to the side.
○ 3. abdomen, with the head slightly turned to the side.
○ 4. back, with the neck slightly extended.

40. The nurse determines that oxygen is being properly administered to the neonate when with each bag compression, the neonate's
○ 1. chest rises.
○ 2. abdomen rises.
○ 3. heart rate increases.
○ 4. efforts to breathe on her own offers resistance.

41. External cardiac massage becomes necessary for the neonate. The nurse should
○ 1. alternate cardiac massage with ventilation.
○ 2. compress the sternum with the heel of the hand.
○ 3. compress the heart 60 to 70 times per minute.
○ 4. displace the chest wall 1 inch.

42. After respirations and heartbeat are established, the neonate is placed in an oxygen hood. While administering oxygen in a hood, the nurse should
○ 1. humidify the air.
○ 2. cover the neonate's eyes.
○ 3. administer calcium bicarbonate.
○ 4. check the neonate's hemoglobin level.

43. The neonate is to be transferred by ambulance to a neonatal care center. To prepare the parents for the transfer, the nurse should include which of the following measures in the nursing care plan?

- ○ 1. Instruct the parents that the neonate's condition is critical.
- ○ 2. Obtain parental consent for the neonate's transfer.
- ○ 3. Allow the parents to see and touch the neonate before transfer.
- ○ 4. Ask the husband if he would like to ride in the ambulance during the transfer.

44. The neonate is diagnosed with respiratory distress syndrome (RDS). The nurse explains to the parents that this syndrome is caused by an alteration in the body's secretion of

- ○ 1. ptyalin.
- ○ 2. surfactant.
- ○ 3. vasopressin.
- ○ 4. aldosterone.

45. The nurse evaluates the adequacy of the neonate's oxygen therapy by

- ○ 1. observing for cyanosis.
- ○ 2. monitoring pulse rate.
- ○ 3. observing arterial blood gas levels.
- ○ 4. monitoring the amount of oxygen received.

A 28-year-old primigravida delivered a viable male neonate at 34 weeks gestation by cesarean section because of a frank breech presentation. The neonate is admitted to the neonatal intensive care nursery.

46. The neonate is diagnosed with respiratory distress syndrome. The nurse plans to instruct the mother about the neonate's condition. The teaching plan should specify that the neonate is at greater risk for respiratory distress syndrome because the

- ○ 1. client had a breech presentation.
- ○ 2. neonate was preterm.
- ○ 3. client had a cesarean delivery.
- ○ 4. neonate had sluggish respiratory activity after delivery.

47. To prevent heat loss in the neonate from conduction, the nurse

- ○ 1. dries the neonate with sterile towels.
- ○ 2. administers warm oxygen to the neonate.
- ○ 3. places the neonate in a warm incubator.
- ○ 4. warms the stethoscope before auscultating the neonate's heart rate.

48. The mother asks why the neonate's oxygen is humidified. The nurse's best response is that oxygen is humidified to help

- ○ 1. promote dilation of the bronchioles.
- ○ 2. decrease bacterial growth in the delivery tube.
- ○ 3. prevent drying of the mucous membranes.
- ○ 4. improve blood circulation in the respiratory system.

49. The neonate is to be fed by a nasal gavage catheter. In planning for this procedure, the nurse should first plan to lubricate the catheter with

- ○ 1. mineral oil.
- ○ 2. sterile water.
- ○ 3. petroleum jelly.
- ○ 4. water-soluble jelly.

50. After a gavage catheter is inserted for feeding, the nurse should

- ○ 1. clamp the catheter momentarily.
- ○ 2. place the free end of the catheter under water.
- ○ 3. aspirate stomach contents through the catheter.
- ○ 4. instill about 5 ml of sterile water into the catheter.

A preterm neonate is admitted to the neonatal intensive care nursery at approximately 32 weeks gestation and is placed in an oxygenated isolette.

51. The mother asks if the neonate can have breast milk for feedings. What is the nurse's best response?

- ○ 1. "No, your baby requires special high-calorie formula."
- ○ 2. "Yes, but not until the baby can suck and swallow better."
- ○ 3. "No, breast milk by gavage feeding is not recommended."
- ○ 4. "Yes, I'll show you how to pump your breasts."

52. The neonate is assessed daily for symptoms of retinopathy of prematurity (ROP). Which of the following findings would warrant further assessment?

- ○ 1. Constricted retinal vessels.
- ○ 2. Nystagmus.
- ○ 3. Lack of response to loud noises.
- ○ 4. Rapidly enlarging head circumference.

53. The neonate's mother asks, "What causes retinopathy of prematurity?" The nurse's best response is that ROP results from

- ○ 1. excessive use of oxygen.
- ○ 2. genetic factors.
- ○ 3. many variable factors.
- ○ 4. congenital anomalies.

54. Before the neonate's discharge, the mother tells the nurse that she is afraid that her 2-year-old daughter will be jealous of the new baby when they get home. After explaining ways to deal with sibling rivalry, the nurse determines that the mother understands the instructions when she says she will

- ○ 1. divide her time equally between the two children.
- ○ 2. ignore signs of jealousy to reduce the behavior.
- ○ 3. let the 2-year-old hold the baby once or twice a day.
- ○ 4. give the 2-year-old undivided attention several times a day.

A neonate is admitted to the neonatal intensive care nursery at approximately 28 weeks gestation, weighing 3 pounds, 4 ounces (1,474 g).

55. The nurse formulates which priority nursing diagnosis for the neonate soon after admission?
- ○ 1. Ineffective Parental Coping related to preterm birth.
- ○ 2. Fluid Volume Deficit related to low birth weight.
- ○ 3. Impaired Gas Exchange related to immature pulmonary vasculature.
- ○ 4. Altered Nutrition related to potential for respiratory distress.

56. When assessing the neonate for symptoms of intraventricular hemorrhage (IVH), the nurse should carefully evaluate
- ○ 1. cardiovascular status.
- ○ 2. neurological status.
- ○ 3. musculoskeletal status.
- ○ 4. respiratory status.

57. In planning care for the neonate experiencing IVH, the nurse prepares for
- ○ 1. lumbar puncture.
- ○ 2. surgical intervention.
- ○ 3. exchange transfusion.
- ○ 4. intravenous administration of nalorphine hydrochloride (Nalline).

58. The neonate develops bronchopulmonary dysplasia. After teaching the mother about the disease, the nurse determines that she needs further instructions when she says that bronchopulmonary dysplasia
- ○ 1. is an acute disease that can be treated with antibiotics.
- ○ 2. can be due to various factors.
- ○ 3. is a chronic condition that may require prolonged hospitalization.
- ○ 4. may limit the neonate's tolerance of activities.

59. When caring for a neonate who develops a pneumothorax, the nurse's first action is to
- ○ 1. prepare the neonate for surgery.
- ○ 2. administer oxygen by hood or mask.
- ○ 3. perform cardiopulmonary resuscitation.
- ○ 4. aspirate air from the lungs with a syringe.

60. The nurse assesses the neonate daily for symptoms of necrotizing enterocolitis. Which of the following symptoms observed by the nurse would require further assessment?
- ○ 1. Absence of residual prior to gavage feedings.
- ○ 2. Minimal changes in abdominal girth.
- ○ 3. Negative blood culture in stool.
- ○ 4. Gastric retention and vomiting.

A neonate is admitted to the neonatal intensive care nursery with a diagnosis of probable meconium aspiration syndrome (MAS). The neonate weighs 9 pounds, 4 ounces (4,196 g) and is at 42 weeks gestation.

61. The neonate has a heart rate of 110 beats per minute and a respiratory rate of 40 breaths per minute with periods of apnea. The nurse should further assess for
- ○ 1. skin flushing.
- ○ 2. cyanosis.
- ○ 3. staining of the nails.
- ○ 4. tachypnea.

62. A priority nursing diagnosis for a neonate experiencing MAS is
- ○ 1. Ineffective Breathing Pattern related to neonate being large for gestational age.
- ○ 2. Altered Nutrition, Less than Body Requirements, related to increased glucose use.
- ○ 3. Immobility related to mechanical ventilation.
- ○ 4. Ineffective Gas Exchange related to the presence of respiratory distress.

63. Which of the following measures should the nurse include in the plan of care for a neonate with MAS?
- ○ 1. Insertion of an umbilical arterial line.
- ○ 2. Vigorous stimulation to increase respiration.
- ○ 3. Breast-feeding as soon as possible.
- ○ 4. Observation for hyperglycemia.

64. The physician orders a blood glucose test for the neonate. The nurse cleanses the site for the puncture, which is usually the
- ○ 1. lateral heel.
- ○ 2. anterior sole.
- ○ 3. fingertip.
- ○ 4. anterior scalp.

A pregnant multigravida has learned that her fetus may be affected by hemolytic disease of the newborn. She is hospitalized for further assessment.

65. The client asks the nurse why the fetus may have hemolytic disease of the newborn. The nurse explains that the combination of parental blood Rh findings that most often leads to the disease is
- ○ 1. both parents are Rh positive.
- ○ 2. both parents are Rh negative.
- ○ 3. the mother is Rh positive and the father is Rh negative.
- ○ 4. the mother is Rh negative and the father is Rh positive.

66. After teaching the client about Rh sensitization, the nurse determines that the client understands why she was not sensitized during her first pregnancy when she says that

○ 1. the first baby is usually Rh negative.
○ 2. most women today are immunized against the Rh factor.
○ 3. antibodies are not ordinarily formed until after exposure to an antigen.
○ 4. the mother's blood is able to neutralize antibodies formed in the first pregnancy.

67. The nurse explains that the most likely reason that the fetus developed hemolytic disease is because the client
○ 1. has an excess of immunoglobulins.
○ 2. had an Rh-positive fetus during an earlier pregnancy.
○ 3. had an Rh-negative fetus during an earlier pregnancy.
○ 4. has an overabundance of hemagglutination inhibition antibodies.

68. The nurse teaches the client about the effects of hemolysis due to Rh sensitization on the neonate at delivery. The nurse determines that the client needs further instruction when she says that the neonate may have
○ 1. edema.
○ 2. anemia.
○ 3. jaundice.
○ 4. heart failure.

69. Following delivery, the neonate is to receive intravenous albumin. The nurse should plan to include which of the following statements about the purpose of the albumin in the teaching plan?
○ 1. Bilirubin production is prevented by maintaining high levels of blood albumin.
○ 2. Bilirubin binds to albumin and is transported to the liver for eventual excretion.
○ 3. Albumin combines with enzymes and couples with bilirubin, which can then be excreted.
○ 4. Albumin acts as a catalyst to convert bilirubin to biliverdin, which can then be excreted.

A 30-year-old gravida IV, para III at 30 weeks gestation is admitted to the hospital for evaluation. The client has experienced three stillbirths due to hemolytic disease of the newborn.

70. An amniocentesis is to be performed to evaluate bilirubin density. In preparing for this procedure, the nurse obtains a specimen container that is
○ 1. dark.
○ 2. warmed.
○ 3. chilled.
○ 4. transparent.

71. Because the client has experienced hemolytic disease of the newborn in previous pregnancies, antibody titers are done during this pregnancy. The nurse assesses the antibody titers by reviewing the laboratory results on the
○ 1. fetal blood.
○ 2. amniotic fluid.
○ 3. maternal urine.
○ 4. maternal blood.

72. The client is to undergo percutaneous umbilical blood sampling (PUBS) to assess fetal hemoglobin and hematocrit. In planning instructions for the client about the procedure, the nurse should include which of the following measures in the teaching plan?
○ 1. The client will be placed in a supine position in a cylindrical unit.
○ 2. Transient fetal bradycardia may occur following the procedure.
○ 3. Fetal bleeding is a common complication of the procedure.
○ 4. A cannula containing a trochar is inserted into the uterus and amniotic fluid.

73. Following delivery, a direct Coombs test is performed on the cord blood. The nurse explains to the client that this test is done to detect
○ 1. fetal red cells in the maternal serum.
○ 2. maternal red cells in the fetal circulation.
○ 3. antibodies coating the neonate's red blood cells.
○ 4. antigens coating the mother's red blood cells.

74. The neonate is to receive an exchange transfusion. After explaining the purpose of the exchange transfusion, the nurse determines that the mother understands when she says that exchange transfusion is done to
○ 1. replenish the body's white blood cells.
○ 2. restore the blood's antigen-antibody balance.
○ 3. lower the blood concentration of bilirubin.
○ 4. replace Rh-negative blood with Rh-positive blood.

75. Before the transfusion, the nurse explains to the mother that treatment of hemolytic disease by exchange transfusion is necessary to prevent damage to the neonate's
○ 1. liver.
○ 2. brain.
○ 3. spleen.
○ 4. kidneys.

A neonate is delivered by cesarean section because the mother is a Class B insulin-dependent diabetic. The neonate weighs 10 pounds, 1 ounce (4,564 g) and is admitted to the neonatal intensive care unit.

76. The mother visits the neonate while on her way to her postpartum room 2 hours after birth. The nurse

explains to the mother that the neonate is being closely monitored for symptoms of hypoglycemia because of
- ○ 1. a reaction to the stresses of labor and the period of increased activity following delivery.
- ○ 2. an interruption in the supply of maternal glucose and continued high production of insulin by the neonate.
- ○ 3. a physical response that normally occurs during transition from intrauterine to extrauterine life.
- ○ 4. an increase in the urine production, which occurs when the kidneys are ridding the body of excess glucose.

77. In planning care for the neonate of a diabetic mother, the nurse plans to treat potential hypoglycemia by preparing a
- ○ 1. 10% glucose intravenous infusion.
- ○ 2. 25% glucose intravenous infusion.
- ○ 3. a bottle of 24-calorie formula.
- ○ 4. a balanced electrolyte infusion.

78. The nurse formulates which priority nursing diagnosis for the neonate?
- ○ 1. Ineffective Family Coping related to hospitalization of the neonate.
- ○ 2. Hypothermia related to delivery by cesarean section.
- ○ 3. Sensory/Perceptual Alteration related to care in an isolette.
- ○ 4. Altered Nutrition, Less than Body Requirements, related to increased glucose metabolism.

79. Following therapy for hypoglycemia, the nurse observes that the neonate's blood glucose level is 60 mg/dl but that the neonate is still exhibiting tremors. The nurse notifies the physician, as these symptoms may indicate
- ○ 1. hyperbilirubinemia.
- ○ 2. polycythemia.
- ○ 3. infection.
- ○ 4. hypocalcemia.

80. At age 36 hours, the neonate is to receive phototherapy. After explaining phototherapy to the parents, the nurse determines that the mother needs further instruction from which statement?
- ○ 1. "The eye patches need to stay on when I feed the baby out of the lights."
- ○ 2. "The eye patches need to stay on during phototherapy."
- ○ 3. "The baby's vital signs will be monitored every 2 hours during phototherapy."
- ○ 4. "The baby's intake and output will be monitored closely during phototherapy."

81. The neonate's mother asks, "Why is my baby in the neonatal intensive care unit?" The nurse's best response is that neonates of Class B diabetic mothers frequently develop
- ○ 1. anemia.
- ○ 2. hypertension.
- ○ 3. hemolytic disease.
- ○ 4. respiratory distress syndrome.

A primigravida at approximately 34 weeks gestation is admitted to the hospital's labor and delivery unit in active labor. The client has had no prenatal care and admits to the nurse that she has been using heroin for 2 years.

82. After learning that the client has been using heroin, the nurse should inform
- ○ 1. the hospital security department as heroin is illegal.
- ○ 2. the head nurse so appropriate steps can be taken.
- ○ 3. no one, as this information is confidential.
- ○ 4. the physician who will deliver the infant.

83. After delivery, the neonate is admitted to the intensive care unit, where the nurse observes her closely for symptoms of heroin withdrawal. The nurse explains to the mother that a typical symptom is
- ○ 1. hoarse cry.
- ○ 2. irritability.
- ○ 3. lethargy.
- ○ 4. hypotonia.

84. In planning the neonate's care, the nurse plans to have which medication available to treat symptoms of withdrawal?
- ○ 1. levallorphan (Lorfan).
- ○ 2. nalorphine hydrochloride (Nalline).
- ○ 3. meperidine hydrochloride (Demerol).
- ○ 4. chlorpromazine hydrochloride (Thorazine).

85. The nurse instructs the mother about likely gastrointestinal symptoms in the neonate. The nurse determines that the instructions have been effective when the mother states that a common symptom is
- ○ 1. colic.
- ○ 2. vomiting.
- ○ 3. constipation.
- ○ 4. paralytic ileus.

86. The nurse plans to instruct the mother to help comfort the neonate when she is fussy by
- ○ 1. offering her a pacifier.
- ○ 2. feeding extra formula.
- ○ 3. allowing her to cry until she gets sleepy.
- ○ 4. positioning her on her abdomen in a cool room.

A male neonate is delivered at 36 weeks gestation by cesarean section. The neonate's mother had prolonged rupture of membranes and an oral temperature of 102°F.

87. The nurse plans to observe the neonate closely for symptoms of infection. Which of the following observations suggesting infection should the nurse report to the physician?
- ○ 1. Elevated white blood count.
- ○ 2. Hypobilirubinemia after 24 hours.
- ○ 3. Lethargy or irritability.
- ○ 4. Flushed, warm skin.

88. The neonate develops sepsis and is treated with intravenous antibiotics. The nurse instructs the parents that because of the neonate's infection, they will
- ○ 1. not be allowed to visit the neonate until the infection is treated.
- ○ 2. be able to visit the neonate but not handle him.
- ○ 3. be allowed to care for the neonate if they perform good handwashing technique.
- ○ 4. be allowed to care for the neonate if they wear a gown, a mask, and sterile gloves.

89. The neonate's condition deteriorates, and death appears imminent. The parents are Roman Catholic, and they request that the neonate be baptized. The nurse should
- ○ 1. ask one of the parents to perform the rites.
- ○ 2. contact a Roman Catholic priest.
- ○ 3. locate another nurse who is Roman Catholic.
- ○ 4. baptise the neonate, regardless of his or her own religious beliefs.

A female neonate delivered vaginally at term with a cleft lip and cleft palate is admitted to the regular nursery.

90. The first time that the parents visit the neonate in the nursery, the nurse should
- ○ 1. explain the surgical procedures that will be required.
- ○ 2. stress that this is not a significant birth defect.
- ○ 3. emphasize the neonate's normal characteristics.
- ○ 4. reassure the parents that everything will be all right once surgery is performed.

91. The nurse teaches the parents about appropriate feeding techniques. The nurse determines that the mother needs further instructions from what statement?
- ○ 1. "I should clean her with water after feeding."
- ○ 2. "She should be fed in an upright position."
- ○ 3. "She needs to be burped frequently."
- ○ 4. "I can use a regular nipple for feeding."

92. The nurse formulates which priority nursing diagnosis for the neonate with a cleft lip and cleft palate?
- ○ 1. Activity Intolerance related to stressors of cleft lip and palate.
- ○ 2. High Risk for Infection related to potential for aspiration during feedings.
- ○ 3. Impaired Mobility related to necessity for restraints before surgery.
- ○ 4. Impaired Skin Integrity related to immobility.

A male neonate born at approximately 36 weeks gestation is admitted to the neonatal intensive care nursery with a diagnosis of probable fetal alcohol syndrome.

93. When instructing the mother about fetal alcohol syndrome, the nurse should include which of the following in the teaching plan?
- ○ 1. Withdrawal symptoms usually do not occur until 3 days after birth.
- ○ 2. Mental retardation is very unlikely with this condition.
- ○ 3. A neonate with fetal alcohol syndrome is usually large for gestational age.
- ○ 4. Symptoms of withdrawal include tremors, sleeplessness, and seizures.

94. The nurse instructs the mother about long-term outcomes for the neonate with fetal alcohol syndrome. An appropriate statement is that neonates with fetal alcohol syndrome
- ○ 1. are often hypoactive and lethargic.
- ○ 2. have average I.Q. scores.
- ○ 3. tend to be hyperactive with speech disorders.
- ○ 4. have a consistent weight gain comparable to nonaffected neonates.

95. The nurse formulates which priority nursing diagnosis for the neonate?
- ○ 1. Altered Growth and Development related to poor parenting abilities of the mother.
- ○ 2. Altered Nutrition, Less than Body Requirements, related to decreased food intake and hyperirritability.
- ○ 3. Altered Mobility related to need for restraints during seizure activity.
- ○ 4. Sleep Pattern Disturbance related to withdrawal symptoms.

96. A neonate has been diagnosed with phenylketonuria at age 4 days. The nurse instructs the parents to feed the neonate a formula low in phenylalanine, such as
- ○ 1. Similac with iron.
- ○ 2. Nutramagen.
- ○ 3. Enfamil without iron.
- ○ 4. Lofenalac.

97. A neonate has been born at 38 weeks gestation to a mother with acquired immune deficiency syndrome

(AIDS). The nurse instructs the mother that neonates born to mothers with AIDS

○ 1. will also have the disorder.
○ 2. will not be allowed to breast-feed.
○ 3. are likely to be stillborn.
○ 4. can be infected early in fetal development.

98. A set of twins born at 34 weeks gestation is admitted to the neonatal intensive care nursery. A twin-to-twin transfusion occurred, and one of the twins has polycythemia. The nurse assesses the neonate for

○ 1. tachycardia and congestive heart failure.
○ 2. umbilical cord and cerebral bleeding.
○ 3. symptoms associated with large-for-gestational age neonates.
○ 4. dehydration and infection.

99. In discussing neonatal behavior with a first-time mother immediately after delivery, the nurse explains that the

○ 1. first period of reactivity occurs 30 to 60 minutes after birth.
○ 2. neonate is usually dozing or sleeping immediately after birth.
○ 3. neonate tends to experience long periods of alertness during the first 2 days.
○ 4. active alert state is most common during the first 24 hours after birth.

100. The nurse rates a neonate using the Apgar scoring method 5 minutes after birth. The neonate has a heart rate of 124 beats per minute, vigorous crying with reflex irritability, some flexion of the extremities, and a pink body with blue extremities. The nurse documents the Apgar score as

○ 1. 7.
○ 2. 8.
○ 3. 9.
○ 4. 10.

CORRECT ANSWERS AND RATIONALE

The letters in parentheses following the rationale identify the step of the nursing process (A, D, P, I, E); cognitive level (K, C, T, N); and client need (S, G, L, H). See the Answer Grid for the key.

The Neonatal Client

1. 2. This neonate's signs and symptoms are normal for the neonate's age. The neonate appears to be regurgitating and choking on mucus, which is common during the second period of reactivity. The recommended procedure in this situation is to change the neonate's position and aspirate mucus as necessary. These symptoms are not indicative of hypoglycemia. Placing the neonate in an incubator will not help expell mucus. Offering formula is not appropriate if the neonate is choking. (I, N, G)

2. 4. If a neonate gags on mucus and becomes cyanotic during the first feeding, the airway is most probably not open. The nurse should clear the airway with gravity (by lowering the infant's head) and/or suction. Administering 100% oxygen is not appropriate. Raising the neonate's head and patting the back are not appropriate actions for removing mucus. (I, N, G).

3. 1. For uncircumcised neonates, efforts should not be made to move the foreskin back any farther than it will retract with ease. Adhesions between the prepuce and the glans are common in the neonate. Current opinion is to wait until separation occurs normally as the male grows. By age 3 to 5 years, the foreskin usually is easily retracted. The foreskin should never be forcibly retracted. Leaving the foreskin in place and using a bulb syringe is not an appropriate way to clean the penis. Notifying the physician is not necessary. (I, N, H)

4. 1. Neonates tend to lose 5% to 15% of their birth weight during the first few days after birth, most likely due to minimal nutritional intake. If breastfeeding, the breasts are not secreting milk for the first few days. If bottle-feeding, the infant's intake varies from one feeding to the next. In addition, the neonate experiences loss of extracellular fluid. This neonate's weight loss falls within a normal range, and therefore, no action is needed at this time. (I, N, H)

5. 1. Assessing for jaundice in the neonate is an important nursing responsibility. The best technique is to blanch the skin over a bony prominence, such as the forehead, chest, or tip of the nose, by applying pressure to the area and observing the area before the normal skin color returns. Until blood returns to the area, the yellow color of the jaundice is relatively obvious. The nurse may also examine the sclera to assess for jaundice. Appropriate lighting is necessary for an accurate assessment. Simply observing the skin will not provide an accurate assessment of the jaundice. (I, N, H)

6. 1. Normally, the posterior fontanel closes by age 2 to 3 months. (I, N, H)

7. 1. Bacteria that inhibit the large intestine synthesize vitamin K, which is then absorbed. Vitamin K is often given to neonates because they lack this bacteria in the intestines. Vitamin K deficiency often results in a bleeding tendency. Neonates are not susceptible to avitaminosis. Hemolysis of fetal red blood cells does not destroy vitamin K. Administration of vitamin K promotes liver formation of clotting factors II, VII, IX, and X. (E, N, G)

8. 3. The neonate is placed under the radiant warmer to prevent unnecessary cold stress, or hypothermia. A neonate with cold stress can develop hypoglycemia and subsequent acidosis. Hyperglycemia is not associated with cold stress. (E, N, G)

9. 3. It is believed that the sense of touch is the most highly developed sense at birth. It is probably for this reason that neonates respond well to touch. (P, N, H)

10. 2. A weak, shrill, or high-pitched cry is not normal and may indicate a neurological problem, such as increased intracranial pressure, drug (e.g., heroin) withdrawal, or hypoglycemia. The neonate's cry should be loud and lusty. The nurse should inform the physician of this observation, so the neonate can be evaluated further. Telling the mother that the cry is normal is inappropriate. Stimulating the neonate to cry more often is not helpful. Assessing for tachypnea is a routine nursing responsibility and is not associated with a high-pitched cry. (I, N, G)

11. 4. Small, shiny white specks on the neonate's gums and hard palate are known as Epstein's pearls. They have no special significance and often disappear within a few weeks. White patches on the mouth may signal thrush due to *Candida albicans,* and they warrant further investigation. The neonate does not need isolation, nor does the physician need to be notified. Sending a sterile specimen to the laboratory is not necessary. (I, N, H)

12. 1. Bluish-colored hands and feet—acrocyanosis—is due to the neonate being cold. The most appropriate action is to wrap the neonate in a warm blanket or place the neonate under a radiant warmer. The nurse should explain to the mother (and father if present) that this is normal. Massaging the extremities, administering oxygen, and notifying the physician are not appropriate actions. (I, N, G)

Physical Assessment of the Neonatal Client

13. 1. If possible, the nurse should examine a neonate about midway between feedings. The hungry neonate is often fussy and irritable, making physical examination difficult. Manipulation after eating may cause the neonate to regurgitate or vomit. The neonate should not be kept NPO for 8 hours because of the potential for hypoglycemia. (P, N, H)

14. 2. Caused by pressure on the head during labor, caput succedaneum is an edematous area over the place where the scalp was encircled by the cervix, possibly crossing the suture line. It usually results from a difficult and long labor or vacuum extraction. Cephalohematoma is caused by blood between the bone and the periosteum. Because bleeding is under the periosteum, it cannot cross the suture line, whereas a caput can. Caput succedaneum is usually reabsorbed within 12 hours or a few days after birth, whereas cephalhematoma may take as long as a few weeks or even months to disappear. This neonate does not have hemorrhagic edema or perinatal caput. (I, N, H)

15. 3. The normal full-term neonate weighs between 6 and 9 pounds, or between 2,700 and 3,500 grams. This infant is normal or average for gestational age. (E, N, H)

16. 2. At birth, the neonate's head circumference is approximately 2 cm larger than the chest circumference. The average normal head circumference is 13 to 14 inches (33 to 35 cm); average normal chest circumference, 12-½ to 14 inches (31 to 35 cm). If the neonate's head has molding, it should be measured again after the molding has been corrected for an accurate measurement. (I, N, H)

17. 4. During vaginal delivery, the cranial bones tend to override when the head accommodates to the size of the mother's birth canal. The amount and length of pressure on the head influences the degree of molding. Molding usually disappears in a few days without any special attention. Molding does not affect the fontanels. (E, N, H)

18. 3. The anterior fontanel is normally diamond-shaped and about 2 to 3 cm wide and 3 to 4 cm long. The measurements may be somewhat smaller from the effects of molding. The posterior fontanel is small and triangle-shaped. (I, N, H)

19. 4. The best way to evaluate patency of the neonate's nostrils is to occlude one nostril at a time and observe respirations while doing so. A neonate initially breathes through the nose and only later learns mouth breathing. Therefore, it is not necessary to cover the neonate's mouth while occluding the nostril. A catheter can cause damage to the nasal mucous membranes. It would be very difficult for the nurse to observe the ciliary movements in the neonate's nares. (I, N, H)

20. 2. An expiratory grunt is significant and should be reported promptly. It may indicate respiratory distress. A heart murmur is not unusual during the neonatal period, although it should be reported. Bronchial breath sounds are normally heard over most of the chest wall. They often sound loud and harsh, because the stethoscope is a very short distance from the interior chest cavity. It is not uncommon to hear fine crackles at the end of deep inspiration when auscultating a neonate's chest. (A, N, G)

21. 3. The tonic neck reflex, also called the fencing position, is present when the neonate turns the head to the left side, extends the left extremities, and flexes the right extremities. This reflex disappears in a matter of months, as the neonatal nervous system matures. (E, N, H)

22. 2. Convergent strabismus is common during infancy until about age 6 months, because of poor oculomotor coordination. The neonate has peripheral vision and can fixate on close objects for short periods. The neonate can also perceive colors, shapes, and faces. (I, N, H)

23. 3. The white cheeselike substance on the neonate's body creases is called vernix caseosa. Unless the vernix is stained with meconium, it should be left on the skin because it serves as a protective coating. It disappears within about 24 hours after birth. It does not need to be removed with oil. The physician does not need to be notified. Brushing the vernix off with a cotton ball will be difficult because of its sticky nature. (I, N, H)

24. 3. A single crease across the palm (simian crease) is most often associated with chromosomal abnormalities, notably Down syndrome. (A, N, G)

25. 3. Normally the anterior fontanel closes between ages 12 and 18 months. Premature closure (craniostenosis or premature synostosis) prevents proper growth and expansion of the brain, resulting in mental retardation. Premature closure of the anterior fontanel is usually treated surgically. (I, N, H)

26. 3. Creases normally are spread over the entire bottoms of the feet in a full-term neonate. An absence of sole creases may indicate less than 40 weeks gestation. (I, N, H)

27. 1. Normal neonatal hemoglobin level ranges from 15 to 20 g/ml blood. After birth, the hemoglobin level gradually decreases. The nurse should document this as a normal finding. The neonate does not demonstrate symptoms of polycythemia, the physician does not need to be notified, and there is no need for the neonate to receive a transfusion. (I, N, G)

28. 2. Corneas of unequal size should be reported, as this may indicate congenital glaucoma. An absence of tears is common because the neonate's lacrimal glands are not yet functioning. The neonate's pupils normally constrict when a bright light is focused on them. The finding implies that light perception and visual acuity are present, as they should be after birth. A red circle on the pupils seen when an ophthalmoscope's light is shining onto the retina is a normal finding. Called the red reflex, this indicates that the light is shining onto the retina. Lens opacity may indicate congenital cataracts. (A, N, H)

29. 2. A positive Babinski reflex in a neonate is a normal finding demonstrating the immaturity of the central nervous system in corticospinal pathways. A neonate's muscle coordination is immature, but the Babinski reflex does not help determine this immaturity. A positive Babinski reflex does not indicate a defect in the spinal cord or an injury to nerves that innervate the feet. A positive Babinski reflex in an adult indicates disease. (E, N, H)

The Postterm Neonate

30. 2. Postterm neonates are born after the 42nd week of gestation. Typical physical characteristics of postterm neonates include a long, thin body; abundant scalp hair; absence of vernix caseosa; dry, thin, cracked, or peeling skin; long, thin nails; and an absence of lanugo. At birth, these neonates tend to look as though they were 1 to 3 weeks old. (I, N, H)

31. 4. Increased respiratory rate and tremors are indicative of hypoglycemia, which frequently affects the postterm neonate because of depleted glycogen stores. There is no indication that the neonate has excessive mucus or decreased cardiac output. Lethargy, not tremors, would be indicative of infection or hyperthermia. Typically, the postterm neonate has difficulty maintaining temperature. So hypothermia, not hyperthermia, is usually more of a problem. (D, N, G)

32. 3. Hypothermia and temperature stability are primary problems in the postterm neonate, so maintaining a normal temperature is an appropriate goal. Postterm neonates have little subcutaneous fat, predisposing them to cold stress. All neonates should have effective parental bonding, so this is not a particular problem with a postterm neonate. A weight gain of 5 ounces before discharge may not be feasible, as the neonate normally loses 5 to 15% of its birth weight during the first few days of life. Postterm neonates often experience polycythemia, which may take a while to resolve, so a normal hemoglobin level may not be a feasible goal before discharge. (P, N, H)

33. 4. If bleeding occurs after circumcision, the nurse should first apply gentle pressure on the area with sterile gauze. Bleeding is not common but requires attention when it occurs. Typically, the neonate's circumcision site is examined every 15 minutes for 1 hour to assess bleeding. Applying pressure with the diaper does not allow the nurse to observe whether bleeding has stopped. The physician needs to be notified when bleeding cannot be stopped by conservative measures. (I, N, G)

34. 4. An infection caused by *Candida albicans*, thrush usually becomes evident 5 to 7 days after birth. The characteristic sign is white patches in the mouth and on the tongue. Frequent hiccups, gray-blue eyes, and a red rash (newborn rash) are normal and do not warrant treatment. (A, N, G)

35. 2. A positive Ortolani's sign indicates probable dislocated hip. Ortolani's maneuver involves flexing the neonate's knees and hips at right angles and bringing the sides of the knees down to the surface of the examining table. A characteristic click felt or heard indicates a positive Ortolani's sign. The nurse should notify the physician promptly, as treatment is needed. The dislocated hip needs to be maintained in a position of flexion and abduction. Methods for this include triple or extra diapers, orthopedic splints, Frejka pillow splint, and hip spica cast. Treatment is usually successful within 3 to 4 months. Wrapping the neonate in a warm blanket and obtaining an order for phototherapy are not appropriate measures (I, N, G)

36. 2. The most commonly recommended procedure is to cleanse the circumcision site with warm water with each diaper change. Other treatments are necessary only if complications develop. (I, N, G)

37. 1. The neonate's soles have pads of fat tissue that make the feet look flat because they obscure the longitudinal arch. This is a normal condition that gradually disappears, so that by about age 3 years the feet appear normal. Flat feet (pes planus) is a deformity caused by a lowering of the longitudinal arch when the bones in the feet are not positioned in proper relation to one another. This condition can rarely, if ever, be detected in infancy. (I, N, H)

38. 4. The first step after cesarean delivery is to aspirate mucus from the neonate's mouth. If this is not done, the neonate will aspirate mucus when it begins to breathe. Later, the neonate may be stimulated to cry, given oxygen, or placed in a resuscitator if necessary. (I, N, G)

39. 4. When being given oxygen by mask with a hand-operated bag, the neonate should be placed on his back with the neck slightly extended, in the sniffing or neutral position. This position provides the most room for lung expansion and puts the upper respiratory tract in the best position for receiving oxygen. Placing a small rolled towel under the neonate's shoulders helps extend the neck properly. Overextension of the neck will block the airway. (I, N, G)

40. 1. Oxygen is being administered properly when it reaches the lungs. When this occurs, the chest rises with each contraction of the hand-operated bag. (A, N, G)

41. 1. Cardiac massage should be alternated with ventilation. A neonate's sternum should be compressed using two fingers, not the heel of the hand. The chest should be compressed 100 to 120 times per minute. The chest wall should be displaced ½ to ¾ inch (1 to 1.5 cm). (I, N, G)

42. 1. Whenever oxygen is administered, it should be humidified to prevent drying of nasal passages and mucous membranes. The neonate's eyes do not need to be covered. Calcium bicarbonate is not indicated. Although the oxygen concentration in the hood should be monitored and blood gases measured, checking hemoglobin level is not necessary. (I, N, G)

43. 3. When a neonate is being transferred to a neonatal care center, the parents should be allowed to see and touch him, if possible, before transfer. The parents should be given the location and telephone number of the unit to which the neonate is being transferred. The parents have signed consent for treatment on admission, and in most states another consent is not necessary. The parents are already aware of the neonate's condition and should recognize that it is critical if the neonate is being transferred to a neonatal care center. The nurse should not ask the husband if he would like to ride in the ambulance with the neonate during transfer. Most ambulances or transferring equipment, such as helicopters or airplanes, do not allow family members to accompany the ill client. Space in the motor vehicle, helicopter, or plane is limited. In addition, most transferring vehicles do not have insurance to cover family members should an accident occur during transfer. (I, N, L)

44. 2. Respiratory distress syndrome (RDS), previously called hyaline membrane disease, is a developmental condition that primarily attacks preterm neonates, although it can also affect term and postterm neonates. When surfactant is decreased, the lung alveoli do not expand properly, leading to RDS. Surfactant comprises a group of surface-active phospholipids, of which one component—lecithin—is the most critical for alveolar stability. Surfactant production peaks at about 35 weeks gestation. (I, N, G)

45. 3. The best way to determine the adequacy of oxygen therapy is to monitor the neonate's arterial blood gas values that indicate oxygen and carbon dioxide tensions. Cyanosis, a late sign, can validate laboratory findings, but using it without laboratory examination is not a sufficiently reliable indicator of the effectiveness of oxygen therapy. Pulse rate likewise does not serve as a good index. Oxygen administration should be monitored carefully and only the amount required for physiological requirements should be given. (E, N, G)

46. 2. Respiratory distress syndrome (RDS) is a developmental condition that primarily attacks preterm infants before 35 weeks gestation. There is little correlation between cesarean section deliveries and RDS. In breech presentations where meconium aspiration has not occurred, there is little correlation between breech presentation and RDS. The neonate's sluggish respiratory activity after delivery is not the likely cause of RDS but may be a sign that the neonate has the condition. (P, N, G)

47. 4. Because a preterm neonate has poor thermal stability, reducing heat loss is very important. Conduction involves the loss of heat to a cooler surface by direct skin contact. Cold stethoscopes, cold hands, and cold scales can all cause heat loss by conduction. Drying the neonate with sterile towels prevents heat loss from evaporation, the loss of heat when water is converted to a vapor. Administering warm oxygen and placing the neonate in a warm incubator prevents heat loss from convection, loss of heat from the warm body surface to cooler air currents. Keeping the neonate away from the walls of an incubator prevents heat loss from radiation. Radiation losses occur when heat is transferred from a heated body surface and objects not in direct contact with the body. (I, N, G)

48. 3. Oxygen should be humidified before administration to help prevent drying of the mucous membranes in the respiratory tract. Drying impedes the normal functioning of cilia in the respiratory tract and predisposes to mucous membrane irritation. (I, N, G)

49. 2. The catheter used for gavaging a neonate should be lubricated with sterile water before introduction. If the catheter is inadvertently introduced into the lungs, oil-based lubricants can cause serious damage. Water-soluble jelly also is not recommended. (P, N, G)

50. 3. After inserting a gavage catheter the nurse should next check that the catheter is in the stomach before instilling nourishment. The best way is to aspirate stomach contents. Another method is to inject a few millimeters of air into the catheter while auscultating over the stomach with a stethoscope to listen for the sound of air entering the stomach. In the past, it was common to place the catheter under water. If bubbles appeared at regular intervals coordinated with respirations, the nurse determined that the catheter was in the airway. This latter procedure is no longer recommended. The catheter does not need to be clamped momentarily, nor should 5 ml of sterile water be instilled. (I, T, S)

51. 4. Many centers that care for high-risk neonates recommend that the mother pump her breasts, store the milk, and bring it to the center so the neonate can be fed with it, even if the neonate is being fed by gavage. As soon as the neonate has developed a coordinated suck and swallow reflex, it can breast-feed. Secretory IgA, found in breast milk, is an important immunoglobulin that can provide immunity to the mucosal surfaces of the gastrointestinal tract. It can protect the neonate from enteric infections, such as those caused by *Escherichia coli* and *Shigella*. Some studies have also shown that preterm neonates tolerate breast-feeding with higher transcutaneous oxygen pressure and maintenance of body temperature better than with bottle-feeding. (I, N, G)

52. 1. Retinopathy of prematurity (ROP) was previously called retrolental fibroplasia. In the early acute stages of ROP, the neonate's immature retinal vessels constrict. If vasoconstriction is sustained, vascular closure follows and irreversible capillary endothelial damage occurs. Until recently, ROP was thought to result from excessive oxygen administration. However, it has been seen in term neonates with cyanotic congenital heart disease and in preterm infants who never received oxygen. The disease is now viewed as having multiple factors. Nystagmus does not require further assessment. Lack of response to loud noise may indicate hearing loss but is not related to ROP. Rapidly enlarging head circumference may indicate hydrocephaly or intraventricular hemorrhage and is not related to ROP. (A, N, G)

53. 3. ROP is thought to be related to multiple factors. Immaturity with its wide range of medical problems and associated therapies, as well as oxygen all can contribute to the disease. (I, N, G)

54. 4. The most appropriate guideline is to suggest that the mother give some undivided time each day to her 2-year-old, who may be jealous of the new baby. Dividing time equally between the two children may not be feasible. Ignoring behavior typical of jealousy will not help meet the youngster's needs. Allowing the older child to hold the baby occasionally is unlikely to help overcome jealousy and may result in the child hurting the baby. (E, N, L)

55. 3. The priority nursing diagnosis for a preterm neonate is Impaired Gas Exchange related to immature pulmonary vasculature. RDS is a primary problem for preterm neonates and a particular problem for neonates of 28 weeks gestation. There is no data to suggest Ineffective Family Coping, although the potential for this diagnosis exists. There is a potential for Fluid Volume Deficit; however, intravenous therapy is usually begun on these low-birth-weight neonates to counteract this deficit. The neonate may have a problem with altered nutrition, but the priority is to establish an airway and adequate respirations. (D, N, G)

56. 2. Neonates weighing less than 1,500 grams or born at less than 34 weeks gestation are susceptible to intraventricular hemorrhage (IVH). The most common site of hemorrhage is the periventricular subependymal germinal matrix, where there is rich blood supply and the capillary walls are thin and fragile. The clinical signs of IVH are variable; however, the most common manifestations are neurologic signs such as hypotonia, lethargy, temperature instability, nystagmus, bulging fontanel, apnea, bradycardia, decreased hematocrit, and increasing hypoxia. Seizures also may occur. Computerized axial tomography (CT) or ultrasonography confirms the diagnosis. Treatment is supportive, and outcome is variable. (A, N, G)

57. 1. The nurse prepares the neonate and assists with a lumbar puncture for spinal fluid analysis if IVH is suspected. Placement of a ventriculoperitoneal shunt may be required if progressive hemorrhage is documented. (P, N, G)

58. 1. Bronchopulmonary dysplasia is a chronic illness that may require prolonged hospitalization. The disease typically occurs in compromised very-low-birth weight neonates who require oxygen therapy and assisted ventilation for treatment of RDS. The cause is multifactorial, and the disease has four stages. Stage 1 is clinically similar to RDS; the alveoli collapse and the resultant ischemia leads to necrosis of the surrounding tissues and capillaries. Stage 2 is marked by opacification of lung fields. Stage 3 involves a transition to chronic lung disease. Emphysematous areas are surrounded by collapsed alveoli, with small amounts of air trapped in the interstitium. Stage 4 involves hypertrophy of the smooth muscles surrounding the bronchi and bronchioles, which leads to a narrowing of the airways. The neonate's activities may be limited by the disease. (E, N, G)

59. 4. Pneumothorax is an accumulation of air in the thoracic cavity between the parietal and visceral pleurae. A life-threatening situation, it requires immediate removal of the accumulated air. The air is aspirated with a syringe attached to an 18 gauge intercath or 23 gauge butterfly and inserted into the second or third intercostal space midclavicular line with the neonate in a supine position. Complete resolution of pneumothorax requires a No. 10 French chest tube connected to continuous negative pressure. The neonate does not need to be prepared for surgery. Administering oxygen by hood and performing cardiopulmonary resuscitation are not appropriate actions. (I, N, G)

60. 4. Signs indicating necrotizing enterocolitis include abdominal distention along with gastric retention and vomiting. Other signs may include lethargy, irritability, positive blood culture in stool, apnea, diarrhea, metabolic acidosis, and unstable temperature. Treatment includes maintaining the neonate on NPO status, providing intravenous therapy and total parenteral nutrition, and surgically removing the necrotic bowel. (A, N, G)

61. 2. Meconium aspiration syndrome (MAS) affects small-for-gestational age, term, and postterm neonates that have experienced long labor. Meconium in the lungs allows inhalation but not exhalation. Clinical manifestations of MAS include fetal hypoxia in utero and signs of distress at birth such as pallor, cyanosis, apnea, slow heart rate, and low Apgar scores (below 6) at 1 and 5 minutes after birth. These neonates often require resuscitative efforts at birth to establish adequate respirations. Pallor and/or cyanosis is often present. Staining of the skin, nails, and umbilical cord is common but does not require further assessment. The staining is evidence that hypoxia has occurred in utero and that MAS is possible. Apnea, rather than tachypnea, is usually present. Treatment for MAS includes oxygen, controlled ventilation, chest physiotherapy, and antibiotics. Bicarbonate may be necessary for severely ill neonates. Mortality rates are high for term and postterm neonates because of the difficulty in maintaining oxygenation. (A, N, G)

62. 4. The priority nursing diagnosis for the neonate with probable MAS is Ineffective Gas Exchange related to respiratory distress. Establishing adequate respirations is the primary goal for these neonates. The neonate's breathing pattern is not ineffective because the neonate is large for gestational age. Nutrition may be altered, but the priority is adequate oxygenation. Immobility may be necessary for ventilation, but this is not a priority problem. (D, N, G)

63. 1. An umbilical arterial line can be used to monitor arterial blood pressures, blood pH, blood gases, and infusion of intravenous fluids, blood, or medications. Vigorous stimulation of the neonate with MAS should be avoided. Breast-feeding as soon as possible may not be feasible, as the health care team focuses interventions on the establishment of adequate oxygenation. The neonate with MAS frequently experiences hypoglycemia, not hyperglycemia. (P, N, G)

64. 1. The lateral heel is the best site because it prevents damage to the posterior tibial nerve and/or artery, plantar artery, and the important longitudinally oriented fat pad of the heel. Toes are acceptable sites if necessary. The nurse should try to select a previously unpunctured site to minimize the risk of infection and scar formation. The anterior sole, fingertip, and anterior scalp are not appropriate sites. (I, N, G)

65. 4. When there are Rh problems, most often the mother is Rh negative and the father is Rh positive. About 13% of white Americans, 7 to 8% of African-Americans, and 1% of Asian-Americans are Rh negative. (I, N, G)

66. 3. The problem of Rh sensitivity arises when the mother's blood develops antibodies when fetal red blood cells enter the maternal circulation. In cases of Rh sensitivity, this usually does not occur until the first pregnancy; hence, hemolytic disease of the newborn is rare in a primigravid client. A mismatched blood transfusion in the past or an unrecognized spontaneous abortion could also result in hemolytic disease, because the transfusion or abortion would have the same effects on the client. (E, N, G)

67. 2. The most common cause of Rh sensitization is delivery of an Rh-positive baby, although transfusion with improperly matched blood or an unrecognized spontaneous abortion can also cause the condition. Although maternal sensitization can be prevented by appropriate administration of RhoGam, neonates still die of hemolytic disease. Concentration of immunoglobulins is unrelated to Rh sensitization. Hemagglutination inhibition tests determine susceptibility or immunity to the rubella virus. (I, N, G)

68. 3. Jaundice is not present at birth because the mother's liver breaks down bilirubin and excretes it. Anemia due to the destruction of red blood cells by antibodies may occur as the severity of hemolytic disease of the neonate increases. Heart failure occurs as the heart decompensates because of the severe anemia. Edema results from the anemia; the severe form is called hydrops fetalis. Congestive heart failure may occur, as may marked jaundice after birth. This jaundice, called icteris gravis, can lead to neurologic damage known as kernicterus. (E, N, G)

69. 2. Intravenous albumin provides binding sites for free or unbound bilirubin, which can cause neurologic damage. Bilirubin production is not inhibited by albumin administration. Albumin does not combine with enzymes, nor does it act as a catalyst to convert bilirubin. (P, N, G)

70. 1. The optical density of the amniotic fluid is evaluated for bilirubin level with a spectrophotometer. The higher the optical density, the more bilirubin is present in the fluid, indicating that fetal red blood cells are being destroyed. From these findings, the severity of the disease can be estimated. Because light destroys bilirubin, specimens should be kept in a dark area. (P, N, G)

71. 4. For the Rh-negative client who may be pregnant with an Rh-positive fetus, an indirect Coombs' test measures antibodies in the maternal blood. Titers should be performed monthly during the first and second trimesters and biweekly during the third trimester and the week before the due date. If an antibody titer of 1:16 or greater is detected, a Delta optical density analysis is performed on the amniotic fluid. It should be noted that titers cannot reliably identify the fetus at risk. In a severely sensitized client, antibody titers may be high and remain at the same level, while the fetus becomes more severely affected. For this reason, fetal assessment should include amniocentesis, amniotic fluid analysis, and ultrasonography. Titers are not performed on fetal blood, amniotic fluid, or urine. (A, N, G)

72. 2. Percutaneous umbilical blood sampling (PUBS) is replacing fetoscopy in major medical centers. This procedure has been used to diagnose hemophilias, hemoglobinopathies, chromosome abnormalities, fetal distress in labor, isoimmune hemolytic disorders, and fetal hemoglobin and hematocrit abnormalities. The client is scanned with a linear-array ultrasound placed in a sterile glove. A 25 gauge spinal needle is inserted into the client's abdomen and into the fetal vein. Fetal blood is aspirated into a syringe containing anticoagulant. Risks include transient fetal bradycardia and potential maternal infection. The client will not be placed in a cylindrical unit; this type of unit is used for magnetic resonance imaging (MRI). Fetal bleeding is not a common problem with PUBS. A cannula containing a trochar is used for fetoscopy. (P, N, G)

73. 3. A direct Coombs test is done on cord blood to detect antibodies coating the neonate's red blood cells. The direct Coombs test does not detect fetal cells in the fetal circulation nor antigens coating the mother's red blood cells. (I, N, G)

74. 3. The goal of care for this neonate is to reduce the blood concentration of bilirubin and to relieve anemia. The exchange transfusion does not replenish the white blood cells nor restore the blood's antigen-antibody balance. Rh-negative blood is used for the transfusion to replace the neonate's Rh-positive blood. (E, N, G)

75. 2. The organ most susceptible to damage from uncontrolled hemolytic disease is the brain. Bilirubin crosses the blood-brain barrier and damages the cells of the CNS. This condition is called kernicterus. (I, N, G)

76. 2. Glucose crosses the placenta, but insulin does not. Hence, high maternal blood glucose level will cause high fetal blood glucose level. This causes the fetal pancreas to secrete more insulin. At birth the neonate loses its maternal glucose source but continues to produce much insulin, which often causes a drop in blood glucose levels, or hypoglycemia. The neonate is not being closely monitored for symptoms of hypoglycemia due to a reaction to the stresses of labor, a normal physical response, or an increase in urine production. (I, N, G)

77. 1. The nurse should plan to give symptomatic neonates of diabetic mothers 10 to 15% glucose intravenously. A rapid infusion of 25 to 50% dextrose is contraindicated, because this may result in severe rebound hypoglycemia. A bottle of 24-calorie formula is not indicated. A balanced electrolyte infusion is not indicated. (P, N, G)

78. 4. A priority nursing diagnosis is Altered Nutrition, Less than Body Requirements, related to increased glucose metabolism. The increased glucose metabolism is a result of the hyperinsulinemia. There are no data to suggest Ineffective Family Coping or Hypothermia. While the neonate may be experiencing Sensory/Perceptual Alterations, this is not a priority diagnosis. (D, N, G)

79. 4. Tremors occurring after therapy for hypoglycemia are clinical signs of hypocalcemia. At term, diabetic women tend to have higher calcium levels, which can cause secondary hypoparathyroidism in their neonates. Other factors that can contribute to hypocalcemia in neonates include hypophosphatemia from tissue metabolism, vitamin D antagonism from elevated cortical levels, and decreased serum magnesium levels. Tremors are not related to hyperbilirubinemia, polycythemia, or infection. (I, N, G)

80. 1. Eye patches should remain in place while the neonate is receiving phototherapy. However, they can be removed when the neonate is taken out for feedings. Vital signs should be monitored every 2 hours during phototherapy. Intake and output should be closely monitored as well. (E, N, G)

81. 4. Neonates born to Class B diabetic women suffer from respiratory distress about seven times more often than neonates born to nondiabetic women. This neonate should be closely monitored for symptoms of respiratory distress, such as apnea, expiratory grunting, nasal flaring, tachypnea, and sternal or subcostal breathing. Neonates of diabetic mothers frequently have polycythemia, not anemia. Hypertension and hemolytic disease are not associated with neonates of diabetic mothers. (I, N, G)

82. 4. The fetus of a heroin-addicted mother is at risk for hypoxia, meconium aspiration, and intrauterine growth retardation (IUGR). It is important to notify the physician of the client's heroin use, as this knowledge will influence the care of the client and neonate. The information is used only in relation to the client's care. With the client's consent, it may be shared with other social service or health agencies that become involved with the client's long-term care. Establishing rapport with the client is an important aspect of care. (I, N, G)

83. 2. Signs of heroin withdrawal in the neonate include a shrill high-pitched cry, irritability, restlessness, fist-sucking, vomiting, and seizures. These signs usually appear within 72 hours and persist for several days. A hoarse cry, lethargy, and hypotonia are not typical symptoms of heroin withdrawal in the neonate. (I, N, H)

84. 4. Chlorpromazine hydrochloride (Thorazine), phenobarbital, diazepam (Valium), or paragoric may be used to treat heroin withdrawal symptoms in a neonate. These drugs help to sedate the neonate; paragoric helps to treat gastrointestinal disorders. Nalorphine hydrochloride (Nalline) and levallorphan (Lorfan) are narcotic antagonists, but they do not help control the symptoms of withdrawal. Meperidine hydrochloride (Demerol) is a narcotic and a depressant and would be inappropriate for this neonate. (P, N, G)

85. 2. Neonates experiencing heroin withdrawal have gastrointestinal problems similar to those of adults withdrawing from heroin. The neonates exhibit poor sucking, vomiting, drooling, diarrhea, regurgitation, and anorexia. In addition, they are difficult to console and difficult to feed. Because of these problems, the neonate withdrawing from heroin needs to be monitored carefully to prevent dehydration. Colic, constipation, and paralytic ileus are not typical problems. (E, N, G)

86. 1. A neonate undergoing heroin withdrawal is irritable, often restless, difficult to console, and often in need of increased activity. It is often helpful to offer the neonate a pacifier and to cuddle and rock her. Environmental stimuli should be kept to a minimum. Offering extra nourishment is not advised, because overfeeding tends to increase gastrointestinal problems, such as vomiting, regurgitation, and diarrhea. Allowing the neonate to cry until sleepy does not console her. Positioning the neonate on her abdomen in a cool room is not appropriate; she should be positioned on her right side in a warm environment when not being held. (P, N, H)

87. 3. Symptoms of infection in a neonate include subtle behavioral changes, lethargy, irritability, and color changes such as pallor or cyanosis. Other symptoms include temperature instability, poor feeding, gastrointestinal disorders, hyperbilirubinemia, and apnea. An elevated white blood cell count ($>30,000/mm^3$) may be normal during the first 24 hours. Flushed, warm skin is not a typical sign of infection in neonates. (I, N, G)

88. 3. The parents of a neonate with an infection should be allowed to participate in daily care as long as they use good handwashing technique. Restricting parental visits has not been shown to have any effect on the infection rate and may have detrimental effects on the neonate's psychological development. Wearing a gown, a mask, and gloves is not necessary. (I, N, G)

89. 4. Tenets of the Roman Catholic Church hold that it would be acceptable for anyone, regardless of his or her religious beliefs, to baptize a neonate. Local practice may vary, and in some situations the parents may prefer to have a Roman Catholic person perform the rites. (I, N, L)

90. 3. On the initial visit, the parents may be shocked, fearful, and anxious. Nursing care should include spending time with the parents to allow them to express their emotions. The nurse should initially emphasize the neonate's normal characteristics. After the parents have had sufficient time to adjust to the neonate's special needs, surgical interventions can be discussed. Telling the parents that this is not a significant defect or that everything will be all right after the surgery is not helpful. (I, N, L)

91. 4. The neonate with a cleft lip and palate should be fed with a special soft nipple that fills the cleft and facilitates sucking. The neonate must be burped frequently and fed in an upright position. After feeding, the mouth should be cleaned with water. The cleft lip should be cleaned with sterile water to prevent crusting before surgical repair. (E, N, G)

92. 2. The priority nursing diagnosis for the neonate with a cleft lip and palate is High Risk for Infection related to potential aspiration. Feeding difficulties are the primary problem before surgical repair. Activity intolerance may occur, but this is not a primary problem. Restraints are not necessary prior to surgery. Problems with skin integrity related to immobility is not a problem for this neonate, who is allowed to engage in normal activity without restraint before surgery. (D, N, G)

93. 4. The long-term prognosis for neonates with fetal alcohol syndrome (FAS) is poor. Symptoms of withdrawal include tremors, sleeplessness, seizures, abdominal distention, hyperactivity, and unconsolable crying. Central nervous system (CNS) disorders are the most common problems associated with FAS. Due to the CNS disorders, children born with FAS are often hyperactive and have a high incidence of speech and language disorders. Symptoms of withdrawal often occur within 6 to 12 hours or, at the latest, within the first 3 days of life. Most neonates with FAS are mildly to severely mentally retarded. The neonate is usually growth deficient at birth. (P, N, H)

94. 3. CNS disorders are common in neonates with FAS. Speech and language disorders and hyperactivity are common manifestations of CNS dysfunction. Mild to severe mental retardation is common. Feeding problems are common, and delayed growth and development is expected. These neonates feed poorly and often have persistent vomiting until age 6 to 7 months. (I, N, H)

95. 2. The priority nursing diagnosis for the neonate with FAS is Altered Nutrition, Less than Body Requirements, related to decreased food intake and hyperirritability. There is no data to suggest that growth and development will be altered because of poor parenting abilities. Restraints are not necessary. The neonate's sleep pattern may be disturbed, but this is not the priority problem. (D, N, G)

96. 4. The infant with phenylketonuria (PKU) is treated with a special diet that limits the ingestion of phenylalanine. Special formulas, such as Lofenalac, are available for these neonates. There is controversy about when, if ever, the special diet should be terminated. (I, N, G)

97. 4. In a pregnant client with AIDS, the fetus can be infected early in development. Currently, the risk to neonates born to HIV-positive women is estimated at 30 to 75%. Infected neonates are usually asymptomatic at birth. Symptoms may not appear until age 12 to 18 months. These symptoms include failure to thrive, recurrent infections, hepatosplenomegaly, neurologic abnormalities, and delayed development. Infected neonates may be born with facial deformities such as microcephaly, a prominent box-like forehead, and flattened nasal bridge. Mortality is high for these neonates. Breast-feeding is controversial, as the AIDS virus has been isolated in breast milk. But this should be the client's decision. (I, N, G)

98. 1. Twins with monochorionic placentas may develop artery-to-artery anastomosis or twin-to-twin transfer. This compromises fetoplacental circulation. One twin is born with excess blood volume and polycythemia, while the other has hypovolemia, anemia, and possibly intrauterine growth retardation. Although many neonates with polycythemia are asymptomatic, symptoms develop in relation to increased blood volume. The most common symptoms include tachycardia and congestive heart failure. Others include respiratory distress, hyperbilirubinemia, decreased peripheral pulses, and seizures, which can result in developmental problems. Umbilical cord and cerebral bleeding are not associated with polycythemia. Twins are often preterm, so large-for-gestational age neonates are not common. Dehydration and infection are not associated with polycythemia. (A, N, G)

99. 1. Most neonates display a quiet, alert state during the first 30 to 60 minutes after birth, characteristic of the first period of reactivity. About 12 to 18 hours after birth, the second period of reactivity occurs, and the neonate becomes alert again. During the first 2 days after birth, the neonate sleeps for long periods in an effort to recuperate from the birth process. (I, N, H)

100. 2. The Apgar score for this neonate would be 8. The neonate receives a score of 2 for a heart rate over 100 beats per minute, a score of 2 for good crying with reflex irritability, a score of 1 for some flexion of the extremities, a score of 2 for a vigorous cry, and a score of 1 for a pink body with blue extremities. (I, N, G)

NURSING CARE OF THE CHILDBEARING FAMILY AND THEIR NEONATE

TEST 5: The Neonate

Directions: Use this answer grid to determine areas of strength or need for further study.

NURSING PROCESS

A = Assessment
D = Analysis, nursing diagnosis
P = Planning
I = Implementation
E = Evaluation

COGNITIVE LEVEL

K = Knowledge
C = Comprehension
T = Application
N = Analysis

CLIENT NEEDS

S = Safe, effective care environment
G = Physiological integrity
L = Psychosocial integrity
H = Health promotion/maintenance

		Nursing Process					Cognitive Level				Client Needs			
Question #	Answer #	A	D	P	I	E	K	C	T	N	S	G	L	H
1	2				I					N		G		
2	4				I					N		G		
3	1				I					N				H
4	1				I					N				H
5	1				I					N				H
6	1				I					N				H
7	1					E				N		G		
8	3					E				N		G		
9	2			P						N				H
10	2				I					N		G		
11	4				I					N				H
12	1				I					N		G		
13	1			P						N				H
14	2				I					N				H
15	3					E				N				H
16	2				I					N				H
17	4					E				N				H
18	3				I					N				H
19	4				I					N				H
20	2	A								N		G		
21	3					E				N				H
22	2				I					N				H
23	3				I					N				H

ANSWER GRID: 1

NURSING PROCESS

A = Assessment
D = Analysis, nursing diagnosis
P = Planning
I = Implementation
E = Evaluation

COGNITIVE LEVEL

K = Knowledge
C = Comprehension
T = Application
N = Analysis

CLIENT NEEDS

S = Safe, effective care environment
G = Physiological integrity
L = Psychosocial integrity
H = Health promotion/maintenance

		Nursing Process					Cognitive Level				Client Needs			
Question #	Answer #	A	D	P	I	E	K	C	T	N	S	G	L	H
24	3	A								N		G		
25	3				I					N				H
26	3				I					N				H
27	1				I					N		G		
28	2	A								N				H
29	2					E				N				H
30	2				I					N				H
31	4		D							N		G		
32	3			P						N				H
33	4				I					N		G		
34	4	A								N		G		
35	2				I					N		G		
36	2				I					N		G		
37	1				I					N				H
38	4				I					N		G		
39	4				I					N		G		
40	1	A								N		G		
41	1				I					N		G		
42	1				I					N		G		
43	3				I					N			L	
44	2				I					N		G		
45	3					E				N		G		
46	2			P						N		G		
47	4				I					N		G		
48	3				I					N		G		
49	2			P						N		G		
50	3				I				T		S			
51	4				I					N		G		
52	1	A								N		G		

ANSWER GRID: 2

NURSING PROCESS

A = Assessment
D = Analysis, nursing diagnosis
P = Planning
I = Implementation
E = Evaluation

COGNITIVE LEVEL

K = Knowledge
C = Comprehension
T = Application
N = Analysis

CLIENT NEEDS

S = Safe, effective care environment
G = Physiological integrity
L = Psychosocial integrity
H = Health promotion/maintenance

		Nursing Process					Cognitive Level				Client Needs			
Question #	Answer #	A	D	P	I	E	K	C	T	N	S	G	L	H
53	3				I					N		G		
54	4					E				N			L	
55	3		D							N		G		
56	2	A								N		G		
57	1			P						N		G		
58	1					E				N		G		
59	4				I					N		G		
60	4	A								N		G		
61	2	A								N		G		
62	4		D							N		G		
63	1			P						N		G		
64	1				I					N		G		
65	4				I					N		G		
66	3					E				N		G		
67	2				I					N		G		
68	3					E				N		G		
69	2			P						N		G		
70	1			P						N		G		
71	4	A								N		G		
72	2			P						N		G		
73	3				I					N		G		
74	3					E				N		G		
75	2				I					N		G		
76	2				I					N		G		
77	1			P						N		G		
78	4		D							N		G		
79	4				I					N		G		
80	1					E				N		G		
81	4				I					N		G		

ANSWER GRID: 3

NURSING PROCESS

A = Assessment
D = Analysis, nursing diagnosis
P = Planning
I = Implementation
E = Evaluation

COGNITIVE LEVEL

K = Knowledge
C = Comprehension
T = Application
N = Analysis

CLIENT NEEDS

S = Safe, effective care environment
G = Physiological integrity
L = Psychosocial integrity
H = Health promotion/maintenance

		Nursing Process					Cognitive Level				Client Needs			
Question #	Answer #	A	D	P	I	E	K	C	T	N	S	G	L	H
82	4				I					N		G		
83	2				I					N				H
84	4			P						N		G		
85	2					E				N		G		
86	1			P						N				H
87	3				I					N		G		
88	3				I					N		G		
89	4				I					N			L	
90	3				I					N			L	
91	4					E				N		G		
92	2		D							N		G		
93	4			P						N				H
94	3				I					N				H
95	2		D							N		G		
96	4				I					N		G		
97	4				I					N		G		
98	1	A								N		G		
99	1				I					N				H
100	2				I					N		G		
Number Correct														
Number Possible	100	11	6	14	54	15	0	0	1	99	1	67	4	28
Percentage Correct														

Score Calculation:

To determine your **Percentage Correct**, divide the **Number Correct** by the **Number Possible**.

ANSWER GRID: 4

BIBLIOGRAPHY

Angelini, D.J., & Whelan Knapp, C.M. (1991). *Case studies in perinatal nursing.* Gaithersburg, MD: Aspen.

Bobak, I. (1992). *Maturity and gynecologic care: The nurse and the family* (5th ed.). St. Louis: Mosby Yearbook.

Bobak, I., & Jensen, M.D. (1991). *Essentials of maternity nursing* (3rd ed.). St. Louis, MO: Mosby Yearbook.

Bobak, I., Jensen, M.D., & Zalar, M.K. (1989). *Maternity and gynecologic care: The nurse and the family.* St. Louis: C.V. Mosby.

Byer, C.O., & Shainberg, L.W. (1991). *Dimensions of human sexuality.* Dubuque, IA: Wm. C. Brown.

Martin, L.L., & Reeder, S.J. (1991). *Essentials of maternity nursing: family-centered care.* Philadelphia: J.B. Lippincott.

May, K.A., & Mahlmeister, L.R. (1990). *Comprehensive maternity nursing* (2nd ed.). Philadelphia: J.B. Lippincott.

Olds, S.B., London, M.L., & Ladewig, P.W. (1992). *Maternal-newborn nursing: A family-centered approach.* Redwood City, CA: Addison-Wesley.

Phillips, C.R. (1992). *Family-centered maternity/newborn care* (3rd ed.). St. Louis: Mosby Yearbook.

Pilliteri, A. (1992). *Maternal and child health nursing care of the childbearing and childbearing family.* Philadelphia: J.B. Lippincott.

Reeder, S.J., Martin, L.L., & Koniak, D. (1992). *Maternity nursing: Family, newborn, and women's health care* (17th ed.). Philadelphia: J.B. Lippincott.

Sherwen, L.N., Scoloveno, M.A., & Weingarten, C.T. (1991). *Nursing care of the childbearing family.* Norwalk, CT: Appleton and Lange.

Part III

Nursing Care of Children

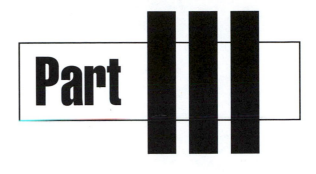

Health Promotion

Test 1

Health Promotion of the Infant and Family
Health Promotion of the Toddler and Family
Health Promotion of the Preschooler and Family
Health Promotion of the School-Aged Child and Family
Health Promotion of the Adolescent and Family
Meetings to Discuss Common Childhood and Adolescent Health Problems
Correct Answers and Rationale

Select the one best answer and indicate your choice by filling in the circle in front of the option.

Health Promotion for the Infant and Family

A nurse works in a children's clinic and helps with care for well and ill children of various ages.

1. A mother brings her 4-month-old infant to the clinic. The mother asks the nurse when she should wean the infant from breast-feeding and begin using a cup. The nurse should explain that the infant will show a readiness to be weaned by
   - ○ 1. taking solid foods well.
   - ○ 2. sleeping through the night.
   - ○ 3. shortening the nursing time.
   - ○ 4. eating on a regular schedule.
2. The mother says that the infant's physician recommends certain foods, but the infant refuses to eat them after breast-feeding. The nurse should suggest that the mother alter the feeding plan by
   - ○ 1. offering dessert followed by vegetables and meat.
   - ○ 2. offering breast milk as long as the infant refuses to eat solid foods.
   - ○ 3. mixing pureed food with cow's milk and feeding it to the infant through a large-hole nipple.
   - ○ 4. giving the infant a few minutes of breast milk and then offering solid foods.
3. Which of the following abilities would the nurse not expect this 4-month-old infant to perform?
   - ○ 1. Sitting up without support.
   - ○ 2. Responding to pleasure with smiles.
   - ○ 3. Grasping a rattle when it is offered.
   - ○ 4. Turning from either side to the back.
4. The nurse plans to administer the Denver Developmental Screening Test (DDST) to a 5-month-old infant. The nurse should explain to the mother that the test measures the infant's
   - ○ 1. intelligence quotient.
   - ○ 2. emotional development.
   - ○ 3. social and physical abilities.
   - ○ 4. predisposition to genetic and allergic illnesses.
5. In addition to immunizing for diphtheria, pertussis, and tetanus (DPT) during the first 6 months of life, the nurse should administer which other immunization?
   - ○ 1. Mumps.
   - ○ 2. Measles.
   - ○ 3. Tuberculosis.
   - ○ 4. Poliomyelitis.
6. A 5-month-old infant's mother asks the nurse, "What about a smallpox vaccination?" The nurse should explain that the current recommendation concerning smallpox immunization is that the vaccination should
   - ○ 1. no longer be given.
   - ○ 2. be given at age 2 years.
   - ○ 3. be delayed until starting school.
   - ○ 4. be postponed until adolescence.
7. When discussing a 7-month-old infant's motor skill development with the mother, the nurse should explain that by age 7 months, an infant most likely will be able to
   - ○ 1. walk with support.
   - ○ 2. eat with a spoon.
   - ○ 3. stand while holding onto furniture.
   - ○ 4. sit alone using the hands for support.
8. A mother brings her 1-month-old infant to the clinic for a checkup. Which of the following developmental achievements would the nurse assess for?
   - ○ 1. Smiling and laughing out loud.
   - ○ 2. Rolling from back to side.
   - ○ 3. Holding a rattle briefly.

○ 4. Turning the head from side to side.

9. A 2-month-old infant is brought to the clinic for the first immunization against DPT. The nurse should administer the vaccine via what route?
○ 1. Oral.
○ 2. Intramuscular.
○ 3. Subcutaneous.
○ 4. Intradermal.

10. The nurse teaches the client's mother about the normal reaction that an infant may experience 12–24 hours after DPT immunization. Which of the following reactions would the nurse discuss?
○ 1. Lethargy.
○ 2. Mild fever.
○ 3. Diarrhea.
○ 4. Nasal congestion.

11. An infant is observed to be competent in the following developmental skills: stares at an object placed in her hand and takes it to her mouth, coos and gurgles when talked to, and sustains part of her own weight when held in a standing position. The nurse correctly assesses this infant's age as
○ 1. 2 months.
○ 2. 4 months.
○ 3. 6 months.
○ 4. 8 months.

12. An infant's mother says, "The soft spot near the front of his head is still big. When will it close?" The nurse's correct response would be at
○ 1. 2 to 4 months.
○ 2. 5 to 8 months.
○ 3. 9 to 12 months.
○ 4. 13 to 18 months.

13. The nurse explains the infant's risk of choking when sucking on a propped bottle of formula or fruit juice. The nurse should also explain that this practice predisposes the infant to
○ 1. obesity.
○ 2. dental caries.
○ 3. prolonged attachment to the bottle.
○ 4. prolonged use of nighttime feedings.

14. A mother states that she thinks her 9-month-old "is developing slowly." When evaluating the infant's development, the nurse would not expect a normal 9-month-old to be able to
○ 1. sit without support.
○ 2. begin to use imitative verbal expressions.
○ 3. put an arm through a sleeve while being dressed.
○ 4. hold a bottle with good hand-mouth coordination.

15. The mother of a 9-month-old says it is difficult to add new foods to his diet. "He spits everything out," she says. The nurse should teach the mother to
○ 1. mix new foods with formula.
○ 2. mix new foods with more familiar foods.
○ 3. offer new foods one at a time.
○ 4. offer new foods after formula has been offered.

Health Promotion for the Toddler and Family

16. A mother brings her 18-month-old to the clinic because he "eats ashes, crayons, and paper." The nurse would first assess whether the toddler is
○ 1. cutting large teeth.
○ 2. experiencing a growth spurt.
○ 3. experiencing changes in the home environment.
○ 4. eating a soft, low-roughage diet.

17. Which of the following tasks typical of an 18-month-old would the nurse assess for?
○ 1. Copying a circle.
○ 2. Pulling toys.
○ 3. Playing tag with other children.
○ 4. Building a tower of eight blocks.

18. A mother brings her normally developed 3-year-old child to the clinic for a checkup. The nurse would expect that the child would be least skilled in
○ 1. riding a tricycle.
○ 2. tying shoelaces.
○ 3. stringing large beads.
○ 4. using blunt scissors.

19. The nurse might use which of the following nursing diagnoses in teaching the mother of a toddler about safety issues?
○ 1. Activity intolerance.
○ 2. Knowledge deficit.
○ 3. Alteration in growth and development.
○ 4. Impaired mobility.

20. A 2-year-old child is brought to the clinic by her mother because she constantly pulls at her ears. The toddler is uncooperative when the nurse tries to look in her ears. Which of the following actions would be best for the nurse to try first?
○ 1. Ask another nurse to assist.
○ 2. Allow the parent to assist.
○ 3. Wait until the child calms down.
○ 4. Restrain the child's arms.

21. Ear drops, instilled twice a day, are prescribed for a toddler. When teaching the mother to instill the drops, the nurse should tell her to pull the toddler's ear lobe
○ 1. up and forward.
○ 2. up and backward.
○ 3. down and forward.
○ 4. down and backward.

22. Before the mother leaves, she tells the nurse that she is having problems toilet-training her 2-year-old child. The nurse would tell the mother that the

number-one reason that toilet-training in toddlers fails is because the
- ○ 1. rewards are too limited.
- ○ 2. training equipment is inappropriate.
- ○ 3. parents ignore "accidents" that occur during training.
- ○ 4. child is not developmentally ready to be trained.

23. A $2\frac{1}{2}$-year-old child is brought to the clinic by his father, who explains that the child is afraid of the dark and always says "no" when asked to do something. The nurse would explain that the negativism demonstrated by toddlers is frequently an expression of
- ○ 1. a quest for autonomy.
- ○ 2. hyperactivity.
- ○ 3. separation anxiety.
- ○ 4. sibling rivalry.

24. The nurse would explain to the father which concept of Piaget's cognitive development as the basis for the child's fear of darkness?
- ○ 1. Reversibility.
- ○ 2. Animism.
- ○ 3. Conservation of matter.
- ○ 4. Object permanence.

25. A father reports that his 2-year-old child often falls when running. The nurse would explain that this may be linked to the fact that a toddler's vision is
- ○ 1. myopic.
- ○ 2. hyperopic.
- ○ 3. presbyopic.
- ○ 4. amblyopic.

26. A mother brings her 2-year-old child to the clinic because of her concerns about the child's nutritional status. She tells the nurse that for the last week the child has refused to eat anything except animal crackers and peanut butter and jelly sandwiches. Which of the following measures would be most appropriate for the nurse to suggest?
- ○ 1. Give the child extra time to play outside if she eats what the family eats at mealtime.
- ○ 2. Consult a physician, because the child's behavior will lead to nutritional deficiency.
- ○ 3. Don't be overly concerned about the child's behavior, because food fads usually last only a short time.
- ○ 4. Insist that the child eat small portions of the family's meal to maintain adequate nutrition.

27. The nurse assesses the child's teeth during the physical examination and teaches the mother to
- ○ 1. brush the child's teeth after every meal and at bedtime.
- ○ 2. brush the child's teeth with a small, soft-bristle toothbrush.
- ○ 3. floss the child's teeth using unwaxed dental floss.
- ○ 4. add a fluoride supplement to the child's milk three times a day.

28. The mother asks the nurse for advice about discipline. The nurse would suggest that the mother first use
- ○ 1. structured interactions.
- ○ 2. spanking.
- ○ 3. reasoning.
- ○ 4. scolding.

29. When a nurse assesses for pain in toddlers, which of the following techniques would be least effective?
- ○ 1. Ask them about the pain.
- ○ 2. Observe them for restlessness.
- ○ 3. Watch their faces for grimaces.
- ○ 4. Listen for pain cues in their cries.

30. The mother of a 15-month-old toddler asks the nurse how much milk her child should receive daily. The nurse's best response would be
- ○ 1. no more than 1 cup.
- ○ 2. 2 to 3 cups.
- ○ 3. 5 to 6 cups.
- ○ 4. 7 to 8 cups.

Health Promotion for the Preschool-Age Child and Family

A mother brings her 4-year-old child to the pediatrician's office for an annual checkup.

31. The mother expresses concern that her child may be hyperactive. She describes the child as always "in motion," constantly dropping and spilling things. Which nursing intervention would be most appropriate at this time?
- ○ 1. Determine if there have been any changes at home.
- ○ 2. Explain that this is not unusual behavior.
- ○ 3. Explore the possibility that the child is being abused.
- ○ 4. Suggest that the child be seen by a pediatric neurologist.

32. Which of the following activities would the nurse recommend to the mother to help channel the child's energy?
- ○ 1. Participate in parallel play.
- ○ 2. Play a game like "Simon says."
- ○ 3. Ride a tricycle.
- ○ 4. String large beads.

33. The mother reports that her child creates quite a scene every night at bedtime and asks what she can do to make bedtime a little more pleasant. The nurse should suggest that the mother

○ 1. allow the child to stay up later one or two nights a week.
○ 2. establish a set bedtime and follow a routine.
○ 3. let the child play tag just before bedtime.
○ 4. give the child a cookie if bedtime is pleasant.

34. The mother asks about dental care for her child. She says that she helps brush the child's teeth daily. Which of the following responses by the nurse would be most appropriate?
○ 1. "Since you help brush her teeth, there's no need to see a dentist now."
○ 2. "You should have begun dental appointments last year, but it's not too late."
○ 3. "Your child doesn't need to see the dentist until she starts school."
○ 4. "A dental checkup is a good idea, even if no noticeable problems are present."

35. The mother says that she will be glad to let her child brush her teeth without help, but at what age should this begin? The nurse should respond, "At
○ 1. 3 years."
○ 2. 5 years."
○ 3. 7 years."
○ 4. 9 years."

36. The mother tells the nurse that her child "doesn't seem to know the difference between right and wrong." In assessing this child, the nurse would explain to the mother that this is typical of which level of moral development as described by Kohlberg?
○ 1. Autonomous.
○ 2. Conventional.
○ 3. Preconventional.
○ 4. Principles.

37. The mother tells the nurse that her other child, a 4-year-old boy, has developed some "strange eating habits," including not finishing meals and eating the same food for several days in a row. She would like to develop a plan to correct this situation. In developing such a plan, the nurse and mother should consider
○ 1. deciding on a good reward for finishing the meal.
○ 2. allowing him to make some decisions about the foods he eats.
○ 3. requiring him to eat the foods served at meal times.
○ 4. not allowing him to play with friends until he eats all the food he's served.

38. Since both parents are nearsighted, the mother is concerned that her 4-year-old may be nearsighted. She says that he likes to look at books and knows most of the alphabet. What assessment technique should the nurse use to evaluate the child's visual acuity?
○ 1. Cover and cross-over test.
○ 2. Allen picture cards.
○ 3. Snellen alphabet chart.
○ 4. Ishihara plates.

39. After having a blood sample drawn, a child insists that the site be covered with a Band-Aid. When the mother tries to remove the Band-Aid before leaving the office, the child screams that all the blood will come out. This behavior indicates
○ 1. a normal fear of injury.
○ 2. a normal fear of compromised body integrity.
○ 3. an abnormal fear of compromised body integrity.
○ 4. an abnormal fear of loss of control.

40. Which nursing intervention would best help prepare a preschool-aged child for an injection?
○ 1. Have an older child explain that shots do not hurt.
○ 2. Suggest diversionary activities such as singing.
○ 3. Give the child a play syringe and a Band-Aid so the child can give a doll injections.
○ 4. Give the child a pounding board to encourage expressions of anger.

Several employees at a flower shop have preschool-age children. At lunch one day, they decide it would be helpful to meet with a pediatric nurse. An employee arranges for a pediatric nurse specialist to meet with them to discuss their children.

41. A mother at the meeting says her 5-year-old seems prone to minor accidents like skinning his elbows and knees and falling off his scooter. The nurse would base further assessment of this child on the knowledge that childhood accidents are more likely to occur when the family
○ 1. consists of only one child.
○ 2. has limited formal education.
○ 3. is experiencing changes.
○ 4. has a high economic status.

42. The nurse knows that one of the most effective strategies that parents can use to teach 4-year-olds about safety is to
○ 1. show them potential dangers to avoid.
○ 2. tell them they are bad when they do something dangerous.
○ 3. provide good examples of safe behavior.
○ 4. show them pictures of children who have been involved in accidents.

43. A mother in the group says that her 5-year-old has had multiple ear infections and asks how preschool-age children perceive illness. The nurse should explain that they generally regard it as
○ 1. a necessary part of life.
○ 2. a test of self-worth.
○ 3. punishment for wrongdoing.

○ 4. the will of God.

44. A father in the group asks if his 5-year-old son should have the Denver Developmental Screening Test. Before answering, the nurse would need additional information about the
- ○ 1. father's understanding of the test.
- ○ 2. reason the father is asking.
- ○ 3. child's developmental level.
- ○ 4. child's performance in kindergarten.

Health Promotion for the School-Age Child and Family

A 9-year-old girl is brought to the pediatrician's office for a camp physical. She has no history of significant health problems.

45. When the nurse asks the child and mother about the child's best friend, the nurse is assessing
- ○ 1. language development.
- ○ 2. motor development.
- ○ 3. neurological development.
- ○ 4. social development.

46. The child proudly tells the nurse that brushing and flossing her teeth is her responsibility. When responding to this information, the nurse should realize that the child
- ○ 1. is too young to be given this responsibility.
- ○ 2. is most likely quite capable of this responsibility.
- ○ 3. should have assumed this responsibility much sooner.
- ○ 4. is probably just exaggerating the responsibility.

47. The mother tells the nurse that the child is continually telling jokes and riddles to the point of driving the other family members crazy. The nurse should explain that this behavior is a sign of
- ○ 1. inadequate parental attention.
- ○ 2. mastery of language ambiguities.
- ○ 3. inappropriate peer influence.
- ○ 4. excessive television watching.

48. The mother relates that the child is beginning to identify behaviors that please others as "good" behaviors. The child's behavior is characteristic of which of Kohlberg's levels of moral development?
- ○ 1. Preconventional morality.
- ○ 2. Conventional morality.
- ○ 3. Postconventional morality.
- ○ 4. Autonomous morality.

49. The mother asks the nurse about the child's apparent need for between-meal snacks, especially after school. The nurse and mother develop a nutritional plan for the child, keeping in mind that the child
- ○ 1. does not need to eat between meals.
- ○ 2. should eat the snacks the mother prepares.
- ○ 3. should help prepare own snacks.
- ○ 4. will instinctively select nutritional snacks.

50. The mother is concerned about the child's compulsion for collecting things. The nurse explains that this behavior is related to the cognitive ability to perform
- ○ 1. concrete operations.
- ○ 2. formal operations.
- ○ 3. coordination of secondary schemata.
- ○ 4. tertiary circular reactions.

51. When the child's height and weight are compared with standard growth charts, she is found to be in the 85th percentile for height and in the 45th percentile for weight. These findings indicate that the child is
- ○ 1. of normal height and weight.
- ○ 2. overweight for height.
- ○ 3. underweight for height.
- ○ 4. taller than average.

52. The nurse explained to the mother that according to Erikson's framework of psychosocial development, play as a vehicle of development can help the school-age child develop a sense of
- ○ 1. initiative.
- ○ 2. industry.
- ○ 3. identity.
- ○ 4. intimacy.

53. The parents of a 6-year-old child tell the nurse that they are very concerned about the child's tonsils. On inspection, the nurse notes that the tonsils are very large but not reddened or inflamed. The nurse explains that these findings most likely indicate
- ○ 1. the need for tonsillectomy.
- ○ 2. acute tonsillitis.
- ○ 3. a normal increase in lymphoid tissue.
- ○ 4. an abnormal growth of lymphoid tissue.

54. The school nurse is planning a series of safety and accident prevention classes for a group of third graders. What preventive measure should the nurse stress during the first class, knowing the leading cause of accidental injury and death in this age group? The use of
- ○ 1. flame-retardant clothing.
- ○ 2. life preservers.
- ○ 3. protective eyewear.
- ○ 4. auto seat belts.

55. The nurse should explain to parents that the immunizations recommended for children between age 4 and 6 years before starting school are
- ○ 1. diphtheria, tetanus, pertussis, and polio.
- ○ 2. measles, mumps, rubella, and polio.
- ○ 3. polio, smallpox, measles, and pertussis.
- ○ 4. tetanus, diphtheria, mumps, and smallpox.

56. The mother of a 10-year-old boy expresses concern that he is overweight. When developing a plan of care with the mother, the nurse should encourage her to

- ○ 1. limit the child's between-meal snacks.
- ○ 2. prohibit the child from playing outside if he eats sweets.
- ○ 3. include the child in meal planning and preparation.
- ○ 4. limit the child's daily caloric intake to 1,200.

Health Promotion for the Adolescent and Family

The school nurse at a high school has the opportunity to counsel many adolescents as they come to talk about various concerns.

57. When interacting with adolescents, the nurse must consider their phase of cognitive development. According to Piaget, this phase of development is characterized by the ability to

- ○ 1. assimilate and accommodate.
- ○ 2. deal with abstract possibilities.
- ○ 3. manipulate concrete materials.
- ○ 4. solve problems of conservation.

58. A 16-year-old female comes to the school nurse complaining of dysmenorrhea. She reports cramps, backache, and nausea with her periods. The nurse recognizes that the basis for these symptoms is most likely

- ○ 1. pathological.
- ○ 2. physiological.
- ○ 3. psychogenic.
- ○ 4. psychosomatic.

59. The nurse develops a plan to provide relief of dysmenorrhea at this time in the adolescent's life because it will help her develop

- ○ 1. positive peer relations.
- ○ 2. positive self-identity.
- ○ 3. a sense of autonomy.
- ○ 4. a sense of control.

60. The adolescent tells the nurse that she would like to use tampons during her period. An appropriate nursing intervention would be to

- ○ 1. assess her understanding of her anatomy.
- ○ 2. determine if she is sexually active.
- ○ 3. provide her with information about toxic shock syndrome.
- ○ 4. refer her to a specialist in adolescent gynecology.

61. The nurse is invited to attend a meeting with several parents. Some parents express frustration with the amount of time their adolescents spend in front of the mirror and the length of time it takes them to get dressed. The nurse should explain that this behavior is

- ○ 1. an indication of an abnormal concern with self.
- ○ 2. a method of procrastination commonly seen in adolescents.
- ○ 3. a method of testing parents' limit-setting.
- ○ 4. a result of rapid body changes and developing self-concept.

62. One mother asks the school nurse if her 16-year-old son still needs immunizations. The nurse should explain that

- ○ 1. children older than age 7 do not need immunizations.
- ○ 2. adolescents should routinely receive a measles vaccination at age 16.
- ○ 3. the last immunization received is a tetanus booster at age 16.
- ○ 4. adolescents and adults should receive a tetanus diphtheria booster every 10 years.

63. Several high school seniors are referred to the nurse because of suspected alcohol misuse. When the nurse assesses the situation, it would be most important to determine

- ○ 1. if they know the legal drinking age.
- ○ 2. the type of alcohol they usually drink.
- ○ 3. the reasons they chose to use alcohol.
- ○ 4. when and with whom they use alcohol.

64. Several parents express concerns about the types and large quantities of food their teenagers eat and their refusal to eat foods served at family meals. It would be most appropriate for the nurse to help parents develop a plan to

- ○ 1. evaluate the adolescent's nutritional intake carefully.
- ○ 2. inform the adolescent about the adverse effects of diets.
- ○ 3. give the adolescent responsibility for grocery shopping for 1 month.
- ○ 4. incorporate the adolescent's preferences into meal planning.

65. An 18-year-old senior tells the nurse, "Everyone does it, so it's all right," to justify rule-breaking behavior. The nurse realizes this is an example of which level of moral reasoning as described by Kohlberg?

- ○ 1. Preconventional level.
- ○ 2. Conventional level.
- ○ 3. Postconventional level.
- ○ 4. Autonomous level.

66. As part of the annual health screening, the nurse visits the 8th grade physical education classes. The nurse asks each student to bend forward at the waist with the back parallel to the floor and the hands together at midline. The purpose of this is to observe for signs of

- ○ 1. slipped epiphysis.
- ○ 2. congenital hip dislocation.

○ 3. idiopathic scoliosis.
○ 4. physical dexterity.

Meetings to Discuss Common Childhood and Adolescent Health Problems

The parents of children attending an elementary school and a high school invite the school nurse to attend Parent-Teacher Association (PTA) meetings to discuss common health problems related to their children.

67. One parent asks about head lice infestation (pediculosis capitis). The nurse discusses the symptoms with the parents. Which of the following symptoms is most common in a child infected with head lice?
○ 1. Itching of the scalp.
○ 2. Scaling of the scalp.
○ 3. Serious weeping on the scalp surface.
○ 4. Pinpoint hemorrhagic spots on the scalp surface.

68. A parent asks, "Can I get head lice too?" The nurse indicates that adults can also be infested with head lice but that pediculosis is more common among school children primarily because
○ 1. an immunity to pediculosis usually is established by adulthood.
○ 2. children of school age tend to be more neglectful of frequent handwashing.
○ 3. pediculosis is most often spread by close contact with infested children in the classroom.
○ 4. the skin of adults is more capable of resisting the invasion of lice.

69. One parent asks what causes ringworm of the scalp (tinea capitis). The nurse explains that the organism is classified as a
○ 1. virus.
○ 2. fungus.
○ 3. bacillus.
○ 4. protozoan.

70. One mother says that her physician ordered griseofulvin (Grisactin) to treat her child's ringworm of the scalp. The physician said, "It is very important to take the medication exactly as ordered for several weeks." The mother asks why it is so important. The nurse should base a response on the knowledge that
○ 1. a sensitivity to the drug is less likely if it is used over a period of time.
○ 2. fewer side effects occur as the body slowly adjusts to a new substance over time.
○ 3. fewer allergic reactions occur if the drug is maintained at the same level long-term.
○ 4. the growth of the causative organism into new cells is prevented when the drug is used long-term.

71. "How did my children get pinworms?," a mother asks. The nurse should respond by explaining that pinworms are most commonly spread by contaminated
○ 1. food.
○ 2. hands.
○ 3. animals.
○ 4. toilet seats.

72. A parent says that her family will soon be traveling abroad, and asks why the drinking water in many regions must be boiled. The nurse would explain that in addition to various types of dysentery, contaminated drinking water is most commonly responsible for the transmission of
○ 1. typhus.
○ 2. brucellosis.
○ 3. poliomyelitis.
○ 4. typhoid fever.

73. A mother says one of her children has chicken pox and asks about care measures. The nurse should explain that the care of a child with chicken pox is directed primarily toward preventing
○ 1. anemia and dehydration.
○ 2. anorexia and malnutrition.
○ 3. infection at the site of the lesions.
○ 4. infection in the respiratory system.

74. Which of the following home regimens should the nurse suggest to relieve itching in children with chicken pox? Applying
○ 1. generous amounts of fine baby powder.
○ 2. a paste of baking soda and water.
○ 3. terrycloth towels moistened with warm water.
○ 4. cool compresses moistened with a weak salt solution.

75. A mother says that a physician described her child as having 20/60 vision and asks the nurse what this means. The nurse should explain that the child
○ 1. has lost approximately one-third of her visual acuity.
○ 2. sees at 60 feet what she should see at 20 feet.
○ 3. sees at 20 feet what she should see at 60 feet.
○ 4. has approximately three times better visual acuity than average.

76. A parent says that her child has hemophilia and she worries whenever the child has a bump or cut. The nurse should explain that after the area is cleansed, the wound should be cared for by applying
○ 1. gentle pressure.
○ 2. warm, moist compresses.
○ 3. a tourniquet above the injured area.
○ 4. dressings moistened with witch hazel.

77. The nurse should also tell this mother to avoid giving her hemophilic child which of the following over-the-counter medications?
○ 1. Acetylsalicylic acid (Aspirin).
○ 2. Magnesium hydroxide (Milk of Magnesia).

○ 3. Acetaminophen (Tylenol).
○ 4. Ibuprofen (Motrin).

78. Some parents ask the school nurse how they can best prepare their children to start school. Which of the following courses of action would be best for the nurse to recommend to the parents?
○ 1. Have an older sibling tell the child about school.
○ 2. Orient the child to the school's physical environment.
○ 3. Offer to stay with the child for the first few days of school.
○ 4. Discuss school with the child if he or she asks questions about it.

79. The nurse should explain that the most common cause for the unhappiness some children experience when first entering school is
○ 1. feelings of insecurity.
○ 2. inability to pay attention.
○ 3. emotional maladjustment.
○ 4. poor language development.

80. Some parents ask about food requirements for school children. The nurse explains that compared to the food requirements of preschoolers and adolescents, the food requirements of school-age children are not as great because they have a lower
○ 1. growth rate.
○ 2. metabolic rate.
○ 3. level of activity.
○ 4. hormonal secretion rate.

81. The nurse discusses the eating habits of school-age children, explaining to the parents that these habits are most influenced by
○ 1. food preferences of their peers.
○ 2. the smell and appearance of the foods offered to them.
○ 3. the atmosphere and examples provided by parents at mealtimes.
○ 4. parents encouraging their children to eat nutritious foods.

82. The nurse discusses adolescent behavior with the parents, explaining that according to Erikson, the central problem of adolescence is establishing a sense of
○ 1. identity.
○ 2. industry.
○ 3. intimacy.
○ 4. initiative.

83. Which of the following statements would be best for the nurse to use when describing the onset of adolescence in boys and girls?
○ 1. "Girls and boys experience the onset of adolescence at approximately the same age."
○ 2. "Boys experience the onset of adolescence approximately 1 to 2 years earlier than girls."
○ 3. "Girls experience the onset of adolescence approximately 1 to 2 years earlier than boys."
○ 4. "Boys experience the onset of adolescence 3 to 4 years later than girls."

84. In discussing safety issues with parents, the nurse would utilize which of the following nursing diagnoses?
○ 1. Ineffective Family Coping.
○ 2. Altered Health Maintenance.
○ 3. High Risk for Injury.
○ 4. Knowledge Deficit.

85. Parents report that their 15-year-old son is moody and rude. The nurse should advise the parents to
○ 1. restrict his activities.
○ 2. discuss their feelings with him.
○ 3. obtain family counseling.
○ 4. talk to other parents of adolescents.

86. Several parents express concern about problems that acne creates in their children and ask the nurse how a teenager with acne should cleanse affected areas. It would be best for the nurse to recommend that teenagers with acne cleanse their skin with
○ 1. witch hazel.
○ 2. soap and water.
○ 3. hydrogen peroxide.
○ 4. lotions and creams.

87. A parent asks the nurse what precautions should be taken to prevent the spread of mononucleosis. Which of the following responses would most accurately reflect current opinion concerning the spread of mononucleosis?
○ 1. No particular precautionary measures are advised.
○ 2. The child's eating utensils should be boiled before being reused.
○ 3. The child's linens should be washed separately in hot, soapy water.
○ 4. Caregivers should wear masks when providing direct personal care.

88. Another parent asks how she would know if her child developed mononucleosis. The nurse should explain that in addition to fatigue, the most typical symptom of mononucleosis is
○ 1. liver tenderness.
○ 2. enlarged lymph glands.
○ 3. persistent nonproductive cough.
○ 4. generalized skin rash resembling a blush.

89. The subject of sexually transmitted diseases (STD's) and their control is discussed at one meeting. The nurse correctly explains that community health measures designed to control STD's are most often directed toward
○ 1. mass screening for STD's.
○ 2. locating the sources of STD's.
○ 3. treating persons who have or are suspected of having an STD.
○ 4. isolating persons who have or are suspected of having an STD.

90. A parent asks why it is recommended that adolescent girls not be given "measles vaccine." The nurse answers that the most important reason why girls after the age of puberty are usually not given rubella vaccine is that

○ 1. risks to the fetus are high, if the girl is pregnant.

○ 2. the chance of contracting the disease is much lower after puberty than before it.

○ 3. dangers associated with a strong reaction to the vaccine are increased after puberty.

○ 4. changes occurring in the immunologic system may affect the rhythm of the menstrual cycle.

CORRECT ANSWERS AND RATIONALE

The letters in parentheses following the rationale identify the step of the nursing process (A, D, P, I, E); cognitive level (K, C, T, N); and client need (S, G, L, H). See the Answer Grid for the key.

Health Promotion for the Infant and Family

1. 3. Readiness for weaning is an individual matter but is usually indicated when an infant begins to decrease the time spent nursing. The infant is then showing independence and will soon be ready to take a cup and learn a new skill. The infant ready for weaning may also demonstrate an ability to take solid foods well, sleep through the night, and eat on a regular schedule, but these behaviors are not necessarily evidence of readiness for weaning. (I, C, H)

2. 4. It is typical for an infant just starting on solid foods to spit them out because the infant does not know how to swallow them. Also, the infant is hungry and is accustomed to having milk to satisfy that hunger. It is generally recommended that an infant be given some milk first and then offered solids. An infant who takes all the milk first will have no interest in the solids. Offering dessert before vegetables and meat, mixing pureed foods with cow's milk, or continuing with breast milk only and delaying offering solid foods are not appropriate approaches. (I, C, H)

3. 1. A 4-month-old infant is not able to sit without support, but will normally display such behaviors as responding with smiles, grasping a rattle, and turning from either side to the back. (A, K, H)

4. 3. The Denver Developmental Screening Test (DDST) measures a child's social and physical abilities. It is not designed to measure intelligence and emotional development, nor predisposition to illnesses. (I, C, H)

5. 4. The United States Public Health Service and the American Academy of Pediatrics have developed recommended guidelines for immunization of children. A series of three injections of diphtheria, pertussis, and tetanus (DPT) and a series of three injections of *Haemophilus influenza* vaccine are recommended during the first year of life. Poliomyelitis protection is administered twice during the first year—unless the disease is prevalent in the area where the child lives, in which case another dose may be given. Measles, mumps, and rubella vaccine and *Haemophilus influenza* administration is recommended when the child reaches age 15 months. (I, T, H)

6. 1. Routine vaccination for smallpox is no longer recommended. The dangers and incidence of complications following vaccination have been determined to be greater than the risk of contracting the disease. (I, T, H)

7. 4. By age 7 months an infant can sit alone, leaning forward on the hands for support. The ability to sit follows progressive head control and straightening of the back. By age 8 months, an infant should be able to sit well unsupported. At about 10 months, an infant can step with one foot and crawl well. At 11 months, an infant can walk while holding onto furniture; by 12 months, an infant can walk with one hand held. At around 18 months, an infant can eat successfully with a spoon. (I, C, H)

8. 4. A 1-month-old infant is able to lift the head and turn it from side to side when lying prone. (The full-term infant with no abnormalities or complications probably has been able to do this since birth.) Smiling and laughing aloud are expected behaviors for a 2- to 3-month old infant. Holding a rattle for a brief time and rolling from the back to the side are characteristic behaviors of a 4-month-old infant. (A, K, H)

9. 2. The diphtheria, pertussis, and tetanus (DPT) vaccine is given by injection deep into the largest muscle available. The best muscle to use in a 2-month-old infant is the vastus lateralis. (I, K, S)

10. 2. Mild fever 12 to 24 hours after administration of a DPT vaccine is common in an infant. The mother should be taught to give the infant acetaminophen for the fever. Fever above 102°F (measured rectally) should be reported to the physician. An infant with a fever tends to be restless rather than lethargic. Diarrhea and nasal congestion are not associated with the DPT vaccine. (I, K, H)

11. 2. Typical behaviors of a 4-month-old infant include holding the head erect when sitting, staring at an object placed in the hand, taking the object to the mouth, cooing and gurgling, and sustaining part of his body weight when in a standing position. (A, N, H)

12. 4. The anterior fontanel usually closes between age 12 and 18 months. The small posterior fontanel usually closes by age 3 months. (I, K, H)

13. 2. Many mothers prop a bottle of formula or fruit juice at bedtime for their infants who are old enough to handle a bottle safely. The infant then awakens periodically to take more formula or juice, constantly bathing the teeth with high-carbohydrate liquid. The practice has been noted to predispose infants to dental caries. Propping a bottle does not necessarily lead to obesity or an abnormally prolonged use of a bottle or nighttime feedings. (I, T, S)

14. 3. Normally, a 9-month-old infant will not be able to put arms through sleeves while being dressed but will be able to perform such activities as sitting with support, holding the nursing bottle, and imitating verbal expressions. (E, K, H)

15. 3. Infants should be offered new foods one at a time. This gives the infant the chance to gradually become familiar with a variety of food tastes and textures and also helps identify any allergies or adverse reactions to a specific food. Mixing new foods with formula or other familiar foods would make it impossible to detect allergic or other unfavorable reactions satisfactorily. This practice may also cause the infant to refuse familiar foods. If a new food is offered after the infant's appetite is satisfied with formula, then the infant is not likely to eat the new food. (I, N, H)

Health Promotion for the Toddler and Family

16. 3. It is important to determine if the child is experiencing any change in the home environment that could cause anxiety, which is relieved through oral gratification. A craving to eat nonfood substances is known as *pica*. Nutritional deficiencies, especially iron deficiency, were once thought to cause pica, but research has not substantiated this theory. Unlikely causes of pica include teething, growth spurts, and a low-roughage diet. (A, N, H)

17. 2. Pulling toys is a typical task of a normally developed 18-month-old child. Copying a circle and building a tower of eight or more blocks are typical behaviors of a 3-year-old. Playing tag with other children requires cooperative play and the ability to follow rules; this behavior develops at about age 5 years. (A, K, H)

18. 2. Tying shoelaces is not expected of a 3-year-old child, because it requires motor skills that remain underdeveloped until the end of the preschool years. A 3-year-old can ride a tricycle, string large beads, and use blunt scissors with one hand. (A, K, H)

19. 2. The most appropriate nursing diagnosis here would be Knowledge Deficit. A normal toddler would not have activity intolerance, altered growth and development, or impaired mobility. Safety issues are part of anticipatory guidance with parents of toddlers. (D, N, S)

20. 2. Parents can be asked to assist when their child becomes uncooperative during a procedure. The child's poor cooperation is commonly due to fright, and he or she will feel more secure with a parent present. Other methods may be necessary, but obtaining a parent's assistance is the recommended first action. (P, T, G)

21. 4. In a child, the ear lobe is pulled down and backward, because the auditory canals are almost straight in children. In an adult, the ear lobe is pulled up and backward because the auditory canals are directed inward, forward, and down. (I, T, S)

22. 4. The most common reason for failed toilet-training is that the child is simply not developmentally ready for training. Even with appropriate rewards and proper equipment, the child who is not ready for training will not be able to learn voluntary control. "Accidents" during training should be ignored. They are usually caused by the child's incomplete sphincter control, along with poor recognition of the impending need to defecate until it is too late to get to the potty chair. (P, T, H)

23. 1. According to Erikson, the developmental task of toddlerhood is acquiring a sense of autonomy while overcoming a sense of doubt and shame. Characteristics of negativism and ritualism are typical of behaviors in this quest for autonomy. The toddler often does the opposite of what others request. Hyperactivity, separation anxiety, and sibling rivalry are behaviors that may be demonstrated by the toddler, but they do not explain a toddler's negativism. (D, C, H)

24. 2. The concept of animism, in which the child attributes the quality of conscious thought to inanimate objects, is a peculiarity of preconceptual thought. The preconceptual phase of cognitive development, which is a part of the preoperational stage, lasts from age 2 to 4 years, according to Piaget's theory. Children in Piaget's concrete operational stage (school age) comprehend the concept of reversibility (an act can be undone by performing an opposite act). Reversibility allows mental action to replace physical action. School-age children also understand the concept of conservation (things remain the same even when their form and shape change). Object permanence, a milestone of the sensorimotor period of Piaget's theory, is demonstrated at age 6 to 9 months when the infant reaches for a hidden object. (D, C, H)

25. 2. Until age 7 years, children are normally hyperopic or farsighted. However, because of accommodative ability, these children usually see objects at close range. Myopia or nearsightedness is the ability to see objects at close range but not at a distance. Presbyopia is a vision defect that occurs in persons over age 40, in which the lens becomes less elastic and near objects are blurred. Amblyopia, or "lazy eye," is reduced visual acuity in one eye despite appropriate optical correction. (D, C, H)

26. 3. Food preferences and appetite are changeable during the toddler years. A child may enjoy one food for several days in a row and suddenly refuse to eat it again for days. Attempts to alter such food fads are met with resentment and obstinacy. It is best to accept such extremes and offer small portions of other foods. Offering extra time to play outside and insisting that the child eat small portions of the family's meal are not appropriate nutritional strategies. Consulting a physician is unnecessary, because food fads are normal and usually temporary. (P, T, G)

27. 3. A parent should clean and floss the toddler's teeth. A toddler does not have the cognitive or motor skills needed for effective cleaning. The parent should brush the toddler's teeth after every meal and at bedtime, using a small toothbrush with soft, rounded nylon bristles that are short and uniform in length. A fluoride supplement is needed only if the child ingests minimal amounts of tap water or the family has well water. (I, C, H)

28. 1. Structuring interactions with 3-year-olds helps minimize unacceptable behavior. This approach involves setting clear and reasonable rules and calling attention to unacceptable behavior as soon as it occurs. Physical punishment (spanking) does cause a dramatic decrease in a behavior but has serious negative effects. However, slapping a child's hand is effective when the child refuses to listen to verbal commands. Reasoning is more appropriate for older children, especially when moral issues are involved. Reasoning combined with scolding often takes the form of shame or criticism. Unfortunately, children take such remarks seriously, believing that they are "bad." (I, T, H)

29. 1. Toddlers usually express pain through such behaviors as restlessness, facial grimaces, irritability, and crying. It is not particularly helpful to ask toddlers about pain; they may not understand or may be unable to describe the nature and location of pain. (A, T, G)

30. 2. Toddlers at this age need 2 to 3 cups of milk per day; 1 cup of milk does not provide enough calcium. More than 3 cups may take the place of other nutrients that are just as important. (I, K, H)

Health Promotion for the Preschooler and Family

31. 2. Preschool-age children have been described as powerhouses of gross motor activity who seem to have endless energy. A limitation of their motor ability is that in moving as quickly as they do, they are not always able to judge distances nor are they able to estimate the amount of strength and balance needed for activities. As a result, they have frequent mishaps. (P, T, H)

32. 2. A game such as "Simon says," which requires the preschooler to use a variety of motor skills, can help channel activity and meet developmental needs. Parallel play and stringing large beads are appropriate for a younger child. Though the preschooler can ride a tricycle well, riding a bicycle requires more skill in balance than a 4-year-old is likely to have. (P, T, H)

33. 2. Bedtime is often a problem with preschoolers. Recommendations for reducing conflicts at bedtime include establishing a set bedtime, having a dependable routine such as story reading, and conveying the expectation that the child will comply. Excitement just before bedtime and the misuse of food should be avoided. (P, T, H)

34. 4. Routine dental exams should begin when a child is young, before any obvious problems develop. Dental caries can occur before age 2 years. Teeth should be brushed after meals and at bedtime. Reprimanding the mother for not taking the child to the dentist is not helpful. (P, T, H)

35. 3. Children under age 7 years do not have the manual dexterity needed for toothbrushing; thus parents should help with this. (I, T, H)

36. 3. The preconventional level of Kohlberg's stages of moral development is typical of the preschool-age child. Stage I behaviors of this preconventional level have a punishment–obedience orientation. Conventional morality pertains to children age 7 to 12. Autonomous and principles are not stages of moral development as described by Kohlberg. (A, T, H)

37. 2. Allowing a child to make some decisions about the foods to eat and not insisting that he finish meals can avoid power struggles. Refusing to finish meals and to eat certain foods is normal behavior for a preschool-age child. It is important to avoid tension at mealtime and to avoid confrontation about food, which can be used as a weapon, a bribe, or a pacificer. (P, T, G)

38. 2. Allen picture cards are used to test visual acuity in children who are not proficient with the alphabet. The Snellen alphabet chart is commonly used by age 8 or 9 years. Ishihara plates are used to test for colorblindness. The cover and cross-over test is used to rule out strabismus. (A, T, H)

39. 2. The preschool-age child does not have an accurate concept of skin integrity and can view medical and surgical treatments as hostile invasions that can destroy or damage the body. The child does not understand that exsanguination will not occur from an injection site. The other fears are unrelated to this behavior. (D, C, H)

40. 3. Allowing the preschool-age child to give play injections can help prepare the child to receive an injection. Giving play injections after the experience and using a pounding board after the experience can help the child feel in control again. Preschool-age children know that injections hurt. Diversionary activities are appropriate during an injection. (I, T, L)

41. 3. Family changes and stresses (such as moving,

having company, taking vacations, or adding new members) can distract parental attention and contribute to accidents. Only children tend to receive more attention than children with siblings. The environment of lower socioeconomic families is more conducive to childhood accidents. (A, T, H)

42. 3. Young children tend to imitate what they see, and parents teach by example, whether intentionally or not. Parents should know where their child plays and should discuss safety with him or her. Even a child who knows safety measures may forget them while playing with friends. A child should not be labeled "bad" or "good" based on behavior; it is the behavior that is undesirable, not the child. As a child matures, parental interventions aimed at preventing accidents progress from protection to education. (I, T, H)

43. 3. Preschool-age children may view illness as punishment for their fantasies. At this age children do not have the cognitive ability to separate fantasies from reality and may expect to be punished for their "evil thoughts." The other options require a higher level of cognition than preschoolers possess. (I, T, H)

44. 1. The father's knowledge and understanding of the test must be assessed, as must the reason for asking the question. The DDST is used to evaluate development in children from age 1 month to 6 years. Gathering information about the other options is premature. (A, C, H)

Health Promotion for the School-age Child and Family

45. 4. During the school-age years, the child learns to socialize with children the same age. The "best friend" stage, which occurs around age 9 or 10 years, is very important in providing a foundation for self-esteem and later relationships. (A, K, H)

46. 2. Children are capable of mastering the skills required for flossing when they reach age 9. By age 9 or 10, many children are able to assume responsibility for personal hygiene. (I, C, H)

47. 2. School-age children delight in riddles and jokes. Mastery of the ambiguities of language and of sentence structure allows the school-age child to manipulate words, and telling riddles and jokes is a way of practicing this skill. (I, T, H)

48. 2. Behaviors characteristic of Kohlberg's conventional level of moral development (level 2) are those related to expectations of others and the desire to conform to social expectations. In stage 3 of the conventional level of moral reasoning, good behavior are seen as those that are approved by others. The other two levels of moral development are preconventional (level 2) and postconventional (level 3). Preconventional morality pertains to children up to age 7 years; postconventional morality pertains to older children, adolescents, and adults. (I, C, H)

49. 3. Snacks are necessary for school-age children; they should help prepare their own snacks. School-age children are in a stage of cognitive development in which they can learn to categorize or classify and can also learn cause and effect. By preparing their own snacks, school-age children can learn the basics of nutrition (for example, what carbohydrates are and what happens when they are eaten). (I, T, G)

50. 1. The school-age child (age 7 to 11) who has achieved the cognitive abilities required to master concrete operations often collects various objects when learning to manipulate and classify these objects. Coordination of secondary schemata and tertiary circular reactions is part of the sensorimotor phase of cognitive development (up to age 2 years). Formal operations do not emerge until later (age 11 to 15 years). (I, T, H)

51. 1. The values of height and weight percentiles are usually similar for an individual child. Marked discrepancies identify overweight or underweight children. Measurements between the 5th and 95th percentile are considered normal. (I, T, H)

52. 2. According to Erikson, industry versus inferiority is the theme of psychosocial development during middle and late childhood. The challenge is mastering skills to create and complete projects; this is often done through play. Sense of initiative is the theme of the preschool-age child. Sense of identity is the theme of early adolescence, and sense of intimacy and solidarity is the theme for late adolescence and young adulthood. (P, K, H)

53. 3. Lymphoid tissue develops rapidly in relative size until age 10 to 11 years. Lymphoid hyperplasia in the form of enlarged tonsils is normal until age 6 to 7 years, after which the tissue slowly atrophies. Enlarged tonsils are not surgically removed unless they become abscessed or compromise physiological functioning. (D, N, G)

54. 4. Motor vehicle accidents are the most common cause of accidental injury and death in children between age 6 and 12 years. Measures that prevent accidents involving motor vehicles, bicycles, or motorized bikes should be emphasized. Other major causes of accidental injury and death in school-age children are drowning, burns, and firearms. Accidents in children up to age 1 year involve falls, poisoning, and burns. (I, T, H)

55. 1. Boosters of diphtheria, tetanus, and pertussis (DPT) and oral polio vaccine (OPV) are the immunizations recommended for children between age 4 and 6 years before entering school. The recommended ages for measles, mumps, and rubella

(MMR) immunizations are 15 months and 12 years. Smallpox vaccinations are no longer routinely given to children. (I, T, H)

56. 3. Children age 9 to 10 years can assume increasing responsibility for their health, and helping in meal preparation is an opportunity to learn about nutrition. The school-age child's food intake cannot be continually monitored by parents due to the child's expanding world. Physical activity should be encouraged, not restricted. A school-age child requires approximately 2,400 calories per day. (P, T, H)

Health Promotion for the Adolescent and Family

57. 2. The ability to deal with abstract possibilities develops in adolescents, but not all adolescents develop this ability. Assimilation and accommodation are characteristics of the sensorimotor development of infants. Problems of conservation are part of concrete operations learned by children between age 4 and 7 years. (P, K, H)

58. 2. The basis for these symptoms is most likely physiological. There are two types of dysmenorrhea: primary and secondary. Primary is the most common type and is believed to be caused by an increased level of prostaglandins. The increased level produces uterine hyperactivity and contractions. Approximately 80% of females who take prostaglandin-inhibitors, such as ibuprofen (Motrin), experience relief of symptoms. (I, C, H)

59. 2. Relieving dysmenorrhea in adolescence is crucial for the female's development of positive self-identity, of which positive body image and sexual identity are parts. Menstruation should not be viewed as painful and debilitating. Sense of autonomy, according to Erikson, is the developmental task of toddlers that, if successfuly mastered, leads to a sense of self-control. (I, C, H)

60. 3. About 95% of cases of toxic shock syndrome occur during menses, and a relationship between tampon use and development of toxic shock syndrome has been identified. Most adolescent females can use tampons safely if they change them frequently. (I, T, H)

61. 4. Adolescence is a time of integrating physical changes into the self-concept, and most teenagers spend much time worrying about their personal appearance. (I, T, H)

62. 4. The only recommended immunization for adolescents and adults is a combined tetanus toxoid and diphtheria toxoid booster every 10 years. Measles vaccination should not be routinely given to adolescent females because of the possible effects on a fetus if the girl was to be pregnant. (I, T, H)

63. 3. Information about why adolescents choose to use alcohol or other drugs can be used to determine whether they are becoming responsible users or problem users. A person may use alcohol out of simple curiosity or as a means of escape. (A, K, L)

64. 4. It is important to prevent food intake from becoming the center of an independence–dependence struggle. Nursing responsibilities include helping parents realize that adolescents require a high caloric intake and need to make individual decisions. Adolescents are subject to peer pressure, which often supersedes family pressure. Responsibility for grocery shopping for a month may encourage independence but does not ensure adequate nutritional status. (I, T, H)

65. 2. Stage 3 behaviors of Kohlberg's conventional level of moral reasoning focus on the approval of others. Moral dilemmas are solved by the group standard, with an emphasis on conformity. Adolescents usually function at this level of moral development. Children up to age 2 years function at the preconventional level; adolescents and adults function at the postconventional level. (I, C, H)

66. 3. When bending forward, a person who had idiopathic scoliosis has an obvious rib hump. The two sides of the back at the hips, ribs, and/or shoulders are not level. Slipped epiphysis is characterized by continuous or intermittent hip pain and a tendency of the leg to externally rotate. Congenital hip dislocation is an abnormality of the hip joint at birth. (A, T, H)

Meetings to Discuss Common Childhood and Adolescent Health Problems

67. 1. The most common characteristic of head lice infestation (pediculosis capitis) is severe itching. Itching also occurs when lice infest other parts of the body. Scratch marks are almost always found when lice are present. The head is the most common site of lice infestation. (A, K, G)

68. 3. Lice are spread by personal contact and contact with infested clothing, bed and bathroom linens, and combs and brushes. Lice are more common in school-age children than in adults because of the close contact in school and the common practice of sharing possessions. Children may be more neglectful of handwashing than adults, but lice are not commonly spread by hand contact. Adults do not have an immunity to lice, nor is their skin resistant to lice. (I, T, G)

69. 2. Ringworm of the scalp is caused by a fungus of the dermatophyte group of species. (I, K, G)

70. 4. Griseofulvin (Grisactin) is an antifungal agent that acts by binding to the keratin that is deposited in the skin, hair, and nails as they grow. This keratin is then resistant to the fungus. But as the keratin is normally shed, the fungus then enters new uninfected cells unless drug therapy continues. Long-term administration does not prevent sensitivity or allergic reactions. (I, T, G)

71. 2. The adult pinworm emerges from the rectum and colon at night onto the perianal area to lay its eggs. Itching and scratching introduces the eggs to the hands, from where they can easily reinfect the child or infect others. Nightclothes and bed linens can also be sources of infection. The eggs can also be transmitted by dust in the home. Transmission through food and water supplies is possible, but rare. (I, K, G)

72. 4. Water is the usual vehicle for spreading typhoid fever. Typhus is spread through insect bites. Brucellosis (undulant fever) is spread by cow's milk. Poliomyelitis is most probably spread through respiratory secretions. (I, K, G)

73. 3. The care of a child with chicken pox focuses primarily on preventing infection in the lesions. The lesions cause severe itching, and organisms are ordinarily introduced into the lesion through scratching. (I, T, G)

74. 2. A paste of baking soda and water often helps relieve the itching associated with chicken pox. Calamine lotion can be used also. Baby powder, a moist terry-cloth towel, or a cool compress is unlikely to relieve itching. (I, T, G)

75. 3. A child with 20/60 vision sees at 20 feet what others with 20/20 vision see at 60 feet. 20/200 is considered the boundary of legal blindness. (I, K, G)

76. 1. In children with hemophilia, an inherited bleeding disorder, a bump, bruise, or cut can cause serious bleeding. After the injured area is cleansed, gentle pressure should be applied over the area to allow clot formation to help stop the bleeding. In addition, the area should be immobilized and elevated. Cold applications are often used to promote vasoconstriction and help control the bleeding. Warmth and moisture do not help promote coagulation. A tourniquet should not be used because of the high risk of tissue hypoxia and resulting necrosis. (I, T, G)

77. 1. Acetylsalicylic acid (aspirin) inhibits platelet aggregation, prolongs bleeding time, and inhibits prothrombin synthesis. It is therefore contraindicated for a child with hemophilia. Acetaminophen (Tylenol) is the recommended alternative for analgesic and antipyretic purposes. Magnesium hydroxide (Milk of Magnesia) and multiple vitamin capsules have no effect on bleeding and are not contraindicated for patients with hemophilia. (I, T, G)

78. 2. To help prepare a child to enter school, it is generally recommended that the child be taken to school to become orientated to the physical surroundings. Older siblings are likely to criticize the younger child, and staying with the child for a few days is not advised. The child may ask questions out of fear, and therefore good preparation probably cannot be accomplished through discussions. (I, T, H)

79. 1. The child entering school is moving into a new environment after having experienced security at home. Unhappiness is a normal response to the lost sense of security with resulting feelings of insecurity. Stronger-than-usual bonds between the child and other members of the family, especially parents, are characteristic of the child with school phobia. Such factors as inability to pay attention, emotional maladjustment, and poor language development suggest psychosocial disturbances and should not be playing a role among normal children who seem unhappy about entering school. (I, T, L)

80. 1. Children between age 6 and 12 years have a slower growth rate than do younger children and adolescents. As a result, their food requirements are comparatively less. (I, K, H)

81. 3. Children are most likely to be influenced by examples and the atmosphere provided by their parents, although at times they may be influenced by their peers. Coaxing and badgering a child to eat most likely will aggravate poor eating habits. (I, K, H)

82. 1. According to Erikson's theory, the central problem confronting adolescents is establishing a sense of identity. The core problem of young adulthood is concerned with intimacy. School-age children are concerned mainly with industry; preschool children, with initiative. (I, K, H)

83. 3. Girls experience the onset of adolescence approximately 1 to 2 years earlier than boys. The reason for this is not understood. (I, K, H)

84. 3. Because the risk for injury is high for children, safety issues should be discussed whenever possible. Nursing diagnoses related to coping and health maintenance are not appropriate here. (D, T, H)

85. 2. Mood swings and rudeness are not abnormal for adolescents. Parents should first discuss their feelings with their adolescent. Family counseling is not indicated as a first intervention. Restricting activities may make the situation worse. Talking to other parents of adolescents may or may not be helpful. (I, T, H)

86. 2. Acne is a disorder of the pilosebaceous follicles (hair follicles and sebaceous gland complex). During adolescence, the secretions of the sebaceous glands increase with alterations of the follicular lining so that the ducts of the sebaceous glands become occluded with accumulated sebum. Bacteria in the follicle then causes an infection. Frequent washing of affected areas with soap and water is recommended to act as a mild peeling agent and reduce secondary infection. Witch hazel is an astringent that can be used after cleansing the skin thoroughly. Lotions and creams aggravate the condition by adding more oily substances to the already oily skin. Hydrogen peroxide is a poor cleansing agent for skin with acne. (I, T, G)

87. 1. The cause of infectious mononucleosis is thought to be the Epstein-Barr virus. No precautionary measures are recommended for patients with mononucleosis. The virus is believed to be spread only by direct intimate contact. (I, T, G)

88. 2. Mononucleosis usually has an insidious onset, with fatigue and the inability to maintain usual activity levels as the most common symptoms. The lymph nodes are typically enlarged, and the spleen also may be enlarged. Fever and a sore throat often accompany mononucleosis. (I, T, G)

89. 2. Public health measures used to control STD's are most often directed toward locating the sources of infection. For a person diagnosed with a STD, an important nursing responsibility is to identify all the person's sexual contacts and urge them to get treatment. Although STD's are prevalent, mass screening is impractical. Isolating persons after they have therapy is unnecessary. Sex education has been found to be an important strategy in the control of STD's. (I, T, S)

90. 1. After receiving the rubella vaccine, the person develops a mild form of the disease, stimulating the body to develop an immunity. Administration to a pregnant woman early in pregnancy puts the fetus at risk for deformity and/or spontaneous abortion. Some authorities recommend withholding the immunization for rubella after puberty because a woman does not always know when she is pregnant, and the fetus will be placed in jeopardy. (I, K, H)

NURSING CARE OF CHILDREN

TEST 1: Health Promotion

Directions: Use this answer grid to determine areas of strength or need for further study.

Nursing Process

A = Assessment
D = Analysis, nursing diagnosis
P = Planning
I = Implementation
E = Evaluation

Cognitive Level

K = Knowledge
C = Comprehension
T = Application
N = Analysis

Client Needs

S = Safe, effective care environment
G = Physiological integrity
L = Psychosocial integrity
H = Health promotion/maintenance

		Nursing Process					Cognitive Level				Client Needs			
Question #	Answer #	A	D	P	I	E	K	C	T	N	S	G	L	H
1	3				I			C						H
2	4				I			C						H
3	1	A					K							H
4	3				I			C						H
5	4				I				T					H
6	1				I				T					H
7	4				I			C						H
8	4	A					K							H
9	2				I		K				S			
10	2				I		K							H
11	2	A								N				H
12	4				I		K							H
13	2				I				T		S			
14	3					E	K							H
15	3				I					N				H
16	3	A								N				H
17	2	A					K							H
18	2	A					K							H
19	2		D							N	S			
20	2			P					T			G		
21	4				I				T		S			
22	4			P					T					H
23	1		D					C						H

ANSWER GRID: 1

NURSING PROCESS

A = Assessment
D = Analysis, nursing diagnosis
P = Planning
I = Implementation
E = Evaluation

COGNITIVE LEVEL

K = Knowledge
C = Comprehension
T = Application
N = Analysis

CLIENT NEEDS

S = Safe, effective care environment
G = Physiological integrity
L = Psychosocial integrity
H = Health promotion/maintenance

		Nursing Process					Cognitive Level				Client Needs			
Question #	Answer #	A	D	P	I	E	K	C	T	N	S	G	L	H
24	2		D					C						H
25	2		D					C						H
26	3			P					T			G		
27	3				I			C						H
28	1				I				T					H
29	1	A							T			G		
30	2				I		K							H
31	2			P					T					H
32	2			P					T					H
33	2			P					T					H
34	4			P					T					H
35	3				I				T					H
36	3	A							T					H
37	2			P					T			G		
38	2	A							T					H
39	2		D					C						H
40	3				I				T				L	
41	3	A							T					H
42	3				I				T					H
43	3				I				T					H
44	1	A						C						H
45	4	A					K							H
46	2				I			C						H
47	2				I				T					H
48	2				I			C						H
49	3				I				T			G		
50	1				I				T					H
51	1				I				T					H
52	2			P			K							H

ANSWER GRID: 2

NURSING PROCESS

A = Assessment
D = Analysis, nursing diagnosis
P = Planning
I = Implementation
E = Evaluation

COGNITIVE LEVEL

K = Knowledge
C = Comprehension
T = Application
N = Analysis

CLIENT NEEDS

S = Safe, effective care environment
G = Physiological integrity
L = Psychosocial integrity
H = Health promotion/maintenance

		Nursing Process					Cognitive Level				Client Needs			
Question #	Answer #	A	D	P	I	E	K	C	T	N	S	G	L	H
53	3		D							N		G		
54	4				I				T					H
55	1				I				T					H
56	3			P					T					H
57	2			P			K							H
58	2				I			C						H
59	2				I			C						H
60	3				I				T					H
61	4				I				T					H
62	4				I				T					H
63	3	A					K						L	
64	4				I				T					H
65	2				I			C						H
66	3	A							T					H
67	1	A					K					G		
68	3				I				T			G		
69	2				I		K					G		
70	4				I				T			G		
71	2				I		K					G		
72	4				I		K					G		
73	3				I				T			G		
74	2				I				T			G		
75	3				I		K					G		
76	1				I				T			G		
77	1				I				T			G		
78	2				I				T					H
79	1				I				T				L	
80	1				I		K							H
81	3				I		K							H

ANSWER GRID: 3

Nursing Process

A = Assessment
D = Analysis, nursing diagnosis
P = Planning
I = Implementation
E = Evaluation

Cognitive Level

K = Knowledge
C = Comprehension
T = Application
N = Analysis

Client Needs

S = Safe, effective care environment
G = Physiological integrity
L = Psychosocial integrity
H = Health promotion/maintenance

		Nursing Process					Cognitive Level				Client Needs			
Question #	Answer #	A	D	P	I	E	K	C	T	N	S	G	L	H
82	1				I		K							H
83	3				I		K							H
84	3		D						T					H
85	2				I				T					H
86	2				I				T			G		
87	1				I				T			G		
88	2				I				T			G		
89	2				I				T		S			
90	1				I		K							H
Number Correct														
Number Possible	90	15	7	11	56	1	23	15	47	5	5	20	3	62
Percentage Correct														

Score Calculation:

To determine your **Percentage Correct**, divide the **Number Correct** by the **Number Possible**.

The Child With Respiratory Health Problems

Test 2

The Client With Tonsillitis
The Client With Chronic Otitis Media
The Client With Foreign Body Aspiration
The Client With Asthma
The Client With Cystic Fibrosis and Bronchopneumonia
The Client With Sudden Infant Death Syndrome
The Client Requiring Cardiopulmonary Resuscitation
Correct Answers and Rationale

Select the one best answer and indicate your choice by filling in the circle in front of the option.

The Client With Tonsillitis

A 4-year-old child is admitted to the pediatric unit for a tonsillectomy and adenoidectomy. The parents plan to stay as much as possible. The child's growth and development are normal.

1. The child asks the nurse if it will hurt to have the tonsils and adenoids out. Which of the following responses would be *best* for the nurse to make?
- ○ 1. "It won't hurt because you'll be asleep."
- ○ 2. "It won't hurt because you're so big."
- ○ 3. "It will hurt because of the incisions made in the throat."
- ○ 4. "It will hurt, but we have medicine to help you feel better."

2. Preoperatively, the nurse discusses with the child and parents the plan of care that will be implemented when the child returns from the recovery room. Which of the following interventions should the nurse emphasize? The child
- ○ 1. should cough frequently.
- ○ 2. can have aspirin for pain, as needed.
- ○ 3. should restrict talking.
- ○ 4. can have sips of clear liquids when awake.

3. Which of the following would the nurse identify as a priority nursing diagnosis preoperatively?
- ○ 1. Anxiety.
- ○ 2. Altered Parenting.
- ○ 3. Anticipatory Grieving.
- ○ 4. Altered Nutrition.

4. Which of the following would the nurse write on the child's care plan as an expected outcome related to the nursing diagnosis of Knowledge Deficit due to impending surgery? The child
- ○ 1. is able to tell about the surgery and recovery.
- ○ 2. plays surgery with dolls.
- ○ 3. appears anxious for the surgery to be over.
- ○ 4. draws a picture of the operating room.

5. The nurse explains to the parents that after surgery and a brief stay in the recovery room, their child will return to the room and be positioned to prevent aspiration. The nurse will place the child in which of the following positions:
- ○ 1. Supine or Trendelenburg.
- ○ 2. Side-lying or supine.
- ○ 3. Side-lying or prone.
- ○ 4. Prone or Trendelenburg.

6. After the child finally awakens, the mother asks the nurse for something for her child to eat or drink. Which of the following would be best for the child *initially?*
- ○ 1. A yellow popsicle.
- ○ 2. Vanilla ice cream.
- ○ 3. Red Kool-aid.

○ 4. Chocolate pudding.

7. The nurse monitors the child frequently for signs and symptoms of hemorrhage. Which of the following would be an *early* indication of hemorrhage?

○ 1. Drooling of bright-red secretions.
○ 2. A pulse rate of 95 beats per minute.
○ 3. Vomiting of 25 ml of dark-brown emesis.
○ 4. Infrequent swallowing.

8. The nurse concludes that the parents understand the discharge instructions when they state that medical attention should be sought for which of the following occurrences?

○ 1. Low-grade fever.
○ 2. Signs of bleeding.
○ 3. Slight ear pain.
○ 4. Objectionable mouth odor.

9. The nurse judges that the parents understand what to feed their child the day after discharge when the mother says

○ 1. steak and corn on the cob.
○ 2. pork chop and noodles.
○ 3. soup and ice cream.
○ 4. hot dog and potato chips.

10. The nurse teaches the parents that the most likely time for hemorrhage to occur is within

○ 1. 2 to 3 days after surgery.
○ 2. 4 to 5 days after surgery.
○ 3. 6 to 7 days after surgery.
○ 4. 9 to 10 days after surgery.

The Client With Chronic Otitis Media

A 15-month-old child is admitted to the pediatric day surgery unit for a bilateral tympanostomy tube insertion. In the past 7 months, the child has had multiple ear infections that have not responded to antibiotic therapy.

11. The nurse judges that the mother understands why children are prone to develop otitis media when she states that the key anatomic difference between adults and children is the

○ 1. nasopharynx.
○ 2. eustachian tubes.
○ 3. external ear canals.
○ 4. tympanic membranes.

12. The nurse would assess whether the parents took which of the following measures to help prevent recurrent otitis media?

○ 1. Cleanse the child's ears thoroughly and often.
○ 2. Administer continuous small-dose antibiotic therapy.
○ 3. Instill ear drops regularly to prevent accumulation of cerumen.
○ 4. Hold the child upright for bottle feedings.

13. The nurse would instruct the parents to report which of the following characteristic signs and symptoms of acute otitis media?

○ 1. Rhinorrhea, fever, and bulging tympanic membranes.
○ 2. Cough, irritability, and inverted tympanic membrane.
○ 3. Pulling at the ears, earache, and gray tympanic membrane.
○ 4. Vomiting, diarrhea, and yellow tympanic membrane.

14. The child has been treated with amoxicillin several times for ear infections. Which of the following side effects of this medication would the nurse have taught the mother to expect?

○ 1. Rash.
○ 2. Bloody diarrhea.
○ 3. Urate crystals.
○ 4. Fever.

15. The nurse instructs the parents to bring their child to the office for a recheck after the child completes a course of antibiotic therapy. The purpose of the recheck is to

○ 1. determine if the ear infection has affected the child's hearing.
○ 2. make certain all the antibiotic has been taken.
○ 3. verify that the infection has completely cleared.
○ 4. obtain a prescription for another course of antibiotics.

16. When approaching this toddler for the first time, the nurse should

○ 1. talk to the mother first so the toddler can get used to the new person.
○ 2. hold the toddler so the toddler becomes more comfortable.
○ 3. walk over to and pick the toddler up right away so the mother can relax.
○ 4. pick up the toddler and take the child to the play area so the mother can rest.

17. Tympanostomy tubes are inserted while the child is under general anesthesia. The nurse should teach the parents that the purpose of the tubes is to

○ 1. distribute antibiotic solution into the middle ear.
○ 2. shrink the mucosal lining of the middle ear.
○ 3. increase pressure in the middle ear.
○ 4. allow ventilation of the middle ear.

18. A goal of postoperative nursing care is to facilitate drainage from the right ear. Which of the following interventions would be most likely to accomplish this goal?

○ 1. Apply external heat to the right ear.
○ 2. Have the child lie on the right side.
○ 3. Apply a gauze pressure dressing to the right ear.
○ 4. Apply cold compresses to the left ear.

19. Two interventions included in the child's postoperative nursing care plan are to apply external heat or cool compresses and to offer liquid or soft foods to keep the child from chewing. Which of the following nursing diagnoses do these interventions address?
- ○ 1. Hyperthermia related to infectious process.
- ○ 2. Potential for Impaired Skin Integrity related to ear drainage.
- ○ 3. Pain related to the inflammatory process.
- ○ 4. Knowledge Deficit related to unfamiliarity with the situation.

20. Before the client's discharge from the day surgery center, the parents ask, "What will happen to the tubes in my child's ears?" The nurse should explain that the tubes will
- ○ 1. dissolve in approximately 6 months.
- ○ 2. probably fall out in about 6 months.
- ○ 3. remain permanently in place.
- ○ 4. be removed in approximately 6 months.

21. The nurse also should teach the parents which of the following before their child is discharged?
- ○ 1. If the child's head will be getting wet, place plugs in the ear canals beforehand.
- ○ 2. Have the child use a nose plug when swimming.
- ○ 3. Administer an antibiotic while the tubes are in place.
- ○ 4. The child will not have another ear infection while the tubes are in place.

22. Ear drops are ordered for the child at home. The nurse teaches the child's parents to instill them. Which of the following statements indicate that the child's father has understood the teaching? "I'll gently pull the ear lobe
- ○ 1. up and forward."
- ○ 2. up and backward."
- ○ 3. down and forward."
- ○ 4. down and backward."

23. Which of the following techniques is best for the nurse to use in evaluating the parents' ability to administer ear drops correctly?
- ○ 1. Observe the parents instilling the drops in the child's ear.
- ○ 2. Listen to the parents as they describe the procedure.
- ○ 3. Ask the parents to list the steps in the procedure.
- ○ 4. Have each parent critique the other's performance of the procedure.

The Client With Foreign Body Aspiration

A 2-year-old child is brought to the emergency department with coughing, shortness of breath, and fever. The parents tell the nurse that the child choked on a peanut about a week ago. They thought that he had coughed it out and had forgotten about the incident until he began to cough and became short of breath. The mother asks the nurse if her child's shortness of breath and fever could be related to aspiration of the peanut.

24. The nurse would choose which one of the following as the priority nursing diagnosis?
- ○ 1. Ineffective Breathing Pattern.
- ○ 2. High Risk for Injury.
- ○ 3. Altered Nutrition.
- ○ 4. Altered Health Maintenance.

25. The mother tells the nurse that her pediatrician said that peanuts are "one of the worst things a child can aspirate" and asks why this is so. The nurse should explain that this is because peanuts
- ○ 1. swell when wet.
- ○ 2. contain a fixed oil.
- ○ 3. decompose when wet.
- ○ 4. contain calcium.

26. The nurse plans to discuss with the parents other foods that are easily aspirated. Which of the following foods are most likely to be aspirated?
- ○ 1. Popcorn and bread.
- ○ 2. Raw vegetables and noodles.
- ○ 3. Round candy and hot dogs.
- ○ 4. Hot dogs and suckers.

27. A goal for a client after bronchoscopy treatment is to stay quiet. Which of the following nursing interventions would help accomplish this goal in this client?
- ○ 1. Have the parents stay at the bedside.
- ○ 2. Allow the child to go to the playroom.
- ○ 3. Have the child play with another child in the room.
- ○ 4. Turn the television set on to cartoons.

28. The child begins to fuss and cry when the parents attempt to leave the hospital for an hour. As the nurse tries to take the child out of the crib, the child pushes the nurse away. The nurse explains to the parents that their child is experiencing what stage of separation anxiety?
- ○ 1. Protest.
- ○ 2. Despair.
- ○ 3. Denial.
- ○ 4. Detachment.

29. To help the client's parents best manage the separation anxiety, the nurse would suggest that they
- ○ 1. Leave while the child is sleeping.
- ○ 2. Bring the child's favorite toys from home.
- ○ 3. Tell the child that they are leaving and explain what time they will return.
- ○ 4. Shorten their visits.

30. After bronchoscopy, which of the following parameters would be most important for the nurse to assess when the child returns to the room?

- ○ 1. Cardiac rate and rhythm.
- ○ 2. Respiratory rate and quality.
- ○ 3. Sputum quantity and color.
- ○ 4. Pulse pressure and deficit.

31. Before the child is discharged, the nurse teaches the parents the three signs that indicate a child is truly choking and needs immediate life-saving interventions. The nurse knows that the parents understand the teaching when they state that a child is choking when he cannot speak, turns

- ○ 1. blue, and vomits.
- ○ 2. red, and gasps.
- ○ 3. blue, and gags.
- ○ 4. blue, and collapses.

32. The mother asks the nurse how long until brain death occurs after a child's airway is completely obstructed. The nurse's correct response is

- ○ 1. 1 to 3 minutes.
- ○ 2. 4 to 6 minutes.
- ○ 3. 7 to 10 minutes.
- ○ 4. More than 10 minutes.

The Client With Asthma

A 6-year-old with bronchial asthma is brought to the hospital's emergency room by the mother. The child is experiencing an acute asthma attack.

33. On initial assessment, the nurse would be most concerned about the child's

- ○ 1. shortness of breath.
- ○ 2. loose cough.
- ○ 3. absence of wheezing.
- ○ 4. expiratory wheezing.

34. The nurse would teach the mother to expect which of the following signs and symptoms to alert her to her child's asthma attack?

- ○ 1. Thin, copious mucus secretions.
- ○ 2. Tight productive cough.
- ○ 3. Whistling sound on expiration.
- ○ 4. Fever of 99.4°F.

35. Which of the following manifestations would the nurse identify as most closely related to the child's probable acid-base imbalance?

- ○ 1. Greatly diminished breath sounds.
- ○ 2. A tingling sensation in the fingertips.
- ○ 3. Heart rate of 68 beats per minute.
- ○ 4. No urination for several hours.

36. The standard dosage of epinephrine (Adrenalin) 1:1,000 to treat asthma is 0.01 ml per kilogram of body weight. The child weighs 45 pounds. Which amount of epinephrine should the nurse administer?

- ○ 1. 0.15 ml.
- ○ 2. 0.02 ml.
- ○ 3. 0.30 ml.
- ○ 4. 0.45 ml.

37. Fifteen minutes after administering a dose of epinephrine (Adrenalin), the nurse would assess the child for evidence that the medication has produced the desired therapeutic effect. Indications that the child is responding to the epinephrine include

- ○ 1. decreased wheezing.
- ○ 2. tachycardia.
- ○ 3. a rise of 0.2°F in temperature.
- ○ 4. paroxysmal wheezing.

38. The nurse would be justified in judging that the client is experiencing a typical side effect of epinephrine (Adrenalin) after observing that the child

- ○ 1. is having tremors.
- ○ 2. feels sleepy.
- ○ 3. is developing a skin rash.
- ○ 4. is experiencing nasal congestion.

39. After the child fails to respond to the epinephrine (Adrenalin), aminophylline (Aminophyllin) is administered intravenously. During the infusion, the nurse should plan to monitor the child for

- ○ 1. hematuria.
- ○ 2. chills.
- ○ 3. circumoral erythema.
- ○ 4. hypotension.

40. The child is receiving both intravenous aminophyllin (Aminophyllin) and hydrocortisone (Solu-medrol). One day, the child vomits breakfast and lunch and is very irritable. Assessment reveals a heart rate of 116 beats per minute but other vital signs within normal ranges. The nurse determines that the child is probably experiencing

- ○ 1. a viral gastroenteritis infection.
- ○ 2. theophylline toxicity.
- ○ 3. a reaction to the hydrocortisone.
- ○ 4. a stress reaction.

41. The nurse explains to the mother that asthma attacks may be triggered by various mechanisms, including certain food allergies, and states that which of the following foods would most likely be responsible for such an allergic reaction?

- ○ 1. Whitefish.
- ○ 2. Tossed salad.
- ○ 3. Hamburger patty.
- ○ 4. Hot-fudge sundae.

42. The mother expresses concern that the child's 6-month-old sibling may also have food allergies. When discussing feeding techniques for the infant, the nurse should suggest that the mother

- ○ 1. avoid giving the infant commercially prepared infant food.
- ○ 2. limit the infant's juice intake to apple juice.
- ○ 3. introduce new foods to the infant one at a time.

○ 4. discontinue formula feedings when the infant begins to eat baby food.

43. The mother asks the nurse what measures she can take to help prevent her child's asthma attacks. Which of the following suggestions by the nurse would be most appropriate?
○ 1. Cover the child's mattress with a sheepskin pad.
○ 2. Use an aerosol spray disinfectant in the child's bedroom.
○ 3. Dust and vacuum the entire house frequently.
○ 4. Have the child sleep with the window open.

44. The nurse would also assess this child for allergic rhinitis, inspecting the child for which of the following to support this diagnosis?
○ 1. Nasal crease and allergic shiners.
○ 2. Abdominal pain and diarrhea.
○ 3. Cough and fever.
○ 4. Rhinorrhea and constipation.

45. The child is about to be discharged from the hospital. During discharge teaching, the nurse would instruct the mother to protect the child from
○ 1. extreme environmental temperatures.
○ 2. chest mobility exercises.
○ 3. other children in the neighborhood.
○ 4. synthetic material in clothing.

46. The mother tells the nurse that the child wants a pet. Which of the following pets should the nurse tell the mother is most appropriate?
○ 1. Cat.
○ 2. Fish.
○ 3. Gerbil.
○ 4. Canary.

47. The nurse discusses the use of cromolyn sodium (Aarane) with the mother. The nurse should teach the mother that the medication will be ineffective if it is administered when the child is
○ 1. about to eat a meal.
○ 2. having an asthmatic attack.
○ 3. being readied for bed.
○ 4. about to engage in strenuous exercise.

48. Which of the following statements best reflects the family's positive adjustment to the child's disorder?
○ 1. "Our child gets what he asks for or else has an asthma attack."
○ 2. "We keep our child away from other children so he's not exposed to cold germs."
○ 3. "Although our child's disease is serious, we try not to let it be the focus of our family."
○ 4. "I'm afraid when my child gets older, I won't be able to supervise what he does."

49. The mother states that the child wants to participate in sports and asks the nurse to suggest appropriate activities. The nurse should teach the mother that
○ 1. physical activities are inappropriate for asthmatic children.
○ 2. asthmatic children should be excluded from team sports.
○ 3. vigorous physical exercise frequently precipitates an asthmatic episode.
○ 4. most asthmatic children can participate in sports if the asthma is controlled.

The Client With Cystic Fibrosis and Bronchopneumonia

A 3-year-old child is admitted to the hospital with bronchopneumonia. This child also has cystic fibrosis.

50. The nurse would assess for which of the following signs and symptoms to help provide pertinent diagnostic data?
○ 1. Weight loss and vomiting.
○ 2. Cough and fever.
○ 3. Constipation and rash.
○ 4. Dysuria and rash.

51. The child is to receive an antibiotic three times in every 24-hour period. Of the following schedules for administering the medication which would be best?
○ 1. Noon, 4 P.M., and 8 P.M.
○ 2. 9 A.M., 2 P.M., and 7 P.M.
○ 3. 10 A.M., 4 P.M., and 10 P.M.
○ 4. 8 A.M., 4 P.M., and midnight.

52. The child is to have postural drainage. The nurse should plan to carry out postural drainage shortly
○ 1. after meals.
○ 2. before meals.
○ 3. after rest periods.
○ 4. before rest periods.

53. The nurse determines that the child's mother understands about the pancreatic enzymes her child receives when she says they
○ 1. should be taken 1 hour before meals.
○ 2. are to help with digestion.
○ 3. are only needed when the child is sick.
○ 4. should be taken 30 minutes after meals.

54. The nurse assesses the type of diet that the child was on before admission. This child should be on a
○ 1. high-fat, moderate-carbohydrate diet.
○ 2. low-fat, high-protein diet.
○ 3. low-protein, low-carbohydrate diet.
○ 4. high-carbohydrate, high-fat diet.

55. In talking to the mother, the nurse would ask the type of stools her child had before the diagnosis of cystic fibrosis was made. The mother most likely would answer
○ 1. hard and almost odorless.
○ 2. bulky and foul-smelling.
○ 3. watery, with an ammonia odor.
○ 4. dry and almost odorless.

56. The nurse plans recreational therapy for the child. Which of the following toys would provide the child with the most support while hospitalized?
- ○ 1. A jigsaw puzzle.
- ○ 2. The child's favorite toy.
- ○ 3. A fuzzy stuffed animal.
- ○ 4. Scissors, paper, and paste.

57. Because of their child's health, the parents do not look forward to the approaching summer weather. They state that the hot weather is hazardous for their child because a child with cystic fibrosis has
- ○ 1. no sweat glands.
- ○ 2. little skin pigment to prevent sunburn.
- ○ 3. a poorly functioning temperature control center.
- ○ 4. abnormally high salt loss through perspiration.

58. The nurse judges that the parents understand the nature of cystic fibrosis when they state that the disease is characterized by
- ○ 1. an abnormality in the body's mucus-secreting glands.
- ○ 2. the formation of fibrous cysts in various body organs.
- ○ 3. the failure of the pancreatic ducts to develop properly.
- ○ 4. an abnormal interaction between the body's antigens and antibodies.

59. Which of the following should the nurse write on the child's care plan as an expected client outcome related to the nursing diagnosis of Ineffective Breathing Pattern due to an infection? The client will
- ○ 1. exhibit no manifestations of respiratory distress.
- ○ 2. have no symptoms of fever such as chills.
- ○ 3. be able to engage in normal activities for age.
- ○ 4. be able to tolerate food without vomiting.

60. The parents ask the nurse what activities their child can become involved in as he becomes older? The nurse should advise such activities as
- ○ 1. swimming and bowling.
- ○ 2. football and track.
- ○ 3. music and soccer.
- ○ 4. basketball and golf.

61. The parents express concerns about how the disease was transmitted to their child. The nurse would explain that
- ○ 1. a disease carrier also has the disease.
- ○ 2. two persons who are carriers may produce a child who has the disease.
- ○ 3. a person who has the disease and an unaffected person will never have children with the disease.
- ○ 4. a disease carrier and an unaffected person will have a child with the disease.

62. The nurse refers the parents to the local chapter of the National Cystic Fibrosis Foundation. The Foundation has been especially helpful for parents of children with cystic fibrosis by helping them
- ○ 1. find tutors to educate their children at home.
- ○ 2. obtain genetic counseling.
- ○ 3. meet with other parents of children with cystic fibrosis for mutual support.
- ○ 4. obtain financial assistance to purchase medications for their children.

63. The nurse judges that the mother knows how to properly administer intravenous antibiotics at home after observing that the mother
- ○ 1. allows the antibiotic to run into the child's vein in 10 minutes.
- ○ 2. flushes the venous access port with heparin 20 minutes after the antibiotic is administered.
- ○ 3. administers the antibiotic 2 hours late because she was shopping.
- ○ 4. calls the nurse because the antibiotic will not infuse.

The Client With Sudden Infant Death Syndrome

A 3-month-old infant is brought into the emergency room by the parents. The infant is not breathing, and a tentative diagnosis of sudden infant death syndrome (SIDS) is made.

64. What would be the best action for the nurse to take in regard to the parents?
- ○ 1. Offer to telephone their pastor.
- ○ 2. Tell them that the doctor will talk with them soon.
- ○ 3. Ask another client to sit with them.
- ○ 4. Accompany them to a private area and stay with them.

65. The emergency room nurse obtains a brief history of events occurring before and after the parents found their infant. Which of the following questions would be most appropriate for the nurse to ask the parents?
- ○ 1. "Was the infant wrapped in a blanket?"
- ○ 2. "Was the infant's sibling jealous?"
- ○ 3. "At what time did you find the infant?"
- ○ 4. "When had you last checked the infant?"

66. The parents have been told that the infant has died. Which of the following interventions should the nurse include in the plan of care to assist the parents with their grieving process?
- ○ 1. Reassure them that the infant's death was not their fault.
- ○ 2. Provide an opportunity for them to see the infant.
- ○ 3. Ask them if they would like to call their pastor.
- ○ 4. Give them a package containing the infant's clothing.

67. Before the parents leave the hospital, the nurse evaluates their understanding of the cause of their infant's death. The parents should know that the etiology of SIDS is

○ 1. unknown.
○ 2. apnea.
○ 3. infection.
○ 4. cardiac dysrhythmias.

68. Which of the following should the nurse write on the parents' care plan as an expected client outcome related to the nursing diagnosis of Anticipatory Grieving related to their child's death? The parents will
○ 1. stay by themselves until 3 months after the baby's death.
○ 2. be able to discuss their feelings with each other.
○ 3. work long hours to pay for the funeral expenses.
○ 4. act as if nothing has happened.

69. Given the crisis associated with the loss of a child from SIDS, the nurse arranges for a community health nurse to visit the parents at home. When should the nurse visit the parents?
○ 1. A few days after the funeral.
○ 2. Two weeks after the funeral.
○ 3. As soon as the parents are ready to talk.
○ 4. As soon after the infant's death as possible.

70. The community health nurse develops nursing goals for the visits with the parents. The primary goal for the second visit would be to help them
○ 1. express their feelings.
○ 2. gain an understanding of the disease.
○ 3. assess the impact of the infant's death on their other children.
○ 4. deal with issues such as having other children.

The Client Requiring Cardiopulmonary Resuscitation

The nurse prepares to discharge a 5-year-old child from the 1-day surgery unit. The nurse leaves the room to get supplies, then, upon returning, finds that the child is not breathing.

71. Which of the following priority nursing measures should the nurse initiate first?
○ 1. Clear the airway.
○ 2. Begin mouth-to-mouth resuscitation.
○ 3. Initiate oxygen therapy.
○ 4. Start chest compressions.

72. Continuing cardiopulmonary resuscitation (CPR), the nurse palpates for a pulse. Which of the following sites is best for checking the pulse during CPR in a 5-year-old child?
○ 1. Femoral.
○ 2. Carotid.
○ 3. Radial.
○ 4. Brachial.

73. Which of the following rescue breathing rates should the nurse administer during CPR for a 5-year-old?
○ 1. 10 breaths/minute.
○ 2. 12 breaths/minute.
○ 3. 15 breaths/minute.
○ 4. 30 breaths/minute.

74. The client is pulseless, and the nurse begins chest compressions. Because effective chest compressions depend on proper technique, the nurse should apply pressure
○ 1. on the lower sternum with the heel of one hand.
○ 2. midway on the sternum with the tips of two fingers.
○ 3. over the apex of the heart with the heel of one hand.
○ 4. on the upper sternum with the heels of both hands.

75. The nurse would plan to administer which of the following rates of external chest compression to a 5-year-old child?
○ 1. 50 to 70 compressions/minute.
○ 2. 60 to 80 compressions/minute.
○ 3. 70 to 80 compressions/minute.
○ 4. 80 to 100 compressions/minute.

76. When providing chest compressions, the nurse should compress the child's chest to a depth of
○ 1. 1" to 1.5".
○ 2. 1.5" to 2".
○ 3. 2" to 2.5".
○ 4. 2.5" to 3".

77. The nurse would know that CPR was effective when the child's
○ 1. skin begins to mottle.
○ 2. pupils dilatate.
○ 3. peripheral pulses are palpable.
○ 4. skin is cool and dry.

78. A 10-month-old infant is choking; the nurse attempts to clear the airway. What should the nurse do next after opening the infant's mouth?
○ 1. Use blind finger sweeps.
○ 2. Deliver four back blows.
○ 3. Apply four subdiaphragmatic abdominal thrusts.
○ 4. Attempt to visualize the object.

79. In which of the following positions should the nurse place an infant to deliver back blows?
○ 1. Face up, with the head lower than the trunk.
○ 2. Face down, with the head lower than the trunk.
○ 3. Face to one side, with the head lower than the trunk.
○ 4. Face up, with the head supported above the trunk.

80. What is the appropriate technique for delivering back blows to an infant?
○ 1. Slowly, with the palm of the hand.
○ 2. Slowly, with the heel of the hand.
○ 3. Rapidly, with the palm of the hand.

○ 4. Rapidly, with the heel of the hand.

81. Suddenly the infant begins to cry. What would be the nurse's most appropriate action?

○ 1. Deliver four chest thrusts.
○ 2. Deliver four back blows.
○ 3. Finger-sweep the mouth.
○ 4. Observe the infant closely.

82. When performing mouth-to-mouth breathing for the infant, the nurse should tilt the infant's head back slightly to

○ 1. prevent airway obstruction.
○ 2. minimize gastric distention.
○ 3. prevent excessive pressure on the neck.
○ 4. inhibit extensor posturing.

CORRECT ANSWERS AND RATIONALE

The letters in parentheses following the rationale identify the step of the nursing process (A, D, P, I, E); cognitive level (K, C, T, N); and client need (S, G, L, H). See the Answer Grid for the key.

The Client With Tonsillitis

1. 4. Preschool-age children are fearful of physical injury. Truthful but simple explanations will minimize distorted fears and reduce anxiety. A detailed explanation may be beyond the child's understanding and add to these fears. (I, T, G)

2. 4. Once the child is alert, he may have sips of clear liquids. Eating enhances the blood supply to the throat, which promotes rapid healing. Coughing is discouraged because it promotes bleeding. Aspirin is contraindicated because it causes bleeding. Talking is not restricted. (I, T, G)

3. 1. A 4-year-old child is very aware of what is happening and may ask many questions. The child would naturally be curious about the impending surgery. The parents would be anxious about how the child will tolerate the surgery and concerned about any complications that may occur. (D, N, G)

4. 1. A 4-year-old child should be able to talk about the surgery and explain what will occur. This would be an expected outcome. Playing with dolls and drawing pictures are interventions to use in teaching the child about the surgery. (I, T, L)

5. 3. Placing the child in a prone or a side-lying position facilitates drainage of secretions and helps prevent aspiration. Trendelenburg position is contraindicated because it decreases effective lung volumes. The supine position is contraindicated due to the risk of aspiration. (I, T, G)

6. 1. The nurse must consider both the color and consistency of foods and fluids given initially. Red or brown-colored foods and fluids should be avoided so that if vomiting occurs, fresh or old blood can be distinguished from the ingested liquids. Ice cream and pudding are not offered until the child can retain clear liquids. (I, T, G)

7. 1. Drooling of bright-red blood indicates hemorrhage. Children tend to avoid swallowing after surgery because of discomfort. Therefore, they drool. It is not unusual for the secretions to be slightly blood-tinged due to the small amount of oozing after surgery. A pulse rate of 95 beats per minute is within the normal range for a 4-year-old child. A small amount of dark-brown blood is often present in postoperative emesis because of the surgical procedure. (I, T, G)

8. 2. The doctor should be notified of any sign of bleeding. It is expected that the child will have a low-grade fever, objectionable mouth odor, and slight ear pain following this surgical procedure. (E, N, G)

9. 3. Liquids and soft foods are better tolerated by the child during the first few days after surgery while the throat is sore. Children do not chew their food thoroughly and solid foods are therefore difficult to swallow. (E, N, G)

10. 3. Hemorrhage might occur about a week after surgery as the tissue where the tonsils were starts to loosen. (I, T, G)

The Client With Chronic Otitis Media

11. 2. In infants and young children, the eustachian tubes are short and lie in a relatively horizontal position. This anatomic position favors the development of otitis media because it is easy for materials from the nasopharynx to enter the tubes. Bacteria may be present in the nasopharynx, but this does not affect middle ear function. An intact tympanic membrane prevents bacteria from entering the middle ear from the external ear canal. The tympanic membrane changes appearance with an ear infection, but its structure does not predispose infants and young children to ear infection. (I, T, G)

12. 4. Sitting or holding a child upright for formula feedings helps prevent pooling of formula in the pharyngeal growth. When the vacuum in the middle ear opens into the pharyngeal cavity, formula (along with bacteria) is drawn into the middle ear. Cleansing the ears will not reduce the incidence of otitis media because the pathogenic bacteria are in the nasopharynx. Continuous low-dose antibiotic therapy is used only in cases of recurrent otitis media. (I, T, G)

13. 1. A bulging, bright-red tympanic membrane (because of increased middle ear pressure) usually indicates otitis media. Other characteristic findings are rhinorrhea, fever, cough, irritability, pulling at the ears, earache, vomiting, and diarrhea. A reddened, nonbulging tympanic membrane may indicate otitis media if the membrane has ruptured. A gray or yellow tympanic membrane may indicate infection, but the most characteristic sign of otitis media is a red and bulging tympanic membrane. (I, T, G)

14. 1. Rash is a common side effect of amoxicillin. Urate crystals can develop during amoxicillin therapy if not enough water is consumed. Bloody diarrhea is not a side effect. A fever may occur but it would be caused by perhaps a viral infection, not as a side effect of amoxicillin. (I, T, H)

15. 3. Because ear infections are sometimes difficult to treat, it is important to determine whether the antibiotic has resolved the infection. If the client is not rechecked, it will be difficult to determine if another infection is a continuation of a previous infection or a separate infection. Studies may be done to determine if an infection has impaired the child's hearing, but they are not done after each course of antibiotics. A visit to the physician's office cannot validate that all the medication was taken. If the infection is resolved with one course of antibiotics, another course will not be prescribed. (I, T, G)

16. 1. Toddlers should be approached slowly. They are wary of strangers and need time to get used to someone they do not know. The best approach is to ignore them initially, but focus on talking to the parents. (I, T, L)

17. 4. Tympanostomy tubes allow ventilation of the middle ear and facilitate drainage of fluid by maintaining the patency of the eustachian tube. The pressure-equalizing tubes do not distribute medication into the ear. Decongestants may be used to shrink mucous membranes and improve eustachian tube function. (I, T, G)

18. 2. Positioning the child on the affected side will promote drainage from the middle ear via gravity. Application of heat may facilitate drainage of exudate from the ear, but only if the child is lying on the affected side. Application of an ice bag may help reduce pressure and edema. A gauze dressing is not applied after surgery, although a loose wick may be inserted in the external ear canal to absorb drainage. (I, T, G)

19. 3. Application of external heat or cool compresses and the avoidance of chewing address the management of pain or discomfort. Approaches for the nursing diagnosis Potential for Impaired Skin Integrity include keeping the skin around the ear clean and dry, cleansing with hydrogen peroxide, and protecting the skin with a protective coating. Interventions for the diagnosis of Hyperthermia include removing bedclothes and extra clothing, reducing environmental temperature, and encouraging fluids. Interventions for Knowledge Deficit include educating parents about follow-up care, the need to avoid activities that allow water to enter the ears, and preventive practices. (I, T, G)

20. 2. The tympanostomy tubes remain in place for approximately 6 months. The tiny tubes are made of a polyurethane material that does not change in structure or composition while in the ear. The tubes are spontaneously ejected from the ear. Parents should be told about the tubes' appearance so they can observe them if they fall out. (I, T, G)

21. 1. Placing ear plugs in the ears will prevent water from entering the middle ear through the tympanoplasty tube. (I, T, S)

22. 4. For children age 3 years and younger, the external auditory canal is straightened by gently pulling the ear lobe down and backward. For the older child and adult, the ear lobe is gently pulled up and backward. (I, T, G)

23. 1. Return demonstrations are the best way to evaluate a person's ability to perform a skill. This technique enables the teacher to observe not only the learner's sequencing of steps of the procedure, but also the learner's ability to perform the skill. (I, T, G)

The Client With Foreign Body Aspiration

24. 1. For a child who has shortness of breath, cough, and fever, the priority nursing diagnosis would be Ineffective Breathing Pattern, which requires immediate intervention. This diagnosis would be the basis for planning and implementing nursing care. (D, N, G)

25. 1. Peanuts swell and become soft when moistened with bronchial secretions, making them difficult to remove. Because peanuts contain a fixed oil, they can cause lipoid pneumonia, but this is not why they are so dangerous when aspirated. Peanuts do begin to decompose when wet and they do contain calcium, but neither of these factors makes them particularly dangerous when aspirated. (I, T, G)

26. 3. Spherical or cylindrical objects are more likely to be aspirated and plug the airway than other-shaped objects. The size, shape, and consistency of foods are important factors in their ability to cause obstruction. (I, T, G)

27. 1. A 2-year-old child is difficult to keep quiet. The parents have a better chance of doing this because they know their child well. Encouraging the parents to stay with the child will help keep the child quiet. A 2-year-old's attention span is short, so watching television would keep the child quiet for only a short time. A 2-year-old does engage in parallel play but does not know how to play with others. Going to the playroom may encourage the child to be quite active. (P, T, H)

28. 1. Young children have specific reactions to separation and hospitalization. In the protest stage, the toddler physically and verbally attacks anyone who attempts to provide care. In the despair stage, the toddler becomes withdrawn and obviously depressed. Denial or detachment occurs if the toddler's stay in the hospital without the parent is prolonged, as the toddler "settles in" to the hospital life and denies the parents' existence. (I, T, G)

29. 2. Bringing a child's favorite toys, security blanket, or familiar objects from home can make the transition from home to hospital less stressful. Leaving without explaining may decrease the child's trust in the parents. The parents should tell their toddler when they are leaving and when they will return, not by time but in relation to the child's usual activities (e.g., by bedtime); 2-year-olds have a very limited sense of time. Short parental visits do not satisfy a toddler's overwhelming need for comfort. (I, T, G)

30. 2. After bronchoscopy, the child should be observed for signs and symptoms of respiratory distress. Laryngeal edema may occur and cause airway obstruction. Signs and symptoms of respiratory distress include tachypnea, increased stridor and retractions, and tachycardia. The sputum may be bloody after bronchoscopy. A change in pulse pressure is not associated with bronchoscopy, but rather with intracranial pressure and shock. Pulse deficit is associated with some dysrhythmias. Assessing cardiac rate and rhythm is important but not the most important assessment step. (I, T, G)

31. 4. The three signs indicating that a child is truly choking and requires immediate life-saving interventions are: inability to speak, blue color (cyanotic), and collapse. (I, T, G)

32. 2. Brain death will begin within 4 to 6 minutes if oxygen is not restored. Complete obstruction of the upper airway results in anoxia to vital organ systems. (I, T, G)

The Client With Asthma

33. 3. Knowing that this child is having an asthma attack, the nurse would expect to hear wheezing and note some shortness of breath. During an asthma attack, the cough usually is dry and sounds tight. The absence of wheezing would indicate that the child is not moving air well through the lungs and would be of great concern to the nurse. (A, C, G)

34. 3. The wheezing sound heard during an asthma attack sounds like a whistle. During an asthma attack, secretions are thick and not usually expelled until the bronchioles are more relaxed. The cough will be tight but nonproductive. A temperature of 99.4°F is low grade in a 6-year-old and not cause for immediate concern. (I, T, G)

35. 2. In respiratory alkalosis, the alkalinity of the body fluids results in a decrease in the ionization of calcium. Low levels of circulating ionized calcium increase the excitability of nerve and muscle tissue. This is manifested by paresthesia (numbness and tingling) of the digits, upper lip, and ear lobes. In mild asthma with respiratory alkalosis, breath sounds are typically loud with expiratory wheezing. The pulse rate is elevated, and urine production is increased because of the increased renal circulation. (I, T, G)

36. 2. Forty-five pounds equals about 20 kilograms (2.2 pounds/kg). 20 kg × 0.01 ml/kg = .02 ml of epinephrine. (I, T, G)

37. 1. Epinephrine relaxes bronchial muscles and reduces congestion and edema in the pulmonary system, resulting in decreased wheezing. Tachycardia is a common side effect of epinephrine. Minor temperature alterations and sneezing are unrelated to the desired improvement in pulmonary status. (I, T, G)

38. 1. Common side effects of epinephrine include tremors or trembling, anxiety or nervousness, nausea and vomiting, headache, palpitations, tachycardia, and dyspnea. (I, T, G)

39. 4. Early signs of possible aminophylline toxicity include hypotension, dysrhythmias, and seizures. Assessment for these manifestations should be made frequently. (I, T, G)

40. 2. Side effects of theophylline include vomiting, headache, and irritability. (E, N, G)

41. 4. In asthma, the airways react to certain external and internal stimuli including allergens, infections, exercise, and emotions. Food allergens commonly associated with asthma include wheat, egg white, dairy products, citrus fruits, corn, and chocolate. (I, T, G)

42. 3. When introducing solid foods to infants, only one new food should be added at a time so that if an allergic reaction occurs, the food allergen can be easily identified. In the absence of evidence of allergy, all foods are appropriate except mixed foods, which should be avoided to facilitate allergen identification. Infant formula is a major source of nutrition for the first year and should not be eliminated when solids are introduced. (I, T, H)

43. 3. Inhaled irritants and allergens are a common trigger for asthmatic episodes. Frequent dusting and vacuuming decrease the amount of inhalable allergens available to the asthmatic child. Wool fibers (from sheepskin), aerosols, and open windows are all potential sources of respiratory irritants. (I, T, G)

44. 1. Allergic reaction to inhaled particles generally causes a nasal crease from frequent nose rubbing. Allergic shiners are dark circles under the eyes caused by nasal congestion. (A, C, G)

45. 1. Parents should be taught that climatic extremes such as excessively cold temperatures, may precipitate an asthmatic episode because of the effect on the airways. Children with asthma should do chest mobility exercises to strengthen respiratory muscles. Children with asthma need to be taught about the disease so they can become active participants in their care. Children with asthma should wear clothing made of synthetic material and cotton, not real fur or wools, which are potential respiratory irritants. (I, T, G)

46. 2. Pets are discouraged when trying to allergy-proof a home for a child with bronchial asthma, unless the pets are kept outside. Pets with hair or feathers are especially likely to trigger asthma attacks. A fish would be a satisfactory pet for this child, but the parents should be taught to keep the fish tank clean to prevent it from harboring mold. (I, T, G)

47. 2. Cromolyn sodium (Aarane) is used as a prophylactic agent to help prevent bronchial asthmatic attacks). The drug is not an anti-inflammatory, bronchodilator, or antihistamine agent. Therefore, it is of no use during an asthma attack. The drug inhibits histamine release and acts locally to prevent the release of mediator substances from mast (connective tissue) cells following exposure to allergens. (I, T, G)

48. 3. Developing a positive family life requires placing the child's illness in its proper perspective. Some parents tend to overprotect the child with a chronic illness. This overprotectiveness may cause a child to have an exaggerated feeling of importance or later, as an adolescent, to rebel against the overprotectiveness. Children with asthma need to be treated as normally as possible within the scope of the limitations imposed by the illness. (I, T, G)

49. 4. Physical activities are beneficial to asthmatic children. Most of these children can engage in school and sports activities with minimal difficulty, if the asthma is kept in check. (I, T, G)

The Client With Cystic Fibrosis and Bronchopneumonia

50. 2. Classic signs of pneumonia include fever and cough. Weight loss may occur in a child with cystic fibrosis because of the energy expenditure needed to fight the infection. Rash, constipation, and dysuria are not associated with pneumonia. Vomiting may occur, especially if the child is coughing frequently and has lots of mucus. (A, C, G)

51. 4. It is important to give antibiotics spaced at equal intervals over a 24-hour period to help maintain therapeutic levels of the medication in the bloodstream. Therefore, if a medication is to be given three times in each 24-hour period, good times to give it are 8 A.M., 4 P.M., and midnight. The client should be awakened to keep such a schedule. (I, T, S)

52. 2. Postural drainage is generally recommended before meals, to avoid the possibility of vomiting or regurgitating food. The need for rest periods is not as important a factor in scheduling postural drainage. (I, T, G)

53. 2. One problem associated with cystic fibrosis is poor digestion and absorption of foods, especially fats. Pancreatic enzymes can help improve digestion and absorption of nutrients. (E, N, S)

54. 2. Cystic fibrosis affects the exocrine glands. Mucus is thick and tenacious, sticking to the walls of the pancreatic and bile ducts and eventually causing obstruction. Because of the difficulty with digestion and absorption, a moderate-fat, high-protein, and high-calorie diet is indicated. (A, K, G)

55. 2. In children with cystic fibrosis, poor digestion and absorption of foods, especially fats, results in frequent bowel movements with bulky, foul-smelling stools. The stools also contain abnormally large quantities of fat, which is called steatorrhea. (I, T, G)

56. 2. The child's favorite doll would be a good choice of toys. The doll provides support and is a familiar toy. In view of the child's lung pathology, a fuzzy stuffed animal would not be advised. Scissors, paper, and paste are not appropriate for a 3-year-old unless the child is supervised. A jigsaw puzzle is not particularly appropriate for an ill 3-year-old child. (I, T, G)

57. 4. One characteristic of cystic fibrosis is the excessive loss of salt through perspiration. Salt supplements are almost always necessary during warm weather or any other time the child perspires more than usual. The absence of sweat glands, little skin pigment, and a poorly functioning temperature control center are conditions unrelated to cystic fibrosis. (I, T, G)

58. 1. Cystic fibrosis is characterized by a dysfunction in the body's mucus-producing exocrine glands. The mucus secretions are very thick and sticky, rather than thin and slippery. The mucus obstructs various passages in the body, especially in the bronchi, bronchioles, and pancreatic ducts. Mucus plugs in the pancreatic ducts can prevent pancreatic digestive enzymes from reaching the small intestine, resulting in poor digestion and poor absorption of various food nutrients. (E, N, G)

59. 1. This is the client outcome that deals directly with the nursing diagnosis Ineffective Breathing Pattern. The child may have vomiting and activity intolerance, but these problems are not directly related to respiratory symptoms. (P, N, G)

60. 1. Swimming and bowling are the best physical activities for a child with cystic fibrosis. They are noncontact sports yet can be team sports. Swimming is excellent because it coordinates breathing and movement of all muscle groups. Bowling is a low-energy-output game that still requires skill. The other sports listed require much energy expenditure, which may become increasingly difficult as the child gets older. (I, C, G)

61. 2. Cystic fibrosis is the most common inherited disease in children. It is inherited as an autosomal recessive trait, meaning the child inherits the defective genes from both parents. The chances are that it will occur in one of four of this couple's children. (P, C, G)

62. 3. An important function of the National Cystic Fibrosis Foundation is to put parents of children with cystic fibrosis in touch with each other. Other parents are often able to offer support and help. In some instances, the Foundation gives parents financial assistance for equipment required for home care of their child with cystic fibrosis (but not for medications). The Foundation does not obtain tutors for children or provide genetic counseling for parents. (I, T, G)

63. 4. Many antibiotics are infused over 30 minutes; 10-minute infusions are irritating to the vein. Heparin should be infused as soon as the antibiotic infusion is finished, so the access will remain patent. The antibiotic is timed to infuse on a schedule to maintain constant blood levels of the antibiotics. Administering an antibiotic 2 hours late affects the drug blood level as well as the schedule. A parent who has difficulty with an infusion should call the nurse to help identify and solve the problem. (E, N, S)

The Client With Sudden Infant Death Syndrome

64. 4. The most important nursing intervention would be to reach out to the anxious parents and stay with them while the infant is being evaluated. (I, T, L)

65. 3. A sensitive approach to the parents can help minimize their guilt and prevent later emotional disturbances. The nurse should never ask any questions that imply parental neglect, wrongdoing, or abuse. (I, T, L)

66. 2. The parents should be given the opportunity to say their final farewell to their infant. This last contact helps them focus on the reality of the infant's death. Reassuring them that they are not at fault does not focus them on the reality of death. The presence of their pastor may be helpful, but enabling them to see their son would be more important. For some parents, clothes may be too painful a reminder of their child's death, and they may not wish to take them home. (I, T, L)

67. 1. One of the main techniques used in crisis intervention in the hospital includes helping parents begin to gain an intellectual understanding of SIDS. Numerous theories have been proposed, but no specific cause of SIDS has been identified. Evidence suggests that infants with SIDS have chronic hypoxia, possibly from prolonged periodic apnea. (I, T, G)

68. 2. The parents need to discuss their feelings with each other to begin the healing process. Avoiding discussing their feelings causes each one to become isolated and to grieve without support. Working long hours is detrimental to the grieving process; there is no time to come to terms with what has occurred. By acting as if nothing has happened, it is avoiding the issue and not dealing with it. (D, T, L)

69. 4. The nurse should visit as soon after the death as possible. The parents need expert counseling to deal not only with the death of their child, but also with a sudden, unexpected, and unexplained tragedy. (I, T, L)

70. 1. The goal of the second visit is to help the parents express their feelings. Gaining an understanding of the disease is a goal of the first visit. Although it is important to assess the impact of SIDS on siblings, this is not the primary goal for the second visit, although plans must be flexible. Parents are unable to deal with decisions such as having other children during the second visit; this should be discussed later. (I, T, L)

The Client Requiring Cardiopulmonary Resuscitation

71. 1. When breathlessness is determined, the priority nursing action is to clear the airway. This action alone may reestablish spontaneous respiration. If the client does not begin breathing, mouth-to-mouth resuscitation is begun. Oxygen therapy would not be initiated at this time. Chest compressions are begun only after the client is determined to be pulseless. (I, T, G)

72. 2. Checking the carotid artery pulse in a child during CPR provides information about perfusion of the brain. The brachial pulse is checked in an infant because the infant's short and often fat neck makes it difficult to palpate the carotid pulse. The femoral and radial arteries might indicate perfusion to the peripheral body sites, but the critical need is for adequate circulation to the brain. (I, T, G)

73. 3. The rescue breathing rate for a child is one every 4 seconds, or 15 times per minute. Rescue breaths should be delivered slowly at a volume that makes the chest rise and fall. (I, T, G)

74. 1. The chest is compressed with the heel of one hand positioned on the lower sternum, two fingerbreadths above the sternal notch. Fingertips are used to compress the sternum in infants, and the heel of two hands is used in adult CPR. (I, T, G)

75. 4. Chest compressions should be delivered at a rate of 80 to 100 times per minute for a 5-year-old child. This rate approximates the resting minimum pulse, which allows for adequate brain perfusion. A rate less than 80 per minute does not provide adequate brain perfusion for a 5-year-old child. (I, T, G)

76. 1. In a 5-year-old child, the chest is compressed to a depth of 1" to 1.5". This depth forces blood out of the heart into the vital organs (lungs and brain).

Deeper compressions could damage the liver, lungs, or other underlying structures. Shallower compressions would not provide adequate circulation to the vital organs. (I, T, G)

77. 3. Signs of recovery from cardiopulmonary arrest include palpable peripheral pulses, the disappearance of mottling and cyanosis, the return of pupils to normal size, and warm dry skin. To determine if the victim of cardiopulmonary arrest has resumed spontaneous breathing and circulation, chest compressions must be stopped for 5 seconds at the end of the first minute and every few minutes thereafter. (I, T, G)

78. 4. After opening the infant's mouth, the nurse attempts to find and remove the object. The nurse should attempt to remove only a visible object; blind finger sweeps are not appropriate in infants and children, because the foreign body may be pushed back into the airway. If the nurse cannot see the foreign body, mechanical force—back blows and chest thrusts—should be used in an attempt to dislodge the object. Subdiaphragmatic abdominal thrusts are not used for infants age 1 year or younger because of the risk of injury to abdominal organs. (I, T, G)

79. 2. The infant is placed face down, straddled over the nurse's arm with the head lower than the trunk and the head supported. This position, together with the back blows, facilitates dislodgement and removal of a foreign object and minimizes aspiration if vomiting occurs. (I, T, G)

80. 4. Back blows are delivered rapidly and forcefully with the heel of the hand between the infant's shoulder blades. Slowly delivered back blows are less likely to dislodge the object. Using the heel of the hand allows more force to be applied, increasing the likelihood of loosening the object. (I, T, G)

81. 4. Crying indicates that the airway obstruction has been relieved and the infant needs close observation. Delivering chest or back blows could jeopardize a patent airway. Blind finger sweeps are contraindicated in infants. (I, T, G)

82. 1. Tilting the head slightly prevents the tongue from obstructing the airway. Gastric distension interferes with diaphragmatic excursion, which occurs when breaths are delivered too rapidly. Excessive pressure on the neck does not directly affect an obstructed airway. Extensor posturing indicates brain damage and is not related to airway obstruction. (I, T, G)

NURSING CARE OF CHILDREN

TEST 2: The Child with Respiratory Health Problems

Directions: Use this answer grid to determine areas of strength or need for further study.

NURSING PROCESS

A = Assessment
D = Analysis, nursing diagnosis
P = Planning
I = Implementation
E = Evaluation

COGNITIVE LEVEL

K = Knowledge
C = Comprehension
T = Application
N = Analysis

CLIENT NEEDS

S = Safe, effective care environment
G = Physiological integrity
L = Psychosocial integrity
H = Health promotion/maintenance

		Nursing Process					Cognitive Level				Client Needs			
Question #	Answer #	A	D	P	I	E	K	C	T	N	S	G	L	H
1	4				I				T			G		
2	4				I				T			G		
3	1		D							N		G		
4	1				I				T				L	
5	3				I				T			G		
6	1				I				T			G		
7	1				I				T			G		
8	2					E			T			G		
9	3					E			T			G		
10	3				I				T			G		
11	2				I				T			G		
12	4				I				T			G		
13	1				I				T			G		
14	1				I				T					H
15	3				I				T			G		
16	1				I				T				L	
17	4				I				T			G		
18	2				I				T			G		
19	3				I				T			G		
20	2				I				T			G		
21	1				I				T		S			
22	4				I				T			G		
23	1				I				T			G		

ANSWER GRID: 1

NURSING PROCESS

A = Assessment
D = Analysis, nursing diagnosis
P = Planning
I = Implementation
E = Evaluation

COGNITIVE LEVEL

K = Knowledge
C = Comprehension
T = Application
N = Analysis

CLIENT NEEDS

S = Safe, effective care environment
G = Physiological integrity
L = Psychosocial integrity
H = Health promotion/maintenance

		Nursing Process					Cognitive Level				Client Needs			
Question #	Answer #	A	D	P	I	E	K	C	T	N	S	G	L	H
24	1		D							N		G		
25	1				I				T			G		
26	3				I				T			G		
27	1			P					T					H
28	1				I				T			G		
29	2				I				T			G		
30	2				I				T			G		
31	4				I				T			G		
32	2				I				T			G		
33	3	A						C				G		
34	3				I				T			G		
35	2				I				T			G		
36	2				I				T			G		
37	1				I				T			G		
38	1				I				T			G		
39	4				I				T			G		
40	2					E				N		G		
41	4				I				T			G		
42	3				I				T					H
43	3				I				T			G		
44	1	A						C				G		
45	1				I				T			G		
46	2				I				T			G		
47	2				I				T			G		
48	3				I				T			G		
49	4				I				T			G		
50	2	A						C				G		
51	4				I				T		S			
52	2				I				T			G		

ANSWER GRID: 2

NURSING PROCESS

A = Assessment
D = Analysis, nursing diagnosis
P = Planning
I = Implementation
E = Evaluation

COGNITIVE LEVEL

K = Knowledge
C = Comprehension
T = Application
N = Analysis

CLIENT NEEDS

S = Safe, effective care environment
G = Physiological integrity
L = Psychosocial integrity
H = Health promotion/maintenance

		Nursing Process					Cognitive Level				Client Needs			
Question #	Answer #	A	D	P	I	E	K	C	T	N	S	G	L	H
53	2					E				N	S			
54	2	A					K					G		
55	2				I				T			G		
56	2				I				T			G		
57	4				I				T			G		
58	1					E				N		G		
59	1			P						N		G		
60	1				I			C				G		
61	2			P				C				G		
62	3				I				T			G		
63	4					E				N	S			
64	4				I				T				L	
65	3				I				T				L	
66	2				I				T				L	
67	1				I				T			G		
68	2		D						T				L	
69	4				I				T				L	
70	1				I				T				L	
71	1				I				T			G		
72	2				I				T			G		
73	3				I				T			G		
74	1				I				T			G		
75	4				I				T			G		
76	1				I				T			G		
77	3				I				T			G		
78	4				I				T			G		
79	2				I				T			G		
80	4				I				T			G		
81	4				I				T			G		

ANSWER GRID: 3

Nursing Process

A = Assessment
D = Analysis, nursing diagnosis
P = Planning
I = Implementation
E = Evaluation

Cognitive Level

K = Knowledge
C = Comprehension
T = Application
N = Analysis

Client Needs

S = Safe, effective care environment
G = Physiological integrity
L = Psychosocial integrity
H = Health promotion/maintenance

		Nursing Process					Cognitive Level				Client Needs			
Question #	Answer #	A	D	P	I	E	K	C	T	N	S	G	L	H
82	1				I				T			G		
Number Correct														
Number Possible	82	4	3	3	66	6	1	5	69	7	4	67	8	3
Percentage Correct														

Score Calculation:

To determine your **Percentage Correct**, divide the **Number Correct** by the **Number Possible.**

Test 3

The Child With Cardiovascular Health Problems

The Child With a Ventricular Septal Defect
The Client With Tetralogy of Fallot
The Client With Down Syndrome
The Client With Rheumatic Fever
The Client With Sickle-Cell Anemia
The Client With Iron-Deficiency Anemia
The Client With Hemophilia and Acquired Immune Deficiency Syndrome
The Client With Leukemia
Correct Answers and Rationale

Select the one best answer and indicate your choice by filling in the circle in front of the option.

The Client With a Ventricular Septal Defect

A 3-year-old child is admitted for a cardiac catheterization. He was born with a ventricular septal defect that has never been repaired.

1. When providing care for this child before the cardiac catheterization, the nurse would designate which of the following nursing diagnosis as priority?
- ○ 1. Altered Comfort.
- ○ 2. Knowledge Deficit.
- ○ 3. Noncompliance.
- ○ 4. Altered Cardiac Output.

2. Which of the following should be included as the nurse teaches this child about the cardiac catheterization?
- ○ 1. A plastic model of the heart.
- ○ 2. A catheter which will be inserted into the artery.
- ○ 3. All the family members.
- ○ 4. Other children undergoing a catheterization.

3. In planning care, the nurse considers the child's stage of development and explains to the parents that a 3-year-old is most likely resolving Erikson's stage of
- ○ 1. autonomy vs. shame and doubt.
- ○ 2. identity vs. identity diffusion.
- ○ 3. initiative vs. guilt.
- ○ 4. industry vs. inferiority.

4. The child is scheduled for a cardiac catheterization tomorrow. The nurse's plan of care should be to tell the parents that this procedure usually involves the use of
- ○ 1. ultra-high-frequency sound waves.
- ○ 2. a right-sided approach.
- ○ 3. a cut-down procedure.
- ○ 4. general anesthesia.

5. The nurse considers the client's need for psychological preparation for cardiac catheterization. The nurse should base interventions on the fact that
- ○ 1. overprotecting a preschooler decreases anxiety considerably.
- ○ 2. preschoolers are cognitively unable to understand the procedure.
- ○ 3. little psychological preparation can be given to preschoolers.
- ○ 4. preparation is a joint responsibility of the physician, parents, and nurse.

6. After the catheterization is performed, the child is returned to the room with a pressure dressing and an I.V. line in place. He is slightly drowsy. The nurse should give highest priority to which of the following postprocedure assessments?
- ○ 1. Vital signs every 4 hours.

○ 2. Pulse checks above the catheterization site.
○ 3. Temperature checks of the right leg.
○ 4. Comparison of color in right and left legs.

7. When preparing the child's parents for his discharge, the nurse should tell them that
○ 1. the child's activities should be limited for 3 weeks.
○ 2. the child should be given sponge baths until the stitches are removed.
○ 3. antibiotics should be given before the child receives any dental work.
○ 4. the stitches will be removed in 2 weeks.

The Client With Tetralogy of Fallot

A 6-year-old child is admitted to the hospital for heart surgery to repair tetralogy of Fallot. The nurse observes that the child is cyanotic at admission.

8. The nurse judges that the parents understand this disorder when they explain that the underlying cause of their child's cyanosis is
○ 1. constriction of the aorta.
○ 2. stenosis of the mitral valve.
○ 3. stenosis of the pulmonary valve.
○ 4. the aorta receiving blood directly from the vena cava.

9. When teaching the parents about the electrocardiogram that their child will undergo, the nurse should explain that the primary reason for this procedure is to determine the
○ 1. electrical activity in the heart muscle.
○ 2. pressure of the blood in the heart.
○ 3. amount of blood entering the heart.
○ 4. various sounds made by each heartbeat.

10. The child asks the nurse if the cardiac catheterization will hurt. Which of the following statements offers the nurse the best guide for responding to the child's question?
○ 1. Some pressure may be felt when the catheter is introduced into the vein.
○ 2. Momentary sharp pain will usually occur when the catheter enters the heart.
○ 3. It is unusual for a 6-year-old to feel discomfort during the procedure.
○ 4. It is a painless procedure, although a tingling sensation may be felt in the extremities.

11. During one of the child's attacks of dyspnea, the nurse makes a typical observation when noting that the child assumes a
○ 1. squatting position.
○ 2. Trendelenburg position.
○ 3. semi-sitting position.
○ 4. left side-lying position.

12. The nurse teaches the child coughing and deep-breathing exercises before corrective heart surgery. Of the following teaching-learning principles to take into account when teaching the client, which should assume first priority?
○ 1. Building the teaching on the child's current level of knowledge.
○ 2. Arranging the order of information to be taught the child in a logical sequence.
○ 3. Arranging to use actual equipment for demonstrations.
○ 4. Presenting the information to be taught in order from simplest to most complex.

13. When planning care for this client before corrective heart surgery, the nurse would choose which of the following as the priority nursing diagnosis?
○ 1. Ineffective Family Coping.
○ 2. Altered Comfort.
○ 3. Knowledge Deficit.
○ 4. Impaired Gas Exchange.

14. After corrective heart surgery is done, the nurse monitors the child for low cardiac output. Which of the following findings would indicate low cardiac output?
○ 1. Cool extremities, bounding pulses, and mottled skin.
○ 2. Altered level of consciousness, cool extremities, and thready pulse.
○ 3. Bounding pulses, cyanosis, and mottled skin.
○ 4. Altered level of consciousness, warm extremities, and cyanosis.

15. The nurse plans to teach the parents about the digoxin (Lanoxin) prescribed for their child. Which of the following would the nurse be sure to include in the teaching plan?
○ 1. Digoxin is absorbed better when given with meals.
○ 2. Digoxin is absorbed better when taken 1 hour before eating.
○ 3. Signs of toxicity include increased heart rate and loss of appetite.
○ 4. If the child vomits 30 minutes after taking the medication, the dose should be repeated.

16. The nurse should teach the mother that digoxin (Lanoxin)
○ 1. can be kept in the medicine chest with other medicines.
○ 2. can be kept in the kitchen for easy administration.
○ 3. should be locked up with the key kept out of reach.
○ 4. should be kept on the kitchen counter so a dose is not forgotten.

17. The nurse should plan to teach the parents that the child will have to
○ 1. receive antibiotics before any invasive procedures.

○ 2. drink lots of liquids before the next appointment.
○ 3. take frequent naps for the first 4 weeks at home.
○ 4. restrict potassium intake.

18. The nurse should teach the parents that when the child returns to the pediatric unit after corrective surgery, he will
○ 1. be on a 2- to 3-gram/day sodium diet.
○ 2. be on absolute bedrest.
○ 3. have restricted visiting.
○ 4. be assigned to an isolation room.

19. The parents express concern that their child wants to be held more frequently than usual postoperatively. Which of the following best describes this behavioral response to stress?
○ 1. Repression.
○ 2. Depression.
○ 3. Regression.
○ 4. Rationalization.

20. The mother asks the nurse why her child has clubbed fingers. The nurse should explain that the clubbing is due to
○ 1. polycythemia.
○ 2. peripheral hypoxia.
○ 3. delayed physical growth.
○ 4. destruction of bone marrow.

21. The nurse should anticipate that the most likely fear that the child's parents will have when they take their child home is fear of
○ 1. allowing the child to lead a normal active life.
○ 2. persuading the child of the need for extra rest.
○ 3. having the child develop postoperative complications.
○ 4. having the child's siblings treat him as handicapped.

22. The child's 3-year-old sibling has become quiet and shy and demonstrates more than the usual amount of sexual curiosity, according to the mother. According to Erikson's description of the central psychosocial problem of preschoolers, the sibling is demonstrating an attempt to resolve a conflict between
○ 1. trust and mistrust.
○ 2. initiative and guilt.
○ 3. industry and inferiority.
○ 4. autonomy and shame or doubt.

The Client With Down Syndrome

A community health nurse has been visiting a home regularly to help with the personal care of a severely retarded child, age 10. The child's mother has a back ailment of recent origin that prevents her from assuming responsibility for the child's care.

23. After talking with the parents, the nurse would determine that the goal for care of this child is to
○ 1. help the parents encourage normal developmental skills in their child.
○ 2. advise the parents to teach the child something new every day.
○ 3. encourage the parents to be more lenient when setting behavior limits for the child.
○ 4. help the parents to be more strict when setting behavior limits for the child.

24. The child's disability was apparent at birth, and her development was slow. Which of the following behaviors is least characteristic of a delay in early development common to mentally retarded children?
○ 1. Not using expressive language.
○ 2. Not responding to verbal commands.
○ 3. Starting to walk at age 20 months.
○ 4. Being able to sit up at age 6 months.

25. Which of the following would be a priority nursing diagnosis for this child?
○ 1. Self-Care Deficit.
○ 2. Knowledge Deficit.
○ 3. Altered Nutrition.
○ 4. Impaired Physical Mobility.

26. The client has an intelligence quotient (IQ) of approximately 40. The kind of environment and interdisciplinary program most likely to benefit this child would be best described as
○ 1. custodial.
○ 2. educational.
○ 3. habit training.
○ 4. sheltered workshop.

27. The nurse discusses with the parents how to best raise their child's IQ. Which of the following means would be most appropriate?
○ 1. Serving hearty, nutritious meals.
○ 2. Giving vasodilating medications as prescribed.
○ 3. Letting the child play with more able children.
○ 4. Providing stimulating, nonthreatening life experiences.

28. The child has no physical defects. The nurse would instruct the parents about which of the following signs are potentially indicative of a physical problem commonly associated with Down syndrome?
○ 1. Weight.
○ 2. Pulse rate.
○ 3. Respirations.
○ 4. Blood pressure.

29. A primary goal of the nurse working with this child's parents is to increase their sense of
○ 1. liking for the child.
○ 2. responsibility for their child's welfare.
○ 3. understanding of their child's disability.
○ 4. confidence in their abilities to care for their child.

30. When discussing plans for genetic counseling for the mother's other daughter, the nurse should teach the mother that the primary role of the genetic team working with a family is to

- ○ 1. provide the parents with the facts about their birth defect risks.
- ○ 2. report to the parents the findings of chromosome analysis of the amniotic cells.
- ○ 3. prepare the parents psychologically for the birth of a defective child.
- ○ 4. prescribe birth control or abortion measures for the parents as needed.

31. The nurse mentions that a group meeting for mothers of retarded children is to be held soon. "Not retarded!," blazes the client's mother, "Exceptional." When responding to this outburst, which of the following replies by the nurse would be best?

- ○ 1. "Why do you prefer the term 'exceptional'?"
- ○ 2. "I'm sorry if I offended you by my thoughtless remark."
- ○ 3. "No matter what it's called, the condition is still the same, isn't it?"
- ○ 4. "I'd like to hear more of your thoughts and feelings on that."

32. In relation to teaching goals, the mother's expressed desire for her child is that she be able to dress herself independently. This would be best written in the nursing care plan as a

- ○ 1. single attainable goal.
- ○ 2. goal that may be postponed.
- ○ 3. series of small, short-term goals.
- ○ 4. part of the overall larger goal of optimal functioning.

33. Sometimes the child seems deliberately to do things that cause her mother to become displeased and upset. The nurse should explain to the mother that the child tends to act this way to

- ○ 1. annoy the mother.
- ○ 2. get attention from the mother.
- ○ 3. express anger toward the mother.
- ○ 4. relieve boredom.

34. The community health nurse observes the family at mealtime and notes that the child is messy and eats noisily. Which of the following approaches that the nurse could recommend to decrease the child's undesirable eating habits would provide the most positive reinforcement for her desirable table manners?

- ○ 1. Praising the child when she chews quietly.
- ○ 2. Scolding the child when she smacks her lips.
- ○ 3. Ignoring the child when she plays with her food.
- ○ 4. Making the child leave the table after she spills milk.

The Client With Rheumatic Fever

A 7-year-old child is admitted to the hospital with the medical diagnosis of acute rheumatic fever.

35. When obtaining a health history from the child's mother, the nurse should ask questions to determine if the child was recently ill with

- ○ 1. mumps.
- ○ 2. measles.
- ○ 3. a viral flu.
- ○ 4. a sore throat.

36. On initial assessment, the nurse determines that the physician should be contacted, based on which of the following signs?

- ○ 1. Heart rate of 150 beats/minute.
- ○ 2. Swollen and painful knee joints.
- ○ 3. Twitching in the extremities.
- ○ 4. Red rash on the trunk.

37. The nurse should plan to talk to the mother about

- ○ 1. encouraging her and her husband to stay at the child's bedside.
- ○ 2. allowing the child to have long periods of rest between activities.
- ○ 3. allowing the child to participate in activities that will not cause fatigue.
- ○ 4. encouraging the child to eat as much as possible.

38. The nurse plans to develop a nursing care plan for the child and family. Which of the following nursing diagnoses would be a priority for this child?

- ○ 1. Altered Comfort.
- ○ 2. Altered Fluid Volume.
- ○ 3. Altered Nutrition.
- ○ 4. Altered Tissue Perfusion.

39. Which of the following laboratory blood findings would confirm that the child likely has rheumatic fever?

- ○ 1. High leukocyte count.
- ○ 2. Low hemoglobin count.
- ○ 3. Elevated antibody level.
- ○ 4. Low erythrocyte sedimentation rate.

40. The nurse determines that the parents understand that their child will need to receive long-term antibiotic therapy when they state

- ○ 1. "It will prevent further streptococcus infections."
- ○ 2. "It will protect against further joint damage."
- ○ 3. "The inflammation will subside with fewer side effects."
- ○ 4. "The inflammation will be reduced with future attacks."

41. Activity is sharply restricted during the acute phase of the child's illness. To evaluate the effectiveness of bedrest, the nurse must recognize that activity restriction is ordered primarily to help

- ○ 1. prevent injury to tender joints.
- ○ 2. reduce the workload on the heart.
- ○ 3. promote the full benefits of drug therapy.
- ○ 4. minimize the severity of the disease's inflammatory process.

42. During the acute phase of the illness, it would be least desirable to interest the child in which of the following diversional activities?

○ 1. Reading a book.
○ 2. Playing with a doll.
○ 3. Listening to the radio.
○ 4. Playing checkers with a roommate.

43. Which of the following physical findings would the nurse assess for as indicative of carditis?
○ 1. Heart murmur.
○ 2. Low blood pressure.
○ 3. Irregular pulse.
○ 4. Pain over the anterior chest wall.

44. The physician prescribes digoxin (Lanoxin) for the child. The nurse teaches the child's mother that the primary reason for giving this drug is that it helps
○ 1. relax the walls of the heart's arteries.
○ 2. improve the strength of the heartbeat.
○ 3. prevent irregularities in ventricular contractions.
○ 4. eliminate dissociation of ventricular and atrial rhythms.

45. The child's daily digoxin (Lanoxin) dose is 0.15 mg p.o. The digoxin is available in liquid form at a concentration of 0.05 mg/ml. How much of the medication should the nurse administer at each dose?
○ 1. 0.2 ml.
○ 2. 0.5 ml.
○ 3. 3.0 ml.
○ 4. 5.0 ml.

46. The nursing care plan specifies that the child's pulse be assessed several times through the night. The nurse teaches the mother that the primary reason for obtaining a sleeping pulse rate is to ensure that the child's pulse rate is free of influence from
○ 1. having had a morning dose of digitalis.
○ 2. carrying out normal activity during waking hours.
○ 3. being in a warmer environment during the day than at night.
○ 4. having various nurses obtaining the pulse rate during day/evening hours.

47. The child is to receive 5 grains of acetylsalicylic acid (aspirin) every 4 hours. The nurse would administer the metric equivalent, which would be
○ 1. 0.032 g.
○ 2. 0.32 g.
○ 3. 3.2 g.
○ 4. 32 g.

48. Which of the following signs or symptoms should lead the nurse to suspect that the child is experiencing early salicylate toxicity?
○ 1. Chest pain.
○ 2. Pink-colored urine.
○ 3. Slow pulse rate.
○ 4. Ringing in the ears.

49. Which of the following measures would the nurse use to help minimize any joint pain the child is experiencing?
○ 1. Massaging the affected joints.
○ 2. Applying ice to the affected joints.
○ 3. Limiting movement of the affected joints.
○ 4. Putting the affected joints through range-of-motion exercises.

50. Which of these other nursing measures would be appropriate to help alleviate joint pain?
○ 1. Changing the child's position in bed frequently.
○ 2. Applying gentle traction to the child's affected joints.
○ 3. Supporting the child's body in proper alignment with rolled pillows.
○ 4. Using a bed cradle to remove the weight of bed linens on the child's joints.

51. If the child develops chorea-like movements, which of the following eating utensils would the nurse remove?
○ 1. Fork.
○ 2. Spoon.
○ 3. Plastic cup.
○ 4. Drinking straw.

52. When discussing long-term care for the child with the parents, the nurse should teach them that a necessary part of this long-term care is
○ 1. physical therapy.
○ 2. antibiotic therapy.
○ 3. psychological therapy.
○ 4. anti-inflammatory therapy.

53. The parents express concern that their other children will develop rheumatic fever. What would be the nurse's best response?
○ 1. "This disease is caused by a special type of streptococcus and is usually not contagious."
○ 2. "Your other children are just as likely to develop rheumatic fever."
○ 3. "There is medicine available to prevent this; check with your doctor."
○ 4. "Your other children are all girls, so there is no need to worry."

The Client With Sickle-Cell Anemia

A 1-year-old boy is admitted to the hospital with sickle-cell crisis.

54. When preparing for the child's admission, the nurse should anticipate and prepare for therapy that most likely will include
○ 1. parenteral iron therapy.
○ 2. exchange transfusion.
○ 3. intravenous fluid therapy.
○ 4. fast-acting anticoagulant therapy.

55. The nurse would explain to the parents that the local tissue damage the child is likely to show at admission is due to
○ 1. a general inflammatory response to an autoimmune reaction complicated by hypoxia.

○ 2. air hunger and resultant respiratory alkalosis due to deoxygenated red blood cells.
○ 3. cell damage with signs of ischemia and necrosis due to circulatory obstruction.
○ 4. hypersensitivity of the central nervous system due to high serum bilirubin levels and adrenocortical imbalance.

56. The nurse notes that the child prefers a side-lying position with the knees sharply flexed. The child's positioning should cause the nurse to assess for further evidence of
○ 1. nausea.
○ 2. backache.
○ 3. abdominal pain.
○ 4. emotional regression.

57. The sickle cell crisis subsides, and the child is to be discharged. The nurse should teach the parents to seek prompt health care if their child develops
○ 1. headaches and nausea.
○ 2. fatigue and lassitude.
○ 3. skin rash and itching.
○ 4. sore throat and fever.

58. The nurse teaches the parents how to care for their child at home. The nurse determines that the parents understand the basic principles of care when they state that they are
○ 1. keeping the child with them at all times.
○ 2. restricting the child's fluids at night.
○ 3. allowing their child to drink as much as he desires.
○ 4. not allowing their child to play with other children.

59. Which of the following statements would the nurse make when teaching the mother that the child was normal at birth and then developed sickle-cell disease?
○ 1. The placenta bars passage of the hemoglobin S from the mother to the fetus.
○ 2. The red bone marrow does not begin to produce hemoglobin S until several months after birth.
○ 3. Antibodies transmitted from the mother to the fetus provide the newborn with temporary immunity.
○ 4. The newborn has a high concentration of fetal hemoglobin in the blood for some time after birth.

60. It has been determined that both parents are carriers of the sickle-cell trait. They ask about the chances of sickle-cell disease occurring in other future children. The nurse should respond to this question based on knowledge that the gene responsible for sickle-cell disease is autosomal recessive and the risk of one of their children having the disease is
○ 1. 25%.
○ 2. 50%.
○ 3. 75%.
○ 4. 100%.

61. The nurse would identify which of the following as the priority nursing diagnosis during the crisis?
○ 1. Ineffective Coping.
○ 2. Altered Cardiac Output.
○ 3. Altered Comfort.
○ 4. Fluid Volume Deficit.

The Client With Iron-Deficiency Anemia

An 11-month-old infant is brought to an outpatient pediatric clinic by her mother. She is very pale, and the mother explains that she drinks more than a quart of cow's milk daily, eats very few solids, and sleeps excessively. A medical diagnosis of iron-deficiency anemia is made.

62. The mother asks the nurse what she could have done to prevent the iron-deficiency anemia. The nurse should respond that solid foods should be introduced into an infant's diet at age
○ 1. 1 to 2 months.
○ 2. 5 to 6 months.
○ 3. 8 to 10 months.
○ 4. 10 to 12 months.

63. The infant's diet needs to be modified. The nurse should teach the mother about which of the following modifications?
○ 1. Equal intake of iron-rich solids and milk.
○ 2. Increased intake of iron-rich solids and decreased milk intake.
○ 3. Near exclusive intake of iron-rich solids.
○ 4. Increased intake of iron-rich solids and maintenance of current milk intake.

64. The nurse teaches the mother about iron-rich foods that are most appropriate for an 11-month-old infant. The mother's selection of which of the following foods would indicate that she understands the teaching?
○ 1. Eggs, fortified cereals, meats, and green vegetables.
○ 2. Fruits, cereals, milk, and yellow vegetables.
○ 3. Eggs, fruits, milk, and mixed vegetables.
○ 4. Juices, fruits, fortified cereals, and milk.

65. The mother asks the nurse about the relationship between iron-deficiency anemia and infection. The nurse should teach the mother that
○ 1. little is known about iron-deficiency anemia and its relationship to infection in children.
○ 2. children with iron-deficiency anemia are more susceptible to infection than are other children.
○ 3. children with iron-deficiency anemia are less susceptible to infection than are other children.
○ 4. children with iron-deficiency anemia are no more susceptible to infection than are other children.

66. The infant is started on iron therapy. The nurse plans to teach the mother how to administer the iron drops. Which of the following instructions would be most appropriate?
○ 1. Mix the iron drops in the infant's milk.
○ 2. Put the iron drops in the infant's mouth, then follow with juice.
○ 3. Put the iron drops in the infant's mouth, then follow with milk.
○ 4. Mix the iron drops in the infant's bedtime water bottle.

The Client With Hemophilia and Acquired Immune Deficiency Syndrome

A neonate is suspected of having hemophilia A (classic hemophilia) because of prolonged bleeding following circumcision.

67. The physician has ordered several laboratory tests to help diagnose the bleeding disorder. The nurse would explain to the parents that which test would most likely be abnormal in a neonate with hemophilia?
○ 1. Bleeding time.
○ 2. Tourniquet test.
○ 3. Clot retraction test.
○ 4. Partial thromboplastin test.

68. Which information that the nurse notes in the neonate's family history would help support the diagnosis of hemophilia?
○ 1. An older brother and sister who are healthy.
○ 2. The ethnic background of the family is Italian and German.
○ 3. The maternal grandfather experienced prolonged bleeding after surgery.
○ 4. The paternal grandmother died from chronic lymphocytic leukemia.

69. A diagnosis of hemophilia A is confirmed. As the child enters the second half of infancy, the nurse should teach the parents to
○ 1. administer one-half of a children's aspirin for a fever above 101°F.
○ 2. sew thick padding into the elbows and knees of the child's clothing.
○ 3. check the child's urine for occult blood every day.
○ 4. expect the eruption of the primary teeth to produce moderate to severe bleeding.

70. The nurse plans to teach the neonate's parents to recognize hemarthrosis, explaining that an early sign of hemarthrosis is
○ 1. the child's reluctance to move a body part.
○ 2. a cool, pale, clammy extremity.
○ 3. petechiae formation around a joint.
○ 4. instability of a long bone on passive movements.

71. The neonate's mother tells the nurse that when her child reaches school age, she is going to do home teaching. She does not want her child in school because the teacher will not watch him as well as she would. The mother's comments represent what common parental reaction to a child's chronic illness?
○ 1. Overprotection.
○ 2. Devotion.
○ 3. Mistrust.
○ 4. Insecurity.

72. The neonate experiences bleeding in the elbow, necessitating a trip to the emergency department. A lyophilized concentrate of Factor VIII is administered intravenously. Besides monitoring the infusion, which of the following nursing interventions would be appropriate to minimize bleeding in the affected area?
○ 1. Apply constant pressure to the elbow.
○ 2. Keep the elbow below the level of the heart.
○ 3. Place a warm, moist pack on the elbow.
○ 4. Immobilize and elevate the elbow.

73. Because of the risks associated with administration of Factor VIII concentrate, the nurse would teach the neonate's family to recognize and report
○ 1. yellowing of the skin.
○ 2. horizontal ridges on the nails.
○ 3. abdominal distension.
○ 4. paroxysmal, nonproductive coughing.

74. The mother tells the nurse she is afraid to allow her child to be very active because of the danger of injury and bleeding. The nurse explains that physical fitness is very important for children with hemophilia and that one ideal activity for them is
○ 1. snow skiing.
○ 2. swimming.
○ 3. football.
○ 4. gymnastics.

75. Which of the following nursing diagnoses would the nurse implement as part of this client's long-term care?
○ 1. Knowledge deficit.
○ 2. Potential for Injury.
○ 3. Self-Esteem Disturbance.
○ 4. Altered Health Maintenance.

76. Laboratory tests confirm the diagnosis of acquired immune deficiency syndrome (AIDS). The nurse should teach the parents that the most likely route of transmission of AIDS to their child was
○ 1. contamination of the Factor VIII replacement received during bleeding episodes.
○ 2. casual contact with a child who tested positive for human immunodeficiency virus (HIV).

○ 3. use of a contaminated needle to obtain a blood sample.
○ 4. ingestion of food prepared by a cook infected with HIV.

77. The nurse plans to teach the family about signs and symptoms of infection, stressing the need to be especially alert for which of the following?
○ 1. Erythema around the infected area.
○ 2. Fever above 100.5°F (measured rectally).
○ 3. Tenderness of the infected area.
○ 4. Warmth of the infected area.

The Client With Leukemia

An acutely ill 10-year-old girl is hospitalized with an upper respiratory infection and right otitis media. She is diagnosed with leukemia.

78. The nurse teaches the parents about leukemia. Which of the following descriptions given by the mother best indicates that she understands the nature of leukemia?
○ 1. The disease is infectious in nature and characterized by increased white blood cell production.
○ 2. The disease is neoplastic in nature and characterized by a proliferation of immature white blood cells.
○ 3. The disease is inflammatory in nature and characterized by solid tumor formation in the lymph nodes.
○ 4. The disease is allergic in nature and characterized by increased circulating antibodies in the bloodstream.

79. Laboratory findings show that the child is anemic. The nurse explains to the parents that the anemia most likely has resulted from blood loss and
○ 1. inadequate dietary iron intake.
○ 2. decreased red blood cell production.
○ 3. increased destruction of red blood cells by lymphocytes.
○ 4. progressive replacement of the bone marrow with scar tissue.

80. Which of the following statements would the nurse use to describe to the parents why their child was prone to infections?
○ 1. Play activities were too strenuous.
○ 2. Vitamin C intake had been inadequate over a period of time.
○ 3. Red blood cells were inadequate for carrying oxygen for tissue nourishment.
○ 4. White blood cells were incapable of handling an infectious process.

81. The nurse notes that the child has petechiae; that her gums, lips, and nose bleed easily; and that she has bruises on various parts of her body. Which of the following laboratory test results would the nurse expect?
○ 1. Low platelet count.
○ 2. Low serum calcium level.
○ 3. Insufficient fibrinogen concentration.
○ 4. High red blood cell count.

82. Which of the following measures should be kept to a minimum, when possible, because the child is prone to bruise and bleed easily?
○ 1. Administering stool softeners.
○ 2. Changing the position in bed.
○ 3. Offering food at frequent intervals.
○ 4. Administering drugs intramuscularly.

83. Which of the following measures would be contraindicated when the nurse provides oral hygiene for the child?
○ 1. Applying petroleum jelly to the lips.
○ 2. Cleaning the teeth with a toothbrush.
○ 3. Swabbing the mouth with moistened cotton swabs.
○ 4. Rinsing the mouth with a nonirritating mouthwash.

84. The nurse observes that an area in the child's mouth is bleeding. Which of the following items would the nurse use because it is most effective for promoting homeostasis over the lesion?
○ 1. Chewing gum.
○ 2. A cotton ball.
○ 3. A gauze sponge.
○ 4. A dry tea bag.

85. Which of the following beverages would the nurse plan to give the child when she feels nauseated?
○ 1. Milk.
○ 2. Weak tea.
○ 3. Plain water.
○ 4. A carbonated beverage.

86. The nurse should question the order if which drug is prescribed for the child to help relieve discomfort?
○ 1. Acetaminophen (Tylenol).
○ 2. Acetophenetidin (phenacetin).
○ 3. Acetylsalicylic acid (aspirin).
○ 4. Propoxyphene hydrochloride (Darvon).

87. The child is scheduled for a bone marrow aspiration. The nurse should prepare her for entry of the needle over which of the following bone sites?
○ 1. The radius.
○ 2. The sternum.
○ 3. A cervical vertebrae.
○ 4. The posterior iliac crest.

88. Which of the following nursing diagnoses would the nurse identify as a priority in dealing with this newly diagnosed leukemic child and family?
○ 1. Potential for Injury.

○ 2. Altered Comfort.
○ 3. Altered Nutrition.
○ 4. Anticipatory Grieving.

89. Mercaptopurine (Purinethol) 75 mg daily is prescribed. Mercaptopurine is marketed in 50-mg tablets for oral administration. How many tablets should the nurse give the child each day?
○ 1. 1/2 of 1 tablet.
○ 2. 1-1/2 tablets.
○ 3. 2 tablets.
○ 4. 2-1/2 tablets.

90. Which of the following signs and symptoms would suggest to the nurse the client is experiencing toxicity to mercaptopurine (Purinethol)?
○ 1. Nausea, vomiting, and diarrhea.
○ 2. Skin rash, constipation, and polyuria.
○ 3. Dry mouth, blurred vision, and headache.
○ 4. Drowsiness, malaise, and low blood pressure.

91. Mercaptopurine (Purinethol) and methotrexate (Amethopterin) are classified as antimetabolites. The nurse explains to the child's mother that antimetabolites function in the body to
○ 1. selectively destroy malignant cells, thereby slowing tumor growth.
○ 2. create a hormonal imbalance within the body that acts to suppress tumor growth.
○ 3. damage deoxyribonucleic acid (DNA) within cell nuclei, which in turn disrupts cell growth and division.
○ 4. imitate nutrients essential for malignant cell growth, thus preventing those cells from using natural nutrients.

92. The child is severely neutropeneic with a low absolute granulocyte count (AGC). The nurse should
○ 1. restrict staff and visitors with active infection.
○ 2. allow the child to play with other hospitalized children.
○ 3. consult with the physician about administering an antiemetic.
○ 4. consult with the physician about the low platelet count.

93. Allopurinol (Zyloprim) is prescribed. Which of the following nursing measures should be observed for a client taking allopurinol?
○ 1. Encouraging a high fluid intake.
○ 2. Omitting carbonated fluids.
○ 3. Giving foods high in potassium.
○ 4. Limiting foods high in natural sugar.

94. Methotrexate (Amethopterin) is prescribed. The nurse should question the order if the physician has not also ordered
○ 1. keeping the child in a state of fasting.
○ 2. a white blood cell count.
○ 3. an X ray examination of the spinal canal.
○ 4. collection of a specimen for urinalysis.

95. Methotrexate (Amethopterin) is administered by injecting it into the spinal canal. The nurse explains to the parents that this type of drug is called
○ 1. subdural.
○ 2. intrathecal.
○ 3. intraosseous.
○ 4. intra-arterial.

96. The child's absolute granulocyte count is now 900. The nurse would teach the mother that
○ 1. the child should stay away from siblings.
○ 2. the child should stay away from crowds.
○ 3. everyone who visits should wear a gown and mask.
○ 4. the child should be in isolation.

97. The child fails to respond to therapy. Which of the following statements offers the nurse the best guide in making plans to assist the parents in dealing with their child's imminent death?
○ 1. Knowing that the prognosis is poor helps prepare relatives for the death of children.
○ 2. Relatives are especially grieved when a child does well at first but then declines rapidly.
○ 3. Trust in health personnel who wish to help relatives in grief is most often destroyed by a death that is considered untimely.
○ 4. It is more difficult for relatives to accept the death of a 10-year-old than the death of a younger child whose family membership has been short.

98. Authorities generally agree that to help others deal with death, a nurse first must have
○ 1. experienced the death of a loved one.
○ 2. worked out a personal philosophy of life and death.
○ 3. taken a course that examined how best to deal with death and grieving.
○ 4. developed a belief that accepts a supreme being and a life after death.

99. Which of the following nursing diagnoses would be a priority for the family at this time?
○ 1. Ineffective Family Coping.
○ 2. Altered Parenting.
○ 3. Anxiety.
○ 4. Grieving.

100. Which of the following courses of action would be most appropriate for the nurse when planning to meet the family's emotional needs during the last days of their child's life?
○ 1. Restrict visitors to the parents so as not to overtax the child.
○ 2. Answer the child's questions about the illness and imminent death honestly.
○ 3. Concentrate nursing efforts on meeting the child's physical needs to help keep her mind on other things.
○ 4. Encourage the child to play quietly with a room-

mate to replace thoughts of sadness with thoughts of pleasurable things.

101. After the child dies, the mother asks the nurse, "What if we had brought her in when she first complained of an earache?" Which of the following would be the nurse's best response to the mother?

○ 1. Explain that everything possible was done for the child.
○ 2. Provide comfort by saying that the child is no longer suffering with an incurable illness.
○ 3. Explain that the child's physician is in the best position to explain what happened.
○ 4. Explain that infections are often the result of leukemia rather than the cause of it.

CORRECT ANSWERS AND RATIONALE

The letters in parentheses following the rationale identify the step of the nursing process (A, D, P, I, E); cognitive level (K, C, T, N); and client need (S, G, L, H). See the Answer Grid for the key.

The Client With a Ventricular Septal Defect

1. 2. The child and family would need to know what the cardiac catheterization is, what to expect, and what care will be provided. Alteration in comfort might be a consideration after the catheterization. There is no evidence that the child or family is noncompliant. Altered cardiac output is not the priority problem here. (D, N, G)
2. 3. Preschoolers are able to understand information that is individualized to their level. Including a plastic model of the heart and a catheter as part of the preoperative preparation may be helpful. The other family members will understand the heart model and catheter better than the preschooler. The most important aspect of teaching a preschooler is to have the family members there for support. (P, T, S)
3. 3. Erikson maintains that the chief psychosocial task of the preschool period is acquiring a sense of initiative. The child's activities center around energetic learning and seeking accomplishment and satisfaction in these activities. The conflict of guilt arises when the child oversteps the limits of abilities and behaves or acts inappropriately. Autonomy vs. shame and doubt is the psychosocial task of toddlers. Identity vs. identity diffusion is the task of early adolescents, and industry vs. inferiority is the task of school-age children. (P, C, L)
4. 2. In children, cardiac catheterization usually involves a right-sided approach because septal defects permit entry into the left side of the heart. The catheter is usually inserted into the femoral vein via a percutaneous puncture; a cutdown procedure is rarely used. The catheterization is usually performed under local anesthesia with sedation. Echocardiography involves the use of ultra-high-frequency sound waves. (P, T, G)
5. 4. Preparation is the joint responsibility of the physician, parents, and nurse. Overprotecting a preschooler can increase anxiety rather than decrease it. Preschoolers are cognitively ready to understand information that is individualized to their level. Little psychological preparation can be given to infants and toddlers. (I, T, L)
6. 4. The involved and uninvolved extremities should be compared in terms of color, temperature, pedal pulses, and capillary filling time. Vital signs, including blood pressure, are checked as often as every 15 minutes after the procedure to detect dysrhythmias and hypotension. Pulses, especially those below the catheterization site, are checked for equality and symmetry. Fluids should be encouraged following the procedure; the dye used during the catheterization procedure causes osmotic diuresis. (P, T, G)
7. 3. Antibiotics are suggested for children with heart defects before dental work is done to reduce the risk of bacterial infection. Activities are not restricted. Stitches are not necessary with a percutaneous approach. The pressure dressing will be removed before the child is discharged, allowing showering or bathing as usual. (P, T, G)

The Client With Tetralogy of Fallot

8. 3. The three congenital defects associated with tetralogy of Fallot are (1) stenosis of the pulmonary artery, (2) interventricular septal defect, and (3) deviation of the aorta. A possible fourth defect is hypertrophy of the right ventricle, which occurs as an adaptive mechanism to help overcome the effects of the three congenital defects. When pulmonary stenosis is severe, the child will be cyanotic because insufficient blood reaches the lungs for good oxygenation. (E, N, G)
9. 1. An electrocardiogram (ECG) records the electrical impulses in heart muscle and provides a graphic tracing of the pattern of the impulses and their sequence and magnitude. An ECG does not provide information about the pressure of the blood in the heart. Cardiac catheterization is used to measure the pressure in the heart chambers and major vessels and to measure the amount of blood entering the heart. Auscultation with a stethoscope is required to detect the various sounds made with each heartbeat. A phonocardiogram provides a graphic presentation of heart sounds. (P, T, G)
10. 1. The nurse's best response when a child asks if cardiac catheterization is painful is to explain that the child will feel some pressure when the catheter is introduced. The child's trust in the nurse will be quickly lost if the nurse is untruthful. Most children are sedated and feel little during the procedure. (I, T, S)
11. 1. Flexing the legs reduces venous flow of blood from the lower extremities. This reduces the volume of blood being shunted through the interventricular septal defect and the overriding aorta in the child with tetralogy of Fallot. As a result, the blood then entering the systemic circulation has a higher oxygen

content, and dyspnea is reduced. Flexing the legs also increases vascular resistance and pressure in the left ventricle. An infant will often assume a knee-chest position in a crib, or the mother learns to put the infant over her shoulder while holding the child in a knee-chest position to relieve dyspnea. (A, K, G)

12. 1. Before planning any teaching program for a child or an adult, the nurse's first step is to assess the child to determine what is already known. Even a 5-year-old child has some understanding of a condition present since birth. The child's interest will soon be lost if familiar material is repeated too often, however. Such techniques as placing information in a logical sequence, presenting the material in a progression from simple to complex, and using actual equipment for demonstrations are recommended, but should be used after obtaining baseline information about what the child already knows. (P, C, S)

13. 3. For planning care for this child, Knowledge Deficit would be the priority nursing diagnosis. The child would need to be prepared for what occurs before and after surgery. There is no evidence of Ineffective Family Coping or Altered Comfort before surgery. The child has been cyanotic since birth, so Impaired Gas Exchange would not be a priority diagnosis. (D, N, G)

14. 2. Clinical signs of low cardiac output and poor tissue perfusion include pale, cool extremities; cyanosis; weak, thready pulses; delayed capillary refill; and altered consciousness. (A, K, G)

15. 2. Taking digoxin 1 hour before meals or 2 hours after meals results in better drug absorption. Signs of digoxin toxicity include decreased heart rate. A digoxin dose is not repeated if the child vomits 30 minutes after ingestion. There would be no way to ascertain how much of the dose had been absorbed. (I, T, G)

16. 3. Digoxin should be kept locked up out of the reach of children. It is toxic and can be harmful, perhaps even fatal, if an overdose is taken. (I, T, G)

17. 1. Children who have undergone open heart surgery with a patch as part of the correction should receive on subacute bacterial endocarditis (SBE) precautions. SBE precautions include receiving an antibiotic before any invasive procedure. Having the child drink a large amount of fluid before a follow-up appointment is not necessary, as is taking frequent naps. Children will gear their rest schedule to their activities. In this situation there are no data to indicate that the child has a high serum potassium; therefore, potassium restriction would not be appropriate. (I, T, G)

18. 1. Because of the hemodynamic changes that occur with repair of the ventricular septal defect and pulmonary valvular stenosis, transient congestive heart failure may develop. The child will not be on bedrest, and in fact should be encouraged to walk in the halls of the unit. The child can be placed in a room with other children who are not contagious. Visitors are not restricted unless the pediatric unit has restrictive visiting. (I, T, G)

19. 3. Regression is defined as the act of moving backward. In psychology the term is used to describe a person who reverts to an earlier stage of behavior or emotion. Depression is characterized by feelings of sadness, gloom, and dispiritedness. Repression is a defense mechanism by which an unacceptable or painful experience is put out of the conscious mind. Rationalization is characterized by constant explanations and excuses for behavior. (D, K, L)

20. 2. The child with persistent hypoxia will eventually experience tissue changes in the body because of the low oxygen content of the blood (hypoxemia). Clubbing of the fingers is one common finding. It apparently results from tissue fibrosis and hypertrophy from the hypoxemia and from an increase in capillaries in the area, which occurs as the body attempts to improve blood supplies. The child may be small for his or her chronological age, but clubbing does not result from slow physical growth. Clubbing of the fingers is also associated with polycythemia, but polycythemia is not a component of tetralogy of Fallot. Destruction of the bone marrow is not related to a cyanotic heart malformation. Instead, bone marrow is actively producing erythrocytes to compensate for the chronic hypoxia. (P, C, G)

21. 1. Most parents find it especially difficult to allow a child who has been unable to be normally active before corrective heart surgery to lead a normal and active life after surgery. These parents are less likely to be apprehensive about persuading the child of the need for rest, having the child develop postoperative complications, and having the child's siblings treat the child as a handicapped person. (P, C, L)

22. 2. The central psychosocial task for the preschool child is to develop a sense of initiative versus guilt, according to Erikson's theory. Any environmental change may affect a child. In this situation, the sibling is very likely feeling less attention from the mother and is attempting to resolve the conflict with inappropriate behavior. (D, K, L)

The Client With Down Syndrome

23. 1. The goal in working with mentally retarded children is to train them to be as independent as possible, focusing on developmental skills. The child may not be capable of learning something new every day, but needs to repeat what has been taught previously.

The parents need to be strict and consistent when setting limits on behavior. (P, T, G)

24. 4. Being able to sit up at age 6 months is a typical developmental skill of a normal infant that could be expected to be delayed in a mentally retarded infant. Mentally retarded children tend to not use expressive language and to not respond to verbal commands at a level appropriate to their chronological age. Walking, which normally occurs at about age 1 year, is almost always delayed in mentally retarded children. (A, K, G)

25. 1. Self-Care Deficit would be the priority diagnosis for this child. The nurse should guide the family toward helping the child become as independent as possible. The child has a knowledge deficit inherent in her medical diagnosis of mental retardation, but this would not be a priority diagnosis. There are no data to support an alteration in nutritional status. The child is developmentally delayed but has no physical impairment. (D, N, G)

26. 3. With recent advances in the care of the mentally retarded, it has been found that most persons with IQ's between about 35 and 50 can learn to take care of their hygienic needs, use acceptable social manners, and manage speech and other simple means of communication. Persons with IQ's between about 50 and 75 are educable. Custodial care is required for the severely and profoundly retarded, those persons with IQ's below about 35. (A, K, G)

27. 4. Nonthreatening experiences that are stimulating and interesting to the child have been observed to help raise IQ. Such practices as serving nutritious meals, administering vasodilating drugs, and letting the child play with more able children have not been demonstrated to increase intelligence. (P, T, G)

28. 3. It is especially important to observe the nature of the child's respirations because children with Down syndrome are prone to develop respiratory infections. (P, T, G)

29. 4. The parents must continue to work daily with their retarded child when the nurse is not there. Instructions and counseling are directed toward increasing their ability to care for the child confidently. A sense of liking for, responsibility for, and understanding of the child tends to grow as this primary goal is accomplished. (P, T, L)

30. 1. The primary aim of genetic counseling is to inform couples of birth defect risks. Reporting results of chromosome analysis of amniotic cells and preparing a couple psychologically for the birth of a defective child are secondary. A decision about birth control methods should be left to the couple. (P, T, L)

31. 4. To respond to a mother who becomes angry when someone calls her child retarded instead of exceptional, the nurse should give the mother a chance to explore her feelings on the subject because she is upset. Trying to use logic, defending the comment, or apologizing are not effective ways to handle the situation. Asking "why" questions may cause the mother to become defensive and does not encourage exploration of feelings. (P, T, L)

32. 3. Goals for a mentally retarded child should be simple and attainable. It is best to break down skills, such as dressing oneself, into many small steps and have the child repeat each step with slowly advancing variations. A series of small, short-term goals would be most appropriate. (P, T, S)

33. 2. The most likely explanation why this mentally retarded child tends to deliberately do things that displease her mother is that she is seeking attention from the mother. Often, the child's need for attention is greater than her fear of being punished and worth risking the mother's displeasure. (A, C, L)

34. 1. Very often, the best reinforcement for desired behavior in children is reward or praise, as described in this situation. Such techniques as scolding the child, ignoring the child, or making the child leave the table when misbehaving do not help reinforce desired behavior. (I, N, H)

The Client With Rheumatic Fever

35. 4. Rheumatic fever is an inflammatory collagen disease that typically follows an infection by Group A beta-hemolytic streptococci. The infection ordinarily occurs in the throat. Rheumatic fever generally follows infection with streptococci within approximately 2 weeks. It is believed that the disease involves an autoimmune or allergic response to the organism. Mumps, measles, and viral influenza are caused by viruses and do not predispose to rheumatic fever. (A, K, G)

36. 1. A heart rate of 150 beats/minute is very high for a 7-year-old child and may indicate carditis. Red, swollen joints, red rash, and twitching or chorea are all findings indicative of rheumatic fever. If present, these signs do not require immediate physician notification, however. (A, N, G)

37. 2. The nurse would encourage and plan to provide long periods of rest for the child with carditis to allow the heart to rest. With carditis, the client will be on bedrest which will curtail many types of activities. There is no reason to encourage the child to eat as much as possible; in fact, overeating should be discouraged, as it will tax the heart muscle. The parents should be made to feel as if they can come and go as they need to. The child is not in critical condition, so the parents do not need to be encouraged to stay at the bedside. (P, T, S)

38. 1. A nursing diagnosis should state a health problem derived from existing evidence about the client and from sound nursing knowledge. The health problem should be amenable to nursing care and should serve as a basis for planning and carrying out client-centered nursing care. Promoting comfort is a nursing responsibility and can serve as a basis for planning and carrying out nursing care. Based on the information given about this client, it is less likely for the child to have impaired fluid volume, tissue perfusion, or nutrition. (D, N, G)

39. 3. Exactly why rheumatic fever follows a streptococcal infection is not known, but it is theorized that an antigen-antibody response occurs to an M protein present in certain strains of streptococci. The antibodies developed by the body attack certain tissues, such as in the heart and joints. Antistreptolysin O (ASO) titer findings show elevated or rising antibody levels. This blood finding is the most reliable evidence indicating a streptococcal infection. (A, K, G)

40. 1. Long-term treatment for rheumatic fever involves monthly penicillin injections to prevent subsequent streptococcal infections, which can cause further heart damage. The current inflammation will subside with bedrest and aspirin or steroids. There is no indication that inflammation will subside with fewer side effects while the child receives long-term antibiotic therapy. (E, N, G)

41. 2. Every effort is made to reduce the work of the heart during the acute phase of rheumatic fever when the heart is inflamed. Bedrest with very limited activity is recommended to help prevent heart failure. Rheumatic fever is among the leading causes of heart failure and death in children between age 5 and 15. (E, K, G)

42. 4. School-age children enjoy board games and are commonly very intense about following rules. Their play can often become emotional. Adequate rest is of utmost importance during the acute stage of rheumatic fever. Therefore, playing a game with another child probably would be too strenuous. Such diversional activities as reading a book, playing with a doll, and listening to a radio would be more satisfactory. (P, C, G)

43. 1. In rheumatic fever, the connective tissue of the heart is inflamed. Signs of carditis indicate inflammation severe enough to compromise heart function. The most common signs of carditis include heart murmurs, tachycardia during rest, cardiac enlargement, and changes in the electrical conductivity of the heart. Heart murmurs are present in about 75% of all clients during the first week of carditis and in 85% of clients by the third week. Low blood pressure, an irregular pulse rate, and pain over the anterior chest wall are not related to the inflammatory process of rheumatic fever. (I, T, S)

44. 2. Digitalis preparations, such as digoxin (Lanoxin), act to improve and strengthen the heartbeat. They increase cardiac output by increasing the strength of the heart's contraction and also decrease the heart rate. Digitalis is not used to relax artery walls, prevent irregularities in ventricular contractions, or eliminate dissociation of ventricular and atrial rhythms. (I, T, G)

45. 3. The following calculation shows how to determine the correct amount of medication when 0.15 mg of a drug is prescribed for each dose and the preparation on hand contains 0.05 mg/ml:

$$0.15 \text{ mg} : x \text{ ml} :: 0.05 \text{ mg} : 1 \text{ ml}$$

$$0.05x = 0.15$$

$$x = \frac{0.15}{0.05} = 3 \text{ ml}$$

The correct dosage will be contained in 3 ml of the drug in solution. (I, T, S)

46. 2. An above-average pulse rate that is out of proportion to the degree of fever present is an early sign of cardiac failure in a client with rheumatic fever. The sleeping pulse is used to determine whether mild tachycardia is present during sleep or whether it is the result of normal daytime activity. (I, T, G)

47. 2. Five grains of a drug are equivalent to 0.32 g or 0.3 g. (I, T, S)

48. 4. Signs and symptoms of early salicylate toxicity include tinnitis, disturbances in hearing and vision, and dizziness. Salicylate toxicity may cause nausea, vomiting, diarrhea, and bleeding from mucous membranes from long-term use. Chest pain, pink-colored urine, and a slow pulse rate are not associated with salicylate toxicity. (P, N, S)

49. 3. In rheumatic fever, the joints—especially the knees, ankles, elbows, and wrists—are painful, swollen, red, and hot to the touch. Pain is typically minimized by limiting movement of the affected joints. Exercise should be avoided, contrary to usual recommendations for clients with other forms of arthritis. Despite joint involvement in rheumatic fever, permanent deformities do not occur. Massaging the joints and applying ice likely will not relieve pain. (I, T, G)

50. 4. For a child with arthritis associated with rheumatic fever, the joints are generally so tender that even the weight of bed linens can cause pain. Using a bed cradle is recommended to help remove the weight of the linens on painful joints. Supporting the body in good alignment and changing the client's position are recommended, but these nursing measures are not likely to relieve pain. Applying traction to the joints is not recommended. Traction is usually used to relieve muscle spasms, and these are not associated with rheumatic fever. (I, T, G)

51. 1. For a child with chorea-like movements, safety is of prime importance. Feeding the child may be difficult. Forks should be avoided because of the danger of injury to the mouth and face with the tines. (P, T, S)

52. 2. A child who has had rheumatic fever is likely to develop the illness again after a future streptococcal infection. Therefore, it is advised that such a child receive antibiotic prophylaxis for at least 5 years and sometimes even longer after the acute attack to prevent recurrence. (I, T, G)

53. 1. Usually other children in the family do not get rheumatic fever. There is no medicine to give the children as prophylactic therapy. They have been exposed to their sibling's rheumatic fever and streptococcal infection. If the other children do not have a streptococcal infection at this time, they probably will not develop it now. Girls are also at risk for developing rheumatic fever. (I, T, G)

The Client With Sickle-Cell Anemia

54. 3. A major therapeutic consideration during a sickle-cell crisis is increasing the transport and availability of oxygen to the body's tissues. Ways to do this include administering a high volume of intravenous fluid and electrolytes to help compensate for the acidosis resulting from hypoxemia associated with sickle-cell crisis. The fluids also help overcome the dehydration with which the patient usually suffers. Rest and analgesics are common components of therapy for sickle-cell crisis. Anticoagulants have been suggested, but they are not included in the general treatment of crisis. Exchange transfusions are used only in certain situations. Iron therapy is contraindicated for this condition. (P, C, G)

55. 3. Characteristic sickle cells tend to cause "log jams" in capillaries. This results in poor circulation to local tissues, leading to ischemia and necrosis. The basic defect in sickle-cell disease is an abnormality in the structure of the red blood cells. The erythrocytes are sickle-shaped, rough in texture, and rigid. (I, T, G)

56. 3. Alerted by the infant's self-positioning on the side with the knees sharply flexed, the nurse should assess for further evidence of abdominal pain. Regression is common in acutely ill hospitalized children, but insufficient data are given in this item to confirm regression to early infancy. Nausea usually causes an infant to refuse nourishment. A backache would most probably cause an infant to lie supine to relieve discomfort. (A, C, G)

57. 4. Children with sickle-cell disease are prone to develop infections as a result of the necrosis of areas within the body and a generalized less-than-optimal health status. The child is often anorexic, gains weight slowly, and exhibits malaise and irritability. Specific signs of infection are sore throat and fever. Fatigue, lassitude, headaches, and nausea could be prodromal signs of infection, but could also be signs of other illnesses. Skin rash and itching usually do not indicate an infection but may be a contact dermatitis. The exception would be varicella; therefore, an assessment should include questions about recent contacts with infected persons. An infection in a child with sickle-cell disease often brings on a crisis and should be treated promptly. (I, T, G)

58. 3. Because sickle cells tend to "log jam" in capillaries, it is important that the child receive adequate fluids. The fluids will increase the blood volume and help prevent the "log jam" action. Children with a chronic illness need to be around other children for normal growth and development. This child should not be around other children with an active infection, however. The parents need to allow the child some independence for normal development. Keeping the child with them at all times will overprotect that child and make the child dependent. (I, T, H)

59. 4. Sickle-cell disease is an inherited disease that is present at birth. However, 60% to 80% of a newborn's hemoglobin is fetal hemoglobin, which has a structure different from hemoglobin S and A. Sickling with symptoms generally occurs about 4 months after birth. Some hemoglobin S is produced by the fetus near term. The fetus produces all its own hemoglobin from the earliest production in the first trimester. Passive immunity conferred by maternal antibodies is not related to sickle-cell disease, but this transmission of antibodies is important to protect the infant from various infections during early infancy. (I, T, G)

60. 1. Sickle-cell disease is an autosomal recessive Mendelian disorder. Therefore, if both parents have the trait, there is a 1 in 4 chance that a child will have the disease and a 1 in 2 chance that a child will have the trait. (I, T, G)

61. 3. Altered comfort is a priority problem that nurses can do something about. Promoting comfort is a nursing responsibility and serves as a basis for planning and carrying out nursing care. Fluid volume deficit is also a problem that the nurse can treat, with intravenous fluids and electrolytes. There is no information here to indicate that ineffective coping is occurring. Altered cardiac output is not a problem with this type of vaso-occlusive crisis. (D, T, G)

The Client With Iron-Deficiency Anemia

62. 2. Solids should be introduced at approximately age 5 to 6 months. Full-term infants use up their prenatal iron stores within 4 to 6 months after birth. Cow's milk contains insufficient iron. (I, C, G)

63. 2. Intake of iron-rich solids needs to be increased and intake of milk needs to be decreased to 1 quart per day. It is impossible to obtain the needed iron from milk alone, but milk does contain essential minerals and vitamins. Decreasing milk intake will increase the child's hunger for and tolerance of solids. Near-exclusive intake of iron-rich solids can cause constipation and inadequate absorption of essential nutrients. (I, T, H)

64. 1. Relatively high amounts of iron are contained in eggs, iron-fortified cereals, meats, and green vegetables. Fruits, nonfortified cereals, milk, yellow vegetables, and juices contain less iron than do eggs, iron-fortified cereals, meats, and green vegetables. (E, N, G)

65. 2. Children with iron-deficiency anemia are more susceptible to infection because of marked decreases in bone marrow functioning with microcytosis. (I, C, G)

66. 2. Iron drops are better absorbed when mixed with fruit juice or followed by fruit juice. Milk tends to decrease iron absorption. Medication should not be mixed in a bottle of fluids. If the child does not drink all the bottle it is not known how much of the medication the child actually received. (I, T, G)

The Client With Hemophilia and Acquired Immune Deficiency Syndrome

67. 4. Partial thromboplastin time (PTT) measures the activity of thromboplastin, which is dependent on intrinsic clotting factors. In hemophilia, the intrinsic clotting Factor VIII (antihemophilic factor) is deficient, resulting in a prolonged PTT. Bleeding time, tourniquet test, and clot retraction test measure platelet function, vasoconstriction, and capillary fragility. These are unaffected in persons with hemophilia. (I, C, G)

68. 3. Hemophilia A is a genetically transmitted X-linked recessive disorder characterized by a deficiency of plasma Factor VIII. A hemophiliac man and a normal woman have normal male children and female children who carry the hemophilia trait. The carrier females pass the abnormal gene to half of their sons. Ethnic background and familial leukemia are unrelated to the development of hemophilia. (A, K, G)

69. 2. As the hemophilic child begins to acquire motor skills, the risk of bleeding increases because of falls and bumps. Such injuries can be minimized by padding vulnerable joints. Aspirin is contraindicated because of its antiplatelet properties. Because genitourinary bleeding is not a typical problem in children with hemophilia, urine testing is not indicated. Tooth eruption does not normally cause bleeding episodes in children with hemophilia. (P, T, G)

70. 1. Bleeding into the joints in the child with hemophilia leads to pain and tenderness, resulting in restricted movement. If the bleeding continues, the area becomes hot, swollen, and immobile. Petechial bleeding is not a problem in hemophilia. (P, T, G)

71. 1. Overprotection is a typical parental reaction to chronic illness. Its characteristics include sacrifice of self and family for the child, failure to recognize the child's capabilities and sense of responsibility, placement of overly stringent restrictions on play and peer friendship, and a lack of confidence in other peoples' capabilities. (D, K, G)

72. 4. When a bleeding episode occurs, the affected area should be immobilized and elevated to slow blood flow to the area and promote hemostasis. Pressure should be applied to the area for 10 to 15 minutes to promote clot formation. Cold packs promote vasoconstriction; warm packs promote vasodilation and bleeding. (I, C, G)

73. 1. Because Factor VIII concentrate is derived from large pools of human plasma, the risk of hepatitis is always present. Clinical manifestations of hepatitis include yellowing of the skin, mucous membranes, and sclera. (P, T, G)

74. 2. Swimming is an ideal activity for a child with hemophilia. Many noncontact sports and physical activities that do not place excessive strain on joints are also appropriate. Such activities strengthen the muscles surrounding joints and help control bleeding in these areas. Noncontact sports also enhance general mental and physical well-being. (I, T, G)

75. 2. The priority long-term nursing diagnosis for this child would be Potential for Injury. This is always a concern for children with hemophilia. As with all children who have chronic illnesses, there is a potential for self-esteem problems. There is no data in this item to support this. The parents should have a good understanding of the disease process and realize the importance of obtaining regular health care for their child. (D, T, G)

76. 1. The AIDS virus is spread by direct contact with blood or blood products and by sexual contact. Children with hemophilia are at particular risk for AIDS because of the factor concentrate infusions they receive. These concentrates are derived from larger quantities of pooled plasma, exposing recipients to thousands of blood donors. There is no evidence that casual contact between infected and uninfected persons transmits the responsible virus. The sterile disposable needles used in all hospitals and clinics to perform venipunctures are not a source of AIDS transmission. (I, C, G)

77. 2. Fever is a cardinal manifestation of infection in persons with AIDS. Because the major physiological alteration in AIDS is generalized immune system dysfunction, typical indicators of the body's response to infection, such as erythema, warmth, and/or tenderness may be absent. (P, T, G)

The Client With Leukemia

78. 2. Leukemia is a neoplastic disorder of blood-forming tissues characterized by a proliferation of immature white blood cells. Leukemia is not an infectious, inflammatory, or allergic disease. (E, N, G)

79. 2. The anemia seen in leukemia is caused by the bone marrow's overproduction of immature white blood cells, at the expense of producing red blood cells and platelets. In this client, anemia is not caused by an inadequate intake of iron, but rather by insufficient red blood cells. The bone marrow is not scarred. (I, C, G)

80. 4. In leukemia, normal white blood cells are decreased (that is, they fail to mature); hence, a child with leukemia is subject to infection. The major morbidity and mortality factor associated with leukemia is infection due to the presence of granulocytopenia. (I, C, G)

81. 1. Megakaryocytes, from which platelets derive, are decreased in leukemia. Platelet counts are low, and the child is subject to easy bruising and bleeding. Low serum calcium, faculty thrombin production, or insufficient fibrinogen concentration are not related to bleeding and bruising in a child with leukemia. (A, C, G)

82. 4. All treatments should be performed gently when caring for a child with leukemia, who is prone to bruising and bleeding. When there is a choice, injections should be avoided or limited. Such measures as administering a stool softener, changing the position in bed, and offering food at frequent intervals are indicated and need not be curtailed because of the increased risk of bleeding. (I, T, S)

83. 2. The oral mucous membranes are easily damaged and are often ulcerated in clients with leukemia. It is better to provide oral hygiene without using a toothbrush, which can easily damage sensitive oral mucosa. Applying petrolatum jelly to the lips, swabbing the mouth with moistened cotton swabs, and rinsing the mouth with a nonirritating mouthwash are appropriate oral care measures for a child with leukemia. (I, T, G)

84. 4. A dry tea bag placed on the bleeding area can be effective to control bleeding from lesions on the oral mucosa. The tannic acid in the tea apparently helps control bleeding. (I, T, G)

85. 4. Carbonated beverages ordinarily are best tolerated when the child feels nauseated. Many children find cola drinks especially easy to tolerate, but noncola beverages are also recommended. (P, T, G)

86. 3. Acetylsalicylic acid (aspirin) prolongs the bleeding time by interfering with proper blood clotting. This drug is contraindicated in clients with leukemia. Nonnarcotic drugs other than aspirin may be prescribed to control pain; narcotic analgesics may be required when pain is severe. (I, T, G)

87. 4. Although bone marrow specimens may be obtained from various sites, the most commonly used site in children is the posterior iliac crest. The area is close to the body's surface but removed from vital organs. The area is large, so specimens can be easily obtained. For infants, the proximal tibia and the posterior iliac crest are used. (P, C, G)

88. 4. The newly diagnosed child and parents are overwhelmed when first informed of the diagnosis. The family and child go through the beginning stages of grieving in anticipation of what may occur. The child may have very little discomfort, some changes in nutritional status, and increased potential for injury, but these would not be priority diagnoses. (D, N, L)

89. 2. The nurse determines the number of 50-mg tablets of a drug to give when the client is to receive 75 mg of the drug for each dosage by using ratios, as follows:

$$1 \text{ tablet}:50 \text{ mg}::x \text{ tablets}:75 \text{ mg}$$

$$50x = 75$$

$$x = 75/50 = 1\tfrac{1}{2} \text{ tablets.}$$

(I, T, S)

90. 1. Toxic doses of mercaptopurine (Purinethol) most likely will produce anorexia, nausea, vomiting, and diarrhea. This drug tends to cause bone marrow suppression; thus, blood counts are especially important. Some of the other signs described in this scenario may be present but are not characteristic of mercaptopurine toxicity. (A, K, S)

91. 4. Antimetabolites have chemical structures resembling those of substances used normally for cell growth and metabolism. These drugs keep cancer cells from using natural nutrients in metabolic processes and therefore interfere with the cellular growth and development of cancer cells. (I, C, G)

92. 1. With a low absolute granulocyte count (AGC), the child will have difficulty fighting off an infection, so staff and visitors are restricted to those without an active infection. The child will be in a private room and will not be allowed to play with other hospitalized children. The physician will not be called, because AGC refers to a specific white blood cell, the granulocyte. (P, T, S)

93. 1. Destruction of malignant cells during chemotherapy produces large amounts of uric acid. The client's kidneys may not be able to eliminate the uric acid, and tubular obstruction from the crystals could result in renal failure and uremia. Allopurinol (Zyloprim) interrupts the process of purine degradation to reduce uric acid buildup. The client should be encouraged to increase fluid intake to further assist in eliminating uric acid. (P, C, G)

94. 2. Methotrexate (Amethopterin) is not highly toxic in low doses but may cause severe leukopenia at higher doses. It is customary and recommended for blood tests to be done before therapy to provide a baseline from which to study the effects of the drug on white blood cell levels. (I, T, G)

95. 2. Methotrexate is administered intrathecally when it is injected into the spinal canal. This route is also called the intraspinal route and the technique is the same as that for a lumbar puncture. The intraosseous route involves injecting a drug in bone tissue. The intraarterial route involves injection into an artery. (I, C, S)

96. 2. The child should avoid crowds because of the risk of exposure to infection. Siblings and others should stay away from the child if they have an active infection. The child's AGC is high enough so that a mask, gown, and isolation are not necessary. (I, N, G)

97. 2. It has been found that parents are more grieved when optimism is followed by defeat. The nurse should recognize this when planning various ways to help the parents of a dying child. It is not necessarily true that knowing about a poor prognosis for years helps prepare parents for a child's death, that trust in health personnel is destroyed when a death is untimely, or that it is more difficult for parents to accept the death of an older child than a younger child. (P, T, L)

98. 2. The nurse caring for terminally ill clients is better prepared to do so when she or he has worked out a personal philosophy of death. Although other experiences, such as having lost a loved one to death, taking classes in caring for dying clients and grieving, and developing a personal belief in a supreme being and a life hereafter may be helpful in assisting the nurse in thinking about death. Most important are the nurse's own feelings about life and death. (P, K, L)

99. 4. Because this family is waiting for the child to die, the most appropriate nursing diagnosis would be Grieving. Families grieve at the time of diagnosis as well as during the illness, as the child is dying, and after death has occurred. This is a normal process and does not indicate ineffective family coping, ineffective parenting, or anxiety. (D, N, L)

100. 2. Most clients, even children, are aware when death appears imminent. The best policy is to answer the child's questions honestly. This helps the child tend to feel less isolated and alone. Such actions as restricting visitors, concentrating on efforts to make the child think of something other than death, and encouraging the child to replace thoughts of sadness with thoughts of pleasurable things are not recommended and tend to increase the dying child's fear, isolation, and feelings of loss of control. (P, T, L)

101. 4. Just as with the child, it is best to answer relatives honestly when they ask questions about their loved one's condition. The nurse answers the questions honestly when explaining that infections are often the result of leukemia rather than a cause of it. It is less satisfactory to tell parents that everything possible has been done for their child, that the child is no longer suffering from the illness, and that the physician is in the best possible position to answer their questions. (I, C, L)

NURSING CARE OF CHILDREN

TEST 3: The Child With Cardiovascular Health Problems

Directions: Use this answer grid to determine areas of strength or need for further study.

NURSING PROCESS

A = Assessment
D = Analysis, nursing diagnosis
P = Planning
I = Implementation
E = Evaluation

COGNITIVE LEVEL

K = Knowledge
C = Comprehension
T = Application
N = Analysis

CLIENT NEEDS

S = Safe, effective care environment
G = Physiological integrity
L = Psychosocial integrity
H = Health promotion/maintenance

		Nursing Process					Cognitive Level				Client Needs			
Question #	Answer #	A	D	P	I	E	K	C	T	N	S	G	L	H
1	2		D							N		G		
2	3			P					T		S			
3	3			P				C					L	
4	2			P					T			G		
5	4				I				T				L	
6	4			P					T			G		
7	3			P					T			G		
8	3					E				N		G		
9	1			P					T			G		
10	1				I				T		S			
11	1	A					K					G		
12	1			P				C			S			
13	3		D							N		G		
14	2	A					K					G		
15	2				I				T			G		
16	3				I				T			G		
17	1				I				T			G		
18	1				I				T			G		
19	3		D				K						L	
20	2			P				C				G		
21	1			P				C					L	
22	2		D				K						L	
23	1			P					T			G		

ANSWER GRID: 1

NURSING PROCESS

A = Assessment
D = Analysis, nursing diagnosis
P = Planning
I = Implementation
E = Evaluation

COGNITIVE LEVEL

K = Knowledge
C = Comprehension
T = Application
N = Analysis

CLIENT NEEDS

S = Safe, effective care environment
G = Physiological integrity
L = Psychosocial integrity
H = Health promotion/maintenance

		Nursing Process					Cognitive Level				Client Needs			
Question #	Answer #	A	D	P	I	E	K	C	T	N	S	G	L	H
24	4	A					K					G		
25	1		D							N		G		
26	3	A					K					G		
27	4			P					T			G		
28	3			P					T			G		
29	4			P					T				L	
30	1			P					T				L	
31	4			P					T				L	
32	3			P					T		S			
33	2	A						C					L	
34	1				I					N				H
35	4	A					K					G		
36	1	A								N		G		
37	2			P					T		S			
38	1		D							N		G		
39	3	A					K					G		
40	1					E				N		G		
41	2					E	K					G		
42	4			P				C				G		
43	1				I				T		S			
44	2				I				T			G		
45	3				I				T		S			
46	2				I				T			G		
47	2				I				T		S			
48	4			P						N	S			
49	3				I				T			G		
50	4				I				T			G		
51	1			P					T		S			
52	2				I				T			G		

ANSWER GRID: 2

Nursing Process

A = Assessment
D = Analysis, nursing diagnosis
P = Planning
I = Implementation
E = Evaluation

Cognitive Level

K = Knowledge
C = Comprehension
T = Application
N = Analysis

Client Needs

S = Safe, effective care environment
G = Physiological integrity
L = Psychosocial integrity
H = Health promotion/maintenance

		Nursing Process					Cognitive Level				Client Needs			
Question #	Answer #	A	D	P	I	E	K	C	T	N	S	G	L	H
53	1				I				T			G		
54	3			P				C				G		
55	3				I				T			G		
56	3	A						C				G		
57	4				I				T			G		
58	3				I				T					H
59	4				I				T			G		
60	1				I				T			G		
61	3		D						T			G		
62	2				I			C				G		
63	2				I				T					H
64	1					E				N		G		
65	2				I			C				G		
66	2				I				T			G		
67	4				I			C				G		
68	3	A					K					G		
69	2			P					T			G		
70	1			P					T			G		
71	1		D				K					G		
72	4				I			C				G		
73	1			P					T			G		
74	2				I				T			G		
75	2		D						T			G		
76	1				I			C				G		
77	2			P					T			G		
78	2					E				N		G		
79	2				I			C				G		
80	4				I			C				G		
81	1	A						C				G		

Answer Grid: 3

Nursing Process

A = Assessment
D = Analysis, nursing diagnosis
P = Planning
I = Implementation
E = Evaluation

Cognitive Level

K = Knowledge
C = Comprehension
T = Application
N = Analysis

Client Needs

S = Safe, effective care environment
G = Physiological integrity
L = Psychosocial integrity
H = Health promotion/maintenance

		Nursing Process					Cognitive Level				Client Needs			
Question #	Answer #	A	D	P	I	E	K	C	T	N	S	G	L	H
82	4				I				T		S			
83	2				I				T			G		
84	4				I				T			G		
85	4			P					T			G		
86	3				I				T			G		
87	4			P				C				G		
88	4		D							N			L	
89	2				I				T		S			
90	1	A					K				S			
91	2				I			C				G		
92	1			P					T		S			
93	1			P				C				G		
94	2				I				T			G		
95	2				I			C			S			
96	2				I					N		G		
97	2			P					T				L	
98	2			P			K						L	
99	4		D							N			L	
100	2			P					T				L	
101	4				I			C					L	
Number Correct														
Number Possible	101	12	11	32	41	5	13	21	53	14	15	68	15	3
Percentage Correct														

Score Calculation:

To determine your **Percentage Correct**, divide the **Number Correct** by the **Number Possible**.

Answer Grid: 4

The Child With Health Problems of the Upper Gastrointestinal Tract

Test 4

The Client With Cleft Lip and Palate
The Client With a Tracheoesophageal Fistula
The Client With Imperforate Anus
The Client With Pyloric Stenosis
The Client With Intussusception
The Client With Inguinal Hernia
The Client With Hirschsprung's Disease
Correct Answers and Rationale

Select the one best answer and indicate your choice by filling in the answer in front of the option.

The Client With Cleft Lip and Palate

An infant born with a cleft lip and palate is transferred from the hospital's newborn nursery to a pediatric unit for care.

1. The infant's parents are shocked when they see their child for the first time. Which of the following nursing actions would most help the parents accept their infant's anomaly?
- ○ 1. Bring the infant to them more often.
- ○ 2. Reassure them that surgery will correct the defect.
- ○ 3. Show them pictures of babies before and after corrective surgery.
- ○ 4. Allow them to complete their grieving process before seeing the infant again.

2. Which of the following goals would the nurse identify as a priority for the infant?
- ○ 1. Preventing infection in the infant's mouth.
- ○ 2. Using techniques to minimize crying.
- ○ 3. Altering the usual method of feeding.
- ○ 4. Preventing the infant from putting fingers in the mouth.

3. Which of the following measures would the nurse use to help the infant retain feedings?
- ○ 1. Bubble the infant at frequent intervals.
- ○ 2. Feed only small amounts at one time.
- ○ 3. Place the nipple on the back of the infant's tongue.
- ○ 4. Hold the infant in a lying position while feeding.

4. The nurse would identify which of the following as a priority nursing diagnosis for the infant and family?
- ○ 1. Impaired Gas Exchange.
- ○ 2. Anticipatory Grieving.
- ○ 3. Ineffective Family Coping.
- ○ 4. Altered Parenting.

5. The infant has surgery to repair the cleft lip. The nurse observes that the infant is having difficulty breathing postoperatively. Which of the following measures would be most helpful in bringing relief?
- ○ 1. Raising the infant's head.
- ○ 2. Turning the infant onto the abdomen.
- ○ 3. Inserting an airway into the infant's mouth.
- ○ 4. Exerting downward pressure on the infant's chin.

6. Which of the following methods would the nurse use to feed an infant following surgical repair of cleft lip?
- ○ 1. Gastric gavage.
- ○ 2. Intravenous infusion.
- ○ 3. A rubber-tipped medicine dropper.
- ○ 4. A bottle with a large-holed nipple.

7. Which of the following nursing diagnoses would the nurse identify as a priority after surgical repair?
- ○ 1. Altered Comfort.
- ○ 2. High Risk for Infection.
- ○ 3. Impaired Physical Mobility.
- ○ 4. Altered Parenting.

8. To keep the surgical suture line clean and free of debris, the nurse should remove formula and drainage with cotton-tipped applicators moistened with
- ○ 1. mineral oil.
- ○ 2. distilled water.
- ○ 3. mild antiseptic solution.
- ○ 4. half-strength hydrogen peroxide.

9. Before the infant is discharged from the hospital, the mother is taught to seek health care if the infant develops an upper respiratory infection because of the risk of which complication?
- ○ 1. Pneumonia.
- ○ 2. Dehydration.
- ○ 3. Otitis media.
- ○ 4. Laryngotracheobronchitis.

10. The parents ask the nurse when their infant's cleft palate likely will be repaired. The nurse should base the response on knowledge that first repair of a cleft palate is usually done
- ○ 1. before the eruption of teeth.
- ○ 2. after the child learns to sit alone.
- ○ 3. before the development of speech.
- ○ 4. after the child learns to drink from a cup.

11. The child is eventually admitted to the hospital for repair of the cleft palate. Which of the following eating utensils would be most appropriate for the child on the second day after the surgery?
- ○ 1. A cup.
- ○ 2. A drinking tube.
- ○ 3. An Asepto syringe.
- ○ 4. A large-holed nipple.

12. Which of the following types of restraints would be best for the nurse to use for the child in the immediate postoperative period after cleft palate repair?
- ○ 1. Safety jacket.
- ○ 2. Elbow restraints.
- ○ 3. Arm and leg restraints.
- ○ 4. Arm and body restraints.

13. In which of the following positions would the nurse place the child to irrigate the mouth after cleft palate repair?
- ○ 1. On the back with the head turned to the side.
- ○ 2. In low Fowler's position with the head straight.
- ○ 3. In a sitting position with the head tilted forward.
- ○ 4. On the abdomen with the head hanging over the side of the bed.

14. The mother is encouraged to stay with her child as much as possible for the first few days after surgery. Which of the following activities by the mother would offer the most support to the child during this time?
- ○ 1. Holding and cuddling the child.
- ○ 2. Helping the child play with some of the toys.
- ○ 3. Reading some of the child's favorite stories.
- ○ 4. Staying at the bedside and holding the child's hand.

15. The nurse will teach the mother that after cleft palate surgery there is a chance that her child may have which of the following problems?
- ○ 1. Weight loss.
- ○ 2. Weight gain.
- ○ 3. Lack of a strong self-concept.
- ○ 4. Speech defect.

The Client With a Tracheoesophageal Fistula

Several hours after birth, assessment reveals that the newborn boy has a tracheoesophageal fistula.

16. The parents express feelings of guilt about their infant's anomaly. Which of the following approaches by the nurse would best support the parents?
- ○ 1. Help the parents accept their feelings as normal.
- ○ 2. Explain that the parents did nothing to cause the infant's defect.
- ○ 3. Encourage the parents to concentrate on long-term plans for the infant.
- ○ 4. Urge the parents to visit their infant as often as possible during hospitalization.

17. The infant is admitted to the pediatric surgical unit. In the initial assessment, the nurse can expect to observe which typical sign of a tracheoesophageal fistula (TEF)?
- ○ 1. Continuous drooling.
- ○ 2. Diaphragmatic breathing.
- ○ 3. Slow response to stimuli.
- ○ 4. Passage of large amounts of frothy meconium.

18. The nurse reports that the infant responds to initial feeding attempts with behavior characteristic of TEF. The nurse has not been able to feed the infant because
- ○ 1. his sucking attempts were too poorly coordinated to be effective.
- ○ 2. his rooting and sucking reflexes were too poor to give formula.
- ○ 3. he coughed after several swallows, choked, and became cyanotic.
- ○ 4. he took about 10 ml of formula, fell asleep, and could not be stimulated to take more formula.

19. The nurse judged that the parents understood their infant's defect when the mother said
- ○ 1. "The muscle below the stomach is too tight and needs to be loosened."
- ○ 2. "There is a blind upper pouch and a tube into the trachea from the lower pouch of the esophagus."
- ○ 3. "There is a telescoping of the lower bowel into the upper bowel."
- ○ 4. "The stomach muscles are not there and part of the stomach and bowel are on the outside."

20. Which of the following nursing diagnoses would the nurse identify as a priority for this infant?
- ○ 1. Altered Parenting.
- ○ 2. High Risk for Aspiration.
- ○ 3. Ineffective Breathing Pattern.
- ○ 4. Altered Nutrition.

21. Before corrective surgery, the infant is placed on his back in a crib with his head and shoulders elevated. The reasons for this positioning are to reduce reflux of gastric secretions into the trachea through the fistula and to
- ○ 1. reduce cardiac workload, which has been increased by the anomaly.
- ○ 2. alleviate the pressure of the distended abdominal contents on the diaphragm.
- ○ 3. enhance pooling of secretions in the bottom of the upper esophageal pouch.
- ○ 4. allow air to escape from the fistula into the trachea to reduce gastric distension.

22. Which of the following signs should indicate to the nurse that the infant needs suctioning?
- ○ 1. Brassy cough.
- ○ 2. Substernal retractions.
- ○ 3. Decreased activity level.
- ○ 4. Increased respiratory rate.

23. The infant is receiving gastrostomy feedings following surgery to correct the TEF. A pressure clamp is placed on the gastrostomy tube, and a syringe barrel is used to instill formula into the tube. While the infant is being fed, which of the following techniques should the nurse use to prevent air from entering the stomach after the syringe barrel is attached to the gastrostomy tube?
- ○ 1. Open the clamp after pouring all the formula into the syringe barrel.
- ○ 2. Open the clamp before pouring all the formula into the syringe barrel.
- ○ 3. Open the clamp and continuously pour the formula down the side of the syringe barrel.
- ○ 4. Open the clamp and allow a small portion of the formula to enter the stomach before pouring additional formula into the syringe barrel.

24. The most appropriate nursing diagnosis for the nurse to identify postsurgery is
- ○ 1. High Risk for Infection.
- ○ 2. Altered Comfort.
- ○ 3. Altered Bowel Elimination.
- ○ 4. Impaired Physical Mobility.

25. After feeding the infant through the gastrostomy tube, the nurse cradles and rocks him for about 15 minutes, primarily to help
- ○ 1. promote relaxation.
- ○ 2. prevent regurgitation of formula.
- ○ 3. relieve pressure on the surgical repair.
- ○ 4. associate eating with a pleasurable experience.

26. When the infant begins receiving oral feedings, the nursing care plan should be based on which of the following principles?
- ○ 1. An infant adjusts to oral feedings better when small, frequent feedings are offered.
- ○ 2. A closely followed feeding schedule helps the infant accept oral feedings more readily.
- ○ 3. Oral feedings following intubation are best accepted when offered by the same nurse repeatedly or by the infant's mother.
- ○ 4. Oral feedings following intubation are best planned in conjunction with observations of the infant's behavior.

27. When preparing for the infant's discharge from the hospital, the nurse teaches the mother about the need for long-term health care because her child has a high probability of developing
- ○ 1. speech problems.
- ○ 2. esophageal stricture.
- ○ 3. delayed psychosocial development.
- ○ 4. recurrent mild diarrhea with dehydration.

28. Which of the following conditions occurring in the mother's pregnancy would have provided a clue that the newborn might have gastrointestinal tract anomaly?
- ○ 1. Meconium in the amniotic fluid.
- ○ 2. Low implantation of the placenta.
- ○ 3. Increased amount of amniotic fluid.
- ○ 4. Premature separation of the placenta.

The Client With Imperforate Anus

Nursing assessment of a newborn reveals an imperforate anal membrane. Based on this and other assessment information, a medical diagnosis of imperforate anus is made.

29. The nurse would expect further physical assessment to reveal
- ○ 1. an absence of meconium stool.
- ○ 2. abdominal distension.
- ○ 3. ribbon-like stools.
- ○ 4. herniation of abdominal viscera.

30. The neonate is to be scheduled for radiographic examination. The nurse explains to the mother that this examination is done to determine the distance between the anal dimple and the
- ○ 1. perineum.
- ○ 2. closed end of the rectum.
- ○ 3. genitalia.
- ○ 4. rectovesical pouch.

31. The nurse establishes which of the following as the priority nursing diagnosis for this newborn?
- ○ 1. Altered Bowel Elimination.

○ 2. Self-Care Deficit.
○ 3. Impaired Gas Exchange.
○ 4. Impaired Physical Mobility.

32. The nurse monitors the neonate's urine output for the presence of meconium, which would indicate what type of fistula?
○ 1. Vesicocervical.
○ 2. Vesicovaginal.
○ 3. Rectourinary.
○ 4. Rectovaginal.

33. The father observes that the neonate's big toe dorsiflexes and the other toes fan when the nurse gently strokes the sole of the foot. The nurse should explain that this is
○ 1. an abnormal tonic foot sign.
○ 2. a normal plantar reflex.
○ 3. a normal Galant reflex.
○ 4. a normal Babinski reflex.

34. The nurse judges that the parents know what a "low" defect is when the father says that the rectum
○ 1. is below the abdominal rectus muscle.
○ 2. is above the abdominal rectus muscle.
○ 3. has descended through the puborectalis muscle.
○ 4. normally ascends through the puborectalis muscle.

35. Before surgery, the neonate is to receive an intramuscular injection of an antibiotic. Which of the following needle sizes should the nurse select?
○ 1. 19G, 1½".
○ 2. 20G, 1".
○ 3. 22G, 2".
○ 4. 25G, ⅝".

36. Based on the knowledge of the preferred intramuscular injection site in infants, the nurse would select what muscle for injection?
○ 1. Deltoid.
○ 2. Dorsogluteal.
○ 3. Ventrogluteal.
○ 4. Vastus lateralis.

37. After successful surgery, the neonate is returned to the crib with only an intravenous infusion. The mother asks whether her child will have normal bowel function. The nurse should answer that infants who have corrective surgery for low anorectal anomalies
○ 1. may or may not be continent.
○ 2. generally achieve social continence.
○ 3. are rarely continent.
○ 4. are generally continent.

38. A postoperative nursing diagnosis for this neonate would be
○ 1. Altered Parenting.
○ 2. Anticipatory Grieving.
○ 3. Altered Nutrition.
○ 4. High Risk for Infection.

39. A postoperative nursing goal is to prevent tension on the perineum. To achieve this goal, the nurse should avoid placing the neonate on his
○ 1. abdomen, with legs pulled up under the body.
○ 2. back, with legs suspended at a 90° angle.
○ 3. left side, with the hips elevated.
○ 4. right side, with the hips elevated.

40. The father asks the nurse how neonates respond to painful stimuli. The nurse's best response would be that neonates generally cry loudly and
○ 1. cannot be distracted into stopping.
○ 2. try to roll away.
○ 3. move the whole body.
○ 4. withdraw the affected part.

41. The neonate's anorectal malformation and subsequent surgery are stressors on the parents. A nursing goal would be to facilitate parent-infant bonding. Which of the following interventions would most likely help achieve this goal?
○ 1. Explain to the parents that they can visit at any time.
○ 2. Encourage them to hold their infant.
○ 3. Ask them to help monitor the intravenous infusion.
○ 4. Help them plan for their child's discharge.

The Client With Pyloric Stenosis

A 4-week-old infant is admitted to the hospital with a history of vomiting. The mother explains that initially her daughter seemed to have a problem with regurgitation then developed nonprojectile vomiting occurring during and after feedings. The vomiting became more forceful until "one time she vomited across the room."

42. The nurse should assess for which of the following serum electrolyte imbalances in an infant with persistent vomiting?
○ 1. K+ 3.2 mEq/L; Cl-92 mEq/L; Na+ 120 mEq/L.
○ 2. K+ 3.4 mEq/L; Cl-120 mEq/L; Na+ 140 mEq/L.
○ 3. K+ 3.5 mEq/L; Cl-90 mEq/L; Na+ 145 mEq/L.
○ 4. K+ 5.5 mEq/L; Cl-110 mEq/L; Na+ 130 mEq/L.

43. For which of the following acid-base imbalances should the nurse monitor most closely?
○ 1. Respiratory alkalosis.
○ 2. Respiratory acidosis.
○ 3. Metabolic alkalosis.
○ 4. Metabolic acidosis.

44. A tentative medical diagnosis of hypertrophic pyloric stenosis is made. Given this diagnosis, the nurse would anticipate that the client's vomitus would contain gastric contents,
○ 1. bile, and streaks of blood.

○ 2. mucus, and bile.
○ 3. mucus, and streaks of blood.
○ 4. bile, and gross blood.

45. The infant's skin is inelastic and the upper abdomen is distended. To feel the pyloric tumor most easily, the nurse should palpate the epigastrium just to the right of the umbilicus
○ 1. just before the infant vomits.
○ 2. while the infant is eating.
○ 3. while the infant is lying on the left side.
○ 4. just after the infant eats.

46. The most appropriate nursing diagnosis at this time would be
○ 1. Fluid Volume Deficit.
○ 2. Knowledge Deficit.
○ 3. Altered Nutrition.
○ 4. Altered Bowel Elimination.

47. Which of the following actions should the nurse take first?
○ 1. Weigh the infant.
○ 2. Begin the intravenous infusion.
○ 3. Measure the infant's head.
○ 4. Orient the mother to the hospital unit.

48. Which of the following statements by the mother would indicate to the nurse that she understands pyloric stenosis?
○ 1. "Pyloric stenosis is an enlarged muscle below the stomach sphincter."
○ 2. "Pyloric stenosis is a telescoping of the large bowel into the smaller bowel."
○ 3. "Pyloric stenosis is caused by overfeeding her."
○ 4. "Pyloric stenosis is caused by feeding her too fast."

49. Before scheduling the infant for surgery, the physician wants to rehydrate the infant and orders the administration of parenteral fluids and electrolytes. Monitoring which of the following parameters would provide the nurse with the least accurate information about the infant's hydrational state?
○ 1. Urine specific gravity.
○ 2. Skin color.
○ 3. Urine output.
○ 4. Daily weight.

50. Which of the following should the nurse write on the infant's care plan as an expected client outcome related to the nursing diagnosis Fluid Volume Deficit related to vomiting? The client
○ 1. exhibits no abdominal distension.
○ 2. exhibits no manifestations of dehydration.
○ 3. does not vomit.
○ 4. breathes easily without dyspnea.

51. Knowing that the infant is at risk due to decreased circulating fluid volume, the nurse should assess for which of the following disorders?
○ 1. Diabetes insipidus.
○ 2. Acute renal failure.
○ 3. Paralytic ileus.
○ 4. Adrenal insufficiency.

52. After undergoing a pyloromyotomy, the infant returns to the room in stable condition. While standing by the crib, the mother says, "Perhaps if I had brought her to the hospital sooner, she wouldn't have needed surgery." What would be the nurse's best response?
○ 1. "Surgery is the most effective treatment for pyloric stenosis."
○ 2. "Try not to worry; she'll be fine."
○ 3. "Do you feel that this problem reflects poorly on your mothering skills?"
○ 4. "Do you think that earlier hospitalization could have avoided surgery?"

53. Which of the following should the nurse write on the infant's care plan as an expected client outcome related to the nursing diagnosis Altered Comfort related to the surgical procedure? The client
○ 1. exhibits no manifestations of pain.
○ 2. has a bowel movement within 2 hours of surgery.
○ 3. has a temperature of 100.0°F measured rectally.
○ 4. retains the first feeding.

54. The mother asks when her baby will be able to take liquids by mouth. The nurse would base the response on knowledge that if the infant does not vomit, feedings of clear liquids will begin
○ 1. 6 hours after surgery.
○ 2. 8 hours after surgery.
○ 3. 10 hours after surgery.
○ 4. 12 hours after surgery.

55. The parents want to be involved in their infant's care postoperatively, and the nurse teaches them proper feeding techniques. The nurse would determine that they understood the teaching if, after a feeding, they positioned the infant in the crib with her head elevated and on her
○ 1. left side.
○ 2. abdomen.
○ 3. right side.
○ 4. back.

56. The infant does not seem satisfied with the first few feedings of formulas. Correctly interpreting the cause of this dissatisfaction, the nurse would
○ 1. encourage the infant's parents to hold her.
○ 2. hang a mobile over the infant's crib.
○ 3. feed the infant more.
○ 4. give the infant a pacificer.

57. The infant's hospitalization and surgery are stressful events for the parents. Which of the following would the nurse correctly interpret as a positive indication of parental coping?
○ 1. They tell the nurse they have to get away for a while.

○ 2. They discuss the infant's care realistically.
○ 3. They discuss the infant's care superficially.
○ 4. They fear that they will disturb the infant.

The Client With Intussusception

A healthy, thriving, 4-month-old boy suddenly experiences episodes of acute abdominal pain. The infant is admitted to the hospital with the diagnosis of intussusception.

58. In an interview with the nurse, the infant's mother describes his behavior before admission. The mother would most likely describe him as crying
○ 1. constantly and extending his legs.
○ 2. intermittently and drawing his knees to his chest.
○ 3. shrilly when ingesting food.
○ 4. intermittently when positioned on his left side.

59. The nurse asks the mother several questions during the initial nursing history. Which of the following questions would be most helpful in obtaining pertinent diagnostic data?
○ 1. "Did his stool look like currant jelly?"
○ 2. "When was the last time he urinated?"
○ 3. "Did he have a fever?"
○ 4. "Has he vomited?"

60. Which of the following would the nurse identify as a priority nursing diagnosis for this infant?
○ 1. Fluid Volume Deficit.
○ 2. Altered Bowel Elimination.
○ 3. Impaired Skin Integrity.
○ 4. Altered Comfort.

61. Which of the following should the nurse write on the infant's care plan as an expected client outcome related to the nursing diagnosis of Altered Comfort related to cramping? The client
○ 1. exhibits no manifestations of pain.
○ 2. is resting quietly.
○ 3. has a normal bowel movement.
○ 4. has not vomited in 3 hours.

62. The infant underwent surgery to reduce the invagination and returns to the room with a nasogastric tube in place. The infant is allowed nothing by mouth and is receiving intravenous fluids. Which of the following parameters would be used to calculate the amount of intravenous fluid and electrolyte solution to be infused over the next 24 hours?
○ 1. Body weight.
○ 2. Urine output.
○ 3. Body weight and gastric output.
○ 4. Body weight and urine output.

63. The nasogastric tube is no longer freely removing gastric secretions. Which troubleshooting technique should the nurse use to determine the position of the tube?
○ 1. Aspirate gastric contents with a syringe.
○ 2. Irrigate the tube with distilled water.
○ 3. Increase the level of suction.
○ 4. Rotate the tube.

64. When fluids by mouth are appropriate for an infant, the nurse most likely would initiate feeding with
○ 1. cereal-thickened formula.
○ 2. full-strength formula.
○ 3. half-strength formula.
○ 4. glucose water.

65. The infant is at risk for an ileus postoperatively. Which observation would the nurse not include in an assessment for this complication?
○ 1. Measurement of urine specific gravity.
○ 2. Assessment of bowel sounds.
○ 3. Documentation of the first stool.
○ 4. Measurement of gastric output.

66. When the infant resumes taking oral feedings after surgery, the parents comment that he seems to suck on the pacifier more since the surgery. Which explanation of this behavior would be most accurate? Sucking
○ 1. provides an outlet for emotional tension.
○ 2. indicates readiness to take solid foods.
○ 3. indicates thirst.
○ 4. is an attempt to get attention from the parents.

67. The nurse teaches the parents at discharge that their infant will
○ 1. have a change in the prehospital schedule.
○ 2. immediately return to the prehospital schedule.
○ 3. need more calories at home than what he consumed in the hospital.
○ 4. continue experiencing abdominal cramping for a few days.

The Client With Inguinal Hernia

A mother brings her 7-month-old daughter to the clinic after noticing a swelling in her right groin. The swelling varies in size. It disappears when the infant is resting but appears when she is crying. A tentative diagnosis of inguinal hernia is made.

68. Which of the following assessment findings should most concern the nurse?
○ 1. The inguinal swelling is reddened and the abdomen is distended.
○ 2. The infant is irritable and a thickened spermatio-cord can be palpated on the right side.
○ 3. The inguinal swelling can be reduced and the infant has a stool in her diaper.

○ 4. The infant's diaper is wet with urine and the abdomen is nontender.

69. The infant is given a warm bath and meperidine hydrochloride (Demerol) to help relax her before the physician attempts to reduce the hernia. The physician then reduces the hernia and schedules the infant for a herniorrhaphy in 2 days. The mother asks the nurse why the surgery is not performed now. The nurse should explain that delaying surgery

○ 1. ensures proper preoperative preparation.
○ 2. ensures the infant will be NPO 24 hours before surgery.
○ 3. allows the edema and inflammation in the area to subside.
○ 4. allows the infant to wear a truss for 24 hours.

70. The mother is concerned about her infant's surgery. She asks the nurse if her infant would have been scheduled for surgery even if the hernia had been asymptomatic. The nurse answers, "Yes." Which of the following statements offers the best explanation why the surgical repair would be done at this time?

○ 1. From a physiological viewpoint, an infant tolerates surgery better than an older child.
○ 2. The experience of surgery is less frightening for an infant than it is for an older child.
○ 3. There is less danger or complications when surgery is an elective procedure rather than an emergency procedure.
○ 4. There is a preference for doing surgery near the genital organs before a child becomes conscious of sexual identity.

71. Which of the following would the nurse identify as a priority nursing diagnosis for this infant and family?

○ 1. Knowledge Deficit.
○ 2. Altered Comfort.
○ 3. Altered Parenting.
○ 4. Fluid Volume Deficit.

72. The infant is scheduled for a herniorrhaphy tomorrow. The nurse's goal should be to prepare the infant and mother psychologically for the surgery. What would be the best method of preparing a 7-month-old infant psychologically for surgery?

○ 1. Explain preoperative and postoperative procedures to the mother.
○ 2. Have the mother stay with the infant.
○ 3. Make sure the infant's blanket is there.
○ 4. Allow the infant to play with sterile dressings.

73. The infant has undergone an inguinal herniorrhaphy and has been on the pediatric unit for several hours. The mother says the surgeon told her that her child can go home today and asks the nurse when they will be able to leave. The nurse would tell her that her infant must be fully recovered from the anesthesia and

○ 1. resume normal activity.
○ 2. have a bowel movement.
○ 3. have a systolic blood pressure reading of 90 mmHg.
○ 4. retain an oral feeding.

74. The nurse prepares the mother for the infant's discharge based on knowledge of the postoperative complication that the infant is most likely to experience. The nurse would teach the mother to

○ 1. change diapers as soon as they become soiled.
○ 2. have the infant wear an abdominal binder.
○ 3. cover the incision with a sterile dressing.
○ 4. keep the infant's hands away from the incision.

75. The mother asks the nurse what to do about bathing her infant. The nurse should tell the mother to provide

○ 1. daily sponge baths for 2 weeks.
○ 2. full tub baths twice a day.
○ 3. daily sponge baths for 1 week.
○ 4. full tub baths every day.

76. A 15-year-old male had an inguinal hernia repaired earlier today and is getting ready to go home. The nurse instructs the client about resumption of physical activities. Which of the following statements would indicate that he has understood the instructions?

○ 1. "I can't ride my bike until next week."
○ 2. "I have to skip phys ed classes for 2 weeks."
○ 3. "I can start wrestling again in 3 weeks."
○ 4. "I'll postpone my weight-lifting class for 6 weeks."

The Client With Hirschsprung's Disease

A 7-month-old infant is admitted to the hospital with a tentative diagnosis of Hirschsprung's disease.

77. As the nurse is obtaining the infant's initial health history from the parents, which of the following statements made by the mother would most likely result in pertinent diagnostic data?

○ 1. "She is constipated often."
○ 2. "She sometimes gets colds."
○ 3. "She sometimes spits up."
○ 4. "She has a temperature of 99.5°F (measured rectally).

78. During physical assessment, the nurse would be most likely to note that the infant

○ 1. exhibits a prominent venous network over her thighs and legs.
○ 2. weighs less than expected for her height and age.
○ 3. has clubbing and cyanosis of the fingers and toes.
○ 4. demonstrates hyperactive deep tendon reflexes.

79. The infant is scheduled for a barium enema to confirm the diagnosis. A primary concern following this procedure is evacuation of barium from the colon. What should the nurse do to identify this evacuation?
- ○ 1. Test the pH of the stool.
- ○ 2. Observe the color of the stool.
- ○ 3. Palpate the left lower abdomen.
- ○ 4. Auscultate for bowel sounds.

80. The nurse assesses the infant's growth and development. Which behavior would the nurse consider *unusual?*
- ○ 1. Grasping a raisin neatly between the index finger and the base of the thumb.
- ○ 2. Raising the chest and upper abdomen off the bed with the hands.
- ○ 3. Imitating sounds that the nurse makes.
- ○ 4. Crying loudly in protest when the mother leaves the room.

81. Diagnostic evaluation confirms the medical diagnosis of Hirschsprung's disease, and a colostomy is planned. When initially discussing the diagnosis and treatment with the parents, it would be most appropriate for the nurse to
- ○ 1. assess the adequacy of their coping skills.
- ○ 2. reassure them that their child will be fine.
- ○ 3. encourage them to ask questions.
- ○ 4. use printed materials.

82. The nurse judges that the parents understand the diagnosis when the father states
- ○ 1. "There is no rectal opening."
- ○ 2. "The small intestine is not fully developed."
- ○ 3. "The nerves to the end of the large colon are missing."
- ○ 4. "The muscle below the stomach is too tight."

83. Before surgery, the infant is to receive oral neomycin for 3 days. The appropriate pediatric dosage of neomycin sulfate is 10.3 mg/kg q 4 hours. The infant weighs 7 kg. Which of the following dosages most closely approximates a safe daily dose?
- ○ 1. 50 mg per day.
- ○ 2. 150 mg per day.
- ○ 3. 280 mg per day.
- ○ 4. 430 mg per day.

84. The nurse anticipates that 24 to 48 hours before surgery, the infant's preoperative preparation will most likely include
- ○ 1. administration of a Fleet's enema.
- ○ 2. insertion of a gastrostomy tube.
- ○ 3. restriction of oral intake to clear liquids.
- ○ 4. preparation of the perineum with povidone-iodine (Betadine).

85. Which of the following nursing diagnoses would be the priority diagnosis for this client and family preoperatively?
- ○ 1. Altered Comfort.
- ○ 2. Altered Elimination.
- ○ 3. Fluid Volume Deficit.
- ○ 4. Impaired Communication.

86. The infant has surgery, and a temporary colostomy is created. The infant's postoperative recovery is uneventful. The nurse prepares the parents for their infant's discharge. Which of the following instructions should the nurse give the parents?
- ○ 1. Position the infant so that there is no pressure on the stoma site.
- ○ 2. Allow the diaper to absorb the colostomy drainage.
- ○ 3. Give the infant plenty of liquids to drink.
- ○ 4. Expect the stoma to become dusky red within 2 weeks.

87. Which of the mother's statements about the colostomy would indicate that she needs further teaching?
- ○ 1. "We'll take care of the colostomy until our child is old enough to do it."
- ○ 2. "The colostomy will give the intestine time to shrink to its normal size."
- ○ 3. "The colostomy may include two separate abdominal openings."
- ○ 4. "Right after the procedure, the stoma will appear big and red."

88. The nurse plans to teach the parents about the appearance of the stoma before discharge. The nurse will teach the parents that the stoma normally will
- ○ 1. become dark brown in 2 months.
- ○ 2. stay deep red in color.
- ○ 3. change to several shades of pink.
- ○ 4. turn very dark red, almost purple.

89. The nurse teaches the mother about the types of foods the child will be able to eat with a colostomy. The nurse would advise
- ○ 1. a high-fiber diet.
- ○ 2. lots of milk and red meats.
- ○ 3. lots of fruits and vegetables.
- ○ 4. a low-residue diet.

90. The child, now age 15 months, has been readmitted to the hospital for colostomy closure. After surgery, the child returns to the pediatric unit with an intravenous line in place. The infusion set delivers 1 ml per 60 drops. A total of 250 ml over the next 3 hours has been ordered. How many drops per minute should the infusion deliver?
- ○ 1. 14 drops/minute.
- ○ 2. 21 drops/minute.
- ○ 3. 60 drops/minute.
- ○ 4. 83 drops/minute.

91. The child is receiving meperidine hydrochloride (Demerol) postoperatively for pain. Which of the following dosages would be a safe dose for the child (who weighs 30 pounds) to receive every 4 hours?
- ○ 1. 15 mg/dose.

○ 2. 35 mg/dose.
○ 3. 40 mg/dose.
○ 4. 45 mg/dose.

92. The nurse is to measure and record the child's abdominal circumference every 8 hours. Which of the following would necessitate calling the physician now?
○ 1. An increase of 3 cm in abdominal circumference.
○ 2. A decrease of 1 cm in abdominal circumference.
○ 3. Absence of bowel sounds 8 hours after surgery.
○ 4. The child's returning appetite.

93. The child will be discharged within a day or two. When evaluating the parent's knowledge of the effects of their child's surgery, the nurse knows that the parents understand when they say that
○ 1. abdominal distension is to be expected.
○ 2. toilet training may be difficult.
○ 3. dairy products should be avoided.
○ 4. vitamin supplements will be needed until adolescence.

CORRECT ANSWERS AND RATIONALE

The letters in parentheses following the rationale identify the step of the nursing process (A, D, P, I, E); cognitive level (K, C, T, N); and client need (S, G, L, H). See the Answer Grid for the key.

The Client With Cleft Lip and Palate

1. 3. Preoperative and postoperative pictures of babies with cleft palates and lips provide a clear and concrete image of expectations of corrective surgery described by health personnel. Providing these pictures is specific to the parents' behavior, because the parents reflect societal values that emphasize an infant's facial appearance and responsive expressiveness. Bringing this infant to the parents more often may be beneficial but would not help the parents accept the infant's anomaly and expectations from surgery. Allowing the completion of the grieving process prior to another interaction between the infant and parents could result in a separation that could last months. (P, T, L)

2. 3. It is important for the infant to have formula prior to corrective surgery for a cleft lip. Methods for feeding will need to be adjusted to fit the infant's needs. Commonly, a rubber-tipped syringe or medicine dropper is used. Infection in the mouth is uncommon, and minimizing crying is of no particular help. There is no special need to keep the infant's fingers out of the mouth preoperatively, and this may upset the infant even further. (P, T, G)

3. 1. An infant with a cleft palate and lip swallows large amounts of air while being fed and therefore should be bubbled frequently. The soft palate defect allows air to be drawn into the pharynx with each swallow of formula. The stomach will become distended with air, and regurgitation, possibly with aspiration, is likely if the infant is not bubbled frequently. Feeding frequently would not prevent swallowing large amounts of air. A nipple is likely to cause the infant to gag and aspirate. Holding the infant in a lying position during feedings can also produce aspiration and regurgitation of formula. (I, C, G)

4. 2. Parents of an infant with a congenital defect are frequently in a state of shock when the child is first born. The parents go through a period of grieving for the normal child they did not have. (D, N, L)

5. 4. Following the repair of a cleft lip, the infant must become accustomed to nasal breathing. However, if the infant is having difficulty breathing, it would be best to open the mouth by exerting downward pressure on the chin. In some instances, an airway is used postoperatively, but when it is not in place it is best to try pressure on the chin first. Raising the infant's head and turning the infant onto the abdomen are likely to aggravate the situation. (I, T, S)

6. 3. A rubber-tipped medicine dropper has been found to be a very satisfactory method for feeding an infant who has had surgical repair of a cleft lip. Gastric gavage is ordinarily not used unless complications develop. Intravenous fluids will not supply complete nutrition for the infant. A large-holed nipple may cause the infant to aspirate because formula enters the mouth too rapidly. Feeding methods should produce the least tension possible on the sutures to promote effective healing of the cleft lip repair. (I, C, G)

7. 2. After surgery the most important nursing diagnosis should be prevention of infection. Surgery involves an incision, which is at risk for infection. The infant with this type of procedure does have discomfort, which can be relieved with acetaminophen. Altered Comfort would be an important nursing diagnosis but not the priority. The infant may be in arm restraints or have the cuff of the sleeve pinned to the diaper or pants. It is important that the infant not touch the incision line so as to disrupt the sutures. There is no indication of Altered Parenting. The parents are reacting normally with the first reaction of shock. (D, N, G)

8. 4. Half-strength hydrogen peroxide is recommended for cleansing the suture line following cleft lip repair. The bubbling action of the hydrogen peroxide is effective for removing debris. Normal saline may be the preferred solution in some agencies. (I, T, G)

9. 3. Inadequate drainage through the eustachian tubes often causes otitis media when an infant with a cleft palate develops an upper respiratory infection. Recurrent otitis media and accumulation of serous drainage in the middle ear prevent normal movement of the tympanic membrane and lead to a resulting hearing deficit. If nutrition is maintained and overall health is good, the child with a cleft palate should have no more respiratory infections than peers of the same age. Although eating is a problem for these children, their intake is not reduced enough to predispose to dehydration unless another condition predisposing to dehydration occurs. (I, T, G)

10. 3. The optimal time for cleft palate repair depends on many factors, but it is best done before speech development and before the child learns faulty speech habits. Such factors as when teeth erupt, when the child can sit alone, and when the child learns to drink from a cup are not ordinarily used to determine the time for palate repair. (I, C, G)

11. 1. A cup is the preferred eating utensil after the repair of a cleft palate. At the age when repair is done, the child is ordinarily able to drink from a cup, and using it avoids having to place a utensil in the mouth, where surgery has just been completed. (I, K, G)

12. 2. Recommended restraints for a child who has had palate surgery would be elbow restraints. They minimize the limitation placed on the child but still prevent the child from injuring the repair with fingers and hands. A safety jacket, arm and leg restraints, and arm and body restraints restrict the child unnecessarily. (I, C, S)

13. 3. A sitting position (that is, with the trunk of the body upright and head tilted forward) is recommended for oral irrigation. This position is best because the child is least likely to choke and aspirate fluid during the irrigation. (I, T, S)

14. 1. The mother should be encouraged to hold and cuddle her child to provide needed emotional support. Such activities as helping the child play with toys, reading stories, and staying with the child would not be contraindicated but do not offer as much emotional support as holding and cuddling. (P, C, L)

15. 4. A speech defect is common following the repair of a cleft palate, and many children require speech therapy following surgery. Such conditions as nutritional inadequacies, obesity, and difficulty in developing a healthy self-concept are uncommon if a child receives adequate care and support. (I, T, G)

The Client With a Tracheoesophageal Fistula

16. 1. The parents of children born with defects often have feelings of guilt and ask what they might have done to cause the condition or how they might have avoided it. It is important to allow parents to express their feelings and to accept these feelings as normal reactions. Encouraging parents to begin long-term planning and having them visit their infant as often as possible would generally be of little help when a nurse is offering emotional support to distraught parents, and it could appear to the parents as though they are being "talked out" of their feelings. Explaining that the parents are not at fault would not be appropriate until they have dealt with their feelings of guilt. (P, T, L)

17. 1. Esophageal atresia prevents the passage of swallowed mucus and saliva into the stomach. After fluid has accumulated in the pouch, it flows from the mouth and the infant then drools continuously. The lack of swallowed amniotic fluid prevents the accumulation of normal meconium; lack of stool results. Responsiveness of the infant to stimuli would depend on the overall condition of the infant and is not considered a classic sign of a tracheoesophageal fistula (TEF). Diaphragmatic breathing is not associated with TEF. (A, C, G)

18. 3. The infant with TEF swallows normally, but the fluids quickly fill the blind pouch. The infant then coughs, chokes, and becomes cyanotic while the fluid returns through the nose and mouth. Poor rooting and sucking reflexes are typical of infants who have neurological dysfunctions; these reflexes may also be depressed by medication giver to the mother during labor. Falling asleep after taking little formula is characteristic of an infant who becomes exhausted with the exertion of feeding and is often caused by a cardiac anomaly. (E, N, G)

19. 2. The type of tracheoesophageal fistula (TEF) in this item is a blind upper pouch and a fistula from the esophagus into the trachea. (E, N, G)

20. 2. Children with TEF frequently have aspiration pneumonia because the blind pouch fills quickly with fluids. Thus, High Risk for Aspiration is a priority nursing diagnosis and a nursing function to prevent aspiration by suctioning or positioning. As a result of the aspiration, the infant may have an Altered Breathing Pattern. There is no evidence here to support the diagnoses Altered Parenting and Altered Nutrition. (D, T, G)

21. 3. Gravity encourages the flow of secretions with pooling in the bottom of the upper pouch when an infant with TEF is placed on the back with the head and shoulders elevated. More effective removal of secretions can be accomplished by positioning a catheter in this pool of secretions. Each breathing cycle forces some air into the stomach, which prevents upward passage of air into the trachea. Although abdominal distension would eventually result from air entering the stomach, this is a much later manifestation of TEF. There is generally no additional cardiac workload and little possibility of cardiac failure unless other anomalies complicate TEF. (A, K, G)

22. 2. Laryngospasms result from the overflow of secretions into the larynx in an infant with TEF. The obstruction to inspiration stimulates the strong contraction of accessory muscles of the thorax to assist the diaphragm in breathing. This produces substernal retractions. A brassy cough is related to a relatively constant laryngeal narrowing, usually due to edema. Decreased activity level and increased respiratory rate are usually due to hypoxia. This is a relatively long-term and constant phenomenon in infants with TEF. The laryngospasms occurring with TEF resolve quickly when secretions are removed from the oropharynx area. (P, C, G)

23. 1. The best way to prevent air from entering the stomach when feeding an infant through a gastrostomy tube is to open the clamp after all the formula has been placed in the syringe barrel. These other techniques will allow air to enter the stomach through the gastrostomy tube. (I, K, G)

24. 1. High Risk for Infection would be a priority nursing diagnosis after surgery. With any type of incision the immediate concern is preventing infection at the site. Altered Comfort is also a diagnosis of concern and would be next in order of priority. The infant would be partially restrained to prevent disturbance of the intravenous infusion, and nasogastric tube. Bowel elimination should begin in a few days. (D, T, G)

25. 4. Helping meet the psychological needs of an infant being fed through a gastrostomy tube can be accomplished by rocking the infant after a feeding. The infant soon learns to associate eating with a pleasurable experience. Holding and rocking an infant may also help accomplish certain other goals, but these are not primary goals in caring for the infant described here. (I, T, L)

26. 4. It is best to follow a care plan based on the principle that oral feedings started after an infant has been fed through a gastrostomy tube are best planned in conjunction with observation of the infant's needs and behavior. When the infant's needs and behavior are overlooked, care plans are likely to be unsatisfactory and are more likely to meet the nurse's needs rather than the infant's needs. (I, C, G)

27. 2. Dilatation at the anastomosis site is needed over the first years of childhood in approximately half of the children who have had corrective surgery for TEF. Speech problems are likely if other abnormalities are present to produce them. The larynx and structures of speech are not affected by TEF. Dysphagia and strictures may decrease food intake and poor weight gain may be noted, but diarrhea and dehydration are not associated with TEF repair. Delayed psychosocial development is possible with long hospitalizations and separation from the parents during TEF treatment. (I, C, G)

28. 3. Maternal hydramnios occurs with infants that have a congenital obstruction of the gastrointestinal tract, such as occurs in the presence of a TEF. The fetus normally swallows amniotic fluid and absorbs the fluid from the gastrointestinal tract. Excretion then occurs through the kidneys and placenta. Most fluid absorption occurs in the colon. Absorption cannot occur when the fetus has a gastrointestinal obstruction. Meconium in the amniotic fluid, low implantation of the placenta, and premature separation of the placenta could occur but are more specifically associated with fetal hypoxia. Meconium in the amniotic fluid is a manifestation of fetal hypoxia. (A, K, G)

The Client With Imperforate Anus

29. 1. The absence of meconium stool is consistent with a diagnosis of imperforate anus. Abdominal distension is a later sign of imperforate anus. Ribbonlike stools are associated with anal stenosis. Herniation of abdominal viscera is not associated with anorectal malformations. (A, K, G)

30. 2. The purpose of the radiographic examination is to ascertain the distance between the anal dimple and the closed end of the rectum. (I, K, G)

31. 1. With the medical diagnosis of imperforate anus, the priority nursing diagnosis would be Altered Bowel Elimination. The other nursing diagnoses are inappropriate. All infants have self-care deficit, and there is no impaired gas exchange or physical mobility with this defect. (D, T, G)

32. 3. Passage of meconium in the urine is a sign of rectourinary fistula, in which the rectum and bladder communicate. In a vesicocervical fistula, the bladder and cervical canal communicate; in a vesicovaginal fistula, the bladder and vagina communicate; and in a rectovaginal fistula, the rectum and vagina communicate. (A, K, G)

33. 4. A normal Babinski reflex involves dorsiflexion of the big toe and fanning of the other toes. Though normal in infants, this response is abnormal after about age 1 year or when walking begins. A plantar reflex is characterized by flexion of the toes. The tonic foot sign does not exist. A normal Galant reflex is initiated by stroking an infant's back alongside the spine; the hips should move toward the stimulated side. (I, K, H)

34. 3. In a low anorectal anomaly, the rectum has descended normally through the puborectalis muscle. In an intermediate anomaly, the rectum is at or below the level of the puborectalis muscle; in a high anomaly, the rectum ends above the puborectalis muscle. (E, N, G)

35. 4. A 25G to 27G, ½" to 1" long needle is appropriate for administering an intramuscular injection to an infant. (I, T, S)

36. 4. The vastus lateralis muscle of the thigh is preferred for administering intramuscular injections to infants because there is less danger of injuring nerves, blood vessels, or bony structures. The deltoid muscle is used for intramuscular injections only when other areas are unavailable. The dorsogluteal site is contraindicated for use in children who have not been walking for at least 1 year. The ventrogluteal site is relatively free of major nerves and blood vessels, but the vastus lateralis remains the preferred intramuscular injection site in infants. (I, K, S)

37. 4. Children who have correction as infants for low anorectal anomalies are generally continent. Fecal continence can be expected after successful correction of anal membrane atresia. Children with high anomalies may or may not achieve continence. (I, K, G)

38. 4. High Risk for Infection is an appropriate priority nursing diagnosis when corrective surgery is performed. This diagnosis is amenable to nursing care and should serve as a basis for planning and carrying out client-centered nursing care. Anticipatory Grieving is an important nursing diagnosis but would not be the priority at this particular time. Altered Parenting and Altered Nutrition may be applicable nursing diagnoses but again, not priority diagnoses. (D, T, G)

39. 1. When placed on the abdomen, a neonate pulls the legs up under the body, which puts tension on the perineum. Therefore, a postoperative neonate should be positioned either supine with the legs suspended at a 90-degree angle or on either side with the hips elevated. (P, T, G)

40. 3. The neonate responds to pain with total body movement associated with brief, loud crying that ceases with distraction. After age 6 months, an infant reacts to pain with intense physical resistance and tries to escape by rolling away. A toddler reacts by withdrawing the affected part. (I, C, L)

41. 2. Encouraging the parents to hold the neonate promotes parent-infant bonding. Explaining that the parents can visit anytime will promote bonding only if they do visit with, talk to, and hold the infant. Asking the parents to help monitor the intravenous infusion may be anxiety-producing. Helping the parents plan for the child's discharge involves them in the child's care. (P, T, L)

The Client With Pyloric Stenosis

42. 1. These serum electrolyte values in an infant with persistent vomiting reflect hypokalemia, hypochloremia, and hyponatremia. (A, K, G)

43. 3. Metabolic alkalosis occurs because of the excessive loss of potassium, hydrogen, and chloride in the vomitus. Chloride loss leads to a compensatory increase in the number of bicarbonate ions. The bicarbonate side of the carbonic acid-base bicarbonate is increased and the pH becomes more alkaline. Metabolic acidosis results from severe diarrhea and starvation. Respiratory acidosis is caused by conditions that result in excessive retention of PaCO2. Respiratory alkalosis is caused by conditions that result in loss of PaCO2. (A, K, G)

44. 3. The vomitus of an infant with hypertrophic pyloric stenosis contains gastric contents, mucus, and streaks of blood. The vomitus does not contain bile because the pyloric constriction is proximal to the ampulla of Vater. (A, K, G)

45. 2. The pyloric tumor is most easily palpated when the abdominal muscles are relaxed during a feeding or immediately after vomiting. (A, K, G)

46. 1. Infants with pyloric stenosis usually have some degree of dehydration because of the vomiting of the stomach contents. A nursing priority would be to restore fluid and electrolyte imbalances. The parents would have knowledge deficit of the medical diagnosis as well as of the necessary nursing care, so this also would be an important, though not the priority, nursing diagnosis. Likewise, Altered Nutrition: Less than Body Requirements could be applicable, but would not be the priority diagnosis. There is no information here to identify Altered Bowel Elimination as the priority diagnosis. (D, T, G)

47. 1. Unless the infant is in hypovolemic shock, obtaining a baseline weight is a very important first action. The intravenous fluid rate and amount of electrolytes to be added to the fluid are based on the infant's weight. The weight will also help determine the infant's degree of dehydration. Measuring the infant's head size would provide important assessment information but could be obtained later. Beginning the intravenous infusion is also important after the weight is obtained. Orientation of the mother could wait until treatment is underway. (P, T, G)

48. 1. Pyloric stenosis is hypertrophy of the pylorus muscle distal to the stomach. Telescoping of the bowel is intussusception. Overfeeding or underfeeding cannot cause pyloric stenosis. (E, N, G)

49. 2. Skin color reflects hemodynamic status. Urine specific gravity, intake and output, and daily weight provide information about hydration status. (A, K, G)

50. 2. An expected client outcome relative to the nursing diagnosis of Fluid Volume Deficit relates to vomiting is that the client exhibits no evidence of dehydration, such as weight loss or decreased skin turgor. (D, N, G)

51. 2. Acute renal failure can occur secondary to a decrease in circulating fluid volume because of renal hypoperfusion. Paralytic ileus, adrenal insufficiency, and diabetes insipidus can result in a fluid volume deficit but do not occur secondary to a decrease in circulating fluid volume, (A, K, G)

52. 4. Restating a mother's response provides the opportunity for clarification and validation. Surgery is the most effective treatment for pyloric stenosis, but this response does not give the mother an opportunity to express her feelings. The nurse should avoid giving premature reassurance and should allow the mother to express her concerns. (I, C, L)

53. 1. An expected client outcome relative to the nursing diagnosis of Altered Comfort related to the surgical procedure is that the client will exhibit no evidence of pain, such as total body movement accompanied by crying. (D, N, L)

54. 1. Clear liquids containing glucose and electrolytes are usually prescribed 4 to 6 hours after surgery. If vomiting does not occur, formula or breast milk can be gradually substituted for clear liquids until the infant is taking normal feedings. (I, C, G)

55. 3. Positioning the infant on the right side with the head elevated facilitates passage of food through the pyloric sphincter into the intestine. (E, N, G)

56. 4. Giving the infant a pacifier would help meet the nonnutritive sucking needs and ensure oral gratification. Encouraging the parents to hold the infant and hanging a mobile over the crib will not meet this need. The postpyloromyotomy infant does not need to be fed more. (I, N, G)

57. 2. The fact that the parents can verbalize the infant's care realistically indicates that they are working through their fears and concerns. Without further data, the fact that the parents "have to get away" could be interpreted as ineffective coping. Superficial discussion of the infant's care does not indicate positive coping, nor does fear of disturbing the infant. (D, N, L)

The Client With Intussusception

58. 2. The infant with intussusception experiences acute episodes of colic-like abdominal pain. Typically, the infant screams and draws the knees to the chest. In between these episodes of acute abdominal pain, the infant appears comfortable and normal. Ingestion of food does not precipitate episodes of pain. Pain that occurs when the infant is positioned on the left side is not associated with intussusception. (A, K, G)

59. 1. Stools in children with intussusception will look like currant jelly due to the intestinal inflammation and hemorrhage because of the intestinal obstruction. The other questions relating to the last time the infant urinated, fever, and vomiting can also elicit important data, but the currant-jelly stools are diagnostic for intussusception. (A, C, G)

60. 4. Due to the colic-like abdominal pain, Altered Comfort would be the priority nursing diagnosis. There are no data to indicate a skin problem or dehydration. Constipation or diarrhea may preceed the appearance of currant-jelly stools. (A, C, G)

61. 1. An expected client outcome relative to the nursing diagnosis of Altered Comfort related to cramping is that the client exhibits no manifestations of discomfort, such as crying or drawing the legs to the abdomen. (D, N, G)

62. 3. The volume of parental fluids needed is based on fluid requirements determined according to body weight and, in this situation, gastric output. If these fluids are not replaced with an appropriate intravenous solution, serious fluid and electrolyte imbalances could develop. Urine output is monitored but is not used to calculate maintenance and replacement needs. (A, K, G)

63. 1. To check tube position, the nurse should aspirate gastric contents or inject a small amount of air while auscultating with a stethoscope over the epigastric area. The tube is irrigated with normal saline, only after the position of the tube is confirmed. The suction level should not be increased; an increased level could damage the mucosa. Rotating the tube could irritate or traumatize the nasal mucosa. (I, C, G)

64. 4. When a child is ready to take fluids by mouth postoperatively, clear liquids are given initially. If clear liquids are tolerated, the concentration and amount of oral feeding are gradually increased. This means advancing half-strength, and then full-strength formula while increasing the amount given with each feeding. (I, C, G)

65. 1. A postoperative ileus is a functional obstruction of the bowel. Assessment of bowel sounds, the first stool, and the amount of gastric output provide information about the return of gastric function. Measurement of urine specific gravity provides information about fluid and electrolyte status. (A, C, G)

66. 1. Sucking provides the infant with a sense of security and comfort. It also is an outlet for releasing tension. The infant should not be discouraged from sucking on the pacifier. Fussiness and irritability after feeding may indicate that the infant's appetite is not satisfied. Sucking is not manipulative in the sense that the infant is seeking parental attention. (D, N, L)

67. 1. Infants who have had an interruption in their normal routine and experiences such as hospitalization and surgery typically manifest behavior changes when discharged. The infant's normal routine has been significantly altered, so it will take time to reestablish another routine. The infant does not need more calories at home than in the hospital. The surgical procedure corrected the problems, so the infant should not continue to have abdominal cramping. (I, T, L)

The Client With Inguinal Hernia

68. 1. A hernia that cannot be reduced, together with abdominal distension, area tenderness, and redness, indicate an incarcerated hernia. An incarcerated hernia can lead to strangulation, necrosis, and gangrene of the bowel. Other findings associated with strangulation include irritability, anorexia, and difficulty in defecation. A palpable thickened spermatic cord on the affected side is diagnostic of inguinal hernia. (A, K, G)

69. 3. If nonoperative reduction is successful, delaying surgery for 2 to 3 days allows the edema and inflammation in the inguinal area to subside. Preoperative preparation is minimal, and the infant is fed until a few hours before surgery to prevent dehydration. Trusses do not prevent incarceration, and there is no reason to use a truss preoperatively. (I, T, G)

70. 3. Inguinal hernia repair is ordinarily done promptly after diagnosis in healthy infants and children. If surgery is delayed, there is a possibility of a partial obstruction when a loop of the bowel protrudes into the inguinal canal. Serious progression with complete obstruction and perhaps strangulation of the bowel requires emergency surgery to prevent gangrene, which could be fatal. The infant does not have a physiological or psychological advantage over older children. Although performing surgery around the genitals prior to the preschool years is recommended, the best reason for performing this surgery now would be to avoid having to perform emergency surgery later. (I, T, G)

71. 1. The mother needs information about the surgical procedure and expected care after surgery. At this time the child does not have problems with comfort or a fluid volume deficit, nor is there any evidence that the mother has any problems related to parenting. (D, N, G)

72. 2. The best way to psychologically prepare a 7-month-old child for surgery is to have the primary caretaker stay with the child. Infants in the second 6 months of life commonly develop separation anxiety. Teaching the mother what to expect may decrease her anxiety; this is important, because infants sense anxiety and distress in parents. Taking a favorite toy or blanket to the operating room provides additional security for the child. Actual play and acting out life experiences are appropriate for preschool-age children. (P, T, L)

73. 4. Before discharge, the infant must be completely recovered from the anesthesia and take and retain an oral feeding. A normal systolic blood pressure reading for a 7-month-old infant is approximately 116 mm Hg. (I, C, G)

74. 1. Changing a diaper as soon as it becomes soiled helps prevent wound infection. This is the most common complication following inguinal hernia repair in an infant because of possible contamination of the wound with urine and stool. The surgical wound is unlikely to dehisce, so an abdominal binder is unnecessary. An infant who is not toilet trained may or may not have the incision covered with a dressing. A topical spray that protects the wound may be applied. (I, T, G)

75. 3. The incision should be kept as clean and dry as possible. Therefore, daily sponge baths are given for about a week postoperatively. (I, C, G)

76. 3. Activities such as bicycle riding, physical education classes, weight-lifting, and wrestling are contraindicated for about 3 weeks because of possible stress on the incision. (E, N, G)

The Client With Hirschsprung's Disease

77. 1. Infants with Hirschsprung's disease typically have a history of abdominal distension, constipation, periodic diarrhea (when liquid stool leaks around the semiobstructed colon), and failure to thrive. Having an occasional cold and spitting up once in a while are normal for infants. A temperature of 99.5°F measured rectally is considered normal. (A, C, G)

78. 2. Infants with Hirschsprung's disease typically display failure to thrive, with poor weight gain, due to malabsorption of nutrients. Prominent thigh and calf veins, clubbing and cyanosis of fingers and toes, and hyperactive deep tendon reflexes are not associated with Hirschsprung's disease. (A, N, G)

79. 2. Barium produces white or clay-colored stools. The passage of white or clay-colored stools after a barium enema indicates that the barium is being expelled. (E, N, G)

80. 1. Infants age 6 to 8 months grasp objects between the index and middle fingers and the base of the thumb. A neat pincer grasp usually develops around age 10 months. At age 6 months, the infant can partially lift his weight on the hands, enjoys imitating sounds, and is developing separation anxiety. (A, K, H)

81. 3. By encouraging parents to ask questions during information-sharing sessions, the nurse can clarify misconceptions and determine their understanding of information. Assessing the adequacy of the parent's coping skills is important, but secondary to encouraging them to express their concerns. The questions they ask and their interaction with the nurse may provide clues to the adequacy of their coping skills. The nurse should never give false reassurance to parents. Written materials are appropriate for augmenting the nurse's verbal communication but also are secondary to encouraging questions. (I, N, L)

82. 3. The primary defect in Hirschsprung's disease is an absence of autonomic parasympathetic ganglion cells in the distal portion of the colon. (E, N, G)

83. 4. The dose is calculated by multiplying 10.3 mg × 7 kg = 72.1 mg. In computing a daily dosage, the dose is multiplied by the number of times it will be given per day (72.1 mg × 6 = 432.6 mg per day). (A, K, S)

84. 3. Dietary intake is limited to clear liquids for 24 to 48 hours before intestinal surgery. A clear liquid diet meets the child's fluid needs and avoids the formation of fecal material in the intestine. Repeated saline enemas are given to empty the bowel, and a nasogastric tube may be inserted for gastric decompression. The perineal area is not prepared because it is not involved in this surgery. (P, C, G)

85. 2. Altered Bowel Elimination would be the priority nursing diagnosis here. The nursing history information of constipation and occasional diarrhea would lead to this diagnosis. In this situation it is not likely that the child would have a fluid volume deficit, problems with communication, or problems with comfort. (D, N, G)

86. 3. Because of decreased fluid reabsorption from the colon, the child with a colostomy benefits from a liberal fluid intake. There is no reason to avoid normal pressure on the stoma; it has a good blood supply and no nerve endings. An appliance should be fitted for stool collection to help prevent skin breakdown. The stoma should always be reddish-pink and moist. A dusk-colored stoma may indicate impaired circulation to the area. (P, T, G)

87. 1. The goal of surgery is to remove the aganglionic bowel and to improve functioning of the internal sphincter. A temporary loop or double-barreled colostomy is usually created to rest the bowel. This enables the normal distal bowel to regain its original tone and size. Final corrective surgery is done when the child is age 6 to 12 months and/or weighs about 10 kg. The colostomy will probably be reversed before the child is old enough to be responsible for its care. A new stoma is swollen and erythematous. (E, N, G)

88. 2. The stoma should remain deep red in color as long as the child has the colostomy. A dark red to purplish color may indicate impaired circulation to the stoma. (I, T, G)

89. 4. A low-residue diet would be recommended for the child with a colostomy. Such a diet causes less bulky stools and facilitates their passage. High-fiber foods such as fruits and vegetables should be minimized, because they increase the bulk in the stool. (I, T, G)

90. 4. The drop rate is determined as follows:

$$\frac{250 \text{ ml fluid}}{3 \text{ hours}} = 83.3 \text{ ml fluid delivered per hour}$$

$$\frac{83 \text{ ml (approximately)} \times 60 \text{ drops/ml}}{60 \text{ minutes}} = \frac{4{,}980}{60} = 83 \text{ drops.}$$

(I, T, S)

91. 1. The dosage for meperidine hydrochloride is ½ to 1 mg per pound per dose. This child weighs 30 pounds, so an appropriate dose would be 15–30 mg. (I, T, S)

92. 1. Abdominal circumference is measured to monitor for abdominal distension. An increase of 3 cm in 8 hours would require notification of the physician. Absence of bowel sounds would be expected following surgery. Even if the child is hungry, fluids will not be offered until bowel sounds are heard. (I, N, G)

93. 2. Toilet-training is commonly more difficult for children who have undergone surgery for Hirschsprung's disease than it is for other children. This is because of the trauma to the area and the associated psychological implications. Distension is an early sign of infection. Dietary restrictions or vitamin supplementation are usually not required. (E, N, G)

NURSING CARE OF CHILDREN

TEST 4: The Child With Health Problems of the Upper Gastrointestinal Tract

Directions: Use this answer grid to determine areas of strength or need for further study.

NURSING PROCESS

A = Assessment
D = Analysis, nursing diagnosis
P = Planning
I = Implementation
E = Evaluation

COGNITIVE LEVEL

K = Knowledge
C = Comprehension
T = Application
N = Analysis

CLIENT NEEDS

S = Safe, effective care environment
G = Physiological integrity
L = Psychosocial integrity
H = Health promotion/maintenance

		Nursing Process					Cognitive Level				Client Needs			
Question #	Answer #	A	D	P	I	E	K	C	T	N	S	G	L	H
1	3			P					T				L	
2	3			P					T			G		
3	1				I			C				G		
4	2		D							N			L	
5	4				I				T		S			
6	3				I			C				G		
7	2		D							N		G		
8	4				I				T			G		
9	3				I				T			G		
10	3				I			C				G		
11	1				I		K					G		
12	2				I			C			S			
13	3				I				T		S			
14	1			P				C					L	
15	4				I				T			G		
16	1			P					T				L	
17	1	A						C				G		
18	3					E				N		G		
19	2					E				N		G		
20	2		D						T			G		
21	3	A					K					G		
22	2			P				C				G		

ANSWER GRID: 1

Nursing Process

A = Assessment
D = Analysis, nursing diagnosis
P = Planning
I = Implementation
E = Evaluation

Cognitive Level

K = Knowledge
C = Comprehension
T = Application
N = Analysis

Client Needs

S = Safe, effective care environment
G = Physiological integrity
L = Psychosocial integrity
H = Health promotion/maintenance

		Nursing Process					Cognitive Level				Client Needs			
Question #	Answer #	A	D	P	I	E	K	C	T	N	S	G	L	H
23	1				I		K					G		
24	1		D						T			G		
25	4				I				T				L	
26	4				I			C				G		
27	2				I			C				G		
28	3	A					K					G		
29	1	A					K					G		
30	2				I		K					G		
31	1		D						T			G		
32	3	A					K					G		
33	2				I		K							H
34	3					E				N		G		
35	4				I				T		S			
36	4				I		K				S			
37	4				I		K					G		
38	4		D						T			G		
39	1			P					T			G		
40	3				I			C					L	
41	2			P					T				L	
42	1	A					K					G		
43	3	A					K					G		
44	3	A					K					G		
45	2	A					K					G		
46	1		D						T			G		
47	1			P					T			G		
48	1					E				N		G		
49	2	A					K					G		
50	2		D							N		G		

Answer Grid: 2

NURSING PROCESS

A = Assessment
D = Analysis, nursing diagnosis
P = Planning
I = Implementation
E = Evaluation

COGNITIVE LEVEL

K = Knowledge
C = Comprehension
T = Application
N = Analysis

CLIENT NEEDS

S = Safe, effective care environment
G = Physiological integrity
L = Psychosocial integrity
H = Health promotion/maintenance

		Nursing Process					Cognitive Level				Client Needs			
Question #	Answer #	A	D	P	I	E	K	C	T	N	S	G	L	H
51	2	A					K					G		
52	4				I			C					L	
53	1		D							N			L	
54	1				I			C				G		
55	3					E				N		G		
56	4				I					N		G		
57	2		D							N			L	
58	2	A					K					G		
59	1	A						C				G		
60	4	A						C				G		
61	1		D							N		G		
62	3	A					K					G		
63	1				I			C				G		
64	4				I			C				G		
65	1	A						C				G		
66	1		D							N			L	
67	1				I				T				L	
68	1	A					K					G		
69	3				I				T			G		
70	3				I				T			G		
71	1		D							N		G		
72	2			P					T				L	
73	4				I			C				G		
74	1				I				T			G		
75	3				I			C				G		
76	3					E				N		G		
77	1	A						C				G		
78	2	A								N		G		

ANSWER GRID: 3

NURSING PROCESS

A = Assessment
D = Analysis, nursing diagnosis
P = Planning
I = Implementation
E = Evaluation

COGNITIVE LEVEL

K = Knowledge
C = Comprehension
T = Application
N = Analysis

CLIENT NEEDS

S = Safe, effective care environment
G = Physiological integrity
L = Psychosocial integrity
H = Health promotion/maintenance

		Nursing Process					Cognitive Level				Client Needs			
Question #	Answer #	A	D	P	I	E	K	C	T	N	S	G	L	H
79	2					E				N		G		
80	1	A					K							H
81	3				I					N			L	
82	3					E				N		G		
83	4	A					K				S			
84	3		D							N		G		
85	2			P				C				G		
86	3			P					T			G		
87	1					E				N		G		
88	2				I				T			G		
89	4				I				T			G		
90	4				I				T		S			
91	1				I				T		S			
92	1				I					N		G		
93	2					E				N		G		
Number Correct														
Number Possible	93	21	14	11	37	10	21	21	28	23	8	68	15	2
Percentage Correct														

Score Calculation:

To determine your **Percentage Correct**, divide the **Number Correct** by the **Number Possible**.

The Child With Health Problems of the Lower Gastrointestinal Tract

Test 5

The Client With Diarrhea/Gastroenteritis
The Client With Appendicitis
The Client With Ingestion of Toxic Substances
The Client With Celiac Disease
The Client With Phenylketonuria
The Client With Colic
The Client With Obesity
The Client With Cow's Milk Sensitivity
Correct Answers and Rationale

Select the one best answer and indicate your choice by filling in the circle in front of the option.

The Client With Diarrhea/Gastroenteritis

A 6-month-old infant is admitted to the hospital with severe diarrhea.

1. The nurse explains to the infant's mother that diarrhea is best defined on the basis of the stools'
- ○ 1. color.
- ○ 2. amount.
- ○ 3. frequency.
- ○ 4. consistency.

2. The nurse should assign the 6-month-old infant with diarrhea to a
- ○ 1. four-bed room with postoperative clients.
- ○ 2. two-bed room with a child with a respiratory disease.
- ○ 3. private room.
- ○ 4. room with other 6-month-olds.

3. On admission the nurse should assess the infant for
- ○ 1. absent bowel sounds and abdominal tenderness.
- ○ 2. pale yellow urine and lethargy.
- ○ 3. normal skin elasticity and sunken eyeballs.
- ○ 4. depressed fontanels and dry mucus membranes.

4. An intravenous infusion is to be administered through a scalp vein on the infant's head. The nurse should prepare the parents for the procedure by explaining that
- ○ 1. a portion of hair will be removed from the infant's scalp.
- ○ 2. a sedative will be given to the infant to help keep him quiet.
- ○ 3. visiting the infant will be delayed until the infusion has been completed.
- ○ 4. holding the infant will be contraindicated while the infusion is being administered.

5. The nurse would plan to perform which of the following nursing interventions?
- ○ 1. Observe the infant at play in the playroom.
- ○ 2. Weigh the infant daily.
- ○ 3. Feed the infant formula.
- ○ 4. Play with the infant and roommate daily.

6. Which of the following nursing measures would the nurse implement to most comfort an irritable 6-month-old infant?
- ○ 1. Offering a pacifier.
- ○ 2. Placing a mobile above the crib.
- ○ 3. Sitting at the crib side and talking to the infant.
- ○ 4. Placing the infant near other infants.

7. Which of the following nursing diagnoses would be appropriate for the nurse to identify as a priority diagnosis?
- ○ 1. Altered Comfort.
- ○ 2. Altered Bowel Elimination.
- ○ 3. Altered Health Maintenance.
- ○ 4. Altered Urinary Elimination.

8. Which of the following should the nurse write on the infant's care plan as an expected client outcome related to the nursing diagnosis of Fluid Volume Deficit related to diarrhea? The client
- ○ 1. exhibits no manifestations of dehydration.
- ○ 2. has a normal bowel movement.
- ○ 3. does not have diarrhea for a 4-hour period.
- ○ 4. tolerates the intravenous fluids well.

9. The nurse explains to the father that initially the infant will
- ○ 1. not receive any liquids by mouth.
- ○ 2. be allowed to go for a ride in the stroller in the hall.
- ○ 3. be placed in a mist tent.
- ○ 4. be given multivitamins.

10. The nurse teaches the father about the next type of treatment. The nurse would determine that the father understands when he explains that
- ○ 1. the infant will receive clear liquids for 24 hours.
- ○ 2. he will offer his infant formula and juice.
- ○ 3. blood will be drawn daily to test for anemia.
- ○ 4. he can take his infant to the playroom.

A 2-year-old girl is admitted to the hospital with gastroenteritis. The mother states that her child vomited seven or eight times in the past 24 hours and has large green liquid stools.

11. The mother says she cannot stay with the child because she has two other children at home. Which response would be best for the nurse to make?
- ○ 1. "You really should stay. Your child is very sick."
- ○ 2. "I understand. You may visit anytime or call to see how your child is doing."
- ○ 3. "It really isn't necessary to stay with your child because we are here to care for her."
- ○ 4. "Is it possible for you to get someone to stay with your children? Your child here needs you because she seems very afraid of us."

12. Enteric precautions are taken with the child. Which of the following precautions would be unnecessary for the nurse to observe in this situation?
- ○ 1. Placing the child in a private room.
- ○ 2. Wearing a gown when providing nursing care.
- ○ 3. Wearing a mask when providing nursing care.
- ○ 4. Wearing gloves when changing soiled diapers.

13. Which of the following signs would the nurse recognize as an indication of moderate (10%) dehydration?
- ○ 1. Vomiting.
- ○ 2. Increased perspiration.
- ○ 3. Absence of tear formation.
- ○ 4. Decreased urine specific gravity.

14. The physician orders that the child receive 500 ml of intravenous fluids every 8 hours. The drop factor on the equipment used for the client is 60 drops per ml. How many drops of fluid should be infused each minute?
- ○ 1. 10.
- ○ 2. 25.
- ○ 3. 42.
- ○ 4. 63.

15. The nurse has an order to add 18 mEq of potassium chloride to the intravenous fluid. The potassium chloride bottle has 40 mEq per 20 ml. How much potassium chloride would the nurse add to the intravenous fluid?
- ○ 1. 4.5 ml.
- ○ 2. 9.0 ml.
- ○ 3. 26 ml.
- ○ 4. 36 ml.

16. Before adding the potassium chloride to the intravenous fluid, the nurse would determine that the child had
- ○ 1. voided.
- ○ 2. a stool.
- ○ 3. no respiratory distress.
- ○ 4. a serum calcium level drawn.

17. The nurse determines that the child is experiencing discomfort and notes swelling in the region where the intravenous needle is inserted. The nurse would explain to the mother that the
- ○ 1. needle has come out of the vein.
- ○ 2. intravenous site has been used too long.
- ○ 3. child is allergic to the metal in the needle.
- ○ 4. rate of fluid administration is too rapid for the size of the vein.

18. After several hours of intravenous fluid therapy, the nurse suspects that the child may have circulatory overload when
- ○ 1. her blood pressure drops.
- ○ 2. her respirations are slow but deep.
- ○ 3. moist crackles are heard with auscultation.
- ○ 4. her urine output has decreased markedly.

19. A culture reveals that the child's diarrhea is due to *Salmonella bacillus.* Which of the following statements would the nurse use to describe the course of *Salmonella* enteritis to the mother?
- ○ 1. Some people become chronic carriers of the organism and remain infectious for a long time.
- ○ 2. After the acute stage of the disease passes, only rarely does the organism continue to be shed from the body.
- ○ 3. The causative organism may live in the body indefinitely, but in time it will be of no danger to anyone.
- ○ 4. For people who excrete the organism for as long

as 2 to 3 months after contracting salmonella, an antitoxin has been found to be helpful in destroying the organism.

20. After the child has been on a clear liquid diet for a time, the nurse helps the mother choose foods for her child. Which of the following foods would be most appropriate?
○ 1. Bacon and eggs.
○ 2. Bananas and toast.
○ 3. Bran Chex and a bagel.
○ 4. Pancakes and sausage.

21. The nurse assesses how the child contracted *Salmonella* diarrhea. Which of the following possible sources would the nurse investigate?
○ 1. A pet dog.
○ 2. A pet canary.
○ 3. Partially cooked eggs.
○ 4. Partially cooked bacon.

22. The mother tells the community health nurse that her child answers "No!" to everything and is difficult to manage. The nurse should explain that the most probable explanation for this behavior is that the child is
○ 1. exhibiting beginning leadership skills.
○ 2. demonstrating an inherited personality trait.
○ 3. beginning to act as an individual.
○ 4. showing a typical 2-year-old's lack of interest in everything.

23. The mother says that when the child cannot have things the way she wants, she throws her legs and arms around, screams and cries. The mother says, "I don't know what to do!" The community health nurse should explain that when a toddler exhibits such behavior, it is probably best for the mother to
○ 1. ignore the behavior.
○ 2. let the child have what she wants occasionally.
○ 3. give the child some of what she demands.
○ 4. tell the child that she is disappointed in her behavior.

24. Of the following courses of action, which would be the best one for the community health nurse to suggest that the parents take when their child is demonstrating regressive behavior?
○ 1. Punishing the child's unacceptable behavior.
○ 2. Accepting the child's behavior as a coping mechanism.
○ 3. Comparing the child's behavior with that of an older sibling.
○ 4. Explaining to the child that it is now time to grow up.

25. After the child returns home, the mother reports that she does not behave as she did before hospitalization and asks the nurse about this. The nurse should reply that
○ 1. "Hospitalization is a traumatic experience for children, and it takes them time to return to former behavior."
○ 2. "Hospitalization is a traumatic experience for children, but usually they have no problems when they return home."
○ 3. "After returning home from being hospitalized, children often still feel that they should be the center of attention."
○ 4. "After returning home from being hospitalized, children usually dislike their home surroundings."

The Client With Appendicitis

A 14-year-old male is brought to the emergency department complaining of right lower quadrant pain. The tentative diagnosis is acute appendicitis.

26. When assessing the client, the nurse would be alert for signs and symptoms of appendicitis. A clinical finding consistent with appendicitis is
○ 1. costovertebral angle tenderness.
○ 2. bradycardia.
○ 3. oral temperature of 100°F.
○ 4. gross hematuria.

27. The nurse asks the client several questions during the initial health history. Which of the following questions would be most helpful in eliciting pertinent diagnostic data?
○ 1. "Where did the pain start?"
○ 2. "What did you do for the pain?"
○ 3. "How many siblings do you have?"
○ 4. "What grade are you in?"

28. While in the emergency department, the client complains of severe abdominal pain. The nurse's most appropriate action to help manage the pain would be to obtain an order for
○ 1. a heating pad.
○ 2. a laxative.
○ 3. an ice bag.
○ 4. an intravenous narcotic.

29. After assessing the client's abdomen, the nurse documents the findings. Which of the following notations would represent a deviation from normal that could indicate appendicitis?
○ 1. The abdomen appears slightly rounded.
○ 2. Bowel sounds are heard twice in 2 minutes.
○ 3. Tympany is heard in all four quadrants.
○ 4. No masses are felt.

30. Which of the client's signs and symptoms would the nurse correctly judge to be unrelated to the sympathetic effects caused by the abdominal pain?
○ 1. Tachycardia.
○ 2. Chills.

○ 3. Rapid breathing.
○ 4. Dilated pupils.

31. A diagnosis of appendicitis is made. The client is scheduled for an emergency appendectomy and is to be transferred directly from the emergency room to the operating room. Which of the following statements by the client would the nurse consider most significant?
○ 1. "It suddenly doesn't hurt at all."
○ 2. "The pain is around my navel."
○ 3. "I feel like I'm going to throw up."
○ 4. "It hurts when you press on my stomach."

32. During surgery, the client was found to have a ruptured appendix. Postoperatively, the client is to receive gentamycin sulfate (Garamycin) for several days. The nurse would recognize that one indication of potential gentamycin toxicity is
○ 1. dizziness.
○ 2. anorexia.
○ 3. hirsutism.
○ 4. constipation.

33. The client is receiving intravenous fluids at a rate of 83 ml/hour. The drop factor on the equipment is 10 drops per ml. How many drops of fluid should be infused each minute?
○ 1. 8.
○ 2. 10.
○ 3. 14.
○ 4. 18.

34. After the client returns from the recovery room, the nurse would first
○ 1. assess the dressing on the surgical site.
○ 2. assess the intravenous fluid infusion site.
○ 3. determine if the nasogastric tube is functioning.
○ 4. determine if the client has to urinate.

35. The client returns from surgery alert and oriented. Parenteral fluids are running and the nasogastric tube is attached to suction. Which of the following nursing measures would be appropriate for the client in the early postoperative period?
○ 1. Irrigate the nasogastric tube every hour.
○ 2. Test the stool for occult blood.
○ 3. Remove the nasogastric tube when the client is fully alert.
○ 4. Encourage the client to urinate frequently.

36. The client complains of nausea. The nurse would first
○ 1. administer an antiemetic.
○ 2. irrigate the nasogastric tube.
○ 3. call the doctor.
○ 4. have the client take deep breaths through the mouth until the feeling passes.

37. The nurse recognizes that the most beneficial position for the client in the early postoperative period is
○ 1. semi-Fowler's
○ 2. supine.
○ 3. left Sims'.
○ 4. prone.

38. Which of the following nursing interventions would most likely be beneficial initially in helping the client's parents deal with the hospitalization?
○ 1. Reassure them that their adolescent will be fine.
○ 2. Assess their current knowledge level before providing information.
○ 3. Encourage them to participate in the client's physical care.
○ 4. Avoid interacting with them if they appear angry or hostile.

39. Which of the following statements by the client reflects a typical concern of adolescents after surgery?
○ 1. "I hope I won't have problems from this surgery when I'm older."
○ 2. "I'm glad no one can see my scar."
○ 3. "I don't want my appendectomy to keep me from playing football."
○ 4. "I wish my scar were located where all my friends could see it."

40. While in the hospital, the client would likely to be most anxious about
○ 1. having an erection when the nurse assesses the incision.
○ 2. being separated from parents and friends.
○ 3. missing school and having to make up the lessons.
○ 4. experiencing potentially painful procedures.

41. Which of the following client actions would the nurse judge to be a healthy coping behavior?
○ 1. Insisting on wearing a shirt and gym shorts rather than pajamas.
○ 2. Avoiding interacting with other adolescents on the unit.
○ 3. Refusing to fill out the menu, allowing the nurse to do so.
○ 4. Discontinuing the intravenous infusion because of fears that "blood will leak out."

42. Which approach would likely be most effective in communicating with the client during hospitalization?
○ 1. Provide only essential information.
○ 2. Offer advice and opinions frequently.
○ 3. Use diagrams when explaining procedures.
○ 4. Use adolescent slang terms.

The Client With Ingestion of Toxic Substances

A nurse works in the children's unit of a hospital emergency room.

43. The nurse checks the drug supplies in the emergency room to ensure that syrup of ipecac is readily available. This drug is used primarily to

○ 1. induce vomiting.
○ 2. promote diuresis.
○ 3. relieve seizure activity.
○ 4. stimulate rapid intestinal elimination.

44. A child is brought to the emergency room after ingesting an undetermined amount of drain cleaner. The nurse plans typical initial care for the child when preparing to assist with
○ 1. administering an emetic.
○ 2. performing a tracheostomy.
○ 3. performing gastric lavage.
○ 4. administering cardiopulmonary resuscitation.

45. The nurse explains to the parents that after the acute stage following the ingestion of drain cleaner, their child is most likely to develop which complication?
○ 1. Esophageal ulcers.
○ 2. Esophageal varices.
○ 3. Esophageal strictures.
○ 4. Esophageal diverticuli.

46. A mother brings her child to the emergency room after the child has taken "some white pills." Which of the following signs, should lead the nurse to judge that the "pills" taken were most probably aspirin?
○ 1. Nosebleed.
○ 2. Seizure activity.
○ 3. Projectile vomiting.
○ 4. Deep, rapid respirations.

47. A child has ingested some kerosene. What complication is this child most likely to experience?
○ 1. Uremia.
○ 2. Hepatitis.
○ 3. Meningitis.
○ 4. Pneumonitis.

48. An 18-month-old child is brought to the urgent care clinic with an upper respiratory infection. Which of the following statements by the mother would indicate to the nurse that the child needs laboratory testing?
○ 1. "My child eats anything on the floor, especially paint chips."
○ 2. "My child drinks 3 cups of milk every day."
○ 3. "My child acts mean and has temper tantrums."
○ 4. "My child is smaller than other kids the same age."

49. It is determined that the child has lead poisoning and needs chelation therapy with edetate disodium. Which of the following would be an important nursing action for this child?
○ 1. Collect the urine in a lead-free container.
○ 2. Assess vital signs every 2 hours during treatment.
○ 3. Test the stool for occult blood.
○ 4. Limit visitors.

50. The nurse would explain to the mother that which of the following complications is most likely to develop if lead poisoning goes untreated?
○ 1. Cirrhosis of the liver.
○ 2. Retarded growth rate.
○ 3. Neurologic changes.
○ 4. Pathologic fractures.

51. The nurse explains to the mother about ways to prevent lead poisoning. Of the following measures, which one has been found to be most effective in preventing lead poisoning?
○ 1. Condemn old housing developments.
○ 2. Educate the public on common sources of lead.
○ 3. Educate the public on the importance of good nutrition.
○ 4. Inoculate children who live in areas where lead poisoning is common.

52. In the emergency department following an accident, a mother asks the nurse, "What's the best way for me to protect my infant when riding in the car?" Which of the following instructions should the nurse provide for using a car's seat belt to protect an infant while traveling?
○ 1. The infant should be lying on the car seat with the seat belt around it, it's better to have the infant facing the driver.
○ 2. The infant seat should sit flat on the car seat with the infant facing the driver. The seat belt is around the infant seat.
○ 3. The infant seat should face forward, with the seat belt around the infant and the seat.
○ 4. The infant seat should face backward, with the infant facing toward the back of the car with the seat belt in place.

53. For a child arriving in the emergency room with aspirin poisoning, the nurse should be prepared to assist with administration of
○ 1. oxygen.
○ 2. an emetic.
○ 3. a diuretic.
○ 4. a sedative.

54. A nurse decides a parent understands typical behavior traits of children who are accident-prone when the parent makes which of the following statements? An accident-prone child
○ 1. is passive and quiet.
○ 2. is quick to mimic elders.
○ 3. is easily frustrated and angered.
○ 4. has a normal attention span for the age.

The Client With Celiac Disease

An 18-month-old child is being treated for celiac disease.

55. The nurse explains to the mother that because the toddler has celiac disease, the stools most likely will be
○ 1. especially dark in color.

- ○ 2. abnormally small in amount.
- ○ 3. unusually hard in consistency.
- ○ 4. particularly offensive in odor.

56. During assessment, the nurse would most likely note which of the following physical findings?
- ○ 1. Enlarged liver.
- ○ 2. Protuberant abdomen.
- ○ 3. Tender inguinal lymph nodes.
- ○ 4. Edema in the lower extremities.

57. The nurse teaches the mother about the child's diet. Which of the following foods should not be included in a gluten-free diet?
- ○ 1. Wheat, oats, rye, and barley.
- ○ 2. Milk, yogurt, cheese, and butter.
- ○ 3. Rice, corn, sorghum, and soybeans.
- ○ 4. Peanuts, almonds, pecans, and walnuts.

58. The nurse should instruct the mother that her child will be on a special diet
- ○ 1. for the rest of the child's life.
- ○ 2. until the disease is well controlled.
- ○ 3. until around puberty.
- ○ 4. until desensitization to offending foods occurs.

59. The child wears reusable diapers at night. The mother asks what safety precautions she should take with wet, soiled diapers. How should the nurse respond?
- ○ 1. The diapers should be boiled after they are washed.
- ○ 2. The diapers should be soaked in an antiseptic solution before they are washed.
- ○ 3. It would be best to use disposable diapers until the diarrhea is under control.
- ○ 4. No special precautions are necessary in the care of this child's diapers.

The Client With Phenylketonuria

A mother brings her 2-year-old child to the physician's office for a routine check-up. The child was diagnosed with phenylketonuria (PKU) as a neonate.

60. For the neonatal screening serum test for phenylketonuria to be reliable, the infant must have
- ○ 1. been asleep for 3 hours before the test.
- ○ 2. had nothing by mouth for 6 hours before the test.
- ○ 3. ingested cow or human milk for 4 days before the test.
- ○ 4. a sibling who has the disease.

61. The child was not screened in the hospital at birth. In screening tests for PKU performed during the first few days of life, false-negative results are most frequently due to the neonate's
- ○ 1. inadequate fluid intake.
- ○ 2. low vitamin K level.
- ○ 3. insufficient protein intake.
- ○ 4. high bilirubin blood level.

62. The goal of care for this child would be to
- ○ 1. meet the child's nutritional needs for optimal growth.
- ○ 2. ensure the special diet is started at age 4 weeks.
- ○ 3. maintain serum phenylalanine level above 15 mg/100 ml.
- ○ 4. maintain serum phenylalanine level below 2 mg/100 ml.

63. When comparing the physical characteristics of a well child with those of this child, the nurse can expect that the child with PKU typically would have
- ○ 1. a shorter stature.
- ○ 2. a larger abdomen.
- ○ 3. a larger head size.
- ○ 4. lighter skin pigmentation.

64. The mother asks how PKU is transmitted. The nurse would reply that the disorder is transmitted by
- ○ 1. a translocation gene.
- ○ 2. a nondisjunction of a gene.
- ○ 3. an autosomal recessive gene.
- ○ 4. a homozygous dominant gene.

65. The client is given Lofenalac, one of several products on the market used to provide an adequate protein intake to a child with PKU. Lofenalac helps maintain low blood levels of what substance?
- ○ 1. Tyrosine.
- ○ 2. Galactose.
- ○ 3. Tryptophan.
- ○ 4. Phenylalanine.

66. The nurse tells the mother that the child must continue to take Lofenalac until age
- ○ 1. 2 years.
- ○ 2. 8 years.
- ○ 3. 12 years.
- ○ 4. 21 years.

67. The nurse reviews the child's diet with the mother. Which of the following foods should be omitted from the child's diet?
- ○ 1. Squash.
- ○ 2. Tapioca.
- ○ 3. Cheese.
- ○ 4. Bananas.

68. Several teaching sessions have been documented in the client's health record. The mother asks the nurse again what caused her child's PKU. Which of the following statements would best explain why the mother keeps asking for information that she has already received?
- ○ 1. Parents of a chronically ill child often want very detailed explanations about the causes of and treatments for their child's disease.
- ○ 2. Parents of a chronically ill child often require a

long time to work through the grieving process for their child's poor health.

○ 3. Parents of a chronically ill child often try to test a health worker's knowledge about the causes of and treatments for their child's disease.

○ 4. Parents of a chronically ill child often deal with their guilt about possibly causing the child's ill health with hostility and challenging questions about their child's disease.

The Client With Colic

A 6-week-old female infant is brought to the health clinic by her parents. They state that she has been crying almost constantly since birth and frequently draws her knees up to her abdomen. Colic is suspected.

69. In collecting data about the infant, the nurse would ask the parents some questions. Which of the following would not provide pertinent diagnostic data about colic?

○ 1. The amount of formula given the infant.
○ 2. The infant's crying pattern.
○ 3. The use of an infant car seat.
○ 4. The position of the infant during burping.

70. Which of the following assessment findings would be consistent with a diagnosis of colic?

○ 1. Failure to gain weight.
○ 2. Expulsion of flatus.
○ 3. Soft abdomen.
○ 4. Frequent vomiting.

71. While obtaining information about the infant's problem, the nurse asks the parents to describe the infant's bowel movements. Which of the following descriptions would the nurse expect if the infant does indeed have colic?

○ 1. Soft, yellow stools.
○ 2. Frequent watery stools.
○ 3. Ribbon-like stools.
○ 4. Mucus-like stools.

72. A diagnosis of colic is made. The mother tells the nurse that the diagnosis upsets her because she knows her infant will continue to have colicky pain. Which of the following responses would be most appropriate for the nurse to make?

○ 1. "I know that your baby's crying upsets you, but she needs your undivided attention for the next few months."
○ 2. "It can be very difficult to listen to your baby cry so often, so try to arrange some free time."
○ 3. "It's distressing to see your baby in pain, but at least she doesn't have an intestinal obstruction."
○ 4. "It will be a rough 3 months, but she will outgrow the colic by then."

73. The nurse develops a teaching plan for the mother after assessing the feeding process. Which of the following observations by the nurse while the mother is feeding the infant would indicate that the mother understood the teaching? The mother

○ 1. holds the infant supine while feeding.
○ 2. burps the infant with her sitting on her lap.
○ 3. places the infant prone after the feeding.
○ 4. burps the infant during and after the feeding.

74. The mother tells the nurse that it is difficult to get her infant comfortable when sleeping. The nurse should suggest that the mother lay the infant on her

○ 1. back.
○ 2. abdomen.
○ 3. right side.
○ 4. left side.

The Client With Obesity

An adolescent male comes to the clinic for a pre-college physical exam. Based upon his appearance, the nurse judges him to be overweight.

75. Which of the following methods would give the nurse an accurate assessment of this client's status in regard to his weight?

○ 1. A food intake diary for 1 week.
○ 2. Height and weight growth charts.
○ 3. A 1-week dietary history.
○ 4. Skinfold thickness measurements.

76. The client is found to be overweight. He is at greatest risk for

○ 1. lifelong obesity.
○ 2. narcolepsy.
○ 3. orthopedic problems.
○ 4. psychosocial problems.

77. The client tells the nurse that he would like to lose weight and asks the nurse's opinion on how to accomplish his goal. The nurse's most appropriate response would be to suggest that the client

○ 1. take appetite-suppressing drugs.
○ 2. severely limit calorie intake.
○ 3. participate in an adolescent weight-reduction program.
○ 4. cut down on sweets and other snacks.

A mother brings her 4-month-old infant to the clinic for a routine checkup. While assessing the infant's nutritional status, the nurse learns that the infant is being fed an 8-ounce bottle five times a day. The nurse realizes that this may be an excessive amount of formula for an infant this age.

78. What other assessment information would support a nursing diagnosis of Altered Nutrition: More than Body Requirements? The child
- ○ 1. wears size 9- to 12-month clothes.
- ○ 2. has a double chin and rolls of fat in the thigh area.
- ○ 3. has not rolled over from the back to the stomach.
- ○ 4. is in the 80th percentile for weight.

79. To decrease the infant's total caloric intake, the nurse should advise the mother to
- ○ 1. change the feeding from formula to skim milk and give the same amount as before.
- ○ 2. decrease the amount of each feeding and add cereal to each bottle.
- ○ 3. decrease the amount of each feeding to 6 ounces and use a smaller-holed and firmer nipple.
- ○ 4. keep the amount of feeding the same but dilute the formula with an equal amount of water.

80. The nurse continues to provide nutritional teaching to the mother, discussing introducing solids into the infant's diet. This teaching plan should include
- ○ 1. decreasing the amount of formula as solids intake increases.
- ○ 2. introducing the infant to the taste of foods by mixing them with formula.
- ○ 3. placing the food on the front of the infant's tongue to allow her to taste it.
- ○ 4. using a large-bowled spoon during the first several months.

81. The nurse would evaluate the teaching as successful when the mother says
- ○ 1. "I can't wait to go to the store! They have such a wonderful variety of fruits and vegetables for babies now."
- ○ 2. "I'll start with green beans tomorrow so the baby doesn't develop a sweet tooth."
- ○ 3. "In 1 to 2 months I can offer my baby rice cereal to start."
- ○ 4. "Since the baby's tongue will push out the food now, I can just add the fruit and cereal to her bottle."

82. The mother's sister, who is pregnant, has also come to the clinic. The nurse discusses ways to prevent overnourishing her infant including
- ○ 1. recognizing clues indicating that a baby is full.
- ○ 2. establishing a regular feeding schedule.
- ○ 3. supplementing feedings with sterile water.
- ○ 4. using commercially prepared formula.

The Client With Cow's Milk Sensitivity

Parents bring their 1-month-old infant to the hospital because he has had diarrhea and cries excessively. The diarrhea usually occurs after feedings, as does the crying. The infant is not dehydrated, and the mother reports that he is an eager nurser, burps well, and does not spit up much after feedings. Based on these findings, the nurse suspects that the child has a milk allergy.

83. The father says that he has heard of cow's milk allergy, but knows nothing about cow's milk sensitivity. The nurse would explain that it is
- ○ 1. a hereditary disorder of carbohydrate metabolism.
- ○ 2. an adverse reaction to cow's milk protein.
- ○ 3. an uncommon nutritional allergy.
- ○ 4. a life-long allergy.

84. The mother asks about the medical plan of care for her infant. The nurse explains that first an evaluation will be done to determine if the baby has a cow's milk sensitivity or lactose intolerance, and teaches the mother about what lactose intolerance means. The nurse would determine that this teaching was effective when hearing the mother explain to a visitor that lactose intolerance is
- ○ 1. a lack of something that breaks down lactose.
- ○ 2. an allergy to lactose.
- ○ 3. an inability to digest proteins.
- ○ 4. a lack of lactose production.

85. The infant undergoes a series of tests to differentiate cow's milk sensitivity from lactose intolerance. Which of the following test results would confirm a diagnosis of lactose intolerance?
- ○ 1. Blood glucose level of 20 mg/dl or less.
- ○ 2. Galactosuria.
- ○ 3. Positive hydrogen breath test.
- ○ 4. Stool pH of 7.5.

86. If a 1-year-old child were lactose-intolerant, what dairy products could the mother plan to include in the child's diet?
- ○ 1. Ice cream.
- ○ 2. Creamed soups.
- ○ 3. Pudding.
- ○ 4. Yogurt.

87. For the 1-month-old infant, lactose intolerance is ruled out and the diagnosis of cow's milk sensitivity is confirmed. If the infant is being breast-fed, the nurse should tell the mother to plan to
- ○ 1. continue to breast-feed but eliminate all milk products from her own diet.
- ○ 2. discontinue breast-feeding and start feeding a predigested formula.
- ○ 3. limit breast-feeding to once per day and begin feeding an iron-fortified formula.
- ○ 4. change to a soy-based formula exclusively and heat it before use.

88. If the child with cow's milk sensitivity is formula-fed, the nurse should advise the parents to buy

○ 1. at least a 1-month supply of goat's milk-based formula.
○ 2. the same brand of meat-based substitute as used in the hospital.
○ 3. only a few cans of soy-based substitute initially.
○ 4. a 3-day supply of predigested milk substitute.

A mother brings her 3-month-old infant to the clinic because he has periodic episodes of crying and drawing his legs up. She reports that the infant eats eagerly when fed and is gaining weight. The nurse assesses the infant to be healthy.

89. Which of the following additional information would be helpful to the nurse in planning interventions for this infant?
○ 1. Whether or not the infant sleeps through the night.
○ 2. The type and length of the mother's labor and delivery.
○ 3. Whether or not anyone in the household smokes.
○ 4. If any other children in the family had similar problems as infants.

90. The mother and the nurse outline a plan to help decrease the infant's crying episodes. Interventions that might be successful include
○ 1. avoiding swaddling the infant in a blanket.
○ 2. providing larger, less frequent feedings.
○ 3. providing movement, such as in a baby swing.
○ 4. keeping the environment as free of stimuli as possible.

91. Certain drugs are sometimes recommended for infants with colic. Which of the following would be acceptable for this infant?
○ 1. Acetaminophen (Tylenol).
○ 2. Dicyclomine hydrochloride (Bentyl).
○ 3. Phenobarbital.
○ 4. Phenytoin (Dilantin).

92. The nurse teaches the mother about feeding techniques that can help decrease colicky pain. When observing the mother feeding her infant, the nurse determines that the teaching was successful when the mother
○ 1. places the infant in an infant seat after the feeding.
○ 2. feeds the infant 7 ounces of formula.
○ 3. allows the infant to finish the bottle before burping her.
○ 4. holds the infant in a horizontal position during feeding.

CORRECT ANSWERS AND RATIONALE

The letters in parentheses following the rationale identify the step of the nursing process (A, D, P, I, E); cognitive level (K, C, T, N); and client need (S, G, L, H). See the Answer Grid for the key.

The Client With Diarrhea/Gastroenteritis

1. 4. Diarrhea is best defined on the basis of the stools' consistency, which is ordinarily liquid in nature. The color of diarrheal stools is usually greenish, but stool color is also affected by food and fluid intake. Estimates of the amount of stool can vary widely; therefore, this is not an accurate criterion by which to define diarrhea. The frequency of stools varies also, although stools occur more frequently than normal when diarrhea is present. (A, C, G)

2. 3. A child with diarrhea of undetermined origin should be placed in a private room until a causative organism can be identified. (P, C, G)

3. 4. A child with severe diarrhea will experience some degree of dehydration. Common signs of dehydration in a child whose fontanels have not closed (younger than age 12–18 months) would be depressed fontanels, dry mucus membranes, lethargy, hyperactive bowel sounds, dark urine, and sunken eyeballs. (A, C, G)

4. 1. Parents are typically quick to notice changes in their infant's physical appearance. The removal of the infant's hair may be very upsetting to them if they have not been told why it is being done. Hair is removed on the scalp at the site of needle insertion for intravenous therapy for better visualization and to provide a smooth surface on which to attach tape to secure the needle. Sedatives are not ordinarily prescribed before intravenous fluid administration. Holding an infant is encouraged to provide comfort. (P, C, L)

5. 2. A child who is dehydrated should be weighed at least once daily to determine if fluid is being restored. Body weight is a good indication of hydration status. The infant would be in a private room and not allowed in the play room. Initially the infant might not be allowed liquids or only clear fluids. (P, T, G)

6. 1. An irritable infant receiving nothing by mouth is usually best comforted by providing a pacifier to satisfy sucking needs. Such activities as placing a mobile over the crib, speaking to the infant, and placing the infant with others (unless the infant has an infectious disease) may not necessarily be contraindicated, but will not offer the comfort provided by a pacifier. (I, K, L)

7. 2. Given this infant's history of diarrhea, the most likely nursing diagnosis would be Altered Bowel Elimination. Sometimes cramping will occur and may cause pain, but this (nor any of the others) would not be the priority diagnosis. (D, N, G)

8. 1. The outcome of exhibiting no manifestations of dehydration focuses on the fluid volume deficit. A normal bowel movement, good tolerance of intravenous fluids, and an increasing time interval between bowel movements are all positive signs but they do not specifically address the nursing diagnosis. (P, T, G)

9. 1. Children hospitalized with acute diarrhea and gastroenteritis are usually not allowed fluids by mouth so as to rest the gut. The child will be in a private room and so would not be allowed to ride in a stroller in the hall. A mist tent would not be needed for this diagnosis; vitamins would be withheld until the child tolerates full-strength formula well (P, C, G)

10. 1. The usual way to treat diarrhea is to provide clear liquids for 24 hours, followed by the BRAT diet (bananas, rice cereal, applesauce, and toast). These foods are easily digested and lack bulk so as not to encourage further diarrhea. In this situation, there is no need to test the infant's blood every day for anemia or to take the infant to the playroom. The infant will remain in a private room until the causative organism can be identified. (E, N, G)

11. 2. The nurse's best course of action would be to support the mother; this is best done by conveying understanding and encouraging the mother to visit or call whenever she wants. Indicating to the mother that she should stay with her ill child seems critical and insensitive. Commenting that the child will be well cared for may suggest that the mother is not needed and may inappropriately direct the mother how to solve her dilemma without sufficient knowledge to warrant the statement. (I, C, L)

12. 3. A mask is unnecessary when enteric precautions are used because the organisms are in the stool and are not transmitted through air droplets. A private room should be provided for a child on enteric precautions. A gown should be worn when the nurse is in direct contact with the client, and gloves are necessary when the nurse is in contact with the client's stools. (A, K, S)

13. 3. The absence of tears is typically found when moderate dehydration is observed. Other typical findings associated with moderate dehydration include a dry mouth, sunken eyes, poor skin turgor, and an increased pulse rate. Perspiration would be decreased with dehydration because the body is attempting to conserve fluids. The specific gravity of urine increases with decreased output in the presence of dehydration. (A, K, G)

14. 4. The number of drops to deliver each minute is determined as follows:

$$\frac{500 \text{ ml}}{8 \text{ hr}} = 63 \text{ ml (approximately) to be infused each hour}$$

$$\frac{63 \text{ ml} \times 60 \text{ (drop factor)}}{60 \text{ min}} = \frac{3{,}780}{60} = 63 \text{ drops/min}$$

The number of drops to be infused each minute is about 63 drops. (I, T, S)

15. 2.

$$\frac{40 \text{ mEq}}{20 \text{ ml}} \times \frac{18 \text{ mEq}}{x} =$$

$$40x = 360$$

$$x = \frac{360}{40}$$

$$x = 9 \text{ ml}$$

Thus, 9 ml of potassium chloride will be added to the intravenous fluids. (I, T, S)

16. 1. Potassium chloride is readily excreted in the urine. Before adding potassium chloride to the intravenous fluid, the nurse should ascertain whether the child can void; if not, potassium chloride may build up in the serum and cause hyperkalemia. (E, N, S)

17. 1. Pain and swelling in the area of needle insertion most likely indicates that the needle has come out of the vein. The swelling occurs as the fluid infuses into subcutaneous tissues. Other typical signs of infiltration include skin pallor and coldness around the insertion site. Inflammation is likely if the intravenous site is used too long. Because an inert metal is used for manufacturing intravenous needles, the risk of an allergic reaction is remote. If fluid is administered too rapidly for the size of the vein, the fluid would most probably leak around the needle at the area of assembly onto the tubing. (E, N, S)

18. 3. Typical signs of circulatory overload include moist rales heard when auscultating over the chest wall; elevated blood pressure; engorged neck veins; a wide variation between fluid intake and output, with a higher intake than output; shortness of breath; increased respiratory rate; dyspnea; and cyanosis. (A, N, G)

19. 1. After having *Salmonella* enteritis, some persons become chronic carriers of the causative organism and remain infectious for a long time as the organism continues to be shed from the body. No antitoxin is available to treat or prevent *Salmonella* infections. (P, C, G)

20. 2. After clear liquids, the foods of choice are bananas, rice cereal, applesauce, and toast. These foods are easily digested, are low in fat, and are not bulk-formers. (Foods high in fat are difficult to digest.) The child is not given high-fiber foods, which will cause more diarrhea. (I, C, G)

21. 3. *Salmonella* bacilli are commonly spread by fowl, eggs, pet turtles, and kittens. (A, C, G)

22. 3. This toddler's behavior is typical for her age as she attempts to be self-assertive as an individual. The negativism reflects the developmental task of establishing autonomy. The toddler is attempting to exert control over her environment. It is too early to assess leadership qualities in a 2-year-old child. Negativism does not show disinterest, nor does it demonstrate an inherited personality characteristic. (D, C, H)

23. 1. Toddlers are busy developing a sense of autonomy. This requires an opportunity to make decisions and express individuality. Temper tantrums occur relatively frequently and are considered normal behavior as toddlers search for autonomy. Ignoring the outbursts is probably the best strategy. However, the mother should intervene in a temper tantrum if the child is likely to injure herself. Allowing the child to have what she wants occasionally, giving her part of what she demands, or expressing disappointment in her behavior would likely add to the problems associated with temper tantrums. (I, C, H)

24. 2. Regression is a method of coping that represents a retreat to an earlier pattern of behavior that preceded the current stresses and discomforts. Conveying acceptance of the child can help increase her feelings of worth and self-esteem, which in turn will enhance her ability to cope with stress. Punishing the child and comparing her behavior with that of an older sibling will tend to reinforce the inappropriate behavior. Shaming a child is detrimental and causes self-doubt. (I, C, L)

25. 1. Hospitalization is a traumatic time for a child, and it takes some time to readjust to the home environment. A child may regress at home for a period until he or she feels comfortable. Children normally do not dislike their home environment; in fact they usually are anxious to get home to familiar surroundings where they feel safe. (I, C, L)

The Client With Appendicitis

26. 3. The most common manifestations of appendicitis are right lower quadrant pain, localized tenderness, and fever of 99° to 102°F. Other signs of inflammation may be present, including increased pulse and respiratory rates. Costovertebral angle tenderness and hematuria are associated with urologic problems. (A, K, G)

27. 1. The pain associated with appendicitis usually begins in the periumbilical area, then progresses to the right lower quadrant. The client's siblings and grade in school may be important information, but is not helpful in making this diagnosis. (A, C, G)

28. 3. An ice bag may help relieve pain. A heating pad is contraindicated, because heat may increase circulation to the appendix and lead to rupture. Laxatives are contraindicated, because they stimulate bowel motility and can exacerbate abdominal pain. Narcotics may mask symptoms and are not given until a diagnosis is made. (P, T, G)

29. 2. Manifestations of appendicitis include decreased or absent bowel sounds. Normally, bowel sounds are heard every 10 to 30 seconds. The contour of the male adolescent abdomen is normally flat to slightly rounded. Tympany is typically heard over most of the abdomen. Masses should be absent. (A, K, G)

30. 2. Chills are a normal response of the body's immune system to infection and are not a response of the sympathetic nervous system to pain. Tachycardia, increased respiratory rate, and dilated pupils are sympathetic effects. (A, N, G)

31. 1. Sudden relief of pain in a client with appendicitis may indicate that the appendix has ruptured. Rupture relieves the pressure within the appendix, but spreads the infection to the peritoneal cavity. Periumbilical pain, vomiting, and abdominal tenderness are common manifestations. (E, N, G)

32. 1. Gentamycin sulfate (Garamycin) is a broad-spectrum aminoglycoside antibiotic that can cause nephrotoxicity and ototoxicity. Manifestations of ototoxicity include hearing problems and vestibular disturbances, such as dizziness. Anorexia, hirsutism, and constipation are not side effects of this antibiotic. (A, K, S)

33. 3.

$$\frac{83\text{ ml} \times 10\text{ (drop factor)}}{60\text{ min}} = \frac{830}{60} = 14\text{ drops/min;}$$

thus, 14 drops/minute should be infused. (I, T, S)

34. 1. Initial assessment should focus on the surgical site to determine if there is drainage. Then the nurse would assess the intravenous infusion site, assess the nasogastric tube to be sure it is functioning, and, finally determine if the client needs to urinate. (P, T, S)

35. 4. After an appendectomy, the client should be encouraged to void frequently to prevent bladder distension, which could cause strain on the incision. There is no reason to irrigate the nasogastric tube unless it ceases to function, and there is no reason to test the stools for occult blood. The nasogastric tube remains in place until peristalsis returns. (P, T, G)

36. 2. The nurse would first ensure that the nasogastric tube is working. If the tube is clogged, it can be irrigated with 20 ml of normal saline. Preparing and administering an antiemetic would take several minutes, and it would not take effect for several more minutes. The physician would not need to be called if irrigating the nasogastric tube relieves nausea. Having the client take deep breaths by itself will probably not relieve the nausea, although doing so while the nurse irrigates the nasogastric tube may help. (P, T, S)

37. 1. After an appendectomy for a ruptured appendix, assuming the semi-Fowler's or a right side-lying position helps localize the infection. These positions promote drainage from the peritoneal cavity and decrease the incidence of subdiaphragmatic abscess. (P, T, L)

38. 2. Before giving information, it is important for the nurse to assess the learner's current level of knowledge. When dealing with parents of an ill child, the nurse considers their emotional strength and the intensity of the situation and deals with it in an accepting, nonthreatening manner. Parents may feel overwhelmed by the events, and they need time to adjust to the situation. (I, T, L)

39. 3. Typically, an adolescent is concerned about the immediate state of his body and its functioning. The adolescent needs to know if any changes, such as illness, trauma, or surgery, will alter his life-style or interfere with his quest for physical perfection. (A, C, L)

40. 1. Fears of the adolescent include body changes and emerging sexual urges. The young adolescent is typically concerned about the inability to control these changes and feelings and about embarrassing himself. The typical adolescent is more concerned about being separated from the peer group than from his family and schoolwork and is not unrealistically worried about experiencing pain. (A, C, L)

41. 1. Adolescents struggle for independence and identity. Typical concerns include peer acceptance, body changes, and sexuality. Adolescents need to feel in control of situations and to conform with peers. Control and conformity are often manifested in appearance, including clothing, and this carries over into the hospital experience. The adolescent feels best when he is able to look and act as he normally does. Adolescents usually understand scientific principles and do not have unrealistic fears of bodily harm. (E, N, L)

42. 3. Adolescents can comprehend scientific rationale and complexity. They appreciate detailed description and explanations using charts, diagrams, and models. They dislike lectures and unsolicited advice and opinions. Jargon is a means to establish the identity of the peer group, and an adult's use of adolescent jargon may be viewed as false or dishonest. (P, T, L)

The Client With Ingestion of Toxic Substances

43. 1. Syrup of ipecac is an emetic that exerts its action by direct stimulation of the vomiting center and by producing irritating effects on the stomach mucosa. It is given with one to two glasses of water or fruit juice. If the child does not vomit within 20 minutes after taking syrup of ipecac, a second dose may be administered. Syrup of ipecac should be removed from the stomach by gavage if emesis does not occur, because it is cardiotoxic and is likely to produce various dysrhythmias. Most authorities recommend that syrup of ipecac be kept in the home for emergency use, stored safely out of reach of children. (A, K, G)

44. 2. Drain cleaner almost always contains lye, which can burn the mouth, pharynx, and esophagus on ingestion. The nurse should be prepared to assist with a tracheostomy, which may be necessary because of swelling around the area of the larynx. Gastric lavage and emetics would be contraindicated because they may cause perforations in the necrotic mucosa. Cardiopulmonary resuscitation would not be indicated, because lye does not interfere with cardiopulmonary function. (P, K, G)

45. 3. As the burn from the lye ingestion heals, scar tissue may cause esophageal strictures. Ulcers, varices, and diverticuli do not ordinarily occur following lye ingestion. (P, C, G)

46. 4. The salicylate ion in aspirin stimulates the respiratory center. Thus, an early sign of aspirin poisoning is deep, rapid respirations. Hyperventilation is the most impressive sign of salicylate poisoning. Other signs, such as vomiting and seizure activity, may occur later in a massive overdose. (A, N, G)

47. 4. Chemical pneumonitis is the most common complication following the ingestion of hydrocarbons, such as in kerosene. The pneumonitis is due to irritation from the hydrocarbons aspirated into the lungs. (P, C, G)

48. 1. Pica, or the eating of nonfood substances, is characteristic of children with lead poisoning. Children who eat lead-containing paint chips commonly develop lead poisoning. Drinking 3 cups of milk per day is normal. Temper tantrums are characteristic of 18-month-old children as they try to assert themselves. Determining whether the child is smaller than other children the same age requires measuring height and weight and plotting them on growth charts. (E, N, G)

49. 1. Collecting urine in lead-free containers is part of the chelation protocol. The urine is then tested for lead concentration. The other measures—taking vital signs every 2 hours, testing the stools, and limiting visitors—are not part of the protocol for chelation therapy. (P, T, G)

50. 3. The most serious and irreversible consequence of lead poisoning is mental retardation due to neurologic changes. It can be expected if lead poisoning is long-standing and goes untreated. Lead poisoning also affects the hematologic and renal systems. (P, C, G)

51. 2. Public education about the sources of lead that could cause poisoning has been found to be the most effective measure to prevent lead poisoning. Condemning old housing developments has been ineffective because lead paint still exists in many other dwellings. Providing education about good nutrition is not an effective preventive measure. There is no agent for inoculating children against lead poisoning. (P, C, G)

52. 4. In a front-end impact, the infant seat will be held securely by the seat belt and the child's head will be protected by the back of the infant seat and the back of the car seat when the infant seat faces backward (with the infant's face toward the back of the car) and the seat belt is secured around the infant seat. Other positions offer less safety. (I, T, H)

53. 2. Emergency treatment for a child who has taken an overdose of aspirin involves inducing vomiting. An emetic, such as syrup of ipecac, is almost always given. Vomiting will stop absorption of the drug by removing it from the stomach. Vomiting is not contraindicated when a child has taken an overdose of aspirin, because the drug causes no damage to tissues in the mouth, pharynx, and esophagus. (P, T, G)

54. 2. Many childhood accidents are believed to result from the child mimicking elders without realizing the dangers associated with such behavior. The accident-prone child tends to be highly curious, daring, and aggressive. The child is unable to wait for desired things and has a short attention span for his or her age. (E, N, S)

The Client With Celiac Disease

55. 4. The stools of a child with celiac disease are characteristically malodorous, pale, large (bulky), and soft (loose). Excessive flatus is common, and bouts of diarrhea may occur. (P, C, G)

56. 2. The intestines of a child with celiac disease fill with accumulated undigested food and flatus, causing the characteristic abdominal protrusion. Celiac disease is not ordinarily complicated with poor liver functioning that may cause the liver to enlarge, or with edema in the extremities. Tender inguinal lymph nodes are often associated with an infection, and celiac disease is not an infectious disease. (A, C, G)

57. 1. Damage to intestinal mucosa in celiac disease is caused by gliadin, a part of the protein found in wheat, rye, barley, and oats. Foods containing these grains must be eliminated entirely from the diet of children with celiac disease and of adults with gluten-induced enteropathy (celiac sprue). (I, T, G)

58. 1. Celiac disease is believed to be inherited. This lifelong disease is most probably due to an inborn error of metabolism or an immunologic error. A child will not outgrow the disease. With good health care, the severity of disease effects can be limited. (I, T, G)

59. 4. For a child with celiac disease, special precautions such as boiling or soaking the diapers in antiseptic are unnecessary. The disease is not infectious. If reusable diapers are used, they should be rinsed well following washing in soap or detergent to minimize skin irritation. (I, C, S)

The Client With Phenylketonuria

60. 3. This neonate must have ingested a diet high in phenylalanine, such as human or cow's milk, for 4 days or more for the serum phenylalanine levels to reach 4 mg/100 ml. (The normal value is below 2 mg/100 ml.) Testing the neonate before that time, excessive vomiting, or poor intake can yield false-negative results. (A, K, G)

61. 3. The result of PKU testing in a neonate likely will be negative even if the neonate has the condition, because the neonate is still not receiving either formula or breast milk, both of which are high in phenylalanine content. Insufficient protein intake causes a false-negative result in a screening test, because the blood level of phenylalanine is not yet elevated. (A, C, G)

62. 1. The goal of care is to prevent mental retardation. The diet is adjusted to meet the infant's nutritional needs for optimal growth. The diet needs to be started as soon as the infant is diagnosed, ideally within a few days of birth. Serum phenylalanine level should be maintained between 3 and 7 mg/100 ml. Significant brain damage usually occurs if the serum phenylalanine level exceeds 10 to 15 mg/100 ml. If the level drops below 2 mg/100 ml, the body begins to catabolize its protein stores, causing growth retardation. (D, N, G)

63. 4. A buildup of phenylalanine in the blood inhibits the proper production of the pigment melanin from tyrosine. As a result, the characteristic skin coloring of a child with PKU is light. The child is also likely to have blue eyes and light hair. Short stature, enlarged abdomen, and large head size are not associated with PKU. (A, K, G)

64. 3. PKU is due to an inborn error of metabolism. It is an autosomal recessive disorder that inhibits the conversion of phenylalanine to tyrosine. (P, C, G)

65. 4. In PKU, amino acid metabolism is abnormal. Phenylalanine is an amino acid contained in many foods. When the hepatic enzyme phenylalanine hydroxylase is missing, phenylalanine cannot be converted to tyrosine. Dietary treatment is directed toward keeping the phenylalanine blood level within a safe range: about 5 to 9 mg/dl in infants and children. (P, C, G)

66. 2. It is not known how long diet therapy must continue for children with PKU. Many experts suggest continuing diet therapy until age 6 to 8 years, by which time 90% of brain growth has occurred. (I, C, G)

67. 3. High-protein foods contain relatively large amounts of phenylalanine. Animal proteins such as milk and cheese are omitted from the diet of a child with PKU. The diet may include fruits and vegetables that are low in protein and phenylalanine; for example, squash, bananas, and tapioca. The only treatment for PKU is dietary. (P, C, G)

68. 2. Parents typically grieve about the loss of health in their child afflicted with a chronic disease. Many times they repeat questions, as though trying to deny what is really happening. This type of behavior represents an attempt to integrate the experience and their feelings with their self-image. Asking for detailed explanations, testing the competence of health workers, and expressing hostility toward health workers may explain the parents' behavior, but viewing the behavior as a part of the grieving process seems the most plausible explanation. (P, N, L)

The Client With Colic

69. 3. Information on the amount of formula ingested, crying pattern, and position for burping all can help verify a diagnosis of colic. Overfeeding may cause discomfort and distension. The colic attack begins abruptly; the cry is loud and continuous and may last for hours. The attack may end when the child is exhausted, or the child may gain some relief after passing a stool or flatus. Holding the infant upright or lying her across the lap may help. (A, K, G)

70. 2. Infants with colic have paroxysmal abdominal pain or cramping caused by the production and accumulation of gas. This causes pain and abdominal distension. They may expel flatus or eructate, but do not vomit. Despite this pain, infants with colic typically tolerate formula well, gain weight, and thrive. (A, C, G)

71. 1. Infants with colic have normal stools, typically soft and yellowish. Abnormal stools may indicate bowel obstruction or infection. (A, K, G)

72. 2. The nurse needs to provide the parents with support. Parents are stressed and need to be encouraged to get out of the house and arrange for some free time. Comparing colic to other problems is inappropriate; parents have the right to be upset. Although colic usually disappears spontaneously by age 3 months, the nurse should not make any guarantees. (P, T, L)

73. 4. Infants with colic should be burped frequently during and after the feeding. Much of the discomfort of colic appears to be associated with the presence of air in the stomach and intestines. Infants with colic should be held fairly upright while being fed, to help air rise. They should be burped using the shoulder position and placed in an infant seat after feedings. (E, N, G)

74. 2. Infants with colic seem to sleep more comfortably on the abdomen than on the back or side. (P, K, G)

The Client With Obesity

75. 4. Measuring skinfold thickness with skinfold calipers is the most common method used to assess obesity. The skinfold thickness test, which determines the amount of subcutaneous fat, determines obesity more accurately than does a height and weight chart. Assessing dietary intake gives no information about whether or not a client is overweight. (A, T, H)

76. 1. The most prevalent complication of adolescent obesity is its persistence into adulthood. The odds are 28 to 1 against an obese adolescent becoming a normal-weight adult. Narcolepsy is the most serious but uncommon effect of severe adolescent obesity. Possible orthopedic and psychological problems would be of concern, but these are not as common as the persistence of obesity into adulthood and its associated problems. (A, K, H)

77. 3. Weight loss treatment modalities that include peer involvement have proven to be the most successful approach with obese adolescents. This is because peer support is critical to adolescents, especially with an all-encompassing problem such as obesity. Use of drugs may lead to habituation. Severe calorie restriction is not recommended, because it can result in use of muscle protein for energy in addition to fat. Although decreased ingestion of nonnutritive snacks is helpful in dietary control, there is no evidence that this is a problem for this adolescent. (P, T, H)

78. 2. The obese infant appears fat, with rolls of fat and flabby skin areas. Height and weight tables are used to compare a child's measurements with norms. A difference between height and weight of one standard deviation is acceptable. Although obesity may cause a delay in motor skills, not rolling over at age 4 months is not a developmental delay. Clothing size is an arbitrary measurement of a child's size. (A, T, H)

79. 3. Six 5-ounce feedings daily is the correct amount for a child this age. Using a firmer and smaller-holed nipple will increase sucking time and help to meet the child's sucking needs. Skim milk is never recommended for infants, because it does not provide the essential fatty acids needed for growth and development. Cow's milk provides excessive protein, which increases renal solute loads and water demands. Cereal should never be mixed in formula and given in a bottle; this does not allow the infant to learn to eat from a spoon. Furthermore, this infant would not be able to digest the cereal for another month or two. Diluting the formula to 50% of its intended calories would result in insufficient caloric intake. (I, N, H)

80. 1. Decreasing the amount of formula as the infant begins to take solids helps prevent excess caloric intake. Mixing the food with formula does not allow the child to become accustomed to new textures. Because of the infant's tendency to push food out with the tongue, it may be helpful to place food at the back of the infant's tongue when feeding. A small bowled spoon is recommended for infants. (I, N, H)

81. 3. Solids are commonly introduced to an infant at around age 5 to 6 months. Before this age, the infant's gastrointestinal tract is unable to block macromolecules from absorption, which can lead to food-protein allergy. It is recommended that foods be introduced one at a time, starting with rice cereal, which is hypoallergenic. This technique enables ready identification of food allergies. After the introduction of cereal, other foods can be given in any order; a common approach is to start with fruits and vegetables and then introduce meats. Mixing food in a bottle does not allow the infant to learn to eat from a spoon. (I, N, H)

82. 1. Infants generally do not overeat unless urged to do so. Parents should watch for clues indicating that the infant is full; for example, stopping sucking and pushing the nipple out of the mouth. Giving a normal-weight infant a regular supplementation of water is unnecessary; the infant's sucking needs can be met by providing a pacifier. A demand schedule, rather than a regulated schedule, allows the infant to regulate intake according to individual needs. Bottle-feeding instead of breast-feeding is more likely to lead to excessive caloric intake. (P, N, H)

The Client With Cow's Milk Sensitivity

83. 2. Cow's milk sensitivity is an adverse local and systemic gastrointestinal reaction to cow's milk protein. This is the most common nutritional allergy in infants. Galactosemia is a hereditary disorder of carbohydrate metabolism. Almost all sensitive children can tolerate cow's milk by age 2 years. (I, C, G)

84. 1. Lactose intolerance is caused by the lack of the digestive enzyme lactase. This enzyme, found in intestinal juice, is necessary for the digestion of lactose, the primary carbohydrate in cow's milk. (E, C, G)

85. 1. A lactose intolerance test is used to confirm the diagnosis of lactose intolerance. A blood glucose level of 20 mg/dl or lower confirms the diagnosis. In lactose intolerance, fecal pH is less than 6 (acidic). A positive hydrogen breath test is associated with, but does not confirm the diagnosis of, lactose intolerance. Hydrogen gas is produced in the intestinal tract of a child who does not digest lactose completely. Galactosuria, or galactose in the urine, indicates galactosemia, a hereditary disorder of carbohydrate metabolism. (A, C, G)

86. 4. Lactose-intolerant persons are usually able to tolerate dairy products in which lactose has been fermented, such as yogurt, cheese, and buttermilk. Pudding, ice cream, and creamed soups contain lactose that has not been fermented. (P, T, G)

87. 1. Mothers of children with cow's milk allergy can continue to breast-feed if they eliminate cow's milk from their diet. It is important to encourage mothers to continue to breast-feed, as mother's milk is usually the least allergenic and most easily digested food for an infant. (P, N, G)

88. 3. Soy protein is the recommended initial milk substitute. Goat's milk is not used because of cross-reactions with cow's milk. If soy milk is not tolerated, then hydrolyzed protein or milk-based formulas may be used. Because the child may be allergic to any formula, it is best not to buy too large a supply until tolerance is verified. (P, N, G)

89. 3. The presence of smokers in the home has been linked to colic symptoms in some infants. Labor and delivery history would not be relevant. The 1-month-old infant is not expected to sleep through the night. A family history of colic is not pertinent information. (A, N, G)

90. 3. Rhythmic movement appears to help reduce crying episodes. Swaddling the child firmly in a stretchy blanket also may be helpful. Feedings for infants with colic should be more frequent and of lesser amounts. Although decreasing noxious stimuli may help, these infants often respond favorably to vibration and rocking movements. (P, T, G)

91. 3. Sedatives such as phenobarbital may be useful in treating colic symptoms. Tylenol and Dilantin would not be helpful. Bentyl can be used in infants older than 6 months, but use in younger infants has led to death. (I, K, G)

92. 1. Effective interventions for colic that center on feeding include placing the infant in an infant seat after feeding, performing frequent burping during feedings, providing small frequent feedings (7 ounces is an excessive amount for a 1-month-old), and holding the infant in a more vertical position when feeding. (E, N, G)

NURSING CARE OF CHILDREN

TEST 5: The Child With Health Problems of the Lower Gastrointestinal Track

Directions: Use this answer grid to determine areas of strength or need for further study.

NURSING PROCESS

A = Assessment
D = Analysis, nursing diagnosis
P = Planning
I = Implementation
E = Evaluation

COGNITIVE LEVEL

K = Knowledge
C = Comprehension
T = Application
N = Analysis

CLIENT NEEDS

S = Safe, effective care environment
G = Physiological integrity
L = Psychosocial integrity
H = Health promotion/maintenance

		Nursing Process					Cognitive Level				Client Needs			
Question #	Answer #	A	D	P	I	E	K	C	T	N	S	G	L	H
1	4	A						C				G		
2	3			P				C				G		
3	4	A						C				G		
4	1			P				C					L	
5	2			P					T			G		
6	1				I		K						L	
7	2		D							N		G		
8	1			P					T			G		
9	1			P				C				G		
10	1					E				N		G		
11	2				I			C					L	
12	3	A					K				S			
13	3	A					K					G		
14	4				I				T		S			
15	2				I				T		S			
16	1					E				N	S			
17	1					E				N	S			
18	3	A								N		G		
19	1			P				C				G		
20	2				I			C				G		
21	3	A						C				G		
22	3		D					C						H

ANSWER GRID: 1

Nursing Process

A = Assessment
D = Analysis, nursing diagnosis
P = Planning
I = Implementation
E = Evaluation

Cognitive Level

K = Knowledge
C = Comprehension
T = Application
N = Analysis

Client Needs

S = Safe, effective care environment
G = Physiological integrity
L = Psychosocial integrity
H = Health promotion/maintenance

		Nursing Process					Cognitive Level				Client Needs			
Question #	Answer #	A	D	P	I	E	K	C	T	N	S	G	L	H
23	1				I			C						H
24	2				I			C					L	
25	1				I			C					L	
26	3	A					K					G		
27	1	A						C				G		
28	3			P					T			G		
29	2	A					K					G		
30	2	A								N		G		
31	1					E				N		G		
32	1	A					K				S			
33	3				I				T		S			
34	1			P					T		S			
35	4			P					T			G		
36	2			P					T		S			
37	1			P					T				L	
38	2				I				T				L	
39	3	A						C					L	
40	1	A						C					L	
41	1					E				N			L	
42	3			P					T				L	
43	1	A					K					G		
44	2			P			K					G		
45	3			P				C				G		
46	4	A								N		G		
47	4			P				C				G		
48	1					E				N		G		
49	1			P					T			G		
50	3			P				C				G		

ANSWER GRID: 2

Nursing Process

A = Assessment
D = Analysis, nursing diagnosis
P = Planning
I = Implementation
E = Evaluation

Cognitive Level

K = Knowledge
C = Comprehension
T = Application
N = Analysis

Client Needs

S = Safe, effective care environment
G = Physiological integrity
L = Psychosocial integrity
H = Health promotion/maintenance

		Nursing Process					Cognitive Level				Client Needs			
Question #	Answer #	A	D	P	I	E	K	C	T	N	S	G	L	H
51	2			P				C				G		
52	4				I				T					H
53	2			P					T			G		
54	2					E				N	S			
55	4			P				C				G		
56	2	A						C				G		
57	1				I				T			G		
58	1				I				T			G		
59	4				I			C			S			
60	3	A					K					G		
61	3	A						C				G		
62	1		D							N		G		
63	4	A					K					G		
64	3			P				C				G		
65	4			P				C				G		
66	2				I			C				G		
67	3			P				C				G		
68	2			P						N			L	
69	3	A						C				G		
70	2	A					K					G		
71	1	A					K					G		
72	2			P					T				L	
73	4					E				N		G		
74	2			P			K					G		
75	4	A							T					H
76	1	A					K							H
77	3			P					T					H
78	2	A							T					H

Answer Grid: 3

NURSING PROCESS

A = Assessment
D = Analysis, nursing diagnosis
P = Planning
I = Implementation
E = Evaluation

COGNITIVE LEVEL

K = Knowledge
C = Comprehension
T = Application
N = Analysis

CLIENT NEEDS

S = Safe, effective care environment
G = Physiological integrity
L = Psychosocial integrity
H = Health promotion/maintenance

		Nursing Process					Cognitive Level				Client Needs			
Question #	Answer #	A	D	P	I	E	K	C	T	N	S	G	L	H
79	3				I					N				H
80	1				I					N				H
81	3				I					N				H
82	1			P						N				H
83	2				I			C				G		
84	1					E		C				G		
85	1	A						C				G		
86	4			P					T			G		
87	1			P						N		G		
88	3			P						N		G		
89	3	A								N		G		
90	3			P					T			G		
91	3				I		K					G		
92	1					E				N		G		
Number Correct														
Number Possible	92	28	3	32	19	10	15	32	23	22	11	57	13	11
Percentage Correct														

Score Calculation:

To determine your **Percentage Correct**, divide the **Number Correct** by the **Number Possible.**

The Child With Health Problems of the Urinary System

Test 6

The Client With Cryptorchidism
The Client With Hydrocele
The Client With Hypospadias
The Client With Urinary Tract Infection
The Client With Glomerulonephritis
The Client With Nephrotic Syndrome
The Client With Acute/Chronic Renal Failure
Correct Answers and Rationale

Select the one best answer and indicate your choice by filling in the circle in front of the option.

The Client With Cryptorchidism

A 1-month-old infant is brought to the clinic by his father for a checkup. The father explains that he is very concerned because the right side of his son's scrotum seems different. The nurse notes that the infant is circumcised and that the left scrotal sac is empty.

1. The father says he is afraid that his son's testicle is missing. The nurse should
- ○ 1. Explain that although the testis should have descended by now, it is not a cause for worry.
- ○ 2. Explain that the testes often do not descend until age 6 months, and examine the child to see if a testis is present.
- ○ 3. Explain that the testis should have been present in the scrotal sac at birth, but surgery can remedy the situation.
- ○ 4. Explain that the testis may not descend until age 6 weeks, and reflect understanding of his concern.

2. While preparing to examine the infant's scrotal sac and testes, the nurse should
- ○ 1. check for recent defecation.
- ○ 2. keep the infant from crying.
- ○ 3. keep the room and his or her hands warm.
- ○ 4. tap lightly on the left inguinal ring.

3. While the nurse is examining the infant, the father paces around the room, shaking his head and teary eyed. Which of the following would be the nurse's best remark at this time?
- ○ 1. "It must be difficult to have a child with a problem."
- ○ 2. "You seem upset; please tell me about how you're feeling."
- ○ 3. "Don't worry; his testes will probably descend on their own."
- ○ 4. "Would you like to talk with a parent of a child who has the same problem?"

4. Because several other conditions are associated with undescended testes, the nurse should also assess the infant for
- ○ 1. an outpouching low on the spine and weakness in the lower extremities.
- ○ 2. difficulty feeding and a history of frequent emesis.
- ○ 3. a reducible or nonreducible bulging in the inguinal area.
- ○ 4. heart murmur and poor weight gain.

5. A diagnosis of undescended testis is confirmed. The father is relieved to learn that surgical intervention will be postponed until the child is 2 or 3 years old. The physician, nurse, and father discuss a nonsurgical treatment consisting of
- ○ 1. a trial of human chorionic gonadotrophic hormone (HCG).

○ 2. frequent stimulation of the cremasteric reflex.
○ 3. frequent warm baths.
○ 4. use of a scrotal support.

6. The nurse planning anticipatory guidance for the child and his family would include
○ 1. teaching the parents and child (when he is developmentally able) to do a testicular self-exam each month.
○ 2. teaching the parents the signs and symptoms of urinary tract infection to watch for and report.
○ 3. informing the parents that the child will probably be sterile.
○ 4. advising the parents of the child's possible future the need for psychological support in adolescence.

7. The child fails to respond to nonsurgical treatment, and when he reaches age 2 years, surgery is scheduled. The nurse plans to do preoperative teaching by
○ 1. telling the child that his penis and scrotum will be "fixed."
○ 2. explaining that the surgeon will make an incision on his scrotum.
○ 3. telling him that he won't be able to see any incisions after surgery.
○ 4. using an anatomically correct doll to show him what will be "fixed" and how it will look.

8. The child returns from surgery, and his postanesthesia recovery period is uneventful. When planning for the child's discharge, the nurse should emphasize which of the following goals to the parents? The child will
○ 1. be free of redness or swelling at the incision site.
○ 2. take clear liquids well within 24 hours.
○ 3. have a normal bowel movement within 48 hours.
○ 4. be ambulatory within 48 hours.

9. If the child returned from surgery with traction applied to the testes, the nurse should teach the parents to
○ 1. remove the traction after 24 hours.
○ 2. maintain the traction consistently.
○ 3. increase the traction by 1/8″ every 24 hours.
○ 4. decrease the traction by 1/8″ every 12 hours.

The Client With Hydrocele

10. A 2-week-old infant is brought to the clinic by his mother for evaluation of fluid accumulation in the scrotal area. This condition is most likely a result of
○ 1. a blockage in the seminal vesicle that allows fluid to accumulate in the epididymis and ductus deferens.
○ 2. a patent processus vaginalis that allows fluid to accumulate in the testicle and peritoneal cavity.
○ 3. a patent vaginalis that results in the collection of fluid along the spermatic cord or tunica vaginalis of the testicle.
○ 4. an obliterated processus vaginalis that allows fluid to accumulate in the scrotal sac.

11. A nurse in the neonatal nursery was the first to notice the infant's problem by differentiating between accumulation of fluid and the presence of intestines in the scrotal sac, noting that
○ 1. the bulge could be reduced.
○ 2. the increase in scrotal size was bilateral.
○ 3. the scrotal sac could be transilluminated.
○ 4. the scrotum was very large.

12. During the clinic visit the mother states that the infant's scrotum is smaller than when he was born. Which further remark by the mother would indicate to the nurse that she understands why this has happened?
○ 1. "I guess keeping his bottom up has helped."
○ 2. "Massaging his groin area is working."
○ 3. "More time is needed for the fluid to be totally reabsorbed."
○ 4. "When will the physician schedule surgery?"

13. When he is 1 year old, the child undergoes surgery to correct the hydrocele. Shortly after returning to his room his mother worriedly approaches the nurse and states that her child's scrotum looks swollen and bruised. The nurse's most appropriate response would be
○ 1. "How much swelling and bruising is there? They told me the surgery was successful."
○ 2. "I'll tell the doctor immediately. Wait in the room while I call."
○ 3. "This happens often after this type of surgery. I'll call the doctor for orders."
○ 4. "This is normal after this type of surgery. Let's look at it together just to be sure."

14. The nurse applies an ice bag to the infant's scrotum. When the mother asks why, the nurse would reply
○ 1. "It increases the blood flow to the area to increase healing."
○ 2. "It's usually ordered for all this surgeon's clients."
○ 3. "The cold decreases circulation to the area and helps prevent further swelling."
○ 4. "The cold initiates a reflex that helps keep the testes in the scrotal sac during healing."

15. The mother says that the surgeon explained that her child may be more susceptible to some problem in the future, but that she was upset at the time and now can't remember what the surgeon said. What would be the nurse's best reply:
○ 1. "I'll call the surgeon if you'd like to speak with him."
○ 2. "A susceptibility to inguinal hernia is associated with this type of condition."

○ 3. "Hydrocele is sometimes associated with sterility."
○ 4. "Your baby might have problems with his bowels."

The Client With Hypospadias

On newborn assessment, a neonate is found to have hypospadias and chordee.

16. Which of the following characteristic signs would the nurse observe?
○ 1. A band of fibrous tissue, pulling the penis ventrally in an arc.
○ 2. The bladder is turned out and the urethral orifices are visible.
○ 3. The urethra opens on the dorsal surface of the penis.
○ 4. The urethra opens on the ventral surface of the penis.

17. The child's parents wish to have him circumcised. Which of the following rationale would underlie the nurse's discussion with the parents concerning the recommendation to delay circumcision?
○ 1. The associated chordee is very difficult to remove during circumcision.
○ 2. The foreskin is used to repair the deformity surgically.
○ 3. The meatus can become stenosed, leading to symptoms of urinary obstruction.
○ 4. The poorly developed penile vasculature makes the surgical procedure too risky at this time.

18. When the child is age 1 year, he is scheduled for surgery to correct the hypospadias and chordee. The nurse would explain to the parents that this is the preferred time for surgical repair because
○ 1. the child will experience less pain at this age.
○ 2. the child is too young to have developed castration anxiety.
○ 3. the reconstructed tissue will grow with the child.
○ 4. the repair is easier before the child is toilet-trained.

19. After surgical repair of the hypospadias, the child is returned to his room on the pediatric unit with an intravenous line and both a urethral catheter and a suprapubic catheter in place. The nurse explains to the parents that the primary purpose for the suprapubic catheter is to provide an
○ 1. accurate measurement of urine output.
○ 2. alternate urine elimination route.
○ 3. entry port for bladder irrigation.
○ 4. opportunity to observe urine color.

20. The nurse would evaluate the preoperative teaching for the parents about the urethral catheter to be successful when the mother states that "The catheter in his penis is there to
○ 1. keep the new tissue in place."
○ 2. keep the new urethra from growing together."
○ 3. measure his urine correctly."
○ 4. prevent bladder spasms."

21. Before the child returns from surgery, the nurse discusses with the parents about how the surgical site will appear, explaining that because this is the first of two surgeries, the child's penis will appear swollen and
○ 1. almost physically perfect.
○ 2. dusky blue at the tip.
○ 3. somewhat misshapen.
○ 4. very pale.

22. A nursing diagnosis for this child is Altered Comfort related to surgical intervention and immobility. An intervention the nurse would carry out in addition to administering an analgesic would be to
○ 1. allow him to play with other children.
○ 2. place a mobile on his crib.
○ 3. allow his parents to stay at the bedside.
○ 4. make sure he sleeps through the night.

23. Considering the child's age and the operative procedure, which of the following postoperative interventions should the nurse teach the parents? To
○ 1. assist the child to become familiar with the catheters by allowing him to manipulate them.
○ 2. encourage the child to ambulate as soon as possible by using a favorite push toy.
○ 3. force fluids, at least 2,500 cc/day, by offering him favorite juices.
○ 4. prevent the child from disrupting the catheters by using soft restraints.

24. The nurse encourages the parents to participate in their son's care. Which of the following nursing diagnoses should be of concern to the parents and nurse at this time?
○ 1. Post-Trauma Response.
○ 2. High Risk for Infection.
○ 3. High Risk for Altered Body Temperature.
○ 4. Feeding Self-Care Deficit.

25. The physician orders a urinalysis for this child. Which of the following results should the nurse report to the physician?
○ 1. Urine specific gravity 1.020.
○ 2. 10 red blood cells per high-powered field.
○ 3. 25 white blood cells per high-powered field.
○ 4. Urine pH of 5.8.

The Client With Urinary Tract Infection

A 3-year-old girl is brought to the clinic by her mother because she has "a fever and is very irritable." Her health history indicates that she has had a urinary tract infection (UTI) within the past year.

26. To complete the assessment, the nurse should also ask the mother whether the child has recently had
- ○ 1. abdominal pain.
- ○ 2. increased appetite.
- ○ 3. skin rash.
- ○ 4. back pain.

27. The nurse obtains a urine specimen for culture. What method of obtaining the specimen results in the least contamination of the specimen?
- ○ 1. Clean-catch midstream void.
- ○ 2. Straight catheterization.
- ○ 3. Suprapubic bladder aspiration.
- ○ 4. Use of a sterile urine collection bag.

28. The nurse collects the specimen and sends it to the lab. Which of the following preliminary results would indicate bacteria in the urine?
- ○ 1. Dark amber color
- ○ 2. Presence of protein
- ○ 3. pH of 3.
- ○ 4. Specific gravity of 1.005

29. The nurse teaches the mother about some measures she can take to help prevent this problem in the future. The nurse would evaluate the teaching as successful when the mother states:
- ○ 1. "She'll like more bubble baths."
- ○ 2. "We'll stop at the store on the way home and buy some of her favorite juice so she'll drink more."
- ○ 3. "We'll try to get her to hold her urine for a longer time."
- ○ 4. "We'll wash her with soap and water each time she has a bowel movement or voids."

30. Co-trimoxazole (Bactrim) is prescribed to treat the child's urinary tract infection. The mother is given a prescription for a 10-day supply. Which of the following information concerning the antibiotic should the nurse provide?
- ○ 1. If the child refuses to take the medication, mix it in some food.
- ○ 2. Keep the child from prolonged exposure to the sun until the medication is finished.
- ○ 3. Do not worry if the medication turns the child's urine red-orange.
- ○ 4. When the symptoms disappear completely, discontinue the medication.

31. Several days later, the child's father calls the clinic. He explains, "My wife and I are concerned because our child refuses to obey us concerning the preventions you told us about. She refuses to take her medication unless we buy her a present. We're reluctant to discipline her because she is sick, but we're worried about her behavior." What would be the nurse's best response?
- ○ 1. "I sympathize with your difficulties, but just ignore her behavior for now and she'll soon return to her pre-illness personality."
- ○ 2. "I understand that it's hard to discipline your child when she's ill, but she needs the family routines, discipline, and rewards to be kept as normal as possible."
- ○ 3. "I understand that things are difficult for you right now, but your child is ill and deserves special treatment."
- ○ 4. "I understand your concern, but this type of behavior happens all the time; she'll get over it when she feels better."

32. The child is found to have vesicoureteral reflux. The nurse explains to the parents that vesicoureteral reflux contributes to the development of urinary infections because it
- ○ 1. prevents complete emptying of the bladder.
- ○ 2. causes urine backflow into the ureter.
- ○ 3. results in painful bladder spasms.
- ○ 4. provides an entryway for bacteria.

The Client With Glomerulonephritis

An acutely ill 14-year-old boy is admitted to the hospital with edema of the ankles and eyelids and complaining of a sore throat. His mother says she noticed that his eyelids are swollen when he gets up in the morning, but that the swelling usually goes away. She became worried when he told her his urine was brown, and she then took him to the doctor. The client's pulse rate is 66 and his blood pressure is 138/95 mm Hg.

33. The nurse knows that another related symptom is a change in voiding, and thus would ask the mother
- ○ 1. "Has he stopped urinating?"
- ○ 2. "Has he been wetting the bed lately?"
- ○ 3. "Has he noticed any decrease in his urine output?"
- ○ 4. "Is it painful when he urinates?"

34. The physician orders a throat culture, which is positive for streptococcus. The client's mother reports that he is allergic to penicillin, and the physician has ordered amoxicillin. The nurse should
- ○ 1. ask the mother if the child is also allergic to amoxicillin.
- ○ 2. do nothing; the client's allergy is to penicillin, not amoxicillin.
- ○ 3. give erythromycin instead; it has the same action as amoxicillin.
- ○ 4. notify the physician of the allergy; the order needs to be changed.

35. The nurse assesses the client's growth. Which of the following principles offers a guideline to help the nurse analyze assessment findings?

- ○ 1. Growth does not normally follow a continuous pattern.
- ○ 2. Normal growth occurs in no particular order.
- ○ 3. The normal rate of growth varies among individuals.
- ○ 4. Various parts of the body grow at about the same rate.

36. During the admission, the nurse notes that the client has a roller-type elastic bandage from his toes to above the ankle. The mother says that he sprained an ankle playing basketball. Noting that the toes are swollen and on the cool side, the nurse would suspect that this is because

- ○ 1. the bandage was applied too loosely.
- ○ 2. the bandage had been applied in a figure-eight movement.
- ○ 3. the direction of bandage application was from the ankle down.
- ○ 4. the direction of bandage application was from the toes up.

37. Later, while talking with the nurse alone, the client says that he has had several "wet dreams" during the past couple of weeks, and he is concerned that this has made him ill. When explaining the significance of nocturnal emissions to the client, the nurse should emphasize that they are

- ○ 1. an early symptom of acute glomerulonephritis.
- ○ 2. a normal occurrence in adolescence.
- ○ 3. a positive sign that the young man is producing live sperm.
- ○ 4. a symptom of a sexual disorder.

38. The client's mouth is dry and his lips are encrusted with mucus (sordes). The most effective agent to cleanse his mouth with would be

- ○ 1. a jelly-type toothpaste.
- ○ 2. a mild white vinegar solution.
- ○ 3. half-strength hydrogen peroxide.
- ○ 4. undiluted mouthwash.

39. The client's fluid intake is restricted to 1,000 ml per 24 hours. Which of the following fluids would the nurse consider to be appropriate for the client's condition and effective at preventing excessive thirst?

- ○ 1. Ginger ale.
- ○ 2. Ice chips.
- ○ 3. Lemonade.
- ○ 4. Tap water.

40. When the client complains about the food served in the hospital, his mother offers to bring him some food from home. Considering the client's nutritional needs at this time, which of the following would the nurse and mother decide not to offer him?

- ○ 1. Apples and strawberries.
- ○ 2. Pancakes and syrup.
- ○ 3. Buttered noodles.
- ○ 4. Bananas and apples.

41. The nurse is planning interventions for the nursing diagnosis Diversional Activity Deficit. Based on his growth and development, which of the following activities would be most useful for this client?

- ○ 1. Playing a card game with a boy his same age.
- ○ 2. Putting together a puzzle with his mother.
- ○ 3. Reading an adventure novel.
- ○ 4. Watching a movie with his younger brother.

42. One of the client's teachers visits him and tells the nurse, "I never worry about him. He always lands on his feet and seems to know where he's going." This description of the client's personality is characteristic of a teenager who, according to psychologist Erik Erikson,

- ○ 1. has a poor relationship with his parents.
- ○ 2. has a sense of identity.
- ○ 3. is of above-average intelligence.
- ○ 4. is emotionally independent of his family at an earlier age than is typical.

43. Which of the following behaviors exhibited by this client would lead the nurse to make a nursing diagnosis of Impaired Thought Processes?

- ○ 1. He lets his mother make all decisions for him.
- ○ 2. He is concerned that his puffy eyes make him look different.
- ○ 3. He has slight mood swings.
- ○ 4. He insists on wearing his own clothes.

The client's condition worsens on the second morning of hospitalization. His blood pressure is elevated, and he has not voided since 7 P.M. the previous evening.

44. The appropriate initial nursing action would be to

- ○ 1. assess his neurological status.
- ○ 2. encourage him to drink more water.
- ○ 3. encourage him to eat a low-sodium breakfast.
- ○ 4. help him to ambulate.

45. The nursing care plan should include

- ○ 1. checking urine pH daily.
- ○ 2. checking vital signs every 8 hours.
- ○ 3. keeping a daily calorie count.
- ○ 4. weighing him daily.

46. The client improves, and the nurse is helping the family plan for his discharge. When developing the plan, the nurse should plan to discuss

- ○ 1. restricting dietary protein.
- ○ 2. monitoring pulse rate and rhythm.
- ○ 3. preventing respiratory infections.
- ○ 4. restricting fluids.

An older adolescent with a history of sickle-cell disease has been admitted to the hospital. His chief complaint is of "losing weight and feeling tired and irritable." He has been diagnosed with chronic glomerulonephritis.

47. Laboratory data for this adolescent most likely would include
- ○ 1. serum sodium 133 mmol/L.
- ○ 2. blood urea nitrogen (BUN) 7 mg/dl.
- ○ 3. serum potassium 4.0 mmol/L.
- ○ 4. blood pH 7.45.

48. Which of the following nursing diagnoses would the nurse most likely formulate for this client?
- ○ 1. Chronic Pain.
- ○ 2. Altered Oral Mucous Membrane.
- ○ 3. Functional Incontinence.
- ○ 4. Anticipatory Grieving.

The Client With Nephrotic Syndrome

A 3-year-old child is hospitalized for observation. He has marked dependent edema and hypoalbuminemia and his urine is frothy, but he is free from infection.

49. When assessing the child's vital signs, the nurse would expect to observe
- ○ 1. blood pressure 100/60 mm Hg.
- ○ 2. body temperature 100.8°F.
- ○ 3. pulse rate 70/minute.
- ○ 4. respiratory rate 16/minute.

50. Urinalysis reveals plus 4 for protein, which would indicate
- ○ 1. decreased production of antidiuretic hormone.
- ○ 2. increased permeability of the glomerular membrane to albumin.
- ○ 3. inhibited tubular reabsorption of sodium and water.
- ○ 4. loss of red blood cells in the urine.

51. The mother reports that the child "has been breathing hard." The child's respiratory rate is 42 and respirations are shallow. What would be the most appropriate nursing diagnosis?
- ○ 1. Ineffective Breathing Pattern related to accumulation of fluid in the alveoli.
- ○ 2. Ineffective Breathing Pattern related to accumulation of fluid in the abdominal cavity.
- ○ 3. Impaired Gas Exchange related to increased fluid in the pulmonary vascular system.
- ○ 4. Impaired Gas Exchange related to right-sided heart failure.

52. In preparing the child to have blood drawn for tests, the nurse would
- ○ 1. explain the procedure in advance and answer any questions the child asks.
- ○ 2. supplement explanations with reasons why the blood needs to be drawn.
- ○ 3. use distraction techniques during the procedure.
- ○ 4. provide verbal explanations about what will occur.

53. When obtaining a health history from the child's mother, the nurse would focus on information concerning which nursing diagnosis?
- ○ 1. Constipation.
- ○ 2. Altered Nutrition: Less than Body Requirements.
- ○ 3. Diversional Activity Deficit.
- ○ 4. Sleep Pattern Disturbance.

54. The parents, nurse, and physician have jointly discussed the child's hospital treatment and care. The nurse would know that the mother had understood the plan when she states
- ○ 1. "He really likes chips and pickles. I guess we'll have to find something else he'll eat."
- ○ 2. "We'll have to encourage him to drink lots more fluids. Did you say about 4,000 cc every day?"
- ○ 3. "We worry about the surgery. Do you think we should do direct donation of blood?"
- ○ 4. "We understand the need for antibiotics. I just wish he could take them by mouth."

55. The parents and the nurse continue to plan for the child's care. In regard to the nursing diagnosis of Fluid Volume Excess, the care plan would include
- ○ 1. limiting visitors to 2 to 3 hours a day.
- ○ 2. observing strict bed rest.
- ○ 3. testing urine for blood every shift.
- ○ 4. weighing the child before breakfast.

56. Which of the following nursing measures would help reduce edema in the child's eyelids?
- ○ 1. Apply cool compresses to the child's eyes.
- ○ 2. Elevate the head of the child's bed.
- ○ 3. Irrigate the child's eyes with warm normal saline.
- ○ 4. Limit the child's television watching.

57. The nurse wishes to evaluate the child's status in relation to fluid retention. Evidence for decreased fluid retention would be
- ○ 1. decreased abdominal girth.
- ○ 2. decreased blood pressure.
- ○ 3. increased caloric intake.
- ○ 4. increased respiratory rate.

58. The child is receiving cyclophosphamide (Cytoxan). During therapy, the nurse would monitor the child's blood
- ○ 1. glucose.
- ○ 2. platelet count.
- ○ 3. sodium.
- ○ 4. white cell count.

59. The child is extremely edematous. Which of the following measures would the nurse take for this child

in regards to the nursing diagnosis Impaired Skin Integrity?
- ○ 1. Ambulate every shift while awake.
- ○ 2. Apply lotion on opposing skin surfaces.
- ○ 3. Pad the bed's side rails.
- ○ 4. Separate opposing skin surfaces with soft cloth.

60. The nurse avoids giving any intramuscular injections to a child who has severe edema secondary to nephrosis, because intramuscular injections
- ○ 1. are more painful when edema is present.
- ○ 2. are more poorly absorbed when edema is present.
- ○ 3. are more rapidly absorbed when edema is present.
- ○ 4. cause more bruising when edema is present.

61. The child responds to treatment and is ready to go home. When helping the family plan for home care, the nurse would instruct the parents to
- ○ 1. administer pain medication whenever necessary.
- ○ 2. keep the child away from anyone with an infection.
- ○ 3. notify the physician of an increase in the child's urine output.
- ○ 4. test the urine daily for blood.

The Client With Acute/Chronic Renal Failure

An adolescent girl is admitted to the hospital with acute renal failure. Two weeks ago she had a Tenckhoff catheter inserted for peritoneal dialysis.

62. The adolescent asks the nurse to reexplain the advantages of peritoneal dialysis over hemodialysis. The nurse should point out that peritoneal dialysis involves
- ○ 1. fewer dietary restrictions.
- ○ 2. less chance of infection.
- ○ 3. less protein loss.
- ○ 4. more rapid fluid removal.

63. As the nurse performs the daily catheter exit site care with the adolescent, an important step would be to
- ○ 1. apply an occlusive dressing after cleansing the site.
- ○ 2. change the dressing when the peritoneal space is empty.
- ○ 3. examine the site for signs of infection while cleansing the area.
- ○ 4. hold the catheter taut while cleansing the skin.

64. The nurse plans discharge teaching for the adolescent and the family. In regarding diet teaching, the nurse would emphasize that which of the following nutrients should be restricted?
- ○ 1. Ascorbic acid.
- ○ 2. Calcium.
- ○ 3. Iron.
- ○ 4. Phosphorus.

65. The nurse has emphasized to the adolescent the importance of maintaining a positive self-concept. An indicator that the plan is working would be that she
- ○ 1. complains about headaches, sore throat, and nausea.
- ○ 2. insists on making her own dietary choices even if the foods she chooses are restricted.
- ○ 3. plans to quit all after-school activities when she returns home.
- ○ 4. wants to do her own dressing changes and take care of her own medications.

66. When evaluating the client's fluid status, the nurse observes that her most recent drain was 500 ml less than the amount instilled. Which of the following would indicate that the recovery of the dialysate was incomplete?
- ○ 1. The client's abdomen appears larger.
- ○ 2. The client's activity increased during the past 8 hours.
- ○ 3. The client complains of abdominal fullness.
- ○ 4. The client's weight increased 0.5 kg in the past 8 hours.

67. The nurse plans to discuss with the adolescent and her family the psychosocial aspects of going home with a peritoneal dialysis catheter in place. A topic of high priority would be the
- ○ 1. advantages of limiting social activities for a few months.
- ○ 2. advisability of not disclosing information about the peritoneal dialysis to persons outside the family.
- ○ 3. possible effect on self-concept of having an abdominal catheter.
- ○ 4. importance of relying on her parents to do the dialysis and dressing changes.

A preschool-age child develops chronic renal failure following vesicoureteral reflux. The child has been receiving intermittent peritoneal dialysis at home for the past year.

68. During a routine home visit, the public health nurse assesses the child's peritoneal catheter exit site. Which of the following findings would lead the nurse to formulate the nursing diagnosis High Risk for Infection?
- ○ 1. Dialysate leakage.
- ○ 2. Granulation tissue.
- ○ 3. Rebound tenderness.
- ○ 4. Tissue swelling.

69. After reviewing the signs and symptoms of peritonitis with the child's mother, the nurse would determine that the mother has understood the teaching when she identifies an important sign as
- ○ 1. cloudy dialysate drainage return.
- ○ 2. distended abdomen.
- ○ 3. shortness of breath.
- ○ 4. weight gain of 3 pounds in 3 days.

70. If peritonitis were suspected, which of the following nursing interventions would be appropriate?
- ○ 1. Check the dialysate drains for occult blood.
- ○ 2. Discontinue peritoneal dialysis until the peritonitis subsides.
- ○ 3. Increase the client's fluid intake.
- ○ 4. Obtain a peritoneal fluid sample for culture and sensitivity.

71. The public health nurse assesses the child for edema. Which of the following findings is associated with edema?
- ○ 1. Absence of pulmonary rales.
- ○ 2. Increased dialysis outflow.
- ○ 3. Lower than normal blood pressure.
- ○ 4. Pallor.

72. The mother tells the public health nurse that she worries about her child's future. She states, "I haven't been able to sleep or eat and have lost 10 pounds over the past month." She has not discussed her concerns with anyone but her husband. Based on this information, the public health nurse would make a tentative nursing diagnosis of
- ○ 1. Altered Parenting.
- ○ 2. Anticipatory Grieving.
- ○ 3. Altered Thought Processes.
- ○ 4. Social Isolation.

73. During the public health nurse's next visit, the mother says that for the past 2 days it has taken 30 minutes to fill the peritoneal space with dialysate and another 30 minutes to drain the dialysate at the end of a run. The nurse would judge that the
- ○ 1. inflow and drain times are normal.
- ○ 2. inflow and drain times are more than twice as long as normal.
- ○ 3. inflow time is normal, but the drain time is slower than normal.
- ○ 4. inflow time is slower than normal, but the drain time is normal.

74. The nurse discusses with the mother factors that can affect inflow and drain times. Kinked or blocked tubing can affect both times. Which of the following factors can decrease drain time?
- ○ 1. Infection of the catheter site.
- ○ 2. Inflammation of the peritoneal tissue.
- ○ 3. Tensing of the abdominal muscles.
- ○ 4. Warming of the dialysate.

75. The mother asks what she can do if both inflow and drain times are increased. The nurse would instruct her to
- ○ 1. assess the child for constipation.
- ○ 2. increase the amount of dialysate infused for each dwell.
- ○ 3. incorporate the increased inflow and drain times into the dialysis schedule.
- ○ 4. monitor the client for shoulder pain during inflow and drain times.

A toddler is admitted to the hospital diagnosed with an abdominal tumor that is the most common type of renal cancer in children. The nurse notes that the tumor does not cross the midline. The child has cryptorchidism, which is highly associated with this type of tumor. Although there is some evidence for genetic inheritance, none of the child's siblings have had this tumor.

76. When assessing the toddler, the nurse could also expect to find
- ○ 1. hypotension.
- ○ 2. hypothermia.
- ○ 3. pallor.
- ○ 4. petechiae.

77. During assessment, the nurse should keep in mind that it is important to avoid
- ○ 1. measuring the child's chest circumference.
- ○ 2. palpating the child's abdomen.
- ○ 3. placing the child in an upright position.
- ○ 4. testing the child's reflex activity.

78. Once the diagnosis is made, the nurse would prepare the family and child for tests and procedures that will be done preoperatively, including
- ○ 1. barium enema.
- ○ 2. bone scan.
- ○ 3. computerized tomography of the abdomen.
- ○ 4. upper gastrointestinal series.

79. The child is scheduled for a nephrectomy the following morning. In planning preoperative care for the child, the nurse should assign lowest priority to
- ○ 1. being very careful and gentle while bathing the child.
- ○ 2. monitoring the child's vital signs frequently.
- ○ 3. providing the child's family with emotional support.
- ○ 4. teaching the parents about the staging of the tumor.

80. The mother tells the nurse that the surgeon has verified that her child has a stage II tumor. The nurse judges that the mother understands staging when she states: "The tumor
- ○ 1. has extended beyond the kidney but was completely removed."

○ 2. is in the kidney and has spread to the lung, liver, bone and brain."
○ 3. is in the kidney but cannot be removed."
○ 4. is in the kidney and was totally removed."

81. After successful surgery, the child is returned to his room. The nurse should place the child in which position?
○ 1. Modified Trendelenburg.
○ 2. Prone.
○ 3. Semi-Fowler's.
○ 4. Supine.

82. When assisting the family in making plans for the child's treatment protocol, the nurse and the physician would discuss the use of chemotherapy and
○ 1. bone marrow transplantation.
○ 2. hyperthermia.
○ 3. leukophoresis.
○ 4. radiation.

83. The nurse would continue to assess the child postoperatively for which common complication of this surgery?
○ 1. increased abdominal distention.
○ 2. elevated blood pressure.
○ 3. increased bowel sounds.
○ 4. increased urine output.

84. The child is to receive dactinomycin (Actinomycin-D) and vincristine. The nurse teaches the parents about side effects of chemotherapy. To evaluate the effectiveness of teaching, the nurse questions them about how many weeks after the initial treatment hair loss usually occurs. Which of the following answers would indicate that they have understood the teaching?
○ 1. 2 weeks.
○ 2. 4 weeks.
○ 3. 6 weeks.
○ 4. 8 weeks.

85. The nurse and parents are planning for the child's discharge. Regarding the prescribed chemotherapy, the nurse should teach the parents to
○ 1. encourage the child to drink plenty of fluids.
○ 2. keep the child out of the sun.
○ 3. monitor the child's urine color.
○ 4. observe the child for drowsiness.

86. Additional discharge planning should involve identifying interventions that will prevent damage to the child's remaining kidney and
○ 1. minimize pain.
○ 2. prevent dependent edema.
○ 3. prevent urinary tract infection.
○ 4. restrict dietary protein intake.

CORRECT ANSWERS AND RATIONALE

The letters in parentheses following the rationale identify the step of the nursing process (A, D, P, I, E); cognitive level (K, C, T, N); and client need (S, G, L, H). See the Answer Grid for the key.

The Client With Cryptorchidism

1. 4. Testes should normally descend by age 6 weeks. Failure to do so may indicate a problem with patency or a hormonal imbalance. By acknowledging the father's concern, the nurse indicates acceptance of his feelings. (I, C, G)

2. 3. A cold environment can cause the testes to retract. Cold and touch stimulate the cremasteric reflex, which cause a normal retraction of the testes toward the body. (A, T, G)

3. 2. The nurse needs more information about the father's perceptions and feelings before providing any information or taking action. It is important that the nurse determine the exact nature of the father's concern rather than making an assumption about it. Telling the father not to worry devalues his concern; the child's testes may in fact not descend spontaneously. (A, T, L)

4. 3. An inguinal hernia, hydrocele, or upper urinary tract anomaly may occur on the same side as the undescended testis. One anomaly in a system warrants a more focused assessment of that system. (A, N, G)

5. 1. A trial of human chorionic gonadotrophin (HCG) may be given to stimulate descent of the affected testis. The cremasteric reflex results in the testis being drawn up; scrotal support or application of warmth would have little or no effect. (P, T, G)

6. 1. Although the involved testis may not produce normal sperm, the child should not be sterile. Because the incidence of testicular cancer is increased in adulthood among children who have had undescended testes, it is important to teach the testicular self-exam (TSE) procedure. Unless there are other anomalies, the incidence of urinary tract infections should not be increased. (P, N, H)

7. 4. A 2-year-old child has a limited vocabulary and will probably not comprehend a totally verbal explanation of the surgery. By using a doll, the nurse gives the child visual cues with which he can identify. Although it will not be very noticeable, an incision will be present. (P, N, L)

8. 1. A priority goal at this time would be to prevent infection at the operative site. The child can usually begin to take fluids and solids shortly after surgery and can usually get up as soon as comfort allows. Defecation is not a usual problem after this type of surgery. (P, N, G)

9. 2. In surgery a rubber band or similar device may be attached by a suture to the testis, then taped to the inner thigh, to maintain a moderate steady tension. This device prevents the testis from ascending. The traction is maintained for 5 to 7 days after surgery. (I, T, G)

The Client With Hydrocele

10. 3. A hydrocele is a collection of fluid in the tunica vaginalis of the testicle or along the spermatic cord. (D, K, G)

11. 3. A distended hydrocele can be transilluminated. A hernia, unless incarcerated, can be reduced. Both hydroceles and hernias can enlarge the scrotal sac and can be either unilateral or bilateral. (A, N, G)

12. 3. Because scrotal size is decreasing, the fluid is being absorbed. Massaging or elevation do not have an effect on fluid reabsorption in hydrocele. Because the fluid is reabsorbing, considering surgery would be premature. (E, N, G)

13. 4. Slight swelling and bruising are normal postoperatively. By assessing the area with the mother, the nurse is conveying acceptance of the mother's concern. (P, N, G)

14. 3. Cold application decreases circulation to an area to prevent edema. Cold initiates the cremasteric reflex, which draws the testis up closer to the body. By referring to surgeon's orders, the nurse avoids answering the mother's question and conveys a lack of knowledge about the intervention. (I, N, G)

15. 2. Hydrocele is often associated with inguinal hernia. It is not associated with sterility or bowel problems and it has few if any sequelae. (I, C, G)

The Client With Hypospadias

16. 4. In hypospadias, the urethra opens on the ventral surface of the penis or perineum. In congenital chordee, a fibrous band of tissue extends from the scrotum up the penis and pulls it ventrally in an arc; congenital chordee may or may not be associated with hypospadias. In epispadias, the urethra opens on the dorsal surface of the penis. In exstrophy of the bladder, the bladder is turned out and the urethral orifices are visible. (A, C, G)

17. 2. The foreskin is often used to reconstruct the urethra. Circulatory development is unimpaired. Circumcision involves removal of the end of the prepuce of the penis, whereas removal of the chordee necessitates straightening out the penis. Urethral meatal stenosis, which can occur in circumcised infants, results from meatal ulceration and can lead to symptoms of urinary obstruction. (P, N, G)

18. 2. The preferred time for surgery is age 6 to 18 months, before the child develops castration and body image anxiety. Pain is different for each client and is not related to the preferred time for repair of the hypospadias and/or chordee. The reconstructed tissue will grow with the child, regardless of the child's age. (I, N, G)

19. 2. An alternate urinary elimination route is important because the surgical site needs to be kept dry, clean, and free from the pressure of a full bladder. Pressure from a full bladder might cause fluid to leak around the urethral catheter or might disrupt the delicate plastic surgery. The bladder is rarely irrigated. Measuring urine output and noting the urine color are important, but not the primary purpose of the suprapubic catheter. (I, N, G)

20. 2. The main purpose of the urethral catheter is to maintain patency of the reconstructed urethra. The catheter prevents the new tissue inside the urethra from healing on itself, but it can cause bladder spasms. Recently, stents have been used instead of catheters. Urine output can be measured through the suprapubic catheter. (E, N, G)

21. 3. The penis may appear somewhat misshapen or bumpy because of the intermediate phase of reconstruction. The penis is unlikely to look entirely normal even after reconstruction. Swelling and local bruising would be normal; however, because the blood supply should be adequate, a dusky blue tip may indicate a problem with circulation. (I, C, G)

22. 3. For a 12-month-old infant, the most important comfort measure would be the presence of his parents. He is too young to participate in play with other children. A mobile would be more appropriate for a younger infant. Sleeping through the night would be an indication that the interventions are effective. (I, N, L)

23. 4. The most important consideration in terms of successful outcome of this surgery is the maintenance of the catheters or stents. The child is on strict bed rest postoperatively. A 12-month-old likes to explore his environment but must be prevented from manipulating his catheters through the use of soft restraints. Although increasing fluids is important, 2,500 ml/day is an excessive amount for a 12-month-old. (I, N, S)

24. 2. Preventing infection is something the parent can do through careful hand-washing. The child may have an altered temperature, but this condition would be related to infection. Post-traumatic Response is a diagnosis related to a traumatic event such as rape and is not appropriate for this child. The child should be able to maintain whatever skills he had in feeding. (D, N, S)

25. 3. A white blood cell count of 25 per high-powered field indicates urinary tract infection. With normal fluid intake, specific gravity should range from 1.002–1.030. Red blood cells are normal in urologic surgery. Normal urine pH is 4.6–8. (A, N, G)

The Client With Urinary Tract Infection

26. 1. Abdominal pain frequently accompanies urinary tract infections in young children. Other associated signs and symptoms include decreased appetite, vomiting, fever, and irritability. Flank or back pain is associated with urinary tract infection in older children and adults. Rash is unrelated to urinary tract infection. (A, N, G)

27. 3. Suprapubic bladder aspiration results in the least opportunity for contamination. (A, K, G)

28. 2. In the presence of bacteria, the urine is usually positive for protein and the pH is greater than 8.0 (alkaline). Dark amber-colored urine indicates concentrated urine. Urine specific gravity is normally 1.002 to 1.030. (A, C, G)

29. 2. Increased fluid intake promotes frequent urination, which flushes bacteria out of the urinary tract. Emptying the bladder frequently and at the first urge to void prevents urine stasis and decreases the risk of infection ascending to the kidneys. Bubble baths and frequent exposure of the vulva and urethra to soap can result in irritation, which may make urination painful and result in inadequate bladder emptying. Wiping from front to back after defecating and voiding helps prevent urethral contamination. (I, N, H)

30. 2. Co-trimoxazole can cause photosensitivity. Mixing unpalatable medications in foods can cause the child to dislike a nutritious food. This medication does not affect urine color. Antibiotic therapy should be continued for the full 10 days to eliminate the bacteria. (I, N, S)

31. 2. A 3-year-old needs to have psychosocial development maintained as much as possible during illness. Family routines and discipline should be kept as normal as possible. (I, N, H)

32. 1. The reason that UTI's are a problem in children with vesicoureteral reflux is that the urine that flows back up the ureter past the incompetent valve drains back into the bladder after the child has finished voiding. It is the incomplete emptying of the bladder that results in stasis of urine and provides a good media for bacterial growth. Vesicoureteral reflex does not cause discomfort. (I, N, G)

The Client With Glomerulonephritis

33. 3. Oliguria (subnormal urine production) is another symptom of glomerulonephritis. Enuresis is bed-wetting. Anuria is total lack of urine output. Dysuria is painful urination. (A, C, G)

34. 4. Persons who are allergic to penicillin are also allergic to amoxicillin. The nurse can not independently change a medication order, although erythromycin is the drug of choice for persons who are allergic to penicillin. (I, T, S)

35. 3. The rate of human growth is complex and varies among individuals. The tempo is uneven and different aspects of growth occur at different rates. Nevertheless, there is an underlying continuous and orderly pattern. Although each individual develops in his or her unique way, certain generalizations can be made concerning all normal human growth. (A, C, H)

36. 3. To facilitate venous drainage of an extremity, it is important to wrap elastic bandages distally to proximally. Edema in the toes, which were not involved in the injury, would indicate poor venous return. The bandage should be wrapped firmly to provide support. A figure-eight application in the ankle area helps keep the bandage in place and is the correct configuration over a flexor joint. (A, N, S)

37. 2. Nocturnal emissions, or "wet dreams," occur in about 85% of men. They occur at any age but usually begin in the teen years. A relatively common misconception is that wet dreams are a sign of sexual disorder. They do not ensure the presence of sperm and are not a sign of disease. (A, C, G)

38. 3. Half-strength hydrogen peroxide is most often recommended for cleansing the mouth and lips of crusted mucus, or sordes. The foaming action that results when the hydrogen peroxide releases oxygen and the moisture of the solution act to remove the debris. Hydrogen peroxide should not be used for regular and frequent mouth cleansing, because repeated exposure to hydrogen peroxide may damage tooth enamel. (I, T, S)

39. 2. Ice chips help moisten the mouth and lips while keeping fluid intake low. Sweet beverages like ginger ale and lemonade tend to increase thirst. Tap water will effectively relieve thirst, but will not help keep fluid intake low. (I, T, S)

40. 4. During periods of oliguria, foods high in potassium, such as bananas and citrus fruits, are restricted. Strawberries and apples are lower in potassium. High carbohydrate foods are encouraged to provide calories. (P, N, S)

41. 1. Generally, teenagers enjoy activities with their peers in preference to socializing with their parents or younger persons. Clannish peer relationships are common and normal during adolescence. They work to help the teenager develop self-identity. (P, N, L)

42. 2. The teenager who handles and solves daily problems with relative ease and seems to have a good idea of where he is going is demonstrating a good sense of self-identity. According to psychologist Erik Erikson, an important aspect of adolescent psychosocial development is developing self-identity. When this does not happen, the adolescent suffers from identity diffusion. An adolescent's success in developing self-identity is not related to intelligence. Although a poor relationship with parents may have an effect on a teenager, the establishment of self-identity is not necessarily affected by such a relationship. The client described here is not demonstrating independence from his family by appearing to develop his self-identity, although teenagers do normally work toward independence from the family. (A, N, L)

43. 1. Teenagers strive to be independent of their families. This client's dependence on his mother may indicate that he has little energy to make decisions. Teenagers are very concerned with their physical appearance and how they dress. They tend to be moody, and slight mood swings should not be of concern. (D, N, L)

44. 1. Neurological status should be assessed and seizure precautions instituted, because hypertensive encephalopathy is a major potential complication of the acute phase of glomerulonephritis. Hypertensive encephalopathy can result in transient loss of vision, hemiparesis, disorientation, and grand mal seizures. A low-sodium diet is encouraged but is not important initially. Bed rest is advocated during the acute phase of glomerulonephritis. Fluids are restricted in clients with oliguria or anuria. (I, N, G)

45. 4. Urine pH, an indication of the renal tubules' ability to maintain normal hydrogen ion concentration in plasma and extracellular fluid, does not need to be measured daily. Glomerulonephritis causes hematuria and proteinuria. The child should be weighed every day. Vital signs need to be assessed more frequently than every 8 hours in a child with an elevated blood pressure. (P, N, G)

46. 3. No diet or fluid restrictions are imposed during convalescence from glomerulonephritis. There is no need for the parents to assess pulse and respiratory rates. Infections of all types should be avoided. (P, N, H)

47. 1. A client with chronic glomerulonephritis is in a permanent salt-loosing state, so the sodium level would be on the low end of normal range. BUN and potassium are usually elevated, and a chronic state of acidosis is usually present. (D, N, G)

48. 4. This adolescent can be expected to be concerned about the loss of kidney function and the result of this loss on his life-style. The other diagnoses are unrelated to this disease process. (D, N, L)

The Client With Nephrotic Syndrome

49. 1. In nephrotic syndrome, blood pressure is characteristically normal or slightly low. The other vital signs are likely to be normal, unless edema causes respiratory distress and the respirations increase and become labored. The blood pressure reading here is within the normal range for a 3-year-old child. Temperature is elevated and pulse and respiratory rates are low for a 3-year-old. (D, N, G)

50. 2. Nephrotic syndrome involves altered glomerular permeability which results in the excretion of large amounts of protein in the urine. Antidiuretic hormone release is increased, resulting in increased tubular reabsorption of sodium and water. Nephrotic syndrome usually does not involve loss of red blood cells in the urine. (A, N, G)

51. 2. In nephrotic syndrome the cause of respiratory distress results from fluid accumulation in the abdominal cavity, which pushes the diaphragm up so it interferes with adequate chest expansion. There is usually a low vascular fluid volume in nephrotic syndrome, so there is no congestive heart failure or fluid accumulation in the pulmonary vascular bed. (D, N, G)

52. 3. A 3-year-old child will respond best to distraction during the procedure. A 3-year-old is too young for verbal teaching alone. Preparation immediately before the procedure is the preferred method for toddlers. (I, T, L)

53. 2. Diet therapy for a child with nephrotic syndrome includes increasing protein intake to replace albumin lost in the urine. During periods of edema, the child's appetite will be poor, so it is important for the nurse to learn about the child's food likes and dislikes. (D, N, G)

54. 1. Sodium intake is restricted in nephrotic syndrome. Potato chips and pickles are high in sodium. Fluid intake is not restricted; however, 4,000 cc is an excessive amount for a 3-year-old child. Surgical intervention and antibiotic therapy are not part of the treatment plan for nephrotic syndrome. (E, N, G)

55. 4. Daily weights help determine fluid losses and gains. Bed rest and limiting visitors would help ensure that the client gets adequate rest. Urine is tested for protein, not blood, in nephrotic syndrome. (P, N, G)

56. 2. Elevating the head of the bed allows gravity to increase the downward flow of fluids in the body and away from the face. Such measures as limiting television, irrigating eyes, and applying cool compresses may be comforting but will not decrease edema. (I, N, G)

57. 1. Decreased abdominal girth is a sign of reduced fluid in the third spaces and tissues. Although increased caloric intake may indicate decreased intestinal edema, it is not the most accurate indicator of fluid retention. Increased respiratory rate might be an indication of increasing ascites. In nephrotic syndrome, as tissue and third space edema increases, intravascular volume decreases; a drop in blood pressure would not necessarily indicate a decrease in fluid retention. (E, N, G)

58. 4. Children with nephrotic syndrome who are sensitive to steroids or have frequent relapses are candidates for therapy with cyclophosphamide. Common side effects include decreased white blood cell count, increased susceptibility to infections, cystitis (from bladder irritation when the drug accumulates in the bladder before excretion) and possibly hair loss and sterility. Because a child with nephrotic syndrome is susceptible to infection, it is very important to monitor white blood cell count and take precautions if it is low. (A, N, S)

59. 4. Placing soft cloth between opposing skin surfaces absorbs moisture. Applying lotion to edematous surfaces that touch increases moisture and can lead to maceration. The child with edema is usually maintained on bed rest. Padding the side rails might be an appropriate safety measure, but it will not prevent skin breakdown. (I, T, S)

60. 2. Intramuscular injections are absorbed more slowly from edematous tissue. Severe edema impedes circulation and interferes with medication absorption. The more edemal present, the less quickly the medication can be absorbed. This fact makes it difficult to maintain consistent drug blood levels. Bruising may be decreased because it occurs when the needle punctures a vessel, and with edema there is less chance of accidently putting the needle through a vein or artery. If the medication is irritating to tissue, the impeded uptake might cause more discomfort, but otherwise the pain level should be about the same as in nonedematous tissue. (I, N, S)

61. 2. A child in remission from nephrotic syndrome should be protected from infection. Pain is not associated with this disorder. The physician should be notified if urine output decreases. There is no reason to test for blood in the urine. (P, T, G)

The Client With Acute/Chronic Renal Failure

62. 1. A client receiving peritoneal dialysis has few dietary restrictions, whereas a client receiving hemodialysis usually has fluid and food restrictions. During peritoneal dialysis, plasma proteins, amino acids, and polypeptides diffuse into the dialysate because of the permeability of the peritoneal membrane. Peritoneal dialysis removes fluid less rapidly than does hemodialysis. Infection is associated with both hemodialysis and peritoneal dialysis. The risk of peritonitis is the major disadvantage of peritoneal dialysis. (I, C, G)

63. 3. Until it heals, the catheter exit site is particularly vulnerable to invasion by pathogenic organisms.

Therefore, the site must be monitored for signs of infection. Holding the catheter taut or pulling on it may cause irritation of the skin at the exit site, which could lead to infection. Site care may be done anytime, but the child may experience abdominal discomfort if the peritoneal space is dry during site care. An occlusive dressing is not needed, because there is no danger of air being sucked in or out of the peritoneal space. Furthermore, the catheter used is designed with a cuff, so the skin grows around the catheter. (I, T, S)

64. 4. With minimal or absent kidney function, the serum phosphate level rises and the ionized calcium level falls in response. This causes increased secretion of parathyroid hormone, which releases calcium from the bones. Renal failure results in decreased erythropoietin production, necessitating increased iron and ascorbic acid intake. (P, N, G)

65. 4. Compliance with the medical regimen indicates a positive self-image. Social withdrawal from activities may indicate depression. Diffuse somatic complaints could indicate anxiety. (A, N, L)

66. 4. Increased weight is the best indicator of unrecovered dialysate. Activity level does not change in direct response to incomplete recovery of fluid. Abdominal distention or fullness could be due to a number of other factors; for example, constipation. (E, N, G)

67. 3. Body image is an important concern to an adolescent, and the client needs opportunities to discuss feelings about altered body image. Other developmental needs of adolescents are increasing appropriate independence and maintaining social activities. The client may choose to confide in friends for both psychological health and physical safety. (P, N, L)

68. 4. Tissue swelling, pain, redness, and exudate indicate infection. Granulation tissue indicates healing around the exit site. Dialysate leakage is associated with improper catheter function, incomplete healing at the insertion site, or excessive instillation of dialysate. Rebound tenderness is a manifestation of peritonitis. (A, T, G)

69. 1. With peritonitis, large numbers of bacteria, white blood cells, and fibrin cause the dialysate to appear cloudy. Weight gain indicates fluid excess rather than infection. Shortness of breath is associated with fluid excess. Abdominal distention is unrelated to peritonitis. (E, N, S)

70. 4. The nurse notifies the physician so that a change in medical management can be made. A sample of the peritoneal fluid is sent for culture and sensitivity; the results guide the choice of an effective antibiotic agent. Discontinuing peritoneal dialysis promotes infection and leads to fluid and electrolyte imbalance. Occult blood in the dialysate is not associated with peritonitis. Peritonitis can cause an ileus; therefore, fluid intake is not increased. (I, N, S)

71. 4. With edema, pallor can occur due to hemodilution. Other indications of edema include elevated blood pressure, pulmonary rales, and decreased dialysate outflow. (A, N, G)

72. 2. Anticipatory Grieving refers to the expectation of the loss of a significant relationship. Symptoms of this state include sleeplessness and altered nutritional patterns. Altered Parenting involves a parent's inability to nurture. Altered Thought Processes refers to inappropriate or nonreality based thinking. Social Isolation is marked by interpersonal interaction below the level desired or required for personal integrity. This mother is confiding in the nurse and in her husband. (D, N, L)

73. 2. Normal inflow and drain times are about 10 minutes. (A, T, S)

74. 3. Tensing the abdominal muscles increases drain time. Peritonitis and catheter site infection do not affect flow. Warming the dialysate to body temperature promotes comfort and minimizes abdominal pain; it does not prevent outflow. (I, T, S)

75. 1. The accumulation of hard stool in the bowel can cause the distended intestine to block the holes of the catheter. Consequently, the dialysate cannot flow freely through the catheter. Increasing the dialysate infusion can cause pain and possible leakage at the exit site. Adjusting the dialysis schedule may make the dialysis less effective. Altering fluid, electrolyte, and waste product removal can cause fluid and electrolyte imbalance and elevated BUN and creatinine levels. Shoulder pain can be caused by air in the peritoneal space and diaphragmatic irritation. (P, N, S)

76. 3. Wilm's tumor, or nephroblastoma, is the most common intra-abdominal tumor of childhood and the most common type of renal cancer. It is highly malignant. Anemia, which is secondary to hemorrhage within the tumor, causes pallor, anorexia, and lethargy. The most common presenting sign is an abdominal mass. Other signs and symptoms are the result of compression from the tumor mass, metabolic alterations secondary to the tumor, or metastasis. Hypertension occurs occasionally, probably due to excessive excretion of renin by the tumor. Other common effects of malignancy include weight loss and fever. Petechiae are not associated with Wilm's tumor. (A, N, G)

77. 2. The abdomen of the child with Wilm's tumor should not be palpated because of the danger of disseminating tumor cells. Techniques such as testing for reflex activity, upright positioning, and measuring chest circumference are not necessarily contraindicated; however, the child with Wilm's tumor should always be handled gently and carefully. (A, N, S)

78. 3. Computerized tomography (CT) scan of the abdomen is done after diagnosis is confirmed to determine the tumor's size and position and its relationship to the involved and uninvolved kidney. Upper and lower gastrointestinal series and bone scan are not indicated. (P, N, G)

79. 4. Teaching the parents about staging of Wilm's tumor is done at the time of diagnosis. Preoperative explanations should be kept simple and focus on what the child will experience. Vital signs, including blood pressure, must be monitored frequently, because hypertension from excess renin production is possible. Careful bathing and handling are essential to prevent trauma to the tumor. As with all diagnoses of cancer, Wilm's tumor is a shock to the family. The parents may feel guilty for not finding the mass sooner, and with the swiftness of the diagnosis will need emotional support. (P, N, G)

80. 1. A stage II tumor extends beyond the kidney but is completely resected. The tumor staging is verified during surgery to maximize treatment protocols. The following criteria for staging are commonly used:
Stage I: Tumor is limited to the kidney and completely resected.
Stage II: Tumor extends beyond the kidney but is completely resected.
Stage III: Residual nonhematogenous tumor is confined to the abdomen.
Stage IV: Hematogenous metastasis occurs; deposits beyond stage III (lung, bone and brain, liver).
Stage V: Bilateral renal involvement is present at diagnosis. (E, C, G)

81. 3. The child who has undergone abdominal surgery is usually placed in a semi-Fowler's position to facilitate draining of abdominal contents and to promote pulmonary expansion. The prone position is likely to be uncomfortable because of the large transabdominal incision. The supine position, without the head elevated, puts the child at increased risk for aspiration. The modified Trendelenburg position is used for clients in shock. (I, T, S)

82. 4. The optimum treatment protocol for Wilm's tumor at stage II is abdominal radiation and chemotherapy. Postoperative radiotherapy is indicated for all children with Wilm's tumor except those with stage I disease and favorable histology. Chemotherapy is indicated for all stages. (P, C, G)

83. 1. Children who have undergone abdominal surgery are at risk for intestinal obstruction from adynamic ileus. Indications of intestinal obstruction include abdominal distention, decreased or absent bowel sounds, and vomiting. Later signs of intestinal obstruction include tachycardia, fever, hypotension, shock, and decreased urinary output. (A, T, G)

84. 1. Hair loss, or alopecia, does not occur until 2 weeks after the initial chemotherapy treatment. Chemotherapy for Wilm's tumor is begun immediately after surgery. (E, C, G)

85. 1. Dactinomycin and vincristine both cause nausea and vomiting. Oral fluids are encouraged and antiemetics are given to prevent dehydration. Avoiding sun exposure is not necessary. Drowsiness and changes in urine color are not associated with either or these drugs. (P, N, S)

86. 3. Because the child only has one kidney, measures should be recommended to prevent urinary tract infection and injury to the remaining kidney. Severe pain and dependent edema are not associated with postoperative Wilm's tumor clients. Dietary protein is not restricted, because function in the remaining kidney is not impaired. (P, N, G)

NURSING CARE OF CHILDREN

TEST 6: The Child With Health Problems of the Urinary System

Directions: Use this answer grid to determine areas of strength or need for further study.

NURSING PROCESS

A = Assessment
D = Analysis, nursing diagnosis
P = Planning
I = Implementation
E = Evaluation

COGNITIVE LEVEL

K = Knowledge
C = Comprehension
T = Application
N = Analysis

CLIENT NEEDS

S = Safe, effective care environment
G = Physiological integrity
L = Psychosocial integrity
H = Health promotion/maintenance

		Nursing Process					Cognitive Level				Client Needs			
Question #	Answer #	A	D	P	I	E	K	C	T	N	S	G	L	H
1	4				I			C				G		
2	3	A							T			G		
3	2	A							T				L	
4	3	A								N		G		
5	1			P					T			G		
6	1			P						N				H
7	4			P						N			L	
8	1			P						N		G		
9	2				I				T			G		
10	3		D				K					G		
11	3	A								N		G		
12	3					E				N		G		
13	4			P						N		G		
14	3				I					N		G		
15	2				I			C				G		
16	4	A						C				G		
17	2			P						N		G		
18	2				I					N		G		
19	2				I					N		G		
20	2					E				N		G		
21	3				I			C				G		
22	3				I					N			L	

Nursing Process

A = Assessment
D = Analysis, nursing diagnosis
P = Planning
I = Implementation
E = Evaluation

Cognitive Level

K = Knowledge
C = Comprehension
T = Application
N = Analysis

Client Needs

S = Safe, effective care environment
G = Physiological integrity
L = Psychosocial integrity
H = Health promotion/maintenance

		Nursing Process					Cognitive Level				Client Needs			
Question #	Answer #	A	D	P	I	E	K	C	T	N	S	G	L	H
23	4				I					N	S			
24	2		D							N	S			
25	3	A								N		G		
26	1	A								N		G		
27	3	A					K					G		
28	2	A						C				G		
29	2				I					N				H
30	2				I					N	S			
31	2				I					N				H
32	1				I					N		G		
33	3	A						C				G		
34	4				I				T		S			
35	3	A						C						H
36	3	A								N	S			
37	2	A						C				G		
38	3				I				T		S			
39	2				I				T		S			
40	4			P						N	S			
41	1			P						N			L	
42	2	A								N			L	
43	1		D							N			L	
44	1				I					N		G		
45	4			P						N		G		
46	3			P						N				H
47	1		D							N		G		
48	4		D							N			L	
49	1		D							N		G		
50	2	A								N		G		

ANSWER GRID: 2

NURSING PROCESS

A = Assessment
D = Analysis, nursing diagnosis
P = Planning
I = Implementation
E = Evaluation

COGNITIVE LEVEL

K = Knowledge
C = Comprehension
T = Application
N = Analysis

CLIENT NEEDS

S = Safe, effective care environment
G = Physiological integrity
L = Psychosocial integrity
H = Health promotion/maintenance

		Nursing Process					Cognitive Level				Client Needs			
Question #	Answer #	A	D	P	I	E	K	C	T	N	S	G	L	H
51	2		D							N		G		
52	3				I				T				L	
53	2		D							N		G		
54	1					E				N		G		
55	4			P						N		G		
56	2				I					N		G		
57	1					E				N		G		
58	4	A								N	S			
59	4				I					N	S			
60	2				I				T		S			
61	2			P					T			G		
62	1				I			C				G		
63	3				I				T		S			
64	4			P						N		G		
65	4	A								N			L	
66	4					E				N		G		
67	3			P						N			L	
68	4	A							T			G		
69	1					E				N	S			
70	4				I					N	S			
71	4	A								N		G		
72	2		D							N			L	
73	2	A							T		S			
74	3				I				T		S			
75	1			P						N	S			
76	3	A								N		G		
77	2	A								N	S			
78	3			P						N		G		

ANSWER GRID: 3

NURSING PROCESS

A = Assessment
D = Analysis, nursing diagnosis
P = Planning
I = Implementation
E = Evaluation

COGNITIVE LEVEL

K = Knowledge
C = Comprehension
T = Application
N = Analysis

CLIENT NEEDS

S = Safe, effective care environment
G = Physiological integrity
L = Psychosocial integrity
H = Health promotion/maintenance

		Nursing Process					Cognitive Level				Client Needs			
Question #	Answer #	A	D	P	I	E	K	C	T	N	S	G	L	H
79	4			P						N		G		
80	1					E		C				G		
81	3				I				T		S			
82	4			P				C				G		
83	1	A							T			G		
84	1					E		C				G		
85	1			P						N	S			
86	3			P						N		G		
Number Correct														
Number Possible	86	23	9	20	26	8	2	12	16	56	20	50	11	5
Percentage Correct														

Score Calculation:

To determine your **Percentage Correct**, divide the **Number Correct** by the **Number Possible**.

The Child With Neurological Health Problems

Test 7

The Client With Myelomeningocele
The Client With Hydrocephalus
The Client With a Seizure Disorder
The Client With Meningitis
The Client With Infectious Polyneuritis (Guillain-Barré Syndrome)
The Client With a Head Injury
The Client With a Brain Tumor
The Client With a Spinal Cord Injury
Correct Answers and Rationale

Select the one best answer and indicate your choice by filling in the circle in front of the option.

The Client With Myelomeningocele

A male neonate is admitted to the neonatal unit following delivery and placed in an isolette. He has a 3 cm by 5 cm sac in the lumbar region of his back. The diagnosis is myelomeningocele.

1. When assessing this neonate, the nurse would expect to see a
- ○ 1. cyst containing serosanguinous fluid and fatty tissue located on any area of the spinal column.
- ○ 2. skin-covered sac containing bits of hair located on the low lumbar or sacral area of the spine.
- ○ 3. soft sac containing fluid and meninges located anywhere on the spine.
- ○ 4. a soft sac containing spinal fluid, meninges, spinal cord, and/or nerve roots protruding through a bony defect in the spine.

2. Given the clinical manifestations associated with upper lumbar myelomeningocele, which of the following findings would the nurse anticipate when assessing this neonate?
- ○ 1. Minimal movement of the lower extremities and dribbling of urine.
- ○ 2. Minimal movement of the lower extremities and dribbling of urine and feces.
- ○ 3. Paralysis of the lower extremities and rectal prolapse.
- ○ 4. Paralysis of the upper and lower extremities and dribbling of feces.

3. The family has been informed of the neonate's diagnosis of myelomeningocele. The nurse is planning to have the parents see the neonate as soon as possible. During the parents' first visit, the nurse would plan to initially
- ○ 1. emphasize the neonate's normal and positive features.
- ○ 2. encourage the parents to discuss their fears and concerns.
- ○ 3. reinforce the doctor's explanation of the defect.
- ○ 4. have the parents hold the neonate.

4. While discussing a plan of care for the neonate, the mother asks if her baby will be at risk for any other defects. The nurse's answer would be based on the fact the myelomeningocele is frequently associated with
- ○ 1. an abnormal increase in cerebrospinal fluid (CSF) within the cranial cavity.
- ○ 2. an abnormally small head.

○ 3. congenital absence of the cranial vault.
○ 4. premature fusion of the cranial sutures.

5. During the planning session, the parents also ask about their child's future mental ability. The nurse's best response would be
○ 1. "Approximately one-third are mentally retarded, but it's too early to tell about your child."
○ 2. "Most infants with this defect are significantly mentally retarded."
○ 3. "Your child will probably be of normal intelligence, because he's so alert now."
○ 4. "You'll need to talk with the doctor about that later."

6. The neonate is experiencing urine retention with overflow incontinence. The nurse should
○ 1. apply gentle pressure to the suprapubic area.
○ 2. initiate an intermittent clean catheterization program.
○ 3. insert an indwelling urinary catheter.
○ 4. perform a suprapubic aspiration.

7. The nurse places the infant in an isolette shortly after birth. The nurse would judge that this intervention was successful when the neonate's
○ 1. arterial pO_2 remains between 90 and 100.
○ 2. axillary temperature remains between 97 to 98°F.
○ 3. bilirubin level remains stable.
○ 4. weight increases by about 1 ounce per day.

8. When planning the nursing care for the neonate before surgical repair of the defect, the nurse should include
○ 1. applying thin layers of tincture of benzoin to the defect.
○ 2. covering the defect with a dry, nonadherent dressing.
○ 3. covering the defect with moist, sterile saline dressings.
○ 4. leaving the defect exposed to air.

9. A nursing goal is to protect the sac from pressure and potential infection before closure. To achieve this goal, the nurse would position the neonate in which position?
○ 1. Low Trendelenburg, with the hips slightly flexed.
○ 2. Supine, with the lower extremities slightly elevated.
○ 3. Side-lying, with support behind the sac.
○ 4. Supine, with the upper body slightly elevated.

10. The neonate undergoes surgery and tolerates the procedure well. When developing a nursing care plan for the neonate, the nurse would include which of the following nursing diagnoses?
○ 1. Activity Intolerance.
○ 2. Self-Care Deficit.
○ 3. Altered Tissue Perfusion.
○ 4. High Risk for Disuse Syndrome.

11. To prevent musculoskeletal deformity, the postoperative nursing care plan for a child with myelomeningocele should include maintaining the
○ 1. feet in a flexed position.
○ 2. hips in an abducted position.
○ 3. knees in hyperextended position.
○ 4. legs in the adducted position.

12. During postoperative assessment of the neonate, the nurse would look for which initial signs of hydrocephalus?
○ 1. Distended scalp veins and vomiting.
○ 2. Frontal bossing and sunset eyes.
○ 3. Increased head circumference and bulging fontanel.
○ 4. Irritability and shrill cry.

13. The nurse and family are preparing for discharge. Appropriate referral(s) for the neonate and the family at this time would include
○ 1. a counselor for ongoing psychological therapy.
○ 2. agencies that can give financial help when medical insurance lapses.
○ 3. a parent group for family support.
○ 4. appropriate residential facilities for future placement.

14. A public health nurse is doing ongoing teaching for the neonate's family. Which of the following statements by the mother would indicate that the parents understand the teaching? "We will
○ 1. apply a heating pad to his lower back."
○ 2. keep him away from other children."
○ 3. notify the doctor if his urine has a bad smell."
○ 4. prevent him from rolling over."

The Client With Hydrocephalus

A mother brings her 6-week-old male infant to the clinic for a well child visit.

15. The nurse weighs the child and measures his length, head circumference, and chest circumference. The child's weight, length, and chest circumference are in the 50th percentile for his age; his head circumference is at the 85th percentile. Next, the nurse should
○ 1. assess motor and sensory function of the legs.
○ 2. examine the fontanel and sutures.
○ 3. advise the mother to bring him back in 1 month for follow-up.
○ 4. obtain a permit for transillumination.

16. The infant is admitted to the hospital and, following diagnostic evaluation, is scheduled to have a ventriculoperitoneal shunt implanted. Preoperatively, the infant is irritable and lethargic and difficult to feed. To maintain his nutritional status, the nurse would

○ 1. feed the infant just before doing any procedures.
○ 2. give the infant small, frequent feedings.
○ 3. leave the infant flat in the crib while feeding.
○ 4. schedule the feedings for every 6 hours.

17. The mother asks the nurse if her child will have any long-term problems because of the hydrocephalus. The nurse should explain that
○ 1. it is impossible to predict the outcome for the child at this point.
○ 2. the child will have some sensory and motor deficits.
○ 3. the child should do very well and have normal intelligence.
○ 4. the physician can answer this question after the shunt is placed.

18. Surgery is to be performed, with a ventroperitoneal shunt inserted on the right side. Immediately after surgery, the nurse would plan to position the infant
○ 1. on the left side, with the foot of the bed elevated.
○ 2. on the right side, with the head of the bed elevated.
○ 3. supine, with the head of the crib elevated.
○ 4. supine, with the head of the crib flat.

19. Postoperative nursing care of an infant with a ventriculoperitoneal shunt should also include
○ 1. administering narcotics for pain control.
○ 2. checking the urine for glucose and ketones.
○ 3. monitoring for increased temperature.
○ 4. testing CSF leakage for protein.

20. Two days after placement of a ventriculoperitoneal shunt, the infant shows signs of increased intracranial pressure. The physician orders the nurse to compress the valve of the shunt. The valve depresses easily but does not refill. The nurse would evaluate this data and judge that
○ 1. the shunt is functioning properly.
○ 2. the shunt is blocked at the distal end of the catheter.
○ 3. the ventricular catheter is blocked.
○ 4. there is a reverse flow of CSF through the catheter.

21. After surgery, the infant is to receive vancomycin prophylactically. The nurse should
○ 1. inject the medication into the gluteus maximus.
○ 2. monitor the child for arrhythmia.
○ 3. give the medication intravenously over 1 hour.
○ 4. check the infant's history for an allergy to penicillin.

22. While planning for the infant's discharge, the nurse teaches the parents the signs of an obstructed shunt. The nurse would evaluate the teaching as successful when the parents identify which of the following as signs of a blocked shunt?
○ 1. Decreased urine output with stable intake.
○ 2. Cold, clammy skin with pale lips.
○ 3. Elevated temperature and reddened areas around the incision site.
○ 4. Irritability and tense fontanels.

23. The mother asks how much acetaminophen (Tylenol) to give the infant when they are at home. The child has an order for 30 mg every 4 hours for pain. The mother indicates that she will use the elixir, which comes in a concentration of 180 mg/5 cc. The nurse would tell her to give the infant
○ 1. $\frac{1}{5}$th of a teaspoon, using a medicine cup.
○ 2. $\frac{1}{5}$th of a teaspoon, using a teaspoon.
○ 3. 0.78 cc, using a 1-cc syringe.
○ 4. 1.5 cc, using a 3-cc syringe.

The Client With a Seizure Disorder

A second-grade girl experiences a generalized tonic-clonic seizure at school. She has no history of seizure disorders nor of any other chronic health problem.

24. The school nurse is called to the classroom and arrives while the child is still in the clonic phase of the seizure. The nurse's first priority would be to
○ 1. have the other children leave the room.
○ 2. move furniture and other objects out of the way.
○ 3. obtain a description of the events preceding the seizure.
○ 4. place a padded tongue blade between the child's teeth.

25. Immediately following the seizure, the nurse notices that the child has been incontinent of urine and is very difficult to arouse. Based on this information, the nurse would
○ 1. ask the teacher if the child has had previous problems with urinary incontinence.
○ 2. awaken the child every 3 to 5 minutes to assess mentation.
○ 3. perform a complete neurologic check every 3 to 5 minutes.
○ 4. place the child in a side-lying position, stay with her, and allow her to sleep.

26. The child is hospitalized for a diagnostic workup. The physician orders phenobarbital. The nurse plans to teach the parents about the drug, stressing the need to
○ 1. pay careful attention to oral hygiene, especially in the gum area.
○ 2. discontinue the drug if the child becomes drowsy.
○ 3. increase the dose by 5 mg per day if breakthrough seizures occur.
○ 4. notify the physician if severe headaches and skin rash occur.

27. The child continues to have seizures. The physician orders phenytoin (Dilantin) in conjunction with the phenobarbital. The nurse and mother discuss the safe and effective use of this drug, including which of the following measure to increase safety and effectiveness?
- ○ 1. Assessing for a pink tinge in the child's urine.
- ○ 2. Not giving phenytoin with over-the-counter medications.
- ○ 3. Limiting the child's exposure to the sun.
- ○ 4. Giving phenytoin on an empty stomach.

28. The child is unable to swallow the phenytoin capsule, and does not like the chewable form of the medication. The mother asks about a liquid form. The nurse would discourage use of the liquid of phenytoin because
- ○ 1. inaccurate dosage can occur more easily with the liquid suspension form.
- ○ 2. liquid suspensions discolor the teeth.
- ○ 3. phenytoin sodium loses potency rapidly when in liquid form.
- ○ 4. the child should learn to swallow capsules.

29. When planning for teaching the child and family about pharmacological treatment of seizures, the nurse should emphasize that the child
- ○ 1. should cut back on the medications when side effects occur.
- ○ 2. should never stop taking his medication abruptly.
- ○ 3. will need less medication as he grows older.
- ○ 4. will need to take the medication for the rest of his life.

30. Which of the following statements made by the mother would indicate that she understands her child's medication therapy for seizures? "I should
- ○ 1. call to refill the prescriptions as soon as the bottles are empty."
- ○ 2. make sure he takes his medication every other day."
- ○ 3. not give him any other medications without asking the doctor."
- ○ 4. not worry about giving him his medication if he's vomiting."

31. While discussing plans for the child's discharge, the nurse teaches the parents about what actions to take when the child has a seizure. The nurse would judge the teaching as effective when the father states, "We'll
- ○ 1. restrain her arms and legs so she won't get hurt."
- ○ 2. tilt her neck forward so that her tongue won't fall back into her throat."
- ○ 3. try to get her to swallow an extra dose of phenobarbital."
- ○ 4. stay with her during the seizure and after it's over."

32. The family and nurse discuss the child's return to school. Based on the nursing goal of promoting the child's growth and development, the nurse would plan to advise the parents that a child with a seizure disorder
- ○ 1. is physically impaired and will benefit from attending a school for handicapped children.
- ○ 2. has a learning disability and needs tutoring to help her reach her grade level.
- ○ 3. most frequently has normal intelligence and can attend regular school.
- ○ 4. suffers from social stigma and should not attend public school.

33. Two years after treatment is started, the child is still having occasional generalized seizures. Her parents want to send her to summer camp and contact the nurse for advice on planning for the camping experience. The nurse should help the family decide which activities the child should avoid, which would include
- ○ 1. archery.
- ○ 2. hiking.
- ○ 3. horseback riding.
- ○ 4. tennis.

A 2-year-old boy experiences a simple generalized seizure that is tentatively diagnosed as a febrile seizure.

34. Which of the following statements from the nursing history would support the medical diagnosis of febrile seizure?
- ○ 1. The child has had a low-grade fever for several weeks.
- ○ 2. The family history is negative for convulsions.
- ○ 3. The seizure resulted in respiratory arrest.
- ○ 4. The seizure occurred when the child had a cough, rhinorrhea, and complaints of ear pain.

35. The child is to be sent home on antibiotic therapy alone, although he has been receiving phenobarbital while hospitalized. The grandmother questions the mother about this situation while the nurse is present. The nurse would judge that the mother understands some of the teaching about febrile seizures when the mother states, "Children who have a seizure with fever
- ○ 1. do not usually need long-term seizure medication."
- ○ 2. need anticonvulsants if they have upper respiratory infections or tonsillitis."
- ○ 3. need anticonvulsants if the seizure lasted for 30 minutes or longer."
- ○ 4. need anticonvulsants if the seizure lasted less than 15 minutes."

36. The nurse teaches the parents about methods to

lower temperature besides medications. The nurse would judge that the teaching was successful when the father states,

- ○ 1. "We'll add extra blankets and clothes if she complains of being cold."
- ○ 2. "We'll wrap her in a blanket if she starts shivering."
- ○ 3. "We'll make the bath water cold enough to make her shiver."
- ○ 4. "We'll use a solution of one-half alcohol and water when sponging the child."

37. An adolescent girl with a seizure disorder that is controlled with phenytoin and carbamazeprine (Tegretol) asks the nurse about someday getting married and having children. After discussing this issue with the client, the nurse would judge that the teaching was effective when the client states

- ○ 1. "I probably shouldn't consider having children until my seizures are cured."
- ○ 2. "My children won't necessarily have an increased risk of seizure disorder."
- ○ 3. "When I decide to have children, I'll ask the doctor to change my medication."
- ○ 4. "Women who have seizure disorders commonly have a difficult time conceiving."

38. When administering phenytoin intravenously to a child with status epilepticus, the nurse would give the drug slowly, because rapid infusion of phenytoin IV can result in

- ○ 1. increased liver enzyme levels.
- ○ 2. blood glucose level below 60 mg/dl.
- ○ 3. asystole.
- ○ 4. venous irritation.

The Client With Meningitis

39. A 4-year-old girl is brought to the hospital by her parents. Her temperature is 39°C. The admitting orders read: Give Tylenol for temperature 102.2°F or higher; sponge for temperature greater than 104.0°F; and obtain blood cultures for temperature 103°F or higher. Based on these orders, the nurse would

- ○ 1. do nothing; the temperature is below 102.2°F.
- ○ 2. give acetaminophen, obtain blood cultures, and sponge the child.
- ○ 3. give acetaminophen and obtain blood cultures.
- ○ 4. give acetaminophen.

40. The nurse weighs the child on admission. It is very important that the weight be accurate, because it will be used to

- ○ 1. calculate drug doses for the child.
- ○ 2. estimate the child's edema status.
- ○ 3. evaluate the child's nutritional status.
- ○ 4. determine the child's developmental status.

41. The physician performs a lumbar puncture, and the CSF sample is sent to the lab for testing. The nurse should then

- ○ 1. assess the child for discomfort at the insertion site.
- ○ 2. encourage the parents to hold the child.
- ○ 3. make sure the child lies flat for at least 12 hours.
- ○ 4. place a sandbag over the puncture site for 3 hours.

42. An intravenous line is inserted, and the child is to receive 500 ml of solution over 12 hours. The tubing delivers microdrips at 60 drops per cc. The nurse should time the drops to be

- ○ 1. 32 drops/minute.
- ○ 2. 42 drops/minute.
- ○ 3. 52 drops/minute.
- ○ 4. 62 drops/minute.

43. The child is restless and irritable during the acute stage of meningitis. The nurse should

- ○ 1. decrease conversation with the child.
- ○ 2. keep extraneous noise to a minimum.
- ○ 3. avoid bathing.
- ○ 4. perform treatments quickly.

44. The nurse knows that it is important to assess the child with meningitis for signs of increasing intracranial pressure. Along with decreased level of consciousness, the nurse would be concerned by

- ○ 1. blood pressure of 122/74 mm Hg.
- ○ 2. pulse of 90/minute.
- ○ 3. respiratory rate of 24/minute.
- ○ 4. temperature of 100.0°F.

45. The nurse would suspect that the child had developed disseminated intravascular coagulation (DIC) based on which of the following signs?

- ○ 1. Hemorrhagic skin rash.
- ○ 2. Swollen glands.
- ○ 3. Cyanosis.
- ○ 4. Dyspnea on exertion.

46. The child's CSF analysis shows growth of pneumococcal meningitis. Which of the following illnesses that can be identified in the child's nursing history would predispose her to this type of meningitis?

- ○ 1. Bladder infection.
- ○ 2. Middle-ear infection.
- ○ 3. Mumps.
- ○ 4. Septic arthritis.

47. When discontinuing the child's intravenous therapy, the nurse allows her to apply a dressing to the area where the needle is removed. The nurse would base this action on the knowledge that a child this age has a need to

- ○ 1. enhance confidence in the personnel caring for him or her.
- ○ 2. find diversional activities.
- ○ 3. protect the image of an intact body.
- ○ 4. relieve the anxiety of separation from home.

48. The child recuperates and discharge is planned. She becomes angry when the discharge is delayed. Which of the following play activities would be appropriate to relieve her pent-up hostilities?
- ○ 1. Being read a story.
- ○ 2. Painting with water colors.
- ○ 3. Pounding a pegboard.
- ○ 4. Stacking blocks.

49. A small infant is admitted with a diagnosis of meningitis. While performing routine ongoing assessment, the nurse notes that the infant is less responsive to stimuli and has bradycardia, slight hypertension, irregular respirations, and a temperature of 103.2°F. The infant's fontanel also seems more tense than at the last assessment. The nurse should immediately
- ○ 1. ask another nurse to verify the findings.
- ○ 2. notify the physician of the findings.
- ○ 3. raise the head of the bed.
- ○ 4. administer an antipyretic.

A school-age child is admitted to the pediatric unit. Two days ago the child developed severe and persistent vomiting and diarrhea and complained of increasing fatigue. Now she is combative. Her pulse and respiratory rates are elevated, and she has a fever.

50. The child's mother tells the nurse all the following facts during history taking. Which fact would the nurse associate with Reye's syndrome? The child
- ○ 1. had an allergic reaction to both penicillin and tetracycline last year.
- ○ 2. had an upper respiratory tract infection 1 week ago.
- ○ 3. had chicken pox 6 months ago.
- ○ 4. was exposed to streptococcus 2 weeks ago.

51. A diagnosis of Reye's syndrome is made, and the child is receiving a 10% glucose infusion. When performing a neurologic assessment, the nurse notes that the child's response to pain is to rigidly flex the arms at the elbows and wrists. Based on this sign, the nurse would suspect that the
- ○ 1. infusion rate is too high.
- ○ 2. infusion rate is too low.
- ○ 3. child is in severe pain.
- ○ 4. child's condition is deteriorating.

52. The nurse should position the child
- ○ 1. left side-lying with the head of the bed elevated 45 degrees.
- ○ 2. side-lying with the head of the bed flat.
- ○ 3. supine with the head of the bed elevated 30 degrees.
- ○ 4. supine with the head of the bed flat.

53. The child's status continues to deteriorate. The nurse would plan to
- ○ 1. keep a tracheostomy set readily available.
- ○ 2. make sure there is oxygen and suction at the bedside.
- ○ 3. prepare the child for a liver biopsy.
- ○ 4. prepare to give the child a fluid challenge.

54. The nurse plans the child's care with the parents. The nurse would know that the parents understood why the child's room should be kept quiet and dimly lit when the mother tells a visitor that "We need to keep the room quiet and dark because
- ○ 1. excessive noise or light can cause agitation."
- ○ 2. excessive light can increase the rash."
- ○ 3. she needs as much rest as possible."
- ○ 4. the nurses are trying to assess her response to sound."

55. The parents tell the nurse that they feel guilty because they didn't bring the child to the hospital sooner. Which of the following remarks by the nurse would be most appropriate?
- ○ 1. "I can understand why you feel guilty, but the onset of this disease is so insidious."
- ○ 2. "Tell me more about your feelings of guilt."
- ○ 3. "You did the best you could."
- ○ 4. "You really shouldn't feel guilty; your child will be all right."

56. If a nurse wishes to decrease the incidence of Reye's syndrome, the best strategy would be to teach parents to
- ○ 1. avoid giving aspirin when treating viral symptoms.
- ○ 2. delay immunizations for children with low-grade fever.
- ○ 3. keep children away from others who have Reye's syndrome.
- ○ 4. treat scrapes and bruises by cleansing carefully and applying antibiotic cream.

The Client With Infectious Polyneuritis (Guillain-Barré Syndrome)

A young school-age child is admitted to the hospital complaining of pain and weakness in the feet and legs for several days. The pain and weakness is symmetrical and appears to be progressing from distal to proximal.

57. During the first 2 days of hospitalization, the child develops motor paralysis of the legs. The nurse asks the child to squeeze the nurse's hand and to raise her arms and legs as high as possible off the bed. The purpose of these requests is to

○ 1. assess the child's ability to follow simple commands.
○ 2. evaluate the child's bilateral muscle strength.
○ 3. make the range-of-motion exercises into a game.
○ 4. provide the child with a diversional activity.

58. When assessing the child's speech for decreased volume and clarity and asking the child to cough, the nurse is assessing for
○ 1. inflammation of the larynx and epiglottis.
○ 2. increased intracranial pressure.
○ 3. involvement of facial and cranial nerves.
○ 4. regression to an earlier developmental phase.

59. The nurse notes that the child is unable to cough and has no gag reflex. In developing a nursing care plan for the child during the acute phase of Guillain-Barré syndrome, the highest priority nursing diagnosis would be
○ 1. Altered Tissue Perfusion.
○ 2. Ineffective Breathing Pattern.
○ 3. Impaired Swallowing.
○ 4. Total Incontinence.

60. The child is transferred to the pediatric intensive care unit, intubated, placed on mechanical ventilation, and placed on a cardiac monitor. The rationale for this level of cardiac assessment is that clients with Guillain-Barré syndrome can experience
○ 1. autonomic dysreflexia.
○ 2. brain stem edema.
○ 3. hypokalemia.
○ 4. hypoglycemia.

61. While being mechanically ventilated, the child should be
○ 1. maintained in a supine position to prevent unnecessary nerve stimulation.
○ 2. moved to a bedside chair twice a day to prevent orthostatic hypotension.
○ 3. receive vigorous passive range-of-motion exercises to prevent loss of muscle function.
○ 4. turned slowly and gently from side to side to prevent respiratory complications.

62. The child is successfully weaned from the ventilator but still requires nasogastric tube feedings. The nurse would judge that the child was ready for oral feedings when she
○ 1. can sit up in a chair without help.
○ 2. gags when the nasogastric tube is repositioned.
○ 3. moves her hands to her mouth.
○ 4. tells her parents that she is hungry.

63. After several weeks, the child is transferred to a general pediatric floor. The parents and nurse would develop a discharge plan that focuses on
○ 1. formulating a rehabilitation plan that includes orthopedic care.
○ 2. enrolling the child in a special education kindergarten class.
○ 3. limiting contact with peers until she has fully recovered.
○ 4. finding a school for handicapped children in the family's neighborhood.

64. After discharge the mother phones the nurse and asks how she can get the child to do her arm exercises. The best advice the nurse can give is to
○ 1. give her candy if she does the exercises.
○ 2. read her a favorite story before she does the exercises.
○ 3. have her watch other children exercising.
○ 4. play a game of catch with her.

The Client With a Head Injury

A school-age child was hit by a car while riding a bicycle. Unconscious at the scene of the accident, he was brought to the hospital emergency department.

65. On the child's arrival at the hospital, the nurse's first priority would be to
○ 1. assess his neurological status.
○ 2. assess for abdominal injuries.
○ 3. establish ventilation.
○ 4. establish intravenous access.

66. If the child had not lost consciousness and was released to his parents from the emergency room, which of the following statements by the parents would indicate they understood when to bring him back for further evaluation? "We'll seek immediate medical advice if he
○ 1. continues to have a headache this evening."
○ 2. doesn't behave normally."
○ 3. sleeps very soundly, but we can arouse him."
○ 4. vomits when we get home."

67. The nurse evaluates the child's neurological status using the Glascow coma scale. Part of the assessment includes eye opening to stimuli. Lack of response to which of the following stimuli would yield the lowest or least desirable score? Having
○ 1. an IV started.
○ 2. his arm moved.
○ 3. his mother stroke his face.
○ 4. the nurse speak to him.

68. The admission orders include inserting a nasogastric tube to
○ 1. administer medications.
○ 2. decompress the stomach.
○ 3. obtain gastric specimens for analysis.
○ 4. provide adequate nutrition.

69. If this child had suffered a basilar skull fracture, the nurse would have
○ 1. asked for the order to be changed to oral-gastric tube.

○ 2. attempted to place the tube into the ileum.
○ 3. tested the gastric aspirate for blood.
○ 4. used extra lubrication when inserting the nasogastric tube.

70. The child is to receive dexamethasone (Decadron) intravenously. The ordered dosage is 7.2 mg, and the drug concentration in the vial is 4 mg/ml. What volume of the drug contains 7.2 mg?
○ 1. 0.4 ml.
○ 2. 0.72 ml.
○ 3. 1.8 ml.
○ 4. 7.2 ml.

71. The child's parents ask the nurse if the child is going to be all right. Which of the following responses by the nurse would be most appropriate?
○ 1. "Children usually don't do very well after head injuries like this."
○ 2. "I'm sure he'll be fine; children can recover rapidly from head injuries."
○ 3. "It's hard to tell this early, but we'll keep you informed of his progress."
○ 4. "That's something you'll have to talk to the doctor about."

72. The physician orders Mannitol for the child. When the parents ask why this drug is being given, the nurse should reply, "Mannitol will
○ 1. help hold fluid in the vascular bed, to prevent shock."
○ 2. help get rid of fluid, to decrease swelling in the brain."
○ 3. increase caloric intake, to aid wound healing."
○ 4. fight off bacteria, to prevent infections."

73. The child is coming out of the coma and is restless, irritable, and confused about where he is. The nurse should
○ 1. apply a chest restraint.
○ 2. ask the parents to leave.
○ 3. encourage the parents to stay.
○ 4. restrain all four extremities.

The Client With a Brain Tumor

A junior high school student has seen the school nurse frequently with complaints of nausea, headache, and difficulty seeing. She has begun to tilt her head to one side and has a wide-based gait.

74. The nurse would decide to talk with the child's parents concerning her behavior, because these symptoms are typical of
○ 1. acute encephalopathy with fatty degeneration of the viscera.
○ 2. an abnormal involuntary neuromuscular activity.
○ 3. a psychological aversion to school.
○ 4. a space-occupying lesion in the cranial vault.

75. The child is later admitted to the hospital with the diagnosis of infratentorial brain tumor. During the child's admission to the pediatric unit, the nurse would plan to
○ 1. alleviate the parents' anxiety.
○ 2. implement seizure precautions.
○ 3. introduce the child to other clients the same age.
○ 4. prepare the child and parents for diagnostic procedures.

76. A diagnosis of probable cerebellar astrocytoma is made, and surgical removal is scheduled. Preoperatively, the nurse should plan to tell the child and her parents about the
○ 1. child's long-term prognosis
○ 2. child's postoperative appearance.
○ 3. long-term therapy for this type of tumor.
○ 4. side effects of the planned chemotherapy.

77. An infratentorial craniotomy is performed and the diagnosis of cerebellar astrocytoma, stage I, is confirmed. The parents want to know what "stage I" means. The nurse should explain that stage I describes a tumor that
○ 1. has extended.
○ 2. has metastasized.
○ 3. is localized.
○ 4. is undifferentiated.

78. After the child is admitted to the intensive care unit, the nurse's first action would be to ensure adequate
○ 1. cardiorespiratory function.
○ 2. fluid and electrolyte balance.
○ 3. pain control.
○ 4. infection protection.

79. The nurse would keep the child in which position?
○ 1. Prone.
○ 2. Reverse Trendelenburg.
○ 3. Side-lying.
○ 4. Trendelenburg.

80. The intubated child shows signs of decreased level of consciousness, and the physician orders manual hyperventilation to keep the PCO_2 between 25 and 29 mm Hg and the PaO_2 between 80 and 100 mm Hg. The nurse would carry out this order to
○ 1. decrease intracranial pressure.
○ 2. ensure a patent airway.
○ 3. lower the arousal level.
○ 4. produce hypercapnia.

81. The nurse notes clear drainage on the child's dressing and on the linen under her head. The nurse
○ 1. changes the dressing.
○ 2. elevates the head of the bed.
○ 3. tests the fluid for glucose.
○ 4. tests the fluid for protein.

82. The child does well after infratentorial tumor removal and is transferred back to the pediatric unit. Although she had been told about having her head shaved for surgery, she is very upset about her bald head. After exploring her feelings, the nurse should

- ○ 1. ask her if she'd like to wear a hat or wig.
- ○ 2. assure her that her hair will grow back.
- ○ 3. explain to her parents that her reaction is normal.
- ○ 4. suggest that the parents buy her a wig as a surprise.

83. Which of the following statements made by the child's mother would warrant further exploration by the nurse?

- ○ 1. "After this, I'll never let her out of my sight again."
- ○ 2. "I hope that she'll be able to go back to school soon."
- ○ 3. "I wonder how long it will be before she can ride her bike."
- ○ 4. "Her best friend is coming to lunch when we get home."

The Client With a Spinal Cord Injury

An adolescent male was involved in a motorcycle accident and thrown about 40 feet from his motorcycle. A nurse arriving at the scene of the accident finds that he is alert.

84. The adolescent is unable to move his legs. While waiting for the emergency medical service to arrive, the nurse should

- ○ 1. flex his knees to relieve stress on his back.
- ○ 2. leave him as is and stay close by.
- ○ 3. remove his helmet as soon as possible.
- ○ 4. roll him onto his left side.

85. The adolescent arrives at the emergency department with a diagnosis of suspected thoracic spinal cord injury. The nurse's first priority would be to

- ○ 1. maintain cardiorespiratory function.
- ○ 2. obtain a signed consent from his parents.
- ○ 3. prevent fluid and electrolyte imbalance.
- ○ 4. provide emotional support.

86. In the emergency department, the adolescent remains conscious and is agitated and anxious. The nurse observes that his pulse and respirations are increasing and that his blood pressure is decreasing. The nurse suspects that the adolescent is developing

- ○ 1. autonomic dysreflexia.
- ○ 2. increased intracranial pressure.
- ○ 3. metabolic acidosis.
- ○ 4. spinal shock.

87. A diagnosis of a T3 spinal cord injury is made. Following insertion of an intravenous line, a nasogastric tube, and a Foley catheter, the adolescent is admitted to the intensive care unit. On noting that his feet and legs are cool to the touch, the nurse should

- ○ 1. cover his legs with blankets.
- ○ 2. report the change to the physician immediately.
- ○ 3. reposition his legs.
- ○ 4. sit him up to aid circulation.

88. During routine assessment, the nurse auscultates the adolescent's abdomen. The nurse explains to the parents that this is necessary because clients with spinal cord injury often develop

- ○ 1. abdominal cramping.
- ○ 2. hyperactive bowel sounds.
- ○ 3. paralytic ileus.
- ○ 4. projectile vomiting.

89. After observing which of the following findings would the nurse decide that spinal shock was resolving?

- ○ 1. Atonic urinary bladder.
- ○ 2. Flaccid paralysis.
- ○ 3. Hyperactive reflexes.
- ○ 4. Return of sensation.

90. The adolescent is moved to the rehabilitation unit. The nurse notes that he tends to refuse to cooperate in care and to be hostile. The nurse recognizes this behavior as a

- ○ 1. normal stage of grief reaction.
- ○ 2. phase of adolescent rebellion.
- ○ 3. reaction to sensory overload.
- ○ 4. severe separation anxiety.

91. Adjustment to paraplegia is especially difficult for an adolescent. The nurse would try to help the adolescent adjust to the situation by fostering

- ○ 1. ego integrity.
- ○ 2. generativity.
- ○ 3. self-definition.
- ○ 4. industriousness.

92. Three months after the adolescent's injury, he complains of a pounding headache, and the nurse notes that his arms and face are flushed and he is diaphoretic. The nurse should

- ○ 1. check the patency of the Foley catheter.
- ○ 2. lower his head.
- ○ 3. place him in a supine position.
- ○ 4. prepare to administer epinephrine.

93. The adolescent is to be discharged to his parent's home and will be living with them. The nurse and family should formulate a short-term goal of

- ○ 1. being able to leave the house.
- ○ 2. being able to maneuver independently inside the house.
- ○ 3. having the activities of daily living met by the parents.
- ○ 4. meeting all self-care needs independently.

CORRECT ANSWERS AND RATIONALE

The letters in parentheses following the rationale identify the step of the nursing process (A, D, P, I, E); cognitive level (K, C, T, N); and client need (S, G, L, H). See the Answer Grid for the key.

The Client With Myelomeningocele

1. 4. A myelomeningocele has three components (bony defect, spinal fluid, and nerve tissue) and protrudes over the vertebrae, usually in the lower back. A meningocele is a soft sac containing only spinal fluid and meninges located anywhere on the spine. A pilonidal cyst is a skin-covered sac containing bits of hair located on the low lumbar or sacral area of the spine. A simple cyst contains serosanguinous fluid and fatty tissue located on any area of the spinal column. (A, C, G)

2. 2. Clinical manifestations of myelomeningocele are related to the anatomic level of the defect and the nerves involved. An upper lumbar (L1–L2) myelomeningocele is associated with minimal movement of the lower extremities and dribbling of urine and feces. The upper lumbar area of the spinal cord controls leg flexion at the hip and adduction of the thigh. The sacral area of the spinal cord controls foot and toe movement, as well as sphincter and perineal muscle contraction. (A, T, G)

3. 1. The parents should see the neonate as soon as possible, and the nurse should emphasize the neonate's normal and positive features. The longer the parents have to wait to see the neonate, the more anxiety they will feel. Since the parents are acutely aware of the deficit, emphasizing the neonate's normal and positive features would be more therapeutic than reinforcing the physician's explanation of the defect. The parents should spend time with or care for the neonate after birth, because parent-infant contact is necessary for attachment. The parents cannot hold the neonate before the defect is repaired, but they can fondle and stroke him. Although the parents need to discuss their fears and concerns, the nurse should initially emphasize the neonate's normal and positive features. (P, N, L)

4. 1. Hydrocephalus, excessive CSF in the cranial cavity, is the most common anomaly associated with myelomeningocele. Microencephaly (abnormally small head) and craniosynostosis (premature fusion of the cranial sutures with skull deformity) are rarely associated with myelomeningocele. Anencephaly (congenital absence of the cranial vault) is a different neural tube defect. (P, T, G)

5. 1. Approximately one-third of infants with myelomeningocele are mentally retarded, but it is particularly difficult to predict intellectual functioning in neonates. The parents are asking for an answer now and should not be told to talk with the physician later. (P, N, G)

6. 1. Overflow incontinence with constant dribbling is common in neonates with myelomeningocele. Applying gentle pressure to the suprapubic area helps empty the neonate's bladder, thus preventing urinary tract infections. Catheterization is done most frequently when a specimen is urgently needed or when the neonate is unable to void. Intermittent clean catheterization is an appropriate technique for management of urine retention in older infants. Suprapubic aspiration is useful in clarifying the diagnosis of suspected urinary tract infection in very ill neonates. (I, T, S)

7. 2. The nurse places the neonate with myelomeningocele in an isolette shortly after birth to help to maintain his temperature. Since the neonate cannot be bundled in blankets, it may be difficult to prevent cold stress. The isolette can be maintained at higher than room temperature, helping maintain the temperature of a neonate who cannot be dressed or bundled. Another use would be for a neonate receiving phototherapy for hyperbilirubinemia. Although preventing cold stress may prevent problems with oxygenation and energy depletion, in this case the isolette is used to keep the infant warm. (E, N, G)

8. 3. If corrective surgery is to be done immediately, the sac is kept moist by covering it with sterile saline dressings. If corrective surgery is delayed, the sac may be exposed to the air or covered with a dry, sterile, nonadherent dressing to facilitate drying and epithelization of the sac, and tincture of benzoin may be applied to make the covering of the sac firmer and more resistant to injury. (I, N, S)

9. 1. A low Trendelenburg position is ideal because it reduces spinal fluid pressure in the sac; slight hip flexion reduces tension on the defect. The side-lying position is also acceptable, but support is placed behind the head and buttocks, not the sac. The supine position is unacceptable because it causes pressure on the defect. (P, T, S)

10. 4. The presence of risk factors for deterioration of body systems as the result of prescribed or unavoidable musculoskeletal inactivity is the definition of High Risk for Disuse Syndrome. The child's weakness and possible paralysis of the lower extremities contributes to the disuse of muscles and possible atrophy and deformation of the extremities. Activity Intolerance relates to the lack of energy (not innervation) needed to carry out desired daily activities. An infant normally needs total care. Altered Tissue Perfusion relates to a chronic deficit in blood supply. (D, N, G)

11. 2. Because of the potential for hip dislocation, the neonate's legs should be slightly abducted, hips maintained in slight to moderate abduction, and feet maintained in a neutral position. Knees cannot be hyperextended without injury. (P, T, S)

12. 3. In a neonate with open cranial sutures, increasing head circumference is the predominant and earliest sign of increased intracranial pressure. Some neonates may exhibit bulging fontanels without head enlargement. Other early but later signs and symptoms are frontal bossing or enlargement with depressed eyes and "setting sun" sign, with the sclera visible above the iris. Distended scalp veins and irritability may also occur. A brief, shrill cry is a later sign. (A, T, G)

13. 3. Local parent support groups, such as the Spina Bifida Association of America, can be helpful to the parents. Although financial problems can influence family functioning, support groups can help parents cope with a wide range of problems that the family may encounter. Referrals for financial aide, counseling, and residential placement are more appropriately made at the time of need. (P, N, L)

14. 3. Children with myelomeningocele are prone to urinary tract infections. Because of sensory impairment, the child is unaware of bladder discomfort. Similarly, the child is insensitive to pressure and other sources of tissue damage, such as heat. Activities that encourage body consciousness, such as rolling over, are encouraged. The child needs the stimulation of others and has a competent immune system. (E, N, G)

The Client With Hydrocephalus

15. 2. Head circumference usually parallels the percentile for length. The discrepancy found requires close and immediate attention because it could indicate hydrocephalus, with its potential for brain damage. In an infant, bulging fontanels and widening cranial sutures are signs of increasing intracranial pressure related to increased CSF in the cranial space. Transillumination is a noninvasive procedure and does not require a permit. Difficulty walking may indicate hydrocephalus in an older child. (A, N, G)

16. 2. Small, frequent feedings given at times when the infant is relaxed and calm are tolerated best. An infant with hydrocephalus is difficult to feed because of poor sucking, lethargy, and vomiting, which are associated with increased intracranial pressure. Ideally, the infant should be held in a slightly vertical position when feeding. (I, N, S)

17. 1. The outcomes for children with hydrocephalus vary from normal growth and development to delayed motor and cognitive development. The degree of impairment is difficult to predict. The nurse should respond now to the inquiry rather than refer the mother to the physician at a later time. (I, N, G)

18. 4. The infant is positioned flat for at least the first 24 hours after surgery. Positioning on the operative side is avoided, because it places pressure on the shunt valve. Elevating the head increases CSF drainage and reduces intracranial pressure; but rapid reduction in the size of the ventricles may cause subdural hematoma. The infant should be kept off the nonoperative side (side opposite the shunt) to help prevent rapid decompression. Elevating the foot of the bed could increase intracranial pressure. (P, T, G)

19. 3. Monitoring temperature allows the nurse to assess for infection, the most common hazardous postoperative complication after ventroperitoneal shunt placement. Neither glucosuria nor ketonuria is associated with shunt placement. Pain should be mild postoperatively, and mild analgesics are given. Narcotics are not given because they alter level of consciousness and make assessment of cerebral function difficult. Any fluid leakage is tested for glucose, an indication of CSF. (A, T, G)

20. 3. Shunts used to treat hydrocephalus consist of a ventricular catheter, a one-way valve, and a distal catheter. The one-way valve prevents reflux of CSF back into the ventricles. When the valve is depressed, CSF flows into the distal end of the catheter. If the ventricular portion of the shunt is patent, the valve should refill when released. (E, N, G)

21. 3. Aminoglycoside antibiotics are usually infused intravenously over ½ to 1 hour. Too-rapid infusion can cause severe hypotension. Intramuscular injections should not be given in the gluteus maximus until the child has been walking for a year. Arrhythmia is not a common side effect of aminoglycosides. There is no relationship between allergy to penicillin and allergy to aminoglycosides. (I, T, S)

22. 4. In an infant, irritability, tense fontanel, increased head circumference, lethargy, poor sucking, vomiting, and decreased level of consciousness are signs of increased intracranial pressure caused by a blocked shunt. Decreased urine output with stable fluid intake indicates fluid loss from a source other than the kidneys. Cold clammy skin with pale lips are shock-like symptoms. Elevated temperature and redness around incisions could indicate infection. (E, N, G)

23. 3. The correct amount is 0.78 cc. A 1-cc syringe

would give the most accurate measurement of this dosage, even though approximately the same amount is in 1/5th of a teaspoon. Using a medicine cup or a teaspoon would necessitate estimating the exact amount and could lead to overdosage or underdosage. (I, N, S)

The Client With a Seizure Disorder

24. 2. During a generalized tonic-clonic seizure, the first priority is to protect the client from injury. Although obtaining information about events surrounding the seizure and providing privacy are important considerations, they are not priority. During a seizure, nothing should be forced into the client's mouth, as this can cause severe damage to the teeth and mouth. The child's classmates will need an opportunity to discuss this incident and learn about seizures. (I, N, S)

25. 4. It is normal for a child to sleep and be difficult to arouse during the postictal period of a generalized tonic-clonic seizure. During this time, the child should be allowed to sleep until he or she awakens. Sleep and drowsiness do not follow other forms of generalized seizures. Obtaining information about neurologic status is important, but awakening the child every 3 to 5 minutes would not be helpful. Urinary incontinence during a seizure is common. (I, N, G)

26. 4. Phenobarbital can cause a skin rash if the child is sensitive to the drug. Headache is an adverse neurologic effect of the drug. Phenobarbital normally causes drowsiness. The dose for children being treated for seizures should never be discontinued, increased, or decreased without physician order. (P, T, H)

27. 2. Phenytoin sodium (Dilantin) interacts with many other drugs and should never be taken in conjunction with over-the-counter medications without first consulting the physician. Dilantin may cause a pink tinge to the urine; although the nurse should warn the parents and child about this effect, it is not important to safe or effective use of the medication. Dilantin does not usually cause photosensitive skin lesions. Dilantin should be taken on a full stomach to decrease gastric upset. (P, T, G)

28. 1. Although many anticonvulsants are available as liquid extracts and emulsions, the drug can be unequally distributed in the solution. This unequal distribution can result in inaccurate dosages, even when the medication is shaken well before pouring. If necessary, the contents of the capsule can be mixed with a sweet substance to make it palatable. (I, T, S)

29. 2. The most common cause of status epilepticus is sudden withdrawal of anticonvulsant medication. Some children may be able to discontinue their medication, but only under supervised conditions and after being completely seizure-free on medication for several years. Physical growth, such as during adolescence, frequently necessitates a dosage increase. The physician should be notified of troublesome side effects. (P, N, H)

30. 3. Many medications, including over-the-counter drugs such as antihistamines, central nervous system stimulants, and alcohol, can lower the seizure threshold. To maintain plasma drug levels within the threshold range, anticonvulsants should be taken at least once daily. When a child is unable to take an oral anticonvulsant, the physician should be notified. Prescriptions should be refilled before the bottle is empty to keep from interrupting the medication regimen. (E, N, H)

31. 4. Safety is the primary concern. It is a common misconception that a person swallows the tongue during a seizure. However, flexing the neck could obstruct the airway. Trying to restrain the child during a seizure or attempting to have him swallow anything, including medications, can result in further injury or aspiration. (E, N, H)

32. 3. Most children who develop seizures after infancy are intellectually normal. A child with seizure disorders needs the same experiences and opportunities to develop his or her intellectual, emotional, and social abilities as any other child. (P, N, H)

33. 3. A child who has generalized seizures should not participate in activities that are potentially hazardous. Even if accompanied by a responsible adult, the child could be seriously injured if he were to have a seizure on horseback. Activities in or on the water should also be avoided. (P, N, H)

34. 4. Most febrile seizures occur in the presence of an upper respiratory infection, otitis media, or tonsillitis. There appears to be increased susceptibility to febrile seizures within families. Febrile seizures, which occur during a temperature rise rather than after prolonged fever, occasionally (but not always) result in respiratory difficulties. (A, N, G)

35. 1. The child who is at low risk for recurrence is usually not treated with anticonvulsant drugs, because drug side effects frequently outweigh the benefits. Without anticonvulsant therapy, the likelihood that a child will experience a second febrile seizure is 30–40 percent; a third seizure, about 15 percent. Prophylactic treatment is indicated for children who experience their first febrile seizure before age 18 months of age, have a family history positive for seizures, and have seizures lasting longer than 15 minutes. (E, T, G)

36. 2. Shivering is the body's defense against rapid temperature decrease; the result is increased body temperature. When caring for a shivering child, the nurse should try to stop the shivering by increasing the room temperature until the shivering stops, and then attempt to lower the temperature more slowly. Alcohol can be absorbed through the skin and is a toxic substance. While attempts are being made to decrease temperature, the child will likely complain of being cold; but as long as the child does not shiver, the treatment can continue. (E, N, H)

37. 3. Phenytoin sodium (Dilantin) is a known teratogenic agent, causing numerous fetal problems, and anticonvulsant requirements usually increase during pregnancy. There is a familial tendency or seizure disorders. Seizures can be controlled, but cannot be cured. Seizure disorders and infertility are not related. (E, N, H)

38. 3. Although phenytoin can produce cardiotoxicity, hepatotoxicity, venous irritation, and hyperglycemia, the most life-threatening side effect during rapid administration is cardiotoxicity. Bradycardia, hypotension, and cardiac arrest (asystole) are possible cardiovascular problems associated with intravenous Dilantin administration. The nurse should monitor the child's vital signs closely during and after intravenous Dilantin administration. (I, T, S)

The Client With Meningitis

39. 4. The nurse would give acetaminophen (Tylenol) for a temperature of 102.2°F. To convert degrees Fahrenheit to degrees centigrade, the nurse subtracts 32 from the Fahrenheit temperature and multiplies the result by 5/9, as follows:

$$102.2°F - 32 = 70.2$$

$$70.2 \times 5/9 = 39°C.$$

To convert centigrade to Fahrenheit, the nurse multiplies the centigrade temperature by 9/5 and adds 32. Using this formula, the conversion is determined as follows:

$$39°C \times 9/5 = 70.2$$

$$70.2 + 32 = 102.2°F.$$

(I, T, G)

40. 1. There is no standard medication dosage for pediatric patients. Medication dosages are most commonly based on a child's weight or total body surface area. The child described in this situation is weighed mainly to help calculate medication dosage. Weighing can also be done to help determine fluid needs, but in this case nutritional needs are not an immediate concern. A child with meningitis is not typically assessed for edema. (A, N, G)

41. 2. The child needs to be comforted after an invasive procedure by people she trusts. There is little discomfort at the insertion site after the lumbar puncture. Narcotics would not be the drugs of choice because they hinder assessment of neurological status. Applying a small bandage after applying pressure for a short time is usually sufficient to stop any leakage and prevent infection of the site. A young child does not need to lay flat for any time after a lumbar puncture. (Besides, laying flat for 12 hours would be difficult, if not impossible, for a 4-year-old.) (I, N, G)

42. 2. The number of drops the client should receive each minute is determined as follows:

$$\frac{500 \text{ ml}}{12 \text{ hours}} = 41 \text{ to } 42 \text{ ml to be infused each hour}$$

$$\frac{42\text{ml} \times 60 \text{ (drop factor)}}{60 \text{ min}} = \frac{2520}{60}$$

$$= 42 \text{ drops to be infused every minute.}$$

(I, T, S)

43. 2. A child in the acute stage of meningitis is irritable and hypersensitive to loud noise and light. The child should be spoken to and bathed gently and calmly; sudden movements should be avoided. (I, T, G)

44. 1. A blood pressure of 122/74 mm Hg is above the 95th percentile for a child age 4. Increased blood pressure is a common sign of increased intracranial pressure. The pulse and respiration rates are within normal limits for a child age 4. A decreased pulse rate and increased or decreased respiratory rate with irregularity may indicate increased intracranial pressure. Temperature of 100.0°F in a child with an infectious process is not related to increased intracranial pressure; but poor temperature control may be a sign of increasing intracranial pressure in older infants and children. (A, N, G)

45. 1. Disseminated intravascular coagulation (DIC) is characterized by skin petechiae and a purpuric skin rash due to spontaneous bleeding into the tissues. An abnormal coagulation phenomenon causes the condition. Heparin therapy is often used to interrupt the clotting process. (A, N, G)

46. 2. Organisms that cause *bacterial meningitis,* such as *pneumococci* or *meningococci* are commonly spread in the body by vascular dissemination from a middle-ear infection. The meningitis may also be a direct extension from the paranasal and mastoid sinuses. The causative organism is a pneumococcus. A chronic draining ear is frequently also found. (A, N, G)

47. 3. Preschool-age children worry about having an intact body and become fearful of any threat to body integrity. Allowing the child to participate with required care helps protect her image of an intact body. Finding diversional activities, relieving the anxiety of separation from the home, and enhancing her confidence in the personnel caring for her are invalid reasons for allowing her to place a dressing on the area where an intravenous needle has been positioned. (I, N, L)

48. 3. An emotionally tense child with pent-up hostilities needs a physical activity that will release energy and frustration. Pounding on a peg board offers this opportunity. Activities such as stacking blocks and painting require concentration and fine movements, which could add to frustration. Listening to a story does not allow the child to express emotions and casts her in a passive role. (I, N, L)

49. 3. The nurse identifies a decreased consciousness, bradycardia, hypertension, irregular respirations, and tense fontanel as signs of increased intracranial pressure. The first action should be to attempt to lower the pressure by raising the head of the bed, which should improve venous return and decrease the pressure. The nurse can then notify the physician and administer the antipyretic. Since temperature, pulse, and respirations are fairly objective data, the nurse does not have to verify these findings. (I, N, G)

50. 2. The etiology of Reye's syndrome is unknown, but symptoms usually develop a few days to several weeks after the onset of a mild viral illness. Upper respiratory tract infections are usually viral in nature. (A, N, G)

51. 4. The physician should be notified, because decorticate posturing in response to pain indicates neurologic deterioration and is characteristic of stage II Reye's syndrome. Pupillary responses provide data about neurologic status, but rechecking them in this situation is not the priority action. The physician determines the rate of the infusion, depending on the fluid being administered and the patient's clinical status. (D, N, G)

52. 3. Elevating the head of the bed 30 degrees and keeping the client's head in midline position help minimize increased intracranial pressure. Neck flexion or rotation can obstruct venous return, which can increase intracranial pressure. (I, T, G)

53. 2. Since the child may progress to stage V Reye's syndrome, the nurse should gather equipment that might be needed to treat seizures. A liver biopsy would have been done earlier to confirm the diagnosis; it is not necessary at this time. If the child needed ventilatory assistance, an endotracheal tube would be used. Increasing fluid intake would increase intracranial pressure. (P, N, S)

54. 1. Minimizing excessive and/or inappropriate stimulation helps minimize the child's agitation. Photosensitivity, hearing loss, and rash are not associated with Reye's syndrome. (E, T, G)

55. 2. Guilt is a common parental response; the parents should be allowed to express their feelings. Reye's syndrome develops quickly, not slowly. Denying the parents' feelings of guilt is not helpful. (I, N, L)

56. 1. Research suggests that giving salicylates (aspirin) to a child with a viral illness can contribute to the development of Reye's syndrome. The disease is not communicable and is not linked to immunizations or bacterial infections. (I, N, H)

The Client With Infectious Polyneuritis (Guillain-Barré Syndrome)

57. 2. Muscle paralysis in Guillain-Barré syndrome is usually progressive and ascending in nature. Assessment of progressive muscle weakness helps determine the extent of involvement. (A, T, G)

58. 3. In a child with Guillain-Barré syndrome, decreased volume and clarity of speech and decreased ability to cough voluntarily indicate ascending progression of neural inflammation. These are not signs of increasing intracranial pressure or regression. A child with laryngeal inflammation retains the ability to cough. (A, T, G)

59. 2. Although Total Incontinence and Impaired Swallowing are both appropriate nursing diagnosis for this child during the acute phase of the illness, addressing Ineffective Breathing Pattern to maintain an adequate oxygen supply takes precedence. Progressive neurological impairment will likely have an effect on the child's ability to maintain respirations. Impaired Gas Exchange relates to a disturbance in oxygen or carbon dioxide exchange in the lungs or at a cellular level. (D, N, G)

60. 1. Impaired autonomic function in Guillain-Barré syndrome can result in cardiac dysrhythmia, possibly leading to cardiovascular shock and death. The vital centers in the medulla oblongata may be affected, not by edema, but by patchy demyelination. Neither hypokalemia nor hypoglycemia is associated with this syndrome. (A, T, G)

61. 4. Even in the absence of respiratory problems or distress, the child must be turned frequently to help prevent the cardiopulmonary complications associated with immobility. During the acute disease phase, vigorous physiotherapy is contraindicated because the child may experience muscle pain and be hypersensitive to touch. The child should be handled extremely gently. (I, N, G)

62. 2. Impaired gag and swallowing reflexes associated with cranial nerve involvement require nasogastric tube feedings in a child with Guillain-Barré syndrome. The presence of a gag reflex indicates the return of normal swallowing. (E, T, G)

63. 1. The family should be involved early in developing a rehabilitation plan. The convalescent period for a child with Guillain-Barré syndrome is lengthy, and full recovery may require 1 to 2 years. Most children recover completely; only 10–15 percent have neurologic sequelae. Maintaining peer relationships during convalescence is important for psychosocial development. Children with Guillain-Barré syndrome can attend regular schools. (P, N, G)

64. 4. Developmentally appropriate activities and therapeutic play should be used as rehabilitation modalities. Inappropriate rewards or threats should not be used to coerce a child into compliance. Significant persons for a child this age are family members. Peer groups are the most significant persons for a young adolescent. (I, N, H)

The Client With a Head Injury

65. 3. The first priority in caring for a child who has sustained a head injury is to establish and maintain ventilation. All other activities are secondary to adequate ventilation. (I, T, G)

66. 2. If the child begins to behave abnormally or is confused, the parents should seek immediate medical attention. Headache is to be expected, if it becomes worse or interferes with sleep, the child should be reevaluated. Vomiting also occurs after head injury; if the child vomits three or more times, medical attention is necessary. Most children sleep soundly, but are arousable. (E, N, G)

67. 1. Lack of response to pain yields the lowest score. From the highest to lowest, the order of eye-opening response to stimuli on the Glascow coma scale is spontaneous opening, response to speech, response to pain, no response. (A, T, G)

68. 2. A nasogastric tube is initially placed following serious head trauma to decompress the stomach and to prevent vomiting and aspiration. (P, T, S)

69. 1. Since a basilar skull fracture can involve the frontal and ethmoid bones, inserting a nasogastric tube carries the risk of introducing the tube into the cranial cavity through the fracture. An oral gastric tube is preferred for a client with basilar skull fracture. (I, T, G)

70. 3. Using the ratio:proportion method, the equation is:

$$\frac{4\text{mg}}{1\text{ ml}} = \frac{7.2\text{ mg}}{x\text{ ml}}$$

$$4x = 7.2$$

$$x = \frac{7.2}{4}$$

$$x = 1.8\text{ ml.}$$

(I, T, G)

71. 3. As a rule children demonstrate more rapid and more complete recovery from coma than do adults. However, it is extremely difficult to predict a specific outcome. Assuring the parents that they will be kept informed helps open lines of communication and establish trust. (I, N, L)

72. 2. Mannitol is an osmotic diuretic used to help decrease intracranial pressure by decreasing cerebral edema. It does contribute to the calorie intake of the child, but is not used for the purpose of increasing caloric intake because of its diuretic effect. (I, N, G)

73. 3. The parents presence may help calm the child. Restraints can frighten and frustrate a child, and straining against them can lead to an increase in intracranial pressure. (I, T, S)

The Client With a Brain Tumor

74. 4. Common signs and symptoms of infratentorial brain tumor in children are headache, visual disturbance, vomiting with or without nausea, and ataxia in the form of gait disturbances. Acute encephalopathy with fatty degeneration of the liver describes Reye's syndrome. Abnormal neuromuscular activity partially describes seizures. A psychological aversion to school describes school phobia. (D, N, G)

75. 4. When a brain tumor is suspected, the child and parents are likely to be very apprehensive and anxious. It is unrealistic to expect to eliminate their fears; rather, the nurse's goal is to decrease them. Preparing both the child and family during hospitalization can help them cope with some of their fears. Children with infratentorial tumors seldom have seizures. Introducing the child to other children is a positive action, but not the most important action at this time. (P, N, L)

76. 2. Both the child and parents should receive preoperative teaching about head shaving, bulky bandages, possible facial edema, and the intensive care unit stay. The prognosis and treatment plan cannot be determined until after surgery, when the type of tumor is diagnosed. (P, N, G)

77. 3. Stage I indicates localized disease without evidence of spread. Such a tumor has a favorable prognosis, if all tumor tissue is removed. Poor prognosis, undifferentiation, extension, and metastasis are characteristics of stage III and IV tumors. (I, K, G)

78. 1. Postoperatively, the child undergoing neurosurgery for brain tumor removal is at risk for cardiopulmonary compromise due to anesthesia, surgical complications, or increased intracranial pressure. The other issues are important, but not the nurse's first priority. (I, N, G)

79. 3. Following surgery for an infratentorial tumor, the child is usually positioned flat on either side with the head and neck in midline with the body slightly extended. Pillows against the back, not the head, help maintain position. Such a position helps avoid pressure on the operative site. Trendelenburg position is usually contraindicated, because keeping the head below the level of the heart increases intracranial pressure. It also increases the risk of hemorrhage. (I, N, G)

80. 1. Hypercapnia, hypoxia, and acidosis are potent cerebral vasodilating mechanisms that can cause increased intracranial pressure. Lowering the CO_2 level and increasing the O_2 level through hyperventilation is the most effective short-term method of reducing intracranial pressure. (I, N, G)

81. 3. Glucose in this clear, colorless fluid indicates the presence of CFS. Excessive fluid leakage should be reported to the physician. The nurse should not change the dressing of a postoperative craniotomy client unless instructed to do so by the surgeon. The head of the bed should already be elevated, and further elevation would have little effect on CSF leakage. (I, T, G)

82. 1. It is not uncommon for a child to be concerned about a change in appearance when the entire head or only part has been shaved. The child should be encouraged to participate in decisions about her care when possible. Assuring her that her hair will grow back does not address the immediate change in appearance; neither does explaining that this type of reaction is normal. (I, N, L)

83. 1. Parents of a child who has undergone neurosurgery can easily become overprotective; yet the parents must foster independence in the convalescing child. It is important for the child to resume age-appropriate activities, and parents play an important role in encouraging this. (D, N, L)

The Client With a Spinal Cord Injury

84. 2. The client's history and symptoms suggest a spinal cord injury. A client with suspected spinal cord injury should not be moved until the spine has been immobilized. Turning the client, removing his helmet, or flexing his knees could aggravate a spinal cord injury. (D, N, G)

85. 1. The first priority in emergency care of the client with spinal cord injury is to maintain cardiovascular and respiratory function. Surgical intervention is usually avoided during the acute phase after injury. Preventing fluid and electrolyte imbalance and providing emotional support are important goals but not priority. (I, N, G)

86. 4. Spinal shock occurs 30 to 60 minutes after a spinal cord injury due to the sudden disruption of central and autonomic pathways. This disruption causes flaccid paralysis, loss of reflexes, vasodilation, hypotension, and increased pulse and respiratory rates. Autonomic dysreflexia occurs only after the return of spinal reflexes and is characterized by hypertension. Increased intracranial pressure is associated with widened pulse pressure and decreased pulse and respiratory rates. Metabolic alkalosis does not occur with spinal shock. (D, N, G)

87. 1. In spinal cord injury, temperature regulation is lost distal to the injury. Body temperature must be maintained by adjusting room temperature and/or bed linens. Changing position does not alleviate the temperature regulation problem and could be harmful, considering the client's diagnosis. Reporting this finding to the physician is unnecessary, because it is an expected development. (I, T, G)

88. 3. A thoracic-level spinal cord injury involves the muscles of the lower extremities, bladder, and rectum. Paralytic ileus often occurs; the nurse evaluates this by auscultating the abdomen. (A, T, G)

89. 3. Spinal cord shock causes a loss of reflex activity below the level of the injury, resulting in bladder atony and flaccid paralysis. When the reflex arc returns, it tends to be overactive, resulting in spasticity. The bladder becomes hypertonic during this phase of spinal shock resolution; sensation does not return. (D, N, G)

90. 1. Initially after a catastrophic injury, denial is a common response. With gradual awareness of the situation, anger commonly occurs. The four major stages of grief are denial, anger, depression, and acceptance. (D, N, G)

91. 3. The adolescent is striving for independence and self-definition. A sudden accident with long-term consequences requires many adjustments in terms of self-concept. Industry is a task of children age 6–12 years; ego integrity and generativity are tasks of adult development. (I, N, H)

92. 1. These are signs of autonomic dysreflexia, a generalized sympathetic response usually caused by bladder or bowel distention. Immediate treatment involves eliminating the cause. Since bladder distention is a common cause of this problem, the nurse should immediately determine the patency of the Foley catheter. The nurse should assist the client to a sitting position to help decrease blood pressure. Epinephrine is contraindicated, because it elevates blood pressure and thus would exacerbate the problem. (D, N, G)

93. 2. A high priority is placed on leaving the house so that the client can participate in his normal activities as much as possible, and a short term goal toward leaving the house is to maneuver inside first. Although independent performance of activities of daily living is important, complete independence may be a long-term goal. (P, N, H)

NURSING CARE OF CHILDREN

TEST 7: The Child with Neurological Health Problems

Directions: Use this answer grid to determine areas of strength or need for further study.

NURSING PROCESS

A = Assessment
D = Analysis, nursing diagnosis
P = Planning
I = Implementation
E = Evaluation

COGNITIVE LEVEL

K = Knowledge
C = Comprehension
T = Application
N = Analysis

CLIENT NEEDS

S = Safe, effective care environment
G = Physiological integrity
L = Psychosocial integrity
H = Health promotion/maintenance

		Nursing Process					Cognitive Level				Client Needs			
Question #	Answer #	A	D	P	I	E	K	C	T	N	S	G	L	H
1	4	A						C				G		
2	2	A							T			G		
3	1			P						N			L	
4	1			P					T			G		
5	1			P						N		G		
6	1				I				T		S			
7	2					E				N		G		
8	3				I					N	S			
9	1			P					T		S			
10	4		D							N		G		
11	2			P					T		S			
12	3	A							T			G		
13	3			P						N			L	
14	3					E				N		G		
15	2	A								N		G		
16	2				I					N	S			
17	1				I					N		G		
18	4			P					T			G		
19	3	A							T			G		
20	3					E				N		G		
21	3				I				T		S			
22	4					E				N		G		
23	3				I					N	S			

ANSWER GRID: 1

Nursing Process

A = Assessment
D = Analysis, nursing diagnosis
P = Planning
I = Implementation
E = Evaluation

Cognitive Level

K = Knowledge
C = Comprehension
T = Application
N = Analysis

Client Needs

S = Safe, effective care environment
G = Physiological integrity
L = Psychosocial integrity
H = Health promotion/maintenance

		Nursing Process					Cognitive Level				Client Needs			
Question #	Answer #	A	D	P	I	E	K	C	T	N	S	G	L	H
24	2				I					N	S			
25	4				I					N		G		
26	4			P					T					H
27	2			P					T			G		
28	1				I				T		S			
29	2			P						N				H
30	3					E				N				H
31	4					E				N				H
32	3			P						N				H
33	3			P						N				H
34	4	A								N		G		
35	1					E			T			G		
36	2					E				N				H
37	3					E				N				H
38	3				I				T		S			
39	4				I				T			G		
40	1	A								N		G		
41	2				I					N		G		
42	2				I				T		S			
43	2				I				T			G		
44	1	A								N		G		
45	1	A								N		G		
46	2	A								N		G		
47	3				I					N			L	
48	3				I					N			L	
49	3				I					N		G		
50	2	A								N		G		
51	4		D							N		G		
52	3				I				T			G		

Answer Grid: 2

NURSING PROCESS

A = Assessment
D = Analysis, nursing diagnosis
P = Planning
I = Implementation
E = Evaluation

COGNITIVE LEVEL

K = Knowledge
C = Comprehension
T = Application
N = Analysis

CLIENT NEEDS

S = Safe, effective care environment
G = Physiological integrity
L = Psychosocial integrity
H = Health promotion/maintenance

		Nursing Process					Cognitive Level				Client Needs			
Question #	Answer #	A	D	P	I	E	K	C	T	N	S	G	L	H
53	2			P						N	S			
54	1					E			T			G		
55	2				I					N			L	
56	1				I					N				H
57	2	A							T			G		
58	3	A							T			G		
59	2		D							N		G		
60	1	A							T			G		
61	4				I					N		G		
62	2					E			T			G		
63	1			P						N		G		
64	4				I					N				H
65	3				I				T			G		
66	2					E				N		G		
67	1	A							T			G		
68	2			P					T		S			
69	1				I				T			G		
70	3				I				T			G		
71	3				I					N			L	
72	2				I					N		G		
73	3				I				T		S			
74	4		D							N		G		
75	4			P						N			L	
76	2			P						N		G		
77	3				I		K					G		
78	1				I					N		G		
79	3				I					N		G		
80	1				I					N		G		
81	3				I				T			G		

ANSWER GRID: 3

Nursing Process

A = Assessment
D = Analysis, nursing diagnosis
P = Planning
I = Implementation
E = Evaluation

Cognitive Level

K = Knowledge
C = Comprehension
T = Application
N = Analysis

Client Needs

S = Safe, effective care environment
G = Physiological integrity
L = Psychosocial integrity
H = Health promotion/maintenance

		Nursing Process					Cognitive Level				Client Needs			
Question #	Answer #	A	D	P	I	E	K	C	T	N	S	G	L	H
82	1				I					N			L	
83	1		D							N			L	
84	2		D							N		G		
85	1				I					N		G		
86	4		D							N		G		
87	1				I				T			G		
88	3	A							T			G		
89	3		D							N		G		
90	1		D							N		G		
91	3				I					N				H
92	1		D							N		G		
93	2			P						N				H
Number Correct														
Number Possible	93	16	10	18	37	12	1	1	32	59	14	58	9	12
Percentage Correct														

Score Calculation:

To determine your **Percentage Correct**, divide the **Number Correct** by the **Number Possible.**

Answer Grid: 4

The Child With Musculoskeletal Health Problems

Test 8

Clients With Musculoskeletal Dysfunction
The Client With Cerebral Palsy
The Client With Duchennés Muscular Dystrophy
The Client With Congenital Hip Dysplasia
The Client With Congenital Clubfoot
The Client With Juvenile Rheumatoid Arthritis
The Client With A Fracture
The Client With Osteomyelitis
Correct Answers and Rationale

Select the one best answer and indicate your choice by filling in the circle in front of the option.

Clients With Musculoskeletal Dysfunction

The nurse works in an orthopedic clinic. The following questions pertain to clients seen in this clinic.

1. A child who limps and complains of pain has been found to have Legg-Calvé-Perthes disease. The right femur is involved. The nurse and family plan for the child's care, which should include
- ○ 1. controlling pain that is especially acute at night.
- ○ 2. encouraging the child to walk despite discomfort in the right hip.
- ○ 3. preventing flexion in the right hip.
- ○ 4. preventing weight-bearing on the head of the right femur.

2. In planning outpatient care for the child with Legg-Calvé-Perthes disease the nurse should emphasize teaching the family
- ○ 1. diet planning for weight reduction.
- ○ 2. gentle stretching exercises for both legs.
- ○ 3. management of the corrective appliance.
- ○ 4. relaxation techniques for pain control.

3. The nurse examines an adolescent who has an abnormally convex angulation in the curvature of the thoracic spine. The nurse would document the findings as
- ○ 1. genu varum.
- ○ 2. kyphosis.
- ○ 3. lordosis.
- ○ 4. scoliosis.

4. The nurse would suspect that a child has torticollis (wry neck) after noting a characteristic abnormality of the
- ○ 1. clavicle.
- ○ 2. cervical vertebrae.
- ○ 3. trapezius muscle.
- ○ 4. sternocleidomastoid muscle.

5. The mother of a child with flat feet asks the nurse why her child needs to wear corrective shoes. The nurse should reply that the shoes help
- ○ 1. keep the legs in proper alignment.
- ○ 2. maintain proper weight-bearing balance on the feet.
- ○ 3. prevent the development of internal tibial torsion.
- ○ 4. strengthen the arches of the feet.

6. The nurse would evaluate her or his teaching about the etiology of muscular dystrophy as successful when the mother of a child with the disease states, "My son's disease is due to the
- ○ 1. effects of the automobile accident."
- ○ 2. genes he inherited from me."
- ○ 3. imbalance in his thyroid hormone."

○ 4. viral infection I had when I was pregnant with him."

7. The nurse would assess a female adolescent for lateral deviation of the spine by having her
○ 1. bend forward at the waist and allow her head and arms to fall freely.
○ 2. lie flat on the floor and extend her legs straight from her trunk.
○ 3. sit in a chair while lifting her feet and legs to a right angle with her trunk.
○ 4. standing against a wall while pressing the length of her back against the wall.

8. The nurse would suspect that the adolescent has scoliosis after observing a skeletal defect that results in a slight limp and
○ 1. a longer-than-average trunk.
○ 2. a rib hump.
○ 3. a forward body thrust while walking.
○ 4. a waddling gait.

9. A child needs to wear a Milwaukee brace for scoliosis, and the nurse teaches his family about when he can remove it. The nurse would evaluate the teaching as successful when the child and parents indicate that the brace will be removed when he
○ 1. bathes, for about 1 hour per day.
○ 2. eats, for about 3 hours a day.
○ 3. is awake, for about 14 hours a day.
○ 4. sleeps, for about 10 hours a day.

10. The nurse would teach exercises to a child wearing the Milwaukee brace primarily to help
○ 1. decrease back muscle spasms.
○ 2. improve the brace's traction effect.
○ 3. prevent spinal contractures.
○ 4. strengthen the torso muscles.

11. The nurse would assess a child with "growing pains" for discomfort in the area of the tuberosity of the
○ 1. calcaneus.
○ 2. femur.
○ 3. fibula.
○ 4. tibia.

The Client With Cerebral Palsy

A mother of a child with cerebral palsy brings the child to the clinic for developmental screening.

12. In teaching the mother about the primary goal of the screening, the nurse would explain the tests are done to recognize primary developmental delays early, in order to
○ 1. encourage health maintenance.
○ 2. facilitate communication.
○ 3. prevent secondary developmental delays.
○ 4. prevent secondary injuries.

13. The mother asks the nurse to define cerebral palsy. The nurse's best response would be, "It's a term applied to impaired nerve and muscle control as a result of
○ 1. injury to the cerebrum due to viral infection."
○ 2. malformation of the blood vessels in the ventricles due to inheritance."
○ 3. nonprogressive brain damage due to injury."
○ 4. progressive brain disease due to metabolic imbalances."

14. The client has a history of neonatal anoxia and the nurse notes increased tone in the calf muscle of the right leg and the right elbow flexor. The nurse would anticipate that this child has
○ 1. ataxic cerebral palsy.
○ 2. atonic cerebral palsy.
○ 3. dyskinetic cerebral palsy.
○ 4. spastic cerebral palsy.

15. The mother and nurse plan goals for this toddler. What would be the primary goal of therapy?
○ 1. Actualization of individual potential.
○ 2. Maintenance of joint mobility.
○ 3. Preparation for corrective surgery.
○ 4. Promotion of general health.

16. The nurse watches as the toddler unsuccessfully attempts to pick up his teddy bear with his right hand. The nurse would document the findings as right-sided
○ 1. diplegia.
○ 2. hemiparesis.
○ 3. paraplegia.
○ 4. quadriparesis.

17. The nurse should encourage the mother to position the child upright and to offer toys to his affected side, to
○ 1. challenge the use of the affected limb.
○ 2. increase strength in the affected limb.
○ 3. keep the infant occupied.
○ 4. test visual acuity.

18. The mother asks the nurse if her child will be able to walk normally, since he can pull himself to a standing position. What would be the nurse's best reply?
○ 1. "Ask the doctor what he thinks at your next appointment."
○ 2. "He might but he might not. How old were you when you first walked?"
○ 3. "It's not easy to predict, but the fact that he's able to bear weight is a positive factor."
○ 4. "That all depends. If he really wants to walk, he'll probably be able to do so eventually."

19. The nurse evaluates the family's ability to cope with the child's cerebral palsy. Which of the following would be indicative of their inability to cope with the disease?

○ 1. Limiting interaction with the extended family and friends.
○ 2. Needing to learn to meet the child's physical needs.
○ 3. Requesting teaching about cerebral palsy in general.
○ 4. Seeking financial help to pay for medical bills.

The Client With Duchenne's Muscular Dystrophy

A family with a child with Duchenne's muscular dystrophy has been referred to a visiting nurse service. The nurse makes the initial visit.

20. When assessing a child who has a sibling with Duchenne's muscular dystrophy, the nurse would suspect that this child also has the disease based on which finding?
○ 1. Abnormal gait on a level surface.
○ 2. Difficulty running.
○ 3. Lack of facial mobility.
○ 4. Small, weak muscles.

21. The child's mother asks the nurse what an X-linked inheritance pattern is. The nurse should explain that it means
○ 1. females are affected almost exclusively.
○ 2. males and females are affected equally.
○ 3. males are affected almost exclusively.
○ 4. males are affected twice as often as females.

22. The nurse observes the child attempt to rise from a sitting position on the floor. After attaining a kneeling position, the child "walks" his hands up his legs to stand. The nurse would document this as an indication of muscular dystrophy referred to as
○ 1. Galleazzi's sign.
○ 2. Goodell's sign.
○ 3. Good enough sign.
○ 4. Gower's sign.

23. The nurse and mother care for the children. The primary nursing goal would be to
○ 1. encourage early wheelchair use.
○ 2. foster social interactions.
○ 3. maintain function in unaffected muscles.
○ 4. prevent circulatory impairment.

24. Taking into consideration the major orthopedic complications associated with muscular dystrophy, the nursing care plan for a child with this disease should include interventions that prevent
○ 1. clubfoot.
○ 2. contractures.
○ 3. multiple fractures.
○ 4. osteomyelitis.

25. When interacting with the child's mother, the nurse observes behavior indicating that she may feel guilty about her children's condition. The nurse would suspect that this guilt stems from the
○ 1. terminal nature of the disease.
○ 2. dependent behavior of the children.
○ 3. genetic mode of transmission.
○ 4. sudden onset of the disease.

26. One of the child's aunts tells the nurse that she understands that the children will not have a normal life span and asks the nurse to explain what the usual cause of death is in children with muscular dystrophy. The nurse replies
○ 1. "Most children die of renal failure."
○ 2. "The usual cause of death is respiratory tract infection or cardiac failure."
○ 3. "You should talk to the children's parents about this subject."
○ 4. "Would you like to talk to our chaplain about this?"

27. The nurse teaches the mother about the course of the disease, therapeutic management, and nursing considerations. Which of the following statements by the mother would indicate that she has understood the teaching?
○ 1. "The boys will probably be unable to walk independently by the time they are 9–11 years old."
○ 2. "Muscle relaxants are effective for some children."
○ 3. "When the children are a little older, they can have surgery to improve their ability to walk."
○ 4. "We'll help the boys be as active as possible to prevent progression of the disease."

The Client With Congenital Hip Dysplasia

The nurse performs a newborn assessment.

28. While gently abducting the hips, the nurse feels the femoral head slip into the acetabulum. The nurse documents this finding as a positive
○ 1. Barlow's test.
○ 2. Jackson's sign.
○ 3. Ortolani's sign.
○ 4. Trendelenburg's sign.

29. The nurse examining a neonate would identify Galleazzi's sign when noting
○ 1. broadening of the perineum.
○ 2. severely limited abduction of the affected side.
○ 3. shortening of the limb on the affected side.
○ 4. symmetric gluteal folds.

A child is fitted with a Pavlik harness to correct congenital hip dysplasia.

30. The nurse would teach the parents to
- ○ 1. keep the clinic appointments for periodic harness readjustment.
- ○ 2. make sure the child's legs are in an adducted position.
- ○ 3. readjust the harness as necessary for comfort.
- ○ 4. remove the harness for cleaning.

31. When teaching the parents about use of orthopedic appliances, the nurse's initial step should be to
- ○ 1. assess their coping strategies.
- ○ 2. determine their knowledge of the device.
- ○ 3. write up the instructions.
- ○ 4. provide the parents with a list of community resources.

A 6-week-old child with congenital hip dysplasia is fitted with a spica cast.

32. The nurse should teach the parents that the abduction stabilizer bar
- ○ 1. can be adjusted to a position of comfort.
- ○ 2. can be used to lift the child.
- ○ 3. is designed to add strength to the cast.
- ○ 4. is removed after the casting material is completely dry.

33. Three weeks after the application of the spica cast, the nurse notes that the child is afebrile and that his toes are swollen and cool to the touch. The nurse would suspect that these findings are due to the fact that the
- ○ 1. child has had his feet in a dependent position.
- ○ 2. child has outgrown the cast.
- ○ 3. cotton wadding lining of the cast has shrunk.
- ○ 4. child has an infection in the tissue under the cast.

34. The mother asks the nurse if she can continue to breast-feed her infant with a spica cast. What would be the nurse's best reply?
- ○ 1. "Do you want to continue to breast-feed?"
- ○ 2. "How would you feel if you couldn't breast-feed?"
- ○ 3. "It's possible, but difficult because of the cast."
- ○ 4. "Yes, let me show you some different nursing positions that may work for you."

35. The nurse notes that the skin on the upper abdomen is being irritated by the cast's rough edges. The nurse should
- ○ 1. add extra plaster material to the edge of the cast.
- ○ 2. file the edges with an orthopedic rasp.
- ○ 3. place overlapping short pieces of tape over the edge of the cast.
- ○ 4. place a transparent protective dressing on the skin.

The Client With Congenital Clubfoot

A neonate is diagnosed as having a congenital clubfoot.

36. When discussing the treatment of congenital clubfoot with the parents, the nurse should tell the parents to expect that initially the neonate will have
- ○ 1. a footboard attached to the crib.
- ○ 2. corrective shoes fitted.
- ○ 3. gentle passive foot exercises.
- ○ 4. the legs elevated above the level of the heart.

37. The parents convey anxiety about how the problem will be treated and express feelings of helplessness and guilt. Initially, the nurse should
- ○ 1. ask them to share these concerns with the physician.
- ○ 2. arrange a meeting with other parents whose infants have undergone successful clubfoot treatment.
- ○ 3. discuss the problem and explains how such deformities are usually corrected.
- ○ 4. suggest that they make an appointment with a counselor.

38. Plaster casts are applied to correct the deformity. In the immediate postapplication period, the nurse should
- ○ 1. change the client's position at least every 2 hours.
- ○ 2. coat the casts with a clear acrylic spray finish.
- ○ 3. dry the casts rapidly with a hair dryer.
- ○ 4. handle the casts with the fingertips only.

39. The nurse has taught the parents about caring for the cast. Which of the following statements would indicate that they have understood the teaching? "We'll
- ○ 1. clean the casts with soap and water carefully when it becomes soiled."
- ○ 2. elevate the casts on pillows, so the legs will be above heart level."
- ○ 3. observe the color and temperature of the toes frequently."
- ○ 4. remove the petals from the edge of the casts after 24 hours."

40. The nurse tells the parents that they will need to bring him to the clinic frequently for cast changes, to
- ○ 1. accommodate the increasing size of his legs.
- ○ 2. measure the circumference of his legs and compare them to norms.
- ○ 3. assess for microorganism growth under the cast.
- ○ 4. facilitate neurovascular assessment of his legs.

41. After clubfoot deformity is overcorrected by serial casting, the client is to wear a Denis Browne splint. The nurse should explain to the parents that the splint is applied to

○ 1. assess the strength of calf and ankle muscles.
○ 2. help maintain the feet in the desired position.
○ 3. prevent kicking.
○ 4. prevent possible bone deformities.

42. The nurse teaches the parents how to maintain the function of the Denis Browne splint. Which of the parents' following actions during the return demonstration would indicate that they have understood the teaching?
○ 1. Repositioning the angle of the shoes on the bar.
○ 2. Slipping the child's feet into the shoes without socks.
○ 3. Tightening a loose shoe against the splint.
○ 4. Using the bar to help lift the child.

43. After the child has been wearing the Denis Browne splint for a while, his mother reports that he is able to wobble across the floor on his hands and knees while wearing the splint. The nurse should tell the mother to
○ 1. notify the physician so corrective shoes can be prescribed.
○ 2. put the child in a playpen to restrict movements.
○ 3. remove the splint so the child can be more mobile.
○ 4. remove tablecloths from all rooms to which the child has access.

The Client With Juvenile Rheumatoid Arthritis

A preschool-age girl is admitted with a tentative diagnosis of juvenile rheumatoid arthritis (JRA).

44. The father asks which test can definitely diagnose JRA. The nurse should explain that
○ 1. a red blood cell electrophoresis is diagnostic.
○ 2. an elevated erythrocyte sedimentation rate is diagnostic.
○ 3. a positive synovial fluid culture is diagnostic.
○ 4. no specific laboratory test is diagnostic.

45. The diagnosis of JRA is confirmed. The parents tell the nurse that the diagnosis frightens them because they know nothing about the prognosis. The nurse should explain that
○ 1. in most children, the disease will be in permanent remission by adolescence.
○ 2. many children go into long remissions but have severe deformities and loss of function.
○ 3. the disease usually progresses to crippling rheumatoid arthritis as the child reaches adulthood.
○ 4. most affected children recover completely within a few years.

46. The child's mother is worried that the child will have to stop attending preschool because of the illness. The nurse should explain that the child
○ 1. may find it difficult to attend school because of the side effects of the prescribed medication regimen.
○ 2. should be encouraged to attend school, but will need time to work out early-morning stiffness.
○ 3. should be kept home from school whenever she experiences joint discomfort.
○ 4. will need to wear splints or knee braces to give her more support.

47. The nurse and family develop a care plan to alleviate joint stiffness in the child. Which of these interventions should be included?
○ 1. Applying moist heat to affected joints.
○ 2. Applying cool compresses to affected joints.
○ 3. Performing repetitive weight-bearing exercises using the affected joints.
○ 4. Restricting the intake of dietary purine.

48. The nurse assesses that the child's family is a close and strong family unit. In planning care for this family, the nurse should
○ 1. contact appropriate community resources.
○ 2. discuss the child's illness with the siblings.
○ 3. ensure that the family has all needed equipment.
○ 4. provide parental education and support.

49. Several months after the diagnosis of JRA is made for their preschool-age child, the mother reports that the child has become withdrawn. The nurse would suspect that the child's withdrawal is
○ 1. a normal stage of development.
○ 2. a side effect of the medication.
○ 3. an indication of sibling rivalry.
○ 4. most likely a reaction to the disease.

50. The nurse should suggest that the mother
○ 1. introduce the child to other children with JRA.
○ 2. spend extra time with the child and less time with her other children.
○ 3. send the child to a counselor.
○ 4. try to be supportive and understanding of the child.

The Client With a Fracture

A 1-year-old child has fractured his left femur. He is placed in Bryant's traction.

51. The nurse should explain to the parent that this traction's primary purpose is to
○ 1. keep the broken bone in proper alignment.
○ 2. maintain muscle strength.
○ 3. minimize demineralization of the femur.
○ 4. prevent infection at the insertion site.

52. When the child is in Bryant's traction, the nurse should make sure that he is positioned on his back with his legs

○ 1. flexed at a 45-degree angle at the hips, with the hips touching the bed.
○ 2. flexed at a 90-degree angle with the hips slightly off the bed.
○ 3. separated, with the affected leg at a right angle to the body and the unaffected leg in any comfortable position.
○ 4. straight in line, with his body resting flat on the bed.

53. The nurse should carefully assess the child for
○ 1. drainage at the pin sites.
○ 2. enuresis.
○ 3. redness over the sacral area.
○ 4. weak pedal pulses.

54. When caring for a child in Bryant's traction, the nurse should
○ 1. allow the weights on the traction to hang freely.
○ 2. change the moleskin used on the legs for obtaining traction each day.
○ 3. decrease the amount of weight on the traction to hang freely.
○ 4. remove the weights while inspecting the legs for evidence of friction over bony prominences.

A 1-year-old child is admitted with a fractured femur. The parents give different explanations for the injury.

55. Which of the following observations by the nurse would strongly suggest that this child has been abused? The child
○ 1. appears happy when personnel work with him.
○ 2. eats his lunch without urging.
○ 3. is physically and emotionally underdeveloped for his age.
○ 4. sucks his thumb.

56. A nurse suspecting that a child has been abused by his or her parents should
○ 1. continue to collect information until there is no doubt that abuse has occurred.
○ 2. ensure that the findings are reported to the proper state authorities.
○ 3. keep the findings confidential, because they are considered legal privileged communication between the nurse and the client.
○ 4. report the findings to the physician, because reporting evidence of child abuse falls within the province of medical practice only.

57. When planning interventions for abusive parents, the nurse should take into account that a very common finding regarding abusive parents is that they
○ 1. are members of a low socioeconomic group.
○ 2. are unemployed.
○ 3. have low self-esteem.
○ 4. have lost emotional attachments in the family.

A preschool-age child is brought to the emergency room with a broken right humerus. The child is fearful and cries, "Mommy, I want to go home. Is the doctor going to cut my arm? I hate the nurse."

58. What would be the nurse's best initial action?
○ 1. Ask the child's parents to leave the room for a while until the nurse has a chance to calm the child.
○ 2. Explain to the child what the physician will be doing during the procedure in language the child can readily understand.
○ 3. Have another nurse care for the child because of the child's reaction to the assigned nurse.
○ 4. Suggest to the child that she will be acting like "a big girl" if she is quiet while the physician fixes her arm.

59. For this normally developing preschooler with an injury the nurse formulates the nursing diagnosis Fear. This fear most likely would be related to
○ 1. being mutilated and disfigured.
○ 2. being separated from the mother.
○ 3. losing control over what is happening.
○ 4. worry about the pain from procedures.

60. The child's arm is casted in the emergency department, and the nurse gives the parents discharge instructions. The nurse would evaluate the teaching as successful when the parents agree to seek medical advice if the child
○ 1. cannot extend the fingers on her right hand.
○ 2. complains of nausea before her evening meal.
○ 3. complains that the cast is cool and damp after 5 hours.
○ 4. is irritable and complains that the cast is heavy.

61. The nurse should teach the mother that while the child sleeps, the drying cast should be supported on a
○ 1. bedside stand.
○ 2. block made from a cardboard box.
○ 3. firm mattress.
○ 4. soft pillow.

The nurse examines a 3-year-old with a history of a recent injury to the left leg who refuses to walk and complains of pain when moving the leg.

62. The nurse would suspect the etiology of the problem to be

- ○ 1. behavioral regression.
- ○ 2. fracture.
- ○ 3. paresthesia.
- ○ 4. traumatic paralysis.

63. The nurse examines the child's leg. When assessing the affected leg, the nurse would expect to find muscles that are
- ○ 1. atrophied
- ○ 2. contracted.
- ○ 3. flabby.
- ○ 4. normal.

64. The nurse notes that the child's left thigh is quite swollen. What should the nurse do next?
- ○ 1. Assess the neurologic status of the toes.
- ○ 2. Determine the circulatory status of the upper thigh.
- ○ 3. Document the findings in the nursing notes.
- ○ 4. Notify the physician immediately.

65. The physician verifies the diagnosis of complete fracture of the femur and orders that the child be placed in Buck's extension. When the mother asks why this treatment is being used, the nurse should explain that it is to
- ○ 1. immobilize the fracture before surgery.
- ○ 2. immobilize the fracture until realignment occurs.
- ○ 3. increase muscle spasms to enhance circulation.
- ○ 4. provide assistance in range-of-motion exercises.

66. The nurse who sets up Buck's traction should use the weights that pull forward on the distal bone fragments, to produce
- ○ 1. countertraction.
- ○ 2. friction.
- ○ 3. pressure.
- ○ 4. traction.

67. Anticipating the immobilized child's diversional needs, the nurse would offer him
- ○ 1. a ball.
- ○ 2. blocks.
- ○ 3. hand puppets.
- ○ 4. marbles.

68. The parents are unable to visit their son for more than an hour a day. (They have five other children and both work outside of the home.) The nurse recognizes expressions of guilt in both parents. To help alleviate this guilt, the nurse would make which of the following remarks?
- ○ 1. "I'm sure you feel very guilty."
- ○ 2. "It's important that you visit as much as you can."
- ○ 3. "Not all parents can stay all the time."
- ○ 4. "Perhaps you could take turns visiting."

A spica cast is applied to a school-age child with a fractured femur.

69. The child seems to adjust to the cast, except that he complains that it is too tight after each meal. The nurse should plan to
- ○ 1. ask the physician to order a laxative.
- ○ 2. give smaller, more frequent meals.
- ○ 3. offer the child a mechanical soft diet.
- ○ 4. offer the child more fruits and grains.

70. The nurse would identify the need to do more teaching concerning skin care with the child's mother if she
- ○ 1. applies lotion to the skin under the cast.
- ○ 2. checks the smoothness of the cast edges.
- ○ 3. covers the cast around the perineum with plastic film.
- ○ 4. inspects inside the cast.

71. The child suddenly develops chest pain, dyspnea, diaphoresis, and tachycardia. The nurse would suspect
- ○ 1. respiratory distress syndrome.
- ○ 2. pneumonia.
- ○ 3. pulmonary edema.
- ○ 4. pulmonary emboli.

72. The nurse planning care for a child placed in a spica cast would identify the highest-priority nursing goal during the immediate post-casting period as preventing
- ○ 1. altered skin integrity.
- ○ 2. neurovascular impairment.
- ○ 3. respiratory impairment.
- ○ 4. urinary stasis.

73. The nurse is helping a family plan for the discharge of their child, who will be going home in a spica cast early in July. Which of the following pieces of information would be of most concern to the nurse?
- ○ 1. The bathrooms are all on the second floor.
- ○ 2. The child's bedroom is on the second floor.
- ○ 3. The child's 16-year-old sister will be responsible for the child during the day hours.
- ○ 4. There are three steps up to the front door.

A child goes home after being casted for an open reduction of the radius. Several hours later, the child's mother phones the hospital and tells the nurse that he is complaining of severe pain, has swollen and pale fingers, and cannot extend his fingers because of discomfort.

74. The nurse should advise the mother to
- ○ 1. administer an extra dose of pain medication.
- ○ 2. bring the child to the emergency room immediately.
- ○ 3. elevate the child's arm over the level of his heart.
- ○ 4. gently exercise his fingers.

The Client With Osteomyelitis

An 8-year-old child is hospitalized with osteomyelitis.

75. During initial assessment of a child with osteomyelitis of the left tibia, the nurse would expect the area over the tibia to have
○ 1. diffuse tenderness.
○ 2. increased pallor.
○ 3. increased warmth.
○ 4. localized edema.

76. The nurse assessing a child diagnosed with osteomyelitis would expect to find
○ 1. bradycardia.
○ 2. bradypnea.
○ 3. fever.
○ 4. pulse deficits.

77. After receiving orders for laboratory tests and antibiotics, the nurse would plan to start the antibiotic after blood is drawn for
○ 1. creatinine.
○ 2. culture.
○ 3. hemoglobin.
○ 4. leukocyte count.

78. On reviewing the preliminary laboratory results, the nurse identifies which of the following findings consistent with the diagnosis of osteomyelitis?
○ 1. Hematocrit 30%.
○ 2. Erythrocyte sedimentation rate 17 mm/hr.
○ 3. Serum potassium 5.0 mEq/L.
○ 4. White blood cell count 12,000/mm^3.

79. The nurse explains the medical care plan to the child's mother. The plan would include long-term antibiotic therapy, bed rest, immobilization of the affected leg, and
○ 1. abduction of the affected leg.
○ 2. application of cool, moist packs to the affected leg.
○ 3. elevation of the affected leg.
○ 4. passive range-of-motion exercises to the unaffected leg.

80. The nurse knows that a child being treated for osteomyelitis will be receiving intravenous antibiotic therapy for 3 to 4 weeks. Therefore, the nurse would plan to monitor the child's
○ 1. blood glucose level.
○ 2. prothrombin times.
○ 3. urine glucose level.
○ 4. urine specific gravity.

81. To meet the developmental needs of a hospitalized 8-year-old with osteomyelitis, the nurse would include which measure in the plan of care?
○ 1. Encouraging the child to communicate with schoolmates.
○ 2. Encouraging the parents to stay with the child.
○ 3. Allowing siblings to visit freely.
○ 4. Talking to the child about his interests daily.

82. The nurse caring for a child on bedrest plans interventions to prevent skin breakdown. The nurse should keep in mind that the most effective way to prevent skin breakdown is
○ 1. attaching a trapeze to the bed.
○ 2. inspecting the skin every 4 hours.
○ 3. giving a back rub at bedtime.
○ 4. repositioning every 2 hours.

83. The nurse would encourage the child with osteomyelitis to choose which of the following meals?
○ 1. Beef and bean burrito with cheese, carrot and celery sticks, and an orange.
○ 2. Buttered wheat bread, cream of broccoli soup, tossed salad with dressing, and an apple.
○ 3. Potato soup; bacon, lettuce, and tomato sandwich; and an orange.
○ 4. Tomato soup, grilled cheese sandwich, and potato chips.

84. After 2 weeks of treatment for osteomyelitis the child responds to the nurse's request to begin her bath by throwing the soap across the room. The nurse should recognize that the child is most likely responding to
○ 1. a dislike for the nurse.
○ 2. lack of control over the situation.
○ 3. separation from her friends and classmates.
○ 4. the doctor's check of her leg a few minutes before.

CORRECT ANSWERS AND RATIONALE

The letters in parentheses following the rationale identify the step of the nursing process (A, D, P, I, E); cognitive level (K, C, T, N); and client need (S, G, L, H). See the Answer Grid for the key.

Clients With Musculoskeletal Dysfunction

1. 4. Legg-Calvé-Perthes disease, also known as coxa plana or osteochondrosis, is characterized by aseptic necrosis at the head of the femur when the blood supply to the area is interrupted. Avoiding weight bearing is especially important to prevent the head of femur from leaving the acetabulum. Devices such as an abduction brace, a leg cast, or a harness sling are used to protect the affected joint while revascularization and bone healing occur. Surgical procedures are used in some cases. (P, N, G)

2. 3. Since most of the child's care takes place on an outpatient basis, the major emphasis for nursing care is to teach the family the care and management of the corrective device. Pain is usually not a problem once therapy has been initiated. There is no need to increase protein or vitamin C intake if the child is eating a well-balanced diet. Weight reduction in an obese child would be recommended, but is not emphasized in normal-weight children. (P, N, G)

3. 2. Kyphosis is an abnormally increased convex angulation in the curvature of the thoracic spine. The most common cause of kyphosis in children is postural. Genu varum refers to "bowlegs." Lordosis is the excessive anterior curvature of the lumbar spine due most often to an underlying neuromuscular disease or spinal deformity. Scoliosis is a lateral curvature of the spine. (A, K, G)

4. 4. In torticollis, the sternocleidomastoid muscle appears contracted, or shortened. Range of motion in the neck is limited. This condition causes the neck to turn laterally to one side with the chin directed to the opposite side. (A, K, G)

5. 1. There is no treatment for flat feet; however, corrective shoes are often prescribed to keep the legs in proper alignment. Toeing in (internal tibial torsion) is not associated with flat feet. Corrective shoes will not strengthen the arches or change weight bearing on the feet. (I, N, H)

6. 2. Muscular dystrophy, a genetically determined, sex-linked condition, is a progressive degenerative disease of the skeletal muscles. There are several different forms of muscle involvement. The various deviations that involve progressive weakness of muscle groups form the largest group of muscular diseases of childhood. (E, N, G)

7. 1. Lateral deviation of the spine (scoliosis) is assessed by having the child bend forward at the waist and allow her arms to hang freely, then looking for lateral curvature of the spine and a rib hump. (A, N, H)

8. 2. A characteristic sign of scoliosis is rib hump. The hump is best observed from the back and front when the child, undressed to the waist, bends over and lets her arms hang freely. The rib hump and flank asymmetry then become obvious. A slight limp, a crooked hemline, and complaints of back pain are other common findings in a child with scoliosis. (D, N, G)

9. 1. One of the most effective spinal braces for correcting scoliosis, The Milwaukee brace should be worn at all times, except when carrying out personal hygiene measures. (E, T, G)

10. 4. Exercises are prescribed for the child with scoliosis wearing a Milwaukee brace to help strengthen muscles that will help overcome the spinal curvature. Exercise also helps improve the correction of the spine and ribs and improves the child's stamina. (I, T, G)

11. 4. The osteochondroses are a group of diseases affecting various parts of the body; the most common one of this group is Osgood–Schlatter disease, frequently referred to as "growing pains." This condition occurs mostly in males between age 13 and 15, when epiphyseal growth is very rapid. This growth places stress on muscles and tendons and eventually produces tendinitis, usually at the tibial tuberosity. Osgood–Schlatter disease is ordinarily self-limiting and usually responds to rest. Warm compresses placed over the painful area can promote comfort. (A, T, G)

The Client With Cerebral Palsy

12. 3. The goal of early recognition of primary developmental delays in children with cerebral palsy is to prevent secondary and tertiary delays. For example, a young infant who is unable to reach or focus on objects would be unable to attain various levels of sensory-perceptual development described by Piaget. Facilitating communication, preventing physical injury, and encouraging health maintenance are all nursing goals for the child with cerebral palsy, but none is the goal of early recognition of primary developmental delays. (I, N, H)

13. 3. Cerebral palsy is a collective term applied to nonprogressive cerebellar damage that results in various alterations in neuromuscular tone and/or function. (I, N, G)

14. 4. Spastic cerebral palsy, the most common clinical type, represents an upper motor neuron muscular impairment that may involve altered tone, persistent reflexes, and a lack or delay of postural control. Dyskinetic movements are involuntary and may be manifested in athetoid movements. Ataxia is the least common type of cerebral palsy, and the atonic type is very uncommon. (D, T, G)

15. 1. The goals of therapy for children with cerebral palsy are early recognition and promotion of optimal development so that the child can realize his potential. (P, N, H)

16. 2. Hemiparesis, partial paralysis of half of the body (in this case, the right side), is the most common form of spastic cerebral palsy. Quadriparesis refers to spastic cerebral palsy in which all four extremities are involved. Paraplegia is pure cerebral paralysis of the lower extremities. In the diplegia type of cerebral palsy, similar parts on both sides of the body are involved. (D, N, G)

17. 1. Challenging the use of the affected limb facilitates increased function. Positioning the child upright and handing toys to his affected side will keep him occupied and may test his visual acuity, but neither of these is the reason for the activity. Similarly, this activity is not done to increase strength of the affected limb. (I, T, G)

18. 3. Most children with hemiparesis spastic cerebral palsy are able to walk. The motor deficit is usually greater in the upper extremity. The nurse should answer the mother's question honestly. The will to walk is important, but without neurological stability the child may be unable to do so. There is no need for the nurse to refer the mother to the physician for an answer to the question. (I, N, G)

19. 1. Lack of interaction with friends and family indicates an inability to cope with others' reactions and responses to the child with cerebral palsy. The need for further teaching and financial problems are of concern but do not indicate the type of response the family is having to the child's problems. (E, N, L)

The Client With Duchenne's Muscular Dystrophy

20. 2. Usually the first clinical manifestations of Duchenne's muscular dystrophy are difficulty running, riding a bicycle, and climbing stairs. Abnormal gait on a level surface becomes apparent later. Occasionally, enlarged calves may be noted. Lack of facial mobility is associated with facioscapulo-humeral dystrophy. (A, C, G)

21. 3. In all X-linked disorders, males are affected almost exclusively, because the mother carries the gene that is expressed in males. (E, C, G)

22. 4. In Gower's sign, the child "walks" the hands up the legs in an attempt to stand. This is the common manner in which children afflicted with Duchenne's muscular dystrophy arise from sitting to standing. Galleazzi's sign refers to the shortening of the affected limb in congenital hip dislocation. Goodenough sign refers to a test of mental age. Goodell's sign refers to the softening of the cervix, considered a sign of probable pregnancy. (D, C, G)

23. 3. The primary goal is to maintain function in unaffected muscles for as long as possible. There is no effective treatment for childhood muscular dystrophy. Children who remain active are able to avoid wheelchair confinement longer. Children with muscular dystrophy become socially isolated as their condition deteriorates and they can no longer keep up with friends. Maintaining function helps prevent social isolation. Circulatory impairment is not associated with muscular dystrophy. (I, N, H)

24. 2. Contractures of the hip, knees, and ankles occur as a result of selective muscle involvement. Fractures are not as common as contractures, and osteomyelitis is not a complication of muscular dystrophy. Clubfoot is associated with muscular dystrophy, but nursing intervention focuses on preventing contractures. (P, N, G)

25. 3. The guilt feelings that mothers of children with muscular dystrophy commonly experience stem from the mother-to-son transmission of the defective gene. Disease onset is usually gradual. Congenital forms of muscular dystrophy are rare. (D, N, G)

26. 2. The usual cause of death in children with muscular dystrophy is respiratory tract infection or cardiac failure. The aunt is asking for information about the disease. The answer is not privileged information, so the nurse does not refer her to the parents. Pastoral care is not warranted at this point. (I, N, G)

27. 1. Muscular dystrophy is a progressive disease; affected children are usually unable to walk independently by age 9–11 years. There is no effective treatment for childhood muscular dystrophy. Children who remain active are able to avoid wheelchair confinement for a longer period, but activity does not prevent disease progression. (E, N, G)

The Client With Congenital Hip Dysplasia

28. 3. Ortolani's sign refers to the feeling of the femoral head slipping forward into the acetabulum when forward pressure is exerted from behind the greater trochanter and the knee is held laterally. This sign indicates hip dislocation. A positive Barlow's test indicates that the hip is unstable with increased risk of dislocation. Jackson's sign refers to a prolonged expiratory sound over the affected area in pulmonary tuberculosis. Trendelenburg's sign refers to a downward tilting of the pelvis toward the normal side when a child with a dislocated hip stands on the affected side with the uninvolved leg elevated. (D, C, G)

29. 3. Shortening of the limb on the affected side, Galeazzi's sign indicates congenital hip dysplasia. Other signs include broadening of the perineum in bilateral dislocation, asymmetric thigh and gluteal folds, and limited abduction of the affected leg. (D, C, G)

30. 1. The Pavlik (or Paulik) harness consists of straps passing from the shoulders and chest to the feet and lower legs. The harness is readjusted to maintain proper alignment of the femur head in the acetabulum. It usually is not removed by the parents, so frequent visits to the clinic may be necessary. The legs should be maintained in an abducted, not adducted position. (I, N, G)

31. 2. Assessing the learner's knowledge is the initial step in teaching. Giving parents written instructions and a list of community resources are appropriate strategies, but neither is the most appropriate initial step. Assessing coping strategies can provide important information to the development of the teaching plan, but is not the initial step. (P, N, H)

32. 3. The abduction bar is incorporated into the cast to increase strength and cannot be removed or adjusted, unless the cast is removed and a new cast applied. The bar should never be used to lift or turn the client. (I, T, S)

33. 2. Neonates grow rapidly, and a cast that was adequate for a neonate may be outgrown in less than 1 month. The cast then becomes too tight, and circulation is impaired. If the child had had surgery, the chances of infection are minimal after a 4-week period and would be accompanied by other symptoms such as fever. The cotton wadding used to line the cast does not shrink over time. (D, N, G)

34. 4. The mother can continue to breast-feed the infant in a spica cast but may need to try alternate nursing positions. Since the mother has been successful in the past, asking whether she wants to continue breast-feeding, or about her feelings about not continuing, is not necessary. Telling her that it is possible but difficult is false and could create anxiety. (I, N, H)

35. 3. Placing short overlapping pieces of tape over the cast edge, commonly referred to as petaling, will protect the skin from the rough plaster and also reinforce the cast edge. It would be difficult to file the edge smooth, and this would weaken the area. It is too difficult and expensive to use special barrier plastic to protect the skin. Placing extra plaster casting material in the area may only increase the roughness. (I, T, S)

The Client With Congenital Clubfoot

36. 3. Management of the infant with a clubfoot deformity starts as soon as possible after birth. Treatment in early infancy is conservative, depending on the severity of the deformity, it may consist of manipulating the feet into a functional position and applying a series of casts until a marked overcorrection is achieved. Corrective shoes may be used once the deformity has been corrected. Elevating the extremities and using a footboard are not done in treating clubfoot. (I, N, G)

37. 3. When an infant is born with an unexpected anomaly, parents are faced with questions, uncertainties, and possible disappointments. They may feel inadequate, helpless, and anxious. The nurse can help the parents initially by assessing their concerns and providing appropriate information to help them clarify and/or resolve the immediate problems. (I, N, L)

38. 1. Complete drying of a plaster cast takes several hours. Turning the child with a newly applied cast at least every 2 hours helps the cast dry uniformly. The drying cast must be handled with the palms only to prevent indentations from the fingers, which could cause pressure areas. Dryers are not used to dry the cast, because the cast dries on the surface but remains wet underneath. Furthermore, heat may be conducted to the tissues through the wet cast, causing burns. The cast must not be coated with any substance that would inhibit the evaporation of moisture from the plaster. (I, T, S)

39. 3. A too-tight cast can cause a tourniquet effect and compromise the neurovascular integrity of the extremity. Manifestations of neurovascular impairment include pain, edema, pulselessness, coolness, altered sensation, and inability to move the distal exposed extremity. The cast should be assessed frequently. Wetting a cast with water and soap softens the plaster, which may alter the cast's effectiveness. Adhesive tape petals are applied to cover the rough edges of the cast and are left in place. There is no reason to elevate the casted extremities when a child is being treated for clubfoot with nonsurgical measures. (E, N, G)

40. 1. Casts may have to be changed every 1 to 2 weeks in an infant with a clubfoot deformity because of the infant's rapid growth. The frequent cast changes have nothing to do with infection. With clubfeet, the legs are neither measured or compared to norms. (I, N, G)

41. 2. The Denis Browne splint is an adjustable metal bar to which special shoes are attached. This splint provides an appropriate degree of eversion, dorsiflexion, and rotation to keep the feet in a slightly overcorrected position. When the infant kicks, the feet are automatically moved into a corrected position. (I, T, G)

42. 3. If the shoes become loose, they are tightened against the Denis Browne splint. The shoes and foot pieces are set at a particular angle to maintain the correction achieved through casting. The angle of the shoes on the bar should not be repositioned. Parents should put socks on the child's feet before applying the splint, to decrease irritation. The splint should not be used as a weight-bearing device when lifting the child. (E, T, S)

43. 4. When an infant begins to become mobile, child-proofing the home is necessary. One important aspect of child-proofing is removing tablecloths, so the child cannot pull on them in an attempt to stand and either fall or pull objects on top of him. The child in the Denis Browne splint needs opportunities to increase mobility to achieve developmental tasks. Increasing mobility is not an indication to remove the splint or to obtain corrective shoes. (I, N, S)

The Client With Juvenile Rheumatoid Arthritis (JRA)

44. 4. There is no definitive test for JRA. Erythrocyte sedimentation rate may or may not be elevated during active disease. Synovial fluid cultures are done to rule out septic arthritis. Red blood cell electrophoresis is done to screen for sickle cell anemia. (I, T, G)

45. 1. In most children with JRA, the disease will be in permanent remission by adolescence. Seventy-five percent of the children go into long remissions without severe deformity or functional loss. Only relatively few children recover completely within a few years. (I, T, G)

46. 2. Socialization is important for this preschool-age child, and activity is important to maintain function. However, because children with JRA have the most trouble in the early-morning after arising, they need more time to "warm up." Splints are worn during periods of rest, not activity, to maintain function. (I, N, G)

47. 1. Applying moist heat to affected joints at any time may facilitate joint movement. Heat increases circulation, decreases pain, and increases mobility. Although exercise is important, weight bearing on affected joints is restricted when joints are affected by the disease, as evidenced by pain and edema. Cool compresses constrict and decrease circulation. Purine restriction is related to gouty arthritis. (P, N, G)

48. 4. Since the family is functioning well, the nurse should foster independence and continued strength through education and support. The parents are capable of arranging for equipment, contacting community resources, and discussing the child's illness with siblings if they are given information and support. (P, N, H)

49. 4. A child with a chronic disease suffers a loss, regardless of the disorder's seriousness or the child's developmental level. Withdrawal and regression are two coping strategies common in young children. Side effects of nonsteroidal anti-inflammatory drugs include nausea, vomiting, and gastrointestinal distress. A 4-year-old is in Erikson's psychological stage of sense of initiative. Sibling rivalry is common in all children, and it is not typically characterized by withdrawal. (D, N, L)

50. 4. Parents need to be supportive and understanding of the child while dealing with the grief and loss associated with chronic illness. The child needs to feel valued, but may experience secondary gain from the illness if the family interaction patterns are altered. Psychological counseling is not needed at this time, because the reaction is normal. Peer support is not effective with a 4-year-old, because a child at this age is developmentally egocentric. (I, N, L)

The Client With a Fracture

51. 1. The primary purpose of traction is to achieve appropriate anatomic alignment. Traction immobilizes bone fragments until sufficient healing has occurred to allow cast application. Muscle strength and mass are not maintained by traction. Bone demineralization occurs with immobility, but traction does not prevent it. Traction has no role in preventing infection. (I, C, G)

52. 2. When placed in Bryant's traction, the child should be on the back with the legs flexed at a 90-degree angle at the hips and the hips raised slightly off the bed. This position provides adequate countertraction to reduce and immobilize the fracture. (I, T, S)

53. 4. Weak pedal pulses are a sign of vascular compromise, which can be caused by pressure on the tissues of the legs by the elastic bandages used to secure this type of skin traction. Bandages and moleskin are used to anchor this type of traction, not pins. Enuresis is bedwetting; a 1-year-old would not be expected to be toilet-trained. Since the hips are kept off the bed in Bryant's traction, decubitus ulcers in the sacral area are unlikely. (A, N, S)

54. 1. Weights for traction must be allowed to hang freely to maintain consistent traction. Changing the moleskins used for securing an infant's traction and decreasing the amount of weight could result in a return of the bone fragments to a misaligned position, with possible resulting soft tissue damage. The bony prominence can be assessed without releasing weights. Traction should be maintained unless a specific order is given with other directions. (I, N, S)

55. 3. An almost universal finding in descriptions of abused children is underdevelopment for age. This may be reflected in small physical size and/or in poor psychosocial development. The child should be evaluated further until a plausible diagnosis can be established. A child sucking his thumb contentedly and eating without urging exhibits normal behavior. Abused children tend to be suspicious of others, especially adults. (A, N, L)

56. 2. Evidence of child abuse is legally reportable by anyone who works with children. The nurse should ensure that the findings are reported. Laws ordinarily provide immunity from legal actions for persons required to report suspicion of child abuse, if the report is done in good faith. Suspicion, not absolute proof, is necessary for reporting abuse. The nurse's primary responsibility is to the primary client, the child. (I, C, S)

57. 3. Parents who are abusive often suffer from poor self-esteem, and the nurse should work to bolster their self-esteem. This can be achieved by praising the parents for appropriate parenting. Employment status and socioeconomic status are not indicators of abusive parents. Abusive parents usually are attached to their children and do not want to give them up to foster care. (P, C, L)

58. 2. Explaining what will happen in language that a child can comprehend commonly is enough to dispel fears of the unknown. The child needs the parents for support. The child's reaction to the nurse is normal for a child this age and does not usually call for a change in staff assignments. Telling the child to act like a "big girl" is shaming and not an appropriate response. (I, N, L)

59. 1. Fears in a preschool child normally center around mutilation and disfigurement. Infants and toddlers most fear separation from parents. School-age children most fear loss of self-control. The child who has little experience with casting may not be worried about pain specifically. (D, N, L)

60. 1. Inability to extend the fingers of the involved arm may indicate neurological impairment caused by pressure on soft tissue. The cast will seem heavy until the child adjusts to the extra weight. Cast drying may take 12 or more hours; the dampness causes the sensation of coolness. It is not unusual for a child to be nauseated after sustaining an injury. (E, N, G)

61. 4. Until the cast dries it should be supported by soft material that will "give" with the weight of the cast. Resting a damp cast on a hard surface may flatten or dent the casting material and cause pressure to the soft tissue under the casting material, which may result in breakdown. (I, T, S)

62. 2. A fracture should be suspected if an injured child who previously walked without problems refuses to walk after the injury. Pseudoparalysis from pain is found in young children with fractures. Paresthesia is characterized by numbness and lack of sensation. Behavioral regression usually does not take the form of refusing to walk. (A, T, G)

63. 2. Immediately after a fracture, the muscles contract and physiologically splint the injured area. This phenomenon also accounts for the deformity that results as the muscles pull the bone ends out of alignment. (A, C, G)

64. 1. Assessing the neurologic and circulatory status of the toes, the tissues distal to the fracture, is important. Soft tissue contusions, which frequently accompany femur fractures, can result in severe hemorrhage into the tissue and subsequent circulatory and neurological impairment. The nurse can document the findings after assessing the leg. There is no need to notify the physician with the finding of edema surrounding the fracture site, unless it is causing problems. (I, N, G)

65. 2. Buck's extension is a type of skin traction used to align and immobilize bone fragments. It is also used to relieve muscle spasms, which enhances circulation and decreases pain. (I, C, G)

66. 4. Traction is the forward force produced by attaching weight to a distal bone fragment. Countertraction is the backward force of the muscle pull. Friction is the force between the client and bed; together with countertraction, it achieves balance. Pressure is not a component of traction. (I, T, G)

67. 3. Hand puppets would enable a 3-year-old child in Buck's traction to act out feelings within the constraints imposed by the traction. Marbles are unsafe at this age because they can be swallowed. Blocks are appropriate for a younger child; besides, there is no flat surface available for the child to set blocks. A ball would encourage more movement than a child in skin traction is allowed. (P, N, H)

68. 2. Stressing that the parents visit when they can will help to alleviate the guilt they feel. Acknowledging the guilt gives the parents an opportunity to talk about it but does not help alleviate it. Suggesting that the parents take turns visiting implies that they should feel guilty because they may not be doing all they could. Comparing them to other parents does not alleviate guilt feelings. (I, N, L)

69. 2. The spica cast encircles the abdomen, and the addition of a large meal to the stomach may cause the cast to become too snug. If the child's appetite was decreased in conjunction with a feeling of fullness, the nurse might suspect that the child was becoming constipated and plan to use laxatives or a higher fiber diet. A soft diet is indicated when the child has difficulty chewing food adequately. (P, N, G)

70. 1. Lotion should not be applied to skin beneath the cast because it can cause irritation and skin breakdown. Checking the smoothness of the cast edges, covering the cast around the perineum, and inspecting inside the cast can help prevent skin breakdown. (E, T, S)

71. 4. Chest pain and dyspnea in an immobilized adolescent with a large bone fracture suggests a fat embolus, in which fat droplets are transferred from the marrow into the general blood stream via the venous arterial route and may eventually reach the lung or brain. Respiratory paralysis is not usually associated with a fracture. Pneumonia can occur, but does not usually develop suddenly with chest pain. Pulmonary edema should not be a problem in a healthy adolescent who has sustained a fracture. (D, N, G)

72. 2. A cast that is too tight (always a possibility in the immediate postcasting period) can cause neurovascular impairment. Respiratory, skin, and urinary problems would not develop in the immediate postcasting period, although their prevention would be long-term nursing goals. (P, N, G)

73. 2. The child will need to have his bed moved to an area that is more central to the family life. The child can be carried up and down the three steps to the house the few times necessary after discharge, but negotiating a flight of steps with a school-age child in a cast at least twice a day would be difficult, if not dangerous. The child will need to use a bedpan or urinal, so the bathrooms can be on any floor. Since the family is involved in the discharge, the 16-year-old should be taught appropriate care with the rest of the family. (P, N, H)

74. 2. Extreme pain (especially when the part distal to the injury is moved), sudden edema, and pale extremities distal to the injury are symptoms of compartment syndrome. Compartment syndrome must be treated immediately to prevent major neurological and circulatory impairment. The first step usually is to split the cast to accommodate the edema. Elevating the arm, administering more medication, and exercising the fingers would not be effective at this time. (I, N, G)

The Client With Osteomyelitis

75. 3. Findings associated with osteomyelitis commonly include increased warmth, localized tenderness, and diffuse swelling over the involved bone. The area over the affected bone is red, not pale. (A, T, G)

76. 3. Elevated temperature and increased pulse and respiratory rates are clinical manifestations of osteomyelitis. Pulse deficit is associated with atrial fibrillation. (A, T, G)

77. 2. Antibiotic therapy starts after blood cultures are drawn. The blood cultures will determine the causative organism. The initial antibiotic therapy may be inappropriate for the causative organism and may need to be altered. (I, T, G)

78. 2. In osteomyelitis, the erythrocyte sedimentation rate (ESR) is elevated (for a child, the normal range is 0–13 mm/hr). The ESR rises in the presence of severe localized or systemic inflammation. The leukocyte count in osteomyelitis is elevated (15,000 to 25,000 mm^3). Hematocrit and potassium levels should be normal. (D, N, G)

79. 3. The affected leg should be elevated and warm moist packs applied to the affected area. This helps decrease the swelling and improves circulation. Good body alignment is maintained; neither leg is abducted. Active range-of-motion exercises are performed on the unaffected leg. (I, T, G)

80. 4. Long-term, high-dose antibiotic therapy can adversely affect renal, hepatic, and hematopoietic function. Therefore, these systems should be assessed carefully. Antibiotics do not usually affect blood glucose level, prothrombin time, or urine glucose level. However, renal impairment may be reflected in the kidneys' decreased ability to concentrate or dilute urine. (A, N, G)

81. 1. Encouraging contact with schoolmates allows the school-age child to maintain and develop socialization with peers, an important developmental task of this age group. Although having family visits and interacting with the child are important, they do not meet developmental needs. (I, N, H)

82. 4. The most effective intervention to prevent skin breakdown is to reposition the client frequently. Although a trapeze might encourage the child to change position, it does not guarantee that the child will do so. Inspecting the skin is not an intervention to prevent skin breakdown, but rather an evaluation strategy. A back rub will increase circulation to the back and sacral areas but is not the most effective intervention to prevent skin breakdown. A high-fiber diet will help prevent constipation. (I, N, S)

83. 1. Children with osteomyelitis need a diet high in protein and calories. Milk, eggs, cheese, meat, fish, and vegetables such as beans are the best sources of these nutrients. (I, N, G)

84. 2. School-age children have an increasing need for independence. Anger and resentment are common responses to dependence and loss of control over the environment, with minimal opportunity to participate in planning and decision making. (D, N, L)

NURSING CARE OF CHILDREN

TEST 8: The Child with Musculoskeletal Health Problems

Directions: Use this answer grid to determine areas of strength or need for further study.

NURSING PROCESS

A = Assessment
D = Analysis, nursing diagnosis
P = Planning
I = Implementation
E = Evaluation

COGNITIVE LEVEL

K = Knowledge
C = Comprehension
T = Application
N = Analysis

CLIENT NEEDS

S = Safe, effective care environment
G = Physiological integrity
L = Psychosocial integrity
H = Health promotion/maintenance

		Nursing Process					Cognitive Level				Client Needs			
Question #	Answer #	A	D	P	I	E	K	C	T	N	S	G	L	H
1	4			P						N		G		
2	3			P						N		G		
3	2	A					K					G		
4	4	A					K					G		
5	1				I					N				H
6	2					E				N		G		
7	1	A								N				H
8	2		D							N		G		
9	1					E			T			G		
10	4				I				T			G		
11	4	A							T			G		
12	3				I					N				H
13	3				I					N		G		
14	4		D						T			G		
15	1			P						N				H
16	2		D							N		G		
17	1				I				T			G		
18	3				I					N		G		
19	1					E				N			L	
20	2	A						C				G		
21	3					E		C				G		
22	4		D					C				G		
23	3				I					N				H

ANSWER GRID: 1

NURSING PROCESS

A = Assessment
D = Analysis, nursing diagnosis
P = Planning
I = Implementation
E = Evaluation

COGNITIVE LEVEL

K = Knowledge
C = Comprehension
T = Application
N = Analysis

CLIENT NEEDS

S = Safe, effective care environment
G = Physiological integrity
L = Psychosocial integrity
H = Health promotion/maintenance

		Nursing Process					Cognitive Level				Client Needs			
Question #	Answer #	A	D	P	I	E	K	C	T	N	S	G	L	H
24	2			P						N		G		
25	3		D							N		G		
26	2				I					N		G		
27	1					E				N		G		
28	3		D					C				G		
29	3		D					C				G		
30	1				I					N		G		
31	2			P						N				H
32	3				I				T		S			
33	2		D							N		G		
34	4				I					N				H
35	3				I				T		S			
36	3				I					N		G		
37	3				I					N			L	
38	1				I				T		S			
39	3					E				N		G		
40	1				I					N		G		
41	2				I				T			G		
42	3					E			T		S			
43	4				I					N	S			
44	4				I				T			G		
45	1				I				T			G		
46	2				I					N		G		
47	1			P						N		G		
48	4			P						N				H
49	4		D							N			L	
50	4				I					N			L	
51	1				I			C				G		
52	2				I				T		S			

ANSWER GRID: 2

NURSING PROCESS

A = Assessment
D = Analysis, nursing diagnosis
P = Planning
I = Implementation
E = Evaluation

COGNITIVE LEVEL

K = Knowledge
C = Comprehension
T = Application
N = Analysis

CLIENT NEEDS

S = Safe, effective care environment
G = Physiological integrity
L = Psychosocial integrity
H = Health promotion/maintenance

		Nursing Process					Cognitive Level				Client Needs			
Question #	Answer #	A	D	P	I	E	K	C	T	N	S	G	L	H
53	4	A								N	S			
54	1				I					N	S			
55	3	A								N			L	
56	2				I			C			S			
57	3			P				C					L	
58	2				I					N			L	
59	1		D							N			L	
60	1					E				N		G		
61	4				I				T		S			
62	2	A							T			G		
63	2	A						C				G		
64	1				I					N		G		
65	2				I			C				G		
66	4				I				T			G		
67	3			P						N				H
68	2				I					N			L	
69	2			P						N		G		
70	1					E			T		S			
71	4		D							N		G		
72	2			P						N		G		
73	2			P						N				H
74	2				I					N		G		
75	3	A							T			G		
76	3	A							T			G		
77	2				I				T			G		
78	2		D							N		G		
79	3				I				T			G		
80	4	A								N		G		
81	1				I					N				H

ANSWER GRID: 3

Nursing Process

A = Assessment
D = Analysis, nursing diagnosis
P = Planning
I = Implementation
E = Evaluation

Cognitive Level

K = Knowledge
C = Comprehension
T = Application
N = Analysis

Client Needs

S = Safe, effective care environment
G = Physiological integrity
L = Psychosocial integrity
H = Health promotion/maintenance

		Nursing Process					Cognitive Level				Client Needs			
Question #	Answer #	A	D	P	I	E	K	C	T	N	S	G	L	H
82	4				I					N	S			
83	1				I					N		G		
84	2		D							N			L	
Number Correct														
Number Possible	84	12	13	12	38	9	2	10	21	51	12	51	10	11
Percentage Correct														

Score Calculation:

To determine your **Percentage Correct**, divide the **Number Correct** by the **Number Possible**.

The Child With Dermatologic, Endocrine, and Other Health Problems

Test 9

The Client Who Is Preterm
The Client Who Is Septic
The Client With Failure to Thrive
The Client With Atopic Dermatitis
The Client With Burns
The Client With Hypothyroidism
The Client With Insulin-Dependent Diabetes Mellitus
Clients Who Are Abused
Correct Answers and Rationale

Select the one best answer and indicate your choice by filling in the circle in front of the option.

The Client Who Is Preterm

A neonate born prematurely and who is small for gestational age is placed in the intensive care nursery.

1. On assessment, the nurse would expect this neonate to display
- ○ 1. firm cartilage to the edge of the ear pinna.
- ○ 2. full areola with breast tissue.
- ○ 3. fine, downy hair over the upper arms and back.
- ○ 4. prominent creases on the soles and heels.

2. During the physical assessment, the nurse would also expect to see
- ○ 1. an abundance of scalp hair.
- ○ 2. a thin, wasted appearance.
- ○ 3. dry, cracked skin.
- ○ 4. numerous rugae on the scrotum.

3. The neonate is suffering from cold stress. The nurse should be especially alert for
- ○ 1. a yellowish undercast to the skin color.
- ○ 2. increased abdominal girth.
- ○ 3. hyperactivity and twitching.
- ○ 4. slow and shallow respirations.

4. Which of the following lab values would the nurse associate with cold stress in a 1-day-old preterm neonate?
- ○ 1. Bilirubin 13 mg/dl.
- ○ 2. Glucose 15 mg/dl.
- ○ 3. Hematocrit 70%.
- ○ 4. Hemoglobin 20.5 g/dl.

5. The infant is subjected to repeated blood withdrawals for laboratory specimens. The nurse should plan to maintain a careful record of the
- ○ 1. amount of blood drawn for each specimen.
- ○ 2. color of each blood specimen.
- ○ 3. neonate's body temperature immediately before each phlebotomy.
- ○ 4. last time the neonate was fed before each specimen is collected.

6. The neonate weighs 1,870 g, and has a respiratory rate of 46 breaths/minute, a pulse rate of 175 beats/minute, and a serum pH of 7.39. He is to receive sodium bicarbonate intravenously. The nurse would know that the sodium bicarbonate is being given to alleviate
- ○ 1. edema.

○ 2. dehydration.
○ 3. metabolic acidosis.
○ 4. respiratory alkalosis.

7. The neonate is being given oxygen as a treatment for cold stress. The nurse would evaluate the oxygen therapy as achieving the desired effect when the child's
○ 1. heart rate is 200 beats/minute at rest.
○ 2. respiratory rate is 48 breaths/minute at rest.
○ 3. axillary temperature is 98°F.
○ 4. blood pressure is 65/55 mm Hg.

8. The nurse is very careful to document the neonate's response to oxygen therapy and to deliver only as much oxygen as is necessary to prevent the development of
○ 1. cataracts.
○ 2. glaucoma.
○ 3. ophthalmia neonatorum.
○ 4. retrolental fibroplasia.

9. The neonate is to be fed by gavage. The nurse should introduce the catheter into the stomach and check placement by
○ 1. aspirating stomach contents through the catheter with a syringe.
○ 2. inserting a small amount of air into the catheter and auscultating for clear breath sounds.
○ 3. introducing water into the catheter and aspirating it back.
○ 4. making sure the measured length has been introduced without resistance.

10. The neonate is receiving his first feeding by nipple. The nurse would plan to first give the neonate a 5 cc feeding of sterile water, to
○ 1. ascertain the patency of the neonate's esophagus.
○ 2. determine whether or not the neonate can retain the feeding.
○ 3. ensure that the neonate's has the energy to take oral feedings.
○ 4. initiate the neonate's peristalsis.

11. The neonate is admitted to the neonatal intensive care unit. The parents express concern about their neonate's condition. To meet the short-term goals of decreasing the parent's fears and fostering bonding, the nurse should plan to
○ 1. allow the parents to see and touch their neonate.
○ 2. arrange for a visit with another couple who have an ill preterm neonate.
○ 3. encourage the parents to participate in the neonate's care.
○ 4. explain to the parents that they need not be concerned because the neonate is doing well.

12. A nurse working in a neonatal intensive care unit is developing policies to help control infection. Which policy would dictate the use of the single most effective means of preventing the spread of infection?
○ 1. Having personnel perform frequent hand and arm washing.
○ 2. Keeping each neonate in an isolette that is opened as infrequently as possible.
○ 3. Maintaining a ventilation system in the unit that provides for continuous clean-air exchange.
○ 4. Requiring all personnel to wear gowns and masks.

The Client Who Is Septic

A 10-day-old neonate is brought to the emergency room by the parents. The neonate is lethargic and tachypneic and has a heart rate of 200 beats/minute.

13. The nurse's initial focus should be on the neonate's
○ 1. history of allergic reactions.
○ 2. number of wet diapers in the past 24 hours.
○ 3. pupillary response.
○ 4. sleep patterns.

14. The mother is very concerned and voices her feelings of guilt for missing signs of the neonate's illness. She asks if there were any signs she should have looked for in her child. What would be the nurse's best response?
○ 1. "You should have inspected for any redness or swelling."
○ 2. "You should have looked for any difficulty in breathing."
○ 3. "You should have noted any decrease or increase in temperature."
○ 4. "You probably would not have been able to see anything special."

15. The nurse makes sure to measure the neonate's baseline abdominal girth because
○ 1. a large abdomen is an indication of brown fat stores the child will need for energy.
○ 2. drugs used to treat sepsis can cause paralytic ileus.
○ 3. it is a good indication of hydration status.
○ 4. the toxins released into the gut by the causative organism may lead to poor absorption of formula.

16. The nurse and doctor plan care for the neonate. The pharmacologic plan of care would likely include
○ 1. ampicillin and gentamicin.
○ 2. furosemide and kanamycin.
○ 3. gentamicin and vitamin K.
○ 4. phenytoin sodium and vancomycin.

17. The nurse caring for the neonate would be worried about the onset of septic shock if the neonate's
○ 1. axillary temperature is 99.8°F.

○ 2. capillary refill is less than 3 seconds.
○ 3. heart rate during sleep is 205 beats/minute.
○ 4. respiratory rate while awake is 32 breaths/minute.

18. The neonate is admitted to the intensive care unit. The tearful mother tells the nurse, "All of this is so difficult to understand. Our other children are so healthy." The nurse's best response would be
○ 1. "Don't worry; we're doing all we can."
○ 2. "Please don't think this is your fault."
○ 3. "Please tell me, what don't you understand?"
○ 4. "You're a good parent; you obviously love your child."

19. The nurse notes that the neonate is using the abdominal muscles to breathe and has a respiratory rate of 30 breaths/minute. The nurse should
○ 1. chart the findings.
○ 2. check oxygen saturation with a pulse oximeter.
○ 3. notify the physician of the findings.
○ 4. elevate the head of the bed.

The Client With Failure To Thrive

A 5-month-old infant is brought to the clinic by his parents because he "cries too much" and "vomits a lot." The infant's birth weight was 6 pounds, 10 ounces, and his current weight is 7 pounds, 4 ounces.

20. After assessing the child, the nurse would suspect a diagnosis of failure to thrive based on what data?
○ 1. History of vomiting and irritability persisting longer than 2 weeks.
○ 2. Weight below the 5th percentile on the growth chart.
○ 3. Weight gain of less than 1 pound per week since birth.
○ 4. Inability to sit upright without support.

21. Which of the following information obtained during a health history is consistent with the diagnosis of failure to thrive? The child
○ 1. fusses during feedings.
○ 2. is very fearful of strangers.
○ 3. is quiet only when being held.
○ 4. sleeps well and has to be awakened for feedings.

22. The nurse formulates the nursing diagnosis Altered Nutrition: Less than Body Requirements related to negative feeding patterns. To meet the short-term goals of the infant's care plan, the nurse would plan to
○ 1. have the parents feed the infant whenever possible.
○ 2. give the infant formula that has 24 calories per ounce.
○ 3. have the same nurse feed the infant whenever possible.
○ 4. have the infant sit in a high chair during feedings.

23. When observing the infant's mother feed the infant, the nurse would be concerned if the mother
○ 1. tries to maintain eye contact with the infant.
○ 2. talks to the infant during the feeding.
○ 3. places the infant in an infant seat for the feeding.
○ 4. sits on the floor to feed the infant.

24. The infant is to be discharged, and the health team believes that the family will need follow-up care. The most effective type of follow-up would be
○ 1. daily phone calls from the primary nurse.
○ 2. enrollment in community parenting classes.
○ 3. twice-weekly clinic appointments.
○ 4. weekly visits by a community health nurse.

25. The mother expresses concern that picking up the infant whenever he cries will "spoil" him. What would be the nurse's best response?
○ 1. "Allow him to cry for no longer than 45 minutes, then pick him up."
○ 2. "Babies need comforting and cuddling; meeting these needs will not spoil him."
○ 3. "Babies this young cry when they're hungry; try feeding him when he cries."
○ 4. "If he isn't soiled or wet, don't pick him up; the crying will stop eventually."

The Client With Atopic Dermatitis

An 11-month-old infant is admitted to the hospital with a persistent puritic eczema. The lesions have become infected, and the physician has ordered intravenous antibiotics.

26. When inserting the reseal for intravenous access, the nurse would best meet the infant's emotional needs by
○ 1. allowing the mother to be present during the procedure.
○ 2. letting the infant become familiar with the equipment.
○ 3. providing the infant with a bottle of formula during the procedure.
○ 4. rocking the infant a few minutes before the procedure.

27. When choosing nightclothes for an infant with atopic dermatitis, which of the following would be best?
○ 1. A nylon nightsack with a drawstring.
○ 2. One-piece cotton pajamas with long sleeves.
○ 3. Two-piece flannel pajamas with short sleeves.
○ 4. A woolen sleeper with feet and mittens.

28. The nurse applies a lotion containing lanolin and urea to the infant's skin lesions. The goal of this treatment is to
- ○ 1. decrease the inflammatory response.
- ○ 2. dry the lesions.
- ○ 3. hydrate the skin.
- ○ 4. prevent infection.

29. A hypoallergenic diet is prescribed for the infant. The nurse would judge that the mother needs more teaching about a hypoallergenic diet when the mother chooses which food from the hospital menu for her child?
- ○ 1. Applesauce.
- ○ 2. Carrots.
- ○ 3. Pears.
- ○ 4. Eggs.

The mother and nurse are planning home care for a 3-year-old child with eczema.

30. The nurse should teach the mother to remove which of the following from the child's environment at home?
- ○ 1. Metal toy trucks.
- ○ 2. Plastic dolls.
- ○ 3. Stuffed animals.
- ○ 4. Wooden blocks.

31. The mother tells the community health nurse that her child usually scratches his lesions to bleeding during the night. The nurse would recommend which medication to sedate the child and help relieve the puritis?
- ○ 1. Acetaminophen.
- ○ 2. Chloral hydrate.
- ○ 3. Diphenhydramine.
- ○ 4. Phenytoin sodium.

The Client With Burns

A 5-year-old boy is admitted to the hospital with severe burns on his legs, head, and lower abdomen and minor burns on other surfaces.

32. The nurse, using the "rule of nines" to estimate the burned area on the body, would allocate a larger percentage of total surface area for this child as compared to a child over age 12, if the burns were on the child's
- ○ 1. head and neck.
- ○ 2. lower extremities.
- ○ 3. upper extremities.
- ○ 4. posterior and anterior chest.

33. The nurse would recognize the need for immediate venous access because the child
- ○ 1. needs antibiotic therapy as soon as possible.
- ○ 2. needs fluid losses replaced immediately.
- ○ 3. needs pain medications delivered through the venous route.
- ○ 4. needs hyperalimentation.

34. The nurse would formulate a plan of care for the child that includes the nursing diagnosis Fluid Volume Deficit related to an initial primary shift in plasma from
- ○ 1. intracellular to intravascular spaces.
- ○ 2. intravascular to interstitial spaces.
- ○ 3. interstitial to intracellular spaces.
- ○ 4. interstitial to intravascular spaces.

35. The nurse inserts an indwelling urinary catheter. The rationale for this action is to help
- ○ 1. decrease the workload of the kidneys.
- ○ 2. ensure adequate urine output measurement.
- ○ 3. obtain regular urine specimens.
- ○ 4. prevent urine retention.

36. The nurse observing which of the following signs would suspect that the child is receiving too much intravenous fluid too rapidly?
- ○ 1. Marked increase in abdominal girth.
- ○ 2. Capillary refill time of 5 seconds.
- ○ 3. Dark-amber urine.
- ○ 4. Moist rales in the lung fields.

37. The child becomes angry and combative when it is time to change the dressings and apply mafenide acetate (Sulfmylon). The nurse would judge that the child would respond best if he
- ○ 1. has parental support during the dressing changes.
- ○ 2. is allowed to assist the nurse in removing the dressings and applying the cream.
- ○ 3. is given permission to cry during the procedure.
- ○ 4. knows the treatment can be delayed until he feels better.

38. The child has a decreased interest in food. The nurse and mother develop a plan of care to increase the child's intake. Which of the following suggestions made by the mother would the nurse reject?
- ○ 1. Allowing the mother to feed the child.
- ○ 2. Explaining that dessert and treats will be withheld unless meals are eaten.
- ○ 3. Offering the child finger-foods that are liked.
- ○ 4. Serving smaller and more frequent meals.

39. On reviewing the child's laboratory results, the nurse notes a serum potassium level of 3.3 mmol/L. The nurse would decide to encourage the child to drink
- ○ 1. cranberry juice.
- ○ 2. ginger ale.

○ 3. grape juice.
○ 4. orange juice.

40. When administering the fifteenth dose of an antibiotic intravenously to the child, the nurse notes that the child is scratching at the IV site on the forearm and also notes small, circumscribed, elevated areas on the same arm. The nurse would
○ 1. apply a cold compress to the area and continue to deliver the antibiotic.
○ 2. assess the IV site for localized edema or redness.
○ 3. remove the IV and restart it in another area.
○ 4. stop the infusion of ampicillin, but continue the IV fluids.

41. The nurse is concerned about the child's fluid balance. The nurse would judge that the child is receiving too little fluid support when he
○ 1. becomes increasingly irritable.
○ 2. has a urine output of 28 ml for the past hour.
○ 3. has a urine specific gravity of 1.033.
○ 4. has had an increase in blood pressure within the past 3 hours.

42. The nurse teaches the child's mother about the importance of specific nutritional support in burn management. The nurse would judge that the teaching needed to be reinforced if the mother chose which of the following from the diet menu for her child?
○ 1. A bacon, lettuce, and tomato sandwich; apple juice; and celery and carrot sticks.
○ 2. A cheeseburger, cottage cheese and pineapple salad, chocolate milk, and a brownie.
○ 3. Chicken nuggets, orange and grapefruit sections, and a vanilla milkshake.
○ 4. A beef, bean, cheese burrito; a banana; fruit-flavored yogurt; and skim milk.

43. The nurse would follow the Centers for Disease Control guidelines concerning sterile gloves by wearing them
○ 1. as an optional but desirable precautionary measure.
○ 2. whenever delivering any care that would necessitate touching the child.
○ 3. whenever entering the child's room.
○ 4. whenever giving direct care to burned areas.

44. The child has infected burns, and the physician orders 250 mg of an antibiotic every 6 hours. The normal dosage for this antibiotic and condition is 20 to 50 mg/kg/24 hours. The child weighs 10 kg. The nurse should
○ 1. carry out the order.
○ 2. give the dose recommended by the pharmacy reference material.
○ 3. question the order because the dose is too low.
○ 4. question the order because the dose is too high.

45. The nurse would be concerned that the child may be hemolyzing red blood cells after noting that the child's
○ 1. eyes appear bloodshot.
○ 2. intact skin appears flushed.
○ 3. stools are black.
○ 4. urine is dark brown.

The Client With Hypothyroidism

A 6-week-old infant was normal at birth but has begun to breast-feed poorly. The infant's skin is dry and scaly, and her tongue protrudes. A diagnosis of cretinism is made.

46. The mother asks the nurse why the child was not diagnosed with this condition at birth. The nurse would reply, "Your child
○ 1. had a normally functioning thyroid as a fetus that has failed to develop properly."
○ 2. had little need for thyroid hormone until 1 month of age."
○ 3. received enough thyroid hormone through your breast milk to get by the first few weeks."
○ 4. received enough thyroid hormone from you while in the womb to delay signs of deficiency."

47. The infant is to receive levothyroxine sodium (Synthroid) orally. The nurse would instruct the mother to observe the infant carefully for signs of overdose, which include
○ 1. anorexia.
○ 2. constipation.
○ 3. insomnia.
○ 4. sleepiness.

48. After teaching the mother about tests performed to monitor the success of the infant's treatment, the nurse would judge that the teaching was effective when the mother states that the child will need frequent blood tests and regular assessment of
○ 1. blood electrolyte levels.
○ 2. metabolic rate.
○ 3. muscular coordination.
○ 4. skeletal growth.

49. The mother asks the nurse what would happen if her child did not receive treatment. The nurse would explain that one of the outcomes of untreated congenital hypothyroidism is
○ 1. blindness.
○ 2. epilepsy.
○ 3. emotional instability.
○ 4. mental retardation.

50. The parents are being taught to administer synthroid to the infant. The nurse would plan to teach the parents to dissolve the pills and mix the medication in

○ 1. a large amount of water.
○ 2. milk, orange juice, or cereal.
○ 3. a small amount of formula.
○ 4. the infant's bottle of formula.

The Client With Insulin-Dependent Diabetes Mellitus

An 8-year-old boy is admitted to the hospital, unconscious due to severe ketoacidosis.

51. The nurse should position the child in which position?
○ 1. Prone.
○ 2. Side-lying.
○ 3. Supine.
○ 4. Trendelenburg.

52. The nurse obtaining a nursing history from the mother would consider which statement by the mother to support a diagnosis of insulin-dependent diabetes mellitus?
○ 1. "He has become almost hyperactive in the past month."
○ 2. "He has begun to wet his bed at night for the first time in 3 years."
○ 3. "He has an increased appetite and is gaining weight."
○ 4. "He has lost his appetite in the past 2 weeks."

53. The nurse may observe which typical sign of ketoacidosis in the child?
○ 1. Slow, bounding pulse rate.
○ 2. Deep, rapid respirations.
○ 3. Diaphoretic, warm skin.
○ 4. Dilated pupils.

54. The child is in ketoacidosis. The mother asks why the child smells like he has been drinking. The nurse would explain that the smell is due to the release of
○ 1. amino acids.
○ 2. glycogen.
○ 3. acetone.
○ 4. urea.

55. The nurse has been teaching the parents about insulin. The nurse would judge the teaching about why insulin needs to be injected as successful when the father states that the child cannot take oral insulin because it
○ 1. can't be digested in the stomach.
○ 2. doesn't come in a pill form.
○ 3. is destroyed in the stomach before it can work.
○ 4. will cause stomach upset.

56. When preparing to give the child his dose of combination regular and NPH humulin insulin, the nurse should
○ 1. premix the insulins in a vial and then withdraw the amount needed in one syringe.
○ 2. use two syringes, one for each type of insulin.
○ 3. withdraw the NPH insulin first, then withdraw the regular insulin into one syringe.
○ 4. withdraw the regular insulin first, then withdraw the NPH insulin into one syringe.

57. A child with newly diagnosed insulin-dependent diabetes mellitus is attending a camp for diabetic children. He is learning to give himself insulin. He gives himself regular and Lente insulin at 8 A.M. The nurse would plan to observe him for pallor, sweating, tachycardia, headache, dizziness, and difficulty speaking as a result of the effects of the Lente insulin between
○ 1. 8:30 and 10:30 P.M.
○ 2. 10 A.M. and noon.
○ 3. noon and 2 P.M.
○ 4. 2 P.M. and 4 P.M.

58. A nurse is called to the arts and crafts room because the child is behaving strangely. The nurse's first action should be to
○ 1. make sure the child receives some form of easily digested simple sugar to prevent brain damage and cardiac arrest.
○ 2. ask the child if he took his insulin this morning to determine if he is ketoacidotic.
○ 3. call the child's physician to check on his medical status before taking any action.
○ 4. have the child run around the camp track to improve insulin utilization.

59. The mother is also learning to help her diabetic child, and is being taught the principles of the diabetic diet. The nurse would judge that the mother understands the place of snacks in the diet when the mother states
○ 1. "By spreading the calories throughout the day in small frequent meals, the risk of hyperglycemia is eliminated."
○ 2. "Most children find it difficult to eat all the calories required on their diets in three main meals."
○ 3. "Snacks are used to keep blood glucose at acceptable levels during times when the insulin level peaks."
○ 4. "Snacks are used to offset the desire for sweets not allowed on the diabetic diet."

60. The nurse and mother are planning interventions that will allow the child to participate in an early morning tennis program at school. The mother has already developed several interventions. Which of the following would the nurse recommend eliminating?
○ 1. Inject the A.M. insulin dose in an area away from major muscles used in playing tennis.
○ 2. Have the child eat more calories for breakfast on "tennis" days.

○ 3. Have the child carry a source of quickly absorbed carbohydrate to the program.
○ 4. Teach the tennis coach the signs and symptoms of hyperglycemia.

61. The client attends nutrition classes at camp. The nurse would judge that the child understands the teaching when he
○ 1. asks the nurse if he can exchange the apple he has been given for an orange.
○ 2. asks to replace his Rice Krispies with Frosted Flakes.
○ 3. requests chocolate milk for dinner.
○ 4. requests that he have a cola instead of milk with his lunch.

62. The client tells the nurse that he does not want his new friends to know about his disease, because "it's weird." The nurse works hard to increase the child's self-esteem and counsel him in ways to present his disability to his friends. The nurse would judge that the hard work had positive results when the child
○ 1. asks the nurse for material on diabetes for a school paper.
○ 2. introduces the nurse to several of his friends as "the nurse who taught me all about my diabetes."
○ 3. says "I'll try to tell my friends, but they'll probably quit hanging out with me."
○ 4. stays out of the hospital for 6 months.

63. The nurse suggests that the nurse and mother meet with the child's teacher before school starts to discuss the teacher's responsibilities in relation to the child's illness. In this meeting, the nurse would plan to discuss
○ 1. how to give an insulin injection.
○ 2. how to perform a glucometer test.
○ 3. signs and symptoms of hypoglycemia.
○ 4. the American Diabetic Association diet.

64. The nurse is teaching the child and his mother what to do when the child has the "stomach flu" and can only tolerate carbonated drinks, jello, and broth. The nurse should explain that the child's insulin regimen will be changed by
○ 1. adding extra-long-acting insulin to the A.M. and P.M. insulin doses.
○ 2. hospitalizing the child and starting a glucose and insulin drip.
○ 3. instituting strict bedrest and use of intermediate-acting insulin only.
○ 4. allowing simple sugars, testing blood glucose more frequently, and using regular insulin only.

A child is brought to the hospital in ketoacidosis. The child is to receive an insulin drip.

65. The nurse would give only which of the following solutions, as ordered?
○ 1. Isophane insulin suspension (NPH) in 0.9% saline.
○ 2. 100 units of regular insulin in 100 cc of 5% dextrose.
○ 3. 100 units of regular insulin in 100 cc of 0.45% saline.
○ 4. 100 units of regular insulin in 100 cc of 0.9% saline.

66. An intravenous solution containing insulin is prepared by the pharmacy. When setting up the solution, the nurse should
○ 1. cover the fluid container with a paper bag.
○ 2. not use an air filter on the tubing.
○ 3. flush the tubing with 40 to 50 cc of the solution.
○ 4. wrap the container and tubing in aluminum foil.

67. An adolescent with diabetes is being taught the importance of rotating the sites of his insulin injections. The nurse would judge the teaching as successful when the adolescent states, "I need to rotate sites because repeated use can result in
○ 1. destruction of the fat tissue and poor absorption."
○ 2. destruction of nerves and painful neuritis."
○ 3. destruction of the tissue and too-rapid insulin uptake."
○ 4. development of resistance to insulin and the need for increased amounts."

68. A diabetic child is overweight for his age, and the parents, child, dietician, and nurse are planning a diet for him. The diet plan should include decreasing intake of
○ 1. calories.
○ 2. carbohydrates.
○ 3. fats.
○ 4. fluids.

69. The mother of a 10-year-old girl with diabetes asks the nurse's advice about whether her child, who has always been very compliant with treatment, should be allowed to go "trick or treating" on Halloween with several of her friends. What would be the nurse's best response?
○ 1. "No, it would be a life-threatening emergency if she eats sweets."
○ 2. "No, she should be sheltered from temptation at all times."
○ 3. "Yes, just give her a little extra insulin before she goes."
○ 4. "Yes, she needs to be with friends and do the things other children do."

70. The nurse plans to start teaching a child with newly diagnosed diabetes about the condition. The child states, "I feel lousy; I didn't get much sleep last night, and my stomach and head hurt." In regard to the teaching, the nurse should

○ 1. begin teaching the signs and symptoms of hypoglycemia.
○ 2. delay the teaching for now.
○ 3. give the child a reading assignment in a nursing text.
○ 4. have the child self-administer the next scheduled insulin dose.

Clients Who Are Abused

A 3-year-old child is seen in the emergency room because of a dislocated shoulder. The child has multiple bruises on the thighs and upper arms, and the nurse suspects child abuse.

71. When obtaining a nursing history from parents who are suspected of abusing their injured child, the nurse would typically find that the parents
○ 1. ask questions about treatment.
○ 2. blame themselves for the injury.
○ 3. give information about the child's developmental achievements.
○ 4. show little concern about the extent of the injury.

72. The nurse would identify which of the following statements made by a mother of a 3-year-old child with unexplained injuries as supporting suspicions of abuse?
○ 1. "A good friend and I meet for coffee twice a week."
○ 2. "I'm disappointed that my child can't tie his shoes."
○ 3. My mother helps me with the children."
○ 4. "My child helps dress himself."

73. When the nurse asks the child how his shoulder was hurt, he replies, "It was my fault; I was bad." What would be the nurse's best response?
○ 1. "Perhaps it wasn't your fault; can we talk about what happened?"
○ 2. "Tell me what you did that made your father hurt you."
○ 3. "We'll help you get better and see that this doesn't happen again."
○ 4. "You'll have to behave better so this won't happen again."

74. The child has blood drawn. The child lies very still and makes no sound during the procedure. What would be the nurse's most appropriate comment?
○ 1. "It's okay to cry when something hurts."
○ 2. "That really didn't hurt, did it?"
○ 3. "We're mean to hurt you that way, aren't we?"
○ 4. "You were very good about the needle."

75. The child is admitted to the hospital and the nurse is aware that a court appearance may be necessary. To plan for this eventuality, the nurse should place priority on
○ 1. remembering the parents behavior when the child was admitted.
○ 2. documenting physical findings and behaviors observed during the child's admission.
○ 3. formulating subjective opinions about the cause of any injuries.
○ 4. preparing answers to questions that may be asked by the attorneys.

76. The nurse develops a plan of care for an abused child who has been hospitalized, keeping the child's needs in mind. The priority of care should focus on
○ 1. a program of restrictive limit setting.
○ 2. consistent management of inappropriate behavior.
○ 3. consistent positive feedback concerning all behavior.
○ 4. limited interaction with the family.

77. A nurse is approached by an adolescent who has been admitted to the hospital for headaches. She confides that she is being sexually abused by a family friend. What would be the nurse's best initial response?
○ 1. "Can you tell me what happened?"
○ 2. "I believe you; you were right to tell me."
○ 3. "I think you should tell your mother and father about this."
○ 4. "Who else have you told about this?"

78. A 3-year-old girl has been sexually abused. While interviewing the child, the nurse should ask her to
○ 1. describe the details of the abusive act.
○ 2. draw a picture and explain what it means.
○ 3. "play out" the event using anatomically correct dolls.
○ 4. use puppets to recreate the sexual abuse and observe the child's reactions.

79. A nurse caring for a 2-year-old girl suspects that she has been sexually abused. The nurse's decision regarding reporting the abuse should be based on the fact that
○ 1. conclusive evidence is needed before abuse can be reported.
○ 2. physicians are primarily responsible for reporting suspected abuse.
○ 3. a nurse can be sued when reporting abuse on suspicions only.
○ 4. a nurse who suspects child abuse is required by law to report these suspicions.

CORRECT ANSWERS AND RATIONALE

The letters in parentheses following the rationale identify the step of the nursing process (A, D, P, I, E); cognitive level (K, C, T, N); and client need (S, G, L, H). See the Answer Grid for the key.

The Client Who Is Preterm

1. 3. Lanugo (fine, downy hair) covers the entire body until about 20 weeks of gestation, when it begins to disappear from the face, trunk, and extremities, in that order. Lanugo is a consistent finding in preterm neonates. Firm cartilage to the edge of the ear pinna, full areola with breast tissue, and creases on the soles and heels are examples of physical characteristics found in neonates born at term. (A, N, G)
2. 2. Common physical characteristics of preterm neonates include a thin, wasted appearance; scarce scalp hair; thin, pink, smooth skin; and in males, absence of rugae on the scrotum and testicles high in the inguinal canal. (A, T, G)
3. 3. Hyperirritability and twitching are signs of hypoglycemia. Preterm neonates, as well as small-for-gestational age and large-for-gestational age neonates, are prone to develop hypoglycemia. A neonate with cold stress must produce heat through increased metabolism, causing oxygen use to increase and glycogen stores to be quickly depleted. Jaundice, abdominal distention, and slow, shallow respirations are not associated with neonatal hypoglycemia. (A, N, G)
4. 2. A common finding in neonates with cold stress is low serum glucose level. The normal range for this infant is 20 to 60 mg/dl. Hemoglobin, bilirubin, and hematocrit determinations are not used to confirm hypoglycemia. (D, N, G)
5. 1. When repeated blood specimens are obtained from a preterm neonate, it is a nursing responsibility to keep a record of the amount of blood taken for each specimen. The total blood volume of a preterm neonate is small, and repeated blood collections can deplete blood volume. A record of the amount of blood taken for specimens is a guide to help determine whether the neonate needs a transfusion. Blood color is not a reliable indicator of blood constituents or volume. (P, N, G)
6. 3. Metabolic acidosis results from the metabolic changes associated with cold stress. End products of metabolism increase the acidity of the blood. Therefore, sodium bicarbonate, a buffer base, is often used. Respiratory alkalosis results from excessive carbon dioxide loss, a condition that would be very unusual in this neonate. Sodium bicarbonate is not used to combat edema or dehydration. (D, N, G)
7. 3. Oxygen is given to a cold-stressed neonate to support an increase in the metabolic rate through a complex process of increasing metabolism. In this situation, both the respiratory rate and heart rate are above the normal range for a neonate at rest, which may reflect the need for more oxygen at the cellular level. Normal blood pressure readings would not indicate that the therapy is effective. (E, N, G)
8. 4. High levels of oxygen delivered to a preterm neonate can result in retrolental fibroplasia. The immature blood vessels in the eye constrict and then overgrow, resulting in edema and hemorrhage, which produces scarring, retinal detachment, and eventual blindness. Cataracts and glaucoma are congenital abnormalities in the neonate. Ophthalmia neonatorum is a gonorrheal infection of the eyes that is likely to occur if a mother has the gonorrheal organism in her birth canal. (I, T, S)
9. 1. The method most often recommended to determine whether the gavage catheter is in the stomach is to aspirate stomach contents with a syringe. The presence of stomach contents indicates that the catheter is in the stomach. Any stomach contents obtained should be reintroduced into the stomach to prevent loss of electrolytes. Water introduced into the catheter before placement is confirmed may end up in the lungs. Air introduced into the catheter can be auscultated as a "whoosh" in the stomach area. Any air introduced in this manner should be removed to prevent overdistention of the stomach. (I, T, S)
10. 1. Sterile water is given to a neonate to ascertain whether the esophagus is patent and to prevent the aspiration of formula if it is not. Assessment of the neonate's ability to retain feedings and energy consumption during feedings takes time. Waiting to give formula would be contraindicated in a neonate who is hypoglycemic from cold stress, because the condition will worsen if calories are withheld. (P, N, G)
11. 1. Permitting the parents to see and touch the neonate allows for visual searching and information gathering, one of the first steps in the bonding process. Fingertip touching also helps promote the bonding process. Seeing and touching the neonate can often help the parents feel less concerned and more comfortable. The nurse should be present to help the parents understand therapeutic measures that may be in use for the neonate. Meeting with parents of another ill neonate may only increase the parents' concerns. Although parents are generally encouraged to care for their ill children, a high-risk neo-

nate's care involves special skills that the parents may lack. A long-term nursing goal would be to instruct the parents in such care. Telling the parents that their concerns are needless ignores their feelings and tends to cut off communication. (P, N, L)

12. 1. Authorities agree that the single most effective way to control the spread of infection is to have personnel perform frequent arm and hand washing techniques. Measures that are beneficial but not as effective include wearing gowns and masks, using isolettes, and providing clean-air exchange. (P, N, S)

The Infant Who is Septic

13. 2. These symptoms in a neonate would lead the nurse to suspect infection. In a neonate who has an immature immunological response, any infection can rapidly become systemic and result in sepsis. The primary focus of assessment is to determine the neonate's hydration status, especially since sepsis can result in shock. The better hydrated the neonate, the better he can handle the septic state. Since a neonate's kidneys are immature, they cannot conserve water as necessary. This fact makes dehydration a rapid process in the ill neonate. The number of wet diapers in 24 hours would provide data on the neonate's hydration status. Other important assessment data would include skin turgor, mucous membrane status, and status of the fontanel. (A sunken fontanel indicates dehydration.) (A, N, G)

14. 4. The signs and symptoms of sepsis in a neonate are almost imperceptible, such as changes in appearance and behavior. Often, the parents' only complaint is that the neonate does not "look right." Respiratory distress is a later sign. Fever or a localized response, which are clues to infections in older children, are often absent in the neonate. (I, N, G)

15. 4. Toxin released by the causative organism can inhibit absorption of fluid and nutrients from the gut. This situation can lead to overdistention, which can push the diaphragm upward, making respiratory effort difficult. It can also lead to emesis or diarrhea, resulting in fluid and electrolyte loss. Abdominal size in a neonate does not reflect brown fat stores. The antibiotics used to treat sepsis do not cause cessation of peristalsis. Abdominal girth is not a good indicator of hydration status. (I, N, G)

16. 1. Sepsis in a neonate is usually treated with a combination of antibiotics that cover a wide spectrum of causative agents. This is done because treatment is begun immediately, before the causative agent is identified. Furosemide is a diuretic and is not indicated for a neonate at risk for septic shock. Phenytoin sodium is an anticonvulsant and is not indicated for this neonate. Vitamin K is a necessary ingredient for blood clotting and is not necessary for this neonate at this time. (P, N, G)

17. 3. A sleeping heart rate of 205 beats/minute is above normal for this age, which is at most 200 beats/minute. Increased heart rate is an early indication of ensuing shock. The neonate's respiratory rate is within normal limits for age. The capillary refill is normal and indicates good peripheral perfusion. The temperature is slightly elevated but is not an indication of shock. A low axillary temperature may indicate shutdown of the peripheral blood supply, which occurs early in shock. (D, N, G)

18. 3. The nurse's best response is an open-ended question that gives the mother an opportunity to share concerns and ask for information. Telling the mother that she loves the child does not respond to her statement; nor does telling her that the situation is not her fault. In this situation the mother is right to be worried, and telling her to not do so would be inappropriate. (I, N, L)

19. 1. It is normal for a neonate to breathe using the abdominal muscles. A respiratory rate of 30 breaths/minute is normal for an infant age 1 month–1 year. The nurse need not do anything but chart the findings. (D, N, G)

The Client With Failure To Thrive

20. 2. Failure to thrive is a term applied to an infant who is not growing at an acceptable rate. One of the accepted parameters for determining whether the growth rate is acceptable is to determine how the infant's weight compares to the weights of other infants the same age. If the infant's weight falls below the 5th percentile, the infant is considered to have failure to thrive. Sitting without support usually occurs around the 6th month. Gaining 1 pound per week steadily would make the infant overweight. Other characteristics of failure to thrive include eating disorders and developmental retardation. (D, T, H)

21. 1. Infants who have failure to thrive often are fussy during feedings. Although they protest being put down, they are often not content while being held. They are typically unafraid of strangers, which would be abnormal for a 5-month-old. These children also have difficulty sleeping for any length of time. (A, T, G)

22. 3. In the short-term care of this infant, it is important that the same person feed the infant at each meal and that this person be able to assess for negative feeding patterns and replace them with positive patterns. Once the diagnosis is made, it is not appropriate for the parents to feed the infant. Once the infant is gaining weight and shows progress in the feeding patterns, the parents can be instructed in proper feeding techniques. This is a long-term goal of nursing care. A 5-month-old infant is still too young to be expected to sit in a high chair for feedings and should still be bottle-fed. Since there is no organic reason for the failure to thrive, it should not be necessary to increase the formula calorie content from 20 to 24 calories. (P, N, H)

23. 3. Engagement with an infant during feeding is important. This is achieved through physical contact, eye contact, and voice contact. Most important of these three is physical contact with the person feeding the infant. Holding the infant in a relaxed manner that provides the most physical contact is important. The locale of feeding is unimportant as long as the infant's need for contact is met. (A, T, H)

24. 4. The most effective follow-up care would occur in the home environment. The community health nurse can be supportive of the parents and observe the parent-infant interactions in a natural environment. The community health nurse can evaluate the infant's progress in gaining weight, offer suggestions to the parents, and help the family solve problems as they arise. (P, N, G)

25. 2. It is a common misconception that picking up an infant whenever he or she cries will make the child "spoiled." Infants need to be cuddled and comforted when they are upset. Comforting may be as simple as feeding or changing a wet diaper. Assuming that the infant is hungry each time he cries could lead to overfeeding. (I, T, L)

The Client With Atopic Dermatitis

26. 1. An 11-month-old infant will not be comforted by rocking before the procedure or allowing him to become familiar with the equipment. Giving the infant a bottle will not distract him and may encourage him to associate eating with an unpleasant experience. The infant will respond best if a person he trusts is allowed to stay with him. Remember, it is important to give emotional support to the mother, so she can support the infant. (I, N, L)

27. 2. Atopic dermatitis results in puritis; the infant's skin should be covered as completely as possible to keep him from scratching himself. Cotton is the preferred material. Flannel may be too warm and cause the child to perspire, which will aggravate the condition. Nylon may be used, but a sack-like garment would allow the infant to rub the skin of the legs with his feet. Since atopic dermatitis is often associated with allergies, wool garments should be avoided. (I, N, G)

28. 3. The goal of treatment for eczema is to hydrate the skin. The lanolin and urea make an occlusive barrier that keeps moisture in the skin. These preparations will not prevent infection or decrease an inflammatory response. (D, N, G)

29. 4. Eggs and cow's milk are responsible for most allergies in infants. Infants with eczema are usually put on hypoallergenic diets that are free of eggs and milk products. Soy-based formula is substituted for cow's milk, and hypoallergenic foods are given to infants eating solids. Other foods are added one at a time, to identify any that are allergens. Hypoallergenic foods include apples, apricots, pears, carrots, and rice cereals. (E, N, G)

30. 3. Suitable toys for a 3-year-old include all of the items listed. However, a child with allergies should not be given stuffed animals because they tend to collect dust and are difficult to clean. Eczema is often related to an allergic response. (P, N, H)

31. 3. Diphenhydramine (Benadryl) has both a sedative and antihistamine effect. Phenytoin sodium (Dilantin) may cause some sedation, but would not relieve puritis. The same is true of chloral hydrate. Acetaminophen (Tylenol) would have an analgesic effect. (I, N, G)

The Client With Burns

32. 1. For a child under age 12 years, 9% plus 1% for each year under 12 is allocated to the head and neck when using the rule of nines. Each lower extremity is allocated 18% minus 0.5% for each year under 12. The upper extremities receive 9% each, and the posterior and anterior chest receive 18% each, regardless of age. The child's head is proportionally larger than an adult's until age 12. (A, T, G)

33. 2. The child will need fluid replacement therapy as soon as possible, primarily due to the shift of plasma from intravascular to interstitial spaces when the burn occurs. Blisters and edema result from this process and lead to fluid and electrolyte loss. Severe burns are usually sterile; antibiotic treatment, if used at all, would not be a priority at this time. Because of the need to assess the child's sensorium, during the first 24 hours after the burn intravenous analgesics would be used judiciously. The child with a burn can usually eat once he is stable, and this is the preferred method for delivering nutrition. Venous access for hyperalimentation would not be a priority at this time. (I, N, G)

34. 2. The primary fluid shift in burns is from the intravascular to interstitial spaces. The first effect of a burn is dilatation of the capillaries and small vessels in the area, leading to increased capillary permeability. Plasma seeps into the surrounding tissues, producing blisters and edema. There is also an exchange for the electrolyte potassium. (D, N, G)

35. 2. Accurate determination of urine output is a crucial factor in the care of a burn victim. The benefits of using an indwelling catheter to measure urine output to the nearest milliliter outweigh the risk of infection and other problems associated with use. An indwelling catheter would not decrease the workload of the kidneys. Unless the burns cover the perineal area, making urination painful, urine retention is usually not a problem. (I, N, G)

36. 4. Moist rales are an indication that fluid is accumulating in the lung field due to overhydration, or too rapid delivery of fluids. Dark urine would be an indication of underhydration. Abdominal girth and capillary refill time would not provide information about fluid status. (D, N, G)

37. 2. Expressions of anger and combativeness are often the result of loss of control and a feeling a powerlessness. Some control over the situation is regained by allowing the child to participate in care. Neither parental support nor permission to cry will give the child a feeling of control over the situation. The treatments are important to the child's physical wellbeing and should not be delayed. (D, N, L)

38. 2. Allowing the mother to feed the child, serving smaller and more frequent meals, and offering finger foods are all acceptable interventions for a 5-year-old child. This is true whether the child is well or ill. Withholding certain foods until the child complies is punitive and rarely successful. (P, T, H)

39. 4. A serum potassium level of 3.3 mmol/L is low for a child; the normal range is 3.4–4.7 mmol/L. Orange juice is the best source of potassium. Grape and cranberry juices have less potassium, and ginger ale has none. Additional sources of potassium for this child would be bananas, cantaloupe, grapefruit juice, tomato juice, honeydew melon, nectarines, and boiled and baked potatoes. (D, N, G)

40. 4. Because it is likely that an allergic reaction is occurring, the nurse should stop the antibiotic. Lesions that are circumscribed, elevated, and puritic (wheals) are a manifestation of a urticarial reaction. The fact that the child has received multiple doses of the drug is important information because the body needs to be exposed to an antigen to develop an allergic response to it. The IV should be maintained in case the child has an anaphylactic reaction, which could occur if the antibiotic is continued, and needs IV access for resuscitation purposes. (D, N, S)

41. 3. The specific gravity of urine increases as the kidneys are forced to conserve water, a sign of dehydration. Normal specific gravity for a child would range from 1.002–1.030. Decreased blood pressure would also indicate too little fluid is being infused. Normal minimal urine output for a child between age 4 and 7 is 24–28 ml/hour. Irritability is not a reliable indicator of the need for more fluids. (D, N, G)

42. 1. Hypoproteinemia is common following severe burns. The child's diet should be high in protein to compensate for protein loss and to promote tissue healing. The child will also require a diet high in calories and rich in iron. The menu of bacon, lettuce, and tomato sandwich, apple juice, and celery sticks is lacking in sufficient protein and calories. The other choices include items that are high in protein and in calories. (E, N, G)

43. 4. The Centers for Disease Control recommends that sterile gloves be worn when giving any care to a burn area. The gloves should be changed after removing soiled dressings and a new pair put on before applying new dressings. Nonsterile gloves should be used for universal precautions, as in any other client. (I, T, S)

44. 4. The ordered dose is 250 mg every 6 hours, which is 1,000 mg in 24 hours. The recommended dose is 20 to 50 mg times the weight of 10 kg in 24 hours, which is 200 to 500 mg in 24 hours. The ordered dose exceeds the recommended dose by at least 100 percent. The order should be questioned. The nurse cannot independently rewrite a medication order. If the physician refuses to change the order and the nurse believes the dose to be incorrect, the nurse can refuse to carry out the order. (I, N, S)

45. 4. A sign of hemolysis is hemoglobinuria, which will cause the urine to appear dark brown. This condition can result from severe trauma. (D, T, G)

The Client With Hypothyroidism

46. 4. Thyroxine can pass through the placenta to the fetus. This exogenous maternal hormone masks the signs of hypothyroidism at birth in most neonates with cretinism. Failure of normal development occurs during the embryonic period, or an inborn error of metabolism prevents the normal synthesis of thyroxine. These conditions are present at birth. The fetus and neonate require thyroxine, but the exogenous maternal hormone seems to be sufficient. Although some thyroxine is present in breast milk, it is an insufficient amount to prevent the onset of symptoms. (I, T, G)

47. 3. Insomnia, rapid pulse, dyspnea, irritability, fever, sweating, and weight loss are all signs indicating Synthroid overdose. Fatigue, sleepiness, decreased or absent appetite (anorexia), and constipation are signs of thyroid insufficiency. (I, T, G)

48. 4. A child with cretinism receiving thyroid replacement therapy should be regularly assessed for blood levels of thyroxine and triiodothyronine. The child also should undergo frequent bone age surveys to ensure optimum growth. Evaluation of metabolic rate, electrolytes, and muscle coordination is not done to evaluate the success of therapy. (E, T, G)

49. 4. The hallmark signs of untreated cretinism (congenital hypothyroidism) are mental retardation and poor physical development. Cretinism is the most preventable cause of mental retardation. Its effects can be prevented by starting therapy early in the first year of life. Blindness, epilepsy, and emotional instability are not associated with cretinism. (I, T, G)

50. 3. Mixing medications in large amounts of fluid is not recommended, because the infant may not take all the liquid. Mixing medication with food is also contraindicated for this infant, who would not be able to digest orange juice, milk, or cereal. Mixing medications with food is also avoided for older children, because food aversions can result. Placing the dissolved pill in a small amount of formula would be acceptable for this infant. Giving honey to an infant is contraindicated because of the possibility that the honey has botulism spores. Sweet-tasting syrups are acceptable for older children who have developed an immunity to the spores. (E, N, S)

The Client With Insulin-Dependent Diabetes Mellitus

51. 2. An unconscious client should always be placed in a side-lying position. The head of the bed can be slightly elevated. This position allows for the best drainage from the mouth and helps prevent aspiration. A comatose client should not be placed on the back unless the head of the bed is elevated. Placing the unconscious client on the abdomen may contribute to suffocation. Placing the client in Trendelenburg position is unnecessary and may cause gravity to contribute to the emesis of gastric contents. (I, T, S)

52. 2. A sign suggesting hyperglycemia is bed-wetting in a previously continent child. The enuresis is due to polyuria, one of the cardinal signs of insulin-dependent diabetes mellitus. Other cardinal signs are polydipsia (excessive thirst) and polyphagia (excessive hunger). The child also loses weight even though he eats more. The hyperglycemic child is usually slightly lethargic. (A, N, G)

53. 2. Ketones, which are organic acids, readily release free hydrogen ions that cause the blood pH to fall. When ketoacidosis is present, the body attempts to compensate by activating the respiratory buffering process. As a result, the child makes an extra effort to rid himself of excess carbon dioxide, taking deep, rapid breaths and breathing as though he is experiencing air hunger. This characteristic breathing pattern is known as Kussmaul's respirations. (A, T, G)

54. 3. In the client with ketoacidosis due to diabetes mellitus, fats break down into fatty acids and glycerol in fat cells and the liver, then convert to ketone bodies. Ketones accumulate in the blood and are expelled by the kidneys into the urine and by the lungs as acetone. (I, T, G)

55. 3. Insulin is rendered inactive by gastric enzymes. (E, T, G)

56. 4. It is recommended that the client taking regular insulin along with an intermediate- or long-acting insulin use only one syringe. Using two syringes is not recommended, because the insulins can be mixed; also, using two syringes is more expensive. NPH does not remain stable for extended periods when mixed with regular insulin, so premixing is rarely recommended. Insulins such as protamine zinc, globin zinc, and NPH contain an additional modifying protein that slows absorption. A vial of insulin that does not contain the protein (i.e., regular insulin) should never be contaminated with insulin that does have the added protein. (I, T, S)

57. 4. The action of an intermediate-acting insulin, such as Lente, begins 2–4 hours after injection and peaks 6–8 hours after injection. This information is important for timing meals and snacks and recognizing when insulin reactions (hypoglycemia) are likely to occur. Symptoms of hypoglycemia include labile mood, confusion, hunger, headache, shakiness, dizziness, pallor, sweating, and tachycardia. (P, N, G)

58. 1. Assessing a child with hypoglycemia can be very difficult. The only sign may be a change in behavior. Because hypoglycemia is a life-threatening condition, the nurse must assume that the child is hypoglycemic and proceed with interventions for that condition. If the child is hyperglycemic, an increase in blood glucose level at this point would not be lethal. Exercise increases the efficiency of insulin and would only aggravate a hypoglycemic reaction. There is no time to confer with a physician. (I, N, G)

59. 3. Snacks are included in the diabetic diet to offset periods of peak insulin action. Because of the lack of pancreatic functioning, the child does not receive differing amounts of insulin in response to the level of glucose available in the blood stream. The child with diabetes mellitus is given insulin at specific times, and dietary intake must be matched to the insulin peaks and troughs. The risk of hyperglycemia is not eliminated through regular snacks, although spreading the calories over the day may help the child achieve a more steady blood glucose level. Snacks are not used to offset hunger for sweets or to decrease the amount of food eaten at meals. (E, N, G)

60. 4. It is not necessary that the coach be able to identify hyperglycemia in this child. Hyperglycemia is not life-threatening, but hypoglycemia can be. The coach should be taught signs and symptoms of hypoglycemia and how to treat the condition. Since exercise increases both the efficiency of insulin and the amount of energy required by the body, the child should eat something before participating in a strenuous activity. In this case, increasing caloric intake at breakfast will offset the increased need for energy and increased insulin efficiency. An easily absorbed carbohydrate should be available in case the child were to experience hypoglycemia. Insulin uptake from the subcutaneous tissue is increased when the circulation is increased in the area, as occurs around large muscle groups when they are used in strenuous exercise. (P, N, G)

61. 1. The diabetic diet is usually based on an exchange system that takes into account the fact that some foods have very similar fat, carbohydrate, and protein components and thus can be exchanged one for another. For instance, an apple is equal to an orange in an exchange diet. The child with diabetes should be taught to avoid simple sugars that have no other nutritive value other than energy. Simple sugars are absorbed quickly into the blood stream and tend to quickly elevate the blood glucose level, and so should be avoided unless the child is hypoglycemic. Frosted Flakes, cola, and chocolate milk are all sources of simple sugars that should be avoided and replaced with plain cereal or milk. (E, N, G)

62. 2. The ability to mention his disability indicates that the child feels good enough about himself to share his problem with his peers. Asking for reference material and staying out of the hospital would not indicate that the nurse's interventions targeted toward improving self-esteem have been successful. Saying that his friends will probably desert him if he tells them about the disability indicates that the child still needs to work on his self-esteem and his feelings about the disease. (E, N, L)

63. 3. An insulin reaction can be a life-threatening event. Since the child may have an insulin reaction in the classroom, the nurse and mother should discuss with the child's teachers the seriousness of the condition and how to evaluate the child for hypoglycemia. The teachers also need to know what measures to take if an insulin reaction occurs. There is no reason why a teacher would need to be able to give an insulin injection, nor does a teacher need to understand the American Diabetic Association diet plan. The child should be responsible for insulin injections, diet, and testing blood glucose levels. (I, N, G)

64. 4. The child who can tolerate oral feedings of simple sugars can be kept at home. The parents should keep careful track of the child's glucose level and confer with the physician and nurse about regular insulin dosages. Using long-acting or intermediate insulin would be risky, since the child's ability to take in food and absorb nutrients can change rapidly. (D, N, G)

65. 4. A client in ketoacidosis receives normal saline as a solution until the blood glucose level approaches the normal range. Only regular insulin can be given intravenously. The insulin concentration is the physician's preference. The rate, or units given per hour, is based on the child's weight. (I, N, S)

66. 3. Because insulin tends to cling to the tubing, the tubing should be flushed before connecting it to the child's venous access. A protective covering for the solution is not needed. An air filter may be used according to the institution policy on air filters on intravenous tubing. (I, T, S)

67. 1. Repeated use of the same infusion site can result in atrophy of the fat in the subcutaneous tissue and lead to poor insulin absorption. The neuritis common in diabetic patients is not related to infusion sites. (E, T, S)

68. 1. The overweight child should be taught to eat a balanced diet as prescribed for him in terms of percentages of nutrients to eat each day, but should also be instructed to decrease his total daily caloric intake. Decreasing intake of fats or carbohydrates only is likely to lead to an unbalanced diet. The child's insulin dosages may have to be decreased; the child should be taught to be especially alert to signs of hypoglycemia when caloric intake is decreased. (P, T, G)

69. 4. The nurse would advise the mother to allow the child to go trick-or-treating. It would not be advisable to give extra insulin, as this action could result in severe hypoglycemia, especially if this usually compliant child remains faithful to the treatment regimen. Eating sweets can result in hyperglycemia, which is not desired but is not life-threatening in this context. Children need to be treated like their peers; sheltering them from all temptation does not allow them the opportunity to develop coping strategies for dealing with the restraints made necessary by their disease. (I, N, G)

70. 2. When teaching, the nurse should remember that the learner needs to be ready to learn. Illness makes it difficult for the child to concentrate on what is being taught. Although some learning may take place, the teaching would be more effective later when the child is feeling better. Before giving any reading material to a learner, it is important to assess the learner's reading level. (I, N, H)

Clients Who Are Abused

71. 4. Parents of an abused child are typically unconcerned about the child's injury. They may blame the child or others for the injury, may not ask questions about treatment, and may not know developmental information. (A, T, L)

72. 2. Parents who are abusive typically lack knowledge of the child's development and needs. A child age 3 can help dress himself but would not be expected to tie his shoes. Abusive parents also usually lack social support from family and friends. (D, N, L)

73. 1. Encouraging the abused child to talk about or play out events surrounding the "accident" can help the child and also provide assessment data. An abused child may feel to blame; even if the parent is accused of abuse, the child may still accept responsibility for the act. The nurse should never make promises that cannot be kept. (I, N, L)

74. 1. It is not normal for a preschooler to be totally passive during a painful procedure. An abused child may become "immune" to pain and find that crying may bring on more pain. The child needs to learn that appropriate emotional expression is acceptable. (I, N, L)

75. 2. It is most important for the nurse to document physical findings and observed behaviors on the client's record. Court proceedings usually occur some-time after the nurse's involvement with the child and family, and memories fade. Thus careful documentation of the facts, not heresay or subjective opinion, is essential. (P, N, S)

76. 2. An abused child needs appropriate attention and affection as well as consistent management of inappropriate behavior. Such a child commonly has learned undesirable behavior to get attention, cope with his or her environment, and relate to others. Behavior modification is used, and anger and aggressive acts are not rewarded. The child still has needs to be a part of the family. Family visits are encouraged so that the nurse can reinforce positive nonabusive parenting as well as meet the child's emotional needs to be a part of the family. It is advisable for the nurse to remain with the child during these visits and not to leave the child alone. (P, N, L)

77. 2. A child who reports abuse must be believed. Often the child has tried to tell the parents about the abuse but has not been believed or has been rejected. The child may be afraid to tell the parents. The nurse should start with neutral questions and later ask the child for an account of the event. (I, N, L)

78. 3. A 3-year-old child has limited verbal skills and should not be asked to describe an event, explain a picture, or respond verbally or nonverbally to questions. More appropriately, the child can act out an event using dolls. (A, N, L)

79. 4. All states have mandatory reporting laws relating to child abuse and neglect. A nurse or other health care professional who fails to report suspected abuse may be charged with a misdemeanor. Nurses who report suspected child abuse have immunity from being sued. (I, T, H)

NURSING CARE OF CHILDREN

TEST 9: The Child with Dermatologic, Endocrine, and Other Health Problems

Directions: Use this answer grid to determine areas of strength or need for further study.

Nursing Process

A = Assessment
D = Analysis, nursing diagnosis
P = Planning
I = Implementation
E = Evaluation

Cognitive Level

K = Knowledge
C = Comprehension
T = Application
N = Analysis

Client Needs

S = Safe, effective care environment
G = Physiological integrity
L = Psychosocial integrity
H = Health promotion/maintenance

		Nursing Process					Cognitive Level				Client Needs			
Question #	Answer #	A	D	P	I	E	K	C	T	N	S	G	L	H
1	3	A								N		G		
2	2	A							T			G		
3	3	A								N		G		
4	2		D							N		G		
5	1			P						N		G		
6	3		D							N		G		
7	3					E				N		G		
8	4				I				T		S			
9	1				I				T		S			
10	1			P						N		G		
11	1			P						N			L	
12	1			P						N	S			
13	2	A								N		G		
14	4				I					N		G		
15	4				I					N		G		
16	1			P						N		G		
17	3		D							N		G		
18	3				I					N			L	
19	1		D							N		G		
20	2		D						T					H
21	1	A							T			G		
22	3			P						N				H
23	3	A							T					H

ANSWER GRID: 1

NURSING PROCESS

A = Assessment
D = Analysis, nursing diagnosis
P = Planning
I = Implementation
E = Evaluation

COGNITIVE LEVEL

K = Knowledge
C = Comprehension
T = Application
N = Analysis

CLIENT NEEDS

S = Safe, effective care environment
G = Physiological integrity
L = Psychosocial integrity
H = Health promotion/maintenance

		Nursing Process					Cognitive Level				Client Needs			
Question #	Answer #	A	D	P	I	E	K	C	T	N	S	G	L	H
24	4			P						N		G		
25	2				I				T				L	
26	1				I					N			L	
27	2				I					N		G		
28	3		D							N		G		
29	4					E				N		G		
30	3			P						N				H
31	3				I					N		G		
32	1	A							T			G		
33	2				I					N		G		
34	2		D							N		G		
35	2				I					N		G		
36	4		D							N		G		
37	2		D							N			L	
38	2			P					T					H
39	4		D							N		G		
40	4		D							N	S			
41	3		D							N		G		
42	1					E				N		G		
43	4				I				T		S			
44	4				I					N	S			
45	4		D						T			G		
46	4				I				T			G		
47	3				I				T			G		
48	4					E			T			G		
49	4				I				T			G		
50	3					E				N	S			
51	2				I				T		S			
52	2	A								N		G		

ANSWER GRID: 2

NURSING PROCESS

A = Assessment
D = Analysis, nursing diagnosis
P = Planning
I = Implementation
E = Evaluation

COGNITIVE LEVEL

K = Knowledge
C = Comprehension
T = Application
N = Analysis

CLIENT NEEDS

S = Safe, effective care environment
G = Physiological integrity
L = Psychosocial integrity
H = Health promotion/maintenance

		Nursing Process					Cognitive Level				Client Needs			
Question #	Answer #	A	D	P	I	E	K	C	T	N	S	G	L	H
53	2	A							T			G		
54	3				I				T			G		
55	3					E			T			G		
56	4				I				T		S			
57	4			P						N		G		
58	1				I					N		G		
59	3					E				N		G		
60	4			P						N		G		
61	1					E				N		G		
62	2					E				N			L	
63	3				I					N		G		
64	4		D							N		G		
65	4				I					N	S			
66	3				I				T		S			
67	1					E			T		S			
68	1			P					T			G		
69	4				I					N		G		
70	2				I					N				H
71	4	A							T				L	
72	2		D							N			L	
73	1				I					N			L	
74	1				I					N			L	
75	2			P						N	S			
76	2			P						N			L	

ANSWER GRID: 3

Nursing Process	Cognitive Level	Client Needs
A = Assessment	K = Knowledge	S = Safe, effective care environment
D = Analysis, nursing diagnosis	C = Comprehension	G = Physiological integrity
P = Planning	T = Application	L = Psychosocial integrity
I = Implementation	N = Analysis	H = Health promotion/maintenance
E = Evaluation		

		Nursing Process					Cognitive Level				Client Needs			
Question #	Answer #	A	D	P	I	E	K	C	T	N	S	G	L	H
77	2				I					N			L	
78	3	A								N			L	
79	4				I				T					H
Number Correct														
Number Possible	79	11	15	14	29	10	0	0	25	54	13	46	13	7
Percentage Correct														

Score Calculation:

To determine your **Percentage Correct**, divide the **Number Correct** by the **Number Possible**.

BIBLIOGRAPHY

Benson, D.S., & Conte, R.S. (1991). *91/92 nursing meds.* Norwalk, CT: Appleton and Lange.

Bernardo, L.M., & Bove, M. (1993). *Pediatric emergency nursing procedures.* Boston: Jones & Bartlett.

Betz, C.L., & Poster, E. (1992). *Mosby's pediatric nursing reference* (2nd ed.). St. Louis: Mosby Yearbook, 1992.

Castiglia, P.Y., & Harbin, R.E. (1992). *Child health care: Process and practice.* Philadelphia: JB Lippincott.

Cox, H.C., Hinz, M.D., Lubno, M.A., Newfield, S.A., Ridenour, N.A., & Sridaromont, K.L. (1989). *Clinical applications of nursing diagnosis.* Baltimore: Williams and Wilkins.

Davis, J., & Sherer, K. (1993). *Applied nutrition and diet therapy for nurses* (2nd ed.). Philadelphia: W.B. Saunders.

Foster, R.L., Hunsberger, M.M., & Anderson, J.J. (1989). *Family-centered nursing care of children.* Philadelphia: W.B. Saunders.

Gordon, M. (1991). *Manual of nursing diagnosis: 1991–1992.* St. Louis: Mosby Yearbook.

Gulanick, M., Puzas, M.K., & Wilson, C.R. (1992). *Nursing care plans for newborns and children: Acute and critical care.* St. Louis: Mosby Yearbook.

Hazinski, M.F. (1992). *Nursing care of the critically ill child* (2nd ed.). St. Louis: Mosby Yearbook.

Hymovich, D.P., and Hagopian, G.A. (1992). *Chronic illness in children and adults: A psychosocial approach.* Philadelphia: W.B. Saunders.

Jackson, D.B., & Saunders, R. (1993). *Child health nursing: A comprehensive approach to the care of children and their families.* Philadelphia: J.B. Lippincott.

Jackson, P.L., & Vessey, J.A. (1991). *Primary care of the child with a chronic condition.* St. Louis: Mosby Yearbook.

James, S., & Mott, S. (1988). *Child health nursing: Essential care of children and families.* Menlo Park, CA: Addison-Wesley.

Kalus, M.H., & Fanaroff, A.A. (1993). *Care of the high–risk neonate.* Philadelphia: W.B. Saunders.

Lewis, S., Grainger, R.D., McDowell, W.A., Gregory, R.J., & Messner, R.L. (1989). *Manual of psychosocial nursing interventions: Promoting mental health in medical-surgical settings.* Philadelphia: W.B. Saunders.

Marlow, D.R., & Redding, B.A. (1988). *Textbook of pediatric nursing.* (6th ed.). Philadelphia: W.B. Saunders.

Mott, S., Frazekas, N., & James, S. (1985). *Nursing care of children and families: A holistic approach.* Menlo Park, CA: Addison-Wesley.

Pillitteri, A. (1992). *Maternal and child health nursing care of the childbearing and childbearing family.* Philadelphia: J.B. Lippincott.

Pipes, P., and Trahms, C.M. (1992). *Nutrition in infancy and childhood* (5th ed.). St. Louis: Mosby Yearbook.

Rose, M., & Thomas, R.B. (1987). *Children with chronic conditions: Nursing in a family and community context.* Philadelphia: W.B. Saunders.

Schuster, C.S., & Ashburn, S.S. (1992). *The Process of Human Development, 3/e: A Holistic Life-Span Approach.* Philadelphia: J.B. Lippincott.

Scipien, G.M., Bernard, M.U., Chard, M.A., Howe, J., & Phillips, P.J. (1986). *Comprehensive pediatric nursing* (3rd ed.). New York: McGraw-Hill.

Scipien, G.M., Chard, M.A., Howe, J., & Barnard, M. (1990). *Pediatric nursing care.* St. Louis: Mosby Yearbook.

Smith, P.S., Nix, K.S., Kemper, J.Y., Ligouri, R., Brantly, D.K., Rollins, J.H., Stevens, N.V., & Clutter, L.B. (1991). *Comprehensive child and family nursing skills.* St. Louis: Mosby Yearbook.

Thompson, S.W. (1990). *Emergency care of children.* Boston: Jones & Bartlett.

Waechter, E., Phillips, J., & Holadaz, B. (1985). *Nursing care of children.* Philadelphia: J.B. Lippincott.

Whaley, L.F., & Wong, D.L. (1991). *Nursing care of infants and children* (4th ed.). St. Louis: Mosby Yearbook.

Part IV

The Nursing Care of Adults With Medical/ Surgical Health Problems

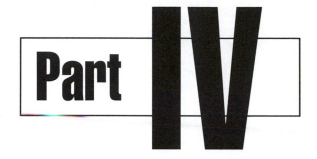

The Client With Respiratory Health Problems

Test 1

The Client With Pneumonia
The Client With Tuberculosis
The Client With Chronic Obstructive Pulmonary Disease (COPD)
The Client With Lung Cancer
The Client With Chest Trauma
General Questions
Correct Answers and Rationale

Select the one best answer and indicate your choice by filling in the circle in front of the option you have chosen.

The Client With Pneumonia

A female client, age 79, is admitted to the hospital with a diagnosis of bacterial pneumonia. She has a temperature of 102.6°F and a productive cough and is experiencing difficulty breathing.

1. When obtaining the client's health history, the nurse learns that she has long-standing osteoarthritis, follows a vegetarian diet, has never been seriously ill, and is very concerned with cleanliness. The client says, "I hope I can take a bath each day. I feel so dirty if I don't bathe every day." Which of the following factors would add most to the danger posed by her illness?

- ○ 1. The client's age.
- ○ 2. History of osteoarthritis.
- ○ 3. Following a vegetarian diet.
- ○ 4. Bathing daily in cold water.

2. A priority nursing diagnosis for this hospitalized client with bacterial pneumonia and difficulty breathing would be

- ○ 1. Altered Cardiopulmonary Tissue Perfusion related to myocardial damage.
- ○ 2. Activity Intolerance related to interrupted sleep/wake cycle.
- ○ 3. Fluid Volume Deficit related to nausea and vomiting.
- ○ 4. Altered Thought Processes related to decreased oxygenation.

3. The client is to be started on IV antibiotics immediately. Which of the following must be completed before antibiotic therapy begins?

- ○ 1. Urinalysis.
- ○ 2. Sputum examination.
- ○ 3. Chest x-ray.
- ○ 4. Red blood cell count.

4. The client is extremely diaphoretic with her high fever. Considering her advanced age, she is at particular risk for developing

- ○ 1. hyponatremia.
- ○ 2. hypokalemia.
- ○ 3. hypercalcemia.
- ○ 4. hyperphosphatemia.

5. Considering the client's symptoms and personality, the nurse should include which of the following measures in her care plan?

- ○ 1. Position changes every 4 hours.
- ○ 2. Nasotracheal suctioning to clear secretions.
- ○ 3. Frequent linen changes.
- ○ 4. Frequent offering of a bedpan.

6. Bedrest is prescribed for the client during the acute phase of her illness. The purpose of bedrest in this situation is to

- ○ 1. reduce the cellular demand for oxygen.
- ○ 2. decrease the basal metabolic rate.
- ○ 3. promote safety.
- ○ 4. promote clearance of secretions.

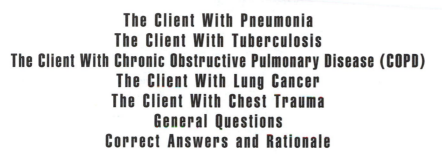

The Client With Tuberculosis

A male client has just been diagnosed with tuberculosis. He had not been feeling well for the past several weeks, and sought medical attention when he began coughing up bloody secretions.

7. Which of the following symptoms are common in clients with active tuberculosis?
- ○ 1. Marked weight loss.
- ○ 2. Increased appetite.
- ○ 3. Dyspnea on exertion.
- ○ 4. Mental status changes.

8. The nurse obtains a sputum specimen from the client for laboratory study. Which of the following laboratory techniques is most commonly used to identify tubercle bacilli in sputum?
- ○ 1. Acid-fast staining.
- ○ 2. Sensitivity testing.
- ○ 3. Agglutination testing.
- ○ 4. Darkfield illumination.

9. Which of the following antituberculosis drugs can damage the eighth cranial nerve?
- ○ 1. Streptomycin.
- ○ 2. Isoniazid (INH).
- ○ 3. Aminosalicylic acid (PAS).
- ○ 4. Ethambutol hydrochloride (Myambutol).

10. The client who experiences eighth cranial nerve damage will most likely report which of the following symptoms?
- ○ 1. Vertigo.
- ○ 2. Facial paralysis.
- ○ 3. Impaired vision.
- ○ 4. Difficulty swallowing.

11. In teaching the client about self-care at home, the nurse will include all of the following measures. Which of the measures would have the highest priority?
- ○ 1. Getting adequate rest.
- ○ 2. Eating a nourishing diet.
- ○ 3. Taking medications as prescribed.
- ○ 4. Living in an area with clean air.

The Client With Chronic Obstructive Pulmonary Disease (COPD)

A client is admitted to the hospital with an acute exacerbation of long-standing chronic obstructive pulmonary disease (COPD) brought on by an upper respiratory infection. He is tachypneic and acutely short of breath. Both he and his wife are extremely anxious.

12. The client is admitted to room 13, but he states that he does not want to remain in the room because the number will bring him bad luck. Personnel in the admitting office say that a change can be made if the nurse feels that it is wise to do so. Which of the following statements offers the best guide for the nurse in this situation?
- ○ 1. Move the client; the client's fears, even when unfounded, can impede recovery.
- ○ 2. Move the client; superstitions have a good chance of coming true for those who believe them.
- ○ 3. Do not move the client; having the client use the room will help him overcome an unwarranted fear.
- ○ 4. Do not move the client; the client may become unmanageable and demanding when he knows he can have his way.

13. Oxygen at the rate of 2L/minute via nasal cannula is prescribed for the client. Which of the following statements best describes why the oxygen therapy is maintained at a relatively low concentration?
- ○ 1. The oxygen will be lost at the client's nostrils if given at a higher level with a nasal cannula.
- ○ 2. The client's long history of respiratory problems indicates that he would be unable to absorb oxygen given at a higher rate.
- ○ 3. The cells in the alveoli are so damaged by the client's long history of respiratory problems that increased oxygen levels and reduced carbon dioxide levels likely will cause the cells to burst.
- ○ 4. The client's respiratory center is so accustomed to high carbon dioxide and low blood oxygen concentrations that changing these concentrations with oxygen therapy may eliminate his stimulus for breathing.

14. The client reports steady weight loss and that he "is too tired from just breathing to eat." Which of the following nursing diagnoses would be most appropriate when planning nutritional interventions for this client?
- ○ 1. Altered Nutrition: Less than Body Requirements related to fatigue.
- ○ 2. Altered Nutrition: Less than Body Requirements related to COPD.
- ○ 3. Weight Loss related to COPD.
- ○ 4. Ineffective Breathing Patterns related to alveolar hypoventilation.

15. When developing the client's discharge plan, the nurse should be guided by an understanding that the client is most likely to
- ○ 1. develop infections easily.
- ○ 2. maintain his current status.
- ○ 3. require less supplemental oxygen.
- ○ 4. show permanent improvement.

16. On hospital discharge, outcome criteria for the client would include
- ○ 1. promises to do pursed-lip breathing.

○ 2. states actions to reduce risk of respiratory infections.
○ 3. exhibits temperature not exceeding 100°F.
○ 4. agrees to call the physician if dyspnea on exertion occurs.

The Client With Lung Cancer

A client was admitted with a diagnosis of lung cancer. She enjoyed good health until 2 months ago, when she developed a persistent cough that became productive of blood-tinged sputum 1 week ago. She has also experienced increasing fatigue over the past month. She reports no anorexia and appears well nourished (5′ 7″ tall, 140 lbs). She has smoked a pack of cigarettes a day for 28 years. A chest x-ray and sputum cytology done a week ago are the basis for the diagnosis.

17. As part of the client's diagnostic work-up, she is to have a bronchoscopy under local anesthesia. Her preoperative medication will be atropine sulfate 0.4 mg and meperidine hydrochloride (Demerol) 100 mg IM. Which of the following interventions should the nurse perform after the test?
○ 1. Irrigate the nasogastric tube with 30 ml of normal saline every 2 hours.
○ 2. Offer 200 ml of oral fluids every hour to liquefy lung secretions.
○ 3. Observe the abdomen for signs of distention and boardlike rigidity.
○ 4. Position the client on her side and keep her NPO for several hours.

18. The client is to have a left lung lobectomy. Certain data are more important than others in planning her postoperative nursing care. Of the following assessment data obtained in the nurse's admission interview and nursing history, which would increase the client's risk of developing postoperative complications?
○ 1. Is 5′ 7″ tall and weighs 140 lbs.
○ 2. Tends to keep her real feelings to herself.
○ 3. Ambulates and can climb one flight of stairs without dyspnea.
○ 4. Has decreased vital capacity.

19. The night before surgery, the nurse remarks to the client that she looks sad and is quieter than usual. The client says, "I'm scared of having cancer. It's so horrible and I brought it on myself. I should have quit smoking years ago." What would be the nurse's best response to the client?
○ 1. "It's okay to be scared. What is it about cancer that you're afraid of?"
○ 2. "It's normal to be scared. I would be, too. We'll help you through it."
○ 3. "Don't be so hard on yourself. You don't know if your smoking caused the cancer."
○ 4. "Do you feel guilty because you smoked?"

20. The client had a left lower lobectomy this morning. She is now alert and responsive. Her vital signs are stable, and her skin is warm and dry. She has two chest tubes to underwater-seal drainage, with 20 cm of water suction applied to the system. The nurse notes that she has a posteriolateral incision. Nursing orders include having the client cough and deep-breathe every hour, turning the client every 2 hours, and administering meperidine hydrochloride (Demerol) 100 mg IM every 4 hours p.r.n. The client complains of moderately severe pain in her left thorax that worsens when she coughs. To help control the client's pain during coughing, the nurse should
○ 1. place the bed in slight Trendelenburg's position and help the client turn onto her operative side to splint the incision.
○ 2. raise the bed to semi-Fowler's position and place one hand on the client's back, on the left side, and one hand under the incision.
○ 3. keep the bed flat and tell the client to place her hands over the incision before taking a deep breath.
○ 4. raise the bed to complete Fowler's position and help the client turn onto her operative side to splint the incision.

21. Postoperatively, the nurse identifies Impaired Gas Exchange as a potential nursing diagnosis. Which of the following factors would contribute to this diagnosis?
○ 1. Anxiety.
○ 2. High amount of chest tube suction.
○ 3. Incisional pain.
○ 4. Advanced age of the client.

22. The goal for the nursing diagnosis Impaired Gas Exchange is to promote optimal ventilation. Which of the following outcome criteria would indicate attainment of this goal?
○ 1. PaO_2 90 mm Hg and $PaCO_2$ 40 mm Hg.
○ 2. Tachypnea.
○ 3. Bilateral crackles on auscultation.
○ 4. Temperature within normal limits.

The Client With Chest Trauma

An elderly male client is transported by ambulance to the emergency department after a serious automobile accident. He complains of severe pain in his right chest where he struck the steering wheel. He also has a compound fracture of his right tibia and fibula and multiple lacerations and contusions.

23. The primary nursing goal at this point should be to
- ○ 1. reduce the client's anxiety.
- ○ 2. maintain effective respirations.
- ○ 3. decrease chest pain.
- ○ 4. maintain adequate circulating volume.

24. The client's respiratory rate is 40 breaths/minute, his blood pressure has fallen to 100/60 mm Hg, and he has a weak, rapid pulse at 96 beats/minute. With a diagnosis of right rib fracture and closed pneumothorax, he should be placed in
- ○ 1. modified Trendelenburg's position with his lower extremities elevated.
- ○ 2. reverse Trendelenburg's position with his head down.
- ○ 3. left side-lying position with his head elevated 15 to 30 degrees.
- ○ 4. semi- to high-Fowler's position, tilted toward his right side.

25. On admission the client's arterial blood gas values were pH 7.20, PaO_2 64 mm Hg, $PaCO_2$ 60 mm Hg, and HCO_3^- 22 mEq/L. A chest tube is inserted, and oxygen at 4 liters/minute is started. Thirty minutes later, his repeat blood gas values are pH 7.30, PaO_2 76, $PaCO_2$ 50, and HCO_3^- 22 mEq/L. This change would indicate
- ○ 1. impending respiratory failure.
- ○ 2. improving respiratory status.
- ○ 3. developing respiratory alkalosis.
- ○ 4. obstruction in the chest tubes.

26. The nurse believes that the client is experiencing an adverse effect from morphine sulfate. Which of the following clinical manifestations would lead the nurse to this conclusion?
- ○ 1. Increased blood pressure.
- ○ 2. Transient visual disturbances.
- ○ 3. Decreased respiratory rate.
- ○ 4. Inhibited mucus secretion.

27. The client's wife arrives on the unit 6 hours after her husband's accident, explaining that she has been out of town. She is distraught because she was not with her husband when he needed her. The most appropriate initial nursing intervention for her would be to
- ○ 1. allow her to verbalize her feelings and concerns.
- ○ 2. describe her husband's medical treatment since admission.
- ○ 3. explain the nature of the injury and reassure her that her husband's condition is stable.
- ○ 4. reassure her that the important fact is that she is here now.

28. Twelve hours after the client's chest tube is removed, his arterial blood gas values include PaO_2 90 mm Hg. The nurse should interpret this value as indicating that
- ○ 1. the client needs additional oxygen.
- ○ 2. the client should be encouraged to cough and deep breathe.
- ○ 3. the client's physician should be notified immediately.
- ○ 4. the client's response is adequate.

General Questions

29. For the client with a productive cough and difficulty breathing, the nurse should obtain the body temperature at what site?
- ○ 1. Mouth.
- ○ 2. Groin fold.
- ○ 3. Rectum.
- ○ 4. Axillae.

30. The cyanosis that accompanies bacterial pneumonia is primarily due to
- ○ 1. cardiac involvement.
- ○ 2. iron deficiency anemia.
- ○ 3. inadequate circulation.
- ○ 4. poor blood oxygenation.

31. A client with pneumonia is experiencing pleuritic chest pain. This type of chest pain is usually described as being
- ○ 1. a mild but constant aching in the chest.
- ○ 2. severe midsternal pain.
- ○ 3. moderate pain that worsens on inspiration.
- ○ 4. muscle spasm pain that accompanies coughing.

32. Which of the following nursing measures would most likely be successful in reducing the client's pleuritic chest pain due to pneumonia?
- ○ 1. Encourage the client to breathe shallowly.
- ○ 2. Have the client practice abdominal breathing.
- ○ 3. Offer the client incentive spirometry.
- ○ 4. Teach the client to splint the rib cage when coughing.

33. Aspirin is administered to clients with pneumonia because of its antipyretic and
- ○ 1. analgesic effects.
- ○ 2. anticoagulant effects.
- ○ 3. adrenergic effects.
- ○ 4. antihistamine effects.

34. A client with bacterial pneumonia is coughing up tenacious, purulent sputum. Which of the following measures would most likely help liquefy these viscous secretions?
- ○ 1. Performing postural drainage.
- ○ 2. Breathing humidified air.
- ○ 3. Clapping and percussing over the affected lung.
- ○ 4. Performing coughing and deep breathing exercises.

35. Which of the following behaviors could indicate that the client with pneumonia is experiencing hypoxia?

○ 1. Anger.
○ 2. Apathy.
○ 3. Anxiety.
○ 4. Aggression.

36. After 1 day of antibiotic therapy, a client's white blood cell count is 14,000/mm^3. In response to this report, the nurse should
○ 1. notify the physician.
○ 2. increase the next dose of the antibiotic.
○ 3. initiate reverse isolation precautions.
○ 4. administer the next scheduled antibiotic dose early.

37. The client with pneumonia develops mild constipation, and the nurse administers docusate sodium (Colace) as ordered. This drug works by
○ 1. softening the stool.
○ 2. lubricating the stool.
○ 3. increasing stool bulk.
○ 4. stimulating peristalsis.

38. Which of the following would be most important to teach an elderly client to prevent a recurrence of bacterial pneumonia?
○ 1. Change current diet habits.
○ 2. Seek prompt antibiotic therapy for viral infections.
○ 3. Receive prophylactic antibiotic therapy.
○ 4. Obtain annual influenza and pneumococcal vaccines.

39. The nurse should teach clients that the most common route of transmitting tubercle bacilli from person to person is through contaminated
○ 1. dust particles.
○ 2. droplet nuclei.
○ 3. water.
○ 4. eating utensils.

40. The single most effective way to decrease the spread of microorganisms is
○ 1. washing the hands frequently.
○ 2. having separate personal care items for each person.
○ 3. using disposable equipment whenever possible.
○ 4. isolating persons known to be harboring disease-causing microorganisms.

41. Many clients with tuberculosis take two antitubercular drugs simultaneously. The primary reason for this is to
○ 1. potentiate the drugs' actions.
○ 2. reduce undesirable drug side effects.
○ 3. allow reduced drug dosages to be given.
○ 4. reduce development of resistant strains of the bacteria.

42. The client with tuberculosis is to be discharged home with community health nursing follow-up. Of the following nursing goals, which would have the highest priority?
○ 1. Offer the client emotional support.
○ 2. Teach the client about the disease.
○ 3. Coordinate various agency services.
○ 4. Assess the client's environment for sanitation.

43. Which of the following techniques for administering the Mantoux test is correct?
○ 1. Hold the needle and syringe almost parallel to the client's skin.
○ 2. Pinch the skin when inserting the needle.
○ 3. Aspirate prior to injection of the medication.
○ 4. Massage the site after injecting the medication.

44. Which member of a family exposed to tuberculosis would be at highest risk for contracting tuberculosis?
○ 1. The 45-year-old mother.
○ 2. The teenaged daughter.
○ 3. The grade-school-age son.
○ 4. The 76-year-old grandmother.

45. Medical therapy for a client with a positive Mantoux skin test who does not have active tuberculosis would involve
○ 1. reevaluating the client's condition every 6 months.
○ 2. performing a repeat skin test every 6 months.
○ 3. administering isoniazid (INH) for approximately 9 months.
○ 4. administering INH until the skin test reverts to negative.

46. The nurse's best evaluation of a client who exhibits a positive Mantoux test would be that the client has
○ 1. clinical tuberculosis.
○ 2. had contact with the tubercle bacilli.
○ 3. developed a resistance to the tubercle bacilli.
○ 4. developed passive immunity to tuberculosis.

47. To prevent development of peripheral neuropathies associated with INH administration, clients taking this drug are usually advised to
○ 1. follow a special foot care regimen.
○ 2. supplement the diet with pyridoxine (vitamin B6).
○ 3. get extra rest.
○ 4. avoid excessive sun exposure.

48. The nurse should caution sexually active female clients taking INH that the drug
○ 1. increases the risk of vaginal infection.
○ 2. has mutagenic effects on ova.
○ 3. decreases the effectiveness of oral contraceptives.
○ 4. inhibits ovulation.

49. Clients who have had active tuberculosis need to be informed that they are at risk for recurrence of tuberculosis during periods of
○ 1. hot and humid and cool and damp weather.
○ 2. active exercise and exertion.
○ 3. physical and emotional stress.
○ 4. rest and inactivity.

50. In which areas of the United States does tuberculosis most commonly occur?
- ○ 1. Rural farming areas.
- ○ 2. Inner city areas.
- ○ 3. Areas where clean water standards are low.
- ○ 4. Suburban areas with significant industrial pollution.

51. Which of the following physical assessment findings is typical in a client with advanced obstructive pulmonary disease?
- ○ 1. Increased anterior–posterior chest diameter.
- ○ 2. Underdeveloped neck muscles.
- ○ 3. Collapsed neck veins.
- ○ 4. Increased chest excursions with respiration.

52. To decrease the risk of chronic obstructive pulmonary disease (COPD), persons should be instructed to
- ○ 1. refrain from drinking more than one alcoholic beverage per day.
- ○ 2. maintain a high-protein diet.
- ○ 3. avoid exposure to persons with known respiratory infections.
- ○ 4. abstain from cigarette smoking.

53. The primary reason to teach pursed-lip breathing to persons with emphysema is to help
- ○ 1. promote oxygen intake.
- ○ 2. strengthen the diaphragm.
- ○ 3. strengthen the intercostal muscles.
- ○ 4. promote carbon dioxide elimination.

54. Theophylline ethylenediamide (aminophylline) is administered to a client with COPD to
- ○ 1. reduce bronchial secretions.
- ○ 2. relax bronchial smooth muscle.
- ○ 3. strengthen myocardial contractions.
- ○ 4. decrease alveolar elasticity.

55. The primary purpose of chest percussion for the client with COPD is to
- ○ 1. stimulate deeper inhalations.
- ○ 2. improve ciliary action in the bronchioles.
- ○ 3. propel secretions along the respiratory tract.
- ○ 4. loosen secretions in congested areas of the lungs.

Questions 56–60 pertain to the following set of arterial blood gas (ABG) values:

pH 7.28; PaO_2 50 mm Hg; $PaCO_2$ 80 mm Hg; HCO_3^- 32 mEq/L.

56. The nurse would interpret these ABG values as indicating
- ○ 1. metabolic acidosis.
- ○ 2. metabolic alkalosis.
- ○ 3. respiratory acidosis.
- ○ 4. respiratory alkalosis.

57. From the client's $PaCO_2$ level, the nurse could safely conclude that the client is
- ○ 1. hypoxemic.
- ○ 2. hypoventilating.
- ○ 3. hyperventilating.
- ○ 4. using oxygen therapy.

58. From the client's PaO_2 level, the nurse could safely conclude that the
- ○ 1. client is hypoxic.
- ○ 2. oxygen level is low but poses no risk for the client.
- ○ 3. client's PaO_2 level is within normal range.
- ○ 4. client requires oxygen therapy with very low oxygen concentrations.

59. Based on these ABG values, the nurse would anticipate that the client will require
- ○ 1. more frequent percussion and postural drainage.
- ○ 2. increased aminophylline and corticosteroid doses.
- ○ 3. intensive teaching to facilitate pursed-lip breathing.
- ○ 4. endotracheal intubation and mechanical ventilation.

60. The nursing care plan for this client should include close monitoring for which of the following signs and symptoms?
- ○ 1. Cyanosis and restlessness.
- ○ 2. Flushed skin and lethargy.
- ○ 3. Weakness and irritability.
- ○ 4. Anxiety and fever.

61. During postural drainage, movement of secretions from the lower respiratory tract to the upper respiratory tract occurs due to
- ○ 1. friction between the cilia.
- ○ 2. the force of gravity.
- ○ 3. the sweeping motion of cilia.
- ○ 4. involuntary muscle contractions.

62. Clients with COPD may be bedridden at home and get little exercise. Which of the following is a normal physiologic reaction to prolonged periods of bedrest and inactivity?
- ○ 1. Increased sodium retention.
- ○ 2. Increased calcium excretion.
- ○ 3. Increased insulin utilization.
- ○ 4. Increased red blood cell production.

63. For a client with COPD who has trouble raising respiratory secretions, which of the following nursing measures would help reduce the tenacity of secretions?
- ○ 1. Ensuring that the client's diet is low in salt.
- ○ 2. Ensuring that the client's oxygen therapy is continuous.
- ○ 3. Helping the client maintain a high fluid intake.
- ○ 4. Keeping the client in a semi-sitting position as much as possible.

64. The nurse teaches the client with COPD measures to conserve energy when performing activities of daily living. The nurse should teach the client to lift objects
- ○ 1. while inhaling through pursed lips.
- ○ 2. while exhaling through pursed lips.
- ○ 3. after exhaling but before inhaling.
- ○ 4. after inhaling but before exhaling.

65. A major nursing intervention to help prevent lung cancer would be to
- ○ 1. encourage cigarette smokers to have yearly chest x-rays.
- ○ 2. emphasize the causative relationship of cigarette smoking to lung cancer.
- ○ 3. recommend that people have their houses and apartments checked for asbestos leakage.
- ○ 4. encourage people to install central air cleaners in their homes.

66. When administering atropine sulfate preoperatively to the client scheduled for lung surgery, the nurse should tell the client which of the following? "This medication will
- ○ 1. make you drowsy."
- ○ 2. help you relax."
- ○ 3. make your mouth feel very dry."
- ○ 4. reduce the risk of postoperative infection."

67. The most appropriate nursing diagnosis for the preoperative client prior to lung surgery would be
- ○ 1. High Risk for Infection related to poor knowledge of postoperative breathing techniques.
- ○ 2. High Risk for Infection related to surgery.
- ○ 3. Future Lobectomy related to lung cancer.
- ○ 4. Altered Nutrition: Less than Body Requirements related to effects of surgery on the bowel.

68. Following lobectomy, clients should be instructed to perform deep breathing exercises to
- ○ 1. elevate the diaphragm, which enlarges the thorax and increases the lung surface available for gas exchange.
- ○ 2. decrease blood flow to the lungs to allow them to rest and increase the surface available for ventilation.
- ○ 3. control the rate of air flow to the remaining lobe so that it will not become hyperinflated.
- ○ 4. expand the alveoli and increase the lung surface available for ventilation.

69. Which of the following signs and symptoms would alert the nurse to possible internal bleeding in a client who has undergone pulmonary lobectomy?
- ○ 1. Increased blood pressure and decreased pulse and respiratory rates.
- ○ 2. Sanguineous drainage from the chest tube at a rate of 50 ml per hour over the past 3 hours.
- ○ 3. Restlessness and shortness of breath.
- ○ 4. Urine output of 180 ml over the past 3 hours.

70. Which of the following is the most important aspect of pain management for the postoperative client following lobectomy?
- ○ 1. Repositioning the client immediately after administering pain medication.
- ○ 2. Reassessing the client 30 minutes after administering pain medication.
- ○ 3. Verbally reassuring the client after administering pain medication.
- ○ 4. Readjusting the pain medication dosage as needed according to the client's condition.

71. While assessing the incisional area from a lobectomy in which a chest tube exits, the nurse feels a crackling sensation under the fingertips along the entire incision. The nurse's first action should be to
- ○ 1. lower the head of the bed and call the physician.
- ○ 2. check the client's blood pressure and ready an aspiration tray.
- ○ 3. mark the area with a skin pencil at the outer periphery of the crackling.
- ○ 4. turn off the suction of the chest drainage system.

72. Which of the following statements contains one of the basic rules to follow when caring for a client with a chest tube and water-seal drainage system?
- ○ 1. Ensure that the air vent on the water-seal drainage system is capped when the suction is off.
- ○ 2. Strip the chest and drainage tubes at least every 4 hours if excessive bleeding occurs.
- ○ 3. Ensure that the collection and suction bottles are at the client's chest level at all times.
- ○ 4. Ensure that the collection and suction bottles are below the client's chest level at all times.

73. In an underwater-seal drainage system, cessation of fluid fluctuation in the chest and drainage tubes generally means that the
- ○ 1. lung has fully expanded.
- ○ 2. lung has collapsed.
- ○ 3. chest tube is in the pleural space.
- ○ 4. mediastinal space has decreased.

74. The nurse observes a constant gentle bubbling in the water-seal bottle of an underwater-seal chest drainage system. This observation should prompt the nurse to
- ○ 1. continue monitoring as usual; this is a normal observation.
- ○ 2. check the connectors between the chest and drainage tubes and where the drainage tube enters the collection bottle.
- ○ 3. decrease the suction to −15 cm H_2O or less and continue observing the system for changes in bubbling over the next several hours.
- ○ 4. drain half the water from the underwater-seal chamber.

75. A client who underwent a lobectomy and has an underwater-seal chest drainage system is breathing with a little more effort and at a faster rate than an hour ago. The client's pulse rate is also increased. Based on knowledge of the pathophysiology involved in a lobectomy and of chest tube function, the nurse should take which of the following actions?

○ 1. Check the tubing to ensure that the client is not lying on it or kinking it.
○ 2. Increase the suction.
○ 3. Lower the drainage bottles 2 to 3 feet below the level of the client's chest.
○ 4. Ensure that the chest tube has two clamps on it to prevent air leaks.

76. Which of the following findings would suggest pneumothorax in a trauma victim?

○ 1. Pronounced crackles.
○ 2. Inspiratory wheezing.
○ 3. Dullness on percussion.
○ 4. Absent breath sounds.

77. Oxygen toxicity results from oxygen concentrations above

○ 1. 21%.
○ 2. 24%.
○ 3. 40%.
○ 4. 60%.

78. For a client with rib fractures and pneumothorax, the physician prescribes morphine sulfate IV, 1 to 2 mg/hour as needed for pain. The primary objective of this order is to provide adequate pain control so the client can breathe effectively. Which of the following outcomes would indicate successful achievement of this objective?

○ 1. Patent chest tube.
○ 2. Decreased client anxiety.
○ 3. Respiratory rate of 26 breaths/minute.
○ 4. Normal arterial blood gas values.

79. A client undergoes surgery to repair lung injuries. Postoperative orders include the transfusion of one unit of packed red cells at a rate of 60 ml/hour. Approximately how long would this transfusion take?

○ 1. 2 hours.
○ 2. 4 hours.
○ 3. 6 hours.
○ 4. 8 hours.

80. The primary reason for infusing blood at a rate of 60 ml/hour is to help prevent

○ 1. emboli formation.
○ 2. pulmonary edema.
○ 3. red blood cell hemolysis.
○ 4. allergic reaction.

81. When teaching a client to cough effectively following a lobectomy, it would be best for the nurse to instruct the client to

○ 1. contract the abdominal muscles.
○ 2. swallow immediately before coughing.
○ 3. exert pressure with the hands on the voice box.
○ 4. hold the breath for a few seconds before coughing.

82. Which of the following items should be readily available at the bedside of a client with a chest tube in place?

○ 1. A tracheostomy tray.
○ 2. Another sterile chest tube.
○ 3. Rubber-capped hemostats.
○ 4. A spirometer.

83. On a client's fourth postoperative day following lung surgery, the nurse auscultates some scattered crackles bilaterally. Which of the following interventions would be most appropriate?

○ 1. Encourage coughing and check the water-seal system.
○ 2. Encourage deep breathing and coughing.
○ 3. Perform endotracheal suctioning once per shift and ask the physician to order an expectorant.
○ 4. Reduce the frequency of pain medication and increase the suction in the water-seal bottle.

84. Which of the following rehabilitative measures should the nurse instruct a client who has undergone chest surgery to perform to prevent a "frozen shoulder?"

○ 1. Turn from side to side.
○ 2. Raise and lower the head.
○ 3. Raise the arm on the affected side over the head.
○ 4. Flex and extend the elbow on the affected side.

85. On the fifth postoperative day following a lobectomy, the water level in the long glass tube in the chest drainage bottle stops fluctuating. The nurse would be justified in judging that the most probable cause for this is that the

○ 1. tubing is kinked.
○ 2. lung has reexpanded.
○ 3. water seal is leaking.
○ 4. tubing is blocked with mucus plugs.

86. A client's chest tube is to be removed by the physician. Which of the following items should the nurse have ready to be placed directly over the wound when the chest tube is removed?

○ 1. Butterfly dressing.
○ 2. Montgomery strap.
○ 3. Fine-mesh gauze dressing.
○ 4. Petrolatum gauze dressing.

87. Complications associated with a tracheostomy tube include

○ 1. decreased cardiac output.
○ 2. damage to the laryngeal nerve.
○ 3. pneumothorax.
○ 4. adult respiratory distress syndrome (ARDS).

88. A priority goal for the hospitalized client with a new tracheostomy would be to

○ 1. decrease secretions.
○ 2. instruct the client in caring for the tracheostomy.

○ 3. relieve anxiety related to the tracheostomy.
○ 4. maintain a patent airway.

89. Which of the following would be a priority nursing diagnosis category for a client with ARDS?
○ 1. Ineffective Breathing Patterns.
○ 2. Pain.
○ 3. Altered Health Maintenance.
○ 4. High Risk for Infection.

90. A characteristic finding in early ARDS is
○ 1. elevated carbon dioxide level.
○ 2. hypoxia refractory to oxygen therapy.
○ 3. metabolic acidosis.
○ 4. severe, unexplained electrolyte imbalance.

CORRECT ANSWERS AND RATIONALE

The letters in parentheses following the rationale identify the step of the nursing process (A, D, P, I, E); cognitive level (K, C, T, N); and client need (S, G, L, H). See the Answer Grid for the key.

The Client With Pneumonia

1. 1. The client described in this item is 79 years old; pneumonia most commonly strikes the elderly and debilitated. Arthritis, vegetarian diet, and cold water bathing are unlikely predisposing factors for pneumonia. (A, T, G)

2. 2. Fatigue from lack of sleep is a major problem for the client with pneumonia who has a productive cough. The hospital environment further contributes to interrupted sleep patterns. Myocardial damage and fluid volume deficit are not typically related to pneumonia. The client's history does not suggest impaired thought processes. (D, N, G)

3. 2. A sputum specimen is obtained for culture to determine the causative organism. After the organism is identified, an appropriate antibiotic can be prescribed. (I, T, S)

4. 1. The electrolyte lost in largest amounts through perspiration is sodium. This accounts for the salty taste of perspiration. (A, T, G)

5. 3. Frequent linen changes take priority for this client, because she has shared her concerns for feeling clean. Diaphoresis may produce general discomfort. Position changes need to be done every 2 hours. Nasotracheal suctioning is not indicated with the client's productive cough. Frequent offering of a bedpan is not indicated in this situation. (I, N, L)

6. 1. Pneumonia interferes with ventilation. It is essential to reduce the body's need for oxygen at the cellular level, and bedrest is the most effective method for doing so. (I, C, G)

The Client With Tuberculosis

7. 1. Tuberculosis typically produces anorexia and weight loss. Other signs and symptoms may include fatigue, afternoon fever, and night sweats. Dyspnea on exertion is not a common symptom of tuberculosis. (A, K, G)

8. 1. The most commonly used technique to identify tubercle bacilli is acid-fast staining. The bacilli have a very waxy surface, which makes them difficult to stain in the laboratory. But when stained, the colorization is very resistant to removal, even with acids. Therefore, tubercle bacilli are often called acid-fast bacilli. (A, C, S)

9. 1. Streptomycin is an aminoglycoside, and eighth cranial nerve damage is a common side effect of aminoglycosides. Common side effects of isoniazid (INH), aminosalicylic acid (PAC), and ethambutol hydrochloride (Myambutol) are peripheral neuritis, gastrointestinal intolerance, and optic neuritis, respectively. (I, C, G)

10. 1. The most common side effect of streptomycin is vertigo, resulting from damage to part of the eighth cranial nerve. Other symptoms of eighth cranial nerve toxicity include tinnitus, hearing loss, and ataxia. (E, T, G)

11. 3. It is essential that a client with tuberculosis takes medications exactly as prescribed. Sufficient rest, a nourishing diet, and clean air are important but do not rate the same high priority as drug therapy. (I, N, H)

The Client With Chronic Obstructive Pulmonary Disease (COPD)

12. 1. Fear, even when unfounded, can stand in the way of recovery. When this client expresses a fear of being in room 13 because he thinks the number would bring him bad luck, it would be best for the nurse to try to eliminate the reason for the client's fears. Refusing to move the client to another room fails to take the client's fears into account. Moving the client because superstitions have a good chance of coming true relies on an unproven phenomenon. A superstition becomes truth only on the basis of chance. (I, N, L)

13. 4. Relatively low concentrations of oxygen are administered to clients with COPD so as not to eliminate their respiratory drive. Carbon dioxide content in the blood normally regulates respirations. But clients with COPD are often accustomed to high carbon dioxide levels, and the low oxygen blood level is their stimulus to breathe. If they receive excessive oxygen and experience a drop in the blood carbon dioxide, they may stop breathing. (P, T, S)

14. 1. The client's problem is altered nutrition—specifically, less than he requires. The etiology, as stated by the client, is the fatigue associated with his disease process. Therefore, option 1 is the most specific nursing diagnosis, which leads the nurse directly to the nursing actions required. COPD is not an appropriate etiology, because nurses cannot treat the disease process. Altered Breathing Patterns may be a problem, but this diagnosis does not specifically address the problem described by the client. Additionally, Weight Loss as such is not a nursing diagnosis. (D, N, G)

15. 1. A client with COPD is subject to respiratory infections. COPD is slowly progressive; therefore, maintaining current status, requiring less supplemental oxygen, and showing permanent improvement are unrealistic expectations. (P, N, G)

16. 2. It is essential that the client understand ways to reduce the risk of infection and rehospitalization. Extracting promises from clients is not an outcome criterion. Fever is not an acceptable outcome criterion. Dyspnea on exertion is not necessarily an indication to call the physician, as the client may experience dyspnea on exertion frequently due to the disease. (E, N, G)

The Client With Lung Cancer

17. 4. Positioning on the side allows any vomitus to roll out by gravity, thereby reducing the risk of aspiration. A nasogastric tube is not placed after a bronchoscopy, because the gastrointestinal tract is not entered. Oral fluids are withheld until the gag and swallow reflexes return. Preoperative sedation and local anesthesia impair swallowing and the laryngeal reflex, which is protective in nature. The trachea can be perforated inadvertently, not the bowel; abdominal distention and rigidity would indicate bowel perforation. (I, N, G)

18. 4. Diminished vital capacity can lead to reduced oxygenation and contribute to postoperative complications. Normal weight does not affect postoperative nursing care. Although keeping feelings inside can be problematic, it probably would not be a major contributing factor in postoperative pulmonary complications. (A, T, G)

19. 1. Acknowledging the basic feeling that the client expressed and asking an open-ended question allows the client to explain her fears. The first option addresses the main feeling expressed—fear of cancer—and attempts to explore it further. The second option does not focus on the client's feelings; it rather, merely gives reassurance. The third option does not acknowledge the client's feelings at all. The fourth option assumes guilt, which might be present, but additional information is needed before taking further action. (I, N, L)

20. 2. Semi-Fowler's position allows for downward displacement of the diaphragm and relaxation of the abdominal muscles, which are needed for good ventilatory excursion. The hand placement supports the operative area and splints it without causing pain from pressure. Trendelenburg's position is contraindicated, because abdominal contents pushing against the diaphragm will decrease effective lung volume. Keeping the bed flat does not allow the diaphragm to descend. Positioning the client on the operative side prevents maximum inflation of the left lung, and placing the hands on the operative area before inhalation can restrict thoracic movement. (I, N, G)

21. 3. Pain causes the client to splint the thorax and makes it difficult to deep breathe and cough, thereby impairing gas exchange. The amount of suction applied to the intrapleural space is normal; its purpose is to reexpand the lung and reestablish normal negative intrapleural pressure. Anxiety does not typically impair gas exchange unless it is severe. Elderly clients over age 65 are at increased risk for impaired gas exchange. (D, N, G)

22. 1. These ABG values indicate good ventilation. Tachypnea and crackles are abnormal findings that may indicate impaired ventilation. Temperature within normal limits is not an outcome specific to the nursing diagnosis Impaired Gas Exchange. (E, N, G)

The Client With Chest Trauma

23. 2. Blunt chest trauma is of special concern in elderly clients with chronic conditions that may decrease vital capacity. Respiratory failure may develop more quickly in these clients. Although pain is distressing to the client and can increase anxiety and decrease respiratory effectiveness, pain control is secondary to maintaining effective respirations. Decreasing the client's anxiety is related to maintaining effective respirations. Maintaining adequate circulatory volume is also secondary to maintaining effective respirations. (P, N, G)

24. 4. Pneumothorax will cause a client to feel extremely short of breath. Semi- or high-Fowler's position will facilitate ventilation by the unaffected lung. A flat or reverse Trendelenburg's position places additional pressure on the chest and inhibits ventilation. Likewise, positioning the client on the unaffected side compromises the remaining functional lung. (I, T, G)

25. 2. The admission ABG values reveal respiratory acidosis and are consistent with a diagnosis of pneumothorax. The ABG values after chest tube insertion are returning to normal, indicating that treatment is effective. The respiratory acidosis would worsen from CO_2 retention if the client were experiencing an asthma attack. The client is not alkalotic, because the pH values are below 7.35. If the chest tubes were obstructed, the client's respiratory status would deteriorate. (E, N, G)

26. 3. Morphine sulfate depresses the respiratory center. Other adverse effects include hypotension, nausea, vomiting, and constipation. Morphine sulfate does not cause transient visual disturbances or inhibit mucus secretion. (A, T, G)

27. 1. Verbalizing feelings and concerns helps decrease anxiety and allows the family member to move on to understanding the current situation. Describing events or explaining equipment is appropriate when the person is not distraught and is ready to learn. Reassuring the family member does not allow verbalization of feelings and discounts the person's feelings. (I, N, L)

28. 4. The normal range for PaO_2 is 80 to 100 mm Hg. The client's current value is within normal limits, and no additional interventions are warranted. This ABG value suggests that the client's lung has remained adequately expanded following chest tube removal and that oxygen delivery to the tissues is adequate. (E, N, G)

29. 3. The recommended site for assessing temperature in a client with pneumonia who is coughing and having difficulty breathing is the rectum. The groin and axilla are usually used when the oral and rectal sites are contraindicated. (A, T, S)

30. 4. A client with pneumonia has a ventilation problem that causes poor blood oxygenation due to infection and lung congestion. This will cause the client to become cyanotic, because blood pumped from the lungs to the heart and thence to the general circulation is being poorly oxygenated. (A, T, G)

31. 3. Chest pain in pneumonia is generally caused by friction between the pleural layers. It is more severe on inspiration than expiration due to chest movement. (A, T, G)

32. 4. The pleuritic pain is triggered by chest movement and is particularly severe during coughing. (Splinting the chest wall will help reduce the discomfort of coughing.) Deep breathing is essential to prevent further atelectasis; an incentive spirometer facilitates effective deep breathing. (I, T, G)

33. 1. Aspirin is administered to clients with pneumonia because it is an analgesic that helps control pain and an antipyretic that helps reduce fever. It is also an anti-inflammatory agent that reduces inflammation. Additionally, it reduces blood platelet aggregation and may be used to help prevent clotting in clients prone to heart attacks and strokes. (I, T, G)

34. 2. Humidified air helps liquefy respiratory secretions, making them easier to raise and expectorate. Postural drainage, vibration and percussion of the chest wall, and coughing and deep breathing exercises may be helpful for respiratory hygiene but will not affect the nature of secretions. (I, T, G)

35. 3. Clients characteristically exhibit anxiety when hypoxia is present. Less frequently will they demonstrate anger, apathy, or aggression. (A, T, L)

36. 1. This client has a white blood cell count of 14,000/mm^3. Normal total white blood cell count is between 5,000 and 10,000/mm^3 in adults. Because this client's white blood cell count is elevated, the physician should be notified. Altering prescribed medication doses is not a nursing responsibility. Initiating isolation is not indicated. (I, T, S)

37. 1. Docusate sodium (Colace) is a stool softener that acts similarly to a detergent; that is, it allows fluid and fatty substances to enter the stool and soften it. (I, K, G)

38. 4. Annual influenza and pneumococcal vaccines are effective in reducing the recurrence of pneumonia. Dietary changes are not indicated. Antibiotic therapy for viral infections does not prevent bacterial infection. Prophylactic antibiotic therapy is not typically prescribed, because of the increasing prevalence of resistant bacterial strains. (P, N, H)

39. 2. Tubercle bacilli may be spread in various ways, most commonly by droplet nuclei carried in air currents. Droplet nuclei are residue of evaporated droplets containing the bacilli, which remain suspended and are circulated in the air. (I, T, S)

40. 1. Unclean hands are thought to spread most organisms. Many techniques can be used to help control the spread of organisms, such as having separate personal care items, using disposable equipment, and isolating persons known to be harboring disease-causing organisms—but the most important technique is washing the hands thoroughly and frequently. (I, K, S)

41. 4. Using a combination of antitubercular drugs slows the rate at which organisms develop resistance to the drugs. Combination therapy also appears to be more effective than single drug therapy. (P, T, G)

42. 2. Offering emotional support, teaching about the disease, coordinating agency services, and assessing environment are all part of care for clients with tuberculosis. However, ensuring that clients are well educated about the disease has the highest priority. (P, N, G)

43. 1. The appropriate technique for an intradermal injection includes holding the needle and syringe almost parallel to the client's skin, keeping the skin slightly taut when the needle is inserted, and inserting the needle with the bevel side up. The area into which an intradermal injection is made is not massaged. (I, N, S)

44. 4. Tuberculosis once affected primarily the young; currently, elderly and immunosuppressed persons are believed to be at higher risk. (A, T, H)

45. 3. Clients with newly positive skin tests are aggressively treated with isoniazid (INH) for approximately 9 months. Repeat skin testing should not be performed, and skin tests do not convert to negative once a positive response has been obtained. (P, N, H)

46. 2. A positive Mantoux skin test indicates that the client has had contact with tubercle bacilli. It does *not* mean that the client has active tuberculosis, nor that the client has developed a resistance to tubercle bacilli or a passive immunity to tuberculosis. (E, N, G)

47. 2. INH competes for the available vitamin B6 in the body and leaves the client at risk for developing neuropathies related to vitamin deficiency. Supplemental B6 is routinely prescribed. (P, T, G)

48. 3. INH interferes with the effectiveness of oral contraceptives, and female clients of childbearing age should be counseled to use an alternate form of birth control while taking the drug. (I, T, H)

49. 3. Tuberculosis can be controlled but never completely eradicated from the body. Periods of intense physical or emotional stress increase the likelihood of recurrence. (I, T, H)

50. 2. Statistics show that of the four geographic areas described in this item, most cases of tuberculosis are found in inner-core residential areas of large cities, where health and sanitation standards tend to be low. These city areas are also generally characterized by substandard housing and poverty. (A, K, S)

51. 1. Increased anterior–posterior chest diameter is characteristic of advanced COPD. Air is trapped in the overextended alveoli, and the ribs are fixed in an inspiratory position. The result is the typical barrel-chested appearance. Other physical changes associated with COPD include overly developed neck muscles, distended neck veins, and diminished chest excursion on respiration. (A, K, G)

52. 4. Cigarette smoking is a major risk factor for COPD. Other risk factors include exposure to environmental pollutants and chronic asthma. Insufficient protein intake and exposure to persons with respiratory infection do not increase the risk of COPD. (I, N, H)

53. 4. Pursed-lip breathing increases pressure within the alveoli and makes it easier to empty the air in the alveoli, thereby promoting carbon dioxide elimination. By decreasing the expiratory rate and helping the client relax, pursed-lip breathing helps the client learn to control the rate and depth of respiration. (I, T, G)

54. 2. Theophylline ethylenediamide (aminophylline) is a xanthine derivative that acts directly on bronchial smooth muscle to relax and dilate the bronchi and relieve bronchial constriction and spasms. When the drug exerts its primary desired effect, dyspnea and shortness of breath decrease. This drug neither reduces bronchial secretions nor decreases alveolar elasticity. It does increase strength of myocardial contractility, but this is not the action for which it is used. (P, T, G)

55. 4. Percussion helps loosen mucus. Deeper inhalation may sometimes result, but this is not the primary purpose of percussion. Percussion itself neither improves ciliary action nor propels secretions along respiratory passages. (I, C, S)

56. 3. The client's pH is acidotic, and $PaCO_2$ is grossly and dangerously elevated, indicating respiratory acidosis. The PaO_2 level has little direct bearing on acid–base status but is very important in evaluating the client's overall condition. (E, N, G)

57. 2. This $PaCO_2$ level indicates that the client is hypoventilating. Normal $PaCO_2$ levels are between 35 and 45 mm Hg. Alveolar hypoventilation occurs when the $PaCO_2$ level exceeds 50 mm Hg. (E, N, G)

58. 1. Normal PaO_2 level ranges between 80 and 100 mm Hg. This range drops with age; between ages 60 and 70, it is 70 to 80 mm Hg. When the PaO_2 value falls to 50 mm Hg, as described in this item, the nurse should be alert for signs of hypoxia and impending respiratory failure. (E, N, G)

59. 4. $PaCO_2$ of 80 mm Hg and PaO_2 of 50 mm Hg both signify acute respiratory failure. The nurse should anticipate aggressive treatment for the client, including endotracheal intubation and mechanical ventilation. More frequent chest physiotherapy and increased medication dosage would probably not be sufficient for this client. A client with these ABG values would not be physically able to learn breathing techniques. (E, N, G)

60. 2. The high $PaCO_2$ level causes flushing due to vasodilatation. The client becomes drowsy and lethargic because CO_2 has a depressant effect on the central nervous system. Restlessness, irritability, and anxiety are not common with a $PaCO_2$ level of 80 mm Hg. (A, T, G)

61. 2. In postural drainage, gravity helps move secretions from smaller to larger airways. Postural drainage is best used after percussion has loosened secretions. (I, T, S)

62. 2. Prolonged inactivity causes the body to excrete excessive calcium. This leads to breakdown of bone tissue; as a result the bones become brittle and fracture easily, a condition known as osteoporosis. (A, C, G)

63. 3. A fluid intake of 2 to 3 L/day, in the absence of cardiovascular or renal disease, helps liquefy bronchial secretions. A low-salt diet, continuous oxygen therapy, and a semi-sitting position will not help reduce the viscosity of mucus. (I, T, G)

64. 2. Exhaling normally requires less energy than inhaling. Therefore, lifting while exhaling saves energy and reduces perceived dyspnea. (I, T, H)

65. 2. Epidermoid cancer involving the larger bronchi is almost entirely associated with heavy cigarette smoking. The American Cancer Society reports that smoking is responsible for more than 80% of lung cancers in men and women. The prevalence of lung cancer is related to the duration and intensity of the smoking, so nurses can best prevent lung cancer by persuading clients to stop smoking. Chest x-rays aid detection of lung cancer; they do not prevent it. Exposure to asbestos has been implicated as a risk factor for lung cancer, but cigarette smoking is the major risk factor. (I, C, H)

66. 3. Atropine sulfate is an anticholinergic drug that decreases mucus secretions in the respiratory tract and dries the mucous membranes of the mouth, nose, pharynx, and bronchi. Atropine does not cause drowsiness; in large doses, it causes excitement and maniacal behavior. It causes the skin to become hot and dry and, in doses less than 0.5 mg, can cause bradycardia. Moderate to large doses cause tachycardia and palpitations. (I, T, G)

67. 1. Teaching the client deep breathing techniques before lung surgery reduces the risk of postoperative infection. Etiologies of surgery and lung cancer are not amenable to nursing intervention. Although altered nutrition may occur, it is not the primary problem for this client. Additionally, lobectomy is not a NANDA diagnosis. (D, N, G)

68. 4. Deep breathing helps prevent microatelectasis and pneumonitis and also helps force air and fluid out of the pleural space into the chest tubes. The diaphragm is the major muscle of respiration; deep breathing causes it to descend, thereby increasing the ventilating surface. More than half the ventilatory process is accomplished by the rise and fall of the diaphragm. Deep breathing increases blood flow to the lungs. The remaining lobe will naturally hyperinflate to fill the space created by the resected lobe. This is an expected phenomenon. (I, T, G)

69. 3. Restlessness indicates cerebral hypoxia due to decreased circulating volume. Shortness of breath occurs because blood collecting in the pleural space faster than suction can remove it prevents the lung from reexpanding. Increased blood pressure and decreased pulse and respiratory rates are classic late signs of increased intracranial pressure. Decreasing blood pressure and increasing pulse and respiratory rates occur with hypovolemic shock. Sanguineous drainage that changes to serosanguineous drainage at a rate less than 100 ml/hour is normal in the early postoperative period. Urine output of 180 ml over the past 3 hours indicates normal kidney perfusion. (A, N, G)

70. 2. It is essential that the nurse evaluates the effects of pain medication after the medication has had time to act. Although the other interventions are appropriate, reassessment is necessary to determine effectiveness and intervene if needed. (I, N, G)

71. 3. Subcutaneous emphysema is not an unusual finding, and it is not dangerous if confined. But progression can be serious, especially if the neck is involved; tracheotomy may be needed. If emphysema progresses noticeably in 1 hour, the physician should be notified. Lowering the head of the bed and assessing blood pressure will not arrest the progress or provide any further information. A tracheotomy tray, not an aspiration tray, would be useful if emphysema progresses to the neck. Emphysema may progress if the chest drainage system does not adequately remove air and fluid; therefore, the system would not be turned off. (I, N, G)

72. 4. The drainage apparatus is always kept *below* the client's chest level to prevent back flow of fluid into the pleural space. The air vent must always be open in the closed chest drainage system to allow air from the client to escape. Stripping a chest tube causes excessive negative intrapleural pressure and is not recommended. (I, T, G)

73. 1. Cessation of fluid fluctuation in the tubing can mean one of several things: the lung has fully expanded and negative intrapleural pressure has been reestablished; the chest tube is occluded; or the chest tube is not in the pleural space. Fluid fluctuation is due to the fact that during inspiration, intrapleural pressure exceeds the negative pressure generated in the water-seal system. Therefore, drainage moves toward the client. During expiration, the pleural pressure exceeds that generated in the water-seal system, and fluid moves away from the client. (A, C, S)

74. 2. There should never be constant bubbling in the water-seal bottle. Constant bubbling in the water-seal bottle indicates an air leak, which means that less negative pressure is being exerted on the pleural space. Decreasing the suction will not reduce the leak, nor will draining part of the water in the water-seal chamber. (I, T, G)

75. 1. Here there may be some obstruction to the flow of air and fluid out of the pleural space, causing air and fluid to collect and build up pressure. This prevents the remaining lung from reexpanding and can cause a mediastinal shift to the opposite side. Increasing the suction is not done without a physician's order. The normal position of the drainage bottles is 2 to 3 feet below chest level. Clamping the tubes obstructs the flow of air and fluid out of the pleural space. (I, T, G)

76. 4. Pneumothorax indicates that the lung has collapsed and is not functioning. The nurse will hear no sounds of air movement on auscultation. (A, C, G)

77. 3. Oxygen concentration greater than 40% has been found to cause oxygen toxicity in adults. (A, K, S)

78. 4. Normal ABG values are the best indicator of effective respiration and achievement of the stated nursing objective. Chest tube patency relates to the client's overall status but does not indicate successful achievement of the objective. Decreased anxiety is not related only to the stated objective; it could also be related to pain relief. Respiratory rate within normal limits is a factor in effective breathing, but ABG values indicate achievement of the objective. (E, N, G)

79. 2. One unit of packed red blood cells is approximately 250 ml. If the blood is delivered at a rate of 60 ml/hour, it will take about 4 hours to infuse the entire unit. (I, T, S)

80. 2. Too-rapid infusion of blood, or any intravenous fluid, is likely to cause pulmonary edema. Emboli formation, red cell hemolysis, and allergic reaction are not related to rapid infusion. (I, T, G)

81. 1. Contracting (pulling in) the abdominal muscles helps produce a forceful and productive cough. The client should cough after taking several short breaths followed by a deep breath. Such measures as swallowing before coughing, exerting pressure on the larynx, and holding the breath before coughing do not produce effective coughing. (I, T, G)

82. 3. Rubber-capped clamps should be readily available and in view when a client has chest drainage. In some institutions, the protocol to follow after accidental disconnection of a chest tube is to clamp the tube close to the client and notify the physician immediately. (P, C, S)

83. 2. Shallow breathing is a common problem after chest surgery due to the pain associated with deep breathing. Assisting the client to cough and deep breathe should clear the lungs regularly and effectively. There is no indication of malfunction in the water-seal system. Reducing pain medication would make effective coughing more difficult. Endotracheal suctioning is not indicated at this time. (I, T, G)

84. 3. A client who has undergone chest surgery should be taught to raise the arm on the affected side over the head to help prevent "frozen shoulder." This exercise helps restore normal shoulder movement, prevents stiffening of the shoulder joint, and improves muscle tone and power. (I, T, G)

85. 2. A fluctuating water level in the long glass tube of a closed chest drainage system is related to the client's inspirations and expirations. When the fluctuations stop on the fifth postoperative day for the client described in this item, the most probable cause is that the client's lung has reexpanded. Other possible reasons for fluid in the tubing to stop fluctuating include an obstruction or a dependent loop in the tube; but for this client, these are less likely causes. (E, N, G)

86. 4. Immediately after chest tube removal, a petrolatum gauze is placed over the wound and covered with a dry sterile dressing, serves as an airtight seal to prevent air leakage or air movement in either direction. Bandages or straps are not applied directly over wounds. Mesh gauze would allow air movement. (I, T, G)

87. 2. Tracheostomy tubes carry several potential complications, including laryngeal nerve damage, bleeding, and infection. They do not cause decreased cardiac output, pneumothorax, or ARDS. (A, C, G)

88. 4. The main goal for a client with a new tracheostomy is to maintain a patent airway. New tracheostomies frequently cause bleeding and excess secretions, and clients may require frequent suctioning to maintain patency. (P, N, G)

89. 1. Ineffective Breathing Pattern is a priority nursing diagnosis category for the client with ARDS. The massive shift of fluid from the capillaries to the alveoli, as well as the reduced surfactant, greatly increase the work of breathing. The lungs become stiff and noncompliant, and the client becomes severely hypoxic. (D, N, G)

90. 2. A hallmark of early ARDS is refractory hypoxemia. The client's PaO_2 level continues to fall, despite higher concentrations of administered oxygen. Elevated carbon dioxide levels and metabolic acidosis occur late in the disorder. Severe electrolyte imbalances are not indicators of ARDS. The client with ARDS usually requires endotracheal intubation and mechanical ventilation. (A, T, G)

THE NURSING CARE OF ADULTS WITH MEDICAL/SURGICAL HEALTH PROBLEMS

TEST 1: The Client With Respiratory Health Problems

Directions: Use this answer grid to determine areas of strength or need for further study.

Nursing Process

A = Assessment
D = Analysis, nursing diagnosis
P = Planning
I = Implementation
E = Evaluation

Cognitive Level

K = Knowledge
C = Comprehension
T = Application
N = Analysis

Client Needs

S = Safe, effective care environment
G = Physiological integrity
L = Psychosocial integrity
H = Health promotion/maintenance

		Nursing Process					Cognitive Level				Client Needs			
Question #	Answer #	A	D	P	I	E	K	C	T	N	S	G	L	H
1	1	A							T			G		
2	2		D							N		G		
3	2				I				T		S			
4	1	A							T			G		
5	3				I					N			L	
6	1				I			C				G		
7	1	A					K					G		
8	1	A						C			S			
9	1				I			C				G		
10	1					E			T			G		
11	3				I					N				H
12	1				I					N			L	
13	4			P					T		S			
14	1		D							N		G		
15	1			P						N		G		
16	2					E				N		G		
17	4				I					N		G		
18	4	A							T			G		
19	1				I					N			L	
20	2				I					N		G		
21	3		D							N		G		
22	1					E				N		G		
23	2			P						N		G		

ANSWER GRID: 1

NURSING PROCESS

A = Assessment
D = Analysis, nursing diagnosis
P = Planning
I = Implementation
E = Evaluation

COGNITIVE LEVEL

K = Knowledge
C = Comprehension
T = Application
N = Analysis

CLIENT NEEDS

S = Safe, effective care environment
G = Physiological integrity
L = Psychosocial integrity
H = Health promotion/maintenance

		Nursing Process					Cognitive Level				Client Needs			
Question #	Answer #	A	D	P	I	E	K	C	T	N	S	G	L	H
24	4				I				T			G		
25	2					E				N		G		
26	3	A							T			G		
27	1				I					N			L	
28	4					E				N		G		
29	3	A							T		S			
30	4	A							T			G		
31	3	A							T			G		
32	4				I				T			G		
33	1				I				T			G		
34	2				I				T			G		
35	3	A							T				L	
36	1				I				T		S			
37	1				I		K					G		
38	4			P						N				H
39	2				I				T		S			
40	1				I		K				S			
41	4			P					T			G		
42	2			P						N		G		
43	1				I					N	S			
44	4	A							T					H
45	3			P						N				H
46	2					E				N		G		
47	2			P					T			G		
48	3				I				T					H
49	3				I				T					H
50	2	A					K				S			
51	1	A					K					G		
52	4				I					N				H

ANSWER GRID: 2

NURSING PROCESS

A = Assessment
D = Analysis, nursing diagnosis
P = Planning
I = Implementation
E = Evaluation

COGNITIVE LEVEL

K = Knowledge
C = Comprehension
T = Application
N = Analysis

CLIENT NEEDS

S = Safe, effective care environment
G = Physiological integrity
L = Psychosocial integrity
H = Health promotion/maintenance

		Nursing Process					Cognitive Level				Client Needs			
Question #	Answer #	A	D	P	I	E	K	C	T	N	S	G	L	H
53	4				I				T			G		
54	2			P					T			G		
55	4				I			C			S			
56	3					E				N		G		
57	2					E				N		G		
58	1					E				N		G		
59	4					E				N		G		
60	2	A							T			G		
61	2				I				T		S			
62	2	A						C				G		
63	3				I				T			G		
64	2				I				T					H
65	2				I			C						H
66	3				I				T			G		
67	1		D							N		G		
68	4				I				T			G		
69	3	A								N		G		
70	2				I					N		G		
71	3				I					N		G		
72	4				I				T			G		
73	1	A						C			S			
74	2				I				T			G		
75	1				I				T			G		
76	4	A						C				G		
77	3	A					K				S			
78	4					E				N		G		
79	2				I				T		S			
80	2				I				T			G		
81	1				I				T			G		

ANSWER GRID: 3

NURSING PROCESS

A = Assessment
D = Analysis, nursing diagnosis
P = Planning
I = Implementation
E = Evaluation

COGNITIVE LEVEL

K = Knowledge
C = Comprehension
T = Application
N = Analysis

CLIENT NEEDS

S = Safe, effective care environment
G = Physiological integrity
L = Psychosocial integrity
H = Health promotion/maintenance

		Nursing Process					Cognitive Level				Client Needs			
Question #	Answer #	A	D	P	I	E	K	C	T	N	S	G	L	H
82	3			P				C			S			
83	2				I				T			G		
84	3				I				T			G		
85	2					E				N		G		
86	4				I				T			G		
87	2	A						C				G		
88	4			P						N		G		
89	1		D							N		G		
90	2	A							T			G		
Number Correct														
Number Possible	90	21	5	11	41	12	6	10	40	34	15	61	5	9
Percentage Correct														

Score Calculation:

To determine your **Percentage Correct**, divide the **Number Correct** by the **Number Possible**.

The Client With Cardiovascular Health Problems

Test 2

The Client With Myocardial Infarction
The Client With Congestive Heart Failure (CHF)
The Client With Valvular Heart Disease
The Client With Hypertension
The Client With Angina
General Questions
The Client With Pernicious Anemia
The Client With Hodgkin's Disease
The Client Requiring Cardiopulmonary Resuscitation
The Client in Shock
The Client With Anemia
The Clients Who Are Dying
General Questions
Correct Answers and Rationale

Select the one best answer and indicate your choice by filling in the circle with a pencil in front of the option.

The Client With Myocardial Infarction

A 60-year-old male client is admitted through the emergency department with crushing substernal chest pain that radiates to the shoulder, jaw, and left arm. He is attached to a bedside monitor, which indicates sinus tachycardia. The admitting diagnosis is acute myocardial infarction (MI). The client is extremely restless and frightened.

1. Immediate admission orders include oxygen by nasal cannula at 4 L/min, blood work, a chest x-ray, a 12-lead electrocardiogram (EKG), and 2 mg of morphine sulfate IV. Which intervention is priority and should be accomplished first?
- ○ 1. Administer the morphine.
- ○ 2. Obtain a 12-lead EKG.
- ○ 3. Obtain the blood work.
- ○ 4. Order the chest x-ray.

2. An intravenous infusion at a "keep open" rate would be ordered primarily to
- ○ 1. help keep him well hydrated.
- ○ 2. help keep him well nourished.
- ○ 3. prevent kidney failure.
- ○ 4. provide a route for emergency drugs.

3. If the client develops cardiogenic shock, which characteristic sign should the nurse expect to observe?
- ○ 1. Oliguria.
- ○ 2. Bradycardia.
- ○ 3. Elevated blood pressure.
- ○ 4. Fever.

4. The client continues to have episodic chest pain during the first 8 hours following admission, despite morphine sulfate administration. He is started on continuous intravenous nitroglycerin (Tridil) infusion. Essential nursing actions would include
- ○ 1. Obtaining an IV infusion pump for the medication.
- ○ 2. Monitoring blood pressure hourly.
- ○ 3. Monitoring urine output hourly.
- ○ 4. Obtaining serum potassium levels daily.

5. After one attack of pain, the client says to the nurse, "My father died of a heart attack when he was 60, and I suppose I will too." Which of the following responses by the nurse would be the most appropriate?

○ 1. "Tell me more about what you are feeling."
○ 2. "Are you thinking that you won't recover from this illness?"
○ 3. "You have a fine doctor. Everything will be all right soon, I'm sure."
○ 4. "Would you agree that this would be very unlikely?"

6. A priority nursing diagnosis during the first 24 hours following an MI is
○ 1. Impaired Gas Exchange.
○ 2. High Risk for Infection.
○ 3. Fluid Volume Deficit.
○ 4. Constipation.

The Client With Congestive Heart Failure (CHF)

A 69-year-old female client has a history of congestive heart failure (CHF). Her physician recently increased her daily digoxin (Lanoxin) and furosemide (Lasix) doses as her condition was deteriorating. Ten days ago, the client stopped taking all her medications, which she blamed for her frequent headaches. She is now admitted to the emergency department with CHF complicated by pulmonary edema. She is edematous and cyanotic, in acute respiratory distress, extremely anxious, and complaining of nausea.

7. The client receives morphine sulfate IV soon after admission. When evaluating the client's response to the morphine sulfate, the nurse should assess the morphine's effect on her
○ 1. nausea.
○ 2. crackles.
○ 3. cyanosis.
○ 4. anxiety.

8. In which of the following positions should the nurse place the client?
○ 1. Semi-sitting (low Fowler's position).
○ 2. Lying on her right side (Sims' position).
○ 3. Sitting nearly upright (high Fowler's position).
○ 4. Lying on her back with her head lowered (Trendelenburg's position).

9. The major goal of therapy for this client would be to
○ 1. increase cardiac output.
○ 2. improve respiratory status.
○ 3. decrease peripheral edema.
○ 4. enhance comfort.

10. Which of the following would be a priority nursing diagnosis for the client with CHF and pulmonary edema?
○ 1. High Risk for Infection related to stasis of secretions in alveoli.
○ 2. Impaired Skin Integrity related to edema and pressure.
○ 3. Activity Intolerance related to imbalance between oxygen supply and demand.
○ 4. Constipation related to immobility.

11. Digoxin (Lanoxin) is administered intravenously to this client, primarily because the drug acts to
○ 1. dilate coronary arteries.
○ 2. strengthen the heartbeat.
○ 3. decrease cardiac dysrhythmias.
○ 4. decrease electrical conductivity in the heart.

12. This client will require careful skin care, primarily because an edematous client is prone to develop
○ 1. itchy skin.
○ 2. decubitus ulcers.
○ 3. electrolyte imbalance.
○ 4. distention of weakened veins.

The Client With Valvular Heart Disease

An elderly female client is scheduled to undergo mitral valve replacement for severely calcific mitral stenosis and mitral regurgitation. Although the diagnosis was made during childhood, she had been asymptomatic until 4 years ago. Recently she noticed increased symptoms despite daily doses of digoxin (Lanoxin) and furosemide (Lasix).

13. During the initial interview with the client, the nurse would most likely learn that the client's childhood health history included
○ 1. scarlet fever.
○ 2. poliomyelitis.
○ 3. rheumatic fever.
○ 4. meningitis.

14. The client undergoes a mitral valve replacement. Postoperatively, she develops multiple premature ventricular contractions (PVCs). The physician orders lidocaine hydrochloride IV, with a 50 mg initial bolus followed by continuous infusion at 2 mg/min. The IV bag contains 2 g of lidocaine in 500 ml of dextrose 5% in water. If the equipment used for administering the drug and solution indicates that 60 microdrops are equal to 1 ml, how many microdrops would provide 2 mg of lidocaine each minute?
○ 1. 15 microdrops.
○ 2. 30 microdrops.
○ 3. 45 microdrops.
○ 4. 60 microdrops.

15. After the client experiences some initial excitation, the nurse would judge that she is demonstrating a typical toxic reaction to lidocaine hydrochloride when she complains of
○ 1. palpitations.
○ 2. tinnitus.
○ 3. urinary frequency.

○ 4. lethargy.

16. The physician orders pulmonary artery pressure monitoring including pulmonary capillary wedge pressure (PCWP) with a pulmonary artery catheter. The purpose of this is to help assess the
○ 1. degree of coronary artery stenosis.
○ 2. blood pressure within the right ventricle.
○ 3. pressure from fluid within the left ventricle.
○ 4. oxygen and carbon dioxide pressure in the blood.

17. As she recovers, the client asks the nurse to adjust the bed so that her knees will be supported in a flexed position and she does not "slide down" in bed. The nurse should explain that the position the client requests is contraindicated, primarily to avoid
○ 1. placing her feet in a dropped position.
○ 2. causing her knees to ankylose ("freeze").
○ 3. causing stagnation of blood in her legs and feet.
○ 4. placing pressure on nerves under her knees.

18. The client's chest tube accidentally disconnects from the drainage tube when she turns onto her side. Which of the following actions should the nurse take first?
○ 1. Notify the physician.
○ 2. Clamp the chest tube.
○ 3. Raise the level of the drainage bottle.
○ 4. Reconnect the tube.

The Client With Hypertension

An industrial health nurse at a large printing plant finds a male employee's blood pressure to be elevated on two occasions 1 month apart and refers him to his private physician. The employee is about 25 pounds overweight and has smoked a pack of cigarettes daily for over 20 years.

19. During a nursing assessment, the client says, "I don't really know why I'm here. I feel fine and haven't had any symptoms." The nurse would recognize the importance of explaining to the client that symptoms of hypertension
○ 1. are seldom present.
○ 2. signify a high risk of stroke.
○ 3. occur only with malignant hypertension.
○ 4. appear after irreversible kidney damage has occurred.

20. The industrial health nurse monitors the client's blood pressure as he begins therapy with methyldopa (Aldomet) and hydrochlorothiazine (HydroDIURIL). The nurse would know that the client must be monitored carefully during the first days of therapy because methyldopa frequently causes
○ 1. drowsiness and inability to concentrate.
○ 2. nausea and facial flushing.
○ 3. tremors and incoordination.
○ 4. hyperexcitability and aggression.

21. The nurse teaches the client about his dietary restrictions, a low-calorie, low-fat, low-sodium diet. Which of the following menu selections would best meet his needs?
○ 1. Mixed green salad with blue cheese dressing, crackers, and cold cuts.
○ 2. Ham sandwich on rye bread and an orange.
○ 3. Baked chicken, an apple, and a slice of white bread.
○ 4. Hot dogs, baked beans, and celery and carrot sticks.

22. The client's job involves working in a warm dry room, frequently bending and crouching to check the underside of a high-speed press, and wearing eye guards. Given this information, for which side effect of hydrochlorothiazide (HydroDIURIL) should the nurse monitor?
○ 1. Muscle aches.
○ 2. Thirst.
○ 3. Lethargy.
○ 4. Postural hypotension.

23. The client asks whether he should begin an exercise program. When teaching him about appropriate exercise, the nurse should emphasize which of the following instructions:
○ 1. Avoid acute exercise; it will increase the heart's workload to a dangerous level.
○ 2. Follow exercise sessions with soaks or steam baths to prevent muscle cramping.
○ 3. Perform isometric exercises to reduce the heart's workload and improve blood flow.
○ 4. Practice muscle pumping exercises for the legs when standing for prolonged periods.

24. The client realizes the importance of quitting smoking, and the nurse develops a plan to help him achieve his goal. Which of the following nursing interventions should be the initial step in this plan?
○ 1. Review the negative effects of smoking on the body.
○ 2. Discuss the effects of passive smoking on environmental pollution.
○ 3. Establish the client's daily smoking pattern.
○ 4. Explain how smoking worsens high blood pressure.

The Client With Angina

Over the past few months a middle-aged woman has felt brief twinges of chest pain while working in her garden and has had frequent episodes of indigestion. She comes to the hospital after experiencing severe anterior chest pain while raking leaves. Her workup confirms a diagnosis of stable angina pectoris.

25. The woman says, "I really thought I was having a heart attack. How can you tell the difference?" Which response by the nurse would provide the client with the most accurate information about the difference between the pain of angina and that of myocardial infarction?
- ○ 1. "The pain associated with a heart attack is much more severe."
- ○ 2. "The pain associated with a heart attack radiates into the jaw and down the left arm."
- ○ 3. "It is impossible to differentiate anginal pain from that of a heart attack without an EKG."
- ○ 4. "The pain of angina is usually relieved by resting or lying down."

26. Following stabilization and treatment, the client is discharged from the hospital. At her follow-up appointment, she is very discouraged because she is experiencing pain with increasing frequency. She states that she visits an invalid friend twice a week and now cannot walk up the second flight of steps to the friend's apartment without pain. Which measure that the nurse could suggest would most likely help the client deal with this problem?
- ○ 1. Visit her friend early in the day.
- ○ 2. Rest for at least an hour before climbing the stairs.
- ○ 3. Take a nitroglycerin tablet before climbing the stairs.
- ○ 4. Lie down once she reaches the friend's apartment.

27. Because of the client's angina pectoris, the nurse should advise her that it would be best for her to avoid weather that is
- ○ 1. dry and hot.
- ○ 2. cold and windy.
- ○ 3. rainy and windy.
- ○ 4. humid and warm.

28. The nurse should teach the client to immediately report which of the following symptoms to her physician?
- ○ 1. A change in the pattern of her pain.
- ○ 2. Pain during sexual activity.
- ○ 3. Pain during an argument with her husband.
- ○ 4. Absence of pain during or after an activity such as lawn-mowing.

29. The physician refers the client for a cardiac catheterization. What is the primary rationale for performing this test for this client?
- ○ 1. To open and dilate blocked coronary arteries.
- ○ 2. To assess the extent of arterial blockage.
- ○ 3. To bypass obstructed vessels.
- ○ 4. To assess the functional adequacy of the valves and heart muscle.

30. The client is scheduled for a percutaneous transluminal coronary angioplasty (PTCA) to treat her angina. Priority goals for the client immediately after PTCA would include
- ○ 1. minimizing dyspnea.
- ○ 2. maintaining adequate urine output.
- ○ 3. decreasing myocardial contractility.
- ○ 4. preventing fluid volume deficit.

General Questions

31. The pain associated with myocardial infarction is due to
- ○ 1. left ventricular overload.
- ○ 2. impending circulatory collapse.
- ○ 3. extracellular electrolyte imbalances.
- ○ 4. insufficient oxygen reaching the heart muscle.

32. Which of the following complications is responsible for the most deaths following acute myocardial infarction?
- ○ 1. Pulmonary embolism.
- ○ 2. Cardiac dysrhythmias.
- ○ 3. Severe anxiety.
- ○ 4. Ventricular septal rupture.

33. While caring for a client who has sustained a myocardial infarction, the nurse notes eight premature ventricular contractions (PVCs) in 1 minute on the cardiac monitor. The client is receiving an IV infusion of 5% dextrose in water and 2 L/minute of oxygen. The nurse's first course of action should be to
- ○ 1. increase the IV infusion rate.
- ○ 2. notify the physician promptly.
- ○ 3. increase the oxygen concentration.
- ○ 4. administer a prescribed analgesic.

34. Which of the following findings is indicative of myocardial infarction?
- ○ 1. Elevated serum cholesterol value.
- ○ 2. Elevated creatinine phosphokinase value.
- ○ 3. Below-normal erythrocyte sedimentation rate.
- ○ 4. Elevated white blood cell count.

35. Which of the following activities would be contraindicated for a client on the second day of hospitalization following a myocardial infarction?
- ○ 1. Filing her fingernails.
- ○ 2. Lying on her stomach for a backrub.
- ○ 3. Using the commode for a bowel movement.
- ○ 4. Reaching across her chest for the bedside table.

36. Nursing measures for the client who has had a myocardial infarction include helping her avoid activity that results in Valsalva's maneuver (bearing down against a closed glottis). Which of the following actions would help prevent Valsalva's maneuver? Have the client
- ○ 1. take fewer but deeper breaths.
- ○ 2. clench her teeth while moving in bed.
- ○ 3. drink fluids through a straw.
- ○ 4. avoid holding her breath during activity.

37. Expected outcomes following IV administration of furosemide (Lasix) include
- ○ 1. increased blood pressure.
- ○ 2. increased urine output.
- ○ 3. decreased pain.
- ○ 4. decreased PVCs.

38. Following a myocardial infarction, the hospitalized client is taught to move his legs about while resting in bed. This type of exercise is recommended primarily to help
- ○ 1. prepare the client for ambulation.
- ○ 2. promote urinary and intestinal elimination.
- ○ 3. prevent thrombophlebitis and blood clot formation.
- ○ 4. decrease the likelihood of decubitus ulcer formation.

39. Which of the following dietary instructions accurately reflects the principles on which a client's diet will most likely be based during the acute phase of myocardial infarction?
- ○ 1. Coffee and other liquids as desired.
- ○ 2. Small frequent feedings.
- ○ 3. Three meals daily that include high-fiber foods.
- ○ 4. Nothing by mouth.

40. A client whose condition remains stable after a myocardial infarction is gradually allowed increased activity. Of the following criteria, the best one on which to judge whether the activity is appropriate is to note the degree of
- ○ 1. edema.
- ○ 2. cyanosis.
- ○ 3. dyspnea.
- ○ 4. weight loss.

41. Which of the following activities would be least appropriate to prevent sensory deprivation during a client's stay in the cardiac care unit?
- ○ 1. Watching television.
- ○ 2. Visiting with her daughter.
- ○ 3. Reading the newspaper.
- ○ 4. Keeping her door closed to provide privacy.

42. Of the following factors, which appears most closely linked to the development of coronary artery disease?
- ○ 1. Diet.
- ○ 2. Climate.
- ○ 3. Air pollution.
- ○ 4. Excessive exercise.

43. A client loses 3.2 kg while hospitalized. How many pounds has the client lost? Approximately
- ○ 1. 1.5 lbs.
- ○ 2. 3 lbs.
- ○ 3. 5.25 lbs.
- ○ 4. 7 lbs.

44. A basic principle of any rehabilitation program, including cardiac rehabilitation, is that rehabilitation begins
- ○ 1. on discharge from the hospital.
- ○ 2. on discharge from the cardiac care unit.
- ○ 3. on admission to the hospital.
- ○ 4. four weeks after the onset of illness.

45. A client is discharged from the hospital following a myocardial infarction. The client is walking and is taught to continue walking gradually progressing distances. Which vital sign should the client be taught to monitor to determine whether to increase or decrease progression?
- ○ 1. Pulse rate.
- ○ 2. Blood pressure.
- ○ 3. Body temperature.
- ○ 4. Respiratory rate.

46. If a client displays behavior detrimental to health such as smoking cigarettes, eating a diet high in saturated fat, or leading a sedentary lifestyle, techniques of behavior modification may be used to help the client change behavior. The nurse can best reinforce new adaptive behaviors by
- ○ 1. explaining how the old behavior leads to poor health.
- ○ 2. withholding praise until the new behavior is well established.
- ○ 3. rewarding the client whenever the acceptable behavior is performed.
- ○ 4. discussing the advantages of developing healthful behavior.

47. Alteplase recombinant (TPA), a thrombolytic enzyme, is administered during the first 6 hours following onset of myocardial infarction to
- ○ 1. control chest pain.
- ○ 2. reduce coronary artery vasospasm.
- ○ 3. control the dysrhythmias associated with myocardial infarction.
- ○ 4. revascularize the blocked coronary artery.

48. A priority nursing assessment measure related to TPA administration is to
- ○ 1. observe for rebound chest pain.
- ○ 2. monitor for increased atrial dysrhythmias.
- ○ 3. monitor the 12-lead EKG every 4 hours.
- ○ 4. observe for signs of spontaneous bleeding.

49. Crackles heard on lung auscultation indicate
- ○ 1. pulmonary edema.
- ○ 2. bronchospasm.
- ○ 3. airway narrowing.
- ○ 4. fluid-filled alveoli.

50. The nurse can best evaluate the effectiveness of oxygen therapy in a client with congestive heart failure (CHF) by observing changes in the client's
- ○ 1. EKG.
- ○ 2. arterial blood gas values.
- ○ 3. central venous pressure.
- ○ 4. serum electrolyte values.

51. Enalapril maleate (Vasotec) is administered in con-

junction with digoxin (Lanoxin) and furosemide (Lasix) to a client with CHF. Enalapril maleate, an angiotensin-converting enzyme inhibitor, acts to improve cardiac output by
- ○ 1. reducing peripheral vascular resistance.
- ○ 2. increasing peripheral vascular resistance.
- ○ 3. reducing fluid volume.
- ○ 4. improving myocardial contractility.

52. Furosemide is administered intravenously to a client with CHF. How soon after IV administration begins should the nurse begin to see evidence of the drug's desired effect?
- ○ 1. 5 to 10 minutes.
- ○ 2. 30 minutes to 1 hour.
- ○ 3. 2 to 4 hours.
- ○ 4. 6 to 8 hours.

53. A client with CHF will take oral furosemide at home. To help the client evaluate the effectiveness of furosemide therapy, the nurse should teach the client to
- ○ 1. take a daily weight.
- ○ 2. take a daily blood pressure.
- ○ 3. take a urine specimen to the laboratory for analysis each week.
- ○ 4. have a specimen of arterial blood obtained each week for blood gas analysis.

54. The nurse teaches a client with CHF to take oral furosemide in the morning. The primary reason for this is to help
- ○ 1. decrease gastrointestinal irritation.
- ○ 2. retard rapid drug absorption.
- ○ 3. excrete fluids accumulated during the night.
- ○ 4. prevent sleep disturbances during the night.

55. Clients with CHF failure are prone to atrial fibrillation. During physical assessment, the nurse would suspect atrial fibrillation when palpation of the radial pulse revealed
- ○ 1. two regular beats followed by one irregular beat.
- ○ 2. an irregular pulse rhythm.
- ○ 3. pulse rate below 60 beats/minute.
- ○ 4. a weak, thready pulse.

56. Complications of atrial fibrillation occur due to
- ○ 1. stasis of blood in the atria.
- ○ 2. increased cardiac output.
- ○ 3. decreased pulse rate.
- ○ 4. elevated blood pressure.

57. Which of the following symptoms should cause the nurse to suspect that a client is experiencing digitalis toxicity?
- ○ 1. Skin rash.
- ○ 2. Constipation.
- ○ 3. Lightheadedness.
- ○ 4. Loss of appetite.

58. The nurse should be especially alert for signs and symptoms of digoxin toxicity if laboratory blood findings indicate that the client has a
- ○ 1. low sodium level.
- ○ 2. high glucose level.
- ○ 3. high calcium level.
- ○ 4. low potassium level.

59. Which of the following foods should the nurse teach the client with CHF to avoid or limit because of the prescribed moderate sodium-restricted diet?
- ○ 1. Apples.
- ○ 2. Tomatoes.
- ○ 3. Hard cheeses.
- ○ 4. Cornish game hen.

60. A client on a moderate sodium-restricted diet should be taught to avoid
- ○ 1. dill.
- ○ 2. wine.
- ○ 3. garlic.
- ○ 4. catsup.

61. To help maintain a normal blood level of potassium, the client on a sodium-restricted diet should be encouraged to eat such foods as bananas, orange juice,
- ○ 1. beans, and celery.
- ○ 2. tomatoes, and asparagus.
- ○ 3. and processed and soft cheeses.
- ○ 4. honeydew melon, and cantaloupe.

62. Which of the following best describes cardiogenic shock? The client experiences
- ○ 1. decreased cardiac output due to hypovolemia.
- ○ 2. shock due to decreased circulating blood volume.
- ○ 3. shock due to decreased myocardial contractility.
- ○ 4. decreased cardiac output due to infection.

63. Which of the following signs and symptoms would least likely be found in a client with combined mitral stenosis and regurgitation?
- ○ 1. Exertional dyspnea.
- ○ 2. Weight gain.
- ○ 3. Fatigue.
- ○ 4. Peripheral edema.

64. The nurse would expect that a client with mitral stenosis would likely demonstrate symptoms associated with congestion in the
- ○ 1. aorta.
- ○ 2. right atrium.
- ○ 3. superior vena cava.
- ○ 4. pulmonary circulation.

65. The client with mitral stenosis has been taking digoxin and furosemide and has been maintained on quinidine sulfate to control atrial dysrhythmias. What problem could the client experience from the quinidine?
- ○ 1. Constipation.
- ○ 2. Hypertension.

○ 3. Digoxin toxicity.
○ 4. Tachycardia.

66. Because a client has mitral stenosis and is a prospective valve recipient, the nurse preoperatively assesses the client's past compliance with medical regimens. Lack of compliance with which of the following regimens would pose the greatest health hazard to this client?
○ 1. Medication therapy.
○ 2. Diet modification.
○ 3. Activity restrictions.
○ 4. Life-style modifications.

67. In preparing a client and the client's family for a postoperative intensive care unit stay, the nurse should explain that
○ 1. the nurses working in the intensive care unit are too busy to answer questions.
○ 2. the client will sleep most of the time while in the intensive care unit.
○ 3. noise and activity within the intensive care unit are minimal.
○ 4. the client may experience transient disorientation and confusion.

68. A client who has undergone a mitral valve replacement experiences persistent bleeding from the surgical incision during the early postoperative period. Which of the following pharmaceutical agents should the nurse be prepared to administer to this client?
○ 1. Vitamin C.
○ 2. Protamine sulfate.
○ 3. Quinidine sulfate.
○ 4. Warfarin sodium (Coumadin).

69. Of the following aseptic practices the nurse should observe when changing a client's dressing after coronary artery bypass surgery, which is usually credited as being the most effective in helping prevent wound infection?
○ 1. Careful handwashing before beginning the procedure.
○ 2. Cleansing the incisional area with an antiseptic.
○ 3. Using prepackaged sterile dressings to cover the incision.
○ 4. Placing soiled dressings in a waterproof bag before disposing of them.

70. For a client who excretes excessive amounts of calcium during the postoperative period following open-heart surgery, which of the following measures should the nurse institute to help prevent complications associated with excessive calcium excretion?
○ 1. Ensure a liberal fluid intake.
○ 2. Provide an alkaline-ash diet.
○ 3. Prevent constipation.
○ 4. Enrich the client's diet with dairy products.

71. To prevent thromboembolic complications associated with mechanical valves, a client with a mechanical heart valve will be maintained indefinitely on warfarin sodium (Coumadin). When teaching the client about warfarin sodium therapy, the nurse should tell the client that
○ 1. partial thromboplastin time (PTT) values determine the dosage of warfarin sodium.
○ 2. protamine sulfate is used to reverse the effects of warfarin sodium.
○ 3. other medications and medical conditions can alter the anticoagulant effect of warfarin sodium.
○ 4. warfarin sodium is started after heparin is discontinued.

72. Good dental care is an important measure in reducing the risk of endocarditis. A teaching plan to promote good dental care in a client with mitral stenosis should include demonstrating the proper use of
○ 1. a manual toothbrush.
○ 2. an electric toothbrush.
○ 3. an irrigation device.
○ 4. dental floss.

73. Before a client's discharge after mitral valve replacement surgery, the nurse should evaluate the client's understanding of postcardiac surgery activity restrictions. Which of the following should the client not engage in until after the 1-month postdischarge appointment with the surgeon?
○ 1. Showering.
○ 2. Lifting anything heavier than 10 pounds.
○ 3. A program of gradual progressive walking.
○ 4. Light housework.

74. A priority goal for the client within 24 hours of insertion of a permanent pacemaker would be to
○ 1. maintain skin integrity.
○ 2. maintain cardiac conduction stability.
○ 3. decrease cardiac output.
○ 4. increase activity level.

75. Which of the following would be a priority nursing diagnosis to include in the discharge plan for a client who has a permanent pacemaker implanted 3 days ago?
○ 1. Self-Care Deficit related to activity restrictions.
○ 2. Immobility related to artificial pacemaker.
○ 3. Anxiety related to lack of knowledge about pacemaker.
○ 4. Ineffective Coping related to fear of pacemaker failure.

76. Essential hypertension would be diagnosed in a 40-year-old man whose blood pressure readings were consistently at or above
○ 1. 120/90 mm Hg.
○ 2. 130/85 mm Hg.
○ 3. 140/90 mm Hg.
○ 4. 160/80 mm Hg.

77. The nurse completes a thorough nursing history and physical examination for a man identified with hypertension by a screening program. The primary purpose of gathering this assessment data is to

○ 1. assess the person's ability to participate in various therapies, such as a stress-reduction class.
○ 2. complete the insurance forms and payment vouchers.
○ 3. develop a baseline for treatment evaluation.
○ 4. identify other current or potential health problems.

78. The plan of care for a client with hypertension taking propranolol hydrochloride (Inderal) would include

○ 1. instructing the client to discontinue the drug if nausea occurs and to monitor blood pressure.
○ 2. monitoring blood pressure every week and adjusting the medication dose accordingly.
○ 3. measuring partial thromboplastin time (PTT) weekly to evaluate blood clotting status.
○ 4. instructing the client to notify the physician of irregular or slowed pulse rate.

79. When teaching a client about propranolol hydrochloride (Inderal), the nurse should base the information on the knowledge that propranolol hydrochloride

○ 1. blocks beta-adrenergic stimulation and thus causes decreased heart rate, myocardial contractility, and conduction.
○ 2. increases norepinephrine secretion and thus decreases blood pressure and heart rate.
○ 3. is a potent arterial and venous vasodilator that reduces peripheral vascular resistance and lowers blood pressure.
○ 4. is an angiotensin-converting enzyme inhibitor that reduces blood pressure by blocking the conversion of angiotensin I to angiotensin II in the kidneys.

80. A priority nursing diagnostic category for the client with hypertension would be

○ 1. Pain.
○ 2. Fluid Volume Deficit.
○ 3. Impaired Skin Integrity.
○ 4. Altered Health Maintenance.

81. Nonpharmacological approaches to hypertension control that the nurse may be involved in teaching the client with hypertension include

○ 1. proper administration of antihypertensive agents.
○ 2. activity restrictions.
○ 3. low-potassium diet therapy.
○ 4. a regular exercise program.

82. The most important long-term goal for a client with hypertension would be to

○ 1. learn how to avoid stress.
○ 2. explore a job change or early retirement.
○ 3. make a commitment to long-term therapy.
○ 4. control high blood pressure.

83. A client with hypertension has been keeping the regularly scheduled appointments for follow-up blood pressure readings. Which of the following factors would best support the nurse's decision to increase the interval between the client's appointments?

○ 1. Regular attendance at stress-reduction classes.
○ 2. Client's scheduling preference.
○ 3. Consistently stable blood pressure.
○ 4. Being symptom-free for 2 consecutive months.

84. Which of the following are generally considered to be risk factors for the development of atherosclerosis?

○ 1. Family history of early myocardial infarction, hypertension, and anemia.
○ 2. Diabetes, smoking, and late onset of puberty.
○ 3. Male gender, total blood cholesterol level above 150 mg/dl, and low protein intake.
○ 4. Physical inactivity, hypertension, and diabetes.

85. Under age about 50 years, many more men than women suffer from coronary artery disease due to atherosclerosis. It is generally believed that this difference is due to the fact that women have

○ 1. life-styles with fewer stressors than men.
○ 2. higher blood levels of estrogen than men.
○ 3. life-styles with more activity and exercise than men.
○ 4. diets that result in lower blood cholesterol levels than men.

86. A client with angina asks the nurse, "What information does an EKG provide?" The nurse would respond that an EKG primarily gives information about the

○ 1. electrical conduction of the myocardium.
○ 2. oxygenation and perfusion of the heart.
○ 3. contractile status of the ventricles.
○ 4. physical integrity of the heart muscle.

87. As an initial step in treating a client with angina, the physician prescribes nitroglycerin tablets, 0.4 mg sublingually. This drug's principal effects are produced by

○ 1. antispasmodic effects on the pericardium.
○ 2. stimulation of alpha and beta receptor sites.
○ 3. vasodilatation of the peripheral vasculature.
○ 4. improved conductivity in the myocardium.

88. The nurse teaches the client with angina about the common expected side effects of nitroglycerin, including

○ 1. headache, hypotension, and dizziness.
○ 2. hypertension, flushing, and dizziness.
○ 3. hypotension, shock, and shortness of breath.
○ 4. stomach cramps, flushing, and dizziness.

89. Sublingual nitroglycerin tablets begin to work within

1 to 2 minutes. How should the nurse instruct the client to use the drug when chest pain occurs?

○ 1. Take one tablet every 2 to 5 minutes until the pain stops.
○ 2. Take one tablet and rest for 10 minutes. Call the physician if pain persists.
○ 3. Take one tablet, then an additional tablet every 5 minutes for a total of three tablets. Call the physician if pain persists.
○ 4. Take one tablet. If pain persists after 5 minutes, take two tablets. If pain still persists 5 minutes later, call the physician.

90. Which of the following points should the nurse include when instructing the client with angina about sublingual nitroglycerin?

○ 1. The drug will cause increased urine output.
○ 2. Store the tablets in a tight, light-resistant container.
○ 3. Use the tablets only when the pain is severe.
○ 4. The shelf life of nitroglycerin is long; it keeps for up to 2 years.

91. Nitroglycerin is also available in ointment or paste form. When applying nitroglycerin ointment, the nurse should be careful to

○ 1. massage it thoroughly into the skin.
○ 2. avoid getting it on her or his own skin.
○ 3. avoid the fumes from it.
○ 4. place it on approximately the same skin area with each application.

92. In explaining the procedure of coronary percutaneous transluminal coronary angioplasty (PTCA) to a client, the nurse should explain that the procedure involves

○ 1. opening a stenosed artery with an inflatable balloon-tipped catheter.
○ 2. increased blood clotting following the procedure.
○ 3. passing a catheter through the coronary arteries to find blocked arteries.
○ 4. inserting grafts to divert blood from blocked coronary arteries.

The Client With Pernicious Anemia

A 75-year-old female comes to the clinic for health care. Based on the symptoms the client reports, the nurse suspects that she may have pernicious anemia. The client is accompanied by her husband, an alert, 75-year-old retired teacher.

93. The nurse prepares the client for a gastric analysis as part of initial assessment. A typical laboratory finding of gastric analysis in a client with pernicious anemia is

○ 1. high bile concentration.
○ 2. absence of hydrochloric acid.
○ 3. low bicarbonate concentration.
○ 4. immature red blood cells.

94. The client is given radioactive B12 in water for a Shilling test. The primary purpose of this test is to measure the client's ability to

○ 1. store vitamin B12.
○ 2. digest vitamin B12.
○ 3. absorb vitamin B12.
○ 4. produce vitamin B12.

95. The client likely will suffer from the symptoms of vitamin B12 deficiency, even though she consumes normal amounts of food containing this vitamin. What is the reason for her vitamin deficiency?

○ 1. Inability to absorb the vitamin because her stomach is not producing sufficient acid.
○ 2. Inability to absorb the vitamin because the stomach is not producing sufficient intrinsic factor.
○ 3. Excessive excretion of the vitamin because of kidney dysfunction.
○ 4. Increased requirement for the vitamin because of rapid red blood cell production.

96. After starting therapy for pernicious anemia, the client asks the nurse how long it will be until she feels better. The nurse should explain that after treatment begins, relief of symptoms for most people with pernicious anemia who are free of complications occurs within

○ 1. hours.
○ 2. days.
○ 3. weeks.
○ 4. months.

97. The client's husband is taught to administer vitamin B12 injections to his wife, using the ventrogluteal site. Which of the following positions would most help to decrease the client's discomfort when her husband injects the vitamin B12. Having the client

○ 1. lie on her side with her legs extended.
○ 2. lie on her abdomen with her toes pointed inward.
○ 3. lean over the edge of a low table with her hips well flexed.
○ 4. stand upright with her feet comfortably apart.

98. The nurse teaches the client's husband to leave a small air bubble in the syringe before injecting the vitamin. The primary purpose of the bubble is to help

○ 1. relieve excessive pressure in the tissue.
○ 2. prevent medication from escaping from the tissue.
○ 3. disperse medication more extensively throughout the tissue.
○ 4. push the medication remaining in the needle into the tissue.

The Client With Hodgkin's Disease

A 47-year-old male client diagnosed with Hodgkin's disease is admitted to the hospital for staging. He is to undergo bone marrow biopsy.

99. The nurse assesses the client's nutritional status to be below adequate. Which of the following blood examinations would be most helpful in determining whether the client's diet contains inadequate protein?
- ○ 1. Red blood cell count.
- ○ 2. Bilirubin level.
- ○ 3. Reticulocyte count.
- ○ 4. Albumin level.

100. Three different chemotherapeutic agents are administered to the client. The nurse explains to the client that three drugs are given over an extended period because
- ○ 1. the second and third drugs increase the effectiveness of the first drug.
- ○ 2. the first two drugs destroy the cancer cells, and the third drug minimizes side effects.
- ○ 3. the three drugs can then be given in lower doses.
- ○ 4. the three drugs have a synergistic effect and different actions.

101. A priority nursing diagnostic category for a client receiving chemotherapy would be
- ○ 1. Fluid Volume Excess.
- ○ 2. Impaired Physical Mobility.
- ○ 3. Altered Nutrition: Less than Body Requirements.
- ○ 4. Altered Health Maintenance.

102. The client experiences episodes of severe nausea and vomiting, with more than 1,000 cc of emesis in 4 hours. The nurse's most appropriate action would be to
- ○ 1. notify the physician.
- ○ 2. maintain the client on a liquid diet.
- ○ 3. continue to monitor the client for another 4 hours.
- ○ 4. administer pain medication as ordered.

103. The chemotherapy is extremely toxic to bone marrow, and the client develops thrombocytopenia (low platelet count). The nurse would recognize that a priority goal of care would be to take precautions to control
- ○ 1. bleeding.
- ○ 2. diarrhea.
- ○ 3. infection.
- ○ 4. hypotension.

104. The client is placed in protective (reverse) isolation. When the nurse describes protective isolation to the family, which of the following statements would best describe the primary purpose? Protective isolation helps prevent the spread of organisms
- ○ 1. to the client from sources outside the client's environment.
- ○ 2. from the client to health care personnel, visitors, and other clients.
- ○ 3. by using special techniques to destroy discharges from the client's body.
- ○ 4. by using special techniques to handle the client's linen and personal items.

The Client Requiring Cardiopulmonary Resuscitation

A nurse is called to a neighbor's home after a 56-year-old man collapses. After quickly assessing the victim, the nurse determines that cardiopulmonary resuscitation (CPR) is necessary. The nurse instructs the man's wife to call the rescue squad.

105. The victim is lying in an upholstered reclining chair when the nurse arrives. Where should the nurse position him for CPR?
- ○ 1. On the sofa.
- ○ 2. On the floor.
- ○ 3. On the tipped-back reclining chair.
- ○ 4. On a mattress pulled onto the floor.

106. After positioning the victim, the nurse's next course of action should be to
- ○ 1. open his airway.
- ○ 2. elevate his head slightly.
- ○ 3. give him four quick breaths.
- ○ 4. administer 15 quick cardiac compressions.

107. The victim's teenage son tells the nurse that he knows CPR and can help. The nurse initiates external cardiac compressions while the son administers artificial ventilations. The nurse should administer cardiac compressions at which rate?
- ○ 1. 40 to 60 per minute.
- ○ 2. 50 to 70 per minute.
- ○ 3. 60 to 80 per minute.
- ○ 4. 80 to 100 per minute.

108. The victim is transported by ambulance to the hospital's emergency room, where the admitting nurse quickly assesses his condition. Of the following observations, the one most often recommended for determining the effectiveness of CPR is noting whether
- ○ 1. pulse rate is normal.
- ○ 2. pupils are reacting to light.
- ○ 3. mucous membranes are pink.
- ○ 4. systolic blood pressure is at least 80 mm Hg.

109. The client receives epinephrine (Adrenalin) in the emergency room. This drug is administered primarily because of its ability to
- ○ 1. dilate bronchioles.

○ 2. constrict arterioles.
○ 3. free glycogen from the liver.
○ 4. enhance myocardial contractility.

110. The client regains consciousness and is breathing spontaneously. He is confused and very anxious. Which of the following courses of action would likely give this client the most support while life-saving measures are being performed?
○ 1. Occasionally hold his hand firmly.
○ 2. Ask him if he knows why he is afraid.
○ 3. Remind him that his wife is in the waiting room.
○ 4. Tell him that he can help most by trying to relax.

The Client in Shock

A 47-year-old woman has had a gastric ulcer for years. After she started vomiting blood today, her neighbor drove her to the emergency room.

111. If the client had blood gases drawn while she was still in the early stage of shock, the nurse would expect the results to indicate
○ 1. respiratory alkalosis.
○ 2. respiratory acidosis.
○ 3. metabolic alkalosis.
○ 4. metabolic acidosis.

112. Fluid resuscitation is ordered for the client. Dextran 70 (Expandex) is started while blood is being typed and matched. A characteristic of this plasma substitute is that it
○ 1. can be administered only once.
○ 2. has no ability to carry oxygen.
○ 3. must be stored in a refrigerator.
○ 4. does not interfere with normal blood clotting.

113. The client receives an IV infusion of packed red blood cells and normal saline solution. Which of the following would be a priority assessment for the client receiving a blood product?
○ 1. Hypovolemia.
○ 2. Anaphylactic reaction.
○ 3. Pain.
○ 4. Altered level of consciousness.

114. The client does not respond adequately to fluid replacement, and an IV infusion of dopamine hydrochloride (Intropin) is started. Dopamine hydrochloride is frequently the drug of choice for treating shock primarily because it
○ 1. is a potent vasodilator.
○ 2. increases myocardial contractility.
○ 3. supports renal perfusion.
○ 4. has no serious side effects.

115. Which of the following would be an essential nursing action for the client receiving dopamine hydrochloride to treat shock?
○ 1. Administer pain medication concurrently.
○ 2. Monitor blood pressure continuously.
○ 3. Evaluate arterial blood gases at least every 2 hours.
○ 4. Monitor for signs of infection.

116. The client's condition stabilizes, but medical intervention fails to stop gastric bleeding. She is scheduled for surgery within the next 6 hours. The nurse ensures that the client is warm but not overheated and that the light in the room is lowered. The nurse gives the client and her family calm, simple answers to their questions about the surgery. What is the primary rationale behind these interventions?
○ 1. To stabilize fluid and electrolyte balance.
○ 2. To minimize oxygen consumption.
○ 3. To increase client and family comfort.
○ 4. To prevent infection.

117. The underlying pathophysiologic alteration in all types of shock is
○ 1. hemorrhage of blood or body fluids.
○ 2. decreased cardiac output.
○ 3. inadequate tissue perfusion.
○ 4. vasodilation of vascular beds.

118. A client is presumed to be in the early stages of hypovolemic shock. All of the following assessment findings indicate early shock except
○ 1. bradycardia.
○ 2. tachypnea.
○ 3. restlessness.
○ 4. cool, clammy skin.

119. If none of the following bed positions is contraindicated, which position would be preferred for the client with hypovolemic shock?
○ 1. Flat in bed.
○ 2. With the head of the bed elevated 45 degrees.
○ 3. Flat with the legs elevated.
○ 4. Flat with the feet elevated and the head below the level of the heart.

120. Which of the following would be the best indication that fluid replacement for the client in hypovolemic shock is adequate?
○ 1. Urine output greater than 30 ml/hour.
○ 2. Systolic blood pressure above 110 mm Hg.
○ 3. Diastolic blood pressure above 90 mm Hg.
○ 4. Urine output of 20 to 30 ml/hour.

121. When assessing a client for early septic shock, the nurse should observe for
○ 1. cool, clammy skin.
○ 2. warm, flushed skin.
○ 3. decreased systolic blood pressure.
○ 4. hemorrhage.

122. The nurse can contribute to preventing septic shock by
○ 1. administering IV fluid therapy replacement as ordered.

○ 2. obtaining vital signs every 4 hours for all clients.
○ 3. monitoring red blood cell counts for elevation.
○ 4. maintaining sterility of indwelling urinary catheters.

The Client With Anemia

123. In relation to the toxic effects of vitamin B12, the nurse should teach the client with pernicious anemia that
○ 1. this vitamin is remarkably free of toxicity.
○ 2. ringing in the ears is a common symptom of toxicity.
○ 3. nausea and vomiting are common symptoms of toxicity.
○ 4. skin rashes and itching are common symptoms of toxicity.

124. A priority nursing problem for a client with iron deficiency anemia would be
○ 1. fluid volume excess.
○ 2. nausea.
○ 3. activity intolerance.
○ 4. immobility.

125. The client with iron deficiency anemia should be instructed to eat which of the following foods high in iron, if it is not contraindicated for other medical reasons?
○ 1. Eggs.
○ 2. Lettuce.
○ 3. Citrus fruits.
○ 4. Cheese.

126. From which of the following foods does the body normally obtain the best supply of vitamin B12?
○ 1. Fresh fruits.
○ 2. Green leafy vegetables.
○ 3. Meats and dairy products.
○ 4. Whole-wheat breads and cereals.

127. A client's Hodgkin's disease was diagnosed early in its course. Which of the following symptoms most likely caused the client to seek health care?
○ 1. Difficulty swallowing.
○ 2. Swollen cervical lymph nodes.
○ 3. Difficulty breathing.
○ 4. A feeling of fullness over the liver.

128. Hodgkin's disease typically affects persons in which of the following age groups?
○ 1. Children (age 6 to 12).
○ 2. Teenagers (age 13 to 20).
○ 3. Young adults (age 21 to 40).
○ 4. Older adults (age 41 to 50).

129. The process of staging Hodgkin's disease provides health care personnel with information useful for all of the following purposes except
○ 1. prescribing therapy.
○ 2. determining the extent of the disease.
○ 3. estimating the activity of the disease.
○ 4. identifying the cell causing the disease.

130. The nurse could anticipate that a bone marrow specimen for a client with Hodgkin's disease most likely will be obtained from the sternum or
○ 1. rib.
○ 2. femur.
○ 3. vertebra.
○ 4. iliac crest.

131. A client with Hodgkin's disease is readmitted to the hospital frequently with exacerbations that prove to be resistant to the aggressive treatment protocol. The client is finally readmitted as death appears imminent. The nurse should be aware that one of the greatest emotional problems that hospitalized terminally ill clients face is
○ 1. fear of pain.
○ 2. fear of further therapy.
○ 3. feelings of isolation.
○ 4. feelings of social inadequacy.

The Clients Who Are Dying

132. Which of the following statements best explains the common observation that health care personnel avoid terminally ill persons?
○ 1. The family members who are present can provide essential care.
○ 2. Health care personnel do not understand their own feelings about death and dying.
○ 3. The dying person requires minimal physical care to be comfortable.
○ 4. It is best to avoid interrupting the person, to protect his right to die with dignity.

133. The nurse caring for a dying client would conclude that the client has accepted impending death from which remark?
○ 1. "I've done all the talking that needs to be done."
○ 2. "I really don't think you're trying to help me anymore."
○ 3. "I'm too young to die, but I guess I have no choice in the matter."
○ 4. "I wish I were well enough to spend one more night with my friends."

134. A terminally ill client slips into a coma. In offering sound advice to the client's family, the nurse explains that the last of the senses to lapse into unconsciousness is thought to be
○ 1. smell.
○ 2. sight.
○ 3. touch.
○ 4. hearing.

135. When the wife of a terminally ill client expresses her anger, the nurse's best response would be to

- ○ 1. offer to call a relative or friend to come be with her.
- ○ 2. remain with her and listen to what she is saying.
- ○ 3. leave her alone so that she can work through her emotions in private.
- ○ 4. explain that everything possible was done for her husband.

General Questions

136. What is the compression-ventilation ratio for two-rescuer cardiopulmonary resuscitation (CPR)?
- ○ 1. 4:2.
- ○ 2. 5:1.
- ○ 3. 5:2.
- ○ 4. 6:3.

137. During CPR, the xiphoid process at the lower end of the sternum should not be deeply compressed when performing external cardiac compression, because of the danger of lacerating the victim's
- ○ 1. lung.
- ○ 2. liver.
- ○ 3. stomach.
- ○ 4. diaphragm.

138. When performing external chest compressions on an adult during CPR, the nurse should depress the sternum
- ○ 1. ½″ to 1″.
- ○ 2. 1″ to 1-½″.
- ○ 3. 1-½″ to 2″.
- ○ 4. 2″ to 2-½″.

139. During CPR, the victim's pulse should be checked at regular intervals using the
- ○ 1. radial artery.
- ○ 2. celiac artery.
- ○ 3. carotid artery.
- ○ 4. brachial artery.

140. If the victim's chest wall fails to rise with each inflation when rescue breathing is administered during CPR, the most likely reason is that the
- ○ 1. airway is not clear.
- ○ 2. victim is beyond resuscitation.
- ○ 3. inflations are being given at too rapid a rate.
- ○ 4. rescuer is using inadequate force for cardiac massage.

141. During rescue breathing in CPR, the victim will exhale by
- ○ 1. normal relaxation of the chest.
- ○ 2. gentle pressure of the rescuer's hand on the upper chest.
- ○ 3. the pressure of cardiac compressions.
- ○ 4. turning the head to the side.

142. What is the estimated maximum time a person can be without cardiopulmonary functioning and still not experience permanent brain damage?
- ○ 1. 1 to 2 minutes.
- ○ 2. 4 to 6 minutes.
- ○ 3. 8 to 10 minutes.
- ○ 4. 12 to 15 minutes.

143. The nurse would know to administer the Heimlich maneuver on a suspected choking victim when the victim
- ○ 1. becomes cyanotic.
- ○ 2. cannot speak due to airway obstruction.
- ○ 3. can make only minimal vocal noises.
- ○ 4. is coughing vigorously.

144. When can the rescuer discontinue CPR?
- ○ 1. When it becomes clear the victim will not recover.
- ○ 2. After 15 minutes of unsuccessful CPR.
- ○ 3. When the rescuer becomes exhausted.
- ○ 4. After 30 minutes of unsuccessful CPR.

CORRECT ANSWERS AND RATIONALE

The letters in parentheses following the rationale identify the step of the nursing process (A, D, P, I, E); cognitive level (K, C, T, N); and client need (S, G, L, H). See the Answer Grid for the key.

The Client With Myocardial Infarction

1. 1. Although obtaining the EKG, chest x-ray, and blood work are all important, the nurse's priority action should be to relieve the crushing chest pain. Thus, administering morphine sulfate is the priority action. (I, T, G)

2. 4. The client with myocardial infarction may develop complications, such as cardiac dysrhythmias, that require prompt intervention. An open IV line allows rapid administration of various agents as needed. (I, T, G)

3. 1. Pulmonary crackles occur as fluid shifts from the intravascular space to the alveoli. Typical signs of cardiogenic shock include low blood pressure, rapid and weak pulse, decreased urine output, and signs of diminished blood flow to the brain, such as confusion and restlessness. Cardiogenic shock is a serious complication of a myocardial infarction, with a mortality rate approaching 90%. (A, T, G)

4. 1. IV nitroglycerin infusion requires an infusion pump for precise control of the medication. Blood pressure monitoring would be done with a continuous system. Hourly urine outputs are not always required for this client. Obtaining serum potassium levels is not associated with nitroglycerin infusion. (I, N, G)

5. 1. When a client makes a comment about their death, it is best for the nurse to help the client express their feelings. Asking a question that requires no more than a "yes" or "no" answer is unlikely to elicit how the client really feels and offers the client no support. Cliches such as "everything will be all right soon" are not helpful because they ignore the client's feelings. Trying to explain away the client's feelings will also be of no help to the client and ignores the way the client feels. (I, T, L)

6. 1. Impaired Gas Exchange related to poor oxygenation and dysrhythmias is a major problem immediately following MI. Therapy is directed toward improving cardiac output and decreasing myocardial workload. High Risk for Infection, Fluid Volume Deficit, and Constipation are not priority problems during the first 24 hours. (D, N, G)

The Client With Congestive Heart Failure

7. 4. Morphine sulfate is given to help alleviate the anxiety common in clients suffering from acute pulmonary edema and associated distress. The drug does not affect nausea, crackles, or cyanosis. (A, T, G)

8. 3. Sitting nearly upright in bed with the feet and legs resting on the mattress decreases venous return to the heart, thus reducing myocardial workload. Also, the sitting position allows maximum space for lung expansion. (I, T, G)

9. 1. Increasing cardiac output is the main goal of therapy for the client with congestive heart failure (CHF) or pulmonary edema. Pulmonary edema is an acute medical emergency requiring immediate intervention. In the client with CHF or pulmonary edema, improved respiratory status will occur when cardiac output is improved. Peripheral edema is not typically associated with pulmonary edema. Comfort will be improved when cardiac output increases to an acceptable level. (P, N, G)

10. 3. Activity intolerance is a primary problem for clients with CHF and pulmonary edema. Clients frequently complain of dyspnea and fatigue. (D, N, G)

11. 2. Digoxin (Lanoxin) is a cardiac glycoside used to help strengthen myocardial contractions and increase output of blood from the left ventricle. As a result, there is less blood shifting from the capillaries into the alveoli. Although digoxin does decrease the electrical conductivity of the myocardium and is used to treat atrial fibrillation, these are not primary reasons for its use in clients with CHF and pulmonary edema. Digoxin does not dilate coronary arteries. (P, T, G)

12. 2. Edematous areas are subject to decubitus ulcers because of interference with the proper blood supply to the skin and underlying tissues. The primary cause of decubitus ulcers is unrelieved pressure over an area, which results in poor oxygenation of cells. (D, N, G)

The Client With Valvular Heart Disease

13. 3. Most clients with mitral stenosis have a history of rheumatic fever or bacterial endocarditis. Such infectious diseases as scarlet fever, poliomyelitis, and meningococcal meningitis are not associated with mitral stenosis. (A, T, G)

14. 2. The solution to this problem is as follows:

$$2 \text{ grams} = 2{,}000 \text{ mg}$$

$$2{,}000 \text{ mg:500ml::2mg:}x \text{ ml}$$

$$2{,}000\, x = 1{,}000$$

$$x = \frac{1{,}000}{2{,}000} = .5 \text{ ml of solution/minute}$$

$$.5 \text{ ml} \times 60 \text{ (microdrops)} = 30 \text{ microdrops/minute.}$$

(I, T, S)

15. 2. The desired effect of lidocaine hydrochloride is to depress automaticity in the His–Purkinje fibers and elevate the stimulation threshold in the ventricles, thereby decreasing ectopic ventricular beats. Common adverse effects of lidocaine hydrochloride include dizziness, tinnitus, blurred vision, tremors, numbness and tingling of extremities, excessive perspiration, hypotension, convulsions, and finally coma may occur. Cardiac effects include slowed conduction and cardiac arrest. (E, T, G)

16. 3. The pulmonary artery pressures are used to assess the heart's ability to receive and pump blood. Pulmonary capillary wedge pressure (PCWP) reflects the left ventricular end diastolic pressure and guides the physician in determining fluid management for clients. Degree of coronary artery stenosis is assessed during a cardiac catheterization. (P, T, G)

17. 3. Every effort should be made to prevent stagnation of blood in the lower extremities during the postoperative period. Having the knees flexed by using a gatched bed or by placing pillows under the knees in the popliteal area promotes stagnation of blood and is contraindicated. If the client wants some support near the knees while lying on her back or while in Fowler's position, a small roll or small pillow may be placed under the lower thigh just above the knees. This placement prevents interference with circulation in the legs. (I, T, G)

18. 2. When a chest tube becomes disconnected, the nurse should take immediate steps to prevent air from entering the chest cavity, which may cause the lung to collapse. Therefore, when a chest tube is accidentally disconnected from the drainage tube, the nurse should either double-clamp the chest tube as close to the client as possible or place the open end of the tube in a container of sterile water or saline solution. Then the physician should be notified. The specific course of action depends on institutional policy and each nurse should be aware of the policy within their institution. (I, T, G)

The Client With Hypertension

19. 1. Most people with hypertension are completely asymptomatic and may continue to be so even with dangerous elevations in blood pressure. Therefore, the presence or absence of symptoms is not an accurate reflection of a person's status. Symptoms are not directly related to the status of the kidney. The severity of the hypertension, rather than the presence of absence of symptoms, determines the risk of complications such as stroke. (I, T, G)

20. 1. Methyldopa (Aldomet) commonly produces drowsiness and an inability to concentrate during the first days of therapy or whenever the dosage is adjusted. These effects can be extremely dangerous for persons who drive or operate machinery and must be closely monitored for. (E, T, G)

21. 3. Processed and cured meat products such as cold cuts, ham, and hot dogs are all high in both fat and sodium and should be avoided on a low-calorie, low-fat, low-salt diet. Dietary restrictions of all types are complex and difficult to implement with clients who are basically asymptomatic. (I, T, H)

22. 4. Possible dizziness from postural hypotension when rising from a crouched or bent position increases the client's risk of being injured by the equipment. The nurse should assess the client's blood pressure in all three positions (lying, sitting, and standing) at all routine visits. The other adverse effects listed could also cause complications in the work environment, but are not as potentially dangerous as postural hypotension. (A, T, G)

23. 4. A regular exercise program will be prescribed for the client to aid weight control and improve cardiac fitness. The program will be initiated slowly to avoid heart damage. Isometric exercises increase muscle tone but do not improve aerobic fitness. Postural hypotension is an ongoing problem that requires muscle pump exercises for standing. Steam baths should be avoided, because they can induce hypotensive fainting and injury. (I, T, H)

24. 3. A plan to reduce or stop smoking begins with establishing the client's personal daily smoking pattern and activities associated with smoking. It is important that the client understand the associated health risks, but this knowledge has not been shown to successfully help clients change their smoking behavior. (I, T, H)

The Client With Angina

25. 4. The characteristic of anginal pain that helps differentiate it from the pain of a heart attack is transient and usually alleviated by resting and/or lying down. However, in unstable angina there is increasing frequency, intensity, or duration of pain. Anginal pain is not always less severe than that of a myocardial infarction, and it may radiate down the arm or into the jaw. (I, C, G)

26. 3. Nitroglycerin may be used prophylactically before stressful physical activities such as stair-climbing to help the client remain pain-free. Resting before or after an activity is not as likely to help prevent an activity-related pain episode. (I, N, G)

27. 2. Cold weather tends to aggravate angina pectoris. Dry, warm, or humid weather has not been noted to affect the condition. (I, T, G)

28. 1. A change in the pattern of chest pain is an essential sign that the client should be instructed to report. It may indicate myocardial deterioration. Pain occurring during stress or sexual activity would not be unexpected. (I, T, G)

29. 2. Cardiac catheterization is done in clients with angina primarily to assess the extent and severity of the coronary artery blockage. A decision about medical management, angioplasty, or coronary artery bypass surgery will be based on the catheterization results. (P, T, G)

30. 4. Because the contrast medium used in PTCA acts as an osmotic diuretic, the client may experience diuresis with resultant fluid volume deficit after the procedure. Additionally, potassium levels must be closely monitored for decreases. Increased myocardial contractility would be a goal, not decreased contractility. Dyspnea would not be anticipated after this procedure. (P, T, G)

General Questions

31. 4. A myocardial infarction interferes with or blocks blood circulation to the heart muscle. This causes ischemia, or poor myocardial oxygenation, producing the characteristic pain. (A, C, G)

32. 2. From 40% to 50% of deaths following an acute myocardial infarction are due to dysrhythmias. Signs and symptoms should be reported promptly when noted. The most common lethal dysrhythmia is premature ventricular contractions (PVCs). Pulmonary embolism may occur, but it is more readily preventable than life-threatening dysrhythmias. Interventricular septal rupture is a rare complication and almost always fatal. Severe anxiety is not attributed as being a cause of death. (E, T, G)

33. 2. Premature ventricular contractions (PVCs) are often a precursor of life-threatening ventricular tachycardia and fibrillations. An occasional PVC is not considered dangerous, but if PVCs occur at a rate greater than five or six a minute, the physician should be notified promptly. More than six PVCs per minute is considered serious, and usually calls for decreasing ventricular irritability by administering lidocaine hydrochloride. (I, T, G)

34. 2. Common laboratory findings in the client who has suffered a myocardial infarction include elevated creatinine phosphokinase (CPK) level. CPK is the first of three enzymes to rise in response to myocardial damage; levels peak within the first 24 hours after myocardial damage. CPK is also released during muscle injury and brain injury. The CPK isoenzyme of CPK-MB elevates only in response to myocardial damage. The other two enzymes that elevate in response to myocardial injury, but after CPK, are lactic dehydrogenase (LDH) and serum glutamic oxaloacetic transaminase (SGOT). White blood cell count and erythrocyte sedimentation rate are typically elevated but not diagnostic for MI. Serum cholesterol level can predict possible risk for MI but is not a diagnostic tool for MI. (A, T, G)

35. 4. Activities that place strain on the heart must be curtailed for the client recovering from a myocardial infarction. Reaching is one such activity and should be avoided. Filing fingernails and lying prone are not necessarily contraindicated. The use of a commode has been found to require less energy and is less fatiguing than using a bedpan. The commode also allows the client to assume a position that promotes elimination. (I, T, G)

36. 4. Bearing down against a closed glottis can best be prevented by instructing the client to avoid holding her breath during activity. For example, the client should avoid bearing down when having a bowel movement, vomiting, coughing, or moving around in bed by exhaling during activity. Valsalva's maneuver may cause a change in the heartbeat, with cardiac dysrhythmias, increased venous pressure, increased intrathoracic pressure, and thrombi dislodgement. Valsalva's maneuver is not prevented by such activities as taking deep breaths (unless they are taken through the mouth), clenching the teeth, or taking fluids through a drinking tube. (I, T, G)

37. 2. Furosemide (Lasix) is a loop diuretic that acts to increase urine output. It does not increase blood pressure, decrease pain, or decrease dysrhythmias. (E, T, G)

38. 3. Exercise helps prevent stasis of blood, which predisposes to thrombophlebitis and blood clot formation. (I, T, H)

39. 2. Recommended dietary principles in the acute phase of myocardial infarction include avoiding myocardial stimulants, such as caffeine; avoiding large meals, because small frequent feedings are better tolerated; and avoiding foods that contribute to constipation. Fluids are given according to the client's needs, and salt restrictions may be prescribed, especially for clients with manifestations of heart failure. (P, T, G)

40. 3. Physical activity is gradually increased following a myocardial infarction while the client is still hospitalized and through a period of rehabilitation. Activity progression requires adjustments if the client has suffered complications, however. One of the recommended ways to evaluate progression of activity is to determine how activity affects the client's degree of fatigue. The client is becoming fatigued and progressing too rapidly if activity causes dyspnea, chest pain, a rapid heartbeat, or feelings of tiredness. When any of these symptoms appear, the client should reduce activity and progress more slowly. (E, T, G)

41. 4. Keeping the client's door closed is likely to contribute to feelings of isolation and sensory deprivation. Such activities as watching television, visiting with a relative, and reading a newspaper help prevent sensory deprivation and do not require physical effort. (I, T, L)

42. 1. Among environmental factors, diet appears most closely linked to coronary heart disease. (A, T, G)

43. 4. There are 2.2 lbs per kg; $3.2 \times 2.2 = 7.04$ lbs. (A, T, G)

44. 3. A basic principle of rehabilitation, including cardiac rehabilitation, is that rehabilitation begins on hospital admission. Early rehabilitation is essential to promote maximum functional ability as the client recovers from an illness. (P, K, S)

45. 1. Clients who continue on a progressive exercise program at home after suffering myocardial infarction should be taught to monitor pulse rate. The pulse rate can be expected to increase with exercise, but exercise should not be increased if pulse rate increases more than about 25 beats/minute from baseline or exceeds 100 to 125 beats/minute. Clients should also be taught to decrease exercise if chest pain or dyspnea occurs. (I, T, H)

46. 3. A basic principle of behavior modification is that behavior that is learned and continued is behavior that has been rewarded. Other reinforcement techniques have not been found to be as effective as reward. (I, T, H)

47. 4. Alteplase recombinant (TPA), a thrombolytic agent administered IV, lyses the clot blocking the coronary artery. The drug is most effective when administered within the first 6 hours following onset of myocardial infarction. (I, T, G)

48. 4. Spontaneous bleeding, such as gastrointestinal bleeding, cerebral hemorrhage, or bruising, is an adverse effect of thrombolytic therapy. Additionally, clients who receive alteplace recombinant (TPA) also receive heparin to prevent closure of the previously obstructed artery. Careful assessment for signs of bleeding, as well as monitoring of partial thromboplastin time (PTT), is essential to detect complications. (A, T, G)

49. 4. Crackles (previously called rales), are auscultated over fluid-filled alveoli. Wheezes are heard when airway narrowing occurs, as with bronchospasm. Pulmonary edema is a medical emergency. Crackles may occur without pulmonary edema. (A, N, G)

50. 2. Oxygen is administered to a client with congestive heart failure to help overcome hypoxia and dyspnea. The best way to evaluate the effectiveness of oxygen therapy is to observe changes in arterial blood gas values. This is most often done by determining the pressure of oxygen dissolved in the blood (PaO_2). When the PaO_2 is high, hemoglobin is carrying large amounts of oxygen, and oxygen therapy should cause the PaO_2 to increase. When the PaO_2 is low, the client has hypoxia. (E, T, G)

51. 1. Angiotensin-converting enzyme (ACE) inhibitors such as enalapril maleate act to decrease levels of angiotensin II, a potent vasoconstrictor. By reducing peripheral vascular resistance, blood pressure is lowered. (P, C, G)

52. 1. After IV injection of furosemide (Lasix), diuresis normally begins in about 5 minutes and reaches its peak within about 30 minutes. Medication effects last 2 to 4 hours. When furosemide is given intramuscularly or orally, drug action begins more slowly and lasts longer than when it is given intravenously. (E, T, G)

53. 1. Monitoring daily weights will help determine the effectiveness of diuretic therapy. A client who gains weight without diet changes most probably is retaining fluids, and the diuretic therapy should be adjusted. Blood pressure monitoring, urinalysis, and arterial blood gas analysis are not used to determine the effectiveness of diuretic therapy. (I, T, G)

54. 4. When diuretics are given early in the day, the client's need to void more frequently will not disturb nighttime sleep. (I, T, G)

55. 2. Characteristics of atrial fibrillation include pulse rate greater than 100 beats/minute, totally irregular rhythm, and no definite P waves on the EKG. During assessment, the nurse is likely to note the irregular rate and should report it to the physician. (A, T, G)

56. 1. Atrial fibrillation occurs when the SA node no longer functions as the heart's pacemaker and impulses are initiated at sites within the atria. Because conduction through the atria is disturbed, atrial contractions are reduced and stasis of blood in the atria occurs, predisposing to emboli. Some estimates predict that 30% of clients with atrial fibrillation will develop emboli. (E, T, G)

57. 4. Anorexia, nausea, and vomiting are common affects of digitalis toxicity. Anorexia and nausea are often the client's first complaints. Other signs of toxicity include dysrhythmias such as atrial fibrillation or bradycardia, seeing yellow spots or colored vision, and diarrhea. (E, T, G)

58. 4. A low serum potassium level predisposes to digoxin toxicity. Thus, the nurse should be especially alert for signs and symptoms of toxicity if the client's blood findings reveal hypokalemia. Because potassium inhibits cardiac excitability, a low serum potassium level increases cardiac excitability. (I, T, G)

59. 3. Hard (processed) cheeses are high in sodium and should be avoided or limited in a diet with moderate sodium restriction. Apples, tomatoes, and Cornish game hens are very low in sodium. (I, T, G)

60. 4. Catsup contains much salt and should not be included in a diet for a client with sodium restrictions. Various herbs, except celery leaves and seeds, may be used; wine and lemon juice are other satisfactory seasoning agents. (I, T, G)

61. 4. Foods rich in potassium include bananas, orange juice, honeydew melon, cantaloupe, and watermelons. Other good sources of potassium are grapefruit juice, nectarines, potatoes, canned tomato juice, dried prunes, raisins, figs, and spinach. (I, T, G)

62. 3. Cardiogenic shock occurs when myocardial contractility diminishes and cardiac output greatly decreases. Cardiogenic shock does not result from hypovolemia; in fact, the circulating blood volume is within normal limits or increased in cardiogenic shock. Infection is not a direct cause of cardiogenic shock. (A, C, G)

63. 2. Although weight gain may signal acute fluid retention and worsening heart failure, weight loss and cachexia more commonly occur in clients with long-standing mitral stenosis and regurgitation. The rise in left atrial pressure that accompanies mitral valve disease is transmitted backward to the pulmonary veins, capillaries, and arterioles, and eventually to the right ventricle. Signs and symptoms of pulmonary and systemic venous congestion follow. (A, T, G)

64. 4. When mitral stenosis is present, the left atrium has difficulty emptying its contents into the left ventricle. Hence, because there is no valve to prevent backward flow into the pulmonary vein, the pulmonary circulation is under pressure. Functioning of the aorta, the right atrium, and the superior vena cava are not immediately influenced by mitral stenosis. (A, T, G)

65. 3. Quinidine sulfate may cause elevated serum digoxin levels. Furosemide (Lasix) may induce hypokalemia, which sensitizes the myocardium to digoxin toxicity. Quinidine sulfate may cause diarrhea and hypotension. Both quinidine sulfate and digoxin (Lanoxin) slow the heart rate. (A, T, G)

66. 1. Preoperatively, anticoagulants may be prescribed for the client with advanced valvular heart disease to prevent emboli. Postoperatively, all clients with mechanical valves, and some clients with bioprostheses, are maintained indefinitely on anticoagulant therapy. Adhering strictly to a dosage schedule and observing specific precautions are necessary to prevent hemorrhage or thromboembolism. Some clients are maintained on life-long antibiotic prophylaxis to prevent recurrence of rheumatic fever. Episodic prophylaxis is required to prevent infective endocarditis following dental procedures or instrumentation or upper respiratory, gastrointestinal, or genitourinary tract surgery. (A, T, G)

67. 4. Altered level of consciousness, including hallucinations, confusion, delusions, depression, excitement, and disorientation, are common after cardiac surgery. Sensory deprivation and overload, high noise levels, and disrupted sleep and rest patterns are some environmental factors implicated in postcardiotomy delirium. Restricting the number of visitors and the amount of time they spend with the client may be necessary to promote sufficient rest. (I, T, S)

68. 2. Protamine sulfate is used to help combat persistent bleeding in a client who has had open-heart surgery. Warfarin sodium (Coumadin) is an anticoagulant, as is heparin, and these two agents would tend to cause the client to bleed even more. Vitamin C and quinidine sulfate do not influence blood clotting. (I, T, G)

69. 1. Many factors help prevent wound infections, including washing hands carefully, using sterile prepackaged supplies and equipment, cleansing the incisional area well, and disposing of soiled dressings properly. However, most authorities say that the single most effective measure in preventing wound infections is to wash the hands carefully before and after changing dressings. Careful handwashing is also important in helping reduce other infections often acquired in hospitals, such as urinary tract and respiratory system infections. (I, T, S)

70. 1. In an immobilized client, calcium leaves the bone and concentrates in the extracellular fluid. When a large amount of calcium passes through the kidneys, calcium can precipitate and form calculi. Nursing interventions that help prevent calculi include ensuring a liberal fluid intake, unless contraindicated; providing a diet rich in acid to keep the urine acid, which increases the solubility of calcium; and limiting foods rich in calcium, such as dairy products. (I, T, S)

71. 3. Hepatic disease, heart failure, vitamin K deficiency, and broad-spectrum antibiotic therapy are only a few of the factors that may increase the effects of warfarin sodium (Coumadin). The drug's anticoagulant action may be decreased by vitamin K, antacids, and many other preparations. Warfarin sodium dosage is determined by prothrombin time (PT) determinations. Because it takes 36 to 72 hours to obtain peak effects, warfarin sodium is usually begun while the client is still receiving heparin. Fresh frozen plasma or vitamin K is used to reverse warfarin sodium's anticoagulant effect. (I, T, H)

72. 1. Daily dental care and frequent checkups by a dentist who is informed about the client's condition are required to maintain good oral health. Using an irrigation device, an electric toothbrush, or dental floss may cause gums to bleed and allow bacteria to enter mucous membranes and the bloodstream, increasing the risk of endocarditis. (I, T, H)

73. 2. Most cardiac surgical clients have median sternotomy incisions, which take about 3 months to heal.

Measures that promote healing include avoiding heavy lifting, performing muscle reconditioning exercises, and using caution when driving. Showering or bathing is allowed as long as the incision is well approximated with no open areas or drainage. Activities should gradually be resumed on discharge. (I, T, G)

74. 2. Maintaining cardiac conduction stability and preventing dysrhythmias is a priority immediately following artificial pacemaker implantation. The client should have continuous EKG monitoring until proper pacemaker function is verified. (P, N, G)

75. 3. Education is a major component of the discharge plan for a client with an artificial pacemaker. Failure to educate the client about how to evaluate pacemaker function can contribute to anxiety and fear. The client needs to learn how to assess pulse rate, when to notify the physician of possible pacemaker malfunction, and when battery changes are needed. Generally, activity restrictions are not required, and immobility is not necessary several days after implantation. (D, N, G)

76. 3. American Heart Association standards define hypertension as a consistent systolic blood pressure level above 140 mm Hg and a consistent diastolic blood pressure level above 90 mm Hg. (A, T, G)

77. 3. Establishing a baseline for treatment evaluation is essential for the nurse monitoring and evaluating the client's progress. Completing insurance forms is secondary to successful treatment. Identifying other problems is a nonspecific reason to gather client history and physical examination data. The data gathered will eventually be used to determine the client's ability to participate in various treatment options. (A, T, G)

78. 4. Propranolol hydrochloride (Inderal) is a beta-adrenergic blocking agent used to treat hypertension. In addition to lowering blood pressure by blocking sympathetic nervous system stimulation, the drug lowers the heart rate. Therefore, the client should be assessed for bradycardia and other dysrhythmias. The client needs to be instructed to not discontinue medication, as sudden withdrawal of propranolol hydrochloride may cause rebound hypertension. Propranolol dosage is not typically adjusted based on weekly blood pressure readings or PTT values. (I, T, G)

79. 1. Actions of propranolol hydrochloride (Inderal) include reducing heart rate, decreasing myocardial contractility, and slowing conduction. (I, T, G)

80. 4. Managing hypertension is a priority for the client with hypertension. Clients with hypertension frequently do not experience other signs and symptoms such as pain, fluid volume deficit, or altered skin integrity. It is this asymptomatic nature that makes hypertension so difficult to treat, since clients may not recognize they are hypertensive or may not perceive the need for aggressive management of the hypertension. (D, N, H)

81. 4. A regular exercise program is a nonpharmacologic approach that aids weight management, an essential component of hypertension control. Activity restrictions are not commonly part of therapy for persons with hypertension. A low-sodium rather than low-potassium diet may be adjunct therapy. Proper administration of antihypertensive agents is a pharmacologic approach. (I, N, H)

82. 3. Compliance is the most critical element of hypertension therapy. Most hypertensive clients require life-long treatment and cannot be managed successfully without drug therapy. Stress and weight management are important components of hypertension therapy, but the priority goal is related to compliance. (P, N, H)

83. 3. Recording actual blood pressure readings is the only accurate way to monitor hypertension. Client compliance is critical in management but is not the only measure of effectiveness. The nurse should consider a client's preference about the monitoring schedule, but the client's physical status is the major factor that determines the schedule. (E, T, S)

84. 4. Risk factors for atherosclerosis include cigarette smoking, hypertension, high blood cholesterol level, male gender, family history of atherosclerosis, diabetes, obesity, and physical inactivity. (A, K, G)

85. 2. It is generally agreed, and increasing evidence supports the theory, that estrogen helps protect females from atherosclerotic changes. Such factors as differing life-styles, exercise and activity levels, and diets have not been found to be significant in determining why more men than women under age 50 have coronary heart disease. Recently, much attention has focused on the lack of research studies dealing with cardiac disease in women and minorities, and work is underway to gain a better understanding of cardiac disease in these populations. (A, K, G)

86. 1. An EKG directly reflects the transmission of electrical cardiac impulses through the heart. This information makes it possible to evaluate indirectly the functional status of the heart muscle and the contractile response of the ventricles. However, these elements are not measured directly. (I, T, S)

87. 3. Nitroglycerin produces peripheral vasodilation, which reduces myocardial oxygen consumption and demand. Vasodilation in coronary arteries and collateral vessels may also increase blood flow to the ischemic areas of the heart. Nitroglycerin affects neither alpha nor beta receptors. It does not affect pericardial spasticity or myocardial conductivity. (I, T, G)

88. 1. Because of its widespread vasodilating effects,

nitroglycerin often produces such side effects as headache, hypotension, and dizziness. The client should sit or lie down to avoid fainting. Nitroglycerin does not cause shortness of breath or stomach cramps. (I, T, G)

89. 3. The correct protocol for nitroglycerin use involves immediate administration with subsequent doses taken at 5-minute intervals as needed, for a total dose of three tablets. Sublingual nitroglycerin appears in the bloodstream within 2 to 3 minutes and is metabolized within approximately 10 minutes. (I, T, G)

90. 2. Clients should be instructed to keep nitroglycerin in a tightly closed, dark container and to replenish it frequently because it deteriorates rather rapidly. Clients should be instructed to use nitroglycerin at the first indication of chest pain and not wait before using the drug. (I, T, G)

91. 2. When applying nitroglycerin ointment to a client's skin, the nurse should be very careful to avoid getting any ointment on her or his own skin. The nurse can absorb the nitroglycerin through the skin and receive medication in the bloodstream the same way the client does. No dangerous fumes arise from the ointment. The ointment should not be massaged into the skin, and application sites should be rotated to avoid irritating the skin in one area. (I, T, S)

92. 1. Percutaneous transluminal coronary angioplasty (PTCA) is best described as insertion of a balloon-tipped catheter into the coronary artery to compress a plaque and thereby open a stenosed artery. PTCA does not directly affect blood clotting mechanisms, even though the client may receive heparin after the procedure to reduce the incidence of recurring obstruction. Inserting grafts to divert blood from blocked arteries describes coronary artery bypass graft surgery. (P, T, G)

The Client With Pernicious Anemia

93. 2. Clients with pernicious anemia demonstrate a lack of hydrochloric acid in gastric secretions. (A, T, S)

94. 3. Pernicious anemia is caused by the body's inability to absorb vitamin B12. This results from a lack of intrinsic factor in the gastric juices. The Shilling test helps diagnose pernicious anemia by determining the client's ability to absorb vitamin B12. (A, C, G)

95. 2. Most clients with pernicious anemia have deficient production of intrinsic factor in the stomach. Intrinsic factor attaches to the vitamin in the stomach and forms of complex that allows the vitamin to be absorbed in the small intestine. (A, N, G)

96. 2. Dramatically quick recovery from symptoms has been observed in clients with pernicious anemia, even those who are very ill, after treatment is initiated. However, symptoms due to permanently damaged tissues will not be relieved. (I, T, G)

97. 2. To promote comfort when injecting at the ventrogluteal site, the position of choice is the client lying on the abdomen with the toes pointing inward. This positioning promotes muscle relaxation, which in turn decreases the discomfort of making an injection into a tense muscle. (I, T, G)

98. 4. Injecting a small air bubble after the medication when giving an intramuscular injection pushes any medication remaining in the needle into muscle tissue. (I, K, S)

The Client With Hodgkin's Disease

99. 4. Serum albumin levels help determine whether protein intake is sufficient. Proteins are broken down into amino acids during digestion. Amino acids are absorbed in the small intestine, and albumin is built from amino acids. (A, T, G)

100. 4. Three chemotherapeutic drugs are given over a period of time. Multiple drug regimens are used because when given in combination, the drugs have a synergistic effect. Additionally, drugs that have different cycles, different actions, and different toxic side effects are given in combination to enhance therapy. (I, T, G)

101. 3. A common priority problem of chemotherapy is Altered Nutrition: Less than Body Requirements related to nausea and vomiting. Aggressive management is indicated for the client to prevent the nutritional deficit from becoming severe. Fluid Volume Deficit is more typical than Fluid Volume Excess. Impaired Physical Mobility and Altered Health Maintenance are not necessarily problems encountered during chemotherapy. (D, N, G)

102. 1. The nurse should notify the physician of extreme amounts of emesis as further treatment may be warranted. Administering pain medication is important but will not relieve the nausea and vomiting. Placing the client on a liquid diet is the physician's decision. (I, N, G)

103. 1. Thrombocytopenia is a low platelet count that leaves the client at risk for potentially life-threatening spontaneous hemorrhage. (I, T, G)

104. 1. The primary purpose of protective (reverse) isolation is to reduce transmission of organisms to the client from sources outside the client's environment. (I, T, G)

The Client Requiring Cardiopulmonary Resuscitation

105. 2. A victim requiring CPR should be placed flat on his back on a firm surface. If the victim is placed on a surface with "give," such as a mattress or sofa, the nurse's efforts to apply sufficient pressure to compress the heart will be ineffective. In a hospital, it is usual to slip a board under a client who is in bed before administering CPR. (I, T, S)

106. 1. The ABCs of CPR are carried out in sequence. The "A" stands for airway, which should be opened *first* by lifting the jaw forward. Any obvious debris in the mouth, such as loosened dentures, should be removed. CPR cannot work unless the airway is open so the victim can receive air. The "B" stands for breathing, and the "C" stands for circulation. Rescue breathing and cardiac compression, if necessary, follow immediately after the airway is opened. (I, T, G)

107. 4. The external cardiac compression rate for two-rescuer CPR is 80 to 100/minute to ensure adequate oxygenation. (I, T, G)

108. 2. Pupillary reaction is the best indication of whether oxygenated blood is reaching the client's brain. Pupils that remain widely dilated and do not react to light likely indicate that serious brain damage has occurred. (A, T, G)

109. 4. Epinephrine is administered during CPR primarily for its ability to improve cardiac activity. Epinephrine has great affinity for adrenergic receptors in cardiac tissue and acts to strengthen and speed the heart rate, as well as increase impulse conduction from atria to ventricles. Epinephrine will constrict arterioles, but this is not the primary reason for administering it during CPR. (I, T, G)

110. 1. Communicating by touch, such as holding hands, is often an effective way to offer the client emotional support. Asking the client why he is fearful, telling him a family member is nearby, and instructing him to relax offer little emotional support to the client in distress. (I, T, L)

The Client in Shock

111. 1. As a compensatory measure in the early stage of shock, the client hyperventilates in response to hypoxemia. Hyperventilation is an attempt to provide more oxygen to the tissues in the face of a decreased circulating volume. It increases minute volume and results in decreased $PaCO_2$, while PaO_2 remains normal. This is the classic picture of respiratory alkalosis. Metabolic acidosis and respiratory acidosis occur in the advanced stage of shock. (A, N, G)

112. 2. A plasma expander such as Dextran 70 (Expandex) cannot carry oxygen. It can be stored without refrigeration and used repeatedly as needed. It can coat blood platelets and interfere with normal blood clotting. Dextran 40 has a lower molecular weight. It does not interfere with blood clotting but is less effective as a volume expander. (I, T, G)

113. 2. The client receiving a blood product requires astute assessment for signs and symptoms of allergic reaction and anaphylaxis, including pruritus (itching), urticaria (hives), facial or glottal edema, and shortness of breath. If such a reaction occurs, the nurse should stop the transfusion immediately and notify the physician. Usually an antihistamine, such as diphenhydramine hydrochloride (Benadryl), is administered. Epinephrine and corticosteroids may be administered in severe reactions. (A, T, G)

114. 2. Dopamine hydrochloride (Intropin) is a potent inotropic agent that increases myocardial contractility. Increased myocardial contractility leads to improved cardiac output and improved tissue perfusion. At moderate doses, dopamine can maintain blood pressure above 90 mm Hg systolic in clients with shock. An added benefit of dopamine is that it dilates the renal and mesenteric arteries, supporting renal perfusion. In high doses, dopamine is a vasoconstrictor and may cause serious side effects; thus it is not administered in high doses. (I, T, G)

115. 2. The client receiving dopamine hydrochloride requires continuous blood pressure monitoring with an invasive or noninvasive device. The nurse may titrate the IV infusion to maintain a systolic blood pressure of 90 mm Hg. (I, T, G)

116. 2. Bedrest decreases the body's need for oxygen and nutrients, substances already deficient in the client in shock. These interventions are not directly related to fluid and electrolyte balance or to infection prevention. These interventions may increase the clients and family's comfort, but this is not the primary goal. (I, N, G)

117. 3. The primary pathophysiological alteration in shock is inadequate tissue perfusion. This alteration may be caused by hemorrhage, as in hypovolemic shock; decreased cardiac output, as in cardiogenic shock; or massive vasodilatation of the vascular bed, as in neurogenic, anaphylactic, and septic shock. (A, N, G)

118. 1. The body responds to the challenge of early hypovolemic shock by increasing adrenergic stimulation. Widespread vasoconstriction conserves fluid, supporting blood pressure and producing the classic cool and clammy skin. Clients are typically anxious, and adrenergic stimulation causes both heart and respiratory rates to increase. Bradycardia would be unexpected. (A, T, G)

119. 3. A client in hypovolemic shock is best positioned flat in bed with the feet elevated to bring peripheral blood into the central circulation. Trendelenburg's position, with the head lower than the heart, was formerly recommended but has been found to inhibit respiratory expansion and possibly to cause increased intracranial pressure. (I, T, G)

120. 1. Urine output provides the most sensitive indication of the client's response to therapy for hypovolemic shock. Urine output should be consistently greater than 30 to 35 ml/hour. Blood pressure is a more accurate reflection of the adequacy of vasoconstriction than of tissue perfusion. (E, N, G)

121. 2. Warm, flushed skin occurs in the hyperdynamic "warm shock" phase of septic shock. Other signs and symptoms of early septic shock include restlessness, confusion, tachypnea, and tachycardia. As the shock stage progresses, the signs and symptoms resemble those of hypovolemic shock, with cool, clammy skin and oliguria. (A, T, G)

122. 4. Preventing septic shock is a major focus of nursing care. Very young and elderly clients (those under 2 years and over 65 years) are at increased risk for septic shock. The mortality rate for septic shock is as high as 90% in some populations. Interventions such as maintaining sterility of indwelling urinary catheters is essential to prevent infection. (I, N, H)

The Client With Anemia

123. 1. Vitamin B12 is remarkably free of toxicity. Allergic reactions that have occurred are believed to be caused by impurities or the preservative in B12 preparations. (I, T, H)

124. 3. Activity intolerance is commonly experienced by clients with iron deficiency anemia due to reduced oxygen-carrying capacity from low hemoglobin. Fluid volume deficit is another possible problem. Nausea and immobility are not necessarily related to iron deficiency anemia. (D, N, G)

125. 1. Eggs are high in iron. Other foods high in iron include organ meats (liver, kidney, heart), muscle meats (dark meat from poultry), shellfish, whole-grain cereals and breads, dark green vegetables, legumes, nuts, and dried fruits (apricots, raisins, dates). (I, N, H)

126. 3. Good sources of vitamin B12 include meats and dairy products. Many fresh fruits are good sources of vitamin A, vitamin B2, and vitamin B9 (folic acid). Whole-wheat breads and cereals are good sources of vitamin B1, vitamin B2, vitamin B3, vitamin B6, and vitamin E. (I, T, G)

127. 2. A characteristic early sign of Hodgkin's disease is swollen cervical lymph nodes. The disease originates in the lymphatic system but its cause is unknown. (A, T, G)

128. 3. Hodgkin's disease most often strikes young adults, usually between age 20 and 40. A resurgence in incidence then occurs after age 50. The disease occurs somewhat more often in men than in women. (A, K, G)

129. 4. Staging of Hodgkin's disease determines the extent and activity of the disease to guide appropriate therapy. The nature of the cell causing the disease is studied microscopically, not by staging. (A, K, G)

130. 4. The iliac crest and the sternum are the most common sites for obtaining bone-marrow specimens in adults. These sites are usually selected because they are easily accessible and are away from major organs. (P, K, G)

131. 3. Terminally ill clients most often describe feelings of isolation because they tend to be ignored, are often left out of conversations (especially those dealing with the future), and sense the attitudes of discomfort that many people feel in their presence. Helpful nursing measures to overcome these feelings include taking the time to be with these clients, offering them opportunities to talk about their feelings, and answering their questions honestly. (P, T, L)

The Clients Who Are Dying

132. 2. Health care personnel may avoid the terminally ill client because they are uncomfortable about death and do not understand their own feelings about dying. Family members should not be expected to assume responsibility for the client's care, but they should be involved in the client's care to the extent they desire. Skilled and knowledgeable nursing care is required to make a dying person comfortable. Interrupting the client does not necessarily interfere with the right to die with dignity. (A, N, S)

133. 1. According to Kubler-Ross, a terminally ill person is generally in a stage of having accepted his finiteness when he shows that he wishes privacy and has said everything that needs saying. This is a period of peace and tranquility. However, the person still needs attention, and the nurse should be alert to comments that may reflect defeat rather than acceptance during this time. Criticism of caretakers typically occurs when a person is in a stage of anger and is asking, "Why me?" The stage of depression is one of sadness, often with crying. The person has not accepted death even though it is imminent. There is an expression of "Yes, me, unfortunately." Trying to bargain for time to do one more thing before dying is common before the acceptance stage. The person may appear to be at peace with death but really is not. (E, N, L)

134. 4. Hearing is thought to be the last sense to leave the body. Although unconscious, the client may still be able to hear. (P, K, G)

135. 2. When a person expresses anger, it is best for the nurse to allow him or her to do so and to listen quietly. The angry behavior can act to relieve a charged emotional situation. Offering to call a relative or friend for the bereaved person turns a nursing responsibility over to others. Allowing the person to remain alone and explaining that everything possible was done for the loved one are of little value in an emotional situation. (I, T, L)

General Questions

136. 2. With two-rescuer CPR, the compression-ventilation ratio is 5:1, with a 1 to 1-½ second pause for ventilation. (I, K, G)

137. 2. Because of its location near the xiphoid process, the liver is the organ most easily damaged from pressure exerted over the xiphoid process during CPR. The pressure on the victim's chest wall should be sufficient to compress the heart but not so great as to damage internal organs. However, injury may result even when CPR is performed properly. (I, K, G)

138. 3. An adult's sternum must be depressed 1-½″ to 2″ with each compression to ensure adequate heart compression. (I, K, G)

139. 3. The carotid artery pulse is assessed to check the effectiveness of CPR. The carotid artery is the nearest to the rescuer, ordinarily is easily accessible, and will usually still have a pulse when more peripheral pulses have diminished and are no longer palpable. (I, K, G)

140. 1. If the airway is not clear, it is impossible to inflate the lungs during CPR. A common sign of airway obstruction is failure of the victim's chest wall to rise with each inflation. (I, C, G)

141. 1. The exhalation phase of ventilation is a passive activity and will occur during CPR as part of the normal relaxation of the victim's chest. No action by the rescuer is necessary. (E, T, G)

142. 2. After a person is without cardiopulmonary function for 4 to 6 minutes, permanent brain damage is almost certain. To prevent permanent brain damage, it is important to begin CPR promptly after a victim suffers cardiopulmonary failure. (E, T, G)

143. 2. The Heimlich maneuver should be administered only to a victim who cannot make *any* sounds due to airway obstruction. If the victim can whisper words, some air exchange is occurring, and the emergency medical system should be called instead of attempting the Heimlich maneuver. (A, T, G)

144. 3. The only acceptable reasons for the rescuer discontinuing CPR are when the rescuer is exhausted, when another trained rescuer is available to take over CPR, and when a physician orders that CPR be discontinued. (I, T, G)

THE NURSING CARE OF ADULTS WITH MEDICAL/SURGICAL HEALTH PROBLEMS

TEST 2: The Client With Cardiovascular Health Problems

Directions: Use this answer grid to determine areas of strength or need for further study.

NURSING PROCESS

A = Assessment
D = Analysis, nursing diagnosis
P = Planning
I = Implementation
E = Evaluation

COGNITIVE LEVEL

K = Knowledge
C = Comprehension
T = Application
N = Analysis

CLIENT NEEDS

S = Safe, effective care environment
G = Physiological integrity
L = Psychosocial integrity
H = Health promotion/maintenance

		Nursing Process					Cognitive Level				Client Needs			
Question #	Answer #	A	D	P	I	E	K	C	T	N	S	G	L	H
1	1				I				T			G		
2	4				I				T			G		
3	1	A							T			G		
4	1				I					N		G		
5	1				I				T				L	
6	1		D							N		G		
7	4	A							T			G		
8	3				I				T			G		
9	1			P						N		G		
10	3		D							N		G		
11	2			P					T			G		
12	2		D							N		G		
13	3	A							T			G		
14	2				I				T		S			
15	2					E			T			G		
16	3			P					T			G		
17	3				I				T			G		
18	2				I				T			G		
19	1				I				T			G		
20	1					E			T			G		
21	3				I				T					H
22	4	A							T			G		
23	4				I				T					H

ANSWER GRID: 1

NURSING PROCESS

A = Assessment
D = Analysis, nursing diagnosis
P = Planning
I = Implementation
E = Evaluation

COGNITIVE LEVEL

K = Knowledge
C = Comprehension
T = Application
N = Analysis

CLIENT NEEDS

S = Safe, effective care environment
G = Physiological integrity
L = Psychosocial integrity
H = Health promotion/maintenance

		Nursing Process					Cognitive Level				Client Needs			
Question #	Answer #	A	D	P	I	E	K	C	T	N	S	G	L	H
24	3				I				T					H
25	4				I			C				G		
26	3				I					N		G		
27	2				I				T			G		
28	1				I				T			G		
29	2			P					T			G		
30	4			P					T			G		
31	4	A						C				G		
32	2					E			T			G		
33	2				I				T			G		
34	2	A							T			G		
35	4				I				T			G		
36	4				I				T			G		
37	2					E			T			G		
38	3				I				T					H
39	2			P					T			G		
40	3					E			T			G		
41	4				I				T				L	
42	1	A							T			G		
43	4	A							T			G		
44	3			P			K				S			
45	1				I				T					H
46	3				I				T					H
47	4				I				T			G		
48	4	A							T			G		
49	4	A								N		G		
50	2					E			T			G		
51	1			P				C				G		
52	1					E			T			G		

ANSWER GRID: 2

NURSING PROCESS

A = Assessment
D = Analysis, nursing diagnosis
P = Planning
I = Implementation
E = Evaluation

COGNITIVE LEVEL

K = Knowledge
C = Comprehension
T = Application
N = Analysis

CLIENT NEEDS

S = Safe, effective care environment
G = Physiological integrity
L = Psychosocial integrity
H = Health promotion/maintenance

		Nursing Process					Cognitive Level				Client Needs			
Question #	Answer #	A	D	P	I	E	K	C	T	N	S	G	L	H
53	1				I				T			G		
54	4				I				T			G		
55	2	A							T			G		
56	1					E			T			G		
57	4					E			T			G		
58	4				I				T			G		
59	3				I				T			G		
60	4				I				T			G		
61	4				I				T			G		
62	3	A						C				G		
63	2	A							T			G		
64	4	A							T			G		
65	3	A							T			G		
66	1	A							T			G		
67	4				I				T		S			
68	2				I				T			G		
69	1				I				T		S			
70	1				I				T		S			
71	3				I				T					H
72	1				I				T					H
73	2				I				T			G		
74	2			P						N		G		
75	3		D							N		G		
76	3	A							T			G		
77	3	A							T			G		
78	4				I				T			G		
79	1				I				T			G		
80	4		D							N				H
81	4				I					N				H

ANSWER GRID: 3

Nursing Process

A = Assessment
D = Analysis, nursing diagnosis
P = Planning
I = Implementation
E = Evaluation

Cognitive Level

K = Knowledge
C = Comprehension
T = Application
N = Analysis

Client Needs

S = Safe, effective care environment
G = Physiological integrity
L = Psychosocial integrity
H = Health promotion/maintenance

		Nursing Process					Cognitive Level				Client Needs			
Question #	Answer #	A	D	P	I	E	K	C	T	N	S	G	L	H
82	3			P						N				H
83	3					E			T		S			
84	4	A					K					G		
85	2	A					K					G		
86	1				I				T		S			
87	3				I				T			G		
88	1				I				T			G		
89	3				I				T			G		
90	2				I				T			G		
91	2				I				T		S			
92	1			P					T			G		
93	2	A							T		S			
94	3	A						C				G		
95	2	A								N		G		
96	2				I				T			G		
97	2				I				T			G		
98	4				I		K				S			
99	4	A							T			G		
100	4				I				T			G		
101	3		D							N		G		
102	1				I					N		G		
103	1				I				T			G		
104	1				I				T			G		
105	2				I				T		S			
106	1				I				T			G		
107	4				I				T			G		
108	2	A							T			G		
109	4				I				T			G		
110	1				I				T				L	

Answer Grid: 4

NURSING PROCESS

A = Assessment
D = Analysis, nursing diagnosis
P = Planning
I = Implementation
E = Evaluation

COGNITIVE LEVEL

K = Knowledge
C = Comprehension
T = Application
N = Analysis

CLIENT NEEDS

S = Safe, effective care environment
G = Physiological integrity
L = Psychosocial integrity
H = Health promotion/maintenance

		Nursing Process					Cognitive Level				Client Needs			
Question #	Answer #	A	D	P	I	E	K	C	T	N	S	G	L	H
111	1	A								N		G		
112	2				I				T			G		
113	2	A							T			G		
114	2				I				T			G		
115	2				I				T			G		
116	2				I					N		G		
117	3	A								N		G		
118	1	A							T			G		
119	3				I				T			G		
120	1					E				N		G		
121	2	A							T			G		
122	4				I					N				H
123	1				I				T					H
124	3		D							N		G		
125	1				I					N				H
126	3				I				T			G		
127	2	A							T			G		
128	3	A					K					G		
129	4	A					K					G		
130	4			P			K					G		
131	3			P					T				L	
132	2	A								N	S			
133	1					E				N			L	
134	4			P			K					G		
135	2				I				T				L	
136	2				I		K					G		
137	2				I		K					G		
138	3				I		K					G		
139	3				I		K					G		

ANSWER GRID: 5

NURSING PROCESS

A = Assessment
D = Analysis, nursing diagnosis
P = Planning
I = Implementation
E = Evaluation

COGNITIVE LEVEL

K = Knowledge
C = Comprehension
T = Application
N = Analysis

CLIENT NEEDS

S = Safe, effective care environment
G = Physiological integrity
L = Psychosocial integrity
H = Health promotion/maintenance

		Nursing Process					Cognitive Level				Client Needs			
Question #	Answer #	A	D	P	I	E	K	C	T	N	S	G	L	H
140	1				I			C				G		
141	1					E			T			G		
142	2					E			T			G		
143	2	A							T			G		
144	3				I				T			G		
Number Correct														
Number Possible	144	35	7	14	74	14	12	6	102	24	12	112	6	14
Percentage Correct														

Score Calculation:

To determine your **Percentage Correct**, divide the **Number Correct** by the **Number Possible**.

ANSWER GRID: 6

The Client With Upper Gastrointestinal Tract Health Problems

Test 3

The Client With Peptic Ulcer Disease
The Client With Cholecystitis
The Client With Cancer of the Stomach
The Client With Pancreatitis
The Client With Hiatal Hernia
General Questions
Correct Answers and Rationale

Select the one best answer and indicate your choice by filling in the circle in front of the option.

The Client With Peptic Ulcer Disease

A 54-year-old male client is admitted through the emergency department with a bleeding duodenal ulcer. He was brought to the hospital after vomiting bright-red blood.

1. While the client is bleeding, it will be essential for the nurse to assess him frequently for signs of early shock. Which one of the following is an important indicator of early shock?
- ○ 1. Tachycardia.
- ○ 2. Dry, flushed skin.
- ○ 3. Increased urine output.
- ○ 4. Loss of consciousness.

2. Which of the following clinical manifestations would most likely indicate that the ulcer has perforated?
- ○ 1. Projectile vomiting.
- ○ 2. Frequent belching.
- ○ 3. Diarrhea.
- ○ 4. Boardlike abdomen.

3. The nurse would correctly evaluate that the client probably ignored an important warning sign of bleeding when he reports that before admission the color of his stools was
- ○ 1. gray.
- ○ 2. black.
- ○ 3. dark green.
- ○ 4. light brown.

4. The client has been taking propantheline bromide (Pro-Banthine) at home. The nurse would prepare a teaching plan for the client that includes the information that the medication acts primarily to
- ○ 1. suppress gastric secretions.
- ○ 2. neutralize acid in the stomach.
- ○ 3. shorten the time required for digestion in the stomach.
- ○ 4. improve the mixing of foods and gastric secretions.

5. The client reports frequent episodes of epigastric pain that awaken him during the night, a feeling of fullness in the abdomen, and anxiety about his health. Based on these data, which nursing diagnosis would be most appropriate?
- ○ 1. Altered Nutrition: Less than Body Requirements related to anorexia.
- ○ 2. Sleep Pattern Disturbance related to epigastric pain.
- ○ 3. Ineffective Individual Coping related to exacerbation of duodenal ulcer.
- ○ 4. Activity Intolerance related to abdominal pain.

6. Which of the following goals would be most appropriate for this client? The client will
- ○ 1. verbalize absence of epigastric pain.
- ○ 2. accept the need to inject himself with vitamin B12 for the rest of his life.
- ○ 3. understand the need to ingest large quantities of milk with his meals.
- ○ 4. eliminate all stress from his life.

7. The client asks, "What type of diet will I have to

follow at home?" The nurse should explain that his diet will most likely consist of
○ 1. full liquids and pureed food.
○ 2. high-fat, high-protein foods.
○ 3. any foods that he can tolerate.
○ 4. six small meals a day.

8. While he is in the hospital, the client is served a modified bland diet. Which of the following items on the dinner tray should the nurse remove before serving the tray?
○ 1. Salt.
○ 2. Sugar.
○ 3. Mayonnaise.
○ 4. Coffee.

9. The nurse should instruct the client to avoid which of the following beverages after discharge?
○ 1. Carbonated mineral water.
○ 2. Low-sodium skim milk.
○ 3. Beer.
○ 4. Fruit juice.

10. Which of the following statements best describes current opinion about diet during the convalescence of clients with peptic ulcer?
○ 1. A bland diet is most effective for clients with peptic ulcer.
○ 2. The type of diet is not as important as including foods that the client can tolerate.
○ 3. Eliminating specific foods from the diet is no longer recommended, as long as the client eats frequently.
○ 4. Dietary restrictions appear to be most helpful for elderly clients but are rarely helpful for young and middle-aged clients.

11. The client is to undergo an upper GI endoscopy to help the physician visualize the ulcer's location and severity. When the client returns to the unit, what should the nurse evaluate besides his vital signs?
○ 1. Return of the gag reflex.
○ 2. Bowel sounds.
○ 3. Breath sounds.
○ 4. Intake and output.

12. The client's treatment plan includes modified bedrest. One afternoon the nurse finds him surrounded by papers from his briefcase and arguing on the telephone with a co-worker. The nurse's interaction with him should be based on knowledge that
○ 1. involvement with his job will keep him from becoming bored in the hospital.
○ 2. rest is an essential component of ulcer healing.
○ 3. not keeping up with his job will increase his stress level.
○ 4. setting limits on a client's behavior is an essential aspect of the nursing role.

13. The client has been instructed to avoid intense physical activity and stress to decrease gastric acid secretion. Which nursing measure would be most effective in helping the client achieve this goal once he returns home?
○ 1. Instructing the client to conduct all physical activity early in the morning so he can rest all afternoon.
○ 2. Having the client's wife agree to perform the necessary yardwork at home.
○ 3. Instructing the client to give up golf.
○ 4. Assisting the client to develop a plan that provides for periods of physical and mental rest.

14. The client will not be able to avoid stress in his job. Therefore, it would be most important for the nurse to encourage him to
○ 1. consider changing jobs.
○ 2. identify stressors at work.
○ 3. set his goals a little lower.
○ 4. improve his ability to cope with stress.

15. Which of the following activities should the nurse encourage the client with a peptic ulcer to avoid?
○ 1. Chewing gum.
○ 2. Smoking cigarettes.
○ 3. Eating chocolate.
○ 4. Taking acetaminophen (Tylenol).

16. The client will take cimetidine (Tagamet) at home. The nurse teaches him about proper drug administration. The nurse would know that the client understands the teaching when he says that he will take the drug
○ 1. before meals.
○ 2. with meals.
○ 3. after meals.
○ 4. when pain occurs.

The Client With Cholecystitis

A 56-year-old female is admitted to the hospital with acute upper right quadrant pain that radiates to her back. She is in obvious distress from the pain, is extremely nauseated, and has vomited several times. The admitting diagnosis is cholecystitis with cholelithiasis.

17. Which of the following symptoms would the nurse most likely observe in a client with cholecystitis from cholelithiasis?
○ 1. Black stools.
○ 2. Nausea after ingestion of high-fat foods.
○ 3. Elevated temperature of 103°F.
○ 4. Decreased white blood cell count.

18. Which of the following nursing interventions should have the highest priority during the first hour after this client's admission?
○ 1. Administering pain medication.
○ 2. Completing the admission history.
○ 3. Maintaining hydration.

○ 4. Teaching about planned diagnostic tests.

19. Propantheline bromide (Pro-Banthine) is ordered for the client. The nurse would understand that this drug is prescribed to
○ 1. relieve pain.
○ 2. decrease biliary contraction.
○ 3. treat infection.
○ 4. relieve nausea.

20. If a gallstone becomes lodged in the common bile duct, the nurse should anticipate that the client's stools would most likely be
○ 1. green.
○ 2. gray.
○ 3. black.
○ 4. yellow.

21. When the common bile duct is obstructed, the nurse should evaluate the client for signs of
○ 1. respiratory distress.
○ 2. circulatory overload.
○ 3. urinary tract infection.
○ 4. prolonged bleeding time.

22. The client is scheduled for cholecystography. In preparation for the test, she is to take iopanoic acid (Telepaque) tablets after her evening meal. Before administering the tablets, the nurse should ask the client if she is allergic to
○ 1. eggs.
○ 2. iodine.
○ 3. food coloring.
○ 4. organ meats.

23. The client undergoes a cholecystectomy and choledochotomy and returns from surgery with an intravenous line, a Penrose drain, and a T-tube in place. To evaluate the effectiveness of the T-tube, the nurse should understand that the primary reason for using it with this client is to
○ 1. promote wound drainage.
○ 2. provide a way to irrigate the biliary tract.
○ 3. minimize the passage of bile into the duodenum.
○ 4. prevent bile from entering the peritoneal cavity.

24. How much bile would the nurse expect the T-tube to drain during the first 24 hours after surgery?
○ 1. 50 to 100 ml.
○ 2. 150 to 250 ml.
○ 3. 300 to 500 ml.
○ 4. 550 to 700 ml.

25. To maintain accurate records, the nurse should measure the amount of drainage from the T-tube and record it by
○ 1. adding it to the client's urine output.
○ 2. charting it separately on the output record.
○ 3. adding it to the amount of wound drainage.
○ 4. subtracting it from the total intake for each day.

26. The presence of the T-tube makes it important for the nurse to develop a plan of care that includes providing extra attention to
○ 1. the skin around the insertion site.
○ 2. intake and output.
○ 3. electrolyte imbalance.
○ 4. acid–base imbalance.

27. Which nursing measure would be most effective in helping the client cough and deep breathe after cholecystectomy?
○ 1. Having the client take rapid, shallow breaths to decrease pain.
○ 2. Having the client lay on the right side while coughing and deep breathing.
○ 3. Teaching the client to use a folded blanket or pillow to splint the incision.
○ 4. Withholding pain medication so the client can be alert enough to follow the nurse's instructions.

28. During the first few weeks after cholecystectomy, the client would probably be more comfortable if the diet was restricted in which of the following ways?
○ 1. Decrease intake of fruits, vegetables, whole grains, nuts, and seeds to increase fiber and minimize pressure within the small intestine.
○ 2. Consume at least four servings of meat, cheese, and peanut butter daily to boost protein and essential amino acids to aid incisional healing.
○ 3. Distribute fat intake in small portions throughout the day so there is not an excessive amount in the intestine at any one time.
○ 4. Take pancreatic extracts with meals to replace the enzymes that would normally have been secreted by the organ that was surgically removed.

29. After cholecystectomy, it is recommended that the client follow a low-fat diet. Which of the following foods would be most appropriate to include in a low-fat diet?
○ 1. Cheese omelet and vanilla pudding.
○ 2. Egg salad sandwich and fresh fruit cup.
○ 3. Ham salad sandwich and baked custard.
○ 4. Roast beef and green beans.

The Client With Cancer of the Stomach

A 70-year-old male client has been diagnosed with adenocarcinoma of the stomach. A subtotal gastric resection is planned.

30. On the client's admission to the hospital, the nurse determines that his nutritional status is severely compromised. Which of the following therapies would be most effective in correcting his nutritional deficits before surgery?
○ 1. High-protein between-meal nourishment four times a day.
○ 2. Tube feedings at 200 ml/hour.
○ 3. Total parenteral nutrition (TPN) for several days.

○ 4. Intravenous infusion of normal saline solution at 125 ml/hour.

31. The client is scheduled to undergo a subtotal gastrectomy (Billroth II procedure). When providing preoperative client teaching, the nurse should explain that the surgical procedure will allow stomach contents to bypass the
○ 1. ileum.
○ 2. duodenum.
○ 3. cardiac sphincter.
○ 4. fundus of the stomach.

32. After surgery, postoperative orders for this client include keep NPO; maintain the nasogastric tube at low intermittent suction; administer IV fluids at 125 ml/hour; have the client turn, cough, and deep breathe every 2 hours; and administer meperidine hydrochloride (Demerol) 100 mg IM every 3 to 4 hours p.r.n. for pain. The client will have a nasogastric tube in place for several days postoperatively to
○ 1. prevent excessive pressure on suture lines.
○ 2. prevent ascites.
○ 3. enable feeding in the immediate postoperative period.
○ 4. enable administration of antacids to promote healing of the anastomosis.

33. The nurse should anticipate that drainage from the nasogastric tube would be what color approximately 12 to 24 hours after surgery?
○ 1. Brown.
○ 2. Green.
○ 3. Bright red.
○ 4. Cloudy white.

34. Following a subtotal gastrectomy, care of the client's nasogastric tube and drainage system should include which of the following nursing interventions?
○ 1. Irrigate the tube with 30 ml of sterile water every hour, if needed.
○ 2. If the tube is not draining well, reposition it.
○ 3. Monitor the client for nausea, vomiting, and abdominal distention.
○ 4. If the drainage is sluggish on low suction, turn the machine to high suction.

35. From an analysis of the data collected about the client and his surgery, the nurse formulates the nursing diagnosis High Risk for Altered Respiratory Function. Which of the following factors would this diagnosis not be related to
○ 1. A high abdominal incision.
○ 2. Weakness and fatigue.
○ 3. Possibility of aspirating gastric contents.
○ 4. Postoperative semi-Fowler's position.

36. The client is monitored for complications common to all surgical clients as well as those specific to gastric resection surgery. Which of the following signs and symptoms would alert the nurse to the development of a leaking anastomosis?
○ 1. Pain, fever, and abdominal rigidity.
○ 2. Diarrhea with fat in the stool.
○ 3. Palpitations, pallor, and diaphoresis after eating.
○ 4. Feelings of fullness and nausea after eating.

37. As part of the client's discharge planning, the nurse has identified Altered Nutrition: Less than Body Requirements as a major nursing diagnosis. To help the client and his family meet nutritional goals, the nurse should develop a plan of care that includes
○ 1. instructing him to increase the amount eaten at each meal by doubling that eaten at the previous meal.
○ 2. encouraging him to eat smaller amounts more frequently and to stop when he feels full.
○ 3. explaining that if he should vomit after a meal, he should eat nothing more that day.
○ 4. informing him that bland foods may cause gastric distress and instructing him to introduce them into his diet gradually.

38. Which of the following outcomes would indicate that the client's nutritional goal is being achieved?
○ 1. Gradual increase in food intake and tolerance.
○ 2. Nausea and vomiting.
○ 3. Ingestion of 2,000 cc of water per day.
○ 4. Rapid weight gain within 1 week.

39. As a result of his gastric resection, the client is at risk for developing dumping syndrome. The nurse would develop a plan of care for this client based on knowledge that this problem primarily stems from
○ 1. excess secretion of digestive enzymes in the intestines.
○ 2. rapid emptying of stomach contents into the small intestine.
○ 3. excess glycogen production by the liver.
○ 4. the loss of gastric juices.

40. Which of the following symptoms would strongly suggest that the client is experiencing dumping syndrome?
○ 1. Constipation.
○ 2. Extreme hunger.
○ 3. Fainting.
○ 4. Abdominal cramps.

41. To reduce the risk of dumping syndrome, the nurse should teach the client which of the following strategies?
○ 1. Sit upright after meals.
○ 2. Drink fluids with meals.
○ 3. Decrease the protein content of meals.
○ 4. Decrease the carbohydrate content of meals.

The Client With Pancreatitis

A 50-year-old woman is admitted with a possible diagnosis of pancreatitis.

42. Which of the following symptoms would the nurse anticipate observing in a client with pancreatitis?
- ○ 1. Hypertension, elevated white blood cell count, and peripheral edema.
- ○ 2. Left upper quadrant abdominal pain, nausea, and vomiting.
- ○ 3. Hypoglycemia, tachycardia, and cyanosis.
- ○ 4. Decreased white blood cell count, clubbing of fingernails, and mid-epigastric discomfort.

43. The initial diagnosis of pancreatitis would be confirmed if the client's blood work showed a significant elevation in serum
- ○ 1. amylase.
- ○ 2. glucose.
- ○ 3. potassium.
- ○ 4. trypsin.

44. The client tells the nurse, "This is the second time this has happened to me and I still don't understand it." The nurse's response would be based on the knowledge that the basic pathophysiology of pancreatitis involves
- ○ 1. spasm of the sphincter of Oddi.
- ○ 2. increased gastric secretions.
- ○ 3. autodigestion of the pancreas.
- ○ 4. severe volume depletion.

45. Because the client rarely drinks, because of her religious convictions, she becomes upset when the physician persists in asking her about alcohol intake. The nurse should explain that the reason for these questions is that
- ○ 1. there is a strong link between alcohol use and acute pancreatitis.
- ○ 2. alcohol intake can interfere with some of the tests used to diagnose pancreatitis.
- ○ 3. alcoholism is a major health problem, and all hospitalized clients are questioned about alcohol intake.
- ○ 4. the physician must obtain the pertinent facts, and religious beliefs cannot be considered.

46. Pain control is an important nursing goal for the client with pancreatitis. Which of the following medications would be the drug of choice in this situation?
- ○ 1. Meperidine hydrochloride (Demerol).
- ○ 2. Cimetidine (Tagamet).
- ○ 3. Morphine sulfate.
- ○ 4. Codeine sulfate.

47. The nurse monitors the client's vital signs frequently, observing for early signs of shock. Shock is extremely difficult to manage in pancreatitis primarily because of the
- ○ 1. frequency and severity of gastrointestinal hemorrhage.
- ○ 2. vasodilating effects of kinin peptides.
- ○ 3. tendency toward congestive heart failure.
- ○ 4. frequent incidence of acute tubular necrosis.

48. Which of the following assessment findings would be unexpected in this client?
- ○ 1. Hypoglycemia.
- ○ 2. Abdominal distention and tenderness.
- ○ 3. Nausea and vomiting.
- ○ 4. Hyperlipidemia.

49. While helping the client change position in bed, the nurse notices muscle twitching in her hands and forearms. The nurse would report these symptoms immediately, because clients with pancreatitis are at serious risk for
- ○ 1. hypermagnesemia.
- ○ 2. hypoglycemia.
- ○ 3. hyperkalemia.
- ○ 4. hypocalcemia.

50. The initial treatment plan for this client most likely would focus on
- ○ 1. resting the gastrointestinal tract.
- ○ 2. ensuring adequate nutrition.
- ○ 3. maintaining fluid and electrolyte balance.
- ○ 4. treating infection.

51. When providing care for a client with pancreatitis, the nurse would anticipate which of the following orders?
- ○ 1. Force fluids to 3,000 ml/24 hours.
- ○ 2. Insert a nasogastric tube and connect it to low suction.
- ○ 3. Place the client in reverse Trendelenburg's position.
- ○ 4. Place the client in enteric isolation.

52. Which of the following medications would most likely be given to the client to augment pain control?
- ○ 1. Ibuprofen (Motrin).
- ○ 2. Magnesium hydroxide (Maalox).
- ○ 3. Propantheline bromide (Pro-Banthine).
- ○ 4. Propranolol (Inderal).

53. Which of the following would most likely be a major nursing diagnosis for a client with acute pancreatitis?
- ○ 1. Ineffective Airway Clearance.
- ○ 2. Fluid Volume Excess.
- ○ 3. Impaired Swallowing.
- ○ 4. Altered Nutrition: Less than Body Requirements.

54. The client's condition becomes chronic. What would be the appropriate diet for a client with chronic pancreatitis?
- ○ 1. A low-protein, high-fiber diet distributed over four to five moderate-sized meals daily.
- ○ 2. A low-fat, bland diet distributed over five to six small meals daily.
- ○ 3. A high-calcium, soft diet distributed over three meals and an evening snack daily.
- ○ 4. A diabetic exchange diet distributed over three meals and two snacks daily.

55. Pancreatic enzyme replacements are ordered for the client. The nurse should instruct the client to take them

○ 1. three times daily between meals.
○ 2. with each meal and snack.
○ 3. in the morning and at bedtime.
○ 4. every 4 hours, at specified times.

56. How should the nurse teach the client to monitor the effectiveness of pancreatic enzyme replacement therapy?
○ 1. Monitor her fluid intake.
○ 2. Perform regular fingerstick tests for glucose.
○ 3. Observe her stools for steatorrhea.
○ 4. Test her urine for ketones.

The Client With Hiatal Hernia

A 45-year-old female client is being evaluated for a possible hiatal hernia.

57. When obtaining the client's health history, the nurse would expect her to report that the symptoms worsen when she is
○ 1. lying down.
○ 2. physically active.
○ 3. upset or angry.
○ 4. sitting.

58. Based on awareness that the primary symptoms of a sliding hiatal hernia are associated with reflux, the nurse should particularly assess the client for
○ 1. heartburn, regurgitation, and dysphagia.
○ 2. jaundice, ascites, and edema.
○ 3. a visible abdominal bulge, diarrhea, and anorexia.
○ 4. vomiting, stomatitis, and board like abdominal rigidity.

59. Which of the following factors most likely would have contributed to the development of the client's hiatal hernia?
○ 1. Her desk job as a secretary.
○ 2. Her height (5′ 3″) and weight (190 lbs.).
○ 3. Frequent laxative use.
○ 4. Her age.

60. Self-care is the cornerstone of hiatal hernia management. Which of the following nursing interventions would most likely promote self-care behaviors in the client?
○ 1. Introduce her to other people who are successfully managing their care.
○ 2. Include her daughter in the teaching so she can help implement the plan.
○ 3. Ask her to identify other situations in which she demonstrated responsibility for herself.
○ 4. Assure her that she will be able to implement all aspects of the plan successfully.

61. The client has been taking magnesium hydroxide (Milk of Magnesia) at home in an attempt to control her symptoms. The nurse should be aware that the most common complaint associated with the ongoing use of magnesium-based antacids is
○ 1. anorexia.
○ 2. weight gain.
○ 3. diarrhea.
○ 4. constipation.

62. Life-style modification is an important aspect of treatment for hiatal hernia. Which of the following behaviors should the nurse encourage the client to include in her daily routine?
○ 1. Daily aerobic exercise.
○ 2. Eliminating smoking and alcohol use.
○ 3. Carefully balancing activity and rest.
○ 4. Avoiding high-stress situations.

63. The nurse assesses the client's understanding of the relationship between body position and gastroesophageal reflux. Which response would indicate that the client understands measures to avoid problems with reflux while sleeping?
○ 1. "I elevate the foot of the bed 4″ to 6″."
○ 2. "I sleep on my stomach with my head turned to the left."
○ 3. "I sleep on my back without a pillow under my head."
○ 4. "I elevate the head of the bed 4″ to 6″."

64. In developing a teaching plan for the client, the nurse's assessment of which work-related factors would be most useful?
○ 1. Number and length of breaks.
○ 2. Body mechanics used in lifting.
○ 3. Temperature in the work area.
○ 4. Cleaning solvents used.

65. The client attends two sessions with the dietitian to learn about diet modifications to minimize gastroesophageal reflux. The teaching would be judged successful if the client says that she will decrease her intake of
○ 1. fats.
○ 2. high-sodium foods.
○ 3. carbohydrates.
○ 4. high-calcium foods.

66. Which of the following dietary measures could also be useful in preventing esophageal reflux?
○ 1. Eating small, frequent meals; avoiding overeating.
○ 2. Belching frequently to reduce abdominal distention.
○ 3. Avoiding air swallowing with meals.
○ 4. Reducing the size of the evening meal and adding a bedtime snack.

67. The nurse instructs the client on health maintenance activities to help control her symptoms from hiatal

hernia. Which of the following statements would indicate the client has understood the instructions?
- ○ 1. "I'll avoid lying down after a meal."
- ○ 2. "I can still enjoy my potato chips and cola at bedtime."
- ○ 3. "I wish I didn't have to give up swimming."
- ○ 4. "If I wear a girdle, I'll have more support for my stomach."

68. The physician prescribes metoclopramide hydrochloride (Reglan) for the client. The nurse would understand that this drug is used in hiatal hernia therapy to
- ○ 1. increase the resting tone of the esophageal sphincter.
- ○ 2. neutralize gastric secretions.
- ○ 3. delay gastric emptying.
- ○ 4. reduce secretion of digestive juices.

69. While the client is taking metoclopramide hydrochloride, the nurse should instruct her to avoid which of the following drugs?
- ○ 1. Antacids.
- ○ 2. Antihypertensives.
- ○ 3. Anticoagulants.
- ○ 4. Alcohol.

70. Cimetidine (Tagamet) may also be used to treat hiatal hernia. The nurse should understand that this drug is used to prevent
- ○ 1. esophageal reflux.
- ○ 2. the feeling of fullness after meals.
- ○ 3. esophagitis.
- ○ 4. ulcer formation.

71. The client asks the nurse whether she will need surgery to correct her hiatal hernia. Which reply by the nurse would be most accurate?
- ○ 1. Surgery is usually required, although medical treatment is attempted first.
- ○ 2. The symptoms of hiatal hernia can usually be successfully managed with diet modifications, medications, and life-style changes.
- ○ 3. Surgery is not performed for this type of hernia.
- ○ 4. A minor surgical procedure to reduce the size of the diaphragmatic opening will probably be planned.

General Questions

72. The physician orders nasogastric tube insertion to irrigate a client's stomach. Which of the following insertion techniques would most likely make it more difficult for the nurse to insert the tube?
- ○ 1. Lubricating the tube with a water-soluble lubricant.
- ○ 2. Asking the client to swallow while the tube is advanced to the stomach.
- ○ 3. Sitting the client upright in a Fowler's position.
- ○ 4. Having the client tilt the head toward the chest while inserting the tube into the nose.

73. Which of the following techniques is considered the best way to determine whether a nasogastric tube is positioned in the stomach?
- ○ 1. Aspirating with a syringe and observing for the return of gastric contents.
- ○ 2. Irrigating with normal saline and observing for the return of solution.
- ○ 3. Placing the tube's free end in water and observing for air bubbles.
- ○ 4. Instilling air and auscultating over the epigastric area for the presence of the tube.

74. The client is scheduled to have an upper gastrointestinal tract series. Which of the following should the nurse plan to administer after the examination?
- ○ 1. A laxative.
- ○ 2. A clear liquid diet.
- ○ 3. An enema.
- ○ 4. An intravenous infusion.

75. Aluminum hydroxide (Amphojel), 30 ml every 2 hours, is prescribed for the client. The nurse would evaluate that the client was likely experiencing a side effect of aluminum hydroxide if he developed
- ○ 1. anorexia.
- ○ 2. nausea.
- ○ 3. constipation.
- ○ 4. belching.

76. The nurse is preparing to start an IV infusion. Before inserting the needle into a vein, the nurse would apply a tourniquet to the client's arm to
- ○ 1. distend the veins.
- ○ 2. stabilize the veins.
- ○ 3. immobilize the arm.
- ○ 4. occlude arterial circulation.

77. Preoperatively, the nurse instructs the client in the correct use of an incentive spirometer. This treatment is essential following surgery in the upper abdominal area because
- ○ 1. the client is maintained on bed rest for several days.
- ○ 2. ambulation is restricted by the presence of drainage tubes.
- ○ 3. the operative incision is near the diaphragm.
- ○ 4. the presence of a nasogastric tube makes it difficult for the client to cough effectively.

78. To evaluate the effectiveness of the incentive spirometer, the nurse should understand that this device is used primarily to
- ○ 1. stimulate circulation.
- ○ 2. prepare for ambulation.
- ○ 3. strengthen abdominal muscles.
- ○ 4. increase respiratory effectiveness.

79. The nurse should understand that the primary rea-

son for withholding food and fluids from a client who has received general anesthesia is to help prevent
- ○ 1. constipation during the immediate postoperative period.
- ○ 2. vomiting and possible aspiration of vomitus during surgery.
- ○ 3. pressure on the diaphragm with poor lung expansion during surgery.
- ○ 4. gas pains and distention during the immediate postoperative period.

80. The nurse administers a preoperative intramuscular medication at the ventrogluteal site. The nurse will inject the medication into which muscle?
- ○ 1. Rectus femoris.
- ○ 2. Gluteus minimus.
- ○ 3. Vastus lateralis.
- ○ 4. Gluteus maximus.

81. Prochloperazine dimaleate (Compazine) is prescribed for postoperative administration. The nurse would evaluate that the drug has had a therapeutic effect when the client no longer complains of
- ○ 1. nausea.
- ○ 2. dizziness.
- ○ 3. abdominal spasms.
- ○ 4. abdominal distention.

82. Preoperatively, a client expresses anxiety and apprehension about having surgery. Which of the following nursing interventions would help achieve the goal of reducing the client's anxiety?
- ○ 1. Provide the client with information, but only if he requests it.
- ○ 2. Tell the client what to expect in the postoperative period.
- ○ 3. Reassure the client by telling him about the high percentage of clients who are not afraid of surgery.
- ○ 4. Stress to the client the importance of following his physician's instructions after surgery.

83. The nurse uses 30 ml of solution to irrigate a nasogastric tube and notes that 20 ml returns promptly into the drainage container. When the nurse records the results of the irrigation, how much solution should be recorded as intake?
- ○ 1. 10 ml.
- ○ 2. 20 ml.
- ○ 3. 30 ml.
- ○ 4. 50 ml.

84. The client complains of sore nostrils while the nasogastric tube is in place. Which of the following nursing measures would be most appropriate to help alleviate the client's discomfort?
- ○ 1. Repositioning the tube in the nares.
- ○ 2. Irrigating the tube with a cool solution.
- ○ 3. Applying a water-soluble lubricant to the nares.
- ○ 4. Having the client change position more frequently.

85. For a client with a nasogastric tube attached to low suction postoperatively, intravenous replacement therapy will be needed primarily to
- ○ 1. maintain bladder function.
- ○ 2. facilitate osmotic diuresis.
- ○ 3. equalize intake and output.
- ○ 4. maintain fluid and electrolyte balance.

86. A major goal of postoperative nursing care is to prevent atelectasis and pneumonia. Which of the following nursing interventions would best accomplish this?
- ○ 1. Give meperidine hydrochloride (Demerol) sparingly to prevent depressing the cough reflex and respirations.
- ○ 2. Offer meperidine hydrochloride (Demerol) 30 minutes before having the client cough and deep breathe.
- ○ 3. Encourage the client to cough, deep breathe, and turn in bed once every 4 hours.
- ○ 4. Maintain the client on bed rest for at least 48 hours to minimize incisional pain and splinting of the chest.

87. The client with a nasogastric tube begins to complain of abdominal distention. Which of the following measures should the nurse implement first?
- ○ 1. Call the physician.
- ○ 2. Irrigate the nasogastric tube.
- ○ 3. Check the function of the suction equipment.
- ○ 4. Reposition the nasogastric tube.

88. The client's serum electrolyte values are obtained postoperatively. The nurse should interpret a potassium level of 4.2 mEq/L as
- ○ 1. above normal.
- ○ 2. within the normal range.
- ○ 3. slightly below normal.
- ○ 4. life-threateningly low.

89. Which of the following signs and symptoms would be an early indication that a client's serum potassium level is below normal?
- ○ 1. Diarrhea.
- ○ 2. Sticky mucous membranes.
- ○ 3. Muscle weakness in the legs.
- ○ 4. Tingling in the fingers.

90. The correct procedure for auscultating a client's abdomen for bowel sounds would include
- ○ 1. palpating the abdomen first to determine correct stethoscope placement.
- ○ 2. encouraging the client to cough to stimulate movement of fluid and air through the abdomen.
- ○ 3. placing the client on the left side to aid auscultation.
- ○ 4. listening for 5 minutes in all four quadrants to confirm absence of bowel sounds.

CORRECT ANSWERS AND RATIONALE

The letters in parentheses following the rationale identify the step of the nursing process (A, D, P, I, E); cognitive level (K, C, T, N); and client need (S, G, L, H). See the Answer Grid for the key.

The Client With Peptic Ulcer Disease

1. 1. In early shock, the body attempts to meet its perfusion needs through tachycardia, vasoconstriction, and fluid conservation. The skin becomes cool and clammy. The client may experience increased restlessness and anxiety from hypoxia, but loss of consciousness is a late sign of shock. Urine output in early shock may be normal or slightly decreased. (A, C, G)

2. 4. The body reacts to perforation of an ulcer by immobilizing the area as much as possible. This results in boardlike abdominal rigidity, usually with extreme tenderness. This may occur over several hours or days. Projectile vomiting, belching, and diarrhea are not associated with perforated ulcer. (A, C, G)

3. 2. Digested blood in the stool causes it to be black. The odor of the stool is very offensive. (E, C, G)

4. 1. Propantheline bromide (Pro-Banthine) is an anticholinergic drug that reduces secretion by the gastric, salivary, bronchial, and sweat glands. Anticholinergic drugs act by blocking ganglionic action in the autonomic nervous system. (P, K, G)

5. 2. Based on the data provided, the most appropriate nursing diagnosis would be Sleep Pattern Disturbance. A client with a duodenal ulcer commonly awakens during the night with pain. There are not enough data to support the other nursing diagnoses. (D, N, G)

6. 1. A realistic goal for this client would be to gain relief from epigastric pain. There is no need for Vitamin B12 injections, as this client has not had any gastric surgery that would lead to vitamin B12 deficiency. Milk in large quantities is not recommended for clients with ulcers, as it actually stimulates further production of gastric acid. It is not possible to eliminate all stress from a client's life. Instead, the client should be assisted to develop effective coping and problem-solving strategies, as necessary. (P, N, H)

7. 3. Diet therapy for ulcer disease is a controversial issue. There is no scientific evidence that diet therapy promotes healing. Most clients are instructed to follow a diet that they can tolerate. Eating six small meals daily is no longer a common treatment for peptic ulcer disease. There is no need for the client to ingest only liquid and pureed food. A high-fat diet would not be healthy or necessary. (I, T, H)

8. 4. Coffee and other caffeinated beverages should be avoided because they seem to stimulate gastric acid production. (I, K, G)

9. 3. Alcohol can stimulate gastric acid secretion and break down the gastric mucosal barrier, resulting in gastritis. If foods that are thought to increase gastric acid (such as cola, coffee, and tea) lead to discomfort, they should be avoided. (I, C, H)

10. 2. Currently accepted nutritional therapy for clients with peptic ulcers is best expressed by the statement, "The type of diet is not as important as including foods the client can tolerate." There is no evidence that special diets promote healing of an uncomplicated peptic ulcer regardless of the client's age. Eating frequent small meals was once suggested, but because eating stimulates acid production, most authorities now recommend eating three meals a day consisting of foods that the client tolerates well. (I, T, H)

11. 1. The client who has had an upper GI endoscopy should be monitored for return of the gag reflex. An upper GI endoscopy does not affect bowel sounds or breath sounds. (E, T, S)

12. 2. Rest is an essential component of ulcer healing. Nurses can help clients understand the importance of rest and find ways to balance work and family demands to promote permanent healing. Nurses cannot demand these changes; clients must choose them. (P, C, L)

13. 4. It would be most effective for the client to develop a health maintenance plan that incorporates regular periods of physical and mental rest. Strategies should be identified that are appropriate to the types of physical and mental stressors that the client needs to cope with in his home and work environments. There is no need for the client to avoid yard work or golf if these activities are not stressful to him. Scheduling all physical activity to occur only in the morning would not be restful. (I, N, H)

14. 4. Although clients cannot eliminate stress, they can improve their ability to cope with it. Identifying stressors at work, setting goals a little lower, and considering a job change may help a client deal with stress, but improving the ability to cope with stress is most important. (I, N, H)

15. 2. The client should avoid cigarette smoking because of its stimulatory effect on gastric secretions. Nicotine also increases the release of epinephrine, which leads to vasoconstriction. A client with peptic ulcer should check with the physician before taking any over-the-counter drug, but acetaminophen does not typically cause gastric irritation. The client may chew gum and eat candy bars if desired. (I, T, G)

16. 2. Cimetidine (Tagamet) decreases gastric acid secretion and should be taken regularly with meals. (E, C, G)

The Client With Cholecystitis

17. 2. A client with cholecystitis with cholelithiasis may experience nausea, vomiting, abdominal discomfort, and other gastrointestinal symptoms after eating high-fat foods. This is due to decreased fat absorption related to lack of normal bile flow from the gallbladder. Clients are more likely to have a low-grade fever and an elevated white blood cell count due to inflammation. Black stools would be unexpected. (A, T, G)

18. 1. Administering pain medication would have the highest priority during the first hour after the client's admission. Completing the admission history, maintaining hydration, and teaching about planned diagnostic tests are aspects of this client's care but are not the highest priority. (I, N, G)

19. 2. Propantheline bromide (Pro-Banthine) is an anticholinergic used to decrease biliary contractions and aid in the reduction of pain. (P, C, G)

20. 2. When bile is not reaching the intestine, the feces will not contain bile pigments. The stool then becomes gray, clay-like, or putty-like in color. Black stool can be caused by upper gastrointestinal bleeding and by certain medications, such as iron supplements. (A, K, G)

21. 4. A client with an obstructed common bile duct should be monitored for prolonged bleeding time. Such an obstruction presents bile from entering the intestinal tract. Absence of bile in this tract prevents absorption of fat-soluble vitamins A, D, E, and K. Vitamin K is necessary for the prothrombin formation. Prothrombin deficiency causes delayed blood clotting, which results in prolonged bleeding time. (E, C, G)

22. 2. Iodine compounds used as radiographic contrast media, such as iopanoic acid (Telepaque), should not be administered to the client with iodine and seafood allergies, because anaphylaxis may occur. (P, C, S)

23. 4. A T-tube is used after exploration of the common duct to help prevent bile from spilling into the peritoneal cavity. The tube also helps maintain patency of the common duct and helps ensure bile drainage out of the body until the edema in the common duct subsides sufficiently for bile to drain into the duodenum. A Penrose drain promotes blood and serosanguineous drainage from a wound. A T-tube is not used to irrigate the biliary tract or to minimize passage of bile into the duodenum. (E, C, G)

24. 3. The T-tube usually drains 300 to 500 ml in the first 24 hours after surgery. After 3 to 4 days, the amount decreases to less than 200 ml per 24 hours. (A, K, G)

25. 2. T-tube drainage is recorded separately on the output record. Adding it to other output makes it difficult to determine the amount of bile drainage. The client's total intake will be incorrect if drainage is subtracted from it. (I, C, G)

26. 1. Bile is erosive and extremely irritating to the skin. Therefore, it is essential that skin around the T-tube be kept clean and dry. (P, T, G)

27. 3. A folded bath blanket or pillow placed over the incision will be most effective in helping the client cough and deep breathe after a cholecystectomy. Taking rapid, shallow breaths would not be effective. Laying on the right side would cause increased incisional pain and decrease lung expansion. The client should be positioned in Fowler's position when possible to promote maximum lung expansion. Withholding pain medication will make the client less likely to cough and deep breathe due to the discomfort. (I, T, S)

28. 3. Bile flows almost continuously into the intestine for the first few weeks after gallbaldder removal. Limiting the amount of fat in the intestine at one time ensures that adequate bile will be available to facilitate digestion. There is no need to eliminate high-fiber foods, and doing so would tend to increase (rather than decrease) pressure within the large intestine (not the small intestine). Eating large amounts of meat, cheese, and peanut butter would be undesirable, because these foods are often high in fat. Removing the gall-bladder does not stop pancreatic secretions. (I, N, H)

29. 4. Lean meats, such as beef, lamb, veal, and well-trimmed lean ham and pork are low in fat. Ham salad and egg salad are high in fat from the fat in salad dressing. Rice, pasta, and vegetables are low in fat when not served with butter, cream, or sauces. Fruits are low in fat. The amount of fat allowed in a client's diet after cholecystectomy will depend on the client's ability to tolerate fat. Typically, the client does not require a special diet. (P, C, G)

The Client With Cancer of the Stomach

30. 3. Total parenteral nutrition bypasses the enteral route and provides total nutrition: protein, carbohydrates, fats, vitamins, minerals, and trace elements. Oral and tube feedings would enter the stomach and could cause the feeling of fullness, nausea, and vomiting that the client had before admission. IV isotonic saline provides incomplete nutrition: water, sodium, and chloride only. (I, N, G)

31. 2. A Billroth II procedure bypasses the duodenum

and connects the stump of the stomach directly to the jejunum. The pyloric sphincter is sacrificed, along with some of the stomach fundus. The cardiac sphincter remains intact. (I, K, G)

32. 1. Nasogastric suctioning is ordered to remove accumulated gas or fluid (secretions). Excessive fluid can cause pressure on suture lines, resulting in injury, rupture, or dislodgement. Ascitic fluid collects in the peritoneal space. The gastrointestinal tract should remain empty (no food or fluids) until peristalsis returns and suture lines have healed adequately, at which time the nasogastric tube is removed. Oral feedings are attempted before resorting to tube feeding. Antacids are not used to promote healing of suture lines. (I, C, G)

33. 1. Approximately 12 to 24 hours after subtotal gastrectomy, gastric drainage is normally brown, which indicates digested blood. Drainage during the first 6 to 12 hours contains some bright-red blood, but large amounts of blood or excessive bloody drainage should be reported to the physician promptly. Green or cloudy-white drainage is not expected during the first 12 to 24 hours after subtotal gastrectomy. (E, C, G)

34. 3. These symptoms indicate that gas and secretions are accumulating within the remaining gastric pouch due to impaired peristalsis or edema at the operative site, and may indicate that the drainage system is not working properly. Saline solution is used to irrigate nasogastric tubes. Hypotonic solutions (e.g., water) would increase electrolyte loss. Following gastric surgery, only the surgeon repositions the nasogastric tube because of the danger of rupturing or dislodging the suture line. In addition, a physician's order is needed to irrigate the nasogastric tube, as this may also disrupt the suture line. The amount of suction varies with the type of tube used and is ordered by the physician. (I, N, S)

35. 4. Semi-Fowler's position facilitates drainage of the remaining stomach contents, thus decreasing the risk of regurgitation, which could result in aspiration of gastric contents. The position also allows for greater chest wall expansion and diaphragm contraction. The other options are factors that contribute to respiratory problems. Breathing and coughing cause pain in clients with high abdominal incisions. Splinting of the chest occurs, which decreases coughing and deep breathing efforts. Shallow breathing leads to hypoventilation and atelectasis. Weak and fatigued clients have a decreased cough effort and cannot move well. Secretions in the gastric stump may collect due to decreased peristalsis and edema around the anastomosis. This increases the risk of regurgitation and aspiration. (D, N, G)

36. 1. Pain, fever, and abdominal rigidity are symptoms of inflammation/peritonitis. Diarrhea with fat in the stool is steatorrhea. Palpitations, pallor, and diaphoresis after eating are vasomotor symptoms of gastric retention. (A, N, G)

37. 2. Because of the client's reduced stomach capacity, frequent small feedings are recommended. Early satiety can result, and large quantities of food are not well tolerated. Each client should progress at his own pace; gradually increasing the amount of food eaten at each meal is the key. The goal is three meals daily if possible, but this can take 6 months or longer to achieve. Nausea can be episodic and can result from eating too fast or eating too much at one time. Eating less and more slowly, rather than not eating at all, can be a solution. Bland foods are recommended as starting foods because they are more easily digested and less irritating to the healing mucosa. (P, T, H)

38. 1. Weight gain will be slow and gradual, because less food can be eaten at one time due to the decreased stomach size. More food and fluid will be tolerated as edema at the suture line decreases and healing progresses. The remaining stomach may stretch over time to accommodate more food. Rapid weight gain may be due to fluid retention (1 pint = 1 pound). Food intake will be greater if nausea and vomiting are absent. Water provides hydration, but not nutrients. (E, T, G)

39. 2. Following gastric resection, ingested food moves rapidly from the remaining stomach into the duodenum or jejunum. The food has not undergone adequate preliminary digestion in the stomach. It is concentrated, distends the intestine, and stimulates significant secretion of insulin by the pancreas. The dumping syndrome results from these factors, which are initiated by the rapid movement of food out of the stomach. (P, K, G)

40. 3. Faintness, weakness, a full feeling, dizziness, excessive perspiration, and diarrhea are characteristic symptoms of the dumping syndrome. (A, C, G)

41. 4. Carbohydrates are restricted, but protein is recommended because it digests more slowly. Fluids are restricted to reduce the bulk of food, and lying on the left side is encouraged to decrease movement of the food bolus. (I, T, G)

The Client With Pancreatitis

42. 2. The most common symptom of pancreatitis is intense abdominal pain in the mid-epigastric area or the left upper quadrant. The pain may radiate to the back. Nausea and vomiting are also common. Hypotension and tachycardia may occur as a result of pancreatic hemorrhage, excessive fluid volume shifting, or enzyme damage. Hyperglycemia and elevated white blood cell count are also common. Peripheral edema, cyanosis, and fingernail clubbing are not typical symptoms of pancreatitis. (A, C, G)

43. 1. The primary diagnostic tests for pancreatitis are serum amylase and lipase and urine amylase. Serum amylase is the most common test; the result may be above 200 Somogyi units/dl. (A, K, G)

44. 3. Premature activation of pancreatic enzymes within the pancreas, rather than in the duodenum, causes the autodigestion process that produces pancreatitis. Spasm of the sphincter of Oddi is not the causative factor. Increased gastric secretions can aggravate pancreatitis by stimulating the pancreas. Volume depletion is a consequence of pancreatitis. (P, K, G)

45. 1. Alcoholism is the major cause of acute pancreatitis in the United States. Because some clients are reluctant to discuss their alcohol use, staff may inquire about it in several ways. Alcohol intake does not interfere with the pertinent tests used to diagnose pancreatitis. However, recent ingestion of large amounts of alcohol may cause an increased serum amylase, and large amounts of ethyl and methyl alcohol may produce elevated urinary amylase levels. All hospitalized clients are asked about alcohol and drug use on admission but are not repeatedly asked about it during hospitalization. Physicians do seek all the facts, but this can be done while considering the client's religious beliefs. Religious beliefs are pertinent to total client care. (I, T, L)

46. 1. Meperidine hydrochloride (Demerol), a strong narcotic analgesic, effectively reduces the pain of acute pancreatitis. Morphine sulfate and codeine sulfate are contraindicated in pancreatitis because they may cause spasm and exacerbate pain. Cimetidine (Tagamet), a histamine receptor antagonist, decreases gastric acidity. (I, T, G)

47. 2. Life-threatening shock is a potential complication of pancreatitis. Kinin peptides activated by the trapped trypsin cause vasodilation and increased capillary permeability. These effects exacerbate shock and are not easily reversed with pharmacologic agents such as vasopressors. (A, K, G)

48. 1. Hypoglycemia would be unexpected in this client. Pancreatitis interferes with beta cell functioning, and clients must be monitored carefully for hyperglycemia. Hyperlipidemia and gastrointestinal distress are also common. (A, C, G)

49. 4. Hypocalcemia is a major potential complication of pancreatitis. Muscle twitching and irritability are primary symptoms of hypocalcemia. Calcium replacement must begin as soon as hypocalcemia is validated. Hypomagnesemia may occur due to vomiting in clients with pancreatitis, especially if they are malnourished. Serum glucose is elevated. Hypokalemia may occur with loss of gastric juice through vomiting or nasogastric suction. (A, C, G)

50. 1. There is little definitive treatment for pancreatitis. It is important to suppress enzymes to reduce pancreatic stimulation. This is done by keeping the client NPO to rest the gastrointestinal tract. Preventing infection and ensuring adequate nutrition and fluid and electrolyte balance are related issues but are not the focus of treatment. (P, N, G)

51. 2. Nasogastric suction is frequently used in the treatment of pancreatitis to decrease pancreatic secretion and gastric distention. Food and fluids are withheld during the acute phase of pancreatitis to rest the pancreas. IV fluids are administered to provide hydration. Placing the client in reverse Trendelenburg's position or maintaining enteric isolation is not appropriate for treating pancreatitis. (P, T, G)

52. 3. Antispasmodic drugs such as proprantheline bromide (Pro-Banthine) may be administered along with narcotics to deal with the intense pain associated with pancreatitis. (I, C, G)

53. 4. Altered Nutrition: Less than Body Requirements is likely to be a priority nursing diagnosis because the abdominal pain, nausea, and vomiting typical of pancreatitis can affect the client's food and fluid intake. Treatment of pancreatitis also frequently involves stopping all oral intake until the inflammation is resolved. Clients with pancreatitis are at risk for developing malnutrition. IV therapy is used for fluid replacement, and total parenteral nutrition may be ordered to prevent malnourishment. (D, N, G)

54. 2. A low-fat bland diet prevents stimulation of the pancreas while providing adequate nutrition. Although calcium is important, the low fat content is more significant. Dietary protein and fiber are not directly related to pancreatitis. The hyperglycemia of acute pancreatitis is usually transient and does not require long-term dietary modification. (I, C, H)

55. 2. Pancreatic enzymes are prescribed to facilitate the digestion of protein and fats and should be taken in conjunction with every meal and snack. Specified hours for administration are ineffective, as the enzymes must be taken in conjunction with food ingestion. (I, C, H)

56. 3. If the dosage and administration of pancreatic enzymes are adequate, the client's stool will be relatively normal. Any increase in odor or fat content would indicate the need for dosage adjustment. Stable body weight would be another indirect indicator. (E, C, H)

The Client With Hiatal Hernia

57. 1. Hiatal hernia produces symptoms of esophageal reflux as the sphincter slides up into the negative-pressure environment of the thorax. The symptoms typically occur when the client is in a recumbent position. Neither emotions nor normal activity influence the incidence of reflux. (A, C, G)

58. 1. Heartburn, the most common symptom of a sliding hiatal hernia, results from reflux of gastric secretions into the esophagus. Regurgitation of gastric contents and dysphagia are other common symptoms. (A, C, G)

59. 2. Any factor that increases intra-abdominal pressure can contribute to the development of hiatal hernia. Such factors include obesity, abdominal straining, and pregnancy. Hiatal hernia is also associated with aging and occurs in both males and females. (A, T, H)

60. 3. Self-responsibility is the key to individual health maintenance. Using examples of situations in which the client had demonstrated responsibility for herself can be very reinforcing and supporting. Meeting other people who are managing their care and involving family members can be helpful, but individual motivation is more important. Reassurance can be helpful but is less important than individualization of care. The client has ultimate responsibility for her personal health habits. (I, T, H)

61. 3. The magnesium salts in magnesium hydroxide (Milk of Magnesia) are related to those found in laxatives and may cause diarrhea. Aluminum salt products can cause constipation. Many clients find that a combination product is required to maintain normal bowel elimination. (P, K, G)

62. 2. Smoking and alcohol use both reduce esophageal sphincter tone and can result in reflux and thus should be avoided or minimized by clients with hiatal hernia. The other factor may increase the client's general health and well-being but are not directly associated with hiatal hernia. (P, T, H)

63. 4. Sleeping with the head of the bed elevated encourages movement of food through the esophagus by gravity. By fostering esophageal acid clearance, gravity helps keep the acidic pepsin and alkaline biliary secretions from contacting the esophagus. Neither elevating the foot of the bed nor sleeping flat without a pillow under the head enhances this clearance. Sleeping on the right side minimizes the problem for some clients. (E, T, G)

64. 2. Bending, especially after eating, can cause gastroesophageal reflux; lifting heavy objects increases intraabdominal pressure. Knowing the client's lifting techniques enables the nurse to assess the client's knowledge of factors contributing to hiatal hernia and of methods that prevent complications. The other factors are not directly related to hiatal hernia. (A, N, H)

65. 1. Fats are associated with decreased esophageal sphincter tone, which increases reflux. Obesity contributes to the development of hiatal hernia, and a low-fat diet might also aid in weight loss. Fat is the most concentrated source of calories. The other options do not affect reflux. (E, T, H)

66. 1. Esophageal reflux worsens when the stomach is overdistended with food. Thus, an important measure is to eat small, frequent meals. Food intake in the evening should be strictly limited to reduce the incidence of nighttime reflux. (I, T, H)

67. 1. A client with a hiatal hernia should avoid the recumbent position immediately after meals to minimize gastric reflux. Wearing tight, constrictive clothing, such as a girdle, can increase intra-abdominal pressure and thus lead to reflux of gastric juices. Bedtime snacks, as well as high-fat foods and carbonated beverages, should be avoided. Excessive vigorous exercise also should be avoided, especially after meals, but there is no reason why the client must give up swimming. (E, N, H)

68. 1. Metoclopramide hydrochloride (Reglan) increases sphincter tone and facilitates gastric emptying; both actions reduce the incidence of reflux. Antacids or histamine receptor antagonists may also be prescribed to help control reflux and esophagitis. (P, K, G)

69. 4. Metoclopramide hydrochloride (Reglan) can cause sedation. Alcohol and other CNS depressants will add to this sedation. A client taking Reglan should be cautioned to avoid driving or other hazardous activities for a few hours after taking the drug. (I, C, G)

70. 3. Cimetidine (Tagamet) is a histamine receptor antagonist that decreases the quantity of gastric secretions. It may be used in hiatal hernia therapy to prevent or treat the esophagitis and heartburn associated with reflux. (P, K, G)

71. 2. Surgery to correct hiatal hernia is extensive and commonly produces complications. It is performed only when medical therapy fails to control the symptoms. Most clients can be successfully treated with a combination of diet restrictions, medications, weight control, and life-style modifications. (I, C, G)

General Questions

72. 4. Having the client look toward the ceiling as the nurse inserts a nasogastric tube facilitates tube insertion. When the tube reaches the nasopharynx, the client should be instructed to bring the head forward a bit by flexing the neck. This technique closes the trachea and opens the esophagus to receive the tube. Correct techniques include having the client assume an upright position, lubricating the tube with a water-soluble lubricant, and having the client swallow as the tube is passed into the stomach. (I, T, S)

73. 1. If the tube is not in the stomach and solution is introduced, the solution will enter respiratory passages and harm the client. The best way to determine whether a nasogastric tube is in the stomach is to apply suction to the tube with a syringe and observe for the return of stomach contents. Another satisfactory method is to instill air into the tube with a syringe while auscultating over the epigastric area. Hearing the air enter the stomach helps ensure proper placement, but the method is not foolproof. Observing for air bubbles when the free end of the tube is placed under water is an unacceptable method of determining tube placement. (I, N, S)

74. 1. A laxative is administered following an upper GI series. This examination involves administration of barium, which must be eliminated from the body because it may harden and cause an obstruction. (P, C, G)

75. 3. Aluminum products, such as aluminum hydroxide, form insoluble salts in the body. These precipitate and accumulate in the intestines, possibly causing constipation. (E, K, G)

76. 1. Applying a tourniquet obstructs venous blood flow and distends the veins. (I, K, G)

77. 3. The incisions made for upper abdominal surgery are near the diaphragm and make deep breathing very painful. Incentive spirometry is essential to prevent the development of atelectasis after surgery. (I, T, G)

78. 4. Incentive spirometry promotes lung expansion and increases respiratory function. When used properly, an incentive spirometer causes sustained maximal inspiration and increases cardiac output. (E, K, G)

79. 2. Oral food and fluids are withheld before surgery when a client receives general anesthesia, primarily to help prevent vomiting and possible aspiration of stomach contents. Withholding food and fluids before surgery does not prevent constipation, gas pains, or abdominal distention in the postoperative period, nor does it relieve pressure on the diaphragm. (I, C, G)

80. 2. When using the ventrogluteal site, the nurse injects the medication into the gluteus minimus muscle. (I, C, S)

81. 1. Prochloperazine dimaleate (Compazine) is administered to control nausea, vomiting, and retching. In doses larger than those needed to control nausea and vomiting, prochlorperazine dimaleate is used in psychotherapy because of its effects on mood and behavior. (E, C, S)

82. 2. If the client understands the reasons for prescribed treatments, he is more likely to participate and cooperate with the plan. Fear of the unknown can increase anxiety. Telling the client to follow his physician's orders or comparing him to others will not decrease anxiety. (I, N, L)

83. 3. The nurse records the total amount of solution used to irrigate a gastric tube as intake and the total amount of return in the drainage bottle as output. (I, T, S)

84. 3. Applying a water-soluble lubricant to the nares helps alleviate sore nares when a gastric tube is in place. Measures such as irrigating and repositioning the tube and changing the client's position will not relieve irritation from the tube. Also, repositioning the tube may cause further problems by dislodging a scab or breaking open an ulceration. (I, T, S)

85. 4. The primary purpose of fluid replacement therapy for a client receiving gastric suction is to maintain fluid and electrolyte balance. Gastric suctioning interrupts the normal intake of fluids; thus, IV replacement therapy is indicated. (I, T, G)

86. 2. Coughing and deep breathing are more effective when pain is minimal. A client in severe pain tends to limit movement and to breathe shallowly to decrease the pain. Enough pain medication should be given to decrease pain without depressing respirations; this allows the client to cough effectively. Deep-breathing exercises should be performed at least every 2 hours. Ambulation to increase ventilation and gas exchange should be encouraged as soon as possible postoperatively (usually on the first postoperative day). (I, N, G)

87. 3. When a client with a nasogastric tube exhibits abdominal distention, the nurse should first check the suction machine. If the equipment is functioning properly, then the nurse should take other steps, such as checking tube patency. (I, N, S)

88. 2. Normal serum potassium level in an adult is 3.5 to 5.5 mEq/L. (A, K, G)

89. 3. An early indication of hypokalemia is muscle weakness in the legs. Potassium is essential for proper neuromuscular impulse transmission. When neuromuscular impulse transmission is impaired, as in hypokalemia, leg muscles become weak and flabby. If hypokalemia progresses, respiratory muscles become involved, and the client becomes apneic. Hypokalemia also causes EKG changes. Diarrhea is common in hyperkalemia. Tingling in the fingers and around the mouth occurs in hypocalcemia. Sticky mucous membranes are common in hypernatremia. (A, K, G)

90. 4. Because of the irregularity of bowel sounds, the nurse should listen for 5 minutes in each quadrant to confirm the absence of bowel sounds. Auscultation is performed before palpation, because palpation may affect peristaltic activity. The client should be positioned supine to provide adequate access to the abdomen. (A, C, G)

THE NURSING CARE OF ADULTS WITH MEDICAL/SURGICAL HEALTH PROBLEMS

TEST 3: The Client With Upper Gastrointestinal Track Health Problems

Directions: Use this answer grid to determine areas of strength or need for further study.

NURSING PROCESS

A = Assessment
D = Analysis, nursing diagnosis
P = Planning
I = Implementation
E = Evaluation

COGNITIVE LEVEL

K = Knowledge
C = Comprehension
T = Application
N = Analysis

CLIENT NEEDS

S = Safe, effective care environment
G = Physiological integrity
L = Psychosocial integrity
H = Health promotion/maintenance

		Nursing Process					Cognitive Level				Client Needs			
Question #	Answer #	A	D	P	I	E	K	C	T	N	S	G	L	H
1	1	A						C				G		
2	4	A						C				G		
3	2					E		C				G		
4	1			P			K					G		
5	2		D							N		G		
6	1			P						N				H
7	3				I				T					H
8	4				I		K					G		
9	3				I			C						H
10	2				I				T					H
11	1					E			T		S			
12	2			P				C					L	
13	4				I					N				H
14	4				I					N				H
15	2				I				T			G		
16	2					E		C				G		
17	2	A							T			G		
18	1				I					N		G		
19	2			P				C				G		
20	2	A					K					G		
21	4					E		C				G		
22	2			P				C			S			

NURSING PROCESS

A = Assessment
D = Analysis, nursing diagnosis
P = Planning
I = Implementation
E = Evaluation

COGNITIVE LEVEL

K = Knowledge
C = Comprehension
T = Application
N = Analysis

CLIENT NEEDS

S = Safe, effective care environment
G = Physiological integrity
L = Psychosocial integrity
H = Health promotion/maintenance

		Nursing Process					Cognitive Level				Client Needs			
Question #	Answer #	A	D	P	I	E	K	C	T	N	S	G	L	H
23	4					E		C				G		
24	3	A					K					G		
25	2				I			C				G		
26	1			P					T			G		
27	3				I				T		S			
28	3				I					N				H
29	4			P				C				G		
30	3				I					N		G		
31	2				I		K					G		
32	1				I			C				G		
33	1					E		C				G		
34	3				I					N	S			
35	4		D							N		G		
36	1	A								N		G		
37	2			P					T					H
38	1					E			T			G		
39	2			P			K					G		
40	3	A						C				G		
41	4				I				T			G		
42	2	A						C				G		
43	1	A					K					G		
44	3			P			K					G		
45	1				I				T				L	
46	1				I				T			G		
47	2	A					K					G		
48	1	A						C				G		
49	4	A						C				G		
50	1			P						N		G		

ANSWER GRID: 2

Nursing Process

A = Assessment
D = Analysis, nursing diagnosis
P = Planning
I = Implementation
E = Evaluation

Cognitive Level

K = Knowledge
C = Comprehension
T = Application
N = Analysis

Client Needs

S = Safe, effective care environment
G = Physiological integrity
L = Psychosocial integrity
H = Health promotion/maintenance

		Nursing Process					Cognitive Level				Client Needs			
Question #	Answer #	A	D	P	I	E	K	C	T	N	S	G	L	H
51	2			P					T			G		
52	3				I			C				G		
53	4		D							N		G		
54	2				I			C						H
55	2				I			C						H
56	3					E		C						H
57	1	A						C				G		
58	1	A						C				G		
59	2	A							T					H
60	3				I				T					H
61	3			P			K					G		
62	2			P					T					H
63	4					E			T			G		
64	2	A								N				H
65	1					E			T					H
66	1				I				T					H
67	1					E				N				H
68	1			P			K					G		
69	4				I			C				G		
70	3			P			K					G		
71	2				I			C				G		
72	4				I				T		S			
73	1				I					N	S			
74	1			P				C				G		
75	3					E	K					G		
76	1				I		K					G		
77	3				I				T			G		
78	4					E	K					G		

Answer Grid: 3

NURSING PROCESS

A = Assessment
D = Analysis, nursing diagnosis
P = Planning
I = Implementation
E = Evaluation

COGNITIVE LEVEL

K = Knowledge
C = Comprehension
T = Application
N = Analysis

CLIENT NEEDS

S = Safe, effective care environment
G = Physiological integrity
L = Psychosocial integrity
H = Health promotion/maintenance

		Nursing Process					Cognitive Level				Client Needs			
Question #	Answer #	A	D	P	I	E	K	C	T	N	S	G	L	H
79	2				I			C				G		
80	2				I			C			S			
81	1					E		C			S			
82	2				I					N			L	
83	3				I				T		S			
84	3				I				T		S			
85	4				I				T			G		
86	2				I					N		G		
87	3				I					N	S			
88	2	A					K					G		
89	3	A					K					G		
90	4	A						C				G		
Number Correct														
Number Possible	90	19	3	17	37	14	17	31	24	18	11	58	3	18
Percentage Correct														

Score Calculation:

To determine your **Percentage Correct**, divide the **Number Correct** by the **Number Possible**.

The Client With Lower Gastrointestinal Tract Health Problems

Test 4

The Client With Cancer of the Colon
The Client With Hepatitis A
The Client With Hepatitis B
The Client With Hemorrhoids
The Client With Inflammatory Bowel Disease
The Client With an Intestinal Obstruction
The Client With Cirrhosis
The Client With an Ileostomy
General Questions
Correct Answers and Rationale

Select the one best answer and indicate your choice by filling in the circle in front of the option.

The Client With Cancer of the Colon

A 66-year-old female client has been experiencing cramping pain in her lower abdomen and has noticed a gradual change in her elimination pattern.

1. The client is scheduled for a barium enema. As part of the preparation for the test she receives 60 ml of castor oil orally. Castor oil facilitates cleansing of the bowel primarily by

○ 1. softening the feces.
○ 2. lubricating the feces.
○ 3. increasing the volume of intestinal contents.
○ 4. irritating the nerve endings in the intestinal mucosa.

2. Following the barium enema, the client will receive which type of medication?

○ 1. A laxative.
○ 2. An emetic.
○ 3. An antacid.
○ 4. A digestant.

3. A diagnosis of colon cancer is confirmed, and the client is scheduled for an abdominoperineal resection with permanent colostomy. When preparing the client for surgery, the nurse would most likely implement which of the following measures?

○ 1. Keep the client NPO for 2 days before surgery.
○ 2. Administer kanamycin (Kantrex) the night before surgery.
○ 3. Inform the client that chest tubes will be in place following surgery.
○ 4. Maintain the client on strict bedrest.

4. The client asks, "Where will my colostomy be placed?" What would be the nurse's best response?

○ 1. "It will allow your stool to pass through the rectum."
○ 2. "It really doesn't matter; you'll have to wear an ostomy pouch anyway."
○ 3. "In the midline of the abdomen near your umbilicus."
○ 4. "A permanent colostomy is usually located on the left side of the abdomen."

5. The client requires a transfusion on her second postoperative day, and two units of packed red blood cells are ordered. The nurse assembles a blood administration setup in which the blood is hung in tandem with which solution?

○ 1. Distilled water.
○ 2. 0.9% saline solution.
○ 3. 5% dextrose in distilled water.
○ 4. 10% dextrose in normal saline.

6. Which of the following actions should the nurse take first when the client complains of headache and a

tingling sensation in her fingers shortly after the blood transfusion is started?
- ○ 1. Notify the physician.
- ○ 2. Check for infiltration.
- ○ 3. Slow the rate of the infusion.
- ○ 4. Stop the blood infusion.

7. Which of the following nursing interventions would be inappropriate during the client's postoperative period?
- ○ 1. Encourage the client to practice diaphragmatic breathing.
- ○ 2. Teach the client to cough against a closed glottis.
- ○ 3. Raise the knee gatch of the bed to prevent the client from sliding down in bed.
- ○ 4. Apply thigh-high antiembolism stockings.

8. The client had a nasogastric tube inserted at the time of surgery. This tube will most likely be removed when the client demonstrates
- ○ 1. absence of nausea and vomiting.
- ○ 2. passage of mucus from the rectum.
- ○ 3. passage of flatus and feces from the colostomy.
- ○ 4. absence of stomach drainage for about 24 hours.

9. The nurse has just removed the client's nasogastric tube and places the client on a clear liquid diet. Which of the following nursing actions would be most appropriate immediately following nasogastric tube removal?
- ○ 1. Provide the client with mouth care.
- ○ 2. Auscultate for bowel sounds.
- ○ 3. Palpate for abdominal distention.
- ○ 4. Give the client some orange sherbet.

10. The client indicates that she is ready to learn about her colostomy. Which of the following nursing interventions would most likely be effective in preparing the client to look at her colostomy?
- ○ 1. Telling the client how normal body functions will continue.
- ○ 2. Encouraging the client to ask questions about the colostomy.
- ○ 3. Asking a member of the local ostomy club to visit the client.
- ○ 4. Using illustrative material during teaching sessions with the client.

11. A colostomy irrigation is ordered for the client on her fifth postoperative day. The primary purpose of this first irrigation is to
- ○ 1. cleanse the colon.
- ○ 2. regulate the bowel.
- ○ 3. dilate the sphincter.
- ○ 4. stimulate peristalsis.

12. If the client complains of abdominal cramping after receiving approximately 150 ml of solution during colostomy irrigation, the nurse should temporarily
- ○ 1. stop the flow of solution.
- ○ 2. have the client sit up in bed.
- ○ 3. remove the irrigating cone or tube.
- ○ 4. insert the cone or tube further into the colon.

13. The nurse evaluates the client's stoma during the initial postoperative period. Which of the following signs would indicate inadequate blood supply to the stoma and should be reported immediately to the physician? A stoma that
- ○ 1. is slightly edematous.
- ○ 2. is dark red to purple.
- ○ 3. oozes a small amount of blood.
- ○ 4. does not expel stool.

14. An indication that the client is ready to participate in her care would be if, while the nurse changes her colostomy bag and dressing, the client
- ○ 1. asks what time her doctor will visit that day.
- ○ 2. asks about the supplies used during the dressing change.
- ○ 3. talks about something she read in the morning newspaper.
- ○ 4. complains about the way the night nurse changed the dressing.

15. Appropriate skin care is an important aspect of teaching for this client. Which of the following preparations would be best to apply around her colostomy?
- ○ 1. Karaya.
- ○ 2. Petrolatum.
- ○ 3. Cornstarch.
- ○ 4. Antiseptic cream.

16. Which of the following measures would most effectively promote wound healing after the client's perineal drains have been removed?
- ○ 1. Taking sitz baths.
- ○ 2. Taking daily showers.
- ○ 3. Applying warm moist dressings to the area.
- ○ 4. Applying a protected heating pad to the area.

17. When planning diet teaching for the client with a colostomy, the nurse should develop a teaching plan based on the knowledge that
- ○ 1. foods containing roughage should be eliminated from the diet.
- ○ 2. liquids are best limited to prevent diarrhea.
- ○ 3. clients with colostomies must experiment to determine the balance of food that is best for them.
- ○ 4. a constipating diet will produce a formed stool that can be passed with more regularity through a colostomy.

The Client With Hepatitis A

A 22-year-old college student is admitted to the hospital acutely ill with hepatitis A (infectious hepatitis).

18. The nurse would expect the client to exhibit which of the following symptoms during the acute phase of hepatitis A?

○ 1. Increased appetite.
○ 2. Yellowed sclera.
○ 3. Shortness of breath.
○ 4. Light, frothy urine.

19. Which of the following precautions would have the lowest priority when the nurse plans appropriate care for the client with hepatitis A?
○ 1. Using disposable dishes.
○ 2. Double-bagging and tagging soiled linens.
○ 3. Assigning him to a private room.
○ 4. Wearing a gown and gloves when giving direct care.

20. The nurse prepares a nursing care plan for the client. Nursing orders should reflect that the primary treatment for the client will be concerned with ensuring that he or she receives
○ 1. adequate bed rest.
○ 2. a generous fluid intake.
○ 3. regular antibiotic therapy.
○ 4. daily IV electrolyte therapy.

21. Which of the following test results would the nurse use to assess the client's liver function?
○ 1. Glucose tolerance.
○ 2. Creatinine clearance.
○ 3. Serum transaminase.
○ 4. Serum electrolytes.

22. Which of the following diets most likely would be prescribed for a client with hepatitis A?
○ 1. High-fat diet.
○ 2. High-protein diet.
○ 3. High-carbohydrate diet.
○ 4. Well-balanced diet.

23. The nurse plans care for the client with hepatitis A with the understanding that the causative virus will be excreted from the client's body primarily through the
○ 1. skin.
○ 2. feces.
○ 3. urine.
○ 4. mucus.

24. Contaminated hands are often responsible for the transmission of hepatitis A. Also, the virus can be spread by
○ 1. infected insects.
○ 2. infected rodents and birds.
○ 3. contaminated foods and fluids.
○ 4. contaminated clothing and eating utensils.

25. The client expresses concern because he fears that members of his fraternity may also acquire hepatitis. Which of the following is most commonly used for prophylactic treatment of persons exposed to hepatitis A?
○ 1. Penicillin.
○ 2. Sulfadiazine (Microsulfon).
○ 3. Immune serum globulin.
○ 4. Hepatitis A vaccine.

26. When preparing the client for extended convalescence, the nurse teaches him about problems that may occur. The nurse knows that the client has understood the teaching when he says that he is most likely to have difficulty
○ 1. controlling pain.
○ 2. maintaining a regular bowel elimination pattern.
○ 3. preventing respiratory complications.
○ 4. maintaining a positive, optimistic outlook.

27. The client who has had hepatitis A should be instructed never to
○ 1. drink alcohol.
○ 2. donate blood.
○ 3. smoke.
○ 4. eat fatty foods.

The Client With Hepatitis B

The client has been admitted to the hospital with a diagnosis of hepatitis B.

28. Which of the following situations would most likely expose the nurse to the hepatitis B virus?
○ 1. Coming in contact with client's feces.
○ 2. Spraying the client's blood into the nurse's eyes.
○ 3. Touching the client's arm with ungloved hands while taking a blood pressure.
○ 4. Disposing of syringes and needles without recapping.

29. Which of the following activities would place a person in a high-risk category for contracting hepatitis B?
○ 1. Frequent use of marijuana.
○ 2. Ingestion of large amounts of acetaminophen (Tylenol).
○ 3. IV drug use.
○ 4. Ingestion of contaminated seafood.

30. Which of the following goals would be appropriate for the client with hepatitis B? The client will
○ 1. adhere to measures to prevent the spread of infection to others.
○ 2. adhere to a low-sodium, low-protein diet.
○ 3. verbalize the importance of using sedatives to provide adequate rest.
○ 4. avoid social activities with friends after discharge from the hospital.

31. The client tells the nurse, "I feel so isolated from my friends and family. Nobody wants to be around me." What would be the nurse's best response?
○ 1. "Don't worry. They'll get over it."
○ 2. "They're probably afraid of contracting hepatitis from you."
○ 3. "I'm sure you're imagining that!"
○ 4. "Tell me more about your feelings of isolation."

The Client With Hemorrhoids

A 36-year-old female has been admitted for an elective hemorrhoidectomy.

32. Which of the following factors in the client's nursing history most likely would be a primary cause of her hemorrhoids?
- ○ 1. Her age.
- ○ 2. Three pregnancies with vaginal deliveries.
- ○ 3. Her job as a schoolteacher.
- ○ 4. Varicosities in her legs.

33. Before surgery, the nurse would expect the physician should prescribe which of the following diets for the client?
- ○ 1. High protein, soft.
- ○ 2. Low roughage, high fiber.
- ○ 3. High roughage, high fiber.
- ○ 4. Bland, soft.

34. Immediately after a hemorrhoidectomy, the priority goal of nursing care for the client should be to
- ○ 1. prevent venous stasis.
- ○ 2. promote ambulation.
- ○ 3. control pain.
- ○ 4. prevent infection.

35. Which position would be ideal for the client in the early postoperative period?
- ○ 1. High Fowler's.
- ○ 2. Supine.
- ○ 3. Prone.
- ○ 4. Trendelenburg's.

36. Warm sitz baths three or four times a day are prescribed for the client after surgery. Implementation should be delayed until at least 12 hours postoperatively to avoid inducing
- ○ 1. hemorrhage.
- ○ 2. rectal spasm.
- ○ 3. urine retention.
- ○ 4. constipation.

37. The client is to continue taking sitz baths after discharge, and the nurse has been teaching her the proper procedure for taking them. The nurse would know that the client has understood the teaching when she says that it is most important to take a sitz bath
- ○ 1. first thing each morning.
- ○ 2. as needed for discomfort.
- ○ 3. after a bowel movement.
- ○ 4. at bedtime.

38. The client says she feels the urge to have her first postoperative bowel movement but is very concerned about the potential pain. Which of the following responses would indicate the nurse's understanding of appropriate pain alleviation techniques?
- ○ 1. "I'll get you a pain pill right away."
- ○ 2. "As soon as you've had a bowel movement, take a warm sitz bath."
- ○ 3. "After the bowel movement, cleanse the rectal area with warm water."
- ○ 4. "You may have some pain, but I'll give you pain medication."

39. The nurse has been teaching the client ways to avoid recurrence of hemorrhoids, including the importance of a high-fiber diet. The client's selection of which of the following breakfast menus would indicate that she understands the instructions?
- ○ 1. Danish pastry, prune juice, coffee, and milk.
- ○ 2. Oatmeal, milk, grapefruit wedges, and bran muffin.
- ○ 3. Corn flakes, milk, white toast, and orange juice.
- ○ 4. Scambled eggs, bacon, English muffin, and apple juice.

The Client With Inflammatory Bowel Disease

A 24-year-old male client has suffered from ulcerative colitis for the past 5 years. He is admitted to the hospital with an exacerbation of his disease, which he has attempted to treat at home for the past 10 days.

40. The nurse assesses the client's bowel elimination pattern. Which of the following signs are most typical of ulcerative colitis?
- ○ 1. Constipation.
- ○ 2. Bloody, diarrheal stools.
- ○ 3. Steatorrhea.
- ○ 4. Alternating periods of constipation and diarrhea.

41. Which of the following factors was most likely of greatest significance in causing an exacerbation of the client's ulcerative colitis?
- ○ 1. He reports that his work is very demanding and he's worried about "measuring up."
- ○ 2. He has recently begun following a modified vegetarian diet.
- ○ 3. He has been working out with weights for the past 3 months.
- ○ 4. He has begun attending a holistic health group with his girlfriend.

42. Which goal for the client's care should take priority during the first days of his hospitalization?
- ○ 1. Promoting self-care and independence.
- ○ 2. Stopping the diarrhea.
- ○ 3. Maintaining adequate nutrition.
- ○ 4. Promoting rest and comfort.

43. The client is following orders for bed rest with bathroom privileges. What would be the primary rationale for his activity restriction?

○ 1. To conserve energy.
○ 2. To reduce intestinal peristalsis.
○ 3. To promote rest and comfort.
○ 4. To prevent injury.

44. The client's symptoms have been present for more than a week. The nurse recognizes that he should be assessed carefully for signs of
○ 1. congestive heart failure.
○ 2. deep vein thrombosis.
○ 3. hypokalemia.
○ 4. hypocalcemia.

45. The client says to the nurse, "I can't take this anymore! I'm constantly in pain, and I can't leave my room because I need to stay by the toilet. I don't know how to deal with this." Based on these comments, an appropriate nursing diagnosis for this client would be
○ 1. Impaired Physical Mobility.
○ 2. Altered Thought Processes.
○ 3. Social Isolation.
○ 4. Ineffective Individual Coping.

46. The nurse should include which of the following measures in this client's care?
○ 1. Encouraging the use of stool softeners.
○ 2. Suggesting sitz baths p.r.n.
○ 3. Keeping the client's bathroom available for use.
○ 4. Wearing a gown to provide direct care.

47. The client's diarrhea persists. He is quite thin and has lost 12 pounds since the exacerbation of his ulcerative colitis. The nurse should anticipate that the physician will order which of the following treatment approaches to help the client meet his nutritional needs?
○ 1. Keeping the client NPO.
○ 2. Encouraging a high-calorie, high-protein diet.
○ 3. Implementing total parenteral nutrition (TPN).
○ 4. Providing six small meals a day.

48. The nurse knows that the site of choice for administering TPN is the
○ 1. subclavian vein.
○ 2. innominate vein.
○ 3. superior vena cava.
○ 4. internal jugular vein.

49. The basic component of the client's TPN solution is most likely to be
○ 1. an isotonic glucose solution.
○ 2. a hypertonic glucose solution.
○ 3. a hypotonic dextrose solution.
○ 4. a low molecular weight dextrose solution.

50. The nurse would regularly assess the client's ability to metabolize the TPN solution adequately by monitoring his
○ 1. pulse rate.
○ 2. blood pressure.
○ 3. temperature.
○ 4. urine glucose.

51. Which of the following interventions should the nurse include in the client's care plan to prevent complications associated with TPN administered via a central line?
○ 1. Use a strict clean technique for all dressing changes.
○ 2. Tape all connections of the system.
○ 3. Encourage bed rest.
○ 4. Cover the insertion site with a moisture-proof dressing.

52. Which of the following would be the best indication that the goals for TPN are being achieved for the client?
○ 1. Urine negative for glucose.
○ 2. Serum potassium level of 4.0 mEg/l.
○ 3. Serum glucose level of 96.
○ 4. Weight gain of ½lb./day.

53. The nurse notices that the client's TPN solution is infusing too slowly. The nurse calculates that the client has received 300 ml less than was ordered for the day. What would be the nurse's most appropriate action at this time?
○ 1. Quickly increase the flow rate to infuse an additional 300 ml over the next hour.
○ 2. Maintain the flow rate at the current rate and document any discrepancy in the chart.
○ 3. Assess the infusion system, note the client's condition, and notify the physician.
○ 4. Discontinue the solution and administer dextrose in 5% water until the infusion problem is resolved.

54. The physician prescribes sulfasalazine (Azulfidine) for the client to continue taking at home. What instructions should the nurse give the client about taking this medication?
○ 1. Avoid taking it with food.
○ 2. Take the total dose at bedtime.
○ 3. Take it with a full glass (240 ml) of water.
○ 4. Stop taking it if urine turns orange-yellow.

55. The client expresses serious concerns about his career as an attorney because of the effects of stress on ulcerative colitis. Which course of action would it be best for the nurse to suggest?
○ 1. Review his current coping mechanisms and develop alternatives, if needed.
○ 2. Consider a less-stressful career in which he would still use his education and experience.
○ 3. Ask his colleagues to help decrease his stress by giving him the easier cases.
○ 4. Prepare family members for the fact that he will have to work part-time.

56. The client is to follow a well-balanced high-protein, high-calorie, low-residue diet. In addition, the nurse should counsel him to avoid which of the following?
○ 1. Eggs and egg products.

○ 2. High-fat foods.
○ 3. Caffeinated beverages.
○ 4. Foods seasoned with salt.

57. Which of the following would be an appropriate expected outcome of nursing care for the client with ulcerative colitis? The client
○ 1. maintains an ideal body weight.
○ 2. verbalizes the importance of restricting fluids.
○ 3. experiences decreased frequency of constipation.
○ 4. accepts that an ileostomy will be necessary.

The Client With an Intestinal Obstruction

A 48-year-old female client is admitted to the hospital complaining of nausea, vomiting, and abdominal pain. Bowel obstruction is suspected.

58. During initial assessment, the nurse hears high-pitched tinkling bowel sounds on auscultation and dull sounds on percussion. What is the reason for the dull sounds?
○ 1. Hyperactive peristalsis.
○ 2. Excessive gas trapped in the intestine.
○ 3. The presence of a mass or tumor in the bowel.
○ 4. Fluid trapped in the intestine.

59. Of the following symptoms of bowel obstruction, which is related primarily to small-bowel obstruction rather than large-bowel obstruction?
○ 1. Profuse vomiting.
○ 2. Cramping abdominal pain.
○ 3. Abdominal distention.
○ 4. High-pitched bowel sounds above the obstruction.

60. The physician orders intestinal decompression for the client using a Cantor tube. The primary purpose of an intestinal tube such as a Cantor tube is to
○ 1. remove fluid and gas from the intestine.
○ 2. prevent fluid accumulation in the stomach.
○ 3. break up the obstruction.
○ 4. provide an alternative route for drug administration.

61. As soon as the Cantor tube has been inserted, the nurse should instruct the client to
○ 1. lie still on her back.
○ 2. lie on her right side.
○ 3. lie on her left side.
○ 4. get up and sit in a chair.

62. Which of the following statements about intestinal tubes, such as the Cantor tube, are correct? The tube
○ 1. cannot be attached to suction.
○ 2. contains a soft rubber bag filled with mercury.
○ 3. is taped securely to the client's cheek after insertion.
○ 4. can have its placement determined only by auscultation.

63. Which of the following measures would most likely be included in the client's care as soon as the Cantor tube has passed into the duodenum?
○ 1. Maintain bedrest with bathroom privileges.
○ 2. Advance the tube 2″ to 4″ at specified times.
○ 3. Provide frequent mouth care.
○ 4. Provide ice chips for the client to suck.

64. Which of the following nursing measures would be inappropriate when caring for a client with a Cantor tube?
○ 1. Injecting 10 ml of air into the tube to facilitate drainage.
○ 2. Applying a water-soluble lubricant to the client's nares.
○ 3. Coiling extra tubing on the client's bed.
○ 4. Irrigating the tube with 50 ml of normal saline solution.

65. Which of the following nursing diagnoses most likely would be appropriate for a client with an intestinal obstruction?
○ 1. Impaired Swallowing related to NPO status.
○ 2. Urinary Retention related to fluid volume depletion.
○ 3. Fluid Volume Deficit related to nausea and vomiting.
○ 4. Chronic Pain related to abdominal distention.

66. The client continues to have pain even though the Cantor tube is patent and draining. The physician wants to delay administering pain medication. When the client asks why, what would be the nurse's best response?
○ 1. "Narcotics trigger the vomiting center and would cause more fluid loss."
○ 2. "Narcotics may mask symptoms of increased obstruction or complications."
○ 3. "There is some risk of becoming addicted to narcotics, so it is best to take them only when necessary."
○ 4. "Narcotics will interfere with the anesthetic if surgery is needed."

67. Intestinal decompression has been successful, but the client needs surgery to relieve the obstruction. The day before surgery, the nurse finds the following set of orders for the client. Which order should the nurse question before performing?
○ 1. Tap water enemas until clear.
○ 2. Out of bed as tolerated.
○ 3. Neomycin sulfate 1 g every 4 hours.
○ 4. Betadine scrub to abdomen b.i.d.

68. The client will be going to surgery soon. The nurse monitors the client's urine output and finds that the total output for the past 2 hours is 35 ml. This would indicate
- ○ 1. successful intestinal intubation.
- ○ 2. inadequate pain relief.
- ○ 3. extension of the obstruction.
- ○ 4. inadequate fluid replacement.

69. The client underwent a bowel resection and was in the postanesthesia recovery unit for 1 hour. She returns from the recovery room with an IV line, a nasogastric tube, and a Foley catheter in place. She complains of pain and asks for medication. What action should the nurse take first?
- ○ 1. Administer the ordered narcotic.
- ○ 2. Establish the location and severity of the pain.
- ○ 3. Determine if she was medicated for pain in the postanesthesia recovery unit.
- ○ 4. Reposition her and give her a back rub.

70. During the evening shift on the day of the client's surgery, her nasogastric tube drains 500 ml of greenish-brown fluid. What action should the nurse take?
- ○ 1. Call the physician immediately.
- ○ 2. Increase the IV infusion rate.
- ○ 3. Record the amount of drainage on the client's chart.
- ○ 4. Irrigate the tube with normal saline solution.

The Client With Cirrhosis

A 55-year-old male factory worker has a long history of cirrhosis related to chronic alcoholism and has been experiencing a slow but steady decline in his general health. Recent blood work reveals hypokalemia, anemia, elevated liver function studies, prolonged prothrombin time, and elevated circulating estrogen level.

71. Because of the elevated circulating estrogen level, the nurse would expect the client to exhibit which of the following symptoms?
- ○ 1. Gynecomastia.
- ○ 2. Increased chest and body hair.
- ○ 3. Testicular hypertrophy.
- ○ 4. Increased libido.

72. The client complains that his skin always feels itchy and he "scratches himself raw" while he sleeps. The nurse should recognize that the itching is the result of which abnormality associated with cirrhosis?
- ○ 1. Folic acid deficiency.
- ○ 2. Prolonged prothrombin time.
- ○ 3. Increased bilirubin levels.
- ○ 4. Hypokalemia.

73. During this stage of his illness, the client should be encouraged to follow which diet?
- ○ 1. High calorie, restricted protein, low sodium.
- ○ 2. Bland, low protein, low sodium.
- ○ 3. Well balanced normal nutrients, low sodium.
- ○ 4. High protein, high calorie, high potassium.

74. The client's wife asks the nurse about health-promoting activities that she could help her husband include in his daily routine. Which one of the following measures would not be appropriate for the nurse to suggest?
- ○ 1. Supplement the diet with daily multivitamins.
- ○ 2. Reinforce all efforts to avoid alcohol.
- ○ 3. Take a sleeping pill at bedtime.
- ○ 4. Avoid contact with ill persons when possible.

75. The client's weight has not changed over the last 6 months, but his abdominal girth has increased. The nurse should recognize that the pathological basis for the development of ascites is portal hypertension and
- ○ 1. excess serum sodium level and increased aldosterone excretion.
- ○ 2. increased aldosterone excretion and decreased serum albumin level.
- ○ 3. decreased colloid osmotic pressure and lymphatic obstruction.
- ○ 4. decreased serum albumin level and decreased colloid osmotic pressure.

76. The position of choice for a client with severe ascites would be
- ○ 1. high Fowler's.
- ○ 2. side-lying.
- ○ 3. modified Trendelenburg's.
- ○ 4. any position, as long as frequent position changes are ensured.

77. The physician decreases the client's dietary sodium restriction to 1 g/day and orders a diuretic. The diuretic that facilitates sodium excretion while conserving body potassium is
- ○ 1. furosemide (Lasix).
- ○ 2. spironolactone (Aldactone).
- ○ 3. hydrochlorothiazide (HydroDIURIL).
- ○ 4. ethacrynic acid (Edecrin).

78. The client receives 100 ml of 25% serum albumin IV. Which assessment finding would best indicate that the albumin was having its desired effect?
- ○ 1. Increased urine output.
- ○ 2. Increased serum albumin level.
- ○ 3. Decreased anorexia and itching.
- ○ 4. Increased ease of breathing.

79. Four months later, the same client is admitted through the emergency department. He is vomiting bright-red blood, and the physician suspects bleeding esophageal varices. An IV infusion and oxygen,

4L/minute via nasal cannula, are started immediately. In addition, the physician decides to insert a Sengstaken–Blakemore tube. The client asks what the purpose of the tube is. The nurse's response should be based on knowledge that the tube acts by

○ 1. providing a large diameter for effective gastric lavage.
○ 2. applying direct pressure to gastric bleeding sites.
○ 3. blocking blood flow to the stomach and esophagus.
○ 4. applying direct pressure to the esophagus.

80. Once the Sengstaken–Blakemore tube is successfully inserted, the client will need constant nursing care. Which of the following nursing interventions would be appropriate?

○ 1. Provide him with an emesis basin to expectorate secretions.
○ 2. Obtain an order for lozenges to counteract dry mouth.
○ 3. Moisten the internal nares with a petroleum-based lubricant.
○ 4. Obtain an order for lidocaine hydrochloride (Xylocaine Viscous) to decrease the discomfort of swallowing.

81. Approximately 30 minutes after the tube is inserted, the nurse observes that the client appears to be having difficulty breathing. The nurse's first action should be to

○ 1. remove the tube.
○ 2. deflate the esophageal portion of the tube.
○ 3. determine whether the tube is obstructing the airway.
○ 4. raise the head of the bed and increase the oxygen flow rate.

82. The client's condition stabilizes, and the Sengstaken–Blakemore tube is removed. The physician orders oral neomycin as well as a neomycin enema. The purpose of this therapy is to

○ 1. reduce abdominal pressure and prevent further bleeding.
○ 2. prevent the client from straining during defecation and stimulating rebleeding.
○ 3. remove intestinal contests and block ammonia formation.
○ 4. reduce the irritating effect of blood on the intestinal mucosa.

83. The nurse monitors the client for the development of portal systemic encephalopathy, being alert for changes in the client's

○ 1. level of consciousness.
○ 2. vital signs.
○ 3. urine output.
○ 4. respiratory status.

84. The client's serum ammonia level begins to rise, and the physician orders 30 ml of lactulose (Cephulac). Which of the following effects of this drug would the nurse expect to see?

○ 1. Increased urine output.
○ 2. Improved level of consciousness.
○ 3. Diarrhea.
○ 4. Nausea and vomiting.

85. The client recovers slowly. He is to be discharged home with a prescription for lactulose (Cephulac). The nurse teaches the client and his wife how to properly administer this medication. Which of the following statements would indicate that the client has understood the teaching?

○ 1. "I'll take it with Maalox."
○ 2. "I'll mix it with apple juice."
○ 3. "I'll take it with a laxative."
○ 4. "I'll mix the crushed tablets in some gelatin."

The Client With an Ileostomy

A 35-year-old female client has been admitted to the hospital for an ileostomy.

86. The client asks the nurse, "Is it really possible to lead a normal life with an ileostomy?" Which action by the nurse would likely be the most effective response to this question?

○ 1. Have the client talk to her clergyman about her concerns.
○ 2. Tell the client to worry about those concerns after surgery.
○ 3. Arrange for a person with an ostomy to visit the client preoperatively.
○ 4. Notify the surgeon of the client's question.

87. The client is learning about caring for her ileostomy. Which of the following statements would indicate that she understands how to care for her ileostomy pouch?

○ 1. "I'll empty my pouch when it's about one-third full."
○ 2. "I can take my pouch off at night."
○ 3. "I should change my pouch immediately after lunch."
○ 4. "I must apply a new pouch system every day."

88. The nurse explains to the client that some form of skin barrier must be used around the stoma at all times. Which of the following statements explains the primary reason for using a skin barrier?

○ 1. A skin barrier helps prevent the formation of odor.
○ 2. A skin barrier helps maintain an accurate output record.
○ 3. A skin barrier protects against irritation from effluent from the ileostomy, which contains high concentrations of digestive enzymes.

○ 4. A skin barrier will allow the client to keep the ostomy pouch on for a longer time.

89. The client is receiving diet instructions from the nurse. Which of the following instructions would be appropriate?
○ 1. "Limit your fluids to 1,000 ml a day."
○ 2. "Chew your food thoroughly."
○ 3. "There's no need to monitor your diet."
○ 4. "Six small meals a day will prevent abdominal distention."

90. The nurse should instruct the client to immediately report which of the following symptoms to the physician?
○ 1. Passage of liquid stool from the stoma.
○ 2. Occasional presence of undigested food in the effluent.
○ 3. Absence of drainage from the ileostomy for 6 or more hours.
○ 4. Temperature of 99.8°F.

General Questions

91. A client is to receive a cleansing enema before surgery. In which of the following positions should the nurse place the client before administering the enema?
○ 1. Prone.
○ 2. Knee-chest.
○ 3. Left lateral.
○ 4. Right lateral.

92. Meperidine hydrochloride (Demerol) and diazepam (Valium) are to be given to a client preoperatively. How should the nurse prepare these drugs for intramuscular injection?
○ 1. Draw up each drug in a separate syringe and give two injections.
○ 2. Draw up the diazepam first in a syringe and then draw up the meperidine hydrochloride in the same syringe.
○ 3. Draw up the meperidine hydrochloride first in a syringe and then draw up the diazepam in the same syringe.
○ 4. Draw up both drugs in one syringe; it makes no difference which drug is drawn up first.

93. The nurse is to administer a preoperative medication to a client who is 5′ 6″ tall and weighs 115 lbs. Which of the following needles would be appropriate for administering the preoperative medications intramuscularly?
○ 1. A 19G, 1-½″ needle.
○ 2. A 20G, 1″ needle.
○ 3. A 22G, 1-½″ needle.
○ 4. A 26g, 1″ needle.

CORRECT ANSWERS AND RATIONALE

The letters in parentheses following the rationale identify the step of the nursing process (A, D, P, I, E); cognitive level (K, C, T, N); and client need (S, G, L, H). See the Answer Grid for the key.

The Client With Cancer of the Colon

1. 4. Castor oil breaks down in the intestines to form ricinoleic acid. This acid irritates nerve endings in the intestinal mucosa, producing evacuation. Mineral oil is a laxative that softens and lubricates the stool. Saline cathartics, such as magnesium sulfate and citrate, increase the volume of intestinal content, thus stimulating evacuation. (I, K, G)

2. 1. Following a barium enema, a laxative is ordinarily prescribed. This is done to promote expulsion of the barium, because retained barium predisposes the client to constipation and fecal impaction. (P, K, G)

3. 2. Antibiotics are administered preoperatively to reduce the bacterial count in the colon. The client will be placed on a low-residue diet to help cleanse the bowel before surgery, but typically is not placed on NPO status until 8 to 12 hours before surgery. Laxatives and enemas may also be administered. Chest tubes would not be expected postoperatively. There is no need to maintain the client on strict bedrest before an abdominoperineal resection. (I, N, S)

4. 4. The preferred site for a permanent colostomy is in the lower portion of the descending colon, when possible; hence, placement is on the left side of the body. Because the colon normally absorbs large quantities of water, placing the colostomy near the end of the colon will result in near-normal stool consistency. Optimal placement of an ostomy is usually determined before surgery by an enterostomal therapist. (I, T, G)

5. 2. The solution of choice for administering blood in a tandem setup is a 0.9% saline solution. This solution is isotonic and will not disturb the electrolyte balance or damage red blood cells. Dextrose solutions are not recommended, because dextrose tends to cause stickiness and clumping of red blood cells. If a hypertonic IV solution is used, crenation is likely. If the solution is hypotonic, hemolysis may occur. (I, C, S)

6. 4. If a client complains of headache and tingling in the fingers while receiving a blood transfusion, the nurse should immediately stop the transfusion. The client may be having an adverse reaction to the blood. The IV line should be kept open. Appropriate personnel (usually the physician and the laboratory personnel) should then be notified. Headache and tingling of the fingers are not symptomatic of infiltration or of too-rapid infusion. (I, N, S)

7. 3. Raising the knee gatch to prevent the client from sliding down in bed is contraindicated, because it contributes to venous stasis. A client who has undergone abdominoperineal resection should practice diaphragmatic breathing, should cough if secretions are present, and may wear antiembolism stockings. (I, T, S)

8. 3. A sign indicating that a client's colostomy is open and ready to function is passage of feces and flatus. When this occurs, gastric suction is ordinarily discontinued, and the client is allowed to start taking fluids and food orally. Absence of bowel sounds would indicate that the tube should remain in place, because peristalsis has not yet returned. Passage of mucus from the rectum will not occur in this client because of the nature of the surgery. Absence of stomach drainage or absence of nausea and vomiting is not a criterion for judging whether or not gastric suction should be continued. (A, C, G)

9. 1. Mouth care should be provided following nasogastric tube removal. Auscultating and palpating the abdomen should have been done before tube removal. After tube removal, the nurse will continue to assess the client's abdomen, but there is no need to do this immediately after removal. Orange sherbet is not allowed on a clear liquid diet. (I, T, S)

10. 4. When a client demonstrates readiness to learn about colostomy, it is usually best to start with simple techniques such as using illustrative material during teaching sessions. This will help the client visualize how the colostomy will appear. Telling the client how normal body functions will continue and encouraging her to ask questions are recommended, but these measures will do less to prepare the client for the sight of a colostomy than will using illustrative material. Visits from members of an ostomy club are also recommended, but these visits usually are more beneficial when the client has knowledge of the colostomy and how it looks and functions. (I, N, L)

11. 4. The primary purpose of colostomy irrigation on the fifth postoperative day is to stimulate peristalsis. It is not done to flush the colon. Stimulating peristalsis so that the colon will empty naturally is an early step in controlling elimination from a colostomy. There is no sphincter to control elimination from the colostomy. (I, N, G)

12. 1. Abdominal cramping that may occur during a colostomy irrigation results from stimulation of the colon by the irrigating solution. The best course of action is to stop the flow of solution temporarily until cramping subsides. Having the client sit up in bed or advancing the cone or tube further will not help stop cramping. There is no need to remove the cone or tube, because it will need to be reinserted when irrigation is continued. (I, T, S)

13. 2. A dark red to purple stoma indicates inadequate blood supply. Mild edema is normal in the early postoperative period, as is slight oozing of blood. The colostomy would typically not begin functioning for 2–4 days after surgery. (E, T, S)

14. 2. A client who asks about supplies used for dressings may be ready to participate in self-care. Inquiring about the physician's visit, discussing news events, and complaining about a dressing change are behaviors that avoid the subject of the colostomy. (E, N, L)

15. 1. Karaya and Stomahesive are both effective agents for protecting the skin around a colostomy. They keep the skin healthy and prevent skin irritation from stoma drainage. Petrolatum, cornstarch, and antiseptic creams do not adequately protect the skin. (I, T, S)

16. 1. Sitz baths are an effective way to cleanse the operative area following an abdominoperineal resection. Sitz baths bring warmth to the area, improve circulation, and promote healing and cleanliness. Most clients find them very comfortable and relaxing. (I, N, G)

17. 3. Experience has shown that it is best to adjust the diet of a client with a colostomy in a manner that best suits the client rather than trying special diets. Limiting roughage and liquids and using a constipating diet are not recommended. (P, K, G)

The Client With Hepatitis A

18. 2. Liver inflammation and obstruction block the normal flow of bile. Excess bilirubin turns the skin and sclera yellow and the urine dark and frothy. Profound anorexia is also common. Shortness of breath would be unexpected. (A, C, G)

19. 3. Enteric precautions are recommended for clients with hepatitis A, but a private room for an adult client is unnecessary. These recommendations are made by the Centers for Disease Control. (P, N, S)

20. 1. Treatment during the acute phase of hepatitis consists primarily of bed rest with bathroom privileges. Bed rest is maintained during the acute phase to reduce metabolic demands on the liver, thus increasing its blood supply and supporting cell regeneration. When activity is gradually resumed, the client should be taught to rest before he feels overly tired. (I, T, G)

21. 3. Bilirubin levels and liver enzymes, such as serum glutamic pyruvic transaminase (SGPT) and serum glutamic oxaloacetic transaminase (SGOT), are carefully monitored during hepatitis. Their levels provide important data about liver function. Blood glucose, creatinine clearance, and serum electrolytes provide no information about liver function. (A, K, G)

22. 4. Unlike the hepatitis of alcoholism, viral forms of hepatitis are not usually associated with nutritional depletion. Therefore, a well-balanced diet is advocated to ensure nutritional status. It is a challenge to ensure that clients with hepatitis A ingest a balanced diet with sufficient calories, because these clients are generally anorexic and have little interest in eating. (P, T, G)

23. 2. The organism causing hepatitis A leaves the body primarily through feces. The respiratory route has not been ruled out entirely as a possible portal but is not considered the most common route of exit. (P, T, S)

24. 3. The hepatitis A virus is transmitted through the fecal–oral route. Common vehicles spreading the virus include contaminated hands, water, and food, especially shellfish growing in contaminated water. Certain animal handlers are at risk for hepatitis A, particularly those handling primates. (A, K, G)

25. 3. Immune serum globulin, an immune serum, is administered prophylactically for persons exposed to hepatitis A. There are no vaccines for hepatitis A, and antibiotics are ineffective. (I, C, H)

26. 4. Convalescence following hepatitis may take weeks or even months. Boredom and depression are common problems that the client should anticipate. Problems with pain, maintaining a regular bowel elimination pattern, and preventing respiratory complications are unlikely. Bed rest is not prescribed, but activity is strictly limited to support healing. (E, T, G)

27. 2. Uncomplicated hepatitis A does not require any particular life-style modifications once healing has occurred. Moderation in alcohol consumption is recommended. Clients should never donate blood, however. (I, T, H)

The Client With Hepatitis B

28. 2. Hepatitis B Virus (HBV) is spread through contact with blood, body fluids contaminated with blood, and such body fluids as cerebrospinal, pleural, peritoneal and synovial fluids, semen, and vaginal secretions. The risk of transmission of HBV through feces is very low. Touching the client without gloves when there is no danger of contact with blood or body fluids is acceptable. Preventive measures for the nurse include using barrier protection (gloves, goggles, and gown) when appropriate and not recapping needles. An HBV vaccine exists and is recommended for high-risk persons. (E, N, S)

29. 3. Persons at high risk for hepatitis B include users of illicit intravenous drugs, persons with multiple sex partners, homosexual males, and health care personnel who have frequent contact with blood. Hepatitis B is not spread through marijuana use or ingestion of contaminated seafood. Acetaminophen taken in large amounts can cause severe hepatic necrosis but does not cause hepatitis B. (A, T, G)

30. 1. The client should be taught how to prevent the spread of hepatitis B to others. It is not necessary for the client to isolate himself from family and friends. Sedatives should be avoided, as these are usually detoxified by the liver. The client should eat a well-balanced, nutritional diet. There is no need to restrict sodium or protein. (P, N, H)

31. 4. The nurse should encourage the client to further verbalize feelings of isolation. Clients with hepatitis frequently feel guilty about possibly exposing others to the disease. Family and friends may experience fear of contracting the disease. Instead of belittling these feelings, the nurse should allow them to verbalize their fears and provide education on how to prevent infection transmission. (I, T, L)

The Client With Hemorrhoids

32. 2. Hemorrhoids are associated with prolonged sitting or standing, portal hypertension, chronic constipation, and prolonged increased intraabdominal pressure, as associated with pregnancy and the strain of vaginal delivery. (A, C, G)

33. 2. A low-roughage, high-fiber diet will produce a soft stool that is not irritating to the inflamed hemorrhoidal area. (P, C, G)

34. 3. Rectal surgery is accompanied by severe pain resulting from spasms of sphincters and muscles. Therefore, controlling pain is a priority goal of posthemorrhoidectomy nursing care. Preventing venous stasis, promoting ambulation, and preventing infection are important goals but not priority goals given the nature of the surgery. (P, T, G)

35. 3. Positioning in the early posthemorrhoidectomy phase should avoid stress and pressure on the operative site. The prone or side-lying positions are ideal from a comfort perspective. Any sitting position is less than ideal, and there is no need for Trendelenburg's position. (I, T, S)

36. 1. Applying heat during the immediate postoperative period may cause hemorrhage at the surgical site. Moist heat may relieve rectal spasms following bowel movements. Urine retention caused by reflex spasm may also be relieved by moist heat. Increasing fiber and fluid in the diet can help prevent constipation. (I, C, S)

37. 3. Adequate cleansing of the anal area is difficult but essential. After rectal surgery, sitz baths assist in this process, so the posthemorrhoidectomy client should take a sitz bath after defecating. Other times are dictated by client comfort. (E, T, H)

38. 2. The first bowel movement after a hemorrhoidectomy is often painful because of sphincter spasm. A warm sitz bath or warm compresses relieve the painful sphincter spasm quickly. Oral analgesics take longer to provide relief. Cleansing the rectal area with warm water after a bowel movement promotes hygiene and comfort, but warm sitz baths relieve sphincter spasm. (I, T, G)

39. 2. Oatmeal, grapefruit wedges, and bran muffins are all high-fiber foods. Processed foods such as pastries, processed cereals, and white bread are low in fiber. Protein foods contain little if any fiber. Prune juice is not high in fiber but has a laxative effect caused by dihydroxyphenyl isatin. (E, K, H)

The Client With Inflammatory Bowel Disease

40. 2. Diarrhea is the primary symptom of ulcerative colitis. It is profuse and severe; the client may pass as many as 15 to 20 watery stools per day. Stools may contain blood, mucus, and pus. The frequent diarrhea is often accompanied by anorexia and nausea. Steatorrhea (fatty stools) is more typical of pancreatitis and cholecystitis. Alternating diarrhea and constipation is associated with irritable bowel syndrome. (A, T, G)

41. 1. Stressful and emotional events have been clearly linked to exacerbations of ulcerative colitis, although their role in the etiology of the disease has been disproved. Diet and exercise are unlikely causes of acute exacerbation. (A, N, G)

42. 2. Diarrhea is the primary symptom, and stopping it is the first goal of treatment. The other goals are ongoing and will be best achieved by halting the exacerbation. The client may receive antidiarrheal agents, antispasmodic agents, bulk hydrophilic agents, and/or antiinflammatory drugs. (P, N, G)

43. 2. Modified bed rest helps conserve energy and promote comfort, but its primary purpose is to help reduce the hypermotility of the colon. (P, C, G)

44. 3. Massive diarrhea causes significant depletion of the body's stores of sodium and potassium, as well as fluid. The client should be closely monitored for hypokalemia and hyponatremia. (A, C, G)

45. 4. It is not uncommon for clients with ulcerative colitis to become apprehensive and upset about the frequency of stools and presence of abdominal cramping. During these acute exacerbations, clients need emotional support and encouragement to verbalize their feelings about their chronic health concerns and assistance in developing effective coping methods. (D, N, L)

46. 2. Anal excoriation is inevitable with profuse diarrhea, and meticulous perianal hygiene is essential. Sitz baths are comforting and cleansing. Diarrhea necessitates the ready availability of a bedpan or bedside commode. It is not appropriate to administer stool softeners to a client with diarrhea. A gown is not indicated, because no infectious agent is involved. (I, T, G)

47. 3. A client with severe symptoms of ulcerative colitis will be kept NPO to rest the bowel. To maintain the client's nutritional status, the client usually is started on total parenteral nutrition (TPN). (P, T, G)

48. 3. The superior vena cava is preferred for introducing hyperalimentation nutrients. It is a large, rapid-flow vein, and the concentrated solution will dilute quickly. The superior vena cava is generally entered through the right or left subclavian vein; it also may be entered through the internal jugular vein. (P, K, S)

49. 2. The TPN solution is usually a hypertonic glucose solution. If a commercial preparation is unavailable, the solution is best prepared in a pharmacy under strict aseptic conditions. Electrolytes may be added to meet a client's particular needs. (I, K, S)

50. 4. During TPN administration, the clients urine should be tested regularly for glycosuria. If the client is not metabolizing the nutrients well, glucose tends to be eliminated in the urine. The client may require small amounts of insulin to improve glucose metabolism. The client should also be observed for signs of hypoglycemia, which may occur if the body overproduces insulin in response to a high glucose intake or if too much insulin is administered to help improve glucose metabolism. (A, T, G)

51. 2. Complications associated with administering TPN via a central line include infection and air embolism. To prevent these complications, strict aseptic technique is used for all dressing changes, the insertion site is covered with an air-occlusive dressing, and all connections of the system are taped. Ambulation and activities of daily living are encouraged. (I, T, S)

52. 4. A steady and progressive weight gain is the best indication that the client's nutritional goals are being met by TPN. These laboratory values are within normal limits but do not indicate attainment of nutritional goals. (E, N, G)

53. 3. The nurse's most appropriate action is to assess the infusion system to determine the cause of the inaccurate flow rate and to note the client's response to the decreased infusion. The physician should be notified of the infusion discrepancy. When adjusted, the flow rate of TPN solution should be gradually increased or decreased to prevent fluid and electrolyte imbalances. It should never be discontinued abruptly. (I, N, S)

54. 3. Adequate fluid intake prevents crystalluria and stone formation during sulfasalazine (Azulfidine) therapy. This drug can cause gastrointestinal distress and is best taken after meals and in equally divided doses. It gives alkaline urine an orange-yellow color. (I, K, G)

55. 1. A client with a chronic disease need not curtail career goals. Self-care is the cornerstone of long-term management, and learning to cope with and modify stressors will enable the client to live with the disease. Giving up a desired career could discourage and even depress the client. Placing the responsibility for minimizing stressors at work in the hands of others leads to a feeling of loss of control and stunts the sense of responsibility needed for sound self-care. Working part-time rather than full-time is unnecessary. (I, N, L)

56. 3. Caffeine, tobacco, and alcohol are gastrointestinal stimulants and should be avoided by clients with ulcerative colitis. (I, K, G)

57. 1. An appropriate expected outcome for a client with ulcerative colitis is maintaining an ideal body weight. It would not be appropriate to restrict fluid intake; the client should strive to remain well hydrated. Ulcerative colitis produces episodic diarrhea, not constipation. It is not inevitable that the client with ulcerative colitis will need an ileostomy. The decision to perform surgery depends on the extent of the disease and the severity of the symptoms. (E, N, G)

The Client With an Intestinal Obstruction

58. 4. On percussion, air produces a resonant sound and fluid produces a dull sound. An intestinal obstruction traps large amounts of fluid in the intestine. Hyperperistalsis would be apparent on auscultation. (A, C, G)

59. 1. Profuse vomiting is the classic sign of small-bowel obstruction. Abdominal distention and discomfort tend to be more pronounced with large-bowel obstruction. High-pitched bowel sounds indicate hyperperistalsis, which occurs early in obstruction. (A, C, G)

60. 1. Intestinal decompression is accomplished with a Cantor, Harris, or Miller-Abbott tube. These 6- to

10-foot tubes are passed through the gastrointestinal tract to the obstruction. They remove accumulated fluid and gas, relieving the pressure. (I, C, S)

61. 2. The client is placed on her right side to facilitate movement of the mercury-weighted tube through the pyloric sphincter. After the tube is in the intestine, the client will be turned from side to side or encouraged to ambulate to facilitate tube movement through the intestinal loops. (I, C, S)

62. 2. An intestinal tube is not taped in position until it has reached the obstruction. A Cantor tube is attached to suction, and the small balloon at its tip is injected with mercury. Because the tube has a radiopaque strip, its progress through the intestinal tract can be followed by fluoroscopy. (I, C, S)

63. 2. Once the intestinal tube has passed into the duodenum, it is usually advanced, as ordered, 2″ to 4″ every 30 to 60 minutes. This enables peristalsis to carry the tube forward. The client is encouraged to walk, which also facilitates tube progression. A client with an intestinal tube needs frequent mouth care to stimulate saliva secretion, to maintain a healthy oral cavity, and to promote comfort. Ice chips are contraindicated, because hypotonic fluid will draw extra fluid into an already distended bowel. (I, T, S)

64. 4. Intestinal tubes are not irrigated. The other nursing measures are appropriate. (I, N, S)

65. 3. A client with an intestinal obstruction is particularly susceptible to fluid volume deficit and electrolyte imbalances. The client's pain is acute in nature, not chronic. The other nursing diagnoses are not appropriate. (D, N, G)

66. 2. Medications that mask symptoms may delay accurate diagnosis and appropriate treatment. Narcotics are thought to stimulate a chemoreceptor emetic trigger zone in the medulla, causing nausea and vomiting. Potential fluid loss is not the reason that such medications are not administered to clients with suspected intestinal obstruction; a patent intestinal tube minimizes vomiting. Addiction is unlikely when pain medication is administered to control pain. Narcotics are often used to facilitate anesthesia induction. (I, C, G)

67. 1. High colonic irrigation can increase the risk of perforation in a distended and inflamed colon. Tap water is hypotonic in the bowel and would draw increased fluid into the area. The other measures are part of standard preparation for intestinal surgery. (I, N, S)

68. 4. The kidney is very sensitive to circulating fluid volume. Urine output below 30 ml/hour indicates that the kidney is concentrating urine and fluid replacement needs to be increased. The intestinal tube removes sequestered fluid in the bowel, not fluid in the general circulation. The effect of pain on renal function is not so dramatic as described here. (E, N, G)

69. 2. Assessing pain, including location and severity, is essential before administering pain medication. Because the client spent an hour in the postanesthesia recovery unit, the nurse would next determine whether she had been medicated for pain in that unit. The pain is most likely incisional but could result from positioning, a too-tight dressing, or anxiety. (I, N, G)

70. 3. Because peristalsis has not been reestablished, this amount of gastric drainage would not be unexpected. The color also would be expected. The appropriate nursing action is to accurately chart the amount and color of output and continue monitoring the client. (I, N, G)

The Client With Cirrhosis

71. 1. The normal liver acts to metabolize and inactivate hormones. Loss of this function increases the levels of circulating hormones. Excess estrogen in a male may cause gynecomastia; loss of axillary, chest, and pubic hair; testicular atrophy; and impotence. It will not increase libido. Palmar erythema and spider angiomas are also common results of hormone excess. (A, K, G)

72. 3. Excess retained bilirubin produces an irritating effect on the peripheral nerves, causing intense itching. Folic acid, prothrombin, and potassium imbalances cause varied symptoms, but itching is not directly related to these imbalances. (E, K, G)

73. 3. Cirrhosis is a slowly progressive disease. Inadequate nutrition is the primary ongoing problem. Clients are encouraged to eat normal, well-balanced diets, restricting sodium to prevent fluid retention. Protein is not restricted until the liver actually fails, which is usually very late in the disease. (I, T, G)

74. 3. General health-promotion measures include maintaining good nutrition, avoiding infection, and abstaining from alcohol. Rest and sleep are essential, but an impaired liver may not be able to detoxify sedatives and barbiturates. Such drugs must be used cautiously, if at all, by clients with cirrhosis. (I, N, H)

75. 4. Ascites results from increased pressure in the venous system, low levels of serum albumin (which contributes to decreased colloid osmotic pressure), and sodium retention, resulting in part from decreased aldosterone clearance. (A, C, G)

76. 1. Ascites can compromise the action of the diaphragm and increase the client's risk of respiratory problems. Frequent position changes are important, but the preferred position is high Fowler's. Ascites also greatly increases the risk of skin breakdown. (I, T, S)

77. 2. Hypokalemia is an ongoing problem for a client with cirrhosis. When a diuretic is needed, the ideal choice is a potassium-sparing agent. Spironolactone (Aldactone) is the diuretic of choice for clients with cirrhosis, because it facilitates sodium excretion while conserving potassium. Furosemide (Lasix), hydrochlorothiazide (HydroDIURIL), and ethacrynic acid (Edecrin) are thiazide diuretics, which cause potassium loss. (I, K, G)

78. 1. Normal serum albumin is administered to reduce ascites. Hypoalbuminemia, a mechanism underlying ascites formation, results in decreased colloid osmotic pressure. Administering serum albumin increases plasma colloid osmotic pressure, which causes fluid to flow from the tissue space into the plasma. Increased urine output is the best indication that the albumin is having the desired effect. A client receiving albumin should be monitored for such complications as fluid overload and pulmonary edema. (I, T, G)

79. 4. The Sengstaken–Blakemore tube has a small gastric balloon that anchors the tube and applies pressure to the area of the cardiac sphincter. The large esophageal balloon applies direct pressure on the bleeding sites in the esophagus. A tube passing through the balloons allows for aspiration and irrigation. (P, C, S)

80. 1. An inflated esophageal balloon prevents swallowing. Therefore, the nurse should provide the client with tissues and encourage him to spit into the tissues or an emesis basin. If the client cannot manage his secretions, gentle oral suctioning is needed. Oral and nasal care is provided every 1 to 2 hours. A water-soluble lubricant is applied to the external nares. (I, T, S)

81. 3. If the gastric balloon should rupture or deflate, the esophageal balloon can move and partially or totally obstruct the airway. The client must be observed closely. No direct action should be taken, however, until the condition is accurately diagnosed. (I, N, S)

82. 3. Neomycin is administered to decrease the bacterial effect on digested blood in the intestines, which results in ammonia production. This ammonia, if not detoxified by the liver, can result in hepatic coma. (P, C, G)

83. 1. Ammonia has a toxic effect on central nervous system tissue and produces altered level of consciousness, marked by drowsiness and irritability. If this process is unchecked, the client may lapse into coma. (A, C, G)

84. 3. Lactulose (Cephulac) increases intestinal motility, thereby decreasing ammonia formation in the intestine. An expected effect, therefore, would be diarrhea. (P, K, G)

85. 2. The taste of lactulose (Cephulac) is a problem for some clients; mixing it with fruit juice can make it more palatable. For clients without dietary sodium restrictions, lactulose can also be mixed with milk. Lactulose should not be given with antacids, which may inhibit its action. Lactulose is a laxative that expels trapped ammonia from the colon. It comes as a syrup for oral or rectal administration. (E, C, G)

The Client With an Ileostomy

86. 3. If the client agrees, having a person who has successfully adjusted to living with an ileostomy visit her would be the most helpful measure. This would let the client actually see that she will be able to pursue typical activities of daily life postoperatively. Her questions can be answered by someone who has felt some of the same concerns. Disregarding the client's concerns is not helpful. Although the physician should know about the client's concerns, this in itself will not reassure the client about life after an ileostomy. A visit from a clergyman may be helpful to some clients, but may not provide this client with the information she is seeking. (I, N, L)

87. 1. The pouch should be emptied when it is about one-third full, to prevent the weight of the pouch from breaking the seal. The client with an ileostomy must wear a pouch at all times to collect stool. A pouch can be worn for 3 to 7 days before being changed. The client should change the pouch at a time when the stoma is least likely to function; 2 to 4 hours after a meal is generally the most appropriate time. (E, N, H)

88. 3. Ileostomy effluent is very irritating to skin and can cause excoriation and ulceration. Some form of protection must be used to keep the effluent from contacting the skin. (I, N, S)

89. 2. The client is instructed to chew food well to aid digestion and prevent obstruction. The client is usually placed on a regular diet, but encouraged to eat high-fiber and high-cellulose foods (e.g., nuts, popcorn, corn, peas, tomatoes) with caution; these foods may swell in the intestine and cause an obstruction. The client should maintain an adequate fluid intake. Eating six small meals a day is not necessary. (I, T, H)

90. 3. The ileostomy drains liquid stool at frequent intervals throughout the day. Any sudden decrease in drainage or onset of severe abdominal pain should be reported to the physician immediately. (A, T, H)

91. 3. To facilitate instillation of enema fluid, the left lateral position is usually recommended, so that the sigmoid colon is below the rectum. (I, C, S)

92. 1. Injectable diazepam (Valium) should not be mixed or diluted with other solutions or drugs and should not be added to IV fluid. Injectable diazepam is a colorless crystalline compound that is insoluble in water. (I, K, S)

93. 3. For a client who is 5′ 6″ tall and weighs 115 lbs., a 22G, 1-½″ needle is preferred for intramuscular injection. A 1″ needle is ordinarily too short to reach deep muscle tissue, and a gauge larger than 22G will tend to cause unnecessary trauma and discomfort. A 26G needle is not recommended for intramuscular injection. (I, N, S)

THE NURSING CARE OF ADULTS WITH MEDICAL/SURGICAL HEALTH PROBLEMS

TEST 4: The Client With Lower Gastrointestinal Tract Health Problems

Directions: Use this answer grid to determine areas of strength or need for further study.

NURSING PROCESS

A = Assessment
D = Analysis, nursing diagnosis
P = Planning
I = Implementation
E = Evaluation

COGNITIVE LEVEL

K = Knowledge
C = Comprehension
T = Application
N = Analysis

CLIENT NEEDS

S = Safe, effective care environment
G = Physiological integrity
L = Psychosocial integrity
H = Health promotion/maintenance

		Nursing Process					Cognitive Level				Client Needs			
Question #	Answer #	A	D	P	I	E	K	C	T	N	S	G	L	H
1	4				I		K					G		
2	1			P			K					G		
3	2				I					N	S			
4	4				I				T			G		
5	2				I			C			S			
6	4				I					N	S			
7	3				I				T		S			
8	3	A						C				G		
9	1				I				T		S			
10	4				I					N			L	
11	4				I					N		G		
12	1				I				T		S			
13	2					E			T		S			
14	2					E				N			L	
15	1				I				T		S			
16	1				I					N		G		
17	3			P			K					G		
18	2	A						C				G		
19	3			P						N	S			
20	1				I				T			G		
21	3	A					K					G		
22	4			P					T			G		

ANSWER GRID: 1

Nursing Process

A = Assessment
D = Analysis, nursing diagnosis
P = Planning
I = Implementation
E = Evaluation

Cognitive Level

K = Knowledge
C = Comprehension
T = Application
N = Analysis

Client Needs

S = Safe, effective care environment
G = Physiological integrity
L = Psychosocial integrity
H = Health promotion/maintenance

		Nursing Process					Cognitive Level				Client Needs			
Question #	Answer #	A	D	P	I	E	K	C	T	N	S	G	L	H
23	2			P					T		S			
24	3	A					K					G		
25	3				I			C						H
26	4					E			T			G		
27	2				I				T					H
28	2					E				N	S			
29	3	A							T			G		
30	1			P						N				H
31	4				I				T				L	
32	2	A						C				G		
33	2			P				C				G		
34	3			P					T			G		
35	3				I				T		S			
36	1				I			C			S			
37	3					E			T					H
38	2				I				T			G		
39	2					E	K							H
40	2	A							T			G		
41	1	A								N		G		
42	2			P						N		G		
43	2			P				C				G		
44	3	A						C				G		
45	4		D							N			L	
46	2				I				T			G		
47	3			P					T			G		
48	3			P			K				S			
49	2				I		K				S			
50	4	A							T			G		

Answer Grid: 2

NURSING PROCESS

A = Assessment
D = Analysis, nursing diagnosis
P = Planning
I = Implementation
E = Evaluation

COGNITIVE LEVEL

K = Knowledge
C = Comprehension
T = Application
N = Analysis

CLIENT NEEDS

S = Safe, effective care environment
G = Physiological integrity
L = Psychosocial integrity
H = Health promotion/maintenance

		Nursing Process					Cognitive Level				Client Needs			
Question #	Answer #	A	D	P	I	E	K	C	T	N	S	G	L	H
51	2				I				T		S			
52	4					E				N		G		
53	3				I					N	S			
54	3				I		K					G		
55	1				I					N			L	
56	3				I		K					G		
57	1					E				N		G		
58	4	A						C				G		
59	1	A						C				G		
60	1				I			C			S			
61	2				I			C			S			
62	2				I			C			S			
63	2				I				T		S			
64	4				I					N	S			
65	3		D							N		G		
66	2				I			C				G		
67	1				I					N	S			
68	4					E				N		G		
69	2				I					N		G		
70	3				I					N		G		
71	1	A					K					G		
72	3					E	K					G		
73	3				I				T			G		
74	3				I					N				H
75	4	A						C				G		
76	1				I				T		S			
77	2				I		K					G		
78	1				I				T			G		

ANSWER GRID: 3

NURSING PROCESS

A = Assessment
D = Analysis, nursing diagnosis
P = Planning
I = Implementation
E = Evaluation

COGNITIVE LEVEL

K = Knowledge
C = Comprehension
T = Application
N = Analysis

CLIENT NEEDS

S = Safe, effective care environment
G = Physiological integrity
L = Psychosocial integrity
H = Health promotion/maintenance

		Nursing Process					Cognitive Level				Client Needs			
Question #	**Answer #**	A	D	P	I	E	K	C	T	N	S	G	L	H
79	4			P				C			S			
80	1				I				T		S			
81	3				I					N	S			
82	3			P				C				G		
83	1	A						C				G		
84	3			P			K					G		
85	2					E		C				G		
86	3				I					N			L	
87	1					E				N				H
88	3				I					N	S			
89	2				I				T					H
90	3	A							T					H
91	3				I			C			S			
92	1				I		K				S			
93	3				I					N	S			
Number Correct														
Number Possible	93	16	2	15	48	12	15	21	29	28	31	47	6	9
Percentage Correct														

Score Calculation:

To determine your **Percentage Correct**, divide the **Number Correct** by the **Number Possible.**

ANSWER GRID: 4

The Client With Endocrine Health Problems

Test 5

The Client With Hyperthyroidism
The Client With Diabetes Mellitus
The Client With Pituitary Adenoma
The Client With Addison's Disease
The Client With Cushing's Disease
General Questions
Correct Answers and Rationale

Select the one best answer and indicate your choice by filling in the circle in front of the option.

The Client With Hyperthyroidism

A 32-year-old homemaker and mother of three children visits her physician complaining of nervousness, irritability, and difficulty sleeping. A tentative diagnosis of hyperthyroidism is made.

1. Another typical symptom of hyperthyroidism is
- ○ 1. anorexia.
- ○ 2. tachycardia.
- ○ 3. weight gain.
- ○ 4. goiter.

2. Which symptom related to the client's menstrual cycle would she likely report during initial assessment?
- ○ 1. Dysmenorrhea.
- ○ 2. Metrorrhagia.
- ○ 3. Oligomenorrhea.
- ○ 4. Menorrhagia.

3. Propylthiouracil (PTU) is prescribed for the client. The nurse should teach the client to immediately report which of the following signs and symptoms?
- ○ 1. Sore throat and fever.
- ○ 2. Painful and excessive menstruation.
- ○ 3. Constipation and abdominal distention.
- ○ 4. Increased urine output and itchy skin.

4. The client's husband has accompanied her to the physician's office. He says to the nurse, "My wife has become so irritable. She's yelling at the children all the time. Our house is in chaos." Which of the following responses by the nurse would give the husband the most accurate explanation of his wife's behavior?
- ○ 1. "Your wife's behavior is caused by temporary confusion brought on by her illness."
- ○ 2. "Your wife's behavior is caused by the excess thyroid hormone in her system."
- ○ 3. "Your wife's behavior is caused by her worry over the seriousness of her illness."
- ○ 4. "Your wife's behavior is caused by the stress of trying to manage your home and cope with illness."

5. This client undergoes a subtotal thyroidectomy. Which of the following techniques would best enable the nurse to assess her wound for bleeding?
- ○ 1. Gently slip a hand behind her neck and check for blood on the back of her neck and on the bed linens.
- ○ 2. Carry out a routine dressing change every 2 hours for at least 12 hours and then every 4 hours for the next 2 days.
- ○ 3. Carefully loosen the dressings on both ends and have the client turn her head to one side while observing for bleeding.
- ○ 4. Check her blood pressure, pulse, and respiratory rate every hour for the first 24 hours and every 2 hours for the next 24 hours.

6. To minimize tension on the incision line, the nurse should teach the client to follow which technique when moving herself to a sitting position?
- ○ 1. Pressing her chin against her chest while moving to the sitting position.
- ○ 2. Supporting her head by placing both hands behind it while moving to the sitting position.
- ○ 3. Rolling to her side and then moving to the sitting position while holding her head perfectly still.
- ○ 4. Grasping her flexed knees with both arms while in the back-lying position and then rocking forward.

The Client With Diabetes Mellitus

A 55-year-old female client has recently been diagnosed with non-insulin-dependent diabetes mellitus (NIDDM) and is being started on the sulfonylurea compound tolbutamide (Orinase). She is very concerned about her diagnosis and says she knows nothing about diabetes. The nurse determines that she needs much teaching and support.

7. Tolbutamide (Orinase) is believed to lower blood glucose level by
- ○ 1. potentiating the action of insulin.
- ○ 2. lowering the renal threshold of glucose.
- ○ 3. stimulating pancreatic cells to release insulin.
- ○ 4. combining with glucose to render it inert.

8. The nurse learns that the client ordinarily wears the articles of clothing listed below. The nurse should recommend that she discontinue wearing
- ○ 1. a girdle.
- ○ 2. pantyhose.
- ○ 3. nylon stockings.
- ○ 4. knee-high stockings.

9. The client asks the nurse to recommend something to remove corns from her toes. The nurse should advise her to
- ○ 1. apply a high-quality corn plaster to the area.
- ○ 2. consult her physician about removing the corns.
- ○ 3. apply iodine to the corns before peeling them off.
- ○ 4. soak her feet in borax solution to peel off the corns.

10. The nurse notes several small bandages covering cuts on the client's hands. The client says, "I'm so clumsy. I'm always cutting or burning myself in the kitchen." Which of the following responses by the nurse would be most appropriate?
- ○ 1. "Don't worry about it, but keep all your cuts clean and covered."
- ○ 2. "Even small cuts can be serious for persons with diabetes and need special care."
- ○ 3. "Why do you think you injure yourself so frequently?"
- ○ 4. "You really should have your doctor check all injuries, even small ones."

11. The client says, "If I could just avoid what you call carbohydrates in my diet, I guess I would be okay." The nurse should base the response to this comment on the knowledge that diabetes affects metabolism of
- ○ 1. carbohydrates only.
- ○ 2. fats and carbohydrates only.
- ○ 3. protein and carbohydrates only.
- ○ 4. proteins, fats, and carbohydrates.

12. The client says her family eats a lot of pasta products, such as macaroni and spaghetti. She asks if she can still eat them. Which of the following would be the nurse's best response?
- ○ 1. "Because you're overweight, it's better to eliminate pasta from your diet."
- ○ 2. "Pasta can be a part of your diet. It's included in the bread and cereal exchange."
- ○ 3. "Pasta can be included in your diet, but it shouldn't be served with sauces."
- ○ 4. "Eating pasta can predispose to various complications, so it's better to eliminate it."

The Client With Pituitary Adenoma

A 42-year-old male client is admitted for surgery to treat a pituitary tumor. On admission, he says that he is "happy the doctor finally discovered what's wrong." He had been experiencing symptoms for the last 5 months.

13. The client reports, with some embarrassment, that he has been experiencing mild galactorrhea. The nurse knows that this problem is caused by overproduction of which hormone?
- ○ 1. Prolactin.
- ○ 2. Adrenocorticotropic hormone (ACTH).
- ○ 3. Growth hormone (GH).
- ○ 4. Thyroid-stimulating hormone (TSH).

14. The nurse would anticipate that the client's primary symptoms were probably
- ○ 1. severe lethargy and fatigue.
- ○ 2. decreased libido and impotence.
- ○ 3. bony proliferation of the hands, jaw, and feet.
- ○ 4. deepening or coarsening of the voice.

15. The client is scheduled for a transsphenoidal hypophysectomy. The nurse would explain that the surgery will be performed through an incision in the
- ○ 1. back of the mouth.
- ○ 2. nose.
- ○ 3. sinus channel below the right eye.
- ○ 4. space between the upper gums and lip.

16. To help minimize the risk of postoperative respiratory complications, the nurse would focus the client's preoperative teaching on the importance of
- ○ 1. using blow bottles.
- ○ 2. making frequent position changes.
- ○ 3. deep breathing.
- ○ 4. coughing.

17. Which of the following would be a major focus of nursing care for the client following transsphenoidal hypophysectomy? Monitoring for
- ○ 1. cerebrospinal fluid leak.
- ○ 2. fluctuating blood glucose level.
- ○ 3. Cushing's syndrome.
- ○ 4. respiratory complications.

18. The client expresses concern about how surgery will affect his sexual ability. Which of the following statements provides the most accurate information about the physiologic effects of hypophysectomy?
- ○ 1. Removing the source of excess hormone will restore the client's natural potency and fertility.
- ○ 2. Potency will be restored, but the client will remain infertile.
- ○ 3. Fertility will be restored, but decreased libido and potency will persist.
- ○ 4. Exogenous hormones will be needed to restore potency after the adenoma is removed.

The Client With Addison's Disease

A 48-year-old salesman came down with what initially appeared to be a routine case of the flu. He awakened during the night extremely ill, anxious, and very weak. Afraid that he was dying, the man's wife drove him to the emergency room, where he is tentatively diagnosed as having Addison's disease and being in crisis.

19. Which of the following would be the priority goal for this client in the emergency room?
- ○ 1. Controlling hypertension.
- ○ 2. Preventing irreversible shock.
- ○ 3. Preventing infection.
- ○ 4. Relieving anxiety.

20. All of the following would be expected findings in this client except
- ○ 1. hypoglycemia.
- ○ 2. nausea.
- ○ 3. edema.
- ○ 4. hypotension.

21. The client is receiving an IV infusion of 5% dextrose in normal saline running at 125 ml/hour. When hanging a new bottle of fluid, the nurse notes swelling and hardness at the infusion site. Which immediate action would be indicated?
- ○ 1. Discontinue the infusion.
- ○ 2. Apply a warm dressing to the site.
- ○ 3. Stop the flow of solution temporarily.
- ○ 4. Irrigate the needle with normal saline.

22. The client's wife asks the nurse if the IV infusion is meeting her husband's nutritional needs, as he has vomited several times. The nurse's response should be based on the knowledge that 1 liter of 5% dextrose in normal saline delivers
- ○ 1. 170 calories.
- ○ 2. 250 calories.
- ○ 3. 340 calories.
- ○ 4. 500 calories.

23. The client is admitted to the medical unit. The nurse formulates the nursing diagnosis Fluid Volume Deficit related to inadequate fluid intake and to fluid loss secondary to inadequate adrenal hormone secretion. As his oral intake increases, which of the following fluids would be most appropriate for him?
- ○ 1. Milk and diet soda.
- ○ 2. Water and eggnog.
- ○ 3. Bouillon and juice.
- ○ 4. Coffee and milkshakes.

24. The client is attending a stress management class, because stress can precipitate Addisonian crisis. Which of the following actions taught by the nurse in the class is based on principles of stress management?
- ○ 1. Remove all sources of stress from the client's life.
- ○ 2. Find alternative relaxation techniques such as music.
- ○ 3. Take anti-anxiety drugs daily.
- ○ 4. Avoid discussing stressful experiences with the client.

The Client With Cushing's Disease

A 42-year-old female client reports that she has gained weight and that her face and body are "rounder," while her legs and arms have become thinner. A tentative diagnosis of Cushing's disease is made.

25. When examining this client, the nurse would expect to find
- ○ 1. orthostatic hypotension.
- ○ 2. muscle hypertrophy in the extremities.
- ○ 3. bruised areas on the skin.
- ○ 4. decreased body hair.

26. The client tells the nurse that the physician said her morning serum cortisol level was within normal limits. She asks, "How can that be? I'm not imagining all these symptoms!" The nurse's response should be based on the knowledge that
- ○ 1. some clients are very sensitive to the effects of cortisol and develop symptoms even with normal levels.
- ○ 2. a single random blood test cannot provide reliable information about endocrine levels.
- ○ 3. the excessive cortisol in Cushing's disease commonly results from loss of the normal diurnal secretion pattern.
- ○ 4. tumors tend to secrete hormones irregularly, and the hormones are often not present in the blood.

27. The woman's diet needs to be modified to control her symptoms. Which diet would be most appropriate?
- ○ 1. High protein, high calorie, and restricted sodium.
- ○ 2. High protein, low calorie, and restricted sodium.

○ 3. High protein, high calorie, and high potassium.
○ 4. Low protein, restricted sodium, and high potassium.

28. The client has been found to have an adrenal tumor and is scheduled for a bilateral adrenalectomy. The nurse begins extensive preoperative teaching, which includes the importance of coughing and deep-breathing. Which of the following would be the most accurate instructions?
○ 1. "Sit in an upright position, take a deep breath, and then cough."
○ 2. "Hold your abdomen firmly, take several deep breaths, and then cough."
○ 3. "Tighten your stomach muscles as you inhale, and then cough forcefully."
○ 4. "Raise your shoulders to expand your chest and then cough deeply."

29. The client undergoes a bilateral adrenalectomy. Which of the following nursing interventions would take priority during the first day of postoperative care?
○ 1. Starting oral nutrition.
○ 2. Teaching dietary restrictions.
○ 3. Monitoring vital signs.
○ 4. Ambulating in the hallway.

30. Which of the following should the nurse include in the client's discharge teaching plan?
○ 1. Emphasizing that the client will need steroid replacement for the rest of her life.
○ 2. Instructing the client about the importance of tapering steroid medication carefully to prevent crisis.
○ 3. Informing the client that steroids will be required only until her body can manufacture sufficient quantities.
○ 4. Emphasizing that the client will need to take steroids whenever her life involves physical or emotional stress.

General Questions

31. A radioactive iodine uptake (RAIU) test and a protein-bound iodine (PBI) test are planned for the client with hyperthyroidism. These two tests would have falsely elevated results if the client has recently taken medications containing
○ 1. iodine.
○ 2. digitalis.
○ 3. ferrous salts.
○ 4. antihistamines.

32. Measures to prevent eye damage from exophthalmos, in which the eyelids do not close completely during sleep, include
○ 1. massaging the eyes at regular intervals.
○ 2. instilling an ophthalmic anesthetic as ordered.
○ 3. taping the eyelids closed with nonirritating tape.
○ 4. covering both eyes with moistened gauze pads.

33. Saturated solution of potassium iodide (SSKI) is prescribed preoperatively for the client with hyperthyroidism. The primary reason for using this drug is that it helps
○ 1. slow progression of exophthalmos.
○ 2. reduce the vascularity of the thyroid gland.
○ 3. decrease the body's ability to store thyroxin.
○ 4. increase the body's ability to excrete thyroxin.

34. Which of the following measures is most often recommended when preparing SSKI for administration?
○ 1. Pour the solution over ice chips.
○ 2. Mix the solution with an antacid.
○ 3. Dilute the solution with water, milk, or fruit juice.
○ 4. Disguise the solution in a pureed fruit or vegetable.

35. The nurse asks the client to state her name as soon as she regains consciousness postoperatively after a subtotal thyroidectomy, then repeats this request from time to time. The nurse does this primarily to monitor for signs of
○ 1. internal hemorrhage.
○ 2. decreasing level of consciousness.
○ 3. laryngeal nerve damage.
○ 4. upper airway obstruction.

36. The client undergoes a subtotal thyroidectomy. Which of the following items should be kept in the client's room to treat any postoperative complications that may develop?
○ 1. Equipment to begin total parenteral nutrition.
○ 2. A cutdown tray.
○ 3. Equipment for tube feedings.
○ 4. Equipment to perform a tracheostomy.

37. Which of the following symptoms might indicate that a client was developing tetany following a subtotal thyroidectomy?
○ 1. Backache and joint pains.
○ 2. Tingling in the fingers.
○ 3. Hoarseness.
○ 4. Retraction of neck muscles with inspiration.

38. Which of the following medications should be available to provide emergency treatment if a client develops tetany following a subtotal thyroidectomy?
○ 1. Sodium phosphate.
○ 2. Calcium gluconate.
○ 3. Echothiophate iodide.
○ 4. Sodium bicarbonate.

39. Signs and symptoms of hypothyroidism include
○ 1. joint pain.
○ 2. weight loss.
○ 3. general fatigue.
○ 4. oily skin.

40. Which of the following nursing diagnoses would most likely be appropriate for the client with hyperthyroidism who has undergone radioactive iodine therapy?

○ 1. High Risk for Injury related to altered level of consciousness.
○ 2. Ineffective Breathing Patterns related to effects of radioactive iodine.
○ 3. Self-Care Deficit related to the need for immobilization after radioactive iodine therapy.
○ 4. Altered Health Maintenance related to lack of knowledge about disease management.

41. Radioactive iodine therapy is administered to a client with hyperthyroidism to

○ 1. limit thyroid hormone absorption by the sympathetic nervous system.
○ 2. limit secretion of thyroid hormone by damaging or destroying thyroid tissue.
○ 3. increase circulating thyroid hormone so that it can be used by the body.
○ 4. reduce the effects of congestive heart failure caused by thyroid hormone.

42. Appropriate nursing diagnoses for the client with hypothyroidism would likely include which of the following?

○ 1. High Risk for Injury: corneal abrasion related to incomplete closure of eyelid.
○ 2. Altered Nutrition: Less than Body Requirements related to hypermetabolism.
○ 3. Fluid Volume Deficit related to diarrhea.
○ 4. Activity intolerance related to fatigue associated with the disorder.

43. When teaching a client with diabetes mellitus about foot care, the nurse should instruct the client to

○ 1. avoid going barefoot.
○ 2. wear hard-soled shoes.
○ 3. apply toenail polish.
○ 4. use bar soap to wash the feet.

44. Which dietary constituent has been observed to minimize a rise in blood glucose level after meals in clients with diabetes mellitus?

○ 1. Dietary fiber.
○ 2. Dairy products.
○ 3. Vitamin-fortified foods.
○ 4. Organ meats.

45. The nurse should caution the client with diabetes mellitus who is taking tolbutamide (Orinase) that alcoholic beverages must be included when calculating total caloric intake and, if used in excess, tend to cause symptoms of

○ 1. hypokalemia.
○ 2. hyperkalemia.
○ 3. hyperglycemia.
○ 4. hypoglycemia.

46. The most important factor predisposing a female to Type II (adult-onset) diabetes mellitus is

○ 1. obesity.
○ 2. cigarette smoking.
○ 3. giving birth to more than two children.
○ 4. sedentary life-style.

47. To which of the following disorders is the client with diabetes mellitus most predisposed?

○ 1. Arthritis.
○ 2. Otitis media.
○ 3. Osteoporosis.
○ 4. Atherosclerosis.

48. In which of the following ways does exercise affect the body's physiologic functioning?

○ 1. Exercise helps avoid hypoglycemia.
○ 2. Exercise stimulates insulin overproduction.
○ 3. Exercise decreases the renal threshold for glucose.
○ 4. Exercise increases the use of glucose by muscles.

49. A client with diabetes mellitus is taught to take NPH insulin at 8:00 A.M. each day. At which time would this client be at greatest risk for hypoglycemia?

○ 1. About 11 A.M., shortly before lunch.
○ 2. About 1 P.M., shortly after lunch.
○ 3. About 5 P.M., shortly before dinner.
○ 4. About 11 P.M., shortly before bedtime.

50. For a client with diabetes mellitus who is being taught to self-administer insulin, learning goals most likely will be attained when they are established by the

○ 1. nurse, because the nurse is responsible for teaching.
○ 2. physician and client, because the physician is the manager of care and the client is the main participant.
○ 3. client, because the client is best able to identify his or her own needs and how to meet those needs.
○ 4. client and nurse, so the client can participate in planning care with the nurse.

51. The most accurate indication that a client has learned how to give an insulin self-injection correctly is the client's ability to

○ 1. perform the procedure faultlessly.
○ 2. critique the nurse's performance of the procedure.
○ 3. explain all steps of the procedure correctly.
○ 4. correctly answer questions about the procedure.

52. The nurse should teach the client that the most common symptoms of hypoglycemia are

○ 1. nervousness and diaphoresis.
○ 2. anorexia and incoherent speech.
○ 3. Kussmaul's respirations and confusion.
○ 4. bradycardia and blurred vision.

53. When teaching a client how to manage diabetes mellitus during episodes of minor illness such as colds or the flu, the nurse should include which of the following measures in the teaching plan?

○ 1. Increase the frequency of blood and urine glucose testing.

○ 2. Try to reduce food intake to reduce nausea.
○ 3. Call the physician if glucose appears in the urine.
○ 4. Stop taking long-acting insulin temporarily.

54. Vascular changes occurring in diabetes mellitus may affect all body organs. Vascular changes will exert their most serious effects when they become prevalent in which body organ?
○ 1. Liver.
○ 2. Lung.
○ 3. Kidney.
○ 4. Pancreas.

55. Of the following eye problems, which is least likely to be related to diabetes mellitus?
○ 1. Cataracts.
○ 2. Blindness.
○ 3. Astigmatism.
○ 4. Blurred vision.

56. What is the most important reason why it is vital to promptly recognize and treat hypoglycemia in the client with diabetes mellitus?
○ 1. The client may become dehydrated quickly.
○ 2. Hypoglycemia may lead to brain damage.
○ 3. Hypoglycemia necessitates increased insulin dosage.
○ 4. The client may become confused, increasing the risk of injury.

57. A priority nursing diagnosis category for a 16-year-old male with newly diagnosed insulin-dependent diabetes mellitus would be
○ 1. Self-Esteem Disturbance.
○ 2. Ineffective Breathing Patterns.
○ 3. Pain.
○ 4. Activity Intolerance.

58. When establishing goals of care for the client with diabetic ketoacidosis, the nurse would identify which of the following nursing diagnosis categories as a priority problem?
○ 1. Sleep Pattern Disturbance.
○ 2. Altered Health Maintenance.
○ 3. Altered Nutrition.
○ 4. Fluid Volume Deficit.

59. Before undergoing a transsphenoidal hypophysectomy for pituitary adenoma, the client asks the nurse how the surgeon closes the incision made in the dura. The nurse would respond based on the knowledge that
○ 1. dissolvable sutures are used to close the dura.
○ 2. the nasal packing provides pressure until normal wound healing occurs.
○ 3. a patch is made with a piece of fascia.
○ 4. a synthetic mesh is placed to facilitate healing.

60. Initial treatment for a cerebrospinal fluid (CSF) leak following a transsphenoidal hypophysectomy for pituitary tumor would most likely involve
○ 1. repacking the nose.
○ 2. returning the client to surgery.
○ 3. enforcing bed rest with the head of the bed elevated.
○ 4. administering high-dose corticosteroid therapy.

61. Diabetes insipidus is a possible complication following pituitary surgery. For which symptom should the nurse observe to aid detection of diabetes insipidus?
○ 1. Urine specific gravity greater than 1.030.
○ 2. Urine output between 5 and 10 L/day.
○ 3. Blood glucose level above 300 mg/100 ml.
○ 4. Urine negative for glucose and ketones.

62. Diabetes insipidus is usually managed conservatively. If the client develops signs of dehydration, the nurse would expect the physician to order which medication?
○ 1. Corticotropin (ACTH).
○ 2. Vasopressin (Pitressin).
○ 3. Oxytocin.
○ 4. Cosyntropin (Cortrosyn).

63. A priority outcome criterion for the client with diabetes insipidus would include which of the following?
○ 1. Responds appropriately to stimuli.
○ 2. Selects ADA diet correctly.
○ 3. States dietary restrictions.
○ 4. Exhibits serum glucose level within normal range.

64. Nursing care of a client recovering from transsphenoidal hypophysectomy would include all of the following except
○ 1. rinsing the mouth with saline solution.
○ 2. performing frequent toothbrushing.
○ 3. cleaning the teeth with toothettes.
○ 4. rinsing the mouth with mouthwash.

65. Following hypophysectomy, the client should be monitored for signs and symptoms of which potential complication?
○ 1. Acromegaly.
○ 2. Cushing's disease.
○ 3. Diabetes mellitus.
○ 4. Hypopituitarism.

66. Which of the following would be a priority goal of care for the client diagnosed with syndrome of inappropriate antidiuretic hormone (SIADH)?
○ 1. Maintain blood glucose level within normal range.
○ 2. Maintain electrolyte balance.
○ 3. Promote a regular sleep pattern.
○ 4. Prevent fluid volume deficit.

67. In planning care for the client with SIADH, the nurse should keep in mind that antidiuretic hormone (ADH) is secreted by the
○ 1. hypothalamus.
○ 2. anterior pituitary gland.
○ 3. posterior pituitary gland.
○ 4. adrenal gland.

68. When teaching the client newly diagnosed with pri-

mary Addison's disease, the nurse should explain that the disease results from
- ○ 1. insufficient secretion of adrenocorticotropic hormone (ACTH).
- ○ 2. dysfunction of the hypothalamic pituitary.
- ○ 3. idiopathic atrophy of the adrenal gland.
- ○ 4. oversecretion of the adrenal medulla.

69. The nurse would expect the client with Addison's disease to exhibit which of the following signs and symptoms?
- ○ 1. Weight gain and irritability.
- ○ 2. Hunger and double vision.
- ○ 3. Lethargy and depression.
- ○ 4. Muscle spasms and tetany.

70. All of the following results from routine blood tests would be typical of Addison's disease except
- ○ 1. hyperkalemia.
- ○ 2. hyponatremia.
- ○ 3. hyperglycemia.
- ○ 4. elevated blood urea nitrogen (BUN) level.

71. The client with Addison's disease who is taking glucocorticoids at home should base medication administration on the principle that
- ○ 1. various circumstances increase the need for glucocorticoids, so dosage adjustments will be needed.
- ○ 2. the need for glucocorticoids stabilizes and a predetermined dose is taken every third day.
- ○ 3. glucocorticoids are cumulative, so a dose is taken every third day.
- ○ 4. a dose is taken every 6 hours because of the pattern of glucocorticoid secretion.

72. Cortisone acetate (Cortone) and fludrocortisone acetate (Florinef) are prescribed as replacement therapy for a client with Addison's disease. What administration schedule should be followed for this therapy?
- ○ 1. Take both drugs three times a day.
- ○ 2. Take the entire dose of both drugs first thing in the morning.
- ○ 3. Take all the Florinef and two-thirds of the Cortone in the morning and take the remaining Cortone in the afternoon.
- ○ 4. Take half of each drug in the morning and the remaining half of each drug at bedtime.

73. The nurse should instruct the client taking oral glucocorticoids to take them
- ○ 1. with a full glass of water.
- ○ 2. on an empty stomach.
- ○ 3. between meals.
- ○ 4. with meals or an antacid.

74. Fluid balance is one important cue for determining whether a client with Addison's disease is receiving the correct amount of glucocorticoid replacement. As part of client teaching, the nurse should instruct the client that the best indicator of fluid balance is
- ○ 1. skin turgor.
- ○ 2. temperature.
- ○ 3. thirst.
- ○ 4. daily weight.

75. Which of the following signs and symptoms would likely indicate that a client with Addison's disease is receiving too much glucocorticoid replacement?
- ○ 1. Anorexia.
- ○ 2. Dizziness.
- ○ 3. Rapid weight gain.
- ○ 4. Poor skin turgor.

76. The nurse should teach a client with Addison's disease to include all of the following measures in his daily routine except
- ○ 1. having his medications available at all times.
- ○ 2. minimizing his daily activities to avoid overstressing his body.
- ○ 3. following a regular activity and sleep pattern to the greatest extent possible.
- ○ 4. monitoring his body's responses to the hormones daily.

77. A client with Addison's disease should anticipate the need for increased glucocorticoid supplementation in which of the following situations?
- ○ 1. Returning to work after a weekend.
- ○ 2. Going on vacation.
- ○ 3. Having dental work performed.
- ○ 4. Having a routine medical checkup.

78. The nurse should teach a client with Addison's disease that the side effect of bronze-colored skin is thought to be due to
- ○ 1. hypersensitivity to sun exposure.
- ○ 2. increased serum bilirubin level.
- ○ 3. side effects of the glucocorticoid therapy.
- ○ 4. increased secretion of adrenocorticotropic hormone (ACTH).

79. A priority nursing diagnosis for a client in Addisonian crisis would most likely be
- ○ 1. Self-Care Deficit related to weakness and fatigue.
- ○ 2. Altered Nutrition: More than Body Requirements related to increased appetite.
- ○ 3. Altered Nutrition: More than Body Requirements related to decreased exercise.
- ○ 4. Fluid Volume Excess related to reduced urinary excretion of fluid.

80. Signs and symptoms of Cushing's disease include
- ○ 1. weight loss.
- ○ 2. thin, fragile skin.
- ○ 3. hypotension.
- ○ 4. abdominal pain.

81. Cushing's disease can result from several different causes. Possible etiologies of Cushing's disease include all of the following except

○ 1. adrenal cortex atrophy.
○ 2. pituitary oversecretion of ACTH.
○ 3. adrenal gland tumor.
○ 4. high-dose steroid therapy.

82. Which of the following test results would be consistent with a diagnosis of Cushing's disease?
○ 1. Postprandial hypoglycemia.
○ 2. Hypokalemia.
○ 3. Hyponatremia.
○ 4. Decreased urinary calcium level.

83. A client's postoperative orders include an order for hydromorphone hydrochloride (Dilaudid) 2 mg subcutaneously every 4 hours p.r.n. for pain. This drug is administered in relatively small doses primarily because it is
○ 1. less likely to cause dependency in small doses.
○ 2. less irritating to subcutaneous tissues in small doses.
○ 3. as potent as most other analgesics in larger doses.
○ 4. excreted before accumulating in toxic amounts in the body.

84. Which of the following factors would be most important in selecting the needle length to use for a subcutaneous injection of Dilaudid?
○ 1. The diameter of the needle.
○ 2. The circumference of the client's arm.
○ 3. The viscosity of the solution to be injected.
○ 4. The amount of medication to be administered.

85. The nurse should recognize that the most probable cause of temperature elevation in the early postoperative period is
○ 1. dehydration.
○ 2. poor lung expansion.
○ 3. wound infection.
○ 4. urinary tract infection.

86. A client recovering from a bilateral adrenalectomy has a patient-controlled analgesia system with morphine sulfate. Priority nursing actions for the client would include
○ 1. observe at regular intervals for narcotic addiction.
○ 2. encourage the client to reduce analgesic use and tolerate the pain.
○ 3. evaluate pain control at least every 2 hours.
○ 4. increase amount of morphine if the client does not administer the medication.

87. Following surgery for bilateral adrenalectomy, a client is kept on bed rest for several days to stabilize the body's need for steroids postoperatively. Which of the following exercises has been found to be especially helpful in preparing a client for ambulation after a period of bed rest? Alternately
○ 1. flexing and extending the knees.
○ 2. abducting and adducting the legs.
○ 3. tensing and relaxing the Achilles tendons.
○ 4. flexing and relaxing the quadriceps femoris muscles.

88. As the nurse helps the postoperative client out of bed, the client complains of gas pains in her abdomen. The most effective nursing intervention to relieve this discomfort would be to
○ 1. encourage the client to ambulate.
○ 2. insert a rectal tube.
○ 3. insert a nasogastric tube.
○ 4. encourage the client to drink carbonated liquids.

89. The nurse frequently observes the client's surgical incisions from a bilateral adrenalectomy. Because of steroid excess, the client is at an increased risk for
○ 1. fistula formation.
○ 2. suture line dehiscence.
○ 3. pulmonary emboli.
○ 4. keloid scar formation.

90. The client who has undergone a bilateral adrenalectomy is nearing discharge. She tells the nurse that she is concerned about persistent body changes and the fact that her moods are still so unpredictable. She says, "I thought surgery was supposed to fix all that." The most appropriate nursing goal for this client would be to help her accept that
○ 1. her body changes are permanent.
○ 2. her body and mood will gradually return to near normal.
○ 3. the physical changes are permanent, but the mood swings will disappear.
○ 4. the physical changes are temporary, but the mood swings are permanent.

91. Bone resorption is a possible complication of Cushing's disease. To counter the damage done by the disease, the nurse should encourage the client to
○ 1. increase the amount of calcium in the diet.
○ 2. maintain a regular program of weight-bearing exercise.
○ 3. limit her dietary phosphate intake.
○ 4. include isometric exercise in her daily routine.

92. Following bilateral adrenalectomy for Cushing's disease, a female client is told by her physician that she needs periodic testosterone injections. She asks the nurse, "What is that for? Did he forget I'm a woman?" What would be the nurse's best response?
○ 1. "Androgens are needed to balance the reproductive cycle."
○ 2. "Androgens are needed to restore the body's sodium and potassium balance."
○ 3. "Androgens are given to stimulate protein anabolism."
○ 4. "Androgens are given to stabilize mood swings."

CORRECT ANSWERS AND RATIONALE

The letters in parentheses following the rationale identify the step of the nursing process (A, D, P, I, E); cognitive level (K, C, T, N); and client need (S, G, L, H). See the Answer Grid for the key.

The Client With Hyperthyroidism

1. 2. Hyperthyroidism is a state of hypermetabolism. The increased metabolic rate generates heat and produces tachycardia and fine muscle tremors. It also causes weight loss and increased appetite. Anorexia and goiter are associated with hypothyroidism. (A, T, G)

2. 3. A change in the menstrual interval, diminished menstrual flow (oligomenorrhea), or even the absence of menstruation (amenorrhea) may result from the hormonal imbalances of hyperthyroidism. Dysmenorrhea is painful menstruation. Metrorrhagia is blood loss between menstrual periods, and menorrhagia is excessive bleeding during menstrual periods. (A, T, G)

3. 1. Two serious side effects of propylthiouracil (Propacil) are leukopenia and agranulocytosis. The client should be taught to promptly report any signs and symptoms of infection, such as a sore throat and fever, because the drug must be discontinued if adverse reactions occur. Other side effects include skin rash, edema, and enlarged salivary and lymph nodes. Painful menstruation, constipation, abdominal distention, increased urine output, and itching are not associated with propylthiouracil therapy. (I, T, S)

4. 2. A typical sign of hyperthyroidism is irritability due to the high level of thyroid hormone in the body. Such behavior decreases as the client responds to therapy. The other explanations for this client's behavior are not satisfactory. (I, N, L)

5. 1. After thyroidectomy, the client is most often placed in Fowler's position. The dressings are rather bulky. To assess for hemorrhage, the nurse should slip the hand behind the client's neck and check for blood on the back of the neck and on bed linens. Considerable bleeding can occur before it is discovered if such measures as changing dressings, loosening dressings, and routinely checking vital signs are relied on to detect bleeding. (I, T, G)

6. 2. To minimize tension on the incision when moving into the sitting position, the post-thyroidectomy client should place both hands behind the head. (I, T, G)

The Client With Diabetes Mellitus

7. 3. Oral hypoglycemic agents of the sulfonylurea group, such as tolbutamide (Orinase), lower blood glucose level by stimulating pancreatic cells to release insulin. These agents also increase insulin's ability to bind to the body's cells, thereby increasing the number of insulin receptors in the body. (P, K, G)

8. 4. Knee-high stockings have circular elastic tops and are contraindicated because they obstruct circulation in the lower legs and feet. A client with diabetes is prone to serious foot problems when circulation is impaired. The client should be taught to wear pantyhose, a garter belt, loose-top anklets, or a girdle with snap garters attached to it. Nylon stockings are not contraindicated, but if the client's feet perspire freely, cotton stockings (which absorb moisture better than nylon) are recommended. Nylon stockings are contraindicated for clients allergic to nylon, however. Good-fitting low-heeled shoes are recommended. (I, T, S)

9. 2. A client with diabetes should be advised to consult the physician for corn removal, because of the danger of traumatizing foot tissue. (I, T, G)

10. 2. Proper and careful first-aid treatment is important when a client with diabetes has a skin break; the client should be taught to consult a physician promptly if any signs of infection, such as redness, swelling, pain, or blistering, occur. The client with diabetes should understand that any skin break, no matter how small, warrants concern. (I, N, G)

11. 4. A disease of glucose intolerance, diabetes mellitus affects the metabolism of carbohydrates, fats, and proteins. The client's diet should contain appropriate amounts of all three nutrients, plus adequate minerals and vitamins. (I, C, G)

12. 2. Special foods are not required for a client with diabetes, nor should certain foods (except refined sugars) be eliminated entirely from the diet. More important is that mealtimes, meal size, and meal composition be consistent. Pasta may be included in the diet as part of the bread and cereal exchange. For example, ½-cup of pasta is equivalent to one slice of bread. Pasta sauces may be used if they are taken into account in the total diet. A client's ethnic, religious, and cultural food preferences should be taken into account in meal planning. If these preferences are not considered, a client may eat foods without making proper adjustments or may reject the diet entirely. (I, N, G)

The Client With Pituitary Adenoma

13. 1. Galactorrhea (abnormal flow of breast milk) results from overproduction of prolactin. Pituitary tumors can cause oversecretion of adrenocorticotropic hormone (ACTH), growth hormone (GH), and thyroid-stimulating hormone (TSH). Prolactin-secreting tumors account for 30% to 50% of pituitary adenomas. (A, T, G)

14. 2. Excessive prolactin secretion in males results in decreased libido and impotence; these are often the only significant symptoms until the tumor becomes quite large. Bony alterations and voice changes are associated with excessive GH. (A, T, G)

15. 4. With transsphenoidal hypophysectomy, the sella turcica is entered from below, through the sphenoid sinus. There is no external incision; the incision is made between the upper lip and gums. (P, C, G)

16. 3. Deep breathing helps prevent atelectasis, but coughing is contraindicated because it increases intracranial pressure. Increased intracranial pressure should be avoided, because it increases pressure on the graft site. The opening made in the dura mater on entering the sella turcica is frequently patched with a piece of fascia from the leg. Blow bottles are not effective in preventing atelectasis because they do not promote sustained alveolar inflation to maximal lung capacity. Frequent position changes help loosen lung secretions, but deep breathing is most important in preventing atelectasis. (I, T, S)

17. 1. A major focus of nursing care following transsphenoidal hypophysectomy is preventing and monitoring for a CSF leak. Hypoglycemia and adrenocortical insufficiency may occur. Monitoring for postoperative respiratory complications is always important but is not related specifically to transsphenoidal hypophysectomy. (P, N, G)

18. 1. The client's sexual problems are directly related to the excessive prolactin level. Removing the source of excessive hormone secretion should allow the client to return gradually to a normal physiologic pattern, but psychological effects may persist. (I, T, L)

The Client With Addison's Disease

19. 2. Addison's disease is caused by a deficiency of adrenocortical hormone. Causes of this deficiency include surgical removal of the adrenal cortex or its destruction from infection, such as histoplasmosis. Immediate treatment for the client in Addisonian crisis is directed toward combating shock by restoring circulating volume and administering hydrocortisone. Hypotension occurs due to shock. Relieving anxiety is appropriate when the client's condition is stabilized, but the calm, competent demeanor of the emergency department staff will be initially reassuring. Preventing infection is not an appropriate goal in this situation. (P, N, G)

20. 3. Adrenal hormone deficiency can cause profound changes. Inhibited gluconeogenesis commonly produces hypoglycemia, and impaired sodium retention causes decreased fluid volume and hypotension. Edema would not be expected. Gastrointestinal disturbances are expected findings in Addison's disease. (A, C, G)

21. 1. Signs of infiltration include slowing of the infusion and swelling, pain, hardness, pallor, and coolness of the skin at the site. If these signs occur, the IV should be discontinued and restarted at another infusion site. (I, T, S)

22. 1. Each liter of 5% dextrose in normal saline solution contains 170 calories. (I, K, G)

23. 3. Electrolyte imbalances associated with Addison's disease include hypoglycemia, hyponatremia, and hyperkalemia. Salted bouillon and fruit juices provide glucose and sodium to replenish these deficits. Water could cause further sodium dilution. Coffee's diuretic effect would aggravate the fluid deficit. Milk contains potassium and sodium, and diet soda does not contain sugar. (D, N, G)

24. 2. Finding alternative methods of dealing with stress, such as relaxation techniques, is a cornerstone of stress management. Removing all sources of stress from one's life is not possible. Avoiding discussion of stressful situations will not necessarily reduce stress. Anti-anxiety drugs are prescribed by physicians, not as a part of stress management classes. (I, N, L)

The Client With Cushing's Disease

25. 3. Skin bruising from increased skin and blood vessel fragility is a classic sign of Cushing's disease. Muscle wasting occurs in the extremities, and fluid retention causes hypertension. Hair on the head typically thins, while body hair increases. (A, T, G)

26. 3. The most prominent feature of Cushing's disease is often the loss of the diurnal cortisol secretion pattern. The client's random morning cortisol level may be within normal limits, but secretion continues at that level throughout the entire day. Twenty-four-hour urine collections are often useful in identifying the cumulative excess. (P, T, G)

27. 2. Primary dietary interventions include reducing weight by restricting total calories and reducing water weight by restricting sodium. Increased protein catabolism necessitates supplemental protein intake. In addition, the client should be encouraged to eat potassium-rich foods, as serum levels are typically depleted. (P, T, G)

28. 2. Effective splinting for a high incision reduces stress on the incision line, reduces pain, and increases the client's ability to cough and deep breathe effectively. Deep breathing should always precede coughing. (I, T, G)

29. 3. The primary concern following adrenalectomy is to identify and prevent adrenal crisis. Monitoring vital signs is the most important evaluation measure; the other interventions are either not a priority or inappropriate during the first postoperative day. (I, N, G)

30. 1. Bilateral adrenalectomy requires lifelong adrenal hormone replacement therapy. If unilateral surgery is performed, most clients gradually reestablish a normal secretion pattern. (P, N, G)

General Questions

31. 1. A client is likely to have falsely elevated radioactive iodine uptake (RAIU) and protein-bound iodine (PBI) tests if he or she has taken a medication containing iodine within the past month or so. Many medications can falsely elevate or depress test results, but medications containing iodine is most commonly used by clients with hyperthyroidism. Digitalis, antihistamines, and ferrous sulfate do not influence these tests. The RAIU and PBI tests are used to evaluate thyroid function. (A, T, S)

32. 3. Because the eyelids tend to not close completely during sleep in exophthalmos, they should be taped shut to prevent drying. Sleeping masks have also proved helpful for some persons. Massaging the eyes, instilling ointment into the eyes, and covering the eyes with moist gauze pads are not satisfactory nursing measures to protect the eyes of a client with exophthalmos during sleep. (I, T, G)

33. 2. Potassium iodide (SSKI) is frequently administered before a thyroidectomy, because it helps decrease the vascularity of the thyroid gland. A highly vascular thyroid gland is very friable, a condition that presents a hazard during surgery. SSKI does not decrease the progression of exophthalmos, decrease the body's ability to store thyroxin, or increase the body's ability to excrete thyroxin. (P, T, G)

34. 3. SSKI should be well diluted in milk, water, juice, or a carbonated beverage before administration, to help disguise the strong, bitter taste. Also, this drug is very irritating to mucosa if taken undiluted. The client should sip the diluted preparation through a drinking straw to help prevent staining of the teeth. (I, T, G)

35. 3. Laryngeal nerve damage is a potential complication of thyroid surgery because of the proximity of the thyroid gland and the recurrent laryngeal nerve. Asking the client to speak helps assess for signs of laryngeal nerve damage. The client's level of consciousness can be partially assessed by asking her to speak, but in this situation this is not the primary reason for doing so. (I, T, G)

36. 4. Equipment for an emergency tracheostomy should be kept in the room, in the event that tracheal edema and airway occlusion occur. The other equipment is not used in the anticipated emergency care. (I, T, S)

37. 2. Tetany may occur following thyroidectomy if the parathyroid glands are accidentally injured or removed during surgery. This would cause a disturbance in calcium metabolism. An early sign of tetany is numbness with tingling of the fingers and the circumoral region. (A, T, G)

38. 2. The client with tetany is suffering from hypocalcemia, which is treated by administering a preparation of calcium, such as calcium gluconate. (I, T, G)

39. 3. Typical symptoms of hypothyroidism include fatigue, apathy, weight gain, brittle nails, dry skin, and numbness and tingling in the fingers. (A, K, G)

40. 4. Management of the disease process is a priority for the client following radioactive iodine therapy. Signs of hyperthyroidism persist until thyroid hormone production stops. At that time, the client will need to be able to monitor herself for symptoms of hypothyroidism. Significant changes in level of consciousness and breathing pattern are not expected. The client does not need to be immobilized following radioactive treatment. (D, N, H)

41. 2. Radioactive iodine therapy is administered to the person with hyperthyroidism to damage the thyroid tissue and thereby limit secretion of thyroid hormones. (P, K, G)

42. 4. A major symptom of hypothyroidism is fatigue. Other signs and symptoms include lethargy, personality changes, generalized edema, impaired memory, slowed speech, cold intolerance, dry skin, muscle weakness, constipation, weight gain, and hair loss. Incomplete closure of the eyelids, hypermetabolism, and diarrhea are associated with hyperthyroidism. (D, N, G)

43. 1. To minimize the risk of foot injury, a client with diabetes mellitus should avoid going barefoot. (I, T, H)

44. 1. Foods high in dietary fiber are recommended by the American Diabetic Association because they tend to blunt the rise in blood glucose levels after meals. Dietary fiber is the part of food not broken down and absorbed during digestion. Most fibers come from plants; good sources include whole grains, legumes, vegetables, fruits, and nuts. Poor sources of fiber include dairy products and meats. Foods fortified with vitamins are satisfactory if they also contain fiber. However, many foods fortified with vitamins contain either no dietary fiber (such as fortified milk) or very little fiber (such as products fortified with vitamins but made with refined grains). (P, C, G)

45. 4. A client with diabetes who takes tolbutamide (Orinase) should be advised to limit alcohol intake. Tolbutamide in combination with alcohol can cause hypoglycemia. (I, T, G)

46. 1. Factors predisposing to the development of Type II dependent diabetes mellitus include obesity and decreased physical activity, which accentuates obesity. Cigarette smoking, multiple births, and a sedentary life-style are not predisposing factors. (A, K, G)

47. 4. The client with diabetes mellitus is especially prone to atherosclerosis. Such atherosclerotic complications as myocardial infarction, cerebrovascular accident, uremia, and gangrene are reported to cause 70% of deaths in persons with diabetes mellitus. Mortality from cardiovascular and renal complications is rising in persons with diabetes mellitus. (E, K, G)

48. 4. Exercise increases the use of blood glucose by the muscles and therefore reduces the body's insulin requirements. Exercise also tends to lower blood cholesterol and triglyceride levels, which is especially important for clients with diabetes mellitus because they are prone to cardiovascular disease. In addition, exercise is a healthful diversional activity, helps control weight, and promotes circulation. The client should be taught the effects of exercise on blood glucose levels and the importance of snacking before exercise, unless the amount and time of exercise is the same every day and has already been taken into account when determining the dosage of hypoglycemic agents. (P, C, G)

49. 3. The client with diabetes mellitus taking NPH insulin is most likely to become hypoglycemic shortly before the evening meal. (I, T, G)

50. 4. Learning goals are most likely to be attained when they are established mutually by the client and the nurse. Learning is motivated by perceived problems or goals arising out of unmet needs. The perception of the unmet needs must be the client's; the nurse helps the client arrive at his own perception of the need or reason to learn. (P, N, H)

51. 1. The nurse would judge that learning has occurred from evidence of a change in the client's behavior. A client who performs a procedure faultlessly demonstrates that he or she has acquired a skill. Evaluating skill acquisition requires performance of that skill. (E, T, H)

52. 1. The four most commonly reported signs and symptoms of hypoglycemia are nervousness, weakness, perspiration, and confusion. Other signs and symptoms include hunger, incoherent speech, tachycardia, and blurred vision. Anorexia and Kussmaul's respirations are clinical manifestations of hyperglycemia or ketoacidosis. (A, C, G)

53. 1. Colds and flu present special challenges to the client with diabetes mellitus because the body's need for insulin increases during illness. Therefore, the client must take the prescribed insulin dose, increase the frequency of blood and urine testing, maintain an adequate fluid intake to counteract the dehydrating effect of hyperglycemia, and contact the physician if urine ketone levels rise significantly. (I, N, H)

54. 3. Renal failure frequently results from the vascular changes associated with diabetes mellitus. Mortality in persons with diabetes mellitus due to renal and cardiovascular diseases is increasing. Heart disease and stroke are twice as common among persons with diabetes mellitus than among persons without the disease. Damage to organs such as the liver, lungs, and pancreas is less life-threatening. (I, C, G)

55. 3. The leading cause of blindness in the United States is diabetes mellitus, and the major cause of blindness in persons with diabetes mellitus is diabetic retinopathy. Corneal problems, cataracts, refractive changes, and extraocular muscle changes are also noted. Astigmatism has not been associated with diabetes mellitus. (E, C, G)

56. 2. Hypoglycemia is dangerous, because it may lead to permanent brain damage. Changes in cerebral function occur because the brain uses glucose for metabolism and is unable to use alternative sources of energy as well as glucose. Prompt treatment of hypoglycemia is essential to prevent cellular damage. Although injury due to confusion is a concern, it is not the most important reason for prompt treatment of hypoglycemia. Dehydration is more frequently associated with hyperglycemia. Hypoglycemia is treated with glucose or glucagon, not insulin. (I, N, G)

57. 1. Disturbed self-esteem is anticipated in the young, newly diagnosed adolescent with diabetes mellitus. It is important to recognize and evaluate this, because it may interfere with the client's ability to manage the complex care regimen involved in diabetes mellitus. (D, N, L)

58. 4. Fluid volume deficit, or dehydration, is the main problem in diabetic ketoacidosis, as increased osmolarity from the glucose leads to a fluid shift from the intracellular to the extracellular space. The fluid shift leads to increased renal excretion of glucose and fluid. Severe dehydration is a medical emergency requiring immediate insulin and fluid administration. (D, N, G)

59. 3. The dural opening is typically repaired with a patch of muscle or fascia taken from the leg. The client should be prepared preoperatively for the presence of a leg incision. (I, T, S)

60. 3. Significant or persistent CSF leaks are treated initially with bed rest, with the head of the bed elevated to decrease pressure on the graft site. Most leaks heal spontaneously, but occasionally surgical repair is needed. (I, T, G)

61. 2. Two major manifestations of diabetes insipidus are polyuria and polydipsia. The client may drink and excrete 5 to 40 L of fluid daily. The urine specific gravity is low (between 1.001 and 1.006). Diabetes insipidus does not affect metabolism. Blood glucose level above 250 mg/100 ml is associated with ketoacidosis. Urine negative for sugar and acetone is normal. (A, T, G)

62. 2. Diabetes insipidus is usually self-limiting and can be managed by fluid replacement. But if a client develops signs of dehydration, vasopressin (Pitressin) is administered to promote fluid retention. Corticotropin (ACTH) and cosyntropin (Cortrosyn) are used to diagnose primary adrenal insufficiency. Oxytocin is used to induce or stimulate labor. (P, T, G)

63. 1. Because diabetes insipidus is caused by neurologic problems (particularly problems of the pituitary), neurologic status is a priority area. Responding appropriately to stimuli is one outcome associated with neurological functioning. Glucose levels and dietary intake are major concerns for the client with diabetes mellitus, not diabetes insipidus. (E, N, S)

64. 2. After transsphenoidal surgery, the client must be careful not to disturb the suture line while healing occurs. Frequent oral care will be provided with rinses of saline, peroxide, or other solutions, and the teeth may be gently cleaned with toothettes, but vigorous tooth-brushing is contraindicated. (P, T, G)

65. 4. Most clients who undergo adenoma removal experience a gradual return of normal pituitary secretion, but the development of hypopituitarism is a possibility that should be monitored. There would be no reason for the excessive secretion of other hormones. (I, T, H)

66. 2. Syndrome of inappropriate antidiuretic hormone (SIADH) is associated with hypervolemia and dilutional hyponatremia due to excessive release of antidiuretic hormone (ADH). Therefore, maintaining electrolyte balance is a priority goal. (P, N, G)

67. 3. ADH is secreted by the posterior pituitary. (A, K, G)

68. 3. Primary disease refers to a problem in the gland itself. Primary Addison's disease occurs from idiopathic atrophy of the glands. The process is believed to be autoimmune in nature. Pituitary dysfunction can cause Addison's disease, but this is not a primary disease process. (A, K, G)

69. 3. The onset of Addison's disease is usually insidious, and clients are relatively asymptomatic until a major stressor such as illness triggers a crisis. Although many of the disease symptoms are vague and nonspecific, most clients experience lethargy and depression as early symptoms. Other early symptoms include irritability, weight loss, nausea, and vomiting. (A, K, G)

70. 3. Hyperkalemia and hyponatremia are characteristic of Addison's disease. There is decreased renal perfusion and excretion of waste products. Decreased hepatic gluconeogenesis and increased tissue glucose uptake cause hypoglycemia, not hyperglycemia, which is associated with cortisol excess. (A, C, G)

71. 1. The need for glucocorticoids changes with circumstances. The basal dose is established when the client is discharged, but this dose covers only normal daily needs and does not provide for additional stressors. As the manager of the medication schedule, the client needs to know signs of excessive and insufficient dosages. Glucocorticoids are not cumulative and must be taken daily. They must never be discontinued suddenly; in the absence of endogenous production, an Addisonian crisis could result. Glucocorticoids are taken daily, with two-thirds of the daily dose taken at about 8 A.M. and the remainder at about 4 P.M. This schedule stimulates the diurnal pattern of normal secretion, with highest levels between 4 and 6 A.M. and lowest levels in the evening. (I, N, H)

72. 3. Florinef can be administered once a day, but Cortone administration should follow the body's natural diurnal pattern of secretion, with greater amounts secreted during the day to meet increased demand. Typically, baseline administration of Cortone is 25 mg in the morning and 12.5 mg in the afternoon. (I, C, G)

73. 4. Oral steroids have pronounced ulcerogenic properties and should be administered with meals, if possible, or otherwise with antacid. They should never be taken on an empty stomach. (I, T, H)

74. 4. Measuring daily weight is a reliable, objective way to monitor fluid balance. Rapid variations in weight reflect changes in fluid volume. Tongue turgor is a more reliable indicator of fluid volume changes than skin turgor in older persons, whose skin is less elastic. Temperature is not a direct measurement of fluid balance. (E, T, H)

75. 3. A client taking glucocorticoids walks a fine line between underdosage and overdosage. Fluid balance is an important indicator of the adequacy of hormone replacement. Rapid weight gain is a warning sign that the client is receiving too much hormone replacement. (A, T, G)

76. 2. Self-care is an essential part of managing Addison's disease. The client must learn to adjust the glucocorticoid dose in response to the normal and unexpected stresses of daily living. Regularity in daily habits will make adjustment easier, but the client should not be encouraged to withdraw from normal activities to avoid stress. (I, T, H)

77. 3. Illness or surgery places tremendous stress on the body, necessitating increased glucocorticoid dosage. Dental work is a good example. Extreme emotional or psychological stress will also necessitate dosage adjustment. (P, T, S)

78. 4. Bronzing, or general deepening of skin pigmentation, is a classic sign of Addison's disease and is due to melanocyte-stimulating hormone produced in response to increased ACTH secretion. The hyperpigmentation is typically found in the distal portion of extremities and areas exposed to sun. Additionally, areas that may not be exposed to sun, such as the nipples, genitalia, tongue, and knuckles, become bronze-colored. Treatment of Addison's disease usually reverses the hyperpigmentation. (I, T, G)

79. 1. Weakness and fatigue are major problems for the client experiencing Addisonian crisis. A client in crisis requires bed rest until the crisis has been resolved. Fluid volume deficit and nausea and vomiting are other problems during crisis. (D, N, G)

80. 2. In Cushing's disease, excessive cortisol secretion causes rapid protein catabolism, depleting the collagen support of the skin. The skin becomes thin and fragile and susceptible to easy bruising. Weight gain, mood swings, and slow wound healing are other symptoms of Cushing's disease. (A, K, G)

81. 1. Cushing's disease is caused by hormone oversecretion, which can be caused by a tumor, overstimulation from the pituitary, or the use of prescription steroid drugs. It does not result from glandular atrophy. (A, T, G)

82. 2. Sodium retention is typically accompanied by potassium depletion. The client with Cushing's disease exhibits postprandial or persistent hyperglycemia, and bone resorption of calcium increases the urine calcium load. Kidney stones also may form. (A, T, S)

83. 3. Dilaudid is about five times more potent than morphine sulfate, from which it is prepared. Thus, it is administered only in small doses. It has the same, but generally less severe, side effects as morphine. (I, C, G)

84. 2. Needle length depends on the amount of adipose tissue at the site and the angle at which the injection is given. The viscosity of the medication determines the needle diameter. The amount of medication could influence the injection site, which in turn could affect the needle length; however, this is not the most important factor in this situation. (I, C, S)

85. 2. Pulmonary problems become evident in the early postoperative period. Poor lung excursion from bed rest, pain, and retained anesthesia are all common causes of slight postoperative temperature elevations. Wound infections typically appear 4 to 7 days after surgery. (A, C, G)

86. 3. Pain control should be evaluated at least every 2 hours for the client with a patient-controlled analgesia system. Addiction is not a common problem for the postoperative client. A client should not be encouraged to tolerate pain; in fact, other nursing actions besides patient-controlled analgesia should be implemented to enhance the action of narcotics. Such nursing actions include providing back rubs, positioning changes, and a calm, restful environment. One of the purposes of patient-controlled analgesia is for the patient to determine frequency of administering the medication; the nurse should not interfere unless the patient is not obtaining pain relief. (I, T, G)

87. 4. Alternately flexing and relaxing the quadriceps muscles helps prepare the client for ambulation. The other exercises listed will do nothing to increase a client's readiness for walking. (I, T, S)

88. 1. Decreased mobility is one of the most common causes of abdominal distention. Ambulation increases peristaltic activity and helps move gas. (I, T, G)

89. 2. Persistent cortisol excess undermines the collagen matrix of the skin, impairing wound healing. It also carries an increased risk of infection and of bleeding. (I, T, G)

90. 2. As the body readjusts to normal cortisol levels, mood and many physical changes will gradually return to a near-normal state. (P, N, L)

91. 2. Osteoporosis is a serious outcome of prolonged cortisol excess, because calcium is resorbed out of the bone. Regular daily weight-bearing exercise is the most effective way to drive calcium back into the bones. (I, T, H)

92. 3. The testosterone is needed not to support sexual functioning but to support protein anabolism. Thus, it is needed by both males and females. (I, T, H)

THE NURSING CARE OF ADULTS WITH MEDICAL/SURGICAL HEALTH PROBLEMS

TEST 5: The Client With Endocrine Health Problems

Directions: Use this answer grid to determine areas of strength or need for further study.

NURSING PROCESS

A = Assessment
D = Analysis, nursing diagnosis
P = Planning
I = Implementation
E = Evaluation

COGNITIVE LEVEL

K = Knowledge
C = Comprehension
T = Application
N = Analysis

CLIENT NEEDS

S = Safe, effective care environment
G = Physiological integrity
L = Psychosocial integrity
H = Health promotion/maintenance

		Nursing Process					Cognitive Level				Client Needs			
Question #	Answer #	A	D	P	I	E	K	C	T	N	S	G	L	H
1	2	A							T			G		
2	3	A							T			G		
3	1				I				T		S			
4	2				I					N			L	
5	1				I				T			G		
6	2				I				T			G		
7	3			P			K					G		
8	4				I				T		S			
9	2				I				T			G		
10	2				I					N		G		
11	4				I			C				G		
12	2				I					N		G		
13	1	A							T			G		
14	2	A							T			G		
15	4			P				C				G		
16	3				I				T		S			
17	1			P						N		G		
18	1				I				T				L	
19	2			P						N		G		
20	3	A						C				G		
21	1				I				T		S			
22	1				I		K					G		
23	3		D							N		G		

ANSWER GRID: 1

Nursing Process

A = Assessment
D = Analysis, nursing diagnosis
P = Planning
I = Implementation
E = Evaluation

Cognitive Level

K = Knowledge
C = Comprehension
T = Application
N = Analysis

Client Needs

S = Safe, effective care environment
G = Physiological integrity
L = Psychosocial integrity
H = Health promotion/maintenance

		Nursing Process					Cognitive Level				Client Needs			
Question #	Answer #	A	D	P	I	E	K	C	T	N	S	G	L	H
24	2				I					N			L	
25	3	A							T			G		
26	3			P					T			G		
27	2			P					T			G		
28	2				I				T			G		
29	3				I					N		G		
30	1			P						N		G		
31	1	A							T		S			
32	3				I				T			G		
33	2			P					T			G		
34	3				I				T			G		
35	3				I				T			G		
36	4				I				T		S			
37	2	A							T			G		
38	2				I				T			G		
39	3	A					K					G		
40	4		D							N				H
41	2			P			K					G		
42	4		D							N		G		
43	1				I				T					H
44	1			P				C				G		
45	4				I				T			G		
46	1	A					K					G		
47	4					E	K					G		
48	4			P				C				G		
49	3				I				T			G		
50	4			P						N				H
51	1					E			T					H
52	1	A						C				G		

ANSWER GRID: 2

Nursing Process

A = Assessment
D = Analysis, nursing diagnosis
P = Planning
I = Implementation
E = Evaluation

Cognitive Level

K = Knowledge
C = Comprehension
T = Application
N = Analysis

Client Needs

S = Safe, effective care environment
G = Physiological integrity
L = Psychosocial integrity
H = Health promotion/maintenance

		Nursing Process					Cognitive Level				Client Needs			
Question #	Answer #	A	D	P	I	E	K	C	T	N	S	G	L	H
53	1				I					N				H
54	3				I			C				G		
55	3					E		C				G		
56	2				I					N		G		
57	1		D							N			L	
58	4		D							N		G		
59	3				I				T		S			
60	3				I				T			G		
61	2	A							T			G		
62	2			P					T			G		
63	1					E				N	S			
64	2			P					T			G		
65	4				I				T					H
66	2			P						N		G		
67	3	A					K					G		
68	3	A					K					G		
69	3	A					K					G		
70	3	A						C				G		
71	1				I					N				H
72	3				I			C				G		
73	4				I				T					H
74	4					E			T					H
75	3	A							T			G		
76	2				I				T					H
77	3			P					T		S			
78	4				I				T			G		
79	1		D							N		G		
80	2	A					K					G		
81	1	A							T			G		

Answer Grid: 3

NURSING PROCESS

A = Assessment
D = Analysis, nursing diagnosis
P = Planning
I = Implementation
E = Evaluation

COGNITIVE LEVEL

K = Knowledge
C = Comprehension
T = Application
N = Analysis

CLIENT NEEDS

S = Safe, effective care environment
G = Physiological integrity
L = Psychosocial integrity
H = Health promotion/maintenance

		Nursing Process					Cognitive Level				Client Needs			
Question #	Answer #	A	D	P	I	E	K	C	T	N	S	G	L	H
82	2	A							T		S			
83	3				I			C				G		
84	2				I			C			S			
85	2	A						C				G		
86	3				I				T			G		
87	4				I				T		S			
88	1				I				T			G		
89	2				I				T			G		
90	2			P						N			L	
91	2				I				T					H
92	3				I				T					H
Number Correct														
Number Possible	92	21	6	17	43	5	10	13	48	21	12	63	5	12
Percentage Correct														

Score Calculation:

To determine your **Percentage Correct**, divide the **Number Correct** by the **Number Possible**.

The Client With Urinary Tract Health Problems

Test 6

The Client With Cancer of the Bladder
The Client With Renal Calculi
The Client With Acute Renal Failure
The Client With Urinary Tract Infection
The Client With Pyelonephritis
The Client With Chronic Renal Failure
General Questions
Correct Answers and Rationale

Select the one best answer and indicate your choice by filling in the circle in front of the option.

The Client With Cancer of the Bladder

A 51-year-old male client is admitted to the outpatient surgery unit for a cystoscopy to rule out cancer of the bladder.

1. The most common symptom associated with bladder cancer is
- ○ 1. painless hematuria.
- ○ 2. decreasing urine output.
- ○ 3. burning on urination.
- ○ 4. frequent infections.

2. Which of the following symptoms would indicate that the client has developed a complication following cystoscopy?
- ○ 1. Dizziness.
- ○ 2. Chills.
- ○ 3. Pink-tinged urine.
- ○ 4. Bladder spasms.

3. If the client develops lower abdominal pain, the nurse should instruct him to
- ○ 1. apply an ice pack to his pubic area.
- ○ 2. massage his abdomen gently.
- ○ 3. ambulate as much as possible.
- ○ 4. sit in a tub of warm water.

4. The diagnosis of bladder cancer is made, and the client is scheduled for an ileal conduit. Preoperatively, the nurse reinforces the client's understanding of the surgical procedure by explaining that an ileal conduit
- ○ 1. is a temporary procedure that can be reversed later.
- ○ 2. diverts urine into the sigmoid colon, where it is expelled through the rectum.
- ○ 3. conveys urine from the ureters to a stoma opening on the abdomen.
- ○ 4. creates an opening in the bladder that allows urine to drain into an external pouch.

5. Which of the following postoperative complications would the nurse particularly anticipate in a client undergoing a pelvic surgical procedure such as an ileal conduit?
- ○ 1. Bleeding.
- ○ 2. Infection.
- ○ 3. Thrombophlebitis.
- ○ 4. Atelectasis.

6. The nurse would expect the client's urine to contain
- ○ 1. pus.
- ○ 2. feces.
- ○ 3. glucose.
- ○ 4. mucus.

7. The nurse assesses the client's stoma regularly for edema. Which of the following signs and symptoms would indicate excessive stomal edema?
- ○ 1. Elevated temperature.
- ○ 2. Urine dribbling from the stoma.
- ○ 3. Complaints of discomfort around the stoma.
- ○ 4. Urine output below 30 ml/hour.

8. When teaching the client to care for his ileal conduit, the nurse instructs him to empty the appliance frequently to help prevent
- ○ 1. tearing of the ileal conduit.
- ○ 2. interruption of urine production.
- ○ 3. forcing urine into the kidneys.

○ 4. separation of the appliance from the skin.

9. The nurse should teach the client to prevent urine leakage when changing the appliance by
- ○ 1. inserting a gauze wick into the stoma.
- ○ 2. closing the opening temporarily with a cellophane seal.
- ○ 3. suctioning the stoma for a few minutes before changing the appliance.
- ○ 4. avoiding oral fluids for several hours before changing the appliance.

10. The client will be using a reusable appliance at home. The nurse should teach him to clean it routinely with
- ○ 1. baking soda.
- ○ 2. soap.
- ○ 3. hydrogen peroxide.
- ○ 4. alcohol.

11. Which of the following solutions will be useful in helping control odor in the collecting bag after it has been cleaned?
- ○ 1. Salt.
- ○ 2. Vinegar.
- ○ 3. Ammonia.
- ○ 4. Bleach.

12. Which of the following preparations would be most effective in protecting the skin around the stoma from irritation?
- ○ 1. Baking soda.
- ○ 2. Cornstarch.
- ○ 3. Stomahesive.
- ○ 4. Karaya.

13. The nurse teaches the client to attach his appliance to a standard urine collection bag at night. The most important reason for doing this is to
- ○ 1. prevent urine reflux into the stoma.
- ○ 2. prevent appliance separation.
- ○ 3. prevent urine leakage.
- ○ 4. eliminate the need to restrict fluids.

14. The nurse teaches the client measures to prevent urinary tract infection. Which of the following measures would likely be most effective?
- ○ 1. Avoiding persons with respiratory tract infections.
- ○ 2. Maintaining a daily fluid intake of 2,000 to 3,000 ml.
- ○ 3. Using sterile technique to change the appliance.
- ○ 4. Irrigating the stoma daily.

15. The nurse evaluates the effectiveness of the client's postoperative plan of care. Which of the following would be an expected outcome for a client with an ileal conduit? The client
- ○ 1. verbalizes the understanding that his physical activity must be significantly curtailed.
- ○ 2. states that he will place an aspirin in the drainage pouch to help control odor.
- ○ 3. demonstrates how to catheterize the stoma.
- ○ 4. states that he will empty the drainage pouch frequently throughout the day.

The Client With Renal Calculi

A 46-year-old-female client is admitted to the hospital with a diagnosis of renal calculi kidney stones. She is experiencing severe flank pain and complains of nausea. Her temperature is 100.6°F.

16. The immediate nursing goal should be to
- ○ 1. prevent urinary tract complications.
- ○ 2. alleviate nausea.
- ○ 3. alleviate pain.
- ○ 4. maintain fluid and electrolyte balance.

17. The client is to have a kidney, ureter, and bladder (KUB) x-ray. Which of the following would be ordered to prepare her for this x-ray?
- ○ 1. Fluid and food will be withheld the morning of the examination.
- ○ 2. A tranquilizer will be given before the examination.
- ○ 3. An enema will be given before the examination.
- ○ 4. No special preparation is required for the examination.

18. Besides nausea and severe flank pain, the client complains of pain in her groin and bladder. The nurse would determine that these symptoms most likely result from
- ○ 1. nephritis.
- ○ 2. referred pain.
- ○ 3. urine retention.
- ○ 4. additional stone formation.

19. The client is scheduled for an intravenous pyelogram (IVP) to determine the location of the stone. Which of the following measures would be most important for the nurse to include in pretest preparation?
- ○ 1. Ensuring adequate fluid intake the day of the test.
- ○ 2. Preparing her for the possibility of bladder spasms during the test.
- ○ 3. Checking her history for allergy to iodine.
- ○ 4. Determining when she had her last bowel movement.

20. After the IVP, the nurse should anticipate incorporating which of the following measures into the client's plan of care?
- ○ 1. Maintaining bed rest.
- ○ 2. Encouraging adequate fluid intake.
- ○ 3. Assessing for hematuria.
- ○ 4. Administering a laxative.

21. The client undergoes renal surgery for removal of a large stone, and returns from surgery with an in-

dwelling Foley catheter attached to a urine drainage system. Postoperative orders specify that a daily urine specimen be sent to the laboratory. What is the procedure for collecting a urine specimen from an indwelling catheter?
- ○ 1. Open the spigot on the collecting bag and allow urine to empty into the specimen container.
- ○ 2. Disconnect the drainage tube from the collecting bag and allow urine to flow from the tubing into the specimen container.
- ○ 3. Disconnect the drainage tube from the indwelling catheter and allow urine to flow from the tubing into the specimen container.
- ○ 4. Remove urine from the drainage tube with a sterile needle and syringe and place urine from the syringe into the specimen container.

22. The nurse finds a container with the client's urine specimen sitting on a counter in the bathroom. The client states that the specimen has been sitting in the bathroom at least 2 hours. What would be the nurse's most appropriate action?
- ○ 1. Discard the urine and obtain a new specimen.
- ○ 2. Send the urine to the laboratory as quickly as possible.
- ○ 3. Add fresh urine to the collected specimen and send the specimen to the laboratory.
- ○ 4. Place the specimen in the refrigerator until it can be transported to the laboratory.

23. The client also has a ureteral catheter in place. A priority nursing action would be to
- ○ 1. irrigate the catheter with 30 ml of normal saline solution every 8 hours.
- ○ 2. ensure that the catheter is draining freely.
- ○ 3. clamp the catheter every 2 hours for 30 minutes.
- ○ 4. ensure that the catheter drains at least 30 ml/hour.

24. To reduce urethral irritation, the nurse should tape the client's Foley catheter to her
- ○ 1. inner thigh.
- ○ 2. gown.
- ○ 3. lower abdomen.
- ○ 4. lower thigh.

25. Paralytic ileus is a common complication of renal surgery. Which of the following interventions would be inappropriate for the client if she develops paralytic ileus?
- ○ 1. Encourage her to ambulate every 2 to 4 hours.
- ○ 2. Offer her 3 to 4 ounces of a carbonated beverage every hour.
- ○ 3. Encourage her to use the incentive spirometer every 2 hours while awake.
- ○ 4. Continue IV fluid therapy with 1,000 ml of 5% dextrose in water every 8 hours.

26. Which of the following best indicates that the client's peristaltic activity is returning to normal?
- ○ 1. The client passes flatus.
- ○ 2. The client says that she is hungry.
- ○ 3. Bowel sounds are absent on auscultation.
- ○ 4. Peristalsis can be felt on abdominal palpation.

27. The day after surgery, the nurse is conducting a postoperative assessment of the client. Which of the following findings would be most important for the nurse to report to the physician?
- ○ 1. Temperature of 99.8°F.
- ○ 2. Urine output of 20 ml/hour.
- ○ 3. Absence of bowel sounds.
- ○ 4. A 2″ by 2″ area of serous sanginous drainage on the flank dressing.

28. Of the following findings in the client's nursing history, which would be the least likely to have predisposed her to renal calculi?
- ○ 1. Having had several urinary tract infections in the past 2 years.
- ○ 2. Having taken large doses of vitamin C over the past several years.
- ○ 3. Drinking less than the recommended amount of milk.
- ○ 4. Having been on prolonged bed rest following an accident the previous year.

29. What instructions should the nurse plan to include in the client's discharge teaching because of her history of stone formation?
- ○ 1. Increase her daily fluid intake to at least 2 to 3 L.
- ○ 2. Strain her urine at home regularly.
- ○ 3. Eliminate dairy products from her diet.
- ○ 4. Follow measures to alkalinize her urine.

30. Because the client's stone was found to be composed of uric acid, a low-purine, alkaline-ash diet was ordered. The nurse has been reinforcing the dietitian's teaching. The client's selection of which of the following food items would indicate that she understands the dietary modification?
- ○ 1. Milk, apples, tomatoes, and corn.
- ○ 2. Eggs, spinach, dried peas, and gravy.
- ○ 3. Salmon, chicken, caviar, and asparagus.
- ○ 4. Grapes, corn, cereals, and liver.

31. Allopurinol (Zyloprim), 200 mg daily, is prescribed for the client. The nurse should teach the client about which of the following side effects of this medication?
- ○ 1. Abdominal pain, retinopathy, and anorexia.
- ○ 2. Drowsiness, maculopapular rash, and anemia.
- ○ 3. Nausea, vomiting, and nasal congestion.
- ○ 4. Dizziness, erythema, and palpitations.

32. The client has a clinic appointment scheduled for 10 days after discharge. Which laboratory finding at that time would indicate that allopurinol (Zyloprim) has had a therapeutic effect?
- ○ 1. Decreased urinary alkaline phosphatase level.

○ 2. Increased urinary calcium excretion.
○ 3. Increased serum calcium level.
○ 4. Decreased serum uric acid level.

The Client With Acute Renal Failure

A 60-year-old client developed shock after a severe myocardial infarction. He now has acute renal failure.

33. The client's family asks the nurse why the client has developed acute renal failure. The nurse should base the response on the knowledge that there is
○ 1. a decrease in the blood flow through the kidneys.
○ 2. an obstruction of urine flow from the kidneys.
○ 3. a prolonged episode of inadequate cardiac output.
○ 4. histologic damage to the kidney resulting in acute tubular necrosis.

34. The most significant sign of acute renal failure is
○ 1. increased blood pressure.
○ 2. elevated body temperature.
○ 3. decreased urine output.
○ 4. increased urine specific gravity.

35. The client's blood urea nitrogen (BUN) level is elevated. This most likely resulted from
○ 1. destruction of kidney cells.
○ 2. hemolysis of red blood cells.
○ 3. below-normal metabolic rate.
○ 4. reduced renal blood flow.

36. The client's potassium blood level is elevated, and the nurse administers sodium polystyrene sulfonate (Kayexalate). This drug is administered because of its ability to
○ 1. increase potassium excretion from the colon.
○ 2. release hydrogen ions for sodium ions.
○ 3. increase calcium absorption in the colon.
○ 4. exchange sodium for potassium ions in the colon.

37. If the client's potassium level continues to rise, the nurse should be prepared for which of the following emergency situations?
○ 1. Cardiac arrest.
○ 2. Pulmonary edema.
○ 3. Circulatory collapse.
○ 4. Hemorrhage.

38. A high-carbohydrate, low-protein diet is prescribed for the client. The rationale for the high-carbohydrate diet is that carbohydrates will
○ 1. act as a diuretic.
○ 2. reduce demands on the liver.
○ 3. help maintain urine acidity.
○ 4. prevent the development of ketosis.

39. The client asks the nurse for a snack. Because the client's potassium level is elevated, which of the following snacks would be most appropriate for the nurse to serve her?
○ 1. A gelatin dessert.
○ 2. Yogurt.
○ 3. An orange.
○ 4. Dried peanuts.

40. The client is on a fluid restriction of 500 ml/day, plus replacement for urine output. Since her 24-hour urine output yesterday was 150 ml, her total fluid allotment for the next 24 hours is 650 ml. What change-of-shift information given by the nurse who worked 7:30 A.M. to 3:30 P.M. would indicate an understanding of how to distribute this fluid? The fluid allotment for this shift was
○ 1. supplemented with gelatin and ice cream.
○ 2. divided equally between breakfast and lunch.
○ 3. given in small amounts throughout the shift.
○ 4. given in its entirety in the morning to minimize the client's thirst.

41. The client has an external cannula inserted in her forearm for hemodialysis. Which of the following measures should the nurse avoid when caring for the client?
○ 1. Using the unaffected arm for blood pressure measurements.
○ 2. Ensuring that clamps are at the bedside at all times.
○ 3. Auscultating the cannula for bruits each shift.
○ 4. Injecting heparin into the cannula each shift.

42. As the client undergoes her first hemodialysis treatment, the nurse should assess her carefully for signs and symptoms of disequilibrium syndrome, including
○ 1. headache, confusion, and nausea.
○ 2. fever, rales, and shortness of breath.
○ 3. fever, chills, and chest pain.
○ 4. hypotension, tachycardia, and shortness of breath.

43. If disequilibrium syndrome occurs during dialysis, the priority nursing action would be to
○ 1. start nasal oxygen administration.
○ 2. slow the rate of dialysis.
○ 3. reassure the client.
○ 4. place the client in Trendelenburg's position.

44. The client receives heparin while on dialysis. Which of the following statements about the anticoagulation that occurs with dialysis is correct?
○ 1. Regional anticoagulation can be achieved through the infusion of heparin for the machine and protamine sulfate for the client.
○ 2. Warfarin sodium (Coumadin) is given to maintain anticoagulation between treatments.
○ 3. Heparin does not enter the body, so there is no risk of bleeding.
○ 4. Clotting time is seriously prolonged for several hours after each treatment.

45. Which of the following abnormal blood values would not be improved by dialysis treatment?
○ 1. Elevated serum creatinine.

○ 2. Hyperkalemia.
○ 3. Low hemoglobin.
○ 4. Hypernatremia.

46. When assessing the shunt for signs of infection, the nurse should note
○ 1. absence of a bruit.
○ 2. sluggish capillary refill time.
○ 3. coolness of the involved extremity.
○ 4. swelling at the shunt site.

47. The client's renal function improves, and she is ready for discharge. She asks the nurse if her kidneys "will ever function normally again." The nurse's response should be based on knowledge that the client's renal status will most likely
○ 1. continue to improve over a period of weeks.
○ 2. result in the need for permanent hemodialysis.
○ 3. improve only if she has a renal transplant.
○ 4. result in end-stage renal failure.

The Client With Urinary Tract Infection

A 24-year-old female client comes to a walk-in clinic in moderate distress with a probable diagnosis of acute cystitis. She is on her honeymoon and is accompanied by her husband.

48. Which of the following symptoms would the nurse expect the client to report during the assessment?
○ 1. Fever and chills.
○ 2. Frequency and burning on urination.
○ 3. Suprapubic pain and nausea.
○ 4. Dark, concentrated urine.

49. A midstream urine specimen is ordered, and the nurse teaches the client how to collect the specimen correctly. Which of the following should the nurse include in the instructions?
○ 1. Void directly into the sterile specimen container.
○ 2. Save the first voided urine.
○ 3. Stop collecting urine after the bladder is empty.
○ 4. Cleanse the urethral meatus after obtaining the specimen.

50. The client asks the nurse, "How did I get this infection?" The nurse should explain that in most instances, cystitis is caused by
○ 1. congenital strictures in the urethra.
○ 2. an infection elsewhere in the body.
○ 3. urine stasis in the urinary bladder.
○ 4. an ascending infection from the urethra.

51. The physician tells the client that the infection has likely been precipitated by sexual intercourse and that an antibiotic will be ordered. Before the physician can continue, the client becomes upset, crying and saying that her "honeymoon is ruined." The nurse helps calm the client, who tearfully asks if this means she should abstain from intercourse for the rest of her honeymoon. What advice should the nurse offer her?
○ 1. "Avoid intercourse until you've completed the antibiotic therapy and then limit intercourse to once a week."
○ 2. "Limit intercourse to once a day in the early morning after your bladder has rested."
○ 3. "As long as you're comfortable, you can have intercourse as often as you wish; but be sure to urinate within 15 minutes after intercourse."
○ 4. "You and your husband can enjoy intercourse as often as you wish. Just make sure he wears a condom and uses a spermicide."

52. The client is afraid to discuss this sexual issue with her husband. She feels that she is a failure because she got sick on her honeymoon and asks the nurse to speak to her husband for her. Which would be the nurse's best approach?
○ 1. Have a group meeting with the client, her husband, the doctor, the nurse, and the pharmacist.
○ 2. Insist that the client talk with her husband alone, as good communication is the basis for a successful marriage.
○ 3. Talk first with the husband alone and then with both of them together to share the husband's reactions.
○ 4. Spend time with the client to increase her comfort and then stay with her while she talks with her husband.

53. The client is given a prescription for co-trimoxazole (Bactrim-DS) for her infection. Which of the following statements would indicate that she understands the principles of antibiotic therapy?
○ 1. "I'll take the pills until I feel better and keep the rest for recurrences."
○ 2. "I'll take all the pills and then return to my doctor."
○ 3. "I'll take the pills until the symptoms go away, and then reduce the dose to one pill a day."
○ 4. "I'll take all the pills and then have the prescription renewed once."

54. The nurse teaches the client methods to relieve her discomfort until the antibiotic takes effect. Which of the following responses by the client would indicate that she understands the nurse's instructions? "I will
○ 1. place ice packs on my perineum."
○ 2. take hot tub baths."
○ 3. drink a cup of warm tea every hour."
○ 4. void every 5 to 6 hours."

55. The client is also given a prescription for phenazopyridine hydrochloride (Pyridium). The nurse should teach the client that this drug is used to treat urinary tract infections by
○ 1. releasing formaldehyde and providing bacteriostatic action.

○ 2. potentiating the action of the antibiotic.
○ 3. providing an analgesic effect on the bladder mucosa.
○ 4. preventing the crystallization that can occur with sulfa drugs.

56. Before the client starts taking phenazopyridine hydrochloride (Pyridium), she should be taught about which of the drug's side effects?
○ 1. Bright orange-red urine.
○ 2. Incontinence.
○ 3. Gastric distress.
○ 4. Slight drowsiness.

57. Which of the following statements by the client would indicate that she is at high risk for a recurrence of cystitis?
○ 1. "I can usually go 8 to 10 hours without needing to empty my bladder."
○ 2. "I shower every morning."
○ 3. "I wipe from front to back after voiding."
○ 4. "I drink a lot of water during the day."

58. To prevent recurrence of cystitis, the nurse should plan to encourage the client to include which of the following measures in her daily routine?
○ 1. Wearing cotton underpants.
○ 2. Wearing tight pants.
○ 3. Douching regularly with 0.25% acetic acid.
○ 4. Using bubble baths and vaginal sprays.

59. The nurse explains to the client the importance of drinking large quantities of fluid. To help her understand, the nurse should tell her to drink
○ 1. twice as much fluid as she usually drinks.
○ 2. at least 1 quart more than she usually drinks.
○ 3. a lot of water, juice, and other fluids throughout the day.
○ 4. at least 3 quarts each day.

The Client With Pyelonephritis

A 45-year-old male client is admitted to the hospital with a diagnosis of acute pyelonephritis.

60. Which of the following symptoms would most likely indicate pyelonephritis?
○ 1. Ascites.
○ 2. Costovertebral angle (CVA) tenderness.
○ 3. Polyuria.
○ 4. Nausea and vomiting.

61. Which of the following factors would put the client at increased risk for pyelonephritis?
○ 1. A 2-year history of hypertension.
○ 2. Ingestion of large quantities of cranberry juice.
○ 3. Average fluid intake of 2,000 cc/day.
○ 4. A 12-year history of diabetes mellitus.

62. The client asks the nurse, "How will I know whether the antibiotics are effectively treating my infection?" The nurse's most appropriate response would be
○ 1. "After you take the antibiotics for 2 weeks, you'll be cured."
○ 2. "The doctor can tell by the color and odor of your urine."
○ 3. "The doctor can determine your progress through urine cultures."
○ 4. "When your symptoms disappear, you'll know that your infection is gone."

The Client With Chronic Renal Failure

A 47-year-old male client has been treated for hypertension since age 22. He developed renal insufficiency 5 years ago and chronic renal failure last year. He had a permanent peritoneal catheter inserted at that time, and so far has been successfully managed with peritoneal dialysis.

63. Common clinical manifestations of uremia include which of the following?
○ 1. Dry, itchy skin.
○ 2. Cyanosis.
○ 3. Bradycardia.
○ 4. Hypotension.

64. Which of the following laboratory results would be unexpected in a client with chronic renal failure?
○ 1. Serum potassium 6.0 mEq/L.
○ 2. Serum creatinine 4.9 mg/dl.
○ 3. Blood urea nitrogen 15 mg/dl.
○ 4. Serum phosphate 5.2 mg/dl.

65. What is the primary disadvantage of using standard peritoneal dialysis for long-term management of chronic renal failure?
○ 1. The danger of hemorrhage is very high.
○ 2. It cannot correct severe imbalances.
○ 3. It is a slow method of treatment.
○ 4. The risk of contracting hepatitis is very high.

66. The client complains that he feels nauseated at least part of every day. The nurse should explain that the nausea is the result of
○ 1. acidosis caused by his medications.
○ 2. accumulation of waste products in his blood.
○ 3. chronic anemia and fatigue.
○ 4. excess fluid load.

67. The dialysis solution is warmed before use in peritoneal dialysis primarily to
○ 1. encourage the removal of serum urea.
○ 2. force potassium back into the cells.
○ 3. add extra warmth to the body.
○ 4. promote abdominal muscle relaxation.

68. Which of the following assessments would be most

appropriate for the nurse to make while the dialysis solution is dwelling within the client's abdomen?
○ 1. Assessing for urticaria.
○ 2. Observing respiratory status.
○ 3. Checking capillary refill time.
○ 4. Monitoring electrolyte status.

69. During the client's dialysis, the nurse observes that the solution draining from his abdomen is consistently blood-tinged. Which interpretation of this observation would be correct? Bleeding
○ 1. is common when the client has a permanent peritoneal catheter.
○ 2. indicates abdominal blood vessel damage.
○ 3. can indicate kidney damage.
○ 4. is caused by too-rapid infusion of the dialysate.

70. During dialysis, the nurse observes that the flow of dialysate stops before all the solution has drained out. What would be the appropriate nursing intervention?
○ 1. Have the client get out of bed and sit in a chair.
○ 2. Turn the client from side to side.
○ 3. Reposition the peritoneal catheter.
○ 4. Have the client get up and walk.

71. Which of the following nursing interventions should be included in the client's care plan during dialysis therapy?
○ 1. Keep him in isolation.
○ 2. Monitor his blood pressure.
○ 3. Pad the siderails of his bed.
○ 4. Keep him NPO.

72. The most potentially dangerous complication of peritoneal dialysis is
○ 1. abdominal pain.
○ 2. gastrointestinal bleeding.
○ 3. peritonitis.
○ 4. muscle cramps.

73. Following completion of dialysis, the nurse would expect the client to exhibit
○ 1. hematuria.
○ 2. weight loss.
○ 3. hypertension.
○ 4. increased urine output.

74. Aluminum hydroxide (Amphojel) is prescribed for the client. The purpose of giving this drug to a client with chronic renal failure is to
○ 1. relieve the pain of gastric hyperacidity.
○ 2. prevent Curling's stress ulcers.
○ 3. bind phosphate in the intestine.
○ 4. reverse metabolic acidosis.

75. The nurse teaches the client when to take the Amphojel. Which of the following statements would indicate that he understands the teaching? "I'll take it
○ 1. every 4 hours around the clock."
○ 2. between meals and at bedtime."
○ 3. when I have a sour stomach."
○ 4. with meals and bedtime snacks."

76. A medication history reveals that the client takes magnesium hydroxide (Milk of Magnesia) for constipation. Why would the nurse suggest that he switch to psyllium hydrophilic mucilloid (Metamucil)?
○ 1. Milk of Magnesia can cause magnesium intoxication.
○ 2. Milk of Magnesia is too harsh on the bowel.
○ 3. Metamucil is more palatable.
○ 4. Milk of Magnesia is high in sodium.

77. In planning teaching strategies for the client, the nurse must keep in mind the neurologic impact of uremia. Which teaching strategy would be most appropriate?
○ 1. Providing all needed teaching in one extended session.
○ 2. Frequently validating the client's understanding of the material.
○ 3. Conducting a one-on-one session with the client.
○ 4. Using videotapes to reinforce the material as needed.

78. The nurse is developing a care plan for the client with the goal of helping him maintain adequate nutritional status. Which of the following diets would be most appropriate for a client with chronic renal failure?
○ 1. High carbohydrate, high protein.
○ 2. High calcium, high potassium, high protein.
○ 3. Low protein, low sodium, and low potassium.
○ 4. Low protein, high potassium.

79. Sexual problems can be very troublesome to clients with chronic renal failure. Which one of the following strategies would not be useful in helping a client cope with such a problem?
○ 1. Using vinegar-and-water mouthwash to control breath odor.
○ 2. Using alternate forms of sexual expression and intimacy during periods of impotence.
○ 3. Planning rest periods before sexual activity.
○ 4. Avoiding sexual activity to prevent the embarrassment of impotence.

80. The client has asked to be evaluated for a home continuous ambulatory peritoneal dialysis (CAPD) program. The nurse should explain that the major advantage of this approach to chronic renal failure is that it
○ 1. is relatively low in cost.
○ 2. allows the client to be more independent.
○ 3. is faster and more efficient than standard peritoneal dialysis.
○ 4. has fewer potential side effects and complications.

81. The client asks if his diet would change on continuous ambulatory peritoneal dialysis (CAPD). Which of the following would be the nurse's best response? "Diet restrictions

○ 1. are more rigid with CAPD, because standard peritoneal dialysis is a more effective technique."
○ 2. are the same for both CAPD and standard peritoneal dialysis."
○ 3. with CAPD are fewer than with standard peritoneal dialysis, because dialysis is constant."
○ 4. with CAPD are fewer than with standard peritoneal dialysis, because it works more quickly."

82. Peritoneal infection is the most serious potential complication of CAPD. Which of the following is the most significant sign of peritoneal infection?
○ 1. Cloudy dialysate fluid.
○ 2. Swelling in the legs.
○ 3. Poor drainage of the dialysate fluid.
○ 4. Redness at the catheter insertion site.

General Questions

83. When starting a client's IV therapy, the nurse applies a tourniquet and selects the site for inserting the needle. When should the nurse remove the tourniquet?
○ 1. When the skin has been cleansed.
○ 2. As soon as the needle is in the vein.
○ 3. As soon as the needle is positioned under the skin.
○ 4. When the needle has been secured with tape.

84. In preparation for starting IV therapy, the nurse selects a site to insert the needle. Which of the following areas should the nurse try first?
○ 1. Back of the hand.
○ 2. Inner aspect of the elbow.
○ 3. Inner aspect of the forearm.
○ 4. Outer aspect of the forearm.

85. Which of the following pharmaceutical agents would most likely be ordered to decrease blood clotting?
○ 1. Folic acid (Folvite).
○ 2. Heparin sodium.
○ 3. Vitamin B12 (cyanocobalamin).
○ 4. Vitamin K (AquaMEPHYTON).

86. Warfarin sodium (Coumadin) is ordered for a client along with the medications listed below. Which of these medications should the nurse question before administering it?
○ 1. Ampicillin (Amcill).
○ 2. Secobarbital (Seconal).
○ 3. Ascorbic acid (vitamin C).
○ 4. Docusate sodium (Colace).

87. Oral ferrous sulfate (Feosol) is prescribed for the client to take at home. The nurse would teach the client to take orange juice with the iron preparation, because orange juice
○ 1. decreases the toxicity of the medication.
○ 2. helps prevent mouth ulcers.
○ 3. masks the bitter taste of the enteric-coated tablet.
○ 4. acts as a reducing agent to increase medication absorption.

88. The nurse's teaching plan also would include telling the client to expect which of the following side effects of oral ferrous sulfate?
○ 1. Bright orange urine.
○ 2. Excessive perspiration.
○ 3. Dark red or black stool.
○ 4. Yellow or light green sputum.

89. When caring for a client after a closed renal biopsy, the nurse would anticipate implementing which of the following nursing measures?
○ 1. Maintaining the client on strict bed rest in a supine position for 6 hours.
○ 2. Inserting an indwelling catheter to monitor urine output.
○ 3. Applying a sandbag to the biopsy site to prevent bleeding.
○ 4. Administering IV narcotic medications to promote comfort.

90. Which of the following laboratory tests is considered the most reliable indicator of renal function?
○ 1. Blood urea nitrogen (BUN).
○ 2. Urinalysis.
○ 3. Serum potassium.
○ 4. Serum creatinine.

91. The nurse should instruct a client receiving heparin therapy to report which of the following symptoms?
○ 1. Constipation.
○ 2. Hematuria.
○ 3. Dyspnea.
○ 4. Pruritis.

CORRECT ANSWERS AND RATIONALE

The letters in parentheses following the rationale identify the step of the nursing process (A, D, P, I, E); cognitive level (K, C, T, N); and client need (S, G, L, H). See the Answer Grid for the key.

The Client With Cancer of the Bladder

1. 1. Painless hematuria is the most common symptom associated with bladder cancer. Bleeding from the lesions occurs fairly early in the disease process, but bladder cancer is basically asymptomatic in early stages. Bladder cancer is not related to infection or renal function. (A, K, G)

2. 2. Pink-tinged urine and bladder spasms are common following cystoscopy, but chills could indicate the onset of acute infection that can progress to septic shock. (E, K, G)

3. 4. Lower abdominal pain following a cystoscopy is frequently caused by bladder spasms. Ice is not effective in relieving spasms. Ambulation may increase bladder irritability. (I, T, G)

4. 3. An ileal conduit is a permanent urinary diversion in which a portion of the ileum is surgically resected and one end of the segment is closed. The ureters are surgically attached to this segment of the ileum, and the open end of the ileum is brought to the skin surface on the abdomen to form the stoma. The client must wear a pouch to collect the urine that continually flows through the conduit. (I, C, G)

5. 3. Clients undergoing pelvic surgery are at increased risk for thrombophlebitis postoperatively. Extensive pelvic surgery, such as involved in an ileal conduit, removes lymph nodes from the pelvis and results in circulatory congestion from edema and stasis. Bleeding, infection, and atelectasis are not unique to this type of surgery. (P, C, G)

6. 4. The urine causes some local irritation to the intestine, and hence the client with an ileal conduit can be expected to excrete urine that contains mucus. Pus or feces in the urine is an abnormal sign that should be reported promptly. There is no reason to expect to find glucose in the client's urine. (P, C, G)

7. 4. Urine output below 30 ml/hour could indicate stomal edema, which obstructs urine output. An elevated temperature should be noted, but it is not related to stomal edema. Discomfort around the stoma is common postoperatively after construction of an ileal conduit. Dribbling of urine from the stoma is normal. (A, N, G)

8. 4. If the appliance becomes too full, it is likely to pull away from the skin completely or leak urine onto the skin. A full appliance will not tear the ileal conduit, interrupt urine production, or force urine into the kidneys. (I, T, H)

9. 1. Inserting a gauze wick into the stoma helps prevent urine leakage when changing the appliance. The stoma should not be sealed or suctioned, and oral fluids should not be avoided. (I, T, H)

10. 2. A reusable appliance should be routinely cleaned with soap and water. (I, T, H)

11. 2. A distilled vinegar solution acts as a good deodorizing agent after an appliance has been cleansed well with soap and water. If the client prefers, a commercial deodorizer may be used. Salt solution does not deodorize. Ammonia and bleaching agents may damage the appliance. (I, T, H)

12. 3. Skin around a urinary stoma can be protected with Stomahesive. Karaya is not used, because urine erodes it. Baking soda and cornstarch are not as effective as Stomahesive. (I, N, S)

13. 1. The most important reason for attaching the appliance to a standard urine collection bag at night is to prevent urine reflux into the stoma and ureters. Using a standard collection bag also keeps the appliance from separating from the skin and resultant urine leakage. A client with an ileal conduit should drink 2,000 to 3,000 ml of fluid each day, unless contraindicated. (I, N, H)

14. 2. Maintaining a fluid intake of 2,000 to 3,000 ml/day is likely to be most effective in preventing urinary tract infection. A high fluid intake results in high urine output, which prevents urinary stasis and bacterial growth. Clean, not sterile, technique is used to change the appliance. An ileal conduit stoma is not irrigated. (I, N, H)

15. 4. It is important that the client empty the drainage pouch throughout the day to decrease the risk of leakage. An ileal conduit stoma is not catheterized by the client. The client does not normally need to curtail physical activity. Aspirin should never be placed in a pouch, because the aspirin can irritate the stoma. (E, T, H)

The Client With Renal Calculi

16. 3. The immediate nursing goal for this client is to alleviate pain, which can be excruciating. The other goals are appropriate throughout the client's hospitalization but are not immediate. (P, N, G)

17. 4. A KUB x-ray examination ordinarily requires no preparation. It is usually done while the client lies supine. It does not involve the use of radiopaque substances. (P, K, S)

18. 2. The pain associated with renal colic due to calculi is often referred to the groin and bladder in females and to the testicles in males. Nausea, vomiting, abdominal cramping, and diarrhea may also be present. Unlikely causes of pain from renal colic in the groin and bladder or testicles include urine retention or nephritis. The type of pain described in this situation is unlikely to be due to additional stone formation. (D, C, G)

19. 3. A client scheduled for an IVP should be assessed for allergies to iodine and shellfish. Clients with such allergies may be allergic to the IVP dye and be at risk for an anaphylactic reaction. Bowel preparation is important before an IVP to allow visualization of the ureters and bladder, but checking for allergies is most important. (I, N, S)

20. 2. After an IVP, the nurse should encourage fluids to decrease the risk of renal complications caused by the contrast agent. There is no need to place the client on bed rest or to administer a laxative. An IVP would not cause hematuria. (I, T, S)

21. 4. To obtain a urine specimen from a client with an indwelling Foley catheter attached to a closed urine drainage system, the nurse removes the specimen from the drainage tube using a sterile needle and syringe. This technique is not likely to predispose to a urinary tract infection, because the drainage system is not opened to the air. Furthermore, this urine specimen would be fresh, unlike the urine collected in the drainage bag. (I, T, S)

22. 1. The appropriate action would be to discard the specimen and obtain a new one. Urine allowed to stand at room temperature will become alkaline. (I, T, S)

23. 2. The ureteral catheter should drain freely without bleeding at the site. The catheter is rarely irrigated and is never clamped. The client's total urine output (ureteral catheter plus voiding or Foley catheter output) should be 30 ml/hour. (I, N, S)

24. 1. To reduce urethral irritation, the nurse should tape the Foley catheter to a female client's inner thigh or a male client's thigh or abdomen. Taping the catheter to the client's gown does not prevent urethral irritation and may lead to accidental removal of the catheter as the client moves. (I, T, S)

25. 2. A client with paralytic ileus is kept NPO until peristalsis returns. Ambulation stimulates the return of peristalsis. IV fluid infusion and incentive spirometry are routine postoperative orders. (I, N, G)

26. 1. Passing flatus indicates the return of peristalsis, as do active bowel sounds. Peristalsis is difficult to palpate, and palpation is not an appropriate method of assessing bowel activity. Hunger is not the best indicator of peristaltic return. (E, N, G)

27. 2. The decrease in urine output may reflect inadequate renal perfusion and should be reported immediately. Urine output of 30 ml/hr or greater is considered acceptable. The other assessment findings are not unusual during the early postoperative period. (E, N, S)

28. 3. A high, rather than low, milk intake predisposes to renal calculi formation. Such conditions as urinary tract infections, low fluid intake, prolonged immobility, and high daily doses of vitamins C and D tend to predispose to stone formation. Men between ages 30 and 50 develop calculi more often than women. Clients who have had renal calculi twice as often experience recurrence. Persons living in hot climates can develop calculi due to an increased insensible fluid loss combined with inadequate fluid intake. This results in concentration of urine and precipitation of urinary salts. (A, C, G)

29. 1. A high daily fluid intake is essential in clients at risk for calculi formation, because it prevents urinary stasis, which can cause crystallization. Depending on the composition of the stone, the client also may be instructed to limit calcium by instituting specific dietary measures aimed at preventing calcium phosphate stone formation. (P, T, H)

30. 1. Because a high-purine diet contributes to the formation of uric acid, a low-purine diet is advocated. An alkaline-ash diet is also advocated, because uric acid crystals are more likely to develop in acid urine. Foods that may be eaten as desired in a low-purine diet include milk, all fruits, tomatoes, cereals, and corn. Foods very high in purines include liver, caviar, and gravy. Foods containing moderate to large amounts of purine include spinach, dried peas, salmon, chicken, and asparagus. Foods allowed on an alkaline-ash diet include milk, fruits (except cranberries, plums, and prunes), vegetables (especially legumes and green vegetables), and small amounts of ham, beef, trout, and salmon. (E, K, H)

31. 2. Side effects of allopurinol (Zyloprim) include drowsiness, maculopapular rash, anemia, abdominal pain, retinopathy, nausea, vomiting, and bone marrow depression. (I, C, G)

32. 4. By inhibiting uric acid synthesis, allopurinol (Zyloprim) decreases its excretion. The drug's effectiveness is assessed by evaluating for decreased serum uric acid level. (E, K, G)

The Client With Acute Renal Failure

33. 4. There are three categories of acute renal failure: prerenal, intrarenal, and postrenal. Causes of prerenal failure occur outside the kidney and include poor perfusion and a decrease in circulating volume due to such factors as trauma, septic shock, and dehydration. Causes of intrarenal failure, such as hypersensitivity (allergic disorders), renal vessel obstruction, and nephrotoxic agents, result in structural damage to the kidney due to acute tubular necrosis. Postrenal failure, or obstruction within the urinary tract, results from kidney stones, tumors, or benign prostatic hypertrophy. (P, C, G)

34. 3. A sudden change in urine output is typical of acute renal failure. Most commonly, the initial change is greatly decreased urine output. Later in the course of acute renal failure, the client may have marked diuresis (nonoliguric failure). Other common signs and symptoms of acute renal failure include lethargy, nausea and vomiting, diarrhea, headaches, muscle twitching, and convulsions. Serum creatinine and BUN levels are elevated. Urine specific gravity usually is within a low-normal range because the kidneys have difficulty concentrating urine. High body temperatures and sudden blood pressure elevation are not typically associated with acute renal failure. (A, C, G)

35. 4. Reduced renal blood flow causes an elevated BUN level. Urea, an end product of protein metabolism, is normally excreted by the kidneys. Any impairment in renal function causes an increase in plasma urea level. (A, C, G)

36. 4. Polystyrene sulfonate (Kayexalate), a cation-exchange resin, causes the body to excrete potassium through the gastrointestinal tract. In the intestines, particularly the colon, the sodium of the resin is partially replaced by potassium. The potassium is then eliminated when the resin is eliminated with feces. Polystyrene sulfonate may be administered orally or rectally and is used specifically to treat hyperkalemia. (I, K, G)

37. 1. Hyperkalemia predisposes to serious cardiac dysrhythmias and cardiac arrest. Therefore, the nurse should be prepared to treat cardiac arrest when caring for a client with hyperkalemia. (P, C, G)

38. 4. High-carbohydrate foods meet the body's caloric needs during acute renal failure. Protein is limited, because its breakdown may result in accumulation of toxic waste products. (I, T, G)

39. 1. Gelatin desserts contain little or no potassium and can be served to a client on a potassium-restricted diet. Foods high in potassium include bran and whole grains; most dried, raw, and frozen fruits and vegetables; most milk and milk products; chocolate, nuts, raisins, coconut, and strong brewed coffee. Highly refined foods, fruits and vegetables cooked in large amounts of water, butter, cream, and hard candies are generally low in potassium content. (I, N, G)

40. 3. Thirst is a strong motivator to drink. Giving small amounts of fluid during an 8-hour shift helps minimize thirst. Gelatin and ice cream are inappropriate supplements because they become liquid at room temperature. Some fluids should be given with meals, but not the entire 8-hour allotment. (I, N, S)

41. 4. Heparin is not injected into the cannula to maintain the patency of a heparin lock. Because it is part of the general circulation, the cannula cannot be heparinized. The external cannula must be handled carefully and protected from damage and disruption. The arm with the cannula is not used for blood pressure measurement, IV therapy, or venipuncture. A tourniquet or clamps should be kept at the bedside, because dislodgement of the cannula would cause arterial hemorrhage. Patency is assessed by auscultating for bruits every shift. (I, T, S)

42. 1. Typical symptoms of disequilibrium syndrome include headache, nausea and vomiting, confusion, and even seizures. Disequilibrium syndrome typically occurs near the end or after the completion of hemodialysis treatment. (A, C, G)

43. 2. If disequilibrium syndrome occurs during dialysis, the most appropriate intervention is to slow the rate of dialysis. The syndrome is believed to result from too-rapid removal of urea and excess electrolytes from the blood; this causes transient cerebral edema, which produces the symptoms. (I, N, G)

44. 1. Regional anticoagulation can be achieved by infusing heparin in the dialyzer and protamine sulfate, its antagonist, in the client. The client's clotting time will not be seriously affected, although some rebound effect may occur. The clotting time is monitored carefully. Coumadin is not used in dialysis treatment. (I, T, G)

45. 3. Dialysis will correct electrolyte imbalances and clear metabolic waste products from the body, but it has no effect on anemia. Because some red cells are injured during the procedure, dialysis aggravates a low hemoglobin concentration. (E, N, G)

46. 4. Signs of an external access shunt infection include redness, tenderness, swelling, and drainage from around the shunt site. (A, T, S)

47. 1. The kidneys have a remarkable ability to recover from serious insult. In view of this client's prompt and effective treatment, her prognosis should be very good. Effective treatment for acute renal failure consists primarily of restoring normal fluid and electrolyte balance so the body can restore renal functioning and repair renal tissue. The client should be taught how to recognize the symptoms of decreasing renal function and to notify the physician if such problems occur. (P, C, G)

The Client With Urinary Tract Infection

48. 2. The classic symptoms of cystitis are severe burning, urgency, and frequent urination. Some clients also develop fever, hematuria, and suprapubic pain. Systemic symptoms are more likely to accompany pyelonephritis than cystitis. (A, K, G)

49. 1. To collect a midstream urine specimen, the client voids directly into a sterile specimen container. Other correct techniques include discarding the first

30 ml, stopping the collection before the bladder is empty, and cleansing the urethral meatus before obtaining the specimen. (I, T, S)

50. 4. Although various conditions may result in cystitis, the most common cause is an ascending infection from the urethra. (I, K, G)

51. 3. Intercourse is not contraindicated in cystitis. Voiding immediately after intercourse flushes bacteria from the urethra, which should help prevent recurrence. There is no reason to wait until the antibiotic therapy is completed or to limit the frequency of intercourse. A condom and spermicide do not prevent cystitis, because cystitis results from the introduction of the client's own organisms (usually *Escherichia coli*) into the urethra. (I, N, H)

52. 4. As newlyweds, the client and her husband need to develop a strong communication base. The nurse can facilitate the development of this base by preparing the client and being there for support. Being present also allows the nurse to intervene, if necessary, to facilitate the discussion of a difficult topic. Given this situation, an interdisciplinary conference is inappropriate and would not promote intimacy for the client and her husband. Insisting that the client talk with her husband alone is not complying with her request. Having the nurse speak first with the husband alone shifts responsibility away from the couple. (I, N, L)

53. 2. Antibiotics are prescribed for a definite treatment period, and all the pills should be taken. A urine culture should be done after the course of antibiotic therapy to ensure that the urine is bacteria free. Stopping the medication early may cause the infection to recur. Tapering the dosage is inappropriate with antibiotics because it lowers the therapeutic blood level. Refilling the prescription would be indicated only after urine culture indicates that the urine is not bacteria free and the physician prescribes another course of antibiotics. (E, T, H)

54. 2. Hot tub baths promote relaxation and help relieve urgency, discomfort, and spasm. Applying heat to the perineum is more helpful than cold, because heat reduces inflammation. Although liberal fluid intake should be encouraged, tea, coffee, and cola can be irritating to the bladder and should be avoided. Voiding at least every 2 to 3 hours should be encouraged, because it reduces urinary stasis. (E, N, H)

55. 3. Phenazopyridine hydrochloride (Pyridium) is a urinary analgesic that works directly on the bladder mucosa to relieve the distressing symptoms of dysuria. (I, C, G)

56. 1. The client should be told that phenazopyridine hydrochloride (Pyridium) turns the urine a bright orange-red, which may stain underwear. It can be quite frightening for a client to see orange-red urine without having been forewarned. (I, C, G)

57. 1. Stasis of urine in the bladder is one of the chief causes of bladder infection, and a client who voids infrequently is at greater risk of reinfection. Liberal fluid intake (unless contraindicated) and scrupulous hygiene are excellent preventive measures, but the client also should be taught to void every 2 to 3 hours during the day. (E, T, H)

58. 1. A woman can adopt multiple health-promotion measures to prevent the recurrence of cystitis, including avoiding too-tight pants, noncotton underpants, and irritating substances such as bubble baths and vaginal soaps and sprays. Regular douching is not recommended; it can alter the pH of the vagina, increasing the risk of infection. (P, T, H)

59. 4. Instructions should be as specific as possible and avoid general statements such as "a lot." A specific goal is most useful. A mix of fluids will increase the likelihood of client compliance. (I, T, H)

The Client With Pyelonephritis

60. 2. Common symptoms of pyelonephritis include CVA tenderness, burning, urinary urgency or frequency, chills, and fever and fatigue. Polyuria, nausea, and vomiting are not indicative of pyelonephritis. (A, C, G)

61. 4. A client with a history of diabetes mellitus, urinary tract infections, or renal calculi are at increased risk for pyelonephritis. Others at high risk include pregnant women and persons with structural alterations of the urinary tract. (A, T, G)

62. 3. Antibiotics are usually prescribed for a 2- to 4-week period. A urine culture is needed to evaluate the effectiveness of antibiotic therapy. (I, T, H)

The Client With Chronic Renal Failure

63. 1. Uremia refers to the accumulation of nitrogenous waste products in the blood. Hypertension, not hypotension, is typical of uremia. Hypertension occurs because renin is secreted in response to renal ischemia and elevates the blood pressure. Uremic clients typically have dry, itchy skin and are troubled by chronic fatigue, anorexia, and even nausea. Cyanosis and bradycardia are not typical manifestations of uremia. (A, C, G)

64. 3. The stated BUN level is within the normal range of 10 to 15 mg/dl and thus would be unexpected in renal failure. BUN level is usually significantly elevated in chronic renal failure, which causes retention of waste products and electrolytes. Elevated serum potassium (normal 3.5 to 5.0 mEq/L), elevated serum creatinine (normal 0.8 to 1.7 mg/dl for males, 0.6 to 1 mg/dl for females), and hyperphosphatemia (normal 2.5 to 4.8 mg/dl) commonly occur in chronic renal failure. (A, K, G)

65. 3. A disadvantage of standard peritoneal dialysis in long-term management of chronic renal failure is that it requires large blocks of time. Peritoneal dialysis is quite effective in maintaining a client's fluid and electrolyte balance. Neither the danger of hemorrhage nor of hepatitis is high with peritoneal dialysis. (E, K, G)

66. 2. Nausea typically results from the chronic presence of retained waste products in the body. The client can control nausea most effectively by following his diet regimen strictly and avoiding wide swings in blood values between treatments. (I, C, G)

67. 1. The main reason for warming the peritoneal dialysis solution is that the warm solution helps dilate peritoneal vessels, which increases urea clearance. Warmed dialyzing solution also contributes to client comfort by preventing chilly sensations, but this is a secondary reason for warming the solution. (I, C, S)

68. 2. During dwell time, the dialysis solution is allowed to remain in the peritoneal cavity for the time ordered by the physician (usually 20 to 45 minutes). During this time, the nurse should monitor the client's respiratory status, as the pressure of the dialysis solution on the diaphragm can create respiratory distress. The client's laboratory values are obtained before beginning treatment and are monitored every 4 to 8 hours during the treatment, not just during the dwell time. (A, N, S)

69. 2. Because the client has a permanent catheter in place, blood-tinged drainage should not occur. Persistent blood-tinged drainage could indicate damage to the abdominal vessels, and the physician should be notified. However, blood-tinged drainage is common with the initial dialysis runs immediately after peritoneal catheter insertion. (A, N, S)

70. 2. Fluid return with peritoneal dialysis is accomplished by gravity flow. Actions that enhance gravity flow include turning the client from side to side, raising the head of the bed, and gently massaging the abdomen. The nurse should not attempt to reposition the catheter. The client is usually confined to a recumbent position during the dialysis. (I, T, S)

71. 2. Because hypotension is a complication associated with peritoneal dialysis, the nurse records intake and output, monitors vital signs, and observes the client's behavior. The nurse also encourages visiting and other diversional activities. A client on peritoneal dialysis need not be kept NPO, placed in isolation, or placed in a bed with padded siderails. (I, T, S)

72. 3. Peritonitis is a very serious risk associated with peritoneal dialysis. Aseptic technique should be maintained during the procedure. Minor abdominal cramping may occur with dialysis, gastrointestinal bleeding is an extremely rare complication. (E, N, G)

73. 2. Weight loss is expected, and blood pressure usually decreases as well. The client's weight before and after dialysis is one measure of the effectiveness of treatment. Dialysis only minimally affects the damaged kidneys' ability to manufacture urine. Hematuria would not occur after completion of peritoneal dialysis. (A, C, G)

74. 3. A client in renal failure develops hyperphosphatemia that causes a corresponding excretion of the body's calcium stores. To decrease this loss, aluminum hydroxide (Amphojel) is prescribed to bind phosphates in the intestine and facilitate their excretion. (P, T, G)

75. 4. Aluminum hydroxide (Amphojel) is administered to bind the phosphates in ingested foods and so must be given with or immediately after meals and snacks. Amphojel is not administered to treat hyperacidity in clients with chronic renal failure and thus is not prescribed between meals or p.r.n. (E, T, G)

76. 1. Magnesium is normally excreted by the kidneys. When the kidneys fail, magnesium can accumulate and cause severe neurologic problems. Milk of Magnesia is harsher than Metamucil, but magnesium toxicity is a more serious problem. A client may find both Milk of Magnesia and Metamucil unpalatable. Milk of Magnesia is not high in sodium. (I, T, G)

77. 2. Uremia can cause decreased alertness, so the nurse needs to validate the client's comprehension frequently. The client's ability to concentrate is limited, so short lessons are most effective. If family members are present at the sessions, they can reinforce material. Written materials that the client can review are superior to videotapes. (P, N, G)

78. 3. Dietary management for clients with chronic renal failure is usually designed to restrict protein, sodium, and potassium intake. The degree of dietary restriction depends on the degree of renal impairment. The client should also receive an adequate caloric intake, along with appropriate vitamins, and mineral supplements. (P, T, G)

79. 4. Altered sexual functioning commonly occurs in chronic renal failure and can stress marriages and relationships. The client should not avoid sexual activity, but instead should modify it. Effective coping strategies include removing uremic fetor and resting before sexual activity. (I, N, L)

80. 2. The major benefit of CAPD is that it frees the client from daily dependence on dialysis centers, health-care personnel, and machines for life-sustaining treatment. This independence is a treasured outcome for some people. (I, C, G)

81. 3. Dietary restrictions with CAPD are fewer than those with standard peritoneal dialysis because dialysis is constant, not intermittent. The constant slow diffusion of CAPD helps prevent accumulation of toxins and allows for a more liberal diet. (I, N, G)

82. 1. Cloudy drainage indicates bacterial activity in the peritoneum. Other signs and symptoms of infection are fever, hyperactive bowel sounds, and abdominal pain. Swollen legs and inadequate dialysate drainage are unrelated to infection. Redness at the insertion site indicates local infection, not peritonitis. If untreated, however, a local infection can progress to the peritoneum. (A, N, G)

General Questions

83. 2. When starting an IV infusion, the nurse should remove the tourniquet as soon as the needle is in the vein. Until then, the tourniquet keeps the vein distended so that it is more visible and easier to enter. After the needle is in the vein, the tourniquet should be removed before applying tape so that fluid will start to enter the vein promptly. (I, T, S)

84. 1. When starting an IV infusion, the nurse initially uses veins low on the hand or arm. Should the vein be damaged, veins higher on the arm are still available for use. After a vein higher up on the arm has been damaged, veins below it on the arm cannot be used. (I, T, S)

85. 2. An anticoagulant such as heparin sodium is the drug of choice when a client develops thrombophlebitis. Anticoagulants prevent thrombi from forming and existing clots from extending, but do not dissolve existing clots. Vitamin K hastens blood clotting and is contraindicated in thrombophlebitis. Vitamin B12 and folic acid do not affect blood clotting. (P, K, G)

86. 2. Barbiturates such as secobarbital (Seconal) decrease anticoagulant activity. They enhance the liver synthesis of enzymes that metabolize anticoagulants. Therefore, if secobarbital must be given, then the client's dosage of warfarin sodium (Coumadin) may need to be increased. (I, N, G)

87. 4. The ascorbic acid in orange juice is believed to act as a reducing agent to promote better absorption of oral iron preparations from the gastrointestinal tract. (P, C, G)

88. 3. Oral iron preparations typically cause the stools to become black or dark red. This is a common side effect that clients should be prepared for. Oral iron preparations do not affect the color of urine or sputum or the amount of perspiration. (A, C, H)

89. 1. After a renal biopsy, the client is maintained on strict bed rest in a supine position for at least 6 hours to prevent bleeding. If no bleeding occurs, the client typically resumes general activity after 24 hours. Narcotics to control pain would not be anticipated; local discomfort at the biopsy site can be controlled with analgesics. Urine output is monitored, but an indwelling catheter is not typically inserted. (I, T, S)

90. 4. Of the tests listed, serum creatinine is the most reliable indicator of renal function. BUN may be influenced by other factors unrelated to renal disease. A urinalysis may indicate the presence of a renal or urologic disorder. Potassium levels are affected by numerous factors. (E, C, G)

91. 2. While receiving anticoagulant therapy, the client should be taught to observe for signs and symptoms of bleeding such as hematuria, blood in the stool, ecchymosis, and petechiae. Such signs of bleeding would indicate that the anticoagulant effect has exceeded the therapeutic level. (I, C, S)

THE NURSING CARE OF ADULTS WITH MEDICAL/SURGICAL HEALTH PROBLEMS

TEST 6: The Client With Urinary Tract Health Problems

Directions: Use this answer grid to determine areas of strength or need for further study.

Nursing Process

A = Assessment
D = Analysis, nursing diagnosis
P = Planning
I = Implementation
E = Evaluation

Cognitive Level

K = Knowledge
C = Comprehension
T = Application
N = Analysis

Client Needs

S = Safe, effective care environment
G = Physiological integrity
L = Psychosocial integrity
H = Health promotion/maintenance

		Nursing Process					Cognitive Level				Client Needs			
Question #	Answer #	A	D	P	I	E	K	C	T	N	S	G	L	H
1	1	A					K					G		
2	2					E	K					G		
3	4				I				T			G		
4	3				I			C				G		
5	3			P				C				G		
6	4			P				C				G		
7	4	A								N		G		
8	4				I				T					H
9	1				I				T					H
10	2				I				T					H
11	2				I				T					H
12	3				I					N	S			
13	1				I					N				H
14	2				I					N				H
15	4					E			T					H
16	3			P						N		G		
17	4			P			K				S			
18	2		D					C				G		
19	3				I					N	S			
20	2				I				T		S			
21	4				I				T		S			
22	1				I				T		S			
23	2				I					N	S			

Answer Grid: 1

NURSING PROCESS

A = Assessment
D = Analysis, nursing diagnosis
P = Planning
I = Implementation
E = Evaluation

COGNITIVE LEVEL

K = Knowledge
C = Comprehension
T = Application
N = Analysis

CLIENT NEEDS

S = Safe, effective care environment
G = Physiological integrity
L = Psychosocial integrity
H = Health promotion/maintenance

		Nursing Process					Cognitive Level				Client Needs			
Question #	Answer #	A	D	P	I	E	K	C	T	N	S	G	L	H
24	1				I				T		S			
25	2				I					N		G		
26	1					E				N		G		
27	2					E				N	S			
28	3	A						C				G		
29	1			P					T					H
30	1					E	K							H
31	2				I			C				G		
32	4					E	K					G		
33	4			P				C				G		
34	3	A						C				G		
35	4	A						C				G		
36	4				I		K					G		
37	1			P				C				G		
38	4				I				T			G		
39	1				I					N		G		
40	3				I					N	S			
41	4				I				T		S			
42	1	A						C				G		
43	2				I					N		G		
44	1				I				T			G		
45	3					E				N		G		
46	4	A							T		S			
47	1			P				C				G		
48	2	A					K					G		
49	1				I				T		S			
50	4				I		K					G		
51	3				I					N				H
52	4				I					N			L	

ANSWER GRID: 2

NURSING PROCESS

A = Assessment
D = Analysis, nursing diagnosis
P = Planning
I = Implementation
E = Evaluation

COGNITIVE LEVEL

K = Knowledge
C = Comprehension
T = Application
N = Analysis

CLIENT NEEDS

S = Safe, effective care environment
G = Physiological integrity
L = Psychosocial integrity
H = Health promotion/maintenance

		Nursing Process					Cognitive Level				Client Needs			
Question #	Answer #	A	D	P	I	E	K	C	T	N	S	G	L	H
53	2					E			T					H
54	2					E				N				H
55	3				I			C				G		
56	1				I			C				G		
57	1					E			T					H
58	1			P					T					H
59	4				I				T					H
60	2	A						C				G		
61	4	A							T			G		
62	3				I				T					H
63	1	A						C				G		
64	3	A					K					G		
65	3					E	K					G		
66	2				I			C				G		
67	1				I			C			S			
68	2	A								N	S			
69	2	A								N	S			
70	2				I				T		S			
71	2				I				T		S			
72	3					E				N		G		
73	2	A						C				G		
74	3			P					T			G		
75	4					E			T			G		
76	1				I				T			G		
77	2			P						N		G		
78	3			P					T			G		
79	4				I					N			L	
80	2				I			C				G		
81	3				I					N		G		

ANSWER GRID: 3

Nursing Process

A = Assessment
D = Analysis, nursing diagnosis
P = Planning
I = Implementation
E = Evaluation

Cognitive Level

K = Knowledge
C = Comprehension
T = Application
N = Analysis

Client Needs

S = Safe, effective care environment
G = Physiological integrity
L = Psychosocial integrity
H = Health promotion/maintenance

		Nursing Process					Cognitive Level				Client Needs			
Question #	Answer #	A	D	P	I	E	K	C	T	N	S	G	L	H
82	1	A								N		G		
83	2				I				T		S			
84	1				I				T		S			
85	2			P			K					G		
86	2				I					N		G		
87	4			P				C				G		
88	3	A						C						H
89	1				I				T		S			
90	4					E		C				G		
91	2				I			C			S			
Number Correct														
Number Possible	91	17	1	14	45	14	11	24	31	25	22	50	2	17
Percentage Correct														

Score Calculation:

To determine your **Percentage Correct**, divide the **Number Correct** by the **Number Possible.**

The Client With Reproductive Health Problems

Test 7

The Client With Uterine Fibroids
The Client With Breast Cancer
The Client With Benign Prostatic Hypertrophy
The Client With a Sexually Transmitted Disease
The Client With Cancer of the Cervix
The Client With Testicular Cancer
General Questions
Correct Answers and Rationale

Select the one best answer and indicate your choice by filling in the circle in front of the option.

The Client With Uterine Fibroids

A 51-year-old female client has been experiencing intermittent vaginal bleeding for the past several months. Her physician tells her that she has uterine fibroids and recommends an abdominal hysterectomy.

1. The nurse is completing the routine admission assessment when the client expresses fear about the surgery. Which of the following statements offers the best guide for the nurse's response?
- ○ 1. The nurse should reassure the client of her physician's competence.
- ○ 2. The nurse should give the client opportunities to express her fears.
- ○ 3. The nurse should teach the client that fear impedes recovery.
- ○ 4. The nurse should change the subject of conversation to pleasantries when the client appears fearful.

2. The nursing care plan includes teaching the client to deep breathe and cough in preparation for the postoperative period. The nurse should teach the client which of the following techniques to use while coughing?
- ○ 1. Lie on her abdomen with her knees flexed.
- ○ 2. Lie flat in bed with her hands behind her head.
- ○ 3. Support her rib cage with her hands.
- ○ 4. Support her abdomen with a pillow or her hands.

3. Which of the following early signs or symptoms will the client most likely experience if she hyperventilates while practicing deep breathing exercises?
- ○ 1. Dyspnea.
- ○ 2. Dizziness.
- ○ 3. Blurred vision.
- ○ 4. Mental confusion.

4. The physician prescribes 0.4 mg of atropine sulfate and 75 mg of meperidine hydrochloride (Demerol) IM 1 hour before surgery. The stock ampule of atropine contains 0.8 mg/ml, and the stock ampule of meperidine hydrochloride contains 100 mg/ml. The two drugs are compatible and can be drawn up in one syringe. How much of the drugs will be in the syringe to give the ordered doses?
- ○ 1. 0.75 ml.
- ○ 2. 1.25 ml.
- ○ 3. 1.50 ml.
- ○ 4. 1.75 ml.

5. The client requires catheterization when she is unable to void. When preparing to insert the catheter into the urinary meatus, the nurse locates the anatomic structures between the labia minora. Starting from the area nearer the pubic bone and moving downward toward the anus, in which of the following order do the clitoris, vaginal opening, and urinary meatus lie?
- ○ 1. Clitoris, vaginal opening, urinary meatus.

○ 2. Urinary meatus, vaginal opening, clitoris.
○ 3. Vaginal opening, clitoris, urinary meatus.
○ 4. Clitoris, urinary meatus, vaginal opening.

6. During the recovery period, the nurse notes that the client is an Orthodox Jew and refuses to eat hospital food. Hospital policy discourages food from outside the hospital. What step should the nurse take first in this situation?
○ 1. Teach the client that it is important for her to eat what she is served.
○ 2. Discuss the situation and possible courses of action with the dietitian.
○ 3. Encourage the client's family to bring food for the client because of the special circumstances.
○ 4. Explain to the client that if she does not eat, the physician will have to order IV therapy.

The Client With Breast Cancer

A lump is discovered in a 50-year-old female client's right breast during a routine physical examination. She is admitted for a breast biopsy and possible surgery.

7. During the admission workup, the client is extremely anxious and asks many questions. Which of the following statements would offer the best guide for the nurse to answer questions raised by this apprehensive preoperative client? It is usually best to
○ 1. tell the client as much as she wants to know and is able to understand.
○ 2. delay discussing the client's questions with her until she is convalescing.
○ 3. delay discussing the client's questions with her until her apprehension subsides.
○ 4. explain to the client that she should discuss her questions first with the physician.

8. The client asks the nurse, "Where is cancer usually found in the breast?" On a diagram of a left breast, the nurse would indicate that most malignant tumors occur in which quadrant of the breast?
○ 1. Upper, outer quadrant
○ 2. Upper, inner quadrant
○ 3. Lower, outer quadrant
○ 4. Lower, inner quadrant

9. The client's biopsy is positive, and her physician recommends a modified radical mastectomy. She agrees to this treatment. Atropine sulfate is included in her preoperative orders. The primary reason for giving this drug preoperatively is that it helps
○ 1. promote general muscular relaxation.
○ 2. decrease pulse and respiratory rates.
○ 3. decrease nausea.
○ 4. inhibit oral and respiratory secretions.

10. Which of the following observations should the recovery room nurse plan to make first when the client returns from the operating room?
○ 1. Obtaining and recording vital signs.
○ 2. Observing that drainage tubes are patent and functioning.
○ 3. Ensuring that the client's airway is free of obstruction.
○ 4. Checking the client's dressings for drainage.

11. Postoperatively, the client has an incisional drainage tube attached to suction. The primary purpose of this tube is to help
○ 1. decrease intrathoracic pressure and facilitate breathing.
○ 2. increase collateral lymphatic flow toward the operative area.
○ 3. remove accumulated serum and blood in the operative area.
○ 4. prevent formation of adhesions between the skin and chest wall in the operative area.

12. On the third postoperative day, the drainage tube is removed and the dressings are changed. The client appears shocked when she sees the operative area and exclaims, "I look horrible! Will it ever look better?" Which of the following responses by the nurse would be most appropriate?
○ 1. "After it heals and you're dressed, you won't even know you had surgery."
○ 2. "Don't worry. You know the tumor is gone, and the area will heal very soon."
○ 3. "Would you like to meet Ms. Paul? She looks just great and she had a mastectomy, too."
○ 4. "You're shocked by the sudden change in your appearance as a result of this surgery, aren't you?"

The Client With Benign Prostatic Hypertrophy

A 72-year-old male client is brought to the emergency room by his son. The client is extremely uncomfortable and has been unable to void for the past 12 hours. He has known for some time that he has an enlarged prostate but has wanted to avoid surgery.

13. During the client's urinary bladder catheterization, the bladder is emptied gradually. The best rationale for the nurse's action is that emptying an overdistended bladder completely at one time tends to cause
○ 1. renal collapse and failure.
○ 2. abdominal cramping and pain.
○ 3. hypotension and possible shock.
○ 4. weakening and atrophy of bladder musculature.

14. While obtaining the client's history, the nurse would anticipate that the client will most likely report having experienced all of the following symptoms except
- ○ 1. voiding at more frequent intervals.
- ○ 2. difficulty starting the flow of urine.
- ○ 3. frequent voiding at night.
- ○ 4. increased force of the urine stream.

15. The client is prepared for admission to the hospital. Which of the following reports by the emergency room nurse would be most helpful to the nurse responsible for admitting the client?
- ○ 1. "A urine specimen was obtained from the client and sent to the laboratory for analysis."
- ○ 2. "The client was catheterized, and 1,100 ml of urine was obtained. The urine appeared cloudy, and a specimen was sent to the laboratory."
- ○ 3. "The client is very cooperative. He is comfortable now that his bladder has been emptied. He had no ill effects from catheterization."
- ○ 4. "The client was in the emergency room for 3 hours because of bladder distention. He is fine now but is being admitted as a possible candidate for surgery."

16. The client is scheduled to undergo a transurethral resection of the prostate gland and a bilateral vasectomy. The procedure is to be done under spinal anesthesia. Postoperatively, the nurse should be particularly alert for early signs of
- ○ 1. convulsions.
- ○ 2. cardiac arrest.
- ○ 3. renal shutdown.
- ○ 4. respiratory paralysis.

17. The client returned from transurethral resection 3 hours ago. In which of the following circumstances would the nurse increase the flow rate of his continuous bladder irrigation?
- ○ 1. When the drainage is continuous but slow.
- ○ 2. When the drainage appears cloudy and dark yellow.
- ○ 3. When the drainage has become brighter red.
- ○ 4. When there is no drainage of urine and irrigating solution.

18. A nursing assistant tells the nurse, "I think the client is confused. He keeps telling me he has to void, but that isn't possible because he has a catheter in place." Which of the following possible responses by the nurse would be most appropriate for the nurse to make?
- ○ 1. "His catheter is probably plugged. I'll irrigate it in a few minutes."
- ○ 2. "That's a common complaint after prostate surgery. The client only imagines the urge to void."
- ○ 3. "The urge to void is usually created by the large catheter, and he may be having some bladder spasms."
- ○ 4. "I think he may be somewhat confused and possibly may be having some internal bleeding."

19. If the client's prostate enlargement had been malignant, which of the following blood examinations should the nurse have anticipated to assess whether metastasis has occurred?
- ○ 1. Serum creatinine level.
- ○ 2. Serum acid phosphatase level.
- ○ 3. Total nonprotein nitrogen level.
- ○ 4. Endogenous creatinine clearance time.

The Client With a Sexually Transmitted Disease

A local public health department operates a sexually transmitted disease clinic twice a week. A nurse does all the basic assessment, screening, and teaching following established protocols for disease management. A newly admitted 25-year-old female client has just been diagnosed with human immunodeficiency virus (HIV); that is, she is HIV positive.

20. The physician prescribes zidovudine (AZT), a drug that acts to help
- ○ 1. destroy the virus.
- ○ 2. enhance the body's antibody production.
- ○ 3. slow replication of the virus.
- ○ 4. neutralize toxins produced by the causative organism.

21. In which of the following ways could the client have contracted HIV?
- ○ 1. Hugging an HIV-positive sexual partner.
- ○ 2. Inhaling cocaine.
- ○ 3. Sharing food utensils with an HIV-positive person.
- ○ 4. Receiving a postoperative blood transfusion.

22. The client develops herpes genitalis and is counseled by the nurse concerning follow-up care. Women who have this disease are at risk for developing
- ○ 1. sterility.
- ○ 2. cervical cancer.
- ○ 3. uterine fibroid tumors.
- ○ 4. irregular menses.

23. The client would most likely require instruction due to which of the following problems associated with the herpes genitalis?
- ○ 1. Sleep disorders.
- ○ 2. Nutritional deficit.
- ○ 3. Pain.
- ○ 4. Activity restrictions.

24. The primary reason that a herpes simplex infection is a serious concern to the client with HIV infection is that herpes simplex
- ○ 1. is an AIDS-defining illness.

- ○ 2. is curable only after 1 year of antiviral therapy.
- ○ 3. leads to cervical cancer.
- ○ 4. causes severe electrolyte imbalances.

25. In providing education to clients, the nurse should take into account the fact that the most effective method known to control the spread of HIV infection is

- ○ 1. premarital serological screening.
- ○ 2. prophylactic treatment of exposed persons.
- ○ 3. laboratory screening of pregnant women.
- ○ 4. ongoing sex education about preventive behaviors.

The Client With Cancer of the Cervix

A 27-year-old female client makes an appointment with a gynecologist for a routine examination and Pap smear. The woman has always been in good health.

26. The woman tells the nurse that she is always very nervous about these examinations because "there's been a lot of cancer in my family." The nurse should be aware that an early sign of cervical cancer is

- ○ 1. a thick, foul-smelling vaginal discharge.
- ○ 2. bleeding after intercourse.
- ○ 3. a change in the menstrual cycle.
- ○ 4. watery vaginal discharge.

27. Following examination and diagnostic testing, the client is diagnosed with cancer of the cervix in situ. A conization is scheduled. Which of the following nursing interventions would take priority during the first 24 postoperative hours?

- ○ 1. Monitoring vital signs hourly.
- ○ 2. Maintaining strict bed rest.
- ○ 3. Monitoring vaginal bleeding.
- ○ 4. Maintaining electrolyte balance.

28. The client's husband says to the nurse, "The doctor told my wife that her cancer is curable. Is he just trying to make us feel better?" Which would be the nurse's most accurate response?

- ○ 1. "When cervical cancer is detected early and treated aggressively, the cure rate is almost 100%."
- ○ 2. "The 5-year survival rate is about 75%, which makes the odds pretty good."
- ○ 3. "Saying a cancer is curable means that 50% of all women with the cancer survive at least 5 years."
- ○ 4. "Cancers of the female reproductive tract tend to be slow growing and respond well to treatment."

29. The client's cancer recurs, and internal radiation treatment with a radium implant is planned. On hospital admission, the client says that she is concerned about being radioactive and has been having nightmares about the treatment. What would be a reasonable explanation for the nurse to give to the client?

- ○ 1. "The radioactive material is controlled and stays with the source; once the material is removed, no radioactivity will remain."
- ○ 2. "The radioactivity will gradually decrease, and you will be discharged when the radioactive material reaches its half-life."
- ○ 3. "These nightmares indicate that you're in the denial phase of accepting the diagnosis."
- ○ 4. "Careful shielding prevents the area above your waist from radioactivity."

30. A lead-lined container and a pair of long forceps are kept in the client's hospital room for

- ○ 1. disposal of emesis or other bodily secretions.
- ○ 2. handling of the dislodged radiation source.
- ○ 3. disposal of client's eating utensils.
- ○ 4. storage of the radiation booster dose.

31. The client's mother asks why so many nurses are involved in her daughter's care and says, "The doctor said I can be in the room for up to 2 hours each day, but the nurses say they're restricted to 30 minutes." The nurse explains that this variation is based on the fact that nurses

- ○ 1. touch the client, which increases their exposure to radiation.
- ○ 2. work with many clients and could carry infection to a client receiving radiation therapy, if exposure is prolonged.
- ○ 3. work with radiation on an ongoing basis, while visitors have infrequent exposure to radiation.
- ○ 4. are at greater risk from the radiation because they are younger than the mother.

The Client With Testicular Cancer

A 28-year-old male client is diagnosed with acute epididymitis.

32. The nurse would expect to find that the classic symptoms of epididymitis that caused the client to seek medical care were

- ○ 1. burning and pain on urination.
- ○ 2. severe tenderness and swelling in the scrotum
- ○ 3. foul-smelling ejaculate and severe scrotal swelling.
- ○ 4. foul-smelling urine and pain on urination.

33. All of the following would be appropriate interventions for this client except

- ○ 1. maintaining bedrest.
- ○ 2. elevating the testes.

○ 3. increasing fluid intake.
○ 4. applying hot packs to the scrotum.

34. A year later the client returns to the physician, saying that he thinks the epididymitis has returned. The physician examines him and makes a preliminary diagnosis of testicular cancer. Which clinical manifestation helps differentiate testicular cancer from epididymitis?
○ 1. The inability to achieve or sustain an erection.
○ 2. Scrotal pain.
○ 3. A dragging sensation in the scrotum.
○ 4. Scrotal swelling.

35. The diagnosis of testicular cancer is confirmed, and the client is scheduled for a right orchiectomy. The day before surgery, the client tells the nurse that he is concerned about the effect that losing a testicle will have on his "manhood." Which of the following facts about orchiectomy should form the basis for the nurse's response?
○ 1. Testosterone levels are decreased.
○ 2. Sexual drive and libido are unchanged.
○ 3. Sperm count increases in the remaining testicle.
○ 4. Secondary sexual characteristics change.

36. Because the client will have a high inguinal incision, a priority problem for the immediate postoperative period would be
○ 1. bladder spasms.
○ 2. urinary elimination.
○ 3. pain.
○ 4. nausea.

37. The orchiectomy is performed, and the pathology report reveals a diagnosis of malignant seminoma. External radiotherapy is ordered. The nurse teaches the client about the potential side effects of radiotherapy to the lower abdomen. Which of the following nursing diagnoses would most likely apply to this client?
○ 1. Body Image Disturbance related to alopecia.
○ 2. Altered Nutrition: Less than Body Requirements related to diarrhea.
○ 3. Altered Nutrition: Less than Body Requirements related to dysphagia.
○ 4. Powerlessness related to metabolic imbalance.

General Questions

38. Eight hours after catheterization, the postoperative abdominal hysterectomy client has the urge to void frequently but voids only a few milliliters of urine each time. This symptom is most commonly associated with
○ 1. bladder damage.
○ 2. kidney infection.
○ 3. inadequate fluid intake.
○ 4. urine retention with overflow.

39. Which nursing measure would most likely relieve postoperative gas pains following abdominal hysterectomy?
○ 1. Offering the client a hot beverage.
○ 2. Providing extra warmth.
○ 3. Applying a snugly fitting abdominal binder.
○ 4. Helping the client walk.

40. What would be the most likely cause of elevated temperature on the second postoperative day following an abdominal hysterectomy?
○ 1. Wound infection.
○ 2. Bladder infection.
○ 3. Atelectasis.
○ 4. Phlebitis.

41. The nursing care plan for a client following gynecological surgery includes nursing orders intended to help reduce the risk of thrombophlebitis. An order that would be contraindicated would be to
○ 1. ambulate the client.
○ 2. massage the client's legs.
○ 3. have the client wear elasticized stockings.
○ 4. have the client exercise her legs in bed.

42. The nurse is changing the dressing of a postoperative client following an abdominal hysterectomy. Which of the following nursing measures would be most appropriate if the dressing sticks to the client's incisional area?
○ 1. Pull off the dressing quickly and then apply slight pressure over the area.
○ 2. Lift an easily moved portion of the dressing and then remove it slowly.
○ 3. Moisten the dressing with sterile normal saline solution and then remove it.
○ 4. Remove part of the dressing and then remove the remainder gradually over a period of several minutes.

43. A priority nursing diagnosis category for the client who experiences wound dehiscence postoperatively after an abdominal hysterectomy would be
○ 1. High Risk for Infection.
○ 2. Fluid Volume Excess.
○ 3. Ineffective Airway Clearance.
○ 4. Altered Nutrition: Less than Body Requirements.

44. What immediate action should the nurse take for the postoperative client who experiences a wound dehiscence following abdominal hysterectomy?
○ 1. Replace the dressing carefully while wearing gloves.
○ 2. Apply a snugly fitting sterile abdominal binder over the wound.
○ 3. Approximate the wound edges by applying strips of adhesive over the wound.

○ 4. Cover the exposed tissues with sterile dressings moistened with normal saline solution.

45. Which of the following hormones may be prescribed for the client following an abdominal hysterectomy and removal of the ovaries and fallopian tubes?
○ 1. Estrogen.
○ 2. Thyroxin.
○ 3. Prolactin.
○ 4. Testosterone.

46. Which of the following nursing diagnoses would be most appropriate for the client being discharged from the hospital 6 days after an abdominal hysterectomy?
○ 1. Altered Nutrition: Less than Body Requirements related to gas pains.
○ 2. Fluid Volume Excess related to surgery.
○ 3. Altered Health Maintenance related to lack of social support resources.
○ 4. Ineffective Individual Coping related to body image disturbance.

47. In preparing discharge instructions for the client following an abdominal hysterectomy, the nurse should first
○ 1. have the client read the discharge instructions.
○ 2. assess the client's available social supports.
○ 3. call the social worker to evaluate the client.
○ 4. read the instructions to the client.

48. All of the following would be considered risk factors for the development of breast cancer except
○ 1. menopause after age 50.
○ 2. a family history of breast cancer.
○ 3. childlessness.
○ 4. breast-feeding.

49. Which of the following positions would be best for the client's right arm when she returns to her room following a right mastectomy?
○ 1. Across her chest wall.
○ 2. At her side at the same level as her body.
○ 3. In the position that affords her the greatest comfort without placing pressure on the incision.
○ 4. On pillows, with her hand higher than her elbow and her elbow higher than her shoulder.

50. In providing discharge teaching for a client following a modified radical mastectomy, the nurse should instruct the client that she may need to modify or avoid which of the following activities?
○ 1. Shampooing her dog.
○ 2. Caring for her tropical fish.
○ 3. Working in her rose garden.
○ 4. Taking a late-evening swim.

51. Priority outcome criteria for the client being discharged after a modified radical mastectomy would include which of the following?
○ 1. Usual arm and shoulder function has returned.
○ 2. Mild swelling of affected arm is noted.
○ 3. Activity level has returned to normal.
○ 4. Fluid and electrolyte levels are within normal limits.

52. A client is to have radiation therapy following a modified radical mastectomy and discharge from the hospital. When caring for the skin at the site of therapy, the client should be taught to avoid all of the following practices except
○ 1. washing the area with water.
○ 2. exposing the area to sunlight.
○ 3. applying an ointment to the area.
○ 4. using talcum powder on the area.

53. The nurse would teach a client that a normal local tissue response to radiation is
○ 1. atrophy of the skin.
○ 2. scattered pustule formation.
○ 3. redness of the surface tissue.
○ 4. sloughing of two layers of skin.

54. The primary purpose of the American Cancer Society's Reach to Recovery program is to
○ 1. help rehabilitate women who have had mastectomies.
○ 2. raise funds to support early breast cancer detection programs.
○ 3. provide free dressings for women who have had radical mastectomies.
○ 4. collect statistics for research from women who have had mastectomies.

55. The nurse should teach female clients that the best time in the menstrual cycle to examine the breasts is during the
○ 1. week that ovulation occurs.
○ 2. week that menstruation occurs.
○ 3. first week after menstruation.
○ 4. week before menstruation occurs.

56. Which of the following positions is the one of choice for palpating tissues during self-breast examination?
○ 1. Sitting.
○ 2. Standing.
○ 3. Flat on the back with a pillow under the head and arms raised over the head.
○ 4. Flat on the back with a pillow under the shoulder on the side being examined.

57. A client states that she has always noticed that her brassiere fits more snugly at certain times of the month. She asks the nurse if this is a sign of breast disease. The nurse should base the reply to this client on the knowledge that
○ 1. benign cysts tend to cause the breasts to vary in size.
○ 2. it is normal for the breasts to increase in size before menstruation begins.
○ 3. a change in breast size warrants further investigation.

○ 4. differences in sizes of the breasts are related to normal growth and development.

58. Nursing interventions to reduce discomfort from benign fibrocystic breast disease include teaching the client to
○ 1. increase her activity level.
○ 2. wear tight supporting garments.
○ 3. avoid caffeine.
○ 4. obtain estrogen therapy from her physician.

59. The best method for the nurse to use when assessing for bladder distention in a male client is to check for
○ 1. a rounded swelling above the pubis.
○ 2. dullness in the lower left quadrant.
○ 3. rebound tenderness below the symphysis.
○ 4. urine discharge from the urethral meatus.

60. The primary reason for lubricating the urinary catheter very generously before inserting it into a male client is that this technique helps reduce
○ 1. spasms at the orifice of the bladder.
○ 2. friction along the urethra when the catheter is being inserted.
○ 3. the number of organisms gaining entrance to the bladder.
○ 4. the formation of encrustations that may occur at the end of the catheter.

61. The primary reason for taping an indwelling catheter laterally to the thigh is to help
○ 1. eliminate pressure at the penoscrotal angle.
○ 2. prevent the catheter from kinking in the urethra.
○ 3. prevent accidental catheter removal.
○ 4. allow the client to turn without kinking the catheter.

62. Following removal of an indwelling catheter originally inserted during a transurethral resection (TUR), the nurse should teach the male client that a temporary symptom he can expect to experience is
○ 1. urine retention.
○ 2. dribbling incontinence.
○ 3. loss of urine while straining.
○ 4. decreased urine output.

63. The report on a urine culture indicates numerous white and red blood cells and a moderate amount of bacterial growth. The nurse evaluating these findings accurately would deduce that the client most likely has a
○ 1. urethral stricture.
○ 2. decreased renal filtration rate.
○ 3. urinary tract infection.
○ 4. prostate gland malignancy.

64. A major goal of care for the client with continuous bladder irrigation following a transurethral resection would be to
○ 1. maintain catheter patency.
○ 2. reduce incisional bleeding.
○ 3. teach signs of prostate cancer.
○ 4. perform activities of daily living.

65. A common nursing diagnosis for clients in the immediate postoperative phase following transurethral resection is
○ 1. Altered Peripheral Tissue Perfusion related to deep vein thrombosis.
○ 2. Self-Care Deficit related to pain of bladder spasms.
○ 3. Body Image Disturbance related to disfiguring surgery.
○ 4. Altered Peripheral Tissue Perfusion related to bleeding at the incision site.

66. A client is to receive bethanechol chloride (Urecholine), as needed, postoperatively after a transurethral resection. The nurse should give the client this drug when he demonstrates signs of
○ 1. painful voiding.
○ 2. urine retention.
○ 3. frequent urination.
○ 4. urinary tract infection.

67. The prostate gland serves primarily to
○ 1. store underdeveloped sperm prior to ejaculation.
○ 2. regulate the acidity/alkalinity environment for proper sperm development.
○ 3. produce a secretion that aids the nourishment and passage of sperm.
○ 4. secrete a hormone that stimulates the production and maturation of sperm.

68. A priority nursing diagnosis category for the client being discharged to home three days after transurethral resection would be
○ 1. Fluid Volume Deficit.
○ 2. Body Image Disturbance.
○ 3. Altered Patterns of Urinary Elimination.
○ 4. Ineffective Airway Clearance.

69. Many older men with prostatic hypertrophy do not seek medical attention until urinary obstruction is almost complete. Investigations have found that the primary reason for this delay in seeking attention is that these men
○ 1. tend to feel too self-conscious to seek help when reproductive organs are involved.
○ 2. expect that it is normal to have to live with some urinary problems as they grow older.
○ 3. are fearful that sexual indiscretions in earlier life may be the cause of their problem.
○ 4. have little discomfort in relation to the amount of pathology, as responses to pain stimuli fade with age.

70. The typical chancre of syphilis appears as
○ 1. a grouping of small, tender pimples.
○ 2. an elevated wart.
○ 3. a painless, moist ulcer.

○ 4. an itching, crusted area.

71. When interviewing a client with newly diagnosed syphilis, the nurse should anticipate that the most difficult problem likely will be

○ 1. motivating the client to undergo treatment.
○ 2. obtaining a list of the client's sexual contacts.
○ 3. increasing the client's knowledge of the disease.
○ 4. assuring the client that records are confidential.

72. Probenecid (Benemid) is prescribed in conjunction with penicillin as treatment for syphilis, because probenecid helps to

○ 1. delay detoxification of penicillin.
○ 2. inhibit excretion of penicillin.
○ 3. maintain sensitivity of organisms to penicillin.
○ 4. decrease the likelihood of an allergic reaction to penicillin.

73. The organism responsible for causing syphilis is classified as a

○ 1. virus.
○ 2. fungus.
○ 3. rickettsia.
○ 4. spirochete.

74. A priority nursing diagnosis for a client with primary syphilis would likely be

○ 1. High Risk for Infection Transmission related to lack of knowledge about mode of transmission.
○ 2. Pain related to cutaneous skin lesions on palms and soles.
○ 3. Altered Skin Tissue Perfusion related to a bleeding chancre.
○ 4. Body Image Disturbance related to alopecia.

75. The most likely presenting symptom of gonorrhea in males is

○ 1. impotence.
○ 2. scrotal pain.
○ 3. urine retention.
○ 4. urethral discharge.

76. In planning an educational program for women, the nurse should emphasize that gonorrhea

○ 1. is often marked by dysuria or bleeding in women.
○ 2. does not lead to serious complications.
○ 3. can be treated but not cured.
○ 4. may not cause symptoms in women until it leads to complications.

77. Which of the following groups has experienced the greatest rise in the incidence of sexually transmitted diseases over the past two decades?

○ 1. Teenagers.
○ 2. Divorced persons.
○ 3. Young married couples.
○ 4. Infants.

78. Which of the following responses by the nurse would be best when a female client says that she is nervous about an upcoming pelvic examination?

○ 1. "Can you tell me more about how you're feeling?"
○ 2. "You're not alone. Most women feel uncomfortable about this exam."
○ 3. "You're not worried about Dr. Smith, are you? He's a specialist in female problems."
○ 4. "We'll do everything we can to avoid embarrassing you."

79. Correct preparation of a client for a Pap smear would include which of the following measures?

○ 1. The test should be scheduled while the client is menstruating.
○ 2. The client should not bathe on the morning before the exam.
○ 3. The woman should not douche on the morning before the exam.
○ 4. The woman should take a laxative the night before the exam.

80. The position of choice for a client undergoing a vaginal examination is the

○ 1. Sims' position.
○ 2. lithotomy position.
○ 3. genupectoral position.
○ 4. dorsal recumbent position.

81. A client asks the nurse to explain the meaning of the Pap smear results. Which of the following concepts should the nurse include in the response?

○ 1. A typical Pap smear means that abnormal—but not necessarily neoplastic—cells were found in the smear.
○ 2. An atypical Pap smear means that cancer cells were found in the smear.
○ 3. A positive Pap smear alone is not very important diagnostically, because there are many false-positive results.
○ 4. Abnormal cells in a Pap smear may be caused by conditions other than cancer.

82. Which of the following is not considered to be a risk factor for cervical cancer?

○ 1. Sexual experiences with multiple partners.
○ 2. History of venereal disease.
○ 3. Positive family history for cervical cancer.
○ 4. Adolescent pregnancy.

83. The American Cancer Society recommends that the average adult woman follow which schedule for Pap smear screening?

○ 1. Annually after age 18.
○ 2. Annually if sexually active; every 5 years if sexually abstinent.
○ 3. Every 3 years after three initial negative tests taken annually.
○ 4. Every 3 years until age 40 and annually thereafter.

84. A priority nursing diagnosis for a client with cervical cancer and an internal radium implant would be

○ 1. Pain related to cervical tumor.
○ 2. Anxiety related to self-care deficit from imposed immobility during radiation.
○ 3. Altered Health Maintenance related to surgery.
○ 4. Sleep Pattern Disturbance related to interruptions of sleep by health care personnel.

85. What activity orders would be appropriate for a client with an internal radium implant for cervical cancer?
○ 1. Out of bed as tolerated within the room.
○ 2. Bedrest with bathroom privileges.
○ 3. Bedrest in position of comfort.
○ 4. Bedrest with the head of the bed flat.

86. Which of the following would be standard nursing care for a client with cervical cancer and an internal radium implant in place?
○ 1. Offer the bedpan every 2 hours.
○ 2. Provide perineal care twice daily.
○ 3. Check the position of the applicator hourly.
○ 4. Offer a low-residue diet.

87. The nurse should carefully observe a client with internal radium implants for typical side effects associated with radiation therapy to the cervix. These effects include
○ 1. cramping pain and severe vaginal itching.
○ 2. confusion and sleep disturbances.
○ 3. high fever in the afternoon or evening.
○ 4. nausea, vomiting, and a foul discharge.

88. A priority nursing diagnosis category for a client diagnosed with pelvic inflammatory disease would be
○ 1. Fluid Volume Deficit.
○ 2. Impaired Physical Mobility.
○ 3. High Risk for Injury.
○ 4. Pain.

89. When teaching a client to perform testicular self-examination, the nurse should explain that the exam should be performed
○ 1. after intercourse.
○ 2. at the end of the day.
○ 3. after a warm bath or shower.
○ 4. after exercise.

90. The normal testis can be described as
○ 1. soft.
○ 2. egg-shaped.
○ 3. spongy.
○ 4. lumpy.

91. Although the cause of testicular cancer is unknown, it is associated with a history of
○ 1. undescended testis.
○ 2. sexual relations at an early age.
○ 3. seminal vesiculitis.
○ 4. epididymitis.

92. A client diagnosed with testicular cancer expresses fear and questions the nurse about his prognosis. The nurse should base the response on the knowledge that
○ 1. testicular cancer is almost always fatal.
○ 2. testicular cancer has a cure rate of 90% when diagnosed early.
○ 3. surgery is the treatment of choice for testicular cancer.
○ 4. testicular cancer has a 50% cure rate when diagnosed early.

CORRECT ANSWERS AND RATIONALE

The letters in parentheses following the rationale identify the step of the nursing process (A, D, P, I, E); cognitive level (K, C, T, N); and client need (S, G, L, H). See the Answer Grid for the key.

The Client With Uterine Fibroids

1. 2. The best approach for a client who is fearful about having surgery is to allow the client opportunities to express her fears. Such courses of action as assuring a client of the physician's competence, saying that fear impedes recovery, and changing the subject are nonsupportive and deny her an opportunity to express her feelings. (I, N, L)

2. 4. The client who has had abdominal surgery is most likely to experience incisional area discomfort postoperatively when she coughs. This discomfort can be minimized by splinting the operative area with a pillow or her hands. (I, T, G)

3. 2. Hyperventilation occurs when the client breathes so rapidly and deeply that she exhales excessive amounts of carbon dioxide. A characteristic symptom of hyperventilation is dizziness. Dyspnea, blurred vision, and mental confusion are not associated with hyperventilation. (A, T, G)

4. 2. The correct amount to administer is determined by using ratios, as follows:

$0.8 \text{ mg} : 1 \text{ ml} :: 0.4 \text{ mg} : x \text{ ml}.$

$0.8\,x = 0.4$

$x = .50$ ml of atropine sulfate

$100 \text{ mg} : 1 \text{ ml} :: 75 \text{ mg} : x \text{ ml}.$

$100\,x = 75$

$x = .75$ ml of meperidine hydrochloride (Demerol)

0.5 ml of atropine + 0.75 ml of meperidine hydrochloride (Demerol) = 1.25 ml total.

(I, C, S)

5. 4. Starting from the area nearer the pubic bone and moving toward the anus, the anatomic order is clitoris, urinary meatus, and vaginal opening. (I, K, G)

6. 2. The best course of action when a client refuses to eat food that is contrary to her religious beliefs is to discuss the situation with a dietitian. Health team members may need to confer about this client's needs. Telling the client that it is important for her to eat what is served is unlikely to help, because she has already refused the food. Encouraging her family to bring suitable food to the hospital for her is ordinarily against agency policy and should not be considered until the situation has been discussed with an agency dietitian. Threatening a client by saying that if she does not eat, intravenous therapy will be necessary is nonsupportive and is unlikely to gain her cooperation. (I, N, G)

The Client With Breast Cancer

7. 1. An important nursing responsibility is preoperative teaching, and the most frequently recommended guide for teaching is to tell the client as much as she wants to know and is able to understand. Delaying discussion of issues, about which the client has concerns is likely to aggravate the situation and cause the client to feel distrust. (I, T, L)

8. 1. Approximately 50% of malignant breast tumors occur in the upper outer quadrant of the breast. Interestingly, but for no known reason, cancer appears in the left breast more often than in the right breast. (A, K, G)

9. 4. Atropine sulfate, a cholinergic blocking agent, is given preoperatively primarily to reduce secretions in the mouth and respiratory tract. It is not used to promote muscle relaxation, decrease pulse and respiratory rates, or decrease nausea and vomiting. (I, C, G)

10. 3. The highest priority when a nurse receives a client from the operating room is to assess airway patency. If the airway is not clear, immediate steps should be taken so that the client is able to breathe. After ensuring that the airway is clear and the client is breathing well, the nurse should proceed with such measures as obtaining the vital signs, assessing that drainage tubes are functioning properly, and checking the client's dressing. (I, T, G)

11. 3. A drainage tube is placed in the wound following a modified radical mastectomy to help remove accumulated blood and fluid in the area. Drainage tubes placed in a wound do not decrease intrathoracic pressure, increase collateral lymphatic flow, or prevent the adhesion formation. (I, T, G)

12. 4. When a client appears shocked by her appearance following surgery, such as after having a mastectomy, the nurse should help her express her feelings and offer supportive care, which she needs at this time. Telling the client not to worry or that her disfigurement will not show when she is dressed are nonsupportive and are likely to cause more concerns. Having the client meet someone who has had breast surgery is often helpful but is better done later, when the client is convalescing and used to the appearance of the operative site. The client needs the nurse's support when the dressings are removed, not sometime later. (I, N, L)

The Client With Benign Prostatic Hypertrophy

13. 3. Rapidly emptying an overdistended bladder may cause hypotension and shock due to the sudden change of pressure within the abdominal viscera. Renal collapse is not likely, nor are abdominal cramping and bladder weakening and atrophy. (I, T, G)

14. 4. It is unlikely that the client with prostatic hypertrophy will report having a more powerful urine than usual. Typical symptoms of prostatic hypertrophy include urinary frequency and hesitancy, decreased in the caliber and force of the urine stream, interruptions in the urine stream when voiding, and frequent voiding at night (nocturia). Collectively, the various symptoms of benign prostatic hypertrophy are often referred to as prostatism. (A, T, G)

15. 2. A report about the client's condition should be as clear, pertinent, and concise as possible, and it should be free of subjective information that could be interpreted differently by different caregivers. In this situation, the nurse should indicate how much urine had been drained from the client's bladder and how the urine appeared. The nurse should also report that a urine specimen has been sent to the laboratory for analysis. (E, T, S)

16. 4. If paralysis of vasomotor nerves in the upper spinal cord occurs when spinal anesthesia is used, the client is likely to develop respiratory paralysis. Artificial ventilation is required until the effects of anesthesia subside. Other possible complications of spinal anesthesia include hypotension, nausea and vomiting, postanesthesia headache, and neurologic complications, such as muscle weakness in the legs. (I, T, G)

17. 3. During continuous bladder irrigation following a prostatectomy, the rate at which the solution enters the bladder should be increased when the drainage becomes brighter red. The color indicates the presence of blood. Increasing the flow of irrigating solution helps flush the catheter well so that clots do not plug it. There would be no reason to increase the flow rate when the return is continuous or appears cloudy and dark yellow. Increasing the flow would be contraindicated if there is no return of urine and irrigating solution. (I, T, G)

18. 3. The Foley catheter creates the urge to void and may also cause bladder spasms. Less likely reasons for the client's urge to void include a plugged catheter, imagining the urge, confusion, and internal bleeding. (I, N, G)

19. 2. The most specific examination to determine whether a malignancy extends outside of the prostatic capsule is a study of the serum acid phosphatase level. The level increases when a malignancy has been metastasized. (A, K, S)

The Client With a Sexually Transmitted Disease

20. 3. Zidovudine (AZT) interferes with replication of HIV and thereby slows progression of HIV to AIDS. There is no known cure for HIV infection. (I, C, G)

21. 4. HIV infection is transmitted through blood and body fluids, particularly vaginal and seminal fluids. A blood transfusion is one way the disease can be contracted. Other modes of transmission are sexual intercourse with an infected partner and sharing needles for intravenous drug injections with an infected person. (A, C, S)

22. 2. Women who have herpes genitalis are more likely to develop cervical cancer than women who have never had the disease. Regular examinations, including Pap tests, are recommended. (I, T, H)

23. 3. Pain is a common problem in women with herpes genitalis. Analgesia may be prescribed for the pain. Sleep disturbances, nutritional deficits, and activity restrictions are not problems frequently experienced by women with herpes genitalis. (D, T, G)

24. 1. Herpes simplex is one of a group of disorders that, when diagnosed in the presence of HIV infection, are considered to be diagnostic for AIDS. Other AIDS-defining illness include Kaposi's sarcoma; cytomegalovirus of the liver, spleen, or lymph nodes; and *Pneumocystis carinii* pneumonia. (A, N, G)

25. 4. Education to prevent behaviors that cause HIV transmission is the primary method of controlling HIV infection. Behaviors that place persons at risk for HIV infection include unprotected sexual intercourse and sharing of intravenous drug needles. Educating clients about using condoms during sexual relations is a priority in controlling HIV transmission. (E, N, H)

The Client With Cancer of the Cervix

26. 4. In its early stages, cancer of the cervix is usually asymptomatic, which underscores the importance of regular Pap smears. A watery vaginal discharge is often the first noticeable symptom. Discomfort, foul-smelling discharge, and weight loss are late signs. (A, T, G)

27. 3. Uncontrolled vaginal bleeding is the priority concern during the first 24 hours after conization of the cervix. This is best monitored by keeping an accurate pad count, which assesses the extent of bleeding. Hourly vital signs and strict bedrest are unnecessary unless complications develop. Electrolyte imbalance is not anticipated with this procedure. (I, T, G)

28. 1. When cervical cancer is detected early and treated aggressively, the cure rate approaches 100%. (I, T, G)

29. 1. The radioactivity comes from a radioactive material such as radium or cesium. Radioactivity affects tissues but does not make them radioactive. Once the radioactive source is removed, no radioactivity remains. Accurate information can help alleviate ungrounded fears. The time required for a radioactive substance to be half-dissipated is called its half-life, but this does not determine discharge time. The client receiving sealed internal radiotherapy is not discharged until the radioactive source is removed. Nightmares probably indicate the client's concern about the therapy. There is no way to shield the area above the waist from radiation with cervical implants. (I, N, L)

30. 2. Dislodged radioactive materials should not be touched with bare or gloved hands. Forceps are used to place the material in the lead-lined container, which shields the radiation. Exposure to radiation can occur only by direct exposure to the encased radioactive substance; it cannot result from contact with emesis or urine or from touching the client. Radioactive materials are kept only in the radiation department. It is not usual to boost an applicator. (I, T, S)

31. 3. The three factors related to radiation safety are time, distance, and shielding. Nurses on the unit work with radiation frequently and so must limit their contact. Nurses are physically closer to clients than are visitors, who are often asked to sit 6 feet away. Touching the client does not increase the amount of radiation exposure; distance does. Aseptic technique and/or isolation prevent the spread of infection. Age is a risk factor for persons involved in reproduction. (I, N, S)

The Client With Testicular Cancer

32. 2. Epididymitis causes acute tenderness and pronounced swelling of the scrotum. It is occasionally, but not routinely, associated with urinary tract infection. (A, T, G)

33. 4. Rest is the foundation of treatment. Elevating the scrotum may increase the client's comfort. Intermittent ice application will enhance comfort and reduce swelling. Hot packs will not be used, as the temperature in the scrotum should remain below body temperature; excessive exposure to heat can cause destruction of sperm cells. (I, T, G)

34. 3. A dragging sensation in the scrotum is associated with testicular cancer, not epididymitis. The manifestations of testicular cancer are less dramatic than those of epididymitis. Other clinical manifestations of testicular cancer include a lump or swelling of the testis, a dull ache in the lower abdomen or inguinal area, and occasional pain. Sexual performance is unaffected. (A, C, G)

35. 2. The remaining testicle undergoes hyperplasia and produces enough testosterone to maintain sexual drive, libido, and secondary sexual characteristics. Sperm count can decrease after a unilateral orchiectomy; this is attributed to the stress of the surgery. (I, N, G)

36. 3. Due to the location of the incision, pain is a major problem during the immediate postoperative period. Bladder spasms and elimination problems are more commonly associated with prostate surgery. (D, N, G)

37. 2. The side effects of radiotherapy to the lower abdomen are related to the treatment site and to the exposure of underlying organs to radiation. Therefore, diarrhea is common with radiation to the retroperitoneal region, because the gastrointestinal tract lies within the treatment field. Alopecia and dysphagia are not associated with radiotherapy to the retroperitoneal area. Nausea is experienced by clients undergoing radiation but is not related to radiotherapy to the retroperitoneal area. (D, N, G)

General Questions

38. 4. The nurse should suspect that a client has retention with overflow when the urge to void is present but the client voids only small amounts of urine at one time. Retention with overflow is not associated with bladder damage, kidney infection, or inadequate fluid intake. (A, T, G)

39. 4. Usually, the discomfort associated with gas pains is likely to be relieved when the client ambulates. The gas will be more easily expelled with exercise. Such techniques as applying an abdominal binder, offering the client a hot beverage, and providing extra warmth are not recommended and may even aggravate the discomfort of gas pains postoperatively. (I, T, G)

40. 3. Elevated temperature on the second postoperative day is most suggestive of a respiratory tract infection. Respiratory infections most often occur during the first 48 hours after surgery. Signs of infection, if present in the wound or urinary tract, are likely to occur later in the postoperative period. So also are signs of phlebitis, which is an inflammatory process in a vein. (A, T, G)

41. 2. Massaging the legs postoperatively is contraindicated because it may dislodge small clots of blood, if present, and cause even more serious problems.

Such measures as ambulating the client, having her wear elasticized stockings, and having her move her legs about in bed have been found to help reduce the incidence of postoperative thrombophlebitis. (I, T, G)

42. 3. When a dressing sticks to a wound, it is best to moisten the dressing with sterile normal saline solution and then remove it carefully. Trying to remove a dry dressing is likely to irritate the skin and wound. (I, T, S)

43. 1. The opening of a wound is called dehiscence. Dehiscence places the client at an immediate increased risk for infection. (D, N, G)

44. 4. The nurse should cover the exposed tissues with sterile dressings moistened with sterile normal saline solutions if the wound opens and tissues are exposed (wound evisceration). The nurse should also cover an eviscerated wound with sterile dressings moistened with sterile normal saline solution. The physician should be notified immediately when a wound dehisces or eviscerates. Such measures as trying to replace the exposed tissues or organs, applying an abdominal binder, or trying to approximate the wound edges with adhesive strips are contraindicated and are likely to aggravate the problem. (I, T, G)

45. 1. The primary ovarian hormone is estrogen. It is likely to be prescribed for a woman whose ovaries, fallopian tubes, and uterus have been surgically removed. Many physicians now use both estrogen and progesterone cyclically in postoperative hormone replacement therapy. (I, C, G)

46. 4. Body image disturbance related to loss of female reproductive organs may lead to ineffective coping in some women. Therefore, interventions to address this problem should be incorporated into discharge planning. Gas pains and fluid volume overload are not problems expected 6 days postoperatively after an abdominal hysterectomy. Lack of social resources is not a problem for all clients and should be diagnosed only after further assessment. (D, N, L)

47. 2. Assessment is the first step in planning client education. Assessing social support resources is a key aspect of discharge planning that begins when the client is admitted to the hospital. Calling the social worker is not the first action the nurse should take. Having the client read the instructions or reading instructions to the client is not the first step of discharge planning. (I, N, S)

48. 4. A family history of breast cancer, early onset of menstruation, delayed onset of menopause, and childlessness all appear to increase a woman's risk of breast cancer. Breast-feeding does not increase the risk. (A, K, G)

49. 4. Lymph nodes are ordinarily removed from the axillary area when a modified radical mastectomy is done. Therefore, to facilitate drainage from the arm on the affected side, the client's arm should be elevated on pillows with her hand higher than her elbow and her elbow higher than her shoulder. The other techniques for positioning the arm on the affected side do not facilitate drainage from the arm. (I, T, G)

50. 3. Following a mastectomy, every effort should be made to avoid cuts, bruises, burns, and the like on the affected arm, because normal circulation has been impaired. Working in a rose or cactus garden is contraindicated because of the danger of skin pricks. Such activities as caring for pets and swimming are not contraindicated for the postmastectomy client. (I, N, H)

51. 1. Return of arm and shoulder function is a priority for the woman following a modified radical mastectomy. Swelling of the affected arm is not a usual expected outcome. The client may not be able to resume her usual activity level after hospital discharge. Fluid and electrolyte balance, while important, is not a common problem at hospital discharge. (E, T, S)

52. 1. A client receiving radiation therapy should avoid lotions, ointments, and anything that may cause irritation to the skin, such as exposure to sunlight and talcum powder. The area may safely be washed with water if it is done gently and if care is taken not to injure the skin. (I, T, S)

53. 3. The most common reaction of the skin to radiation therapy is redness of the surface tissues. Dryness, desquamation, tanning, and capillary dilation are also common. (I, T, H)

54. 1. The American Cancer Society's Reach to Recovery is a rehabilitation program for women who have had breast surgery. It is designed to meet their physical, psychological, and cosmetic needs but does not provide funds or dressings. Research is not part of the program. (I, T, L)

55. 3. It is generally recommended that the breasts be examined during the first week after menstruation. During this period the breasts are least likely to be tender or swollen, since the secretion of estrogen, which prepares the uterus for implantation, is at its lowest level. (I, T, H)

56. 4. For a self-breast examination, placing a pillow or towel under the shoulder on the side being examined elevates the chest wall while the woman lies flat on her back. This positioning allows for better distribution of breast tissue over the chest wall and allows for the most thorough examination of tissues by palpation. A standing position, facing a mirror, is used to examine the breasts for changes in size and shape, for skin dimpling, and for nipple changes. The standing or sitting positions are not appropriate for palpating breast tissues. (I, C, H)

57. 2. The breasts normally are approximately the same size. They may vary in size somewhat before menstruation, due to breast engorgement caused by hormonal changes. A woman may then note that her brassiere fits more tightly than usual. (I, T, H)

58. 3. Avoiding caffeine is thought to alleviate discomfort associated with fibrocystic breast disease. Wearing tighter garments could increase discomfort. Activity level is not associated with fibrocystic breast disease. A nurse should not recommend estrogen therapy as an intervention for discomfort from fibrocystic breast disease. (I, T, G)

59. 1. The best way to assess for a distended bladder is to check for a rounded swelling above the pubis. This swelling represents the distended bladder rising above the pubis into the abdominal cavity. (A, C, G)

60. 2. Lubricating the catheter liberally before catheterizing a male decreases friction along the urethra and reduces irritation and trauma to urethral tissues. Because the male urethra is tortuous, a liberal amount of lubrication is advised to ease catheter passage. The female urethra is not tortuous, and although the catheter should be lubricated before insertion, not as much lubricant is necessary as for a male. (I, C, S)

61. 1. The primary reason for taping an indwelling catheter to a male client so that the penis is held in a lateral position is to prevent pressure at the penoscrotal angle. Prolonged pressure at the penoscrotal angle can cause a ureterocutaneous fistula. (I, T, S)

62. 2. After an indwelling catheter is removed, the client will likely experience some dribbling incontinence. This is normal and temporary. The problem usually resolves itself as perineal muscles are strengthened by exercise. (I, T, H)

63. 3. The presence of red and white blood cells in the urine is most typical of a urinary tract infection. (E, T, G)

64. 1. Maintaining catheter patency during the immediate postoperative period following a transurethral resection is a priority. Incisional bleeding is not expected unless a complication occurs. Performing activities of daily living, such as bathing, is not a priority immediately following surgery. The client in the immediate postoperative period is not ready for teaching. (P, T, S)

65. 2. The pain of bladder spasms frequently necessitates intervention. Deep vein thrombosis and bleeding at the incisional site are not common after a transurethral resection. The surgery is not disfiguring. (D, N, G)

66. 2. Bethanechol chloride (Urecholine) is a cholinergic drug that stimulates the parasympathetic nervous system. It acts to increase the tone and motility of the smooth muscles of the urinary and gastrointestinal tracts. The drug is frequently used when the client lacks bladder tone and cannot empty the bladder completely. It is contraindicated when urine retention is caused by a urinary tract obstruction. Following transurethral resection, the drug is administered to overcome urine retention and decrease the risk of urinary tract infection due to catheterization. (I, T, G)

67. 3. The prostate gland serves one primary purpose: It produces a secretion that aids the nourishment and passage of sperm. (A, K, G)

68. 3. Altered patterns of urinary elimination, such as dribbling, may persist for several months following transurethral resection. Fluid volume deficit, bleeding, and ineffective airway clearance are postoperative complications that should be resolved before discharge. (D, N, H)

69. 2. It has been found that older men tend to believe that it is normal to live with some urinary problems. As a result, these men often overlook symptoms and simply attribute them to aging. (E, K, H)

70. 3. The chancre of syphilis is characteristically a painless, moist ulcer. Its serous discharge is very infectious. The chancre most often occurs on the penis but may also occur on the anus, rectum, lips, and mouth. It also occasionally occurs on the skin where the causative organism entered the body. (A, K, G)

71. 2. An important aspect of controlling the spread of sexually transmitted diseases is obtaining a list of the sexual contacts of an infected client. These contacts in turn should be encouraged to obtain immediate care. Many persons with a sexually transmitted disease are reluctant to reveal their sexual contacts, which makes controlling sexually transmitted diseases difficult. There are fewer reported difficulties in motivating persons with sexually transmitted diseases to seek treatment, increasing their knowledge of the disease, and assuring them that their records are confidential. (P, N, S)

72. 2. Normally, the kidneys effectively clear penicillin from the blood. Probenecid (Benemid) inhibits excretion of penicillin and thereby helps maintain high blood levels of penicillin. (I, C, G)

73. 4. *Treponema pallidum,* the organism that causes syphilis, is classified as a spirochete because of its corkscrew appearance. (A, K, G)

74. 1. A client with primary syphilis is at risk of transmitting the disease to sexual partners if he or she is not knowledgeable about how the disease is spread. Cutaneous lesions on the palms and soles and alopecia are signs of secondary syphilis. Chancres do not bleed sufficiently to alter tissue perfusion. (D, N, H)

75. 4. Gonorrhea in the male is characterized by a mucopurulent urethral discharge and dysuria. (A, T, G)

76. 4. Many females are unaware that they have gonorrhea because they are symptom-free or experience only very mild symptoms until the disease progresses to pelvic inflammatory disease. (I, T, H)

77. 1. Statistics reveal that the incidence of sexually transmitted diseases is rising more rapidly in teenagers than in any other age group. Many reasons have been given for this trend, including a change in societal mores and increasing sexual activity among teenagers. (E, N, H)

78. 1. Asking the client to describe her nervousness gives her the opportunity to express her concerns and allows the nurse to understand her better. Responses that make assumptions about the source of the concern or offer cliched reinforcement are nonsupportive and block successful communication. (I, N, L)

79. 3. Douching within 24 to 48 hours before a Pap smear may wash away cells and secretions needed for accurate test results. The test should be scheduled for a time when the client is not menstruating. No bowel preparation is needed, and the client may bathe as desired. (I, C, S)

80. 2. Although other positions may be used, the preferred position for a vaginal examination is the lithotomy position, because it is convenient for the examiner and offers the best visualization. (I, T, S)

81. 4. The Pap smear identifies atypical cervical cells that may be present for various reasons. Cancer is the most common possible cause, but not the only one. An adequate smear provides quite accurate diagnostic data; the false-positive rate is only about 5%. (I, T, G)

82. 4. The incidence of cervical cancer is closely linked to sexual experience with multiple partners and a history of sexually transmitted disease (i.e., syphilis, gonorrhea, herpes genitalis). A positive family history is an associated risk. Pregnancy at an early age alone does not increase the risk. (A, T, G)

83. 3. Current American Cancer Society guidelines advocate Pap smears every 3 years after an initial negative pattern is established and the woman is deemed to be at low risk for development of cervical cancer. Annual screening is recommended for any woman in the high-risk category. (P, C, H)

84. 2. A client may experience anxiety since she is immobilized on strict bedrest and is unable to care for herself while the implant is in place. The other diagnoses are not priorities; typically the tumor is surgically removed before the implant is placed. (D, N, L)

85. 4. The client with a cervical implant is kept on strict bedrest, flat in bed. Limitation of movement is designed to prevent accidental displacement or even dislodgement of the implant. Client knowledge and understanding are critical to compliance with these restrictions. (I, T, S)

86. 4. Bowel movements can be difficult with the radium applicator in place. The purpose of the low-residue diet is to decrease the need for a bowel movement. To prevent dislodging the applicator, the client is maintained on strict bedrest and allowed only to turn from side to side. Perineal care is omitted during radium implant therapy, although any vaginal discharge should be reported to the doctor. It is rare for the applicator to extrude, so this need not be checked every hour. (I, T, G)

87. 4. Nausea, vomiting, and foul vaginal discharge are common side effects of internal radiation therapy for cervical cancer. Cramping pain is also common, but itching is uncommon. Fever and confusion would not be expected, although sleep disturbances may occur. (A, T, G)

88. 4. Pain is a major problem for most women diagnosed with pelvic inflammatory disease. Fluid balance disturbances, falls, and impaired mobility are not typically associated with the disorder. (D, N, G)

89. 3. After a warm bath or shower, the testes hang low and relaxed and are in ideal position for manual evaluation and palpation. (I, T, H)

90. 2. Normal testes feel smooth, egg-shaped, and firm to the touch, without lumps. They should not be soft or spongy to the touch. (A, K, G)

91. 1. Cryptorchidism (undescended testis) carries a greatly increased risk for testicular cancer. Other possible causes include chemical carcinogens, trauma, orchitis, and environmental factors. Testicular cancer is not associated with early sexual relations in men, although cervical cancer is associated with early sexual relations in women. (E, C, H)

92. 2. When diagnosed early and treated aggressively, testicular cancer has a cure rate of approximately 90%. Surgery is only one mode of treatment and is combined with chemotherapy and radiation therapy. The chemotherapeutic regimen used today is responsible for the successful treatment of testicular cancer. (P, T, G)

THE NURSING CARE OF ADULTS WITH MEDICAL/SURGICAL HEALTH PROBLEMS

TEST 7: The Client With Reproductive Health Problems

Directions: Use this answer grid to determine areas of strength or need for further study.

NURSING PROCESS

A = Assessment
D = Analysis, nursing diagnosis
P = Planning
I = Implementation
E = Evaluation

COGNITIVE LEVEL

K = Knowledge
C = Comprehension
T = Application
N = Analysis

CLIENT NEEDS

S = Safe, effective care environment
G = Physiological integrity
L = Psychosocial integrity
H = Health promotion/maintenance

		Nursing Process					Cognitive Level				Client Needs			
Question #	Answer #	A	D	P	I	E	K	C	T	N	S	G	L	H
1	2				I					N			L	
2	4				I				T			G		
3	2	A							T			G		
4	2				I			C			S			
5	4				I		K					G		
6	2				I					N		G		
7	1				I				T				L	
8	1	A					K					G		
9	4				I			C				G		
10	3				I				T			G		
11	3				I				T			G		
12	4				I					N			L	
13	3				I				T			G		
14	4	A							T			G		
15	2					E			T		S			
16	4				I				T			G		
17	3				I				T			G		
18	3				I					N		G		
19	2	A					K				S			
20	3				I			C				G		
21	4	A						C			S			
22	2				I				T					H
23	3		D						T			G		

ANSWER GRID: 1

Nursing Process

A = Assessment
D = Analysis, nursing diagnosis
P = Planning
I = Implementation
E = Evaluation

Cognitive Level

K = Knowledge
C = Comprehension
T = Application
N = Analysis

Client Needs

S = Safe, effective care environment
G = Physiological integrity
L = Psychosocial integrity
H = Health promotion/maintenance

		Nursing Process					Cognitive Level				Client Needs			
Question #	Answer #	A	D	P	I	E	K	C	T	N	S	G	L	H
24	1	A								N		G		
25	4					E				N				H
26	4	A							T			G		
27	3				I				T			G		
28	1				I				T			G		
29	1				I					N			L	
30	2				I				T		S			
31	3				I					N	S			
32	2	A							T			G		
33	4				I				T			G		
34	3	A						C				G		
35	2				I					N		G		
36	3		D							N		G		
37	2		D							N		G		
38	4	A							T			G		
39	4				I				T			G		
40	3	A							T			G		
41	2				I				T			G		
42	3				I				T		S			
43	1		D							N		G		
44	4				I				T			G		
45	1				I			C				G		
46	4		D							N			L	
47	2				I					N	S			
48	4	A					K					G		
49	4				I				T			G		
50	3				I					N				H
51	1					E			T		S			
52	1				I				T		S			

Answer Grid: 2

Nursing Process	**Cognitive Level**	**Client Needs**
A = Assessment	K = Knowledge	S = Safe, effective care environment
D = Analysis, nursing diagnosis	C = Comprehension	G = Physiological integrity
P = Planning	T = Application	L = Psychosocial integrity
I = Implementation	N = Analysis	H = Health promotion/maintenance
E = Evaluation		

		Nursing Process					Cognitive Level				Client Needs			
Question #	Answer #	A	D	P	I	E	K	C	T	N	S	G	L	H
53	3				I				T					H
54	1				I				T				L	
55	3				I				T					H
56	4				I			C						H
57	2				I				T					H
58	3				I				T			G		
59	1	A						C				G		
60	2				I			C			S			
61	1				I				T		S			
62	2				I				T					H
63	3					E			T			G		
64	1			P					T		S			
65	2		D							N		G		
66	2				I				T			G		
67	3	A					K					G		
68	3		D							N				H
69	2					E	K							H
70	3	A					K					G		
71	2			P						N	S			
72	2				I			C				G		
73	4	A					K					G		
74	1		D							N				H
75	4	A							T			G		
76	4				I				T					H
77	1					E				N				H
78	1				I					N			L	
79	3				I			C			S			
80	2				I				T		S			
81	4				I				T			G		

ANSWER GRID: 3

Nursing Process

A = Assessment
D = Analysis, nursing diagnosis
P = Planning
I = Implementation
E = Evaluation

Cognitive Level

K = Knowledge
C = Comprehension
T = Application
N = Analysis

Client Needs

S = Safe, effective care environment
G = Physiological integrity
L = Psychosocial integrity
H = Health promotion/maintenance

		Nursing Process					Cognitive Level				Client Needs			
Question #	Answer #	A	D	P	I	E	K	C	T	N	S	G	L	H
82	4	A							T			G		
83	3			P				C						H
84	2		D							N			L	
85	4				I				T		S			
86	4				I				T			G		
87	4	A							T			G		
88	4		D							N		G		
89	3				I				T					H
90	2	A					K					G		
91	1					E		C						H
92	2			P					T			G		
Number Correct														
Number Possible	92	20	10	4	51	7	9	13	47	23	17	51	8	16
Percentage Correct														

Score Calculation:

To determine your **Percentage Correct**, divide the **Number Correct** by the **Number Possible**.

The Client With Neurological Health Problems

Test 8

The Client With a Head Injury
The Client With Seizures
The Client With Cerebrovascular Accident
The Client With Parkinson's Disease
The Client With Multiple Sclerosis
The Unconscious Client
The Client in Pain
Correct Answers and Rationale

Select the one best answer and indicate your choice by filling in the circle in front of the option.

The Client With a Head Injury

A 22-year-old male is brought to the emergency room with an apparent head injury after being involved in a serious motor vehicle accident. He is unconscious on arrival and exhibits signs of increasing intracranial pressure. He is accompanied by his fiancee and an adult friend.

1. Which of the following methods would be best, from a legal standpoint, for obtaining permission to treat the unconscious client?
- ○ 1. Having his fiancee sign the consent form.
- ○ 2. Having three physicians agree on treatment he needs.
- ○ 3. Obtaining a verbal consent by telephone from a responsible relative.
- ○ 4. Obtaining written consent from the adult friend who accompanied the client to the emergency room.

2. When the client arrives in the emergency room, to which of the following considerations should the nurse give highest priority in his care?
- ○ 1. Establishing an airway.
- ○ 2. Replacing blood losses.
- ○ 3. Stopping bleeding from open wounds.
- ○ 4. Determining whether he has a neck fracture.

3. The client's initial blood pressure is 124/80 mm Hg. As his condition worsens, pulse pressure increases. Which of the following blood pressure readings indicates a pulse pressure greater than the initial pulse pressure?
- ○ 1. 102/60 mm Hg.
- ○ 2. 110/90 mm Hg.
- ○ 3. 140/100 mm Hg.
- ○ 4. 160/100 mm Hg.

4. The nurse assesses the client frequently for signs of increasing intracranial pressure, including
- ○ 1. unequal pupils.
- ○ 2. decreasing systolic blood pressure.
- ○ 3. tachycardia.
- ○ 4. decreasing body temperature.

5. Which of the following respiratory signs would indicate increasing intracranial pressure in the brain stem?
- ○ 1. Slow, irregular respirations.
- ○ 2. Rapid, shallow respirations.
- ○ 3. Asymmetrical chest excursion.
- ○ 4. Nasal flaring.

6. The nurse checks the client's gag reflex. The recommended technique for testing the gag reflex is to
- ○ 1. touch the back of the client's throat with a tongue depressor.
- ○ 2. observe the client for evidence of spontaneous swallowing when the neck is stroked.

○ 3. place a few milliliters of water on the client's tongue and note whether he swallows.
○ 4. observe the client's response to the introduction of a catheter for endotracheal suctioning.

7. Which of the following nursing assessments of the client's eyes would be least helpful when assessing for signs of increased intracranial pressure?
○ 1. The color of the sclera.
○ 2. The size of the pupils.
○ 3. The pupils' reaction to light.
○ 4. The reaction of the corneas to touch.

8. The nurse obtains a specimen from clear fluid that is draining from the client's nose. To determine whether this fluid is mucus or cerebrospinal fluid, it should be tested for
○ 1. pH level.
○ 2. specific gravity.
○ 3. glucose.
○ 4. microorganisms.

9. Which of the following positions would be most appropriate for a client with a head injury?
○ 1. Head of the bed elevated 30 to 45 degrees.
○ 2. Trendelenburg's position.
○ 3. Left Sim's position.
○ 4. Head elevated on two pillows.

10. The client receives mannitol (Osmitrol) during surgery to help decrease intracranial pressure. Which of the following nursing observations would most likely indicate that the drug is having the desired effect?
○ 1. Urine output increases.
○ 2. Pulse rate decreases.
○ 3. Blood pressure decreases.
○ 4. Muscular relaxation increases.

11. Which of the following comments by the nurse would most help the client become oriented following surgery when he regains consciousness?
○ 1. "I'm your nurse, and I'll take care of you."
○ 2. "Can you tell me your name and where you live?"
○ 3. "Can you move your hands and feet a few inches from side to side?"
○ 4. "You are in a hospital, where you had an operation after your accident."

12. As the client gradually regains consciousness, he becomes very restless and attempts to pull out his IV. Which action should the nurse take to protect the client without increasing his intracranial pressure?
○ 1. Place him in a jacket restraint.
○ 2. Wrap his hands in soft "mitten" restraints.
○ 3. Hold his hands firmly in place at his sides.
○ 4. Apply a wrist restraint to each arm.

13. When the client is fully conscious, the nurse would best assess his motor strength by having him
○ 1. squeeze the nurse's hands.
○ 2. feed himself with a spoon.
○ 3. demonstrate his ability to move his legs.
○ 4. signal as soon as he can feel pressure applied to the soles of his feet.

14. Which of the following postoperative care measures would be contraindicated for a client at risk for increased intracranial pressure?
○ 1. Deep breathing.
○ 2. Turning.
○ 3. Coughing.
○ 4. Passive range-of-motion exercises.

15. Of the following nursing orders on the client's care plan, which would be most helpful in determining whether he may be developing diabetes insipidus?
○ 1. Obtain vital signs every 2 hours.
○ 2. Measure urine specific gravity hourly.
○ 3. Determine arterial blood gas values every other day.
○ 4. Test a urine specimen for glucose every morning.

16. The client is suffering from short-term memory loss. Which of the following nursing actions would be appropriate to help him cope with his memory loss?
○ 1. Instruct family members to ignore his behavior.
○ 2. Place a single-date calendar where he can view it.
○ 3. Tell him every morning what activities he will be expected to perform that day.
○ 4. Explain that he will have to try harder to remember things.

17. During the client's recovery period, the nurse notes at 4 P.M. that he seems uninterested in his visitors and is more lethargic than usual. Of the following notations on the client's record, which would indicate the most likely reason for his lethargy?
○ 1. 12:30 P.M.: Refused lunch; drank a glass of milk only.
○ 2. 3 P.M.: Placed in side-lying position after being in semi-sitting position for 2 hours.
○ 3. 3 P.M.: Meperidine hydrochloride (Demerol) 75 mg given IM for pain.
○ 4. 3:30 P.M.: Intake 800 ml and output 300 ml since 8 A.M.

The Client With Seizures

A young adult has had several episodes of seizures. He is admitted to the hospital for diagnostic studies.

18. The client is placed on seizure precautions. Which of the following measures would be contraindicated?
○ 1. Encourage him to perform his own personal hygiene.

○ 2. Allow him to wear his own clothing.
○ 3. Assess oral temperature with a glass thermometer.
○ 4. Encourage him to be out of bed.

19. Which of the following statements would best describe the seizure activity of a tonic-clonic (grand mal) seizure?
○ 1. Seizure activity begins in one extremity and spreads gradually to adjacent areas.
○ 2. The client's eyes become vacant with an abrupt cessation of all activity.
○ 3. The client exhibits facial grimaces, patting motions, and lip smacking.
○ 4. The seizure activity is marked by sudden loss of consciousness and stiffening of the body, followed by violent muscle contractions.

20. The nurse plans to teach the client about the computed tomography (CT) scan that will be done at noon the next day. Which of the following statements by the nurse would be most accurate?
○ 1. "You must shampoo your hair tonight to remove all oil and dirt."
○ 2. "You may drink fluids until about 8 A.M. Then we will give you a cleansing enema."
○ 3. "We will partially shave your head tonight so that electrodes can be securely attached to your scalp."
○ 4. "There is no special preparation necessary. You will need to hold your head very still during the examination."

21. An electroencephalogram (EEG) is ordered for the client. What action should the nurse take when the client is served a breakfast consisting of a soft-boiled egg, toast with butter and marmalade, orange juice, and coffee on the morning of the EEG?
○ 1. Remove all the food.
○ 2. Remove the coffee.
○ 3. Remove the toast, butter, and marmalade only.
○ 4. Substitute vegetable juice for the orange juice.

22. The client asks the nurse, "What caused me to have a seizure? I've never had one before." The nurse's reply should be based on the knowledge that a primary cause of tonic-clonic seizures in adults over age 20 is
○ 1. head trauma.
○ 2. electrolyte imbalance.
○ 3. a congenital defect.
○ 4. an episode of high fever.

23. The nurse enters the client's room as the client, who is sitting in a chair, begins to have a seizure. Which of the following actions should the nurse take first?
○ 1. Lift the client onto his bed.
○ 2. Ease the client to the floor.
○ 3. Restrain the client's body movements.
○ 4. Insert an airway into the client's mouth.

24. In which position in bed should the nurse place the client after the seizure has subsided?
○ 1. Side-lying.
○ 2. Supine.
○ 3. Low Fowler's.
○ 4. Modified Trendelenburg's.

25. After the client's seizure has subsided, the nurse would judge that the client is behaving in a typical manner if he
○ 1. becomes restless and agitated.
○ 2. sleeps for a long time.
○ 3. says he is thirsty and hungry.
○ 4. is most comfortable walking and moving about.

26. During the seizure, which of the following would be appropriate for the nurse to note?
○ 1. Heart rate and blood pressure.
○ 2. When the last dose of anticonvulsant medication was administered.
○ 3. What type of aura the client had.
○ 4. Movement of the extremities.

27. Which of the following observations would the nurse not expect in a client who has experienced a tonic-clonic (grand mal) seizure? The client
○ 1. was drowsy after the seizure.
○ 2. was unable to talk after the seizure.
○ 3. was incontinent of urine during the seizure.
○ 4. failed to respond to stimuli during the clonic phase of the seizure.

28. Phenytoin (Dilantin) is prescribed for the client. He asks the nurse how the medication will help him. The nurse's best response should be based on knowledge that the drug is thought to act by
○ 1. correcting the abnormal synthesis of norepinephrine in the body.
○ 2. depressing transmission of abnormal impulses in the spinal cord.
○ 3. reducing the responsiveness of neurons in the brain to abnormal impulses.
○ 4. interrupting the flow of abnormal impulses from the viscera to the brain.

29. The nurse plans to teach the client about prescribed phenytoin (Dilantin) therapy. It is important that the client understand that the medication must not be stopped suddenly, because
○ 1. a physical dependency on the drug develops over time.
○ 2. this can precipitate the development of status epilepticus.
○ 3. this would lead to a hypoglycemic reaction.
○ 4. phenytoin is the only effective drug for tonic-clonic seizures.

30. The client states that he is afraid he will not be able to drive again because of his seizures. The nurse should respond by telling him that driving will depend on local laws but that most laws require

- ○ 1. that a person with a history of seizures drive only during daytime hours.
- ○ 2. evidence that the seizures are under medical control.
- ○ 3. evidence that seizures occur no more often than every 6 months.
- ○ 4. that the person with a history of seizures carry a medical identification card at all times when driving.

31. The client tells the nurse that he is unclear about what an aura is. The nurse would correctly define an aura as

- ○ 1. a postseizure state of amnesia.
- ○ 2. hallucinations occurring during a seizure.
- ○ 3. a symptom that occurs just before a seizure.
- ○ 4. a feeling of relaxation as the seizure begins to subside.

32. When the client is discharged from the hospital, the nurse instructs him to continue taking the phenytoin (Dilantin) as prescribed. One week after discharge, the client reports a skin rash. The nurse should tell the client to

- ○ 1. come to the office that day for consultation with the physician.
- ○ 2. decrease the amount of medication by taking one less pill each day.
- ○ 3. stop taking the medication but keep his regular appointment next week.
- ○ 4. continue taking the prescribed dosage of the medication but increase his fluid intake to at least 3,000 ml/day.

33. Which of the following findings should suggest to the nurse that a client is having a typical reaction to long-term phenytoin therapy? The client

- ○ 1. has gained considerable weight.
- ○ 2. reports insomnia.
- ○ 3. exhibits an excessive growth of his gum tissue.
- ○ 4. says that he now needs to wear eyeglasses.

The Client With a Cerebrovascular Accident

A 72-year-old retired male experiences a thrombotic cerebrovascular accident and is admitted to the hospital. The diagnosis is a left cerebrovascular accident with flaccid hemiplegia of his right side.

34. When planning the client's care, the nurse should keep in mind that rehabilitation begins

- ○ 1. as soon as anticoagulant therapy is started.
- ○ 2. when the client is admitted to the hospital.
- ○ 3. when the client is first able to work cooperatively with health care personnel.
- ○ 4. as soon as a physical therapist can be brought into the client's health care team.

35. Regular oral hygiene is an essential intervention for the client. Which of the following nursing measures would be inappropriate when providing oral hygiene?

- ○ 1. Placing the client on his back with a small pillow under his head.
- ○ 2. Keeping portable suctioning equipment at the bedside.
- ○ 3. Opening the client's mouth with a padded tongue blade.
- ○ 4. Cleansing the client's mouth and teeth with a toothbrush.

36. Nursing assessment data include: inability to move the right arm and leg; absence of muscle tone in the right arm and leg; and lack of knowledge about how to turn in bed. Based on this data, which of the following would be the most appropriate nursing diagnosis for this client?

- ○ 1. Activity Intolerance.
- ○ 2. Body Image Disturbance.
- ○ 3. Impaired Physical Mobility.
- ○ 4. Unilateral Neglect.

37. The nurse changes the client's position in bed regularly. Which of the following techniques would most likely cause friction and predispose to decubitus ulcer formation?

- ○ 1. Rolling the client onto his side.
- ○ 2. Sliding the client to move him up in bed.
- ○ 3. Lifting the client on a drawsheet when moving him up in bed.
- ○ 4. Having the client help by lifting himself off the bed using a trapeze.

38. The nurse is concerned about the possible development of plantar flexion (footdrop). Which of the following measures has been found to be the most effective means of preventing plantar flexion in a stroke client?

- ○ 1. Placing the client's feet against a firm footboard.
- ○ 2. Repositioning the client every 2 hours.
- ○ 3. Having the client wear ankle-high tennis shoes at intervals throughout the day.
- ○ 4. Massaging the client's feet and ankles regularly.

39. Because the cerebrovascular accident affected the left side of the client's brain, the nurse should anticipate that the client will most likely experience

- ○ 1. expressive aphasia.
- ○ 2. dyslexia.
- ○ 3. apraxia.
- ○ 4. agnosia.

40. For the client experiencing expressive aphasia, which of the following nursing actions would be most helpful in promoting communication?

- ○ 1. Speaking loudly.
- ○ 2. Using short sentences.

○ 3. Writing all directions so the client can read them.
○ 4. Correcting all of the client's speech errors.

41. For the client with dysphagia, which of the following measures would be ineffective in decreasing the risk of aspiration while eating?
○ 1. Maintaining an upright position.
○ 2. Restricting the diet to liquids until swallowing improves.
○ 3. Introducing foods on the unaffected side of the mouth.
○ 4. Keeping distractions to a minimum.

42. The client experiences urinary incontinence following the cerebrovascular accident. Which of the following nursing interventions would likely be most successful in helping reestablish urinary continence?
○ 1. Obtain an order for a Foley catheter.
○ 2. Apply an external urinary catheter.
○ 3. Make sure the urinal is within the client's reach.
○ 4. Help the client stand to void every 2 hours.

43. When helping the client learn self-care skills, the nurse should use which of the following interventions to help him learn to dress himself?
○ 1. Encourage the client to wear clothing designed especially for persons who have had a stroke.
○ 2. Dress the client, explaining each step of the process as it is completed.
○ 3. Teach the client to put on clothing on the affected side first.
○ 4. Encourage the client to ask his wife for help when dressing.

44. Which of the following techniques would help the nurse successfully communicate with a client experiencing expressive aphasia?
○ 1. Speak in a clear, normal voice.
○ 2. Use gestures instead of words to communicate.
○ 3. Speak more loudly than usual.
○ 4. Use pictures as cue cards for communication.

45. The cerebrovascular accident has caused homonymous hemianopsia (blindness in half of the visual field). Homonymous hemianopsia would probably manifest itself in which of the following food-related behaviors?
○ 1. Increased preference for foods high in salt.
○ 2. Eating food on only one-half of the plate.
○ 3. Forgetting the names of foods.
○ 4. Inability to swallow liquids.

46. Although all of the following measures might be useful in reducing the client's visual disability, which measure should the nurse teach him primarily as a safety precaution?
○ 1. Wear a patch over one eye.
○ 2. Place personal items on his sighted side.
○ 3. Lie in bed with the unaffected side toward the door.
○ 4. Turn his head from side to side when walking.

47. The client is experiencing mood swings and often has "crying jags" that are very distressing to his family. It would be best for the nurse to instruct family members to do which of the following when these "crying jags" occur?
○ 1. Sit quietly with the client until the episode is over.
○ 2. Ignore the behavior and continue what they were doing.
○ 3. Attempt to divert the client's attention.
○ 4. Tell the client that this behavior is unacceptable.

48. The client is aware of and discouraged by his physical handicaps. The nurse can best help him overcome a negative self-concept by conveying
○ 1. helpfulness and sympathy.
○ 2. concern and charity.
○ 3. direction and firmness.
○ 4. encouragement and patience.

49. The nurse is preparing the client for discharge to home. Which of the following factors would most likely influence the client's continuing progress in rehabilitation at home?
○ 1. The family's ability to provide support to the client.
○ 2. The client's ability to ambulate.
○ 3. The availability of a home health aide to care for the client.
○ 4. The frequency of follow-up visits with the physician.

The Client With Parkinson's Disease

A 67-year-old male is admitted to the hospital for a diagnostic workup for probable Parkinson's disease.

50. When assessing the client, the nurse would anticipate which of the following signs and symptoms?
○ 1. Dry mouth.
○ 2. Aphasia.
○ 3. An exaggerated sense of euphoria.
○ 4. A stiff, masklike facial expression.

51. The nurse who admits the client to the hospital documents that he has a "shuffling and propulsive" gait. The client's gait is characterized by
○ 1. slumping forward while walking.
○ 2. walking erect on the balls of the feet.
○ 3. moving with increasingly quicker steps.
○ 4. leaning backward while walking.

52. The nurse observes that the client's upper arm tremors disappear as he unbuttons his shirt. Which of the following statements would best guide the nurse when analyzing these observations about the client's tremors?

- ○ 1. The tremors are probably psychological and can be controlled at will.
- ○ 2. The tremors sometimes disappear with purposeful and voluntary movements.
- ○ 3. The tremors often increase in severity when the client's attention is diverted by some activity.
- ○ 4. There is no explanation for the observation, which is probably a chance occurrence.

53. Clients with Parkinson's disease are prone to hypokinesia. To minimize the effects of hypokinesia, the client should be taught to schedule his most demanding physical activities

- ○ 1. early in the morning, when his energy level is high.
- ○ 2. to coincide with the peak action of drug therapy.
- ○ 3. immediately after a rest period.
- ○ 4. when family members will be available.

54. Which of the following goals would be most realistic and appropriate when planning the client's nursing care?

- ○ 1. To cure the disease.
- ○ 2. To stop progression of the disease.
- ○ 3. To begin preparations for terminal care.
- ○ 4. To maintain optimal body function.

55. The physical therapy regimen developed for a client with Parkinson's disease is aimed primarily at

- ○ 1. maintaining joint flexibility and relaxing muscles.
- ○ 2. building muscle strength.
- ○ 3. improving muscle endurance.
- ○ 4. reducing ataxia.

56. The client is started on levodopa (L-Dopa) therapy. The nurse would evaluate that the drug is exerting its desired effect when the client experiences an improvement in

- ○ 1. mood.
- ○ 2. muscle rigidity.
- ○ 3. appetite.
- ○ 4. alertness.

57. To maintain the therapeutic effects of levodopa (L-Dopa), most clients require gradually increasing dosages. The nurse should teach the client's family that important symptoms of levodopa toxicity are

- ○ 1. lethargy and sleepiness.
- ○ 2. anorexia and nausea.
- ○ 3. diarrhea and cramping.
- ○ 4. delusions and hallucinations.

58. The client may be able to function effectively with less levodopa if he follows a

- ○ 1. high-fiber diet.
- ○ 2. low-fiber diet.
- ○ 3. high-protein diet.
- ○ 4. low-protein diet.

59. The client needs a long time to complete his morning hygiene, but he becomes quite annoyed when the nurse offers assistance and refuses all help. Which would be the nurse's best initial response in this situation?

- ○ 1. Tell him firmly that he needs assistance and help him with his care.
- ○ 2. Praise him for his desire to be independent and give him extra time and encouragement.
- ○ 3. Tell him that he is being unrealistic about his abilities and must accept the fact that he needs help.
- ○ 4. Suggest that if he insists on self-care, he should at least modify his routine.

60. The nurse asks the client to read the menu aloud each day. What is the purpose of this intervention?

- ○ 1. To develop control of the tongue.
- ○ 2. To decrease rigidity in the facial muscles.
- ○ 3. To exercise the temporomandibular joint.
- ○ 4. To increase awareness of voice intonation.

The Client With Multiple Sclerosis

A 48-year-old female is admitted to the hospital with a bladder infection and incontinence. She has had multiple sclerosis for 15 years.

61. Which of the following factors is least likely to cause an exacerbation of multiple sclerosis?

- ○ 1. Fatigue.
- ○ 2. A hot bath or shower.
- ○ 3. Stress.
- ○ 4. A high-protein diet.

62. Clients with multiple sclerosis experience many different symptoms. Which of the following symptoms is atypical of multiple sclerosis?

- ○ 1. Double vision.
- ○ 2. Sudden bursts of energy.
- ○ 3. Weakness in the extremities.
- ○ 4. Muscle tremors.

63. The client's care plan includes nursing measures to help prevent complications commonly associated with multiple sclerosis. Which of the following complications would be least likely?

- ○ 1. Ascites.
- ○ 2. Contractures.
- ○ 3. Decubitus ulcer.
- ○ 4. Respiratory infection.

64. Baclofen (Lioresal) is prescribed for the client. The nurse would evaluate that the drug is accomplishing its intended purpose when it

- ○ 1. induces sleep.
- ○ 2. stimulates the client's appetite.
- ○ 3. relieves muscular spasticity.
- ○ 4. reduces the urine bacterial count.

65. The client has received various drug therapies for

multiple sclerosis over the years. It is difficult to evaluate the effectiveness of any particular drug, because clients with multiple sclerosis tend to

○ 1. exhibit intolerance to many drugs.
○ 2. experience spontaneous remissions from time to time.
○ 3. require multiple drugs that are used simultaneously.
○ 4. endure long periods of exacerbation before the illness responds to a particular drug.

66. The client has slurred speech. When the nurse talks with her, which of the following techniques would be contraindicated?

○ 1. Encouraging her to speak slowly.
○ 2. Encouraging her to speak distinctly.
○ 3. Asking her to repeat indistinguishable words.
○ 4. Asking her to speak louder when tired.

67. The client's right hand trembles severely whenever she attempts a voluntary action. She spills her coffee twice at lunch and cannot get her dress fastened securely. Which of the following nurse's notes offers the best account of these observations?

○ 1. "Has an intention tremor of the right hand."
○ 2. "Right-hand tremor worsens with purposeful acts."
○ 3. "Needs assistance with dressing and eating due to severe trembling and clumsiness."
○ 4. "Slight shaking of right hand increases to severe tremor when client tries to button her clothes or drink from a cup."

68. The client may eventually lose control of her bowels and require bowel retraining. If this occurs, which of the following measures would likely be least helpful?

○ 1. Eating a diet high in roughage.
○ 2. Setting a regular time for elimination.
○ 3. Raising the toilet seat for easy access by wheelchair.
○ 4. Limiting fluid intake to 1,000 ml/day.

69. The client sometimes exhibits signs or symptoms of emotional distress. The nurse should be aware that clients with multiple sclerosis are most likely to exhibit

○ 1. mood disorders.
○ 2. thought disorders.
○ 3. psychosomatic illnesses.
○ 4. drug dependency problems.

70. As part of the rehabilitation program planned for the client, therapy and hobbies would be used to help develop her

○ 1. diligence and persistence.
○ 2. muscles and motivation.
○ 3. intellect and imagination.
○ 4. productivity and personality.

71. As the client prepares for discharge, the nurse should encourage her to

○ 1. accept the necessity for a quiet and inactive lifestyle.
○ 2. keep active while avoiding emotional upset and fatigue.
○ 3. follow good health habits to change the course of the disease.
○ 4. practice using the mechanical aids that she will need when future disabilities arise.

72. The client has various sensory impairments associated with her disease. Which of the following would not be an appropriate safety precaution for this client?

○ 1. Carefully testing the temperature of bath water.
○ 2. Avoiding kitchen activities due to the high risk of injury.
○ 3. Avoiding hot-water bottles or heating pads.
○ 4. Inspecting the skin daily for injury or pressure points.

73. Which of the following nursing interventions would most likely be used to help the client avoid episodes of urinary incontinence?

○ 1. Maintain a fluid intake of 1,500 ml/day.
○ 2. Insert an indwelling urinary catheter.
○ 3. Establish a regular voiding schedule.
○ 4. Administer prophylactic antibiotics, as ordered.

74. The client's daughter and 3-year-old granddaughter live with her. The daughter asks the nurse what she can do to most help her mother at home. From which of the following measures would the client probably benefit most at home?

○ 1. A course of psychotherapy.
○ 2. A regular program of daily activities.
○ 3. A day-care center for the granddaughter.
○ 4. A weekly visit by another person with multiple sclerosis.

The Unconscious Client

A 38-year-old male is admitted to the emergency room after being found unconscious at the wheel of his car in the hospital parking lot. The client is comatose and does not respond to stimuli. A drug overdose is suspected.

75. Which of the following assessment findings would lead the nurse to suspect that the coma is a result of a toxic drug overdose?

○ 1. Hypertension.
○ 2. Fever.
○ 3. Dilated pupils.
○ 4. Facial asymmetry.

76. Blood and urine analysis confirm a diagnosis of salicylate overdose. The client is treated with gastric lavage. Which of the following positions would be

most appropriate for the client during this procedure?
- ○ 1. Lateral.
- ○ 2. Supine.
- ○ 3. Trendelenburg's.
- ○ 4. Lithotomy.

77. In anticipation of further emergency treatment for the client, which of the following medications should the nurse have available?
- ○ 1. Vitamin K (AquaMEPHYTON).
- ○ 2. Dextrose 50%.
- ○ 3. Activated charcoal powder.
- ○ 4. Sodium thiosulfate.

78. The client's wife and sister arrive at the hospital, distraught about his comatose condition as well as the possibility that this seems to be an intentional overdose. Which of the following would be an appropriate initial nursing intervention with this family?
- ○ 1. Explain that since the client was found on hospital property, he was probably asking for help and did not intentionally overdose.
- ○ 2. Give the wife and sister a big hug and assure them that he is in good hands.
- ○ 3. Encourage the wife and sister to ventilate their feelings and concerns and listen carefully.
- ○ 4. Allow the wife and sister to help care for the client by rubbing his back when he is turned.

79. The nurse would base the frequency of the client's turning schedule primarily on an evaluation of
- ○ 1. his weight.
- ○ 2. his skin condition.
- ○ 3. his level of consciousness.
- ○ 4. his age.

80. The client is at risk for developing a decubitus ulcer. The first warning of an impending decubitus ulcer is when pressure applied to skin turns it
- ○ 1. bluish.
- ○ 2. reddish.
- ○ 3. whitish.
- ○ 4. yellowish.

81. The client's skin care includes frequent massage over bony prominences. The primary reason for this massage is to help
- ○ 1. relax tense muscles.
- ○ 2. improve blood circulation.
- ○ 3. keep the skin dry.
- ○ 4. reduce the number of organisms on the skin.

82. The client has been positioned on his side. The nurse would anticipate that which of the following areas would be a pressure point in this position?
- ○ 1. Sacrum.
- ○ 2. Occiput.
- ○ 3. Ankles.
- ○ 4. Heels.

83. The client is placed in a right side-lying position. Which of the following techniques to position the client is incorrect? The client's
- ○ 1. head is placed on a small pillow.
- ○ 2. right leg is extended without pillow support.
- ○ 3. left arm is rested on the mattress with the elbow flexed.
- ○ 4. left leg is supported on a pillow with the knee flexed.

84. To prevent external rotation of the client's hips while he is lying on his back, it would be best for the nurse to place
- ○ 1. firm pillows under the length of his legs.
- ○ 2. sandbags alongside his legs from knees to ankles.
- ○ 3. trochanter rolls alongside his legs from ilium to midthigh.
- ○ 4. a footboard that supports his feet in the normal anatomic position.

85. The nurse's goal for performing passive range-of-motion exercises on an unconscious client would be to
- ○ 1. preserve muscle mass.
- ○ 2. prevent bone demineralization.
- ○ 3. increase muscle tone.
- ○ 4. maintain joint mobility.

86. When the nurse performs oral hygiene for the unconscious client, which of the following actions would be most appropriate?
- ○ 1. Keep a suction machine available.
- ○ 2. Place the client in a prone position.
- ○ 3. Wear sterile gloves while brushing the client's teeth.
- ○ 4. Use gauze wrapped around the fingers to cleanse the client's gums.

87. The nurse observes that the client's right eye does not close totally. Based on this finding, which of the following nursing interventions would be most appropriate?
- ○ 1. Making sure the client wears his eyeglasses at all times.
- ○ 2. Placing an eye patch over his right eye.
- ○ 3. Instilling artificial tears once every shift.
- ○ 4. Cleansing the eye with a clean washcloth every shift.

88. The nurse is assessing the client's respiratory status. Which of the following symptoms may be an early indicator of hypoxia in the unconscious client?
- ○ 1. Cyanosis.
- ○ 2. Decreased respirations.
- ○ 3. Restlessness.
- ○ 4. Hypotension.

89. Intermittent enteral tube feedings are ordered for the client. When administering the feeding, the nurse should implement which of the following actions?
- ○ 1. Heat the formula in a microwave.
- ○ 2. Place the client in semi-Fowler's position.

○ 3. Obtain a sterile gavage bag and tubing for use.
○ 4. Weigh the client before administering the feeding.

90. The client is to receive 200 ml of tube feeding every 4 hours. The nurse checks the client's gastric residual before administering the feeding and obtains 40 ml of gastric residual. What should the nurse do next?
○ 1. Withhold the tube feeding and notify the physician.
○ 2. Dispose of the residual and continue with the feeding.
○ 3. Delay feeding the client for 1 hour and then recheck the residual.
○ 4. Readminister the residual to the client and continue with the feeding.

91. Of the following actions the nurse could take when providing catheter care, which should have the highest priority?
○ 1. Cleansing the area around the urethral meatus.
○ 2. Clamping the catheter periodically to maintain muscle tone.
○ 3. Irrigating the catheter with several ounces of normal saline solution.
○ 4. Changing the location where the catheter is taped to the client's leg.

The Client in Pain

A 34-year-old male of Chinese descent is admitted to the hospital after experiencing multiple trauma as a result of an automobile accident. He has three fractured ribs, a hairline fracture of the pelvis, a compound fracture of his right tibia and fibula, and soft tissue injuries. He is in severe pain when he arrives on the unit after emergency surgery.

92. The client reports severe pain and requests frequent medication. A nursing assistant expresses her surprise, saying, "I thought Oriental people were very stoic about pain." Which of the following statements about pain is correct. The level of pain
○ 1. perception varies widely from person to person.
○ 2. tolerance is about the same in all people.
○ 3. tolerance is determined by a person's genetic makeup.
○ 4. perception is about the same in all people.

93. The nurse finds it difficult to satisfactorily relieve the client's pain. Which of the following measures should the nurse take into consideration when continuing efforts to promote comfort?
○ 1. Improving the nurse–client relationship.
○ 2. Enlisting the help of the client's family.
○ 3. Allowing the client additional time for privacy to work through his responses to pain.
○ 4. Arranging to have the client share a room with a client who has little pain.

94. After 5 days of hospitalization, the client asks for pain medication with increasing frequency and exhibits increased anxiety and restlessness. What is the probable cause of his behavior?
○ 1. His physical condition is deteriorating.
○ 2. He is becoming addicted to the narcotic.
○ 3. His coping mechanisms are exhausted.
○ 4. He has developed tolerance to his narcotic dosage.

95. The client tells the nurse, "If I could be among my people, I could receive acupuncture for this pain." The nurse should understand that acupuncture in the Oriental culture is based on the theory that it
○ 1. eliminates evil spirits.
○ 2. promotes tranquility with God.
○ 3. restores the balance of energy.
○ 4. blocks nerve pathways to the brain.

96. When the client complains of pain at the site of his surgical incision, where in the brain is he perceiving the pain?
○ 1. Thalamus.
○ 2. Brain stem.
○ 3. Cerebellum.
○ 4. Cerebral cortex.

97. The client's physician decides to change the medication to oral meperidine hydrochloride (Demerol). His current dose is ordered as 75 mg IM q 4 h p.r.n. What dosage of oral meperidine hydrochloride will be required to provide an equivalent analgesic dose?
○ 1. 25 to 50 mg.
○ 2. 75 to 100 mg.
○ 3. 125 to 150 mg.
○ 4. 250 to 300 mg.

98. Meperidine hydrochloride (Demerol) is an effective in pain reliever because of its ability to
○ 1. reduce the perception of pain.
○ 2. decrease the sensitivity of pain receptors.
○ 3. interfere with pain impulses traveling along sensory nerve fibers.
○ 4. block the conduction of pain impulses along the central nervous system.

99. The nurse bases interventions to reduce pain on the gate-control theory of pain. This theory holds that a regulatory process controls impulses reaching the brain. This regulatory process is believed to be located in the
○ 1. brain stem.
○ 2. cerebellum.
○ 3. spinal cord.
○ 4. hypothalamus.

100. Common behavioral responses to pain occur. The body typically and automatically responds to pain first with attempts to improve its ability to

○ 1. tolerate the pain.
○ 2. decrease the perception of pain.
○ 3. escape the source of pain.
○ 4. divert attention from the source of pain.

101. Ergotamine tartrate (Gynergen) is prescribed for the client's migraine headaches. The nurse would judge correctly that the desired effect of the drug is being accomplished when the client reports that it
○ 1. aborts the migraine attacks.
○ 2. reduces the severity of migraine attacks.
○ 3. relieves the sleeplessness experienced in the past after a migraine attack.
○ 4. decreases the visual problems experienced in the past after a migraine attack.

102. The pain associated with migraine headaches is believed to be due to
○ 1. dilation of the cranial arteries.
○ 2. a temporary decrease in intracranial pressure.
○ 3. irritation and inflammation of the openings of the sinuses.
○ 4. sustained contraction of muscles around the scalp and face.

103. The client is evaluated at the pain center, and biofeedback therapy is suggested. The purpose of biofeedback is to enable the client to exert control over physiologic processes by
○ 1. regulating the body processes through electrical control.
○ 2. shocking himself when an undesirable response is elicited.
○ 3. monitoring his body processes for the therapist to interpret.
○ 4. translating signals of his body processes into observable forms.

104. According to current pain theory, the primary reason a back rub effectively relieves pain is because it
○ 1. stimulates large-diameter cutaneous fibers to block the pain impulses from the spinal cord to the brain.
○ 2. stimulates small-diameter cutaneous fibers and blocks the pain impulses from the brain to the spinal cord.
○ 3. stimulates the release of endorphins.
○ 4. distracts the client from focusing on the source of the pain.

105. Research studies have demonstrated that patient-controlled analgesia is more effective than intermittent narcotic administration. Which response by the nurse to a client asking about patient-controlled analgesia reflects knowledge of these research findings? "Patient-controlled analgesia is more effective because
○ 1. a different narcotic is used."
○ 2. two narcotics are administered simultaneously."
○ 3. the client controls the amount of pain medication administered."
○ 4. the nurse interrupts the client less frequently and the client can get more sleep."

106. Nursing responsibilities for the client with a patient-controlled analgesia system would include
○ 1. reassuring the client that pain will be relieved.
○ 2. documenting the client's response to pain medication on a routine basis.
○ 3. instructing the client to continue pressing the system's button whenever pain occurs.
○ 4. titrating pain medication as necessary until the client is free of pain.

107. Which of the following statements represents a major principle of chronic pain management?
○ 1. A physiological approach is most effective.
○ 2. A psychological approach is most effective.
○ 3. Medication is the mainstay of therapy.
○ 4. A multidisciplinary approach is most effective.

108. For a client with pernicious anemia, the nurse would anticipate which of the following clinical manifestations?
○ 1. Incontinence.
○ 2. Sore tongue.
○ 3. Impaired vision.
○ 4. Itchy skin.

109. A client with pernicious anemia asks why she cannot take vitamin B12 orally. The nurse should explain that oral administration is unsatisfactory because
○ 1. gastric juices destroy oral vitamin B12 preparations.
○ 2. oral vitamin B12 preparations are rapidly excreted from the body.
○ 3. a lack of intrinsic factor prevents absorption of vitamin B12.
○ 4. intestinal secretions impede the absorption of oral vitamin B12 preparations.

110. When locating the ventrogluteal site before giving an intramuscular injection, the nurse should place her or his hand on the client's
○ 1. iliac crest.
○ 2. greater trochanter.
○ 3. anterior superior iliac spine.
○ 4. posterior superior iliac spine.

111. The nurse holds the gauze pledget against an intramuscular injection site while removing the needle from the muscle. This technique helps
○ 1. seal off the track left by the needle in the tissue.
○ 2. speed the spread of the medication in the tissue.
○ 3. avoid the discomfort of the needle pulling on the skin.
○ 4. prevent organisms from entering the body through the skin puncture.

112. A client asks why the nurse does not give the intramuscular injection into the upper arm. The nurse should explain that the deltoid muscle is rarely used because the muscle

○ 1. is small.
○ 2. is difficult to locate.
○ 3. has many pain receptors.
○ 4. has a poor blood supply.

113. After administering an intramuscular injection with a disposable needle and syringe, the nurse should dispose of the needle and syringe by

○ 1. cutting the needle at the hilt in a needle cutter before disposing of it in the universal precaution container.
○ 2. leaving the needle uncapped and disposing of the needle and syringe in the universal precaution container.
○ 3. recapping the needle and placing the needle and syringe in the universal precaution container.
○ 4. separating the needle and syringe and placing both in the universal precaution container.

CORRECT ANSWERS AND RATIONALE

The letters in parentheses following the rationale identify the step of the nursing process (A, D, P, I, E); cognitive level (K, C, T, N); and client need (S, G, L, H). See the Answer Grid for the key.

The Client With a Head Injury

1. 3. An operative permit must be signed before any surgical procedure is performed. If the client is unable to sign a permit because of his condition, a responsible relative should be obtained to sign the permit. When a relative is not readily available and when time is of the essence, a letter, telephone call, or telegram may be used to obtain permission. (I, N, S)

2. 1. The highest priority for a client with multiple injuries is to establish an open airway to enable effective ventilation and brain oxygenation. Unless the client is breathing, other care measures will be futile. (I, N, S)

3. 4. The pulse pressure is determined by subtracting the diastolic pressure from the systolic pressure. For example, a client with a blood pressure of 102/60 mm Hg has a pulse pressure of 42 mm Hg. Widening pulse pressure is a sign of increased intracranial pressure. (A, T, G)

4. 1. Increasing intracranial pressure causes unequal pupils from pressure on the third cranial nerve, rising body temperature from hypothalmic damage, and rising systolic pressure, which reflects the additional pressure needed to perfuse the brain. Pressure on the vagus nerve produces bradycardia, not tachycardia. (A, T, G)

5. 1. Neural control of respiration takes place in the brain stem. Deterioration and pressure produce irregular respiratory patterns. Rapid, shallow respirations; asymmetrical chest movements; and nasal flaring are more characteristic of respiratory distress or hypoxia. (A, T, G)

6. 1. The best technique for assessing the gag reflex is to touch the back of the client's throat in the pharyngeal area with a tongue depressor or cotton swab. The reflex is absent if the client does not gag. Reflexes are typically absent or sluggish in the presence of increased intracranial pressure. It is dangerous to place liquids in the mouth of an unconscious client, because of the danger of aspiration. (A, N, S)

7. 1. In a client with increased intracranial pressure, the pupils are likely to be of unequal size and nonreactive to light, and there is no response when the corneas are touched. Altered color of the sclera is not a significant assessment finding in increased intracranial pressure. (A, T, G)

8. 3. The constituents of cerebrospinal fluid (CSF) are similar to those of blood plasma. An examination for glucose content is done to determine whether body fluid is mucus or CSF. Mucus does not contain glucose; CSF does. (A, T, G)

9. 1. The client should be positioned to avoid extreme neck flexion or extension. The head of the bed is usually elevated 30 to 45 degrees to help prevent increased intracranial pressure. (I, T, S)

10. 1. Mannitol (Osmitrol) is an osmotic diuretic that helps decrease intracranial pressure through its dehydrating effects. The drug is acting in the desired manner when urine output increases. It may be desirable to decrease pulse rate, decrease blood pressure, and relax the muscles in certain situations, but mannitol is not used to accomplish these goals. (A, N, G)

11. 4. Explaining where a client is and why he is there helps him become oriented after a period of unconsciousness. Asking the client his name and instructing him to move his hands and feet are done to help determine his level of orientation. (I, T, G)

12. 2. It would be best to wrap the client's hands in washcloths or to have him wear mitts when he becomes restless while regaining consciousness after brain surgery. Restraining him tends to increase activity and restlessness and thus increase intracranial pressure. (I, T, S)

13. 1. Having a client squeeze the nurse's hand is a technique used to assess his motor strength. Noting that the client can feed himself verifies coordination as well as motor ability but does not help the nurse determine muscle strength. The ability to move the legs demonstrates motor ability but not strength. Having the client signal when pressure is applied to his feet tests sensory function. (A, T, G)

14. 3. Coughing is contraindicated for a client at risk for increased intracranial pressure, because coughing increases intracranial pressure. Deep breathing, turning, and passive range-of-motion exercises can be continued. (I, T, S)

15. 2. Diabetes insipidus results from deficiency of antidiuretic hormone (ADH). The condition may occur in conjunction with head injuries as well as with other disorders. In ADH deficiency, the client is extremely thirsty and excretes large amounts of highly diluted urine. The degree of urine concentration is best assessed by measuring the specific gravity of urine samples. (A, C, G)

16. 2. It is not unusual for a client to be disoriented and suffer short-term memory loss after a head injury. Explanations of activities should be simple and given immediately before the procedure. Family members should be encouraged to bring familiar objects from home for the client to see. Clocks, single-date calendars, and other items to help orient the client should be provided. Frequent reassurance and orientation by the nurse and family members will help the client understand the reason for his hospitalization and recognize that he is in a safe environment. Ignoring the client's behavior would not provide the client with the reassurance and assistance that he needs. (I, N, G)

17. 3. Meperidine hydrochloride (Demerol) is a narcotic analgesic. After an IM injection of 100 mg, an adult client would be lethargic an hour later. (E, N, G)

The Client With Seizures

18. 3. In a client subject to seizure activity, temperature should be assessed by a route other than oral when using a mercury thermometer. A glass thermometer could break in the client's mouth if a seizure occurred. (I, T, S)

19. 4. Tonic-clonic (grand mal) seizures characteristically begin with a sudden loss of consciousness and generalized tonic muscle contractions. During this phase, which usually lasts less than 1 minute, the client is apneic. The clonic phase of the seizure then begins, characterized by violent, rhythmic muscle contractions. Respirations resume at this time. Most tonic-clonic seizures last a total of 2 to 5 minutes. (A, C, G)

20. 4. In general, there is no special preparation for a computed tomography (CT) scan. The client will be asked to hold the head very still during the examination, which lasts about 30 to 60 minutes. In some instances, food and fluids may be withheld for 4 to 6 hours before the procedure if a contrast medium is used, because the radiopaque substance sometimes causes nausea. (I, C, S)

21. 2. Beverages containing caffeine, such as coffee, tea, and cola drinks, are withheld before an electroencephalogram (EEG) because of the stimulating effects of the caffeine. A meal should not be omitted before an EEG, because low blood sugar could alter brain wave patterns. (I, C, S)

22. 1. Trauma is one of the primary causes of brain damage and seizure activity in adults. This condition is referred to as posttraumatic epilepsy. Other common causes of seizure activity in adults include neoplasms, withdrawal from drugs and alcohol, and vascular disease. (P, C, G)

23. 2. If a client has a seizure while sitting in a chair, it would be best to ease him to the floor and place a pillow under his head. No effort should be made to restrain him. The strong muscle contractions may cause the client to injure himself if he is restrained. The nurse is likely to be hurt, as well as the client, if the nurse tries to lift him to a bed. Placing an airway in the client's mouth during a seizure is not necessary or recommended. (I, N, S)

24. 1. The position of choice during and following a seizure is the side-lying position, because it facilitates drainage from the mouth and helps prevent aspiration. (I, T, S)

25. 2. A brief period of confusion usually follows a seizure. After this period, the client typically sleeps for a long period. (P, C, G)

26. 4. During a seizure, the nurse should note movement of the client's head, eyes, and extremities, especially when the seizure first begins. Other important assessments would include noting the progression and duration of the seizure; respiratory status; loss of consciousness; pupil size; and incontinence of urine and stool. It is typically not necessary to assess the client's pulse and blood pressure during a tonic-clonic seizure. The nurse should focus on maintaining an open airway and preventing injury to the client. (A, N, G)

27. 2. A client is rarely able to respond to even painful stimuli during a seizure. The client may be incontinent during the seizure and will be quite drowsy after the seizure. Despite drowsiness, however, the client's physical ability to speak should be preserved, and its loss would be unexpected. (A, N, G)

28. 3. Exactly how phenytoin (Dilantin) helps control seizures is unclear. The most common theory posits that it reduces the responsiveness of neurons in the brain to abnormal impulses—that is, it depresses neural activity. (P, C, G)

29. 2. Anticonvulsant drug therapy should never be stopped suddenly; doing so can lead to the life-threatening status epilepticus. Phenytoin (Dilantin) does not carry a risk of physical dependency. It is one of many drugs used to effectively treat tonic-clonic seizure disorders. (P, C, G)

30. 2. Specific motor vehicle regulations and restrictions for persons who experience seizures vary locally. Most commonly, evidence that the seizures are under medical control is required before the person is given permission to drive. It is recommended that a person subject to seizures carry a card or wear an identification bracelet describing the illness so that in an emergency the condition can be quickly identified. (I, C, H)

31. 3. An aura is a premonition of an impending seizure. Auras usually are of a sensory nature (i.e., an olfactory, visual, gustatory, or auditory sensation); some may be of a psychic nature. Evaluating an aura may help identify the area of the brain from which the seizure originates. (I, K, G)

32. 1. Skin rash may indicate a toxic effect of phenytoin (Dilantin). The client should be instructed to come to the physician's office that day for a consultation. The nurse should not instruct the client to adjust or stop the medication; decreasing or stopping the drug dosage may lead to increased seizure activity. (I, N, G)

33. 3. A common side effect of long-term phenytoin therapy is an overgrowth of gingival tissues. Problems may be minimized with good oral hygiene, but in some cases overgrown tissues may have to be removed surgically. (E, C, G)

The Client With a Cerebrovascular Accident

34. 2. Rehabilitation for a client who has sustained a cerebrovascular accident should begin at the time the client is admitted to the hospital. The first goal of rehabilitation should be to help prevent the client from developing deformities. This goal is achieved through such techniques as positioning the client properly in bed, changing his position frequently, and supporting all parts of his body in proper alignment. Passive range-of-motion exercises may also be started, unless contraindicated. (P, C, G)

35. 1. A helpless client should be positioned on the side, not on the back, with the head over a small pillow. This positioning helps secretions escape from the throat and mouth and minimizes the risk of aspiration. Suctioning equipment should be available, the client's mouth should be opened with a padded tongue blade, and the mouth and teeth can be cleaned with a toothbrush. (I, N, S)

36. 3. Based on the data provided, the most appropriate nursing diagnosis is Impaired Physical Mobility. There are no data to indicate that this client is suffering from a disturbance in body image or an inability to tolerate activity. There also is no indication that the client is neglecting the right side of his body. (D, N, G)

37. 2. Sliding a client on a sheet causes friction and should be avoided. Friction tends to injure skin tissues and predispose to decubitus ulcer formation. Rolling the client, lifting him on a drawsheet, and having him help lift himself off the bed with a trapeze all help prevent friction from being moved in bed. (I, T, G)

38. 3. Regular repositioning and range-of-motion exercises are important interventions, but the use of ankle-high tennis shoes has been found to be most effective in preventing plantar flexion (footdrop). Foot boards stimulate spasms and are not routinely recommended. (I, N, S)

39. 1. Broca's area, which controls expressive speech, is located on the left side of the brain. Therefore, a client with a cerebrovascular accident in this area is likely to exhibit expressive or motor aphasia. Dyslexia, the inability of a person with normal vision to interpret written language, is thought to be due to a central nervous system defect in the ability to organize graphic symbols. Apraxia is the inability to perform purposeful movements in the absence or loss of motor power, sensation, or coordination. Agnosia is the loss of comprehension of auditory, visual, or other sensations despite an intact sensory sphere. (P, C, G)

40. 2. Although the client with expressive aphasia is unable to communicate verbally, he can understand what is being said to him. The client's communication with others may be helped by a communication or picture board on which he can point to objects or activities he desires. (I, T, S)

41. 2. A client with dysphagia (difficulty swallowing) frequently has the most difficulty ingesting liquids, which are easily aspirated. Measures that minimize the risk of aspiration in a client with dysphagia include maintaining an upright position while eating (unless contraindicated), introducing foods on the unaffected side of the mouth, and keeping distractions to a minimum. (I, N, S)

42. 4. Reestablishing urinary continence is a realistic goal for most stroke clients. The client should be assisted to a normal voiding position and instructed to try to urinate. Foley catheters pose a serious infection risk, and neither indwelling nor external catheters address the goal of reestablishing urinary continence. (I, N, G)

43. 3. When dressing, the client should put clothing on the affected side first. He should wear normal clothing, if possible. Other people may help the client dress, but the emphasis should be on self-care. (I, T, H)

44. 1. Expressive aphasia involves a problem with speaking. Reception remains intact, and the nurse does not need to use other cues for communication or to adjust voice level. (I, T, G)

45. 2. Although many eating behaviors may be disturbed after a cerebrovascular accident, eating food on only half the plate would result from an inability to coordinate visual images and spatial relationships. (E, C, G)

46. 4. To expand the visual field, the partially sighted client should be taught to turn his head from side to side when walking. Neglecting to do so may result in accidents. This technique helps maximize the use of remaining sight. A patch does not address the problem of hemianopsia. Appropriate positioning of the client and personal items will increase his ability to cope with the problem, but will not affect his safety. (I, T, S)

47. 3. A client who has brain damage may be emotionally labile and may cry or laugh for no explainable reason. "Crying jags" are best dealt with by attempting to divert the client's attention. Ignoring the behavior or attempting to deal with it behaviorally will not affect it. (I, N, L)

48. 4. When offering emotional support to a client who is discouraged and has a negative self-concept because of physical handicaps, the nurse should display encouragement and patience. The client should be praised when he shows progress in his efforts to overcome handicaps. Sympathy, charity, and firm discipline have little supportive value. (I, N, L)

49. 1. The strong support of family members is frequently identified as an important factor that influences a stroke client's continuing progress in rehabilitation after discharge. Discharge planning should prepare the client and family for the many changes that will be necessary when the client returns home. Family support groups can be beneficial in guiding and supporting families in the care of the client. An effective discharge plan will coordinate the resources of the client, family, and community. (P, N, H)

The Client With Parkinson's Disease

50. 4. Typical signs of Parkinson's disease include drooling; a low-pitched, monotonous voice; and a stiff, masklike facial expression. Aphasia is not a symptom of Parkinson's disease. An exaggerated sense of euphoria would not be typical; more likely, the client will exhibit depression, probably related to the progressive nature of the disease and the client's difficulties in dealing with it. Many clients also begin to show a decline in cognitive, memory, and perceptual abilities. (A, C, G)

51. 3. A propulsive gait, a typical disorder of locomotion noted in Parkinson's disease, is characterized by a tendency to take increasingly quicker steps while walking. This type of gait often causes the client to fall or to have trouble stopping. (A, C, G)

52. 2. Voluntary and purposeful movements will often temporarily decrease or stop the tremors associated with Parkinson's disease. However, in some clients tremors may increase with voluntary effort. Tremors are not psychological in nature and cannot be willfully controlled. (E, C, G)

53. 2. Demanding physical activity should be performed during the peak action of drug therapy. Clients should be encouraged to maintain independence in self-care activities to the greatest extent possible. Adequate time should be allowed to perform these self-care activities. (I, N, G)

54. 4. Parkinson's disease progresses in severity, and there is no known cure or way to stop its progression. However, many clients live for years with the disease, and it would not be appropriate to start planning terminal care at this time for this client. The most appropriate and realistic goal is to help the client function at his best. (P, N, G)

55. 1. Muscle rigidity, which can lead to contracture, is a major symptom of Parkinson's disease. Physical therapy is aimed at maintaining joint flexibility and relaxing muscles. (P, C, G)

56. 2. Levodopa (L-Dopa) is prescribed to decrease severe muscle rigidity. Its effectiveness is primarily measured by the client's response in this area. (E, C, G)

57. 4. Increasing doses of levodopa put a client at serious risk for toxicity. Severe mental deterioration such as delusions or hallucinations frequently occur in the toxic state, and family members must be instructed about this possibility. (I, K, G)

58. 4. A high-protein diet reduces the effectiveness of levodopa. Limiting dietary protein intake may improve the drug's effectiveness, especially during the daytime hours, when the drug action is most critical to normal functioning. (I, C, H)

59. 2. Ongoing self-care is a major goal for clients with Parkinson's disease. The client should be given additional time as needed and praised for his efforts to remain independent. (I, N, L)

60. 4. The primary reason for having a client with Parkinson's disease read aloud is to help him increase his awareness of the typical low-pitched, monotonous tone of his voice. Doing so makes it easier for the client to modify intonation and speak more clearly. (P, N, G)

The Client With Multiple Sclerosis

61. 4. Factors that may aggravate the symptoms of multiple sclerosis include fatigue, hot baths or showers, overexertion, exposure to climatic temperature extremes, and stress. There is no evidence that a high-protein diet will cause an exacerbation of multiple sclerosis. (A, C, G)

62. 2. Visual disturbances, speech impairment, problems with walking associated with loss of muscle tone and tremors, spastic weakness in the extremities, and dizziness with nausea and vomiting are some common symptoms of multiple sclerosis. Hyperexcitability and euphoria may occur, but, because of muscle weakness, sudden bursts of energy are unlikely. (A, C, G)

63. 1. Typical complications of multiple sclerosis include contractures, decubitus ulcers, and respiratory infections. Nursing care should be directed toward the goal of preventing these complications. Ascites is not associated with multiple sclerosis. (P, C, G)

64. 3. Baclofen (Lioresal) is a centrally acting skeletal muscle relaxant that helps relieve the muscle spasms common in multiple sclerosis. Methocarbamol (Robaxin) is another skeletal muscle relaxant used to treat multiple sclerosis; the nurse may encounter others in practice. (E, C, G)

65. 2. Evaluating drug effectiveness is difficult, because a high percentage of clients with multiple sclerosis exhibit unpredictable episodes of remission, exacerbation, and steady progress without apparent cause. (E, C, G)

66. 4. Such practices as asking a client with slurred speech to speak slowly and distinctly and to repeat indistinguishable words tend to improve her ability to communicate effectively. Asking a client to speak louder even when tired may aggravate the problem. (I, N, G)

67. 4. Nurse's notes should be concise, objective, clearly stated, and relevant. This client trembles when she attempts voluntary action such as drinking a beverage or fastening clothing. This activity should be described exactly as it occurs so that others reading the note will have no doubt about the nurse's observation of the client's behavior. (I, N, S)

68. 4. Limiting fluid intake is likely to aggravate rather than relieve symptoms when a bowel-training program is being implemented. Furthermore, water imbalance, as well as electrolyte imbalance, tends to aggravate symptoms of multiple sclerosis. (I, T, H)

69. 1. Clients with multiple sclerosis often experience psychological disturbances that are best described as mood disorders. Emotional instability is typical. Thought disorders, psychosomatic illnesses, and drug dependency are not typical of clients with multiple sclerosis, unless these disorders are present independently. (P, T, L)

70. 2. Care for the client with multiple sclerosis is directed toward muscle rehabilitation and client motivation. The disease is chronic; thus, goals should be those with the most benefit over a prolonged period. (P, T, H)

71. 2. The nurse's most positive approach is to encourage a client with multiple sclerosis to keep active while avoiding emotional upset and fatigue. A quiet, inactive life-style is not necessarily indicated. Good health habits will not likely alter the course of the disease, although they may help minimize complications. Practicing using aids that will be needed for future disabilities may be helpful, but also possibly discouraging. (I, N, L)

72. 2. Safety concerns are essential for a client with sensory impairment. Water temperature should be tested carefully, hot water bottles should be avoided, and the skin should be inspected regularly. Independence and self-care are also important; the client should not be instructed to avoid kitchen activities out of fear of injury. (I, N, H)

73. 3. Establishing a regular fluid intake of 2,000 to 3,000 ml/day and maintaining a regular voiding pattern would be the most appropriate measure to help the client avoid urinary incontinence. Inserting an indwelling catheter would be a treatment of last resort, because of the increased risk for infection. If catheterization is required, intermittent self-catheterization is preferred because of its lower risk of infection. (P, T, G)

74. 2. A client with multiple sclerosis usually does best and is least frustrated at home when a regular program of daily activities is planned. There is no information given in this item suggesting that psychological counseling is necessary or that it would be helpful to have the granddaughter attend a day-care center. A weekly visit by another person with multiple sclerosis may not be contraindicated, but it is less likely to benefit the client as much as a regular program of planned activities. (I, N, L)

The Unconscious Client

75. 3. Equal, normally reactive pupils indicate adequate neurologic functioning. Progressive pupil dilation indicates increased intracranial pressure, and fixed dilated pupils indicate injury at the midbrain. Overdose of amphetamines, alcohol, or cocaine also causes dilated pupils; overdose of morphine and barbiturates results in constricted pupils. Blood pressure is regulated by various factors, and a finding of hypertension would not pinpoint a toxic disorder. Fever is related either to infection or dehydration. Facial asymmetry indicates paralysis. (A, T, G)

76. 1. An unconscious client is best positioned in a lateral or semiprone position because these positions allow the jaw and tongue to fall forward, facilitate drainage of secretions, and prevent aspiration. Positioning the client supine carries a major risk of airway obstruction from the tongue, vomitus, or nasopharyngeal secretions. Trendelenburg's position, with the head lower than the heart, decreases effective lung volume and increases the risk of cerebral edema. The lithotomy position has no purpose in this situation. (I, N, S)

77. 3. Activated charcoal powder is administered to absorb remaining particles of salicylate. Vitamin K (AquaMEPHYTON) is an antidote for warfarin (Coumadin). Dextrose 50% is an antidote for insulin. Sodium thiosulfate is an antidote for cyanide. (P, K, G)

78. 3. The initial response to crisis is high anxiety. Anxiety must dissipate before a person can deal with the actual situation. Allowing family members to ventilate their feelings can help this dissipation. The reasons for the client's actions are unknown; assumptions must be validated before they become facts. Touch can be appropriate, but not when used as false reassurance. Helping with the client's care is appropriate at a later time. (I, N, L)

79. 2. The frequency of turning depends primarily on the condition of the client's skin. Every 2 hours is usually sufficient; however, some clients may need to be turned as often as every 30 to 60 minutes. (E, T, G)

80. 3. When pressure is applied to the skin, the area first becomes blanched, or whitish. When pressure is relieved, the circulation tends to carry excess blood to the area to make up for the temporary decrease in blood supply. This effect, called reactive hyperemia, causes the skin to redden. Such a reddened area is a precursor of a pressure sore. (A, C, G)

81. 2. Decubitus ulcers are caused by prolonged pressure on an area, which in turn decreases circulation to that area. The poorly oxygenated tissues then tend to break down, causing a decubitus ulcer. The primary reason for massaging areas at risk for decubitus ulcers is to improve circulation in the area. The massage may help relax muscles and dry the skin, but these are of less importance in this situation. (I, C, G)

82. 3. Common pressure points in the side-lying position include the ears, shoulders, ribs, greater trochanter, medial and lateral condyles, and the ankles. (P, T, G)

83. 3. The client will not be in proper body alignment if, when in the right side-lying position, his left arm rests on the mattress with the elbow flexed. This positioning of the arm pulls the left shoulder out of good alignment, restricting respiratory movements. The arm should be supported on a pillow. (I, T, G)

84. 3. Trochanter rolls placed alongside the client's legs from the ilium to midthigh are recommended to prevent external rotation of the hips. Placing sandbags from the knees to the ankle will not effectively support the hips in proper alignment. Pillows can be used only as a temporary measure, because they cannot hold the legs and hips in proper alignment over a prolonged period. A footboard does not help keep the legs and hips in proper alignment. (I, T, G)

85. 4. Passive range-of-motion exercises are performed to maintain joint mobility. They will not have a positive affect on the client's muscle tone or bone structure. Active exercise is needed to preserve bone and muscle mass. (P, C, S)

86. 1. The nurse should keep suction equipment available to remove secretions, and should place the client in a side-lying position. Performing oral hygiene is a clean procedure, therefore, the nurse wears clean gloves, not sterile gloves. The nurse should never place any fingers in an unconscious client's mouth; the client may bite down. Padded tongue blades, swabs, or a toothbrush should be used instead. (I, T, S)

87. 2. When the blink reflex is absent or the eyes do not close completely, the cornea may become dry and irritated. Placing a patch over the eye is the most appropriate intervention to prevent eye injury. (I, N, S)

88. 3. Restlessness is an early indicator of hypoxia. The nurse should suspect hypoxia in the unconscious client who becomes restless. The most accurate method for determining the presence of hypoxia is to evaluate arterial blood gas values. Cyanosis and decreased respirations are late indicators of hypoxia. Hypertension, not hypotension, is a sign of hypoxia. (A, T, G)

89. 2. The client should be placed in a semi-Fowler's position to reduce the risk of aspiration. The formula should be at room temperature, not heated. Administering enteral tube feedings is a clean procedure, not a sterile one; thus, sterile supplies are not required. Clients receiving enteral feedings should be weighed regularly, but not necessarily before each feeding. (I, T, S)

90. 4. Gastric residuals are checked before administration of enteral feedings to determine whether gastric emptying is delayed. A gastric residual of less than 50% of the previous feeding volume is usually considered acceptable. If the amount of gastric residual is excessive, the nurse notifies the physician and holds the feeding. If only a small amount of gastric residual is obtained, the nurse reinstills it through the tube and then administers the feeding. Reinstilling the residual helps prevent electrolyte and fluid losses. (I, N, S)

91. 1. It is generally agreed that bladder infections in a client with an indwelling catheter result from infections that ascend from the urethra into the bladder. Good catheter care, including meticulous cleansing of the area around the urethral meatus, is of the highest priority for the client with an indwelling catheter. Clamping an indwelling catheter is not recommended. (I, N, S)

The Client in Pain

92. 1. Pain perception is an individual experience. Research indicates that pain tolerance and perception varies widely among people due to individual differences. (P, C, G)

93. 1. Experience has demonstrated that clients who feel confidence in the personnel caring for them do not require as much therapy for pain relief as those who have less confidence. Without the client's confidence, developed in an effective nurse-client relationship, other interventions may be less effective. (P, N, L)

94. 4. Physical tolerance to a regular narcotic dose develops rapidly with frequent use. The client experiences increased discomfort, asks for medication more frequently, and exhibits anxious and restless behavior, which is often misinterpreted as indicative of developing dependence or addiction. (A, N, G)

95. 3. Acupuncture, like acumassage and acupressure, is performed in certain Oriental cultures to help restore the energy balance within the body. Pressure, massage, and fine needles are applied to "energy pathways" to help restore the body's balance. In the Western world, many researchers think that the gate-control theory of pain may be applicable to acupuncture, acumassage, and acupressure. (P, K, L)

96. 4. Pain is perceived in the cerebral cortex. (A, K, G)

97. 4. The equianalgesic dose of oral meperidine hydrochloride (Demerol) is up to four times the intramuscular dose. Although meperidine hydrochloride can be given orally, it is more effective when given intramuscularly. (I, K, G)

98. 1. Narcotic analgesics relieve pain by reducing or altering the perception of pain. They do not decrease the sensitivity of pain receptors, interfere with pain impulses traveling along sensory nerve fibers, or block the conduction of pain impulses in the central nervous system. (P, C, G)

99. 3. According to the gate-control theory, the regulatory process that controls pain impulses reaching the brain most probably occurs in the spinal cord. (P, C, G)

100. 3. Responses to pain are directed initially toward the body's ability to escape or flee the source of pain. The response is typical of the fight-or-flight phenomenon, first described by Walter B. Cannon when working on theories of homeostasis and fear. (A, C, G)

101. 1. Ergotamine tartrate (Gynergen) is used to help abort a migraine attack. The drug acts as a vasoconstrictor. It should be taken as soon as prodromal symptoms of migraine appear. The drug is not used to reduce severity of headaches, relieve sleeplessness after an attack, or decrease visual problems after an attack. (A, T, G)

102. 1. A vascular disturbance involving branches of the carotid artery is believed to cause migraine attacks. Vasoconstriction of blood vessels apparently occurs first. The extracranial and intracranial arteries then dilate, causing the headache. Family history of migraine is present in more than half of all persons with migraine. (A, K, G)

103. 4. Biofeedback aims to translate body processes into observable signs, which the client can use to exercise some control over certain body processes. For example, a biofeedback machine measures a client's pulse rate and displays the information. The client is then instructed to try to lower the pulse rate, using such techniques as listening to relaxing music or thinking of a pleasant scene. If any action lowers the pulse rate, the client learns to continue to do whatever it was that decreased the pulse rate. The reinforcement of learning is immediate, because the client can see the results of his actions. (P, T, G)

104. 1. Massage stimulates the large-diameter cutaneous fibers, which block transmission of pain impulses from the spinal cord to the brain. Although massage may have other positive effects, such as distracting the client, the physiological process of fiber stimulation supports using massage as therapy for pain relief. (A, C, G)

105. 3. Studies have supported that one reason patient-controlled analgesia is effective is because the client has control over the narcotic administration. Morphine is the most commonly used narcotic in patient-controlled analgesia. Only one narcotic is administered at a time. Nursing assessments and actions remain basically the same for the client using patient-controlled analgesia. (I, T, G)

106. 2. It is essential that the nurse documents the client's response to pain medication on a routine, systematic basis. Through careful assessment and documentation, the effectiveness of pain relief interventions can be evaluated and modified, if necessary. Reassuring the client that pain will be relieved is often not realistic. A client who continually presses the patient-controlled analgesia button may not be getting adequate pain relief. Pain medication is not titrated. (I, T, S)

107. 4. A multidisciplinary approach to pain relief is needed for greatest effectiveness. In addition to the client, the nurse, and the physician, others that may be needed on the team include a social worker, an occupational therapist, a dietician, and a psychologist or a psychiatrist. Pain relief interventions based on physiological and psychological principles can be used simultaneously to obtain greater pain relief. Medication administration is only one option for reducing pain. (E, N, S)

108. 2. Clients with pernicious anemia almost always complain of a sore tongue. The tongue appears smooth and red. (A, T, G)

109. 3. Pernicious anemia is caused by the absence of intrinsic factor, which is necessary for the absorption of vitamin B12 in the gastrointestinal tract. In the absence of intrinsic factor, orally administered vitamin B12 cannot be absorbed in the body. (I, N, G)

110. 2. To locate the ventrogluteal site, the nurse places the palm on the client's greater trochanter with the index finger on the anterior superior iliac spine. The posterior iliac spine is a landmark for locating the dorsogluteal site. The site should be carefully and correctly identified to avoid tissue or nerve damage. (I, K, S)

111. 3. Holding a pledget against an injection site while removing the needle helps prevent the needle from pulling on the skin. The technique makes any injection more comfortable. (I, K, S)

112. 1. Because the deltoid muscle is small, any injection into it is relatively uncomfortable. The muscle is very easy to locate. It has pain receptors and a good blood supply, just as do the other muscles in the body. (I, K, S)

113. 2. Universal precautions for care of needles and syringes involve *never* recapping used needles. Immediately after giving an injection, the nurse should place the entire needle and syringe set in the universal precautions container in the client's room. (I, K, S)

THE NURSING CARE OF ADULTS WITH MEDICAL/SURGICAL HEALTH PROBLEMS

TEST 8: The Client With Neurological Health Problems

Directions: Use this answer grid to determine areas of strength or need for further study.

Nursing Process

A = Assessment
D = Analysis, nursing diagnosis
P = Planning
I = Implementation
E = Evaluation

Cognitive Level

K = Knowledge
C = Comprehension
T = Application
N = Analysis

Client Needs

S = Safe, effective care environment
G = Physiological integrity
L = Psychosocial integrity
H = Health promotion/maintenance

		Nursing Process					Cognitive Level				Client Needs			
Question #	Answer #	A	D	P	I	E	K	C	T	N	S	G	L	H
1	3				I					N	S			
2	1				I					N	S			
3	4	A							T			G		
4	1	A							T			G		
5	1	A							T			G		
6	1	A								N	S			
7	1	A							T			G		
8	3	A							T			G		
9	1				I				T		S			
10	1	A								N		G		
11	4				I				T			G		
12	2				I				T		S			
13	1	A							T			G		
14	3				I				T		S			
15	2	A						C				G		
16	2				I					N		G		
17	3					E				N		G		
18	3				I				T		S			
19	4	A						C				G		
20	4				I			C			S			
21	2				I			C			S			
22	1			P				C				G		
23	2				I					N	S			

ANSWER GRID: 1

Nursing Process

A = Assessment
D = Analysis, nursing diagnosis
P = Planning
I = Implementation
E = Evaluation

Cognitive Level

K = Knowledge
C = Comprehension
T = Application
N = Analysis

Client Needs

S = Safe, effective care environment
G = Physiological integrity
L = Psychosocial integrity
H = Health promotion/maintenance

		Nursing Process					Cognitive Level				Client Needs			
Question #	Answer #	A	D	P	I	E	K	C	T	N	S	G	L	H
24	1				I				T		S			
25	2			P				C				G		
26	4	A								N		G		
27	2	A								N		G		
28	3			P				C				G		
29	2			P				C				G		
30	2				I			C						H
31	3				I		K					G		
32	1				I					N		G		
33	3					E		C				G		
34	2			P				C				G		
35	1				I					N	S			
36	3		D							N		G		
37	2				I				T			G		
38	3				I					N	S			
39	1			P				C				G		
40	2				I				T		S			
41	2				I					N	S			
42	4				I					N		G		
43	3				I				T					H
44	1				I				T			G		
45	2					E		C				G		
46	4				I				T		S			
47	3				I					N			L	
48	4				I					N			L	
49	1			P						N				H
50	4	A						C				G		
51	3	A						C				G		
52	2					E		C				G		

Answer Grid: 2

NURSING PROCESS

A = Assessment
D = Analysis, nursing diagnosis
P = Planning
I = Implementation
E = Evaluation

COGNITIVE LEVEL

K = Knowledge
C = Comprehension
T = Application
N = Analysis

CLIENT NEEDS

S = Safe, effective care environment
G = Physiological integrity
L = Psychosocial integrity
H = Health promotion/maintenance

		Nursing Process					Cognitive Level				Client Needs			
Question #	Answer #	A	D	P	I	E	K	C	T	N	S	G	L	H
53	2				I					N		G		
54	4			P						N		G		
55	1			P				C				G		
56	2					E		C				G		
57	4				I		K					G		
58	4				I			C						H
59	2				I					N			L	
60	4			P						N		G		
61	4	A						C				G		
62	2	A						C				G		
63	1			P				C				G		
64	3					E		C				G		
65	2					E		C				G		
66	4				I					N		G		
67	4				I					N	S			
68	4				I				T					H
69	1			P					T				L	
70	2			P					T					H
71	2				I					N			L	
72	2				I					N				H
73	3			P					T			G		
74	2				I					N			L	
75	3	A							T			G		
76	1				I					N	S			
77	3			P			K					G		
78	3				I					N			L	
79	2					E			T			G		
80	3	A						C				G		
81	2				I			C				G		

ANSWER GRID: 3

Nursing Process

A = Assessment
D = Analysis, nursing diagnosis
P = Planning
I = Implementation
E = Evaluation

Cognitive Level

K = Knowledge
C = Comprehension
T = Application
N = Analysis

Client Needs

S = Safe, effective care environment
G = Physiological integrity
L = Psychosocial integrity
H = Health promotion/maintenance

		Nursing Process					Cognitive Level				Client Needs			
Question #	Answer #	A	D	P	I	E	K	C	T	N	S	G	L	H
82	3			P					T			G		
83	3				I				T			G		
84	3				I				T			G		
85	4			P				C			S			
86	1				I				T		S			
87	2				I					N	S			
88	3	A							T			G		
89	2				I				T		S			
90	4				I					N	S			
91	1				I					N	S			
92	1			P				C				G		
93	1			P						N			L	
94	4	A								N		G		
95	3			P			K						L	
96	4	A					K					G		
97	4				I		K					G		
98	1			P				C				G		
99	3			P				C				G		
100	3	A						C				G		
101	1	A							T			G		
102	1	A					K					G		
103	4			P					T			G		
104	1	A						C				G		
105	3				I				T			G		
106	2				I				T		S			
107	4					E				N	S			
108	2	A							T			G		
109	3				I					N		G		
110	2				I		K				S			

ANSWER GRID: 4

NURSING PROCESS

A = Assessment
D = Analysis, nursing diagnosis
P = Planning
I = Implementation
E = Evaluation

COGNITIVE LEVEL

K = Knowledge
C = Comprehension
T = Application
N = Analysis

CLIENT NEEDS

S = Safe, effective care environment
G = Physiological integrity
L = Psychosocial integrity
H = Health promotion/maintenance

		Nursing Process					Cognitive Level				Client Needs			
Question #	Answer #	A	D	P	I	E	K	C	T	N	S	G	L	H
111	3				I		K				S			
112	1				I		K				S			
113	2				I		K				S			
Number Correct														
Number Possible	113	26	1	23	54	9	11	32	34	36	30	67	9	7
Percentage Correct														

Score Calculation:

To determine your **Percentage Correct**, divide the **Number Correct** by the **Number Possible**.

ANSWER GRID: 5

The Client With Musculoskeletal Health Problems

Test 9

The Client With Arthritis
The Client With a Hip Fracture
The Client With a Herniated Disc
The Client With Peripheral Vascular Disease
The Client With a Femoral Fracture
The Client With a Spinal Cord Injury
Correct Answers and Rationale

Select the one best answer and indicate your choice by filling in the circle in front of the option.

The Client With Arthritis

A 60-year-old female with the diagnosis of rheumatoid arthritis has been hospitalized for an evaluation of her increasingly impaired physical mobility.

1. The client asks the nurse to explain why her joints are becoming increasingly painful. The nurse's response should be based on knowledge that rheumatoid arthritis

- ○ 1. results from degenerative joint damage.
- ○ 2. affects only the weight-bearing joints of the body.
- ○ 3. begins with inflammation of joint synovial tissue.
- ○ 4. is usually caused by aging.

2. The client has been taking large doses of aspirin to relieve her joint pain. The nurse should assess the client for which important symptom of aspirin toxicity?

- ○ 1. Dysuria.
- ○ 2. Tinnitus.
- ○ 3. Chest pain.
- ○ 4. Drowsiness.

3. Which statement by the client would indicate that she needs additional teaching to safely receive the maximum benefit of her aspirin therapy?

- ○ 1. "I always take aspirin with food to protect my stomach."
- ○ 2. "Once I learned to take my aspirin with meals, I was able to start using the inexpensive generic brand."
- ○ 3. "I always watch for bleeding gums or blood in my stool."
- ○ 4. "I try to take aspirin only on days when the pain seems particularly bad."

4. Based on analysis of the client's symptoms, the nurse formulates a nursing diagnosis Activity Intolerance related to lack of energy conservation. Which of the following activities would the nurse likely choose to implement in response to this nursing diagnosis?

- ○ 1. Encourage the client to perform all tasks early in the day.
- ○ 2. Encourage the client to alternate periods of rest and activity throughout the day.
- ○ 3. Administer narcotics to promote pain relief and rest.
- ○ 4. Instruct the client to not perform daily hygienic care until activity tolerance improves.

5. Which of the following symptoms of arthritis is unique to rheumatoid arthritis?

- ○ 1. Joint pain.
- ○ 2. Joint stiffness.
- ○ 3. Limited joint movement.
- ○ 4. Joint swelling.

6. The client tells the nurse, "I have a friend who took gold shots and had a wonderful response. Why didn't my doctor let me try that?" Which of the following replies by the nurse would be best?

○ 1. "It would be best if you asked the doctor."
○ 2. "Tell me more about your friend's arthritic condition. Maybe I can answer that question for you."
○ 3. "That drug is used for cases that are worse than yours. It wouldn't help you."
○ 4. "You shouldn't try to compare your condition with anyone else's. Every patient is different."

7. The physician recommends that the client undergo a right total knee replacement. In planning the client's postoperative care, the nurse should consider that clients with rheumatoid arthritis should usually be positioned so as to
○ 1. decrease edema around the joints.
○ 2. promote maximum comfort.
○ 3. prevent venous stasis.
○ 4. prevent flexion deformities of the joints.

8. In the postoperative period, the client finds it very painful to move, and she resists efforts to change her position in bed. Which nursing action would be most appropriate?
○ 1. Admonish the client for her negative attitude toward therapy.
○ 2. Explain to the client why turning and realignment are necessary.
○ 3. Remind the client that she is to blame if she develops complications.
○ 4. Point out to the client that she is not following her doctor's directions.

9. Postoperatively, the client's right leg is placed in a continuous passive motion (CPM) machine. Nursing responsibilities when caring for a client with this apparatus would include all of the following except:
○ 1. adjusting the settings as needed to prevent client discomfort.
○ 2. checking the range-of-motion settings at least every 8 hours.
○ 3. maintaining proper positioning of the joint on the CPM machine.
○ 4. evaluating the client's response to the CPM therapy.

10. The nurse teaches the client to perform isometric exercises to strengthen her leg muscles after surgery. Isometric exercises are particularly effective for clients with rheumatoid arthritis because they
○ 1. cost little in terms of time and money.
○ 2. strengthen the muscles while keeping the joints stationary.
○ 3. involve clients in their own care and thus improve morale.
○ 4. prevent joint stiffness.

11. When preparing the client to ambulate after her surgery, the nurse should explain the quadriceps-setting exercises. These exercises are accomplished by
○ 1. bending the knee to form a right angle.
○ 2. rotating the leg slowly around in circles.
○ 3. pressing the back of the knee into the mattress.
○ 4. turning the leg inward toward the opposite thigh.

12. The client wants to protect herself from "quack" treatments for her arthritis and asks the nurse, "How can I tell what is valid and good for me and what isn't?" The nurse's reply should be based on the fact that genuine and reputable products are most often available through
○ 1. testimonials inserted in leading magazines.
○ 2. advertisements in circulars received in the mail.
○ 3. prescriptions and treatments individually prescribed by health care professionals.
○ 4. special clinics that promote curative remedies.

A 70-year-old male has been diagnosed with degenerative joint disease (osteoarthritis) of the left hip.

13. In osteoarthritis, it would be reasonable to expect that which of the following joints would least likely be affected by the disease?
○ 1. Hip.
○ 2. Knee.
○ 3. Finger.
○ 4. Shoulder.

14. Which of the following factors would be most likely to increase joint symptoms of osteoarthritis?
○ 1. A long history of smoking.
○ 2. Excessive alcohol use.
○ 3. Obesity.
○ 4. Emotional stress.

15. The client's physician orders ibuprofen (Motrin) to treat the left hip pain. To minimize gastric mucosal irritation, the nurse should teach the client to take this medication
○ 1. at bedtime.
○ 2. on arising.
○ 3. immediately after a meal.
○ 4. when her stomach is empty.

16. The client reports increasingly severe pain in the left hip; the physician recommends a total hip replacement. Preoperative nursing care for this client should begin with
○ 1. teaching how to prevent hip flexion.
○ 2. demonstrating coughing and deep breathing techniques.
○ 3. displaying an actual hip prosthesis.
○ 4. assessing the client's understanding of the procedure.

The Client With a Hip Fracture

A 73-year-old female is admitted to the hospital with a diagnosis of a right hip fracture. She complains of right hip pain and cannot move her right leg.

17. The nurse assesses correctly that the client has a typical sign of a hip fracture after observing that the client's right leg is
- ○ 1. rotated internally.
- ○ 2. held in a flexed position.
- ○ 3. adducted.
- ○ 4. shorter than the leg on the unaffected side.

18. The nurse assesses the area of fracture. Which of the following phenomena results from broken fragments in the client's hip rubbing against each other?
- ○ 1. Crepitation.
- ○ 2. Subluxation.
- ○ 3. Proliferation.
- ○ 4. Consolidation.

19. The client's fracture is corrected by surgical internal fixation with the insertion of a pin. The nurse develops a plan of care that incorporates the understanding that, in contrast to other surgical procedures, internal fixation with a pin is the treatment of choice for most older persons because it
- ○ 1. is a simpler procedure.
- ○ 2. promotes rapid healing.
- ○ 3. carries less danger of infection.
- ○ 4. makes earlier mobilization possible.

20. The client returns from surgery with a drainage tube in her incision that is attached to suction. The nurse's plan of care should reflect an understanding that the primary purpose of this apparatus is to help
- ○ 1. detect a wound infection.
- ○ 2. eliminate the need for wound irrigation.
- ○ 3. prevent fluid accumulation in the wound.
- ○ 4. provide a way to instill antibiotics into the wound.

21. Which of the following signs or symptoms would be of least importance when the nurse evaluates the client for postoperative peripheral nerve damage?
- ○ 1. Pain.
- ○ 2. Sensation.
- ○ 3. Bleeding.
- ○ 4. Pulselessness.

22. Which of the following pieces of equipment should the nurse use to help prevent external rotation of the client's right leg postoperatively?
- ○ 1. Sandbags.
- ○ 2. A high footboard.
- ○ 3. A rubber air ring.
- ○ 4. A metal bed cradle.

23. Which of the following nursing measures would be most important to implement to decrease the risk of a surgical wound infection in this client?
- ○ 1. Inserting an indwelling urinary catheter to prevent possible soiling of the dressing.
- ○ 2. Accurately measuring drainage from the surgical drainage tube.
- ○ 3. Changing the surgical dressings using sterile technique.
- ○ 4. Monitoring the incision for signs of redness, swelling, and warmth.

24. Before turning the client onto her left side, two nurses first plan to move the client as far as possible to the right side of the bed. The nurses can increase their own stability before moving the client by
- ○ 1. bending at the waist.
- ○ 2. widening their bases of support.
- ○ 3. leaning against the edge of the bed.
- ○ 4. moving the client in a rocking manner.

25. When the client is lying on her side, the nurse should place a pillow between her legs to prevent
- ○ 1. flexion of the knees.
- ○ 2. abduction of the thighs.
- ○ 3. adduction of the hip joint.
- ○ 4. hyperextension of the knees.

26. In which of the following chairs would it be best for the client to sit postoperatively?
- ○ 1. A desk-type swivel chair.
- ○ 2. A padded upholstered chair.
- ○ 3. A high-backed chair with armrests.
- ○ 4. A recliner with an attached footrest.

27. The nurse should teach the client that which of the following leg positions is contraindicated for her while sitting in a chair?
- ○ 1. Crossing her legs.
- ○ 2. Elevating her legs.
- ○ 3. Flexing her ankles.
- ○ 4. Extending her knees.

28. The client is being considered as a candidate for crutch walking. When assessing her, the nurse should take into account that for some elderly people, crutch walking is an impractical goal primarily because of decreased
- ○ 1. visual acuity.
- ○ 2. reaction time.
- ○ 3. motor coordination.
- ○ 4. level of comprehension.

29. Which of the following activities should the nurse plan to teach the client to strengthen her hand muscles in preparation for using crutches?
- ○ 1. Brushing her hair.
- ○ 2. Squeezing a rubber ball.
- ○ 3. Flexing and extending her wrists.
- ○ 4. Pushing her hands into the mattress while raising herself in bed.

30. The nurse assesses the client's home environment for the safe use of crutches and finds the home contains all of the following items. Which one would pose the greatest hazard to the client's safe use of crutches at home?
- ○ 1. A 4-year-old cocker spaniel.
- ○ 2. Scatter rugs.
- ○ 3. Snack tables.
- ○ 4. Rocking chairs.

31. The client has been instructed to take psyllium hydrophilic mucilloid (Metamucil) at home for occasional constipation. In planning to teach the client how to properly take the medication, the nurse would need to understand that this agent acts to stimulate peristalsis by
- ○ 1. moistening fecal material.
- ○ 2. lubricating fecal material.
- ○ 3. increasing the bulk within the intestinal tract.
- ○ 4. irritating the nerve endings in the intestinal mucosa.

32. If the client failed to maintain an adequate fluid intake while using psyllium hydrophilic mucilloid (Metamucil), this preparation could
- ○ 1. cause dehydration.
- ○ 2. ulcerate the duodenum.
- ○ 3. cause a fecal impaction.
- ○ 4. produce an allergic reaction.

The Client With a Herniated Disc

A 45-year-old male is hospitalized for a herniated lumbar disc at the L4–L5 interspace. The physician has explained that surgery will probably be necessary to correct the problem.

33. During the initial client interview, the nurse would most likely learn that the symptom that first caused the client to seek health care was
- ○ 1. loss of bladder control.
- ○ 2. loss of voluntary muscle control.
- ○ 3. back pain that is relieved with resting.
- ○ 4. back pain that radiates to the shoulders.

34. Because hyperextension of the back causes discomfort, which of the following positions would be contraindicated for this client?
- ○ 1. Prone.
- ○ 2. Supine.
- ○ 3. Low Fowler's.
- ○ 4. Right or left Sims'.

35. The client is scheduled for a myelogram and asks the nurse about the procedure. The nurse would explain that x-rays will be taken of the client's spine after an injection of
- ○ 1. sterile water.
- ○ 2. normal saline solution.
- ○ 3. liquid nitrogen.
- ○ 4. radiopaque dye.

36. The client returns from the myelogram, for which an iodized oil (Pantopaque) was used. Which one of the following nursing measures would not be included in his care?
- ○ 1. Bed rest.
- ○ 2. Unrestricted fluid intake.
- ○ 3. Head of the bed elevated 45 degrees.
- ○ 4. Assessment of lower extremity movement and sensation.

37. The client is scheduled for a laminectomy. He asks the nurse to explain again what this surgery involves. The nurse's response should be based on knowledge that the herniated disc will be removed, as will
- ○ 1. the nerve roots affected by the cord compression.
- ○ 2. a major portion of the vertebra in the affected area.
- ○ 3. a portion of the involved vertebra's posterior arches.
- ○ 4. the spinous processes of the vertebra in the affected areas.

38. Which of the following would most likely be a priority nursing diagnosis for this client in the postoperative phase?
- ○ 1. Impaired Physical Mobility related to fear of back pain.
- ○ 2. Altered Nutrition: Less than Body Requirements related to inability to eat in supine position.
- ○ 3. Bowel Incontinence related to decreased physical activity.
- ○ 4. Body Image Disturbance related to fear of disfiguring surgical scar.

39. Postoperatively, the nurse administers trimethobenzamide hydrochloride (Tigan) to the client. The nurse would correctly evaluate that the drug is accomplishing its intended purpose if it controls the client's
- ○ 1. muscle spasms and anxiety.
- ○ 2. nausea and vomiting.
- ○ 3. shivering and dizziness.
- ○ 4. palpitations and dry mouth.

40. The client asks to be turned onto his side. The nurse would be correct in
- ○ 1. asking the client to help by using an overhead trapeze to turn himself.
- ○ 2. turning the client's shoulders first, followed by his hips and legs.
- ○ 3. informing the client that because of his laminectomy he may only lie supine.
- ○ 4. getting another nurse to help logroll the client into position.

41. The nurse helps the client apply the back brace he is to wear. Which of the following positions should the client assume before the brace is applied?
- ○ 1. Standing.
- ○ 2. Lying on his side in bed.
- ○ 3. Lying on his abdomen in bed.
- ○ 4. Sitting in a straight chair.

42. To protect the client's skin under the brace, the nurse should
- ○ 1. place padding as necessary for a snug fit.

○ 2. have the client wear a thin cotton shirt under the brace.
○ 3. lubricate the areas where the client's brace will contact skin surfaces.
○ 4. apply powder to the areas where the client's brace will contact skin surfaces.

43. When the client ambulates for the first time after surgery, he begins to feel faint. Which nursing action would be best until help arrives?
○ 1. Have the client close his eyes for a few minutes.
○ 2. Maneuver the client to a sitting position on the floor.
○ 3. Separate her or his feet to form a wide base of support and have the client rest against her or his hip.
○ 4. Have the client separate his feet to form a wide base of support and then bend at the waist to place his head near his knees.

44. The nurse would know that the client understood his postoperative instructions when he places his feet in which of the following positions when sitting in a chair?
○ 1. Flat on the floor.
○ 2. On a low footstool.
○ 3. In any position of comfort while keeping his legs uncrossed.
○ 4. On a high footstool so that his feet are approximately at the same level as the chair seat.

45. Which of the following activities would not be suitable for the client in the first postoperative days?
○ 1. Assisting with his daily hygiene.
○ 2. Lying flat on his back in bed.
○ 3. Walking in the hall.
○ 4. Sitting in his room to read or watch television.

46. The client complains of abdominal distention in the postoperative period. Of the following medications, which would best help relieve distention?
○ 1. Codeine sulfate.
○ 2. Diazepam (Valium).
○ 3. Neostigmine bromide (Prostigmin).
○ 4. Psyllium hydrophilic mucilloid (Metamucil).

The Client With Peripheral Vascular Disease

A 65-year-old male is admitted with peripheral vascular disease of the lower extremities.

47. Which of the following would not be considered a typical symptom of peripheral arterial disease?
○ 1. Ankle edema.
○ 2. Intermittent claudication.
○ 3. Decreased or absent pulses.
○ 4. Cool skin.

48. During the admission assessment, the nurse palpates the client's peripheral pulses. To assess the dorsalis pedis pulse, the nurse should palpate the
○ 1. medial surface of the ankle.
○ 2. area behind the ankle.
○ 3. ventral aspect of the top of the foot.
○ 4. medial aspect of the dorsum of the foot.

49. The nurse notes the following assessment findings regarding the client's peripheral vascular status: cramping leg pain relieved by rest; cool, pale feet; and delayed capillary refilling. Based on this data, the nurse would make a nursing diagnosis of
○ 1. Impaired Skin Integrity.
○ 2. Impaired Gas Exchange.
○ 3. Altered Peripheral Tissue Perfusion.
○ 4. Impaired Physical Mobility.

50. The client says, "I've really tried to manage my condition well." Which of the following routines would the nurse evaluate as having been appropriate for him?
○ 1. Resting with his legs elevated above the level of his heart.
○ 2. Walking slowly but steadily for 30 minutes twice a day.
○ 3. Minimizing activity.
○ 4. Wearing antiembolism stockings at all times when out of bed.

51. An examination reveals that the arterial obstruction in the client's left leg is complete. Early signs of gangrene are developing, and the physician informs him that amputation will probably be necessary. Which of the following clinical manifestations would the nurse most likely find on assessment?
○ 1. Aching pain.
○ 2. Burning sensations.
○ 3. Numbness and tingling.
○ 4. Coldness.

52. While the nurse is providing preoperative teaching, the client says, "I hate the idea of being an invalid after they cut off my leg." The nurse's most therapeutic response would be
○ 1. "You'll still have one good leg to use."
○ 2. "Tell me more about how you're feeling."
○ 3. "Let's finish the preoperative teaching."
○ 4. "You're fortunate to have a wife who can take care of you."

53. The client asks the nurse, "Why can't the doctor tell me exactly how much of my leg he's going to take off? Don't you think I should know that?" The nurse should respond based on knowledge that the final decision on the level of the amputation will depend primarily on
○ 1. the need to remove as much of the leg as possible.
○ 2. the adequacy of the blood supply to the tissues.
○ 3. the ease with which a prosthesis can be fitted.
○ 4. the client's ability to walk with a prosthesis.

54. The client returns from surgery for a below-the-knee amputation with the residual limb covered with dressings and a woven elastic bandage. At first the bandage was dry, but now, 30 minutes later, the nurse notices a small amount of bloody drainage. What should be the priority action?
- ○ 1. Notify the physician.
- ○ 2. Mark the area of drainage.
- ○ 3. Change the dressing.
- ○ 4. Reinforce the dressing.

55. The client's room should contain which emergency equipment when he returns from surgery?
- ○ 1. Suction equipment.
- ○ 2. Emergency cart.
- ○ 3. Airway.
- ○ 4. Tourniquet.

56. What would be the most important nursing intervention in caring for the client's residual limb during the first 24 hours after surgery?
- ○ 1. Keeping the residual limb flat on the bed.
- ○ 2. Abducting the residual limb on a scheduled basis.
- ○ 3. Applying traction to the residual limb.
- ○ 4. Elevating the residual limb on a pillow.

57. Which of the following nursing goals would take priority when planning for the client's physical mobility following amputation?
- ○ 1. Preventing contractures.
- ○ 2. Promoting comfort.
- ○ 3. Preventing edema.
- ○ 4. Preventing phantom-limb pain.

58. The second morning after surgery, the client says, "This sounds crazy, but I feel my left toes tingling." This statement would indicate to the nurse that he is experiencing a
- ○ 1. denial reaction.
- ○ 2. phantom-limb sensation.
- ○ 3. hallucination.
- ○ 4. body image disturbance.

59. The client is to be fitted with a functioning prosthesis. The nurse has been teaching him how to care for his residual limb. Which behavior would demonstrate that the client has an understanding of proper residual limb care? The client
- ○ 1. applies powder to the residual limb.
- ○ 2. inspects the residual limb weekly with a mirror.
- ○ 3. removes the prosthesis whenever he sits down.
- ○ 4. washes and dries the residual limb daily.

60. The client will use crutches while his prosthesis is being adjusted. Which of the following exercises would best prepare him for using crutches?
- ○ 1. Range-of-motion exercises of the shoulders.
- ○ 2. Isometric exercises of the shoulders.
- ○ 3. Quadriceps and gluteal setting exercises.
- ○ 4. Triceps exercises.

61. When using crutches, the client should be taught to support his weight primarily on his
- ○ 1. axillae.
- ○ 2. elbows.
- ○ 3. upper arms.
- ○ 4. hands.

62. The client is to be discharged on a low-fat, low-cholesterol, low-sodium diet. What would be the nurse's first step in planning the dietary instructions?
- ○ 1. Determine the client's knowledge level about cholesterol.
- ○ 2. Ask the client to name foods high in fat, cholesterol, and salt.
- ○ 3. Explain the importance of complying with the diet.
- ○ 4. Assess the family's food preferences.

63. The nurse has been instructing the client on how to prepare meals that are low in fat, cholesterol, and sodium. Which of these comments would indicate that he needs additional teaching?
- ○ 1. "I'll eat only water-packed tuna."
- ○ 2. "I'll use a Teflon-coated pan when cooking."
- ○ 3. "I'll eat more liver with onions."
- ○ 4. "I'll avoid using steak sauce and catsup."

The Client With a Femoral Fracture

A 28-year-old male construction worker is brought to the hospital emergency room following a fall from a beam. He has a fractured right femur and multiple cuts and bruises on his upper body and right arm and hand.

64. A booster injection for tetanus is administered in the emergency room after it is determined that the client has not had any immunizations since childhood. Which of the following biologic products would be used to provide the client with passive immunity for tetanus?
- ○ 1. Tetanus toxoid.
- ○ 2. Tetanus antigen.
- ○ 3. Tetanus vaccine.
- ○ 4. Tetanus antitoxin.

65. Providing immunologic protection for this client would be essential to prevent which pathologic condition?
- ○ 1. Tetany.
- ○ 2. Lockjaw.
- ○ 3. Meningitis.
- ○ 4. Gas gangrene.

66. The client is admitted to the orthopedic unit in balanced skeletal traction using a Thomas splint and Pearson attachment. The primary purpose of traction in this case is to
- ○ 1. prevent neurologic damage.
- ○ 2. realign fracture fragments.
- ○ 3. control internal bleeding.
- ○ 4. maintain skin integrity.

67. The nurse is responsible for maintaining effective traction. Which of the following conditions is necessary for effective traction?
- ○ 1. The weights rest securely on the bed frame.
- ○ 2. The ropes are in the wheel grooves of the pulleys.
- ○ 3. The client is positioned low in the bed.
- ○ 4. The weights are increased by ½ pound each shift.

68. When a client is placed in balanced skeletal traction, which of the following nursing actions would be appropriate?
- ○ 1. Ensuring that the traction weights hang freely from the bed at all times.
- ○ 2. Gradually increasing the traction weight as the client's tolerance increases.
- ○ 3. Applying and removing the traction weights at regular intervals throughout the day.
- ○ 4. Removing the weights briefly as necessary to reposition the client in bed.

69. What is the purpose of the Pearson attachment on the traction setup.
- ○ 1. To support the lower portion of the leg.
- ○ 2. To support the thigh and upper leg.
- ○ 3. To attach the skeletal pin.
- ○ 4. To prevent flexion deformities in the ankle and foot.

70. Because of the nature of his fracture, the client is at risk for fat emboli. Which of the following manifestations would the nurse most likely note if this complication occurs?
- ○ 1. Mental confusion.
- ○ 2. Migraine-like headaches.
- ○ 3. Numbness in the right leg.
- ○ 4. Muscle spasms in the right thigh.

71. Which of the following treatments would most likely be used to reduce the surface tension of the fat globules if emboli occur?
- ○ 1. Hypothermia.
- ○ 2. Supplemental oxygen.
- ○ 3. Intravenous heparin.
- ○ 4. Anticholesterol drugs.

72. The client is quite upset and agitated about his injury and its treatment. He says, "How can I stay like this for weeks? I can't even move!" The nurse should explain that while he is in traction, he
- ○ 1. can turn from side to side in bed and sit up.
- ○ 2. must lie flat in bed and cannot turn at all.
- ○ 3. can sit up straight in bed but cannot turn.
- ○ 4. can turn slightly from side to side and sit up at a 30-to 40-degree angle.

73. Because of the Thomas splint, the nurse would need to assess the client regularly for
- ○ 1. signs of skin pressure in the groin area.
- ○ 2. decreased breath sounds.
- ○ 3. skin breakdown behind the heel.
- ○ 4. urine retention.

74. The nurse plans to teach the client about the traction. What would be the most appropriate plan?
- ○ 1. Give cursory explanations for the first few days so as not to overwhelm him.
- ○ 2. Initiate teaching just before administering pain medication, to ensure that he is alert.
- ○ 3. Use medical terminology exclusively so that he will recognize the terms when the doctors use them.
- ○ 4. Relate the information about the traction to his knowledge of construction when possible.

75. The client has the nursing diagnosis Self-Care Deficit related to the confinement of traction. Which of the following would indicate a successful outcome for this diagnosis? The client
- ○ 1. assists as much as possible in his care, and his participation increases over time.
- ○ 2. allows the nurse to complete his care in an efficient manner and does not interfere.
- ○ 3. allows his wife to assume total responsibility for his care.
- ○ 4. allows his wife to complete his care because he knows she needs to feel useful.

76. To prevent infection and osteomyelitis, the nurse provides pin site care and inspects the site daily for evidence of infection. Which of the following clinical manifestations at the pin site would alert the nurse to infection?
- ○ 1. Slight serous oozing.
- ○ 2. Lack of scab formation.
- ○ 3. Itching.
- ○ 4. Pain.

77. The client has a nursing diagnosis of Constipation related to the decreased mobility imposed by traction. A care plan that incorporates which of the following breakfasts would be most helpful in reestablishing a normal bowel routine?
- ○ 1. Eggs and bacon, buttered toast, orange juice, and coffee.
- ○ 2. Corn flakes with sliced banana, milk, and English muffin and jelly.
- ○ 3. Orange juice, breakfast pastries (doughnut and danish), and coffee.
- ○ 4. An orange, raisin bran and milk, and wheat toast with butter.

The Client With a Spinal Cord Injury

The client, a 25-year-old female, fell during a rock-climbing trip. She is alert and conscious but cannot move her arms or legs on command.

78. The priority concern when planning to move a person with a possible spinal cord injury is to
- ○ 1. wrap and support the extremities, which can be easily injured.

○ 2. move the person gently to help reduce pain.
○ 3. immobilize the head and neck to prevent further injury.
○ 4. cushion the back with pillows to ensure comfort.

79. It is determined that the client suffered a C7 spinal cord injury. Which of the following would be the most important nursing intervention during the acute stage of her care?
○ 1. Turning and repositioning every 2 hours.
○ 2. Maintaining proper alignment.
○ 3. Maintaining a patent airway.
○ 4. Monitoring vital signs.

80. The nurse recognizes that spinal shock is likely to persist for the first several weeks after the injury. Which of the following symptoms would be unexpected during the period of spinal shock?
○ 1. Tachycardia.
○ 2. Rapid respirations.
○ 3. Hypertension.
○ 4. Dry, warm skin.

81. During the period of spinal shock, the nurse should expect the client's bladder function to be
○ 1. spastic.
○ 2. normal.
○ 3. atonic.
○ 4. uncontrolled.

82. Passive range-of-motion exercises for the legs and assisted range-of-motion exercises for the arms are part of the client's care regimen. Which observation by the nurse would indicate a successful outcome of this treatment?
○ 1. Free, easy movement of the joints.
○ 2. Absence of paralytic footdrop.
○ 3. External rotation of the hips at rest.
○ 4. Absence of tissue ischemia over bony prominences.

83. The client's fracture is surgically repaired. Once healing has begun, daily physical therapy sessions are scheduled that include using a tilt table. After the therapist places the client at a 45-degree angle, the nurse should monitor her for which of the following?
○ 1. Hypertension.
○ 2. Pedal edema.
○ 3. Facial flushing.
○ 4. Dizziness.

84. After a month of therapy, the client begins to experience muscle spasms in her legs. She calls the nurse in excitement to report the leg movement. Which response by the nurse would be the most accurate?
○ 1. "These movements indicate that the damaged nerves are healing."
○ 2. "This is a good sign. Keep trying to move all the affected muscles."
○ 3. "The return of movement means that eventually you should be able to walk again. The damage is not permanent."
○ 4. "The movements occur from muscle reflexes. They can't be initiated or controlled by the brain."

85. The nurse realizes that the client is at risk for autonomic dysreflexia. Which of the following symptoms would indicate this condition?
○ 1. Sudden, severe hypertension.
○ 2. Bradycardia.
○ 3. Paralytic ileus.
○ 4. Hot, dry skin.

86. If autonomic dysreflexia occurs, what would be the priority nursing intervention?
○ 1. Administer nitroprusside sodium (Nipride) intravenously.
○ 2. Call the physician.
○ 3. Place the client in Fowler's position.
○ 4. Send a urine sample for culture.

87. The nurse assesses the client to determine the cause of the autonomic dysreflexia. The nurse would prioritize assessment based on the knowledge that the most common stimulus for an autonomic dysreflexia episode is
○ 1. bowel distention.
○ 2. bladder distention.
○ 3. anxiety.
○ 4. rising intracranial pressure.

88. The orthotics department makes a custom trunk brace for the client. The nurse would plan to apply this brace at which time?
○ 1. While the client is sitting in a chair.
○ 2. Before the client gets out of bed.
○ 3. As soon as the client becomes fatigued.
○ 4. When the client is standing on the tilt table.

89. Urinary tract infection is a serious problem following spinal cord injury. Which of the following would be the most important measure to prevent this?
○ 1. Drink a glass of citrus fruit juice at every meal.
○ 2. Drink at least 2,000 ml of fluid daily.
○ 3. Add extra protein to the daily diet.
○ 4. Ensure that the urine remains alkaline.

90. The client asks the nurse why the dietitian has recommended that she decrease her total daily intake of calcium. Which of the following responses by the nurse would provide the most accurate information?
○ 1. "Excessive intake of dairy products makes constipation more common."
○ 2. "Immobility increases calcium absorption from the intestine."
○ 3. "Lack of weight-bearing causes demineralization of the long bones and increases the kidneys' calcium load."
○ 4. "Dairy products likely will contribute to weight gain."

91. As a first step in teaching the client about her sexual health, the nurse assesses her understanding of the sexual functioning of a quadriplegic. Which of the following statements by the client would indicate good understanding?

○ 1. "I won't be able to have sexual intercourse until the Foley catheter is removed."
○ 2. "I can participate in sexual activity but might not experience orgasm."
○ 3. "I won't be able to have sexual intercourse because it causes hypertension, but other sexual activity is allowed."
○ 4. "I'll be able to participate in sexual activity but will be infertile."

92. The client had been very active in sports and outdoor activities, and she talks almost obsessively about her past activities. In tears, one day she asks the nurse, "Why can't I stop talking about these things? I know those days are gone forever." Which response by the nurse would convey the best understanding of the client's behavior?

○ 1. "Be patient. It takes time to adjust to such a massive loss."
○ 2. "Talking about the past is a form of denial. We have to help you focus on today."
○ 3. "Reviewing your losses is a way of working through your grief. Someday soon you'll be able to let go."
○ 4. "It's a simple escape mechanism to go back and live again in happier times."

CORRECT ANSWERS AND RATIONALE

The letters in parentheses following the rationale identify the step of the nursing process (A, D, P, I, E); cognitive level (K, C, T, N); and client need (S, G, L, H). See the Answer Grid for the key.

The Client With Arthritis

1. 3. Synovial joints are characteristically affected by rheumatoid arthritis. Rheumatoid arthritis is an inflammatory disorder that most commonly affects middle-aged women. Osteoarthritis is a degenerative joint disease that affects weight-bearing joints and is associated with aging. (I, K, G)

2. 2. Tinnitus (ringing in the ears) is a common symptom of aspirin toxicity. Dysuria, drowsiness, and chest pain are not associated with aspirin toxicity. (A, K, G)

3. 4. Aspirin therapy in rheumatoid arthritis involves continuous ongoing administration to establish and maintain therapeutic blood levels. Aspirin should not be used on a p.r.n. basis. It should always be buffered with food, and clients should be instructed to observe for symptoms of bleeding. (E, C, H)

4. 2. The client with rheumatoid arthritis should be encouraged to alternate periods of activity and rest throughout the day. Neither encouraging the client to perform all activities of daily living at once nor encouraging her to cease all participation in daily activities will increase activity tolerance; instead, these actions may further decrease activity tolerance. Narcotics are not typically administered to control arthritic pain. (I, N, G)

5. 4. Both osteoarthritis and rheumatoid arthritis cause joint pain, joint stiffness, and movement limitations. Inflammation, a characteristic feature of rheumatoid arthritis, produces pronounced swelling, which is not a common feature of osteoarthritis. (A, N, G)

6. 4. When a client compares her therapy with someone else's, it is best for the nurse to explain truthfully and point out that there are various forms of arthritis. What helps one person may not help another. Avoiding the question or suggesting that the client should not ask a particular question is nontherapeutic. (I, N, L)

7. 4. Proper positioning to prevent flexion deformities of the joints is an ongoing need for clients with rheumatoid arthritis and should be included in the postoperative care plan. Positioning to promote comfort and avoid venous stasis is important but not unique to clients with rheumatoid arthritis. (P, T, S)

8. 2. Postoperative care following total knee replacement can be extremely painful. The client must have a firm commitment to active participation in the rehabilitation process. Scolding or blaming the client is useless. The nurse should help the client understand why the care is necessary and reinforce this understanding as necessary. (I, N, S)

9. 1. Using a continuous passive motion (CPM) machine will likely produce initial discomfort for the client. If the client cannot tolerate the discomfort, the physican should be notified for an order to adjust the settings. (The settings for the machine are determined by the physician and cannot be changed without an order.) The nurse must frequently evaluate the positioning of the client's leg, the range-of-motion setting, and the client's response to the therapy. (I, T, S)

10. 2. An exercise program is recommended to strengthen muscles following arthroplasty. Isometric (or muscle-setting) exercises strengthen muscles but keep the joint stationary during the healing process. Isometric exercise costs little in terms of time and money, and may help improve a client's morale by involving her in her own care, but these are not necessarily primary reasons for using it. Isometric exercise will not help prevent joint stiffness; the joint is kept stationary. (I, N, G)

11. 3. The quadriceps-setting exercises strengthen the quadriceps femoris, leg muscles important for proper walking. These muscles can be exercised in bed by pushing the back of the knee into the mattress. (I, T, S)

12. 3. Using only medications and treatments presented by reputable health care professionals is the best way to avoid "quack" therapy. Relying on testimonials and advertisements is a poor way to select therapy. Widespread abuse and misuse of drugs makes it important for nurses to teach clients about the importance of using only drugs recommended and prescribed by a physician and about the dangers of relying on others' opinions. The client described here has rheumatoid arthritis. Because of its chronicity and discomfort, many such clients unfortunately succumb to so-called cures. The client should be taught that there currently is no cure for the disease, and many advertised "remedies" may be potentially hazardous. (P, T, H)

13. 4. Osteoarthritis is a degenerative joint disease. The weight-bearing joints, such as the knees and hips, and finger joints, are most commonly affected. The shoulder joints are the least likely to be involved in osteoarthritis. (A, K, G)

14. 3. Osteoarthritis most commonly results from "wear

and tear," excessive and prolonged mechanical stress on the joints. Increased weight increases stress on weight-bearing joints. Therefore, an obese client with osteoarthritis should be encouraged to lose weight. (A, C, G)

15. 3. Drugs that cause gastric irritation are best taken after or with a meal, when stomach contents help minimize the local irritation. (I, T, H)

16. 4. All of the information provided is important. However, before implementing any teaching plan, the nurse should first determine the client's level of understanding about the procedure. Only then could the nurse develop an individualized teaching plan designed to meet the needs of this client. (A, N, L)

The Client With a Hip Fracture

17. 4. After a hip fracture, the leg on the affected side is characteristically shorter than the unaffected leg. Typically, it is also abducted and rotated externally. Pain is usually present. (A, T, G)

18. 1. Crepitation is the grating sensation produced when broken bone fragments rub against each other. Subluxation is the dislocation of a joint. Proliferation is growth by cell multiplication. Consolidation is the conversion of a substance into a solid mass. (A, K, G)

19. 4. Using a pin for the internal fixation of a fractured hip has various advantages. This procedure is especially favored for older clients because it enables earlier postoperative ambulation and provides good fixation at the fracture site. (P, N, G)

20. 3. The primary reason for applying suction to a wound drainage tube is to prevent fluid from accumulating in the wound. This greatly enhances wound healing and helps prevent abscess formation. (P, C, G)

21. 3. Nerve damage may be indicated by the presence of any of the "five P's": pain, pallor, pulselessness, paresthesia, and paralysis. Bleeding does not indicate peripheral nerve damage. Peripheral nerve damage can occur after almost any orthopedic surgery. (E, N, G)

22. 1. It is best to support the client's leg in its proper anatomic position and to prevent external rotation by supporting the leg with sandbags. A trochanter roll can also be used. Sandbags should be placed along the length of the thigh and lower leg. Neither a footboard, a rubber air ring, nor a metal frame bed cradle will help prevent external rotation of the leg. (I, T, S)

23. 3. Wound infection can best be prevented by using strict sterile technique during dressing changes. Accurately measuring drainage and monitoring the incision for signs of infection are important nursing actions, but will not prevent a wound infection. Inserting a Foley catheter is an unnecessary action in this case and would predispose the client to a urinary tract infection. (I, N, G)

24. 2. Before moving a client, the nurse should spread her or his feet apart to provide a wide base of support and increase stability. Assuming this stance, flexing the knees, coming close to the client, and using the weight of the client's body as a force to reduce the amount of strain on the nurse's body are recommended techniques for moving a client. (I, C, S)

25. 3. Following hip surgery for a fractured femur, the client should be positioned on the nonoperative side with a pillow between the legs to help prevent adduction of operative leg. This positioning places the hip in proper alignment. Dislocation of the hip can occur if the leg on the affected side is allowed to adduct. (I, C, S)

26. 3. A high-backed straight chair with armrests is recommended to help keep the client in the best possible alignment following surgery for a hip fracture. Soft, low, and swivel chairs do not promote good body alignment or good security. (I, N, H)

27. 1. Leg crossing causes adduction of the hips; following hip surgery, this may result in a dislocation of the operated hip. This client should not cross her legs. Elevating the legs, flexing the ankles, and extending the knees are not necessarily contraindicated. (I, T, H)

28. 3. Some elderly persons are not good candidates for crutch walking because they are not strong enough to use crutches or are not coordinated enough to crutch walk safely. Such factors as visual acuity, reaction time, and level of comprehension may influence the ability to learn crutch walking but are not as important as motor coordination. (A, T, S)

29. 2. A client being prepared for crutch walking should be taught to support her weight with her hands when crutch walking. Supporting weight in the axillae is contraindicated due to the risk of possible nerve damage and circulatory obstruction. The client should be taught to squeeze a ball vigorously to help strengthen her hands in preparation for weight bearing with the hands. Such activities as brushing the hair, flexing and extending the wrists, and doing push-ups may be indicated, but they are not likely to strengthen the hands. (P, C, S)

30. 2. Scatter rugs are the single greatest hazard in the home, especially for elderly people who are unsure of walking. Falls have been found to account for nearly half the accidental deaths that occur in the home. (A, N, S)

31. 3. Psyllium hydrophilic mucilloid (Metamucil) stimulates peristalsis by increasing bulk within the intestinal tract. It causes the formation of a soft, gelatinous, water-retaining substance in the bowel to produce bulk. An example of a laxative that lubricates the stool is mineral oil. An example of a laxative that moistens the stool by increasing the water content of the feces is magnesium citrate. An example of a laxative that stimulates peristalsis by irritating nerve endings in the intestinal mucosa is castor oil. (P, K, S)

32. 3. Bulk-producing laxatives pick up moisture in the gastrointestinal tract. These laxatives may cause a fecal implication if the person using such laxatives does not maintain a generous fluid intake. (I, N, H)

The Client With a Herniated Disc

33. 3. A typical symptom of a herniated lumbar disc is low back pain that is usually relieved by rest and aggravated by activity that causes an increase in fluid pressure in the spine, such as sneezing, coughing, lifting, and bending. Muscle weakness and sensory losses may occur, and there is generally a change in tendon reflexes. Pain radiating to the shoulders that often causes a person to believe he is having a heart attack is a typical symptom of cervical disc herniation. Loss of voluntary muscle control, which may cause chorea-like movements, and loss of urinary control are not typical early symptoms of lumbar disc problems. (A, C, G)

34. 1. Hyperextension of the spine occurs when a client lies on the abdomen (that is, in the prone position). Hyperextension of the spine causes discomfort for a client with a herniated disc; thus, the prone position is contraindicated for this client. This client will be most comfortable in the supine, low Fowler's, or left or right Sims' position. (I, T, G)

35. 4. A radiopaque dye (usually an iodized oil, but in some instances a water-soluble compound) is used for a myelogram. Air may be used for an air–contrast study. Myelography is used to determine the exact location of a herniated disc. (I, K, G)

36. 3. Nursing care of the client after a myelogram depends in part on the type of dye used. For example, if an oil contrast such as Pantopaque was used, the client will usually lie flat for 8 to 12 hours. If a water-soluble contrast was used, the head of the bed is elevated 45 degrees for 8 to 24 hours. This position reduces the rate of upward dispersion of the contrast medium. Regardless of the type of dye used for the test, bedrest is required for several hours after a myelogram. Fluid intake is encouraged to replace cerebrospinal fluid, to reduce headache, and to facilitate absorption of retained contrast media. Neurologic status in the lower extremities is assessed frequently. (I, N, G)

37. 3. To reach the disc, a portion of the vertebra's lamina is removed to explore the involved nerve root and to remove disc fragments. The laminae help form the posterior arches of the vertebrae. (P, K, G)

38. 1. Postoperative back pain related to the surgical incision and muscle spasms is common after laminectomy. The client may avoid movement to prevent pain if nursing measures are not implemented to control pain. Depending on the activity order, the client may be turned to his side or have the head of the bed elevated for meals. Constipation is more likely to be a problem postoperatively due to inactivity. Surgical laminectomy scars are small and typically do not cause fear of disfigurement. (D, N, G)

39. 2. Trimethobenzamide hydrochloride (Tigan) is a centrally acting antiemetic that helps control nausea and vomiting. It does not control muscle spasms, anxiety, shivering, dizziness, palpitations, or dry mouth. (E, C, G)

40. 4. After a laminectomy, the client's spine must be maintained in proper alignment. The client who had a laminectomy may be turned to his side by logrolling him in one unit while keeping his back straight. It takes at least two people to perform this procedure correctly. Having the client turn himself, or moving his shoulders and hips separately, does not allow the back to remain in straight alignment. (I, N, S)

41. 2. A back brace should be applied before the client who has had back surgery is out of bed and placing weight on the legs and back. The brace is placed on the bed while the client assumes a side-lying position. The client is then rolled onto the brace. Hyperextension of the back following back surgery is contraindicated. (I, T, S)

42. 2. Having the client wear a thin cotton shirt under a brace helps protect the skin and keep the brace free of skin oils and perspiration. Using padding may increase pressure points. Lubricating and powdering the skin under the brace do not provide the best protection from irritation by the brace. (I, N, S)

43. 3. A client who feels faint while walking with the nurse should rest on the nurse's hip. This maneuver is relatively easy and can be maintained until help is available. Having the client close his eyes is unlikely to relieve symptoms of fainting. Maneuvering the client to the floor requires considerable strength and may injure the client, especially when done quickly. This client should not bend at the waist because of his recent back surgery. (I, N, S)

44. 1. A client who has had back surgery should place the feet flat on the floor. This ordinarily provides the greatest comfort because it places no strain on the operative area. A client who is allowed to choose his or her own position may choose one that places strain on the back. The nurse teaches and explains that placing the feet flat on the floor is recommended. (E, N, G)

45. 4. After a laminectomy, a client should either lie flat in bed in good alignment or should walk. Sitting for long periods is contraindicated, as pressure is increased to the operative area and alignment is compromised. (I, T, G)

46. 3. Neostigmine bromide (Prostogmin) stimulates peristalsis through its effects on the smooth muscles in the intestinal tract. Psyllium hydrophilic mucilloid (Metamucil) helps relieve constipation, and constipation predisposes to distention. However, the first choice for early relief of distention is to use the neostigmine bromide. Codeine sulfate and diazepam (Valium) may relieve discomfort and anxiety but will not relieve distention. (I, C, G)

The Client With Peripheral Vascular Disease

47. 1. Inadequate arterial circulation produces symptoms of hypoxia. The skin is cool to the touch, pulses are difficult or impossible to palpate, and exercise causes moderate to severe cramping pain. Ankle edema is associated with venous insufficiency and stasis. (A, C, G)

48. 4. The dorsalis pedis pulse is found on the medial aspect of the dorsal surface of the foot in line with the big toe. The posterior tibial pulse is on the medial surface of the ankle just behind the medial malleolus. The popliteal pulse is behind the knee. (A, K, S)

49. 3. The data obtained by the nurse are major defining characteristics for the nursing diagnosis Altered Peripheral Tissue Perfusion. The data do not indicate that the client's skin integrity or physical mobility has been impaired at this time. The diagnosis Impaired Gas Exchange is used to describe clients with respiratory insufficiency. (D, N, G)

50. 2. Slow, steady walking is a recommended activity for clients with peripheral arterial disease because it stimulates the development of collateral circulation. The client with peripheral arterial disease should not remain inactive. Elevating the legs above the heart and wearing antiembolism stockings are strategies for venous congestion and may worsen peripheral arterial disease. (E, T, G)

51. 4. Coldness is the assessment finding most consistent with complete arterial obstruction. Other expected findings would include paralysis and pallor. Aching pain, burning sensations, and numbness and tingling are earlier signs of tissue hypoxia and ischemia and are associated with incomplete obstruction. (A, C, G)

52. 2. Encouraging the client undergoing amputation to verbalize feelings is the most therapeutic nursing intervention. By eliciting information, the nurse may be able to provide information to help the client cope. The nurse should avoid value-laden responses that may make the client feel guilty or hostile and block further communication. The nurse should not ignore the client's expressed concerns. The nurse should not reinforce the client's concern about invalidism and dependency or assume that his wife is willing to care for him. (I, T, L)

53. 2. The level of amputation often cannot be accurately determined until surgery, when the surgeon can directly assess the adequacy of the circulation of the residual limb. A longer residual limb facilitates prosthesis-fitting and this aspect will be considered in the final decision, but it is not the primary factor. (P, C, G)

54. 2. The nurse should mark the blood stain and observe it again in 10 minutes. There is no need to notify the physician immediately, since some oozing and bloody drainage are expected. Given the slight amount of drainage, there is no need either to replace the dressing or reinforce it. (I, N, S)

55. 4. Hemorrhage is an unexpected, but possible, complication of radical surgery such as amputation. A tourniquet should be available at the bedside during the early postoperative period to deal with such a complication. (P, K, S)

56. 4. Elevating the residual limb on a pillow for the first 24 hours after surgery helps prevent edema and promotes comfort by increasing venous return. Elevating the residual limb for longer than the first 24 hours is contraindicated, because of the potential for developing contractures. Adducting the residual limb on a scheduled basis prevents abduction contracture. (I, N, G)

57. 1. Preventing joint contractures is essential to physical mobility. Promoting comfort and preventing edema are appropriate immediate postoperative nursing goals, but attaining them does not affect physical mobility in the immediate and extended postoperative periods. Phantom-limb pain begins from 2 weeks to 2 months after amputation. It occurs briefly in about 30% of clients, but only about 2% experience persistent pain. (P, T, G)

58. 2. Descriptions of sensations, painful and otherwise, in the amputated part are common and are known as phantom-limb sensations. The client should be reassured that these sensations are normal and are not a sign of a mental problem. Denial may be present following amputation; signs include refusal to look at and/or talk about the amputation. Hallucinations indicate a serious, possibly psychotic condition and should be thoroughly assessed. Referral to an appropriate health care provider is in order. Body image disturbances can develop after amputation due to fear, grief, loss of locomotion, and decreased self-esteem related to the loss of the body part. (D, K, G)

59. 4. Washing and thoroughly drying the residual limb daily are important hygiene measures to prevent infection. Nothing should be applied to the residual limb after it is cleansed. Powder may cause excessive drying and cracking of the skin, and cream may soften the skin excessively. The residual limb should be inspected daily with a mirror for early signs of skin breakdown. To reduce residual limb swelling, the prosthesis should be removed only at night. (E, T, G)

60. 4. Using crutches requires significant strength from the triceps muscles, and efforts should be focused on strengthening these muscles in anticipation of crutch walking. Bed and wheelchair pushups are excellent exercises targeted at the triceps muscles. (I, N, G)

61. 4. Using crutches properly requires supporting body weight primarily on the hands. Using crutches improperly can cause nerve damage from excess pressure. Careful instruction and evaluation of crutch use is essential. (I, K, S)

62. 4. Before beginning dietary interventions, the nurse must assess the client's pattern of food intake, life cycle, food preferences, and ethnic, cultural, and financial influences. (P, N, H)

63. 3. Liver and organ meats are high in cholesterol and saturated fat and should be limited. Water-packed tuna is one of the leanest fish available. Using a Teflon-coated pan when cooking reduces the need for shortening. Steak sauce and catsup are high in sodium. (E, N, G)

The Client With a Femoral Fracture

64. 4. Passive immunity for tetanus is provided in the form of tetanus antitoxin or tetanus immune globulin. An antitoxin is an antibody to the toxin of an organism. Toxoids, antigens, and vaccines all provide active immunity by stimulating the body to produce its own antibodies. (I, K, G)

65. 2. The antitoxin is specific for preventing tetanus, also called lockjaw. The etiologic agent is *Clostridium tetani.* Tetany, characterized by intermittent tonic spasms, is caused by hypocalcemia. Meningitis, or inflammation of the membranes of the spinal cord or brain, can be caused by bacteria, viruses, or other organisms that reach the meninges. Gas gangrene is caused by *Clostridium perfringens.* (I, K, H)

66. 2. Traction promotes realignment of the bone fragments. This will facilitate subsequent internal fixation. Traction immobilizes the fracture site and may increase the client's comfort. Mobilization could result in further damage. Traction increases circulation to the affected part but does not control internal bleeding. Traction may create, rather than prevent, a problem with skin integrity. (P, K, G)

67. 2. For the weights to maintain the therapeutic effect of the traction, they must be properly positioned and free hanging and should be removed only in life-threatening situations. Effective traction depends on the client being positioned at the head of the bed. Sufficient weight is applied initially to overcome spasm in affected muscles. As the muscles relax, the weight may be reduced. (I, T, S)

68. 1. In balanced skeletal traction, the appropriate pressures and counterpressures are applied to the fracture site with the traction weights hang freely at all times. These weights are in place continuously and should never be lifted, reduced, or eliminated. Skin traction may be applied intermittently, but balanced skeletal traction is continuous. (I, T, S)

69. 1. The Pearson attachment supports the lower leg and provides increased stability in the overall traction setup. It also makes it easier to maintain correct alignment. (P, C, G)

70. 1. Fat emboli usually result in cerebral disturbances that cause mental confusion or agitation from hypoxia. If severe, hypoxia can produce delirium and coma. (A, C, G)

71. 2. Respiratory failure is a common cause of death following fat emboli. Oxygen therapy appears to reduce the surface tension of the fat globules and supports respiratory function by reducing hypoxia. (P, C, G)

72. 1. Although normal movement is not possible in skeletal traction, the balanced weights ensure that changes in position do not alter or interfere with the traction pull. Therefore, a client can turn and sit up in bed while the traction is in place. (I, T, L)

73. 1. The Thomas splint is secured by rings that slip over the thigh. They are placed tight up into the groin and may cause discomfort, pressure, or skin irritation. (A, T, S)

74. 4. Understanding is enhanced when the learner can relate new information to existing knowledge. Linking the common principles of construction and traction would be a perfect way to help this client learn. It is unwise to overload the client with information, but complete, simple teaching will facilitate relaxation. Teaching is best done when pain is minimal, because discomfort impairs concentration. The client may not understand medical terminology, and the nurse should always tailor teaching to the client's level of understanding. (P, N, H)

75. 1. Self-care minimizes sensory deprivation and allows the client to gain a sense of control. Passivity can indicate denial or depression. Family members can assist, but giving them primary responsibility undermines the client's self-esteem. (E, N, H)

76. 4. Inflammation, evidenced by pain, swelling, and redness, is one of the early signs of infection and needs prompt intervention. Slight oozing at the pin site is expected and decreases bacteria in the pin tract. Crusting or scab formation should be prevented, as it may trap bacteria in the pin tract. Itching at the pin site may be due to dryness or irritation. (A, C, G)

77. 4. High-fiber foods provide bulk and decrease water absorption in the bowel. Whole grains and fruits (not juices, which often are strained) are recommended. Processed foods and breads contain little fiber. (P, T, G)

The Client With a Spinal Cord Injury

78. 3. The immediate concern is to immobilize the head and neck to prevent further trauma when the fractured vertebra may be unstable and easily displaced. Pain is usually not a significant consideration with this type of injury. (P, N, S)

79. 3. Initial care is focused on establishing and maintaining a patent airway and supporting ventilation. Innervation to the intercostals is affected; if spinal edema extends to the C4 level, paralysis of the diaphragm usually occurs. The effects and extent of edema are unpredictable in the first hours, and respiratory status must be closely monitored. Suction equipment should be readily available. (I, N, G)

80. 3. Spinal shock produces massive vasodilation and subsequent pooling of blood in the peripheral circulation. The client is relatively hypovolemic and exhibits tachycardia, tachypnea, anxiety, and flushed but dry skin. Hypertension would not be expected. (A, C, G)

81. 3. During the period of spinal shock, the bladder is completely atonic and will continue to fill passively unless the client is catheterized. No reflex activity occurs during this period, so reflex emptying does not occur. (P, C, G)

82. 1. Range-of-motion exercises help preserve joint motion and stimulate circulation. Contractures develop rapidly in clients with spinal cord injuries, and the absence of this complication indicates treatment success. Footdrop is prevented by using a footboard. External rotation of the hips is prevented by using trachanter rolls. Local ischemia over bony prominences is prevented by following a regular turning schedule. (E, T, G)

83. 4. Lack of vasomotor tone in the lower extremities causes venous pooling, and the client may become hypotensive and dizzy when positioned upright. The tilt table is used to help the client overcome vasomotor instability and tolerate an upright position. Some pedal edema could occur, but it would develop gradually and would be less problematic than the hypotension. Elastic stockings are sometimes used to facilitate venous return from the legs. Signs and symptoms of insufficient cerebral circulation are pallor, diaphoresis, tachycardia, and nausea. (A, T, G)

84. 4. After the period of spinal shock, the muscles gradually become spastic due to an increased sensitivity of the lower motor neurons. The movement is not voluntary and cannot be brought under voluntary control. It is expected, but does not indicate that healing is taking place. (I, C, G)

85. 1. With a cervical injury, the client has sympathetic fibers that can be stimulated to fire reflexively. The firing is cut off from brain control and is both reflexive and massive. It classically produces pounding headache and dangerously elevated blood pressure, "goose bumps," and profuse sweating. Hot and dry skin, bradycardia, and paralytic ileus typically occur during spinal shock, not during autonomic dysreflexia. (A, C, G)

86. 3. Autonomic dysreflexia is a medical emergency. Although notifying the physician is important, it is more essential that the nurse intervene immediately in the situation. The rising blood pressure can cause cerebrovascular accident, blindness, or even death. Placing the client in the Fowler's position lowers blood pressure. Administering nitroprusside sodium (Nipride) intravenously is appropriate if the conservative measures are ineffective. A urine sample for culture should be obtained if the client has an elevated temperature and no other cause for the dysreflexia is found. A urinary tract infection may be causing symptoms. (I, N, G)

87. 2. The dysreflexia occurs from a sympathetic response to autonomic nervous system stimulation. A distended bladder is the most common cause; bowel fullness may also trigger the syndrome. After placing the client in a Fowler's position, the nurse should check the Foley catheter for patency and the rectum for fecal impaction. (A, T, G)

88. 2. Braces are designed to be applied while the client is lying down. They are custom-designed to fit contours of the chest and buttocks and may not fit properly if applied with the client in other positions. A poor fit could result in pressure areas and/or inadequate support. (P, C, S)

89. 2. As soon as the client's vasomotor status stabilizes, it is essential that she drink at least 2,000 ml of fluid daily, unless contraindicated. Increased fluid intake helps flush out bacteria and prevents urinary stasis.

Ingesting an acid-ash diet forms acid urine, which helps prevent urinary tract infection. Most citrus fruits are not metabolized as acids in the body. (I, N, H)

90. 3. Long-bone demineralization is a serious consequence of the loss of weight bearing. An excessive calcium load is brought to the kidneys and precipitation may occur, predisposing to stone formation. Absorption is not altered. (I, K, G)

91. 2. There are no contraindications to sexual activity in a woman with spinal cord injury, although she may not be able to experience orgasm. A Foley catheter may be left in place during intercourse in both male and female clients. Because a spinal cord injury does not affect fertility, the client should have access to family planning information so that an unplanned pregnancy can be avoided. (E, T, G)

92. 3. Spinal cord injury represents a physical loss; grief is the normal response to this loss. Working through grief entails reviewing memories and eventually letting go of them. The process may take as long as 2 years. (I, N, L)

THE NURSING CARE OF ADULTS WITH MEDICAL/SURGICAL HEALTH PROBLEMS

TEST 9: The Client With Musculoskeletal Health Problems

Directions: Use this answer grid to determine areas of strength or need for further study.

NURSING PROCESS

A = Assessment
D = Analysis, nursing diagnosis
P = Planning
I = Implementation
E = Evaluation

COGNITIVE LEVEL

K = Knowledge
C = Comprehension
T = Application
N = Analysis

CLIENT NEEDS

S = Safe, effective care environment
G = Physiological integrity
L = Psychosocial integrity
H = Health promotion/maintenance

		Nursing Process					Cognitive Level				Client Needs			
Question #	Answer #	A	D	P	I	E	K	C	T	N	S	G	L	H
1	3				I		K					G		
2	2	A					K					G		
3	4					E		C						H
4	2				I					N		G		
5	4	A								N		G		
6	4				I					N			L	
7	4			P					T		S			
8	2				I					N	S			
9	1				I				T		S			
10	2				I					N		G		
11	3				I				T		S			
12	3			P					T					H
13	4	A					K					G		
14	3	A						C				G		
15	3				I				T					H
16	4	A								N			L	
17	4	A							T			G		
18	1	A					K					G		
19	4			P						N		G		
20	3			P				C				G		
21	3					E				N		G		
22	1				I				T		S			
23	3				I					N		G		

ANSWER GRID: 1

Nursing Process

A = Assessment
D = Analysis, nursing diagnosis
P = Planning
I = Implementation
E = Evaluation

Cognitive Level

K = Knowledge
C = Comprehension
T = Application
N = Analysis

Client Needs

S = Safe, effective care environment
G = Physiological integrity
L = Psychosocial integrity
H = Health promotion/maintenance

		Nursing Process					Cognitive Level				Client Needs			
Question #	Answer #	A	D	P	I	E	K	C	T	N	S	G	L	H
24	2				I			C			S			
25	3				I			C			S			
26	3				I					N				H
27	1				I				T					H
28	3	A							T		S			
29	2			P				C			S			
30	2	A								N	S			
31	3			P			K				S			
32	3				I					N				H
33	3	A						C				G		
34	1				I				T			G		
35	4				I		K					G		
36	3				I					N		G		
37	3			P			K					G		
38	1		D							N		G		
39	2					E		C				G		
40	4				I					N	S			
41	2				I				T		S			
42	2				I					N	S			
43	3				I					N	S			
44	1					E				N		G		
45	4				I				T			G		
46	3				I			C				G		
47	1	A						C				G		
48	4	A					K				S			
49	3		D							N		G		
50	2					E			T			G		
51	4	A						C				G		
52	2				I				T				L	

Answer Grid: 2

NURSING PROCESS

A = Assessment
D = Analysis, nursing diagnosis
P = Planning
I = Implementation
E = Evaluation

COGNITIVE LEVEL

K = Knowledge
C = Comprehension
T = Application
N = Analysis

CLIENT NEEDS

S = Safe, effective care environment
G = Physiological integrity
L = Psychosocial integrity
H = Health promotion/maintenance

		Nursing Process					Cognitive Level				Client Needs			
Question #	Answer #	A	D	P	I	E	K	C	T	N	S	G	L	H
53	2			P				C				G		
54	2				I					N	S			
55	4			P			K				S			
56	4				I					N		G		
57	1			P					T			G		
58	2		D				K					G		
59	4					E			T			G		
60	4				I					N		G		
61	4				I		K				S			
62	4			P						N				H
63	3					E				N		G		
64	4				I		K					G		
65	2				I		K							H
66	2			P			K					G		
67	2				I				T		S			
68	1				I				T		S			
69	1			P				C				G		
70	1	A						C				G		
71	2			P				C				G		
72	1				I				T				L	
73	1	A							T		S			
74	4			P						N				H
75	1					E				N				H
76	4	A						C				G		
77	4			P					T			G		
78	3			P						N	S			
79	3				I					N		G		
80	3	A						C				G		
81	3			P				C				G		

ANSWER GRID: 3

Nursing Process

A = Assessment
D = Analysis, nursing diagnosis
P = Planning
I = Implementation
E = Evaluation

Cognitive Level

K = Knowledge
C = Comprehension
T = Application
N = Analysis

Client Needs

S = Safe, effective care environment
G = Physiological integrity
L = Psychosocial integrity
H = Health promotion/maintenance

		Nursing Process					Cognitive Level				Client Needs			
Question #	Answer #	A	D	P	I	E	K	C	T	N	S	G	L	H
82	1					E			T			G		
83	4	A							T			G		
84	4				I			C				G		
85	1	A						C				G		
86	3				I					N		G		
87	2	A							T			G		
88	2			P				C			S			
89	2				I					N				H
90	3				I		K					G		
91	2					E			T			G		
92	3				I					N			L	
Number Correct														
Number Possible	92	20	3	19	40	10	15	21	25	31	24	52	5	11
Percentage Correct														

Score Calculation:

To determine your **Percentage Correct**, divide the **Number Correct** by the **Number Possible**.

The Client With Sensory Health Problems

Test 10

The Client With Cataracts
The Client With a Retinal Detachment
The Client With Glaucoma
The Client Undergoing Nasal Surgery
The Clients With Hearing Disorders
The Client With Ménière's Disease
The Client With Cancer of the Larynx
The Client With Burns
Correct Answers and Rationale

Select the one best answer and indicate your choice by filling in the circle in front of the option.

The Client With Cataracts

A 76-year-old female client is admitted to outpatient surgery for a cataract extraction on her right eye. The procedure is to be done under a local anesthetic. The client lives alone in an isolated location and has no one to help her at home.

1. The client asks the nurse, "What causes cataracts in old people?" Which of the following statements should form the basis for the nurse's response? Cataracts
- ○ 1. usually result from chronic systemic disease.
- ○ 2. are thought to be a result of aging.
- ○ 3. are believed to result from eye injuries sustained early in life.
- ○ 4. usually result from the prolonged use of toxic substances.

2. The client says, "The doctor told me that he'll remove the lens of my eye. What does the lens do, anyway?" The nurse should explain that the lens of the eye
- ○ 1. produces aqueous humor.
- ○ 2. holds the rods and cones.
- ○ 3. focuses light rays onto the retina.
- ○ 4. regulates the amount of light entering the eye.

3. The client tells the nurse that she does not like the idea of being awake during the eye surgery. Which of the following responses by the nurse would be the most appropriate?
- ○ 1. "Have you ever had any reactions to local anesthetics in the past?"
- ○ 2. "What is it that disturbs you about the idea of being awake?"
- ○ 3. "By using a local anesthetic, you won't have nausea and vomiting after the surgery."
- ○ 4. "There's really nothing to fear about being awake. You'll be given a medication that will help you relax."

4. The client becomes disoriented postoperatively. Which of the following nursing measures would most likely help the client become reoriented?
- ○ 1. Reminding her where she is frequently.
- ○ 2. Calling her by familiar family names, such as "Granny."
- ○ 3. Dimming her room lights.
- ○ 4. Asking friends to make more frequent visits.

5. An essential aspect of the plan of care for the client following cataract removal surgery would be to
- ○ 1. increase cardiac output.
- ○ 2. prevent fluid volume excess.
- ○ 3. maintain a darkened environment.
- ○ 4. promote safety.

6. The client will be discharged to home on the same day as the surgery. What information about her vision would be most important for the nurse to include in her discharge plan?
- ○ 1. She will need to wear glasses or contact lenses to correct her vision.

○ 2. She will need to wear her glasses only until her eye heals.
○ 3. Cataract glasses correct vision by magnifying objects.
○ 4. She will need to relearn to judge distances accurately.

7. A client with a cataract would most likely complain of which symptoms?
○ 1. Halos and rainbows around lights.
○ 2. Eye pain and irritation that worsens at night.
○ 3. Blurred and hazy vision.
○ 4. Eyestrain and headache when doing close work.

8. Preoperatively before cataract surgery, the nurse is to instill several types of eye drops into a client's right eye. The accepted abbreviation for the right eye is
○ 1. OD.
○ 2. OS.
○ 3. OU.
○ 4. RE.

9. The nurse is to instill drops of phenylephrine hydrochloride (Neo-Synephrine) into a client's right eye before cataract removal surgery. This preparation acts in the eye to produce
○ 1. dilation of the pupil and blood vessels.
○ 2. dilation of the pupil and constriction of blood vessels.
○ 3. constriction of the pupil and constriction of blood vessels.
○ 4. constriction of the pupil and dilation of blood vessels.

10. After instilling eye drops in the client's eye, the nurse should apply slight pressure against the nose at the inner angle of the client's closed eye. What is the rationale for this action?
○ 1. It prevents the medication from entering the tear duct.
○ 2. It prevents the drug from running down the client's face.
○ 3. It allows the sensitive cornea to adjust to the medication.
○ 4. It facilitates distribution of the medication over the eye surface.

11. A short time after surgery, the client says, "I am sick to my stomach." The nurse's best course of action would be to
○ 1. instruct the client to take a few deep breaths until the nausea subsides.
○ 2. explain that this is a very common feeling that will pass quickly.
○ 3. tell the client to call the nurse promptly if vomiting occurs.
○ 4. medicate the client with an antiemetic, as ordered.

12. Which of the following would be an appropriate postoperative goal of decreasing intraocular pressure following eye surgery? The client will avoid
○ 1. lying supine.
○ 2. coughing.
○ 3. deep breathing.
○ 4. ambulation.

13. Following cataract removal surgery, the nurse teaches the client about activities that she can do postoperatively. Which of the following activities would be contraindicated?
○ 1. Walking down the hall unassisted.
○ 2. Lying in bed on the nonoperative side.
○ 3. Performing isometric exercises.
○ 4. Bending from the hips to pick up a pair of slippers.

14. Following cataract removal surgery, the client suddenly complains of a sharp pain in the operative eye and becomes restless. The nurse's actions should be guided by the knowledge that the client has very possibly developed which of the following postoperative complications?
○ 1. Detached retina.
○ 2. Prolapse of the iris.
○ 3. Extracapsular erosion.
○ 4. Intraocular hemorrhage.

15. Outcome criteria for the client following cataract removal surgery would include the client states
○ 1. her vision is clear.
○ 2. her infection is under control.
○ 3. methods to decrease intraocular pressure.
○ 4. she is able to maintain IV home infusion for pain management.

16. On reviewing the health record of a client admitted for cataract removal surgery, the nurse notes a long history of hypertension. With this knowledge, the nurse would correctly plan client teaching to include information about other eye problems the client may experience, because chronic hypertension tends to damage the eye's
○ 1. iris.
○ 2. sclera.
○ 3. retina.
○ 4. cornea.

The Client With a Retinal Detachment

A 70-year-old man is admitted through the emergency department with a diagnosis of detached retina in the right eye. His eyes are patched bilaterally on admission. He is accompanied by his wife, and they are extremely anxious.

17. As the nurse completes the admission history, the client reports that before the physician patched his eye, he saw many spots or "floaters." The nurse should explain to the client that these spots were caused by

○ 1. pieces of the retina floating in the eye.
○ 2. blood cells released into the eye by the detachment.
○ 3. contamination of the aqueous humor.
○ 4. spasms of the retinal blood vessels traumatized by the detachment.

18. The client's wife says that she does not understand what happened to her husband's eye. Which of the following explanations by the nurse would most accurately describe the pathology of retinal detachment?

○ 1. "A tear in the retina permits the escape of vitreous humor from the eye."
○ 2. "The optic nerve is damaged when it is exposed to vitreous humor."
○ 3. "The two layers of the retina separate, allowing fluid to enter between them."
○ 4. "Retinal injury produces inflammation and edema, which increase intraocular pressure."

19. The client asks the nurse why his eyes have to be patched. He finds the enforced blindness very frightening and rather disorienting. The nurse's reply should be based on the knowledge that eye patches serve to

○ 1. reduce rapid eye movements.
○ 2. decrease the irritation of light entering the damaged eye.
○ 3. protect the injured eye from infection.
○ 4. rest the eyes to promote healing.

20. The client remains extremely apprehensive. He states, "I'm afraid of going blind. It would be so hard to live that way." What factor should the nurse consider before responding to his statement?

○ 1. Repeat surgery is impossible, so if this procedure fails, vision loss is inevitable.
○ 2. The surgery will only delay blindness in the right eye, but vision is preserved in the left eye.
○ 3. More and more services are available to help newly blind persons adapt to daily living.
○ 4. Optimism is justified, because surgical treatment is 70% to 90% successful.

21. In the immediate postoperative period following scleral buckling, the client's nursing care should include all of the following except

○ 1. encouraging deep breathing every 2 hours.
○ 2. providing meaningful stimuli.
○ 3. applying pressure dressings to both eyes.
○ 4. performing range-of-motion exercises.

22. Which of the following statements would provide the best guide for activity for the client during his rehabilitation period?

○ 1. Activity is resumed gradually, and he can resume his usual activities in 5 to 6 weeks.
○ 2. Activity level is determined by the client's tolerance, and he can be as active as he wishes.
○ 3. Activity levels will be restricted for several months, so he should plan on being sedentary.
○ 4. Activity resumption is controlled by a graduated series of "buckle" exercises.

23. Which of the following clinical manifestations commonly occur in retinal detachment?

○ 1. Sudden, severe eye pain and colored halos around lights.
○ 2. Inability to move the eye and loss of light accommodation.
○ 3. A tearing sensation and increased lacrimation.
○ 4. Flashing lights and visual field loss.

24. Which of the following would be a priority goal for a client who has undergone surgery for retinal detachment?

○ 1. Control pain.
○ 2. Increase intraocular pressure.
○ 3. Promote a low-sodium diet.
○ 4. Maintain normothermia.

25. Following admission to the hospital and before surgical repair of a detached retina, the client is placed on flat bedrest. What is the rationale for this position?

○ 1. It helps reduce intraocular pressure.
○ 2. It facilitates drainage from the eye.
○ 3. It will keep the client safe while confined to bed.
○ 4. It helps prevent further retinal detachment or tearing.

26. Cryosurgery, a technique used to treat retinal detachment, uses extreme cold to

○ 1. seal the margins of the tear.
○ 2. stimulate an inflammatory response and scarring.
○ 3. attach the separated layers of the retina.
○ 4. reduce the metabolic demands of the retina.

27. Scleral buckling, another procedure used to treat retinal detachment, involves

○ 1. removing the torn segment of the retina and stitching down the remaining segment.
○ 2. replacing the torn segment of the retina with a strip of retina from a donor.
○ 3. stitching the retina firmly to the optic nerve to give it support.
○ 4. creating a splint to hold the retina together until a scar can form and seal off the tear.

28. In discharge planning following scleral buckling, the nurse should ensure that the client understands the need for initial activity restriction. Which of the following activities would be contraindicated during the early recovery period?

○ 1. Watching television.
○ 2. Reading.
○ 3. Talking on the telephone.
○ 4. Walking in the yard.

29. As part of discharge teaching following scleral buck-

ling for a detached retina, the nurse should instruct the client to
- ○ 1. avoid abrupt or jarring movement of the head.
- ○ 2. exercise the eye muscles each day.
- ○ 3. turn the entire head rather than just the eyes for sight.
- ○ 4. avoid activities requiring good depth perception.

The Client With Glaucoma

A 74-year-old male client is admitted to the hospital for diagnostic tests. He has been treated for chronic open-angle glaucoma for 5 years

30. The client asks the nurse, "How does glaucoma damage my eyesight?" The nurse's reply should be based on the knowledge that chronic open-angle glaucoma
- ○ 1. results from chronic eye inflammation.
- ○ 2. causes increased intraocular pressure.
- ○ 3. leads to detachment of the retina.
- ○ 4. is caused by decreased blood flow to the retina.

31. If the client experienced any symptom of glaucoma, it would most likely be
- ○ 1. eye pain.
- ○ 2. excessive lacrimation.
- ○ 3. colored light flashes.
- ○ 4. decreasing peripheral vision.

32. The nurse instructs the client on how to instill his eye drop medication. The client would perform the procedure correctly when he
- ○ 1. blows his nose immediately after administering the eye drops.
- ○ 2. positions himself on his right side to instill the eye drops.
- ○ 3. instills the eye drops into the conjunctival sac.
- ○ 4. wipes the tip of the eye drop applicator with a disposable tissue.

33. Miotics are frequently used in the basic treatment of glaucoma. The nurse should understand that miotics work by
- ○ 1. paralyzing ciliary muscles.
- ○ 2. constricting intraocular vessels.
- ○ 3. constricting the pupil.
- ○ 4. relaxing ciliary muscles.

34. The nurse would plan to administer which of the following drugs to the client with open-angle glaucoma?
- ○ 1. Pilocarpine hydrochloride.
- ○ 2. Atropine sulfate.
- ○ 3. Scopolamine hydrobromide.
- ○ 4. Acetazolamide (Diamox).

35. Glaucoma is a progressive disease that can be easily and effectively treated and yet can lead to blindness if not identified and treated. The most effective health-promotion measure related to glaucoma is
- ○ 1. prompt treatment of all eye infections.
- ○ 2. avoidance of extended-wear contact lenses by older persons.
- ○ 3. annual intraocular pressure measurements for all persons over age 40.
- ○ 4. appropriate blood pressure control.

36. The client's workup includes tonometry. Which of the following information should the nurse give the client when preparing him for the procedure?
- ○ 1. Oral pain medication will be given before the procedure.
- ○ 2. It is a painless procedure with no side effects.
- ○ 3. Blurred or double vision may occur after the procedure.
- ○ 4. Medication will be given to dilate the pupils prior to the procedure.

37. The nurse learns that the client uses timolol maleate (Timoptic) eye drops. The nurse would understand that this beta-adrenergic blocker helps control glaucoma by
- ○ 1. constricting the pupils.
- ○ 2. dilating the canals of Schlemm.
- ○ 3. reducing aqueous humor formation.
- ○ 4. improving ciliary muscle contractability.

38. The nurse observes the client instill his eye drops. The client says, "I just try to hit the middle of my eyeball so the drops don't run out of my eye." The nurse should teach him to instill the eye drops into the lower conjunctival sac and explain that the method he is now using may cause
- ○ 1. scleral staining.
- ○ 2. corneal injury.
- ○ 3. excessive lacrimation.
- ○ 4. systemic drug absorption.

39. When reviewing the discharge plan with the client, the nurse should encourage him to implement which of the following measures?
- ○ 1. Reducing daily fluid intake.
- ○ 2. Wearing dark glasses in the bright sun.
- ○ 3. Minimizing active exercise.
- ○ 4. Adding extra lighting to his home.

40. Acute narrow-angle glaucoma is a medical emergency that can quickly lead to blindness. Which of the following clinical manifestations would the nurse associate with this condition?
- ○ 1. Sudden loss of vision in one eye and headache.
- ○ 2. Acute light sensitivity and blurred vision.
- ○ 3. Double vision and headache.
- ○ 4. Sudden eye pain and colored halos around lights.

41. The client is scheduled for a minor surgical procedure. Which of the following orders would require clarification or correction before the nurse would carry it out?

○ 1. Administer morphine sulfate.
○ 2. Administer atropine sulfate.
○ 3. Teach deep breathing exercises.
○ 4. Teach leg exercises.

42. The client asks when he can stop taking the eye medication for his chronic open-angle glaucoma. The nurse's best response would be to tell the client that he

○ 1. can stop using the eye drops when his vision improves.
○ 2. needs to use the eye drops only when he has symptoms.
○ 3. must ask his physician that question.
○ 4. must use the eye medication for the rest of his life.

43. At 3 A.M., the client is awake. He has not received the sedative that had been ordered on a p.r.n. basis, nor does he routinely take sedatives at home. Which of the following nursing measures to promote sleep should receive the lowest priority in this situation?

○ 1. Offering him a bedpan.
○ 2. Giving him a backrub.
○ 3. Changing his position in bed.
○ 4. Administering the sedative.

44. The client has been diagnosed with an acute episode of narrow-angle glaucoma. The nurse would anticipate planning the client's nursing care based on an understanding that acute narrow-angle glaucoma

○ 1. frequently resolves itself without treatment.
○ 2. is typically treated with sustained bedrest.
○ 3. is a medical emergency that can rapidly lead to blindness.
○ 4. is most commonly treated with steroid therapy.

45. The client reports difficulty sleeping at night. The nurse explores the issue with the client and finds that he rarely sleeps more than 5 hours each night but takes a nap almost every morning and afternoon. The nurse evaluates the client's sleeping habits as poor. Which of the following statements most accurately describes the nurse's evaluation? The evaluation

○ 1. is correct; frequent short naps interfere with the overall quality of sleep.
○ 2. is correct; the total number of hours the client is sleeping is insufficient for a person his age.
○ 3. is incorrect; the total number of hours the client sleeps in each 24-hour period is more important than when he sleeps.
○ 4. is incorrect; sleeping for short periods usually is more healthful than sleeping for one long period in each 24-hour cycle.

The Client Undergoing Nasal Surgery

A 27-year-old female is admitted for elective nasal surgery.

46. The client returns from surgery after a submucosal resection for a deviated septum with nasal packing in place. Which of the following assessments would be a priority for the nurse at this time?

○ 1. Determining the degree of pain the client is experiencing.
○ 2. Assessing for airway obstruction.
○ 3. Observing for ecchymosis in the periorbital region.
○ 4. Assessing the client's appetite.

47. Which of the following techniques is the most appropriate way to assess for posterior nasal bleeding?

○ 1. Change the client's nasal drip pad frequently and note the amount of drainage.
○ 2. Monitor the client's hemoglobin and hematocrit values every 8 hours.
○ 3. Frequently ask the client if she feels nauseated.
○ 4. Use a penlight to inspect the back of the pharynx for bleeding.

48. After the client returns from surgery, the nurse would anticipate placing her in what position?

○ 1. Supine.
○ 2. Left side-lying.
○ 3. Semi-Fowler's.
○ 4. Reverse Trendelenburg's.

49. In addition to the prescribed analgesic, which of the following interventions would likely be most effective in managing the discomfort of rhinoplasty during the first 24 hours after surgery?

○ 1. Applying warm, moist compresses.
○ 2. Keeping the client in the prone position.
○ 3. Instructing the client to blow the nose gently.
○ 4. Applying ice compresses.

50. The client's postoperative orders include monitoring for bleeding. Which of the following would be an important initial clue that bleeding was occurring even if the nasal drip pad remained dry and intact?

○ 1. Complaints of nausea.
○ 2. Repeated swallowing.
○ 3. Rapid respiratory rate.
○ 4. Anxiety.

51. On the night of surgery, the client complains that the nasal packing is uncomfortable and asks when it will be removed. What information should the nurse give her about removing the packing?

○ 1. The nurse can remove it later that evening.
○ 2. The physician will remove it the next morning.
○ 3. The physician will remove it at the follow-up visit.
○ 4. The client can remove it after it has been in place for a week.

52. Because the packing blocks the client's nose, the nurse would need to include which of the following measures in her postoperative care?
- ○ 1. Frequent mouth care.
- ○ 2. Frequent lung auscultation.
- ○ 3. Increased frequency of vital sign measurement.
- ○ 4. Accurate intake and output records.

53. To promote adequate nutrition in the early postoperative period, the nurse would encourage the client to
- ○ 1. increase her fluid intake.
- ○ 2. drink through a straw.
- ○ 3. request an antiemetic before eating.
- ○ 4. limit intake of high-fiber foods.

54. The nurse would teach the client to implement which of the following nasal care measures after the nasal packing is removed?
- ○ 1. Irrigate the nares with normal saline solution daily.
- ○ 2. Remove old blood from inside the nares with cotton-tipped applicators.
- ○ 3. Lubricate the membranes for comfort with a water-soluble lubricant.
- ○ 4. Avoid cleaning the nares for at least 2 days.

55. The nurse should include which of the following information in the client's discharge teaching?
- ○ 1. She should expect tarry stools for several days at home.
- ○ 2. Nausea is an expected outcome of surgery and may persist for several days.
- ○ 3. Brief episodes of epistaxis are expected after the surgery.
- ○ 4. The pain from surgery should be resolved by the time of discharge.

56. The client is ready for discharge. Which of the following discharge instructions would be appropriate for the client?
- ○ 1. Avoid activities that elicit the Valsalva maneuver.
- ○ 2. Take aspirin to control nasal discomfort.
- ○ 3. Avoid brushing teeth until the nasal packing is removed.
- ○ 4. Apply heat to the nasal area to control swelling.

57. The nurse would include which of the following in the client's discharge instructions?
- ○ 1. Take aspirin to relieve pain.
- ○ 2. Use stool softeners and follow diet modifications to prevent constipation.
- ○ 3. Cough vigorously every 2 hours to prevent respiratory complications.
- ○ 4. Blow the nose forcefully each day to prevent the accumulation of dried secretions.

58. A woman tells the nurse that her 6-year-old daughter has severe nosebleeds. She says, "We both get so scared that I'm not sure I do anything right." Which of the following instructions should the nurse give this woman about managing nosebleeds?
- ○ 1. Help the child assume a comfortable position with her head tilted backward.
- ○ 2. Tilt the child's head backward and place firm pressure on the nose.
- ○ 3. Help the child lie on her stomach and collect the blood on a clean towel.
- ○ 4. Place the child in a sitting position with her neck bent forward and apply firm pressure on the nasal septum.

The Clients With Hearing Disorders

These are a variety of different situations.

59. Which of the following nursing interventions would be most appropriate for facilitating communication with a client who has a hearing impairment?
- ○ 1. Stand to one side of the client when speaking, to direct the voice directly into the client's ear.
- ○ 2. Speak loudly; shout if necessary.
- ○ 3. Stand close to the client and speak slowly and clearly.
- ○ 4. Ask only questions that the client can answer with a "yes" or "no" response.

60. A 75-year-old client who has been taking furosemide (Lasix) regularly for 4 months tells the nurse that he is having trouble hearing. What would be the nurse's best response to this statement?
- ○ 1. Tell the client that because he is 75, it is inevitable that his hearing should begin to deteriorate.
- ○ 2. Have the client immediately report the hearing loss to his physician.
- ○ 3. Schedule the client for audiometric testing and a hearing aid.
- ○ 4. Tell the client that the hearing loss is only temporary; when his system adjusts to the furosemide, his hearing will improve.

61. Which of the following techniques is appropriate for irrigating an adult client's ear to move cerumen?
- ○ 1. Allow the irrigating solution to run down the wall of the ear canal.
- ○ 2. Use sterile solution and equipment.
- ○ 3. The irrigating solution should be cool.
- ○ 4. After instilling the solution, pack the ear canal tightly with cotton pledgets.

62. Which of the following best describes the effects of a hearing aid for a client with sensorineural hearing loss?
- ○ 1. It will make sounds louder and clearer.
- ○ 2. It will have no effect on hearing.

○ 3. It will make sounds louder but not clearer.
○ 4. It improves the client's ability to separate words from background noises.

The Client With Ménière's Disease

A 58-year-old male client is undergoing a workup by an otolaryngologist for a diagnosis of Ménière's disease.

63. The classic triad of symptoms associated with Ménière's disease is vertigo,
○ 1. nausea, and headache.
○ 2. tinnitus, and hearing loss.
○ 3. headache, and double vision.
○ 4. hearing loss, and vomiting.

64. The client reports that he has noticed progressively worsening hearing problems over the last 5 years. Which one of the following symptoms is not a characteristic of sensorineural hearing loss?
○ 1. Greater loss of ability to hear high-pitched tones.
○ 2. Inability to distinguish and understand speech.
○ 3. Ability to hear better in a noisy environment.
○ 4. Speaking more loudly than normal.

65. The symptoms of dizziness and vertigo are both subjective experiences. Which of the following is the most accurate description of the experience of vertigo?
○ 1. A feeling that the environment is in motion.
○ 2. An episode of blackout.
○ 3. Light-headedness.
○ 4. Narrowed vision preceding fainting.

66. The client would be experiencing a typical symptom of Ménière's disease if, prior to an attack, he experienced
○ 1. a severe headache.
○ 2. nausea.
○ 3. blurred vision.
○ 4. a feeling of intra-ear fullness.

67. In Ménière's disease, diet modification is part of the client's treatment plan. The nurse would explain that the most frequently recommended modification is
○ 1. low sodium.
○ 2. high protein.
○ 3. low carbohydrate.
○ 4. low fat.

68. Which of the following statements by the client would indicate that he understands the expected course of the disease?
○ 1. The disease process will gradually extend to the eyes.
○ 2. Control of the episodes is usually possible, but a cure is not yet available.
○ 3. Continued medication therapy will cure the disease.
○ 4. Bilateral deafness is an inevitable outcome of the disease.

69. The potential for injury during an attack of Ménière's disease is great. The nurse should instruct the client to take which immediate action when experiencing vertigo?
○ 1. Place his head between his knees.
○ 2. Concentrate on rhythmic deep-breathing.
○ 3. Close his eyes tightly.
○ 4. Assume a reclining or flat position.

70. The client's wife expresses concern because during the past year, her husband has curtailed family activities and evenings out. Based on this information, which of the following would be the most appropriate nursing diagnosis?
○ 1. Social Isolation related to attacks of vertigo and hearing loss.
○ 2. Anxiety related to concern about progressive hearing loss.
○ 3. Self-Care Deficit related to labyrinth dysfunction.
○ 4. Altered Sensory Perception related to labyrinth dysfunction.

71. The nurse would anticipate that all of the following drugs may be used in the attempt to control the client's symptoms except
○ 1. antihistamines.
○ 2. anticholinergics.
○ 3. diuretics.
○ 4. glucocorticoids.

72. The client finds the chronic tinnitus extremely irritating. Which of the following strategies would be best for the nurse to suggest?
○ 1. Maintain a quiet, restful environment.
○ 2. Mask the tinnitus with background music.
○ 3. Ensure adequate levels of vitamin B6 in his diet.
○ 4. Explore the use of a hearing aid.

73. The primary goal of medical management for the client would be to
○ 1. save his hearing.
○ 2. prevent environmental injury.
○ 3. control his symptoms.
○ 4. help him cope with the disease.

The Client With Cancer of the Larynx

A 63-year-old male with intrinsic laryngeal cancer is admitted to the hospital for a total laryngectomy.

74. Because the intrinsic laryngeal cancer was identified early, the nurse would anticipate that the client's primary symptom was most likely

○ 1. difficulty in swallowing.
○ 2. persistent mild hoarseness.
○ 3. chronic foul breath.
○ 4. nagging unproductive cough.

75. The client is scheduled for radical neck surgery and a total laryngectomy. For which of the following postoperative possibilities should the nurse prepare the client preoperatively?
○ 1. Endotracheal intubation.
○ 2. Minimal postoperative pain.
○ 3. Immediate speech therapy.
○ 4. Normal oral and nasal breathing.

76. A priority nursing diagnosis category for the client with a laryngectomy would be
○ 1. Fluid Volume Excess.
○ 2. Impaired Communication.
○ 3. Decreased Cardiac Output.
○ 4. Powerlessness.

77. The priority nursing goal for the client during the immediate postoperative period should be to
○ 1. maintain a patent airway.
○ 2. provide nutrition.
○ 3. prevent strain on suture lines.
○ 4. prevent hemorrhage.

78. A nasogastric tube was inserted during surgery, and the client receives tube feedings to meet his fluid and nutrition needs. The primary rationale for tube feedings in this situation would be to
○ 1. prevent pain from swallowing.
○ 2. ensure adequate intake.
○ 3. prevent fistula development.
○ 4. allow for adequate suture line healing.

79. The client appears withdrawn and depressed. He keeps the curtain drawn, refuses visitors, and says he wants to be left alone. Which nursing intervention would most likely be therapeutic for the client?
○ 1. Discussing his behavior with his wife to determine the cause.
○ 2. Exploring his future plans.
○ 3. Respecting his need for privacy.
○ 4. Encouraging him to express his feelings nonverbally and in writing.

80. The development of laryngeal cancer is most clearly linked to which of the following factors?
○ 1. High-fat, low-fiber diet.
○ 2. Heavy alcohol use.
○ 3. Low socioeconomic status.
○ 4. Overuse of artificial sweeteners.

81. Which of the following measures should the nurse perform in relation to suctioning a tracheostomy tube?
○ 1. Apply suction while inserting the suction catheter into the tube.
○ 2. Change the tracheostomy tube after suctioning the client.
○ 3. Select a suction catheter that approximates the diameter of the tracheostomy tube.
○ 4. Administer high concentrations of oxygen before suctioning the client.

82. To more easily remove thick, tenacious secretions when suctioning a tracheostomy, the nurse would liquefy the secretions before suctioning by instilling the tracheostomy tube with 1 to 2 ml of sterile
○ 1. water.
○ 2. normal saline solution.
○ 3. bacteriostatic water.
○ 4. diluted hydrogen peroxide.

83. While suctioning a client's laryngectomy tube, the nurse should insert the catheter
○ 1. approximately 1″ to 2″.
○ 2. until resistance is met.
○ 3. until resistance is met, and then withdraw it 1 to 2 cm.
○ 4. until the client begins coughing.

84. The longest period the nurse should suction a client at one time is
○ 1. 5 to 10 seconds.
○ 2. 11 to 15 seconds.
○ 3. 21 to 25 seconds.
○ 4. 26 to 30 seconds.

85. After suctioning a client's tracheostomy tube, the nurse waits a few minutes before suctioning again. The nurse would use intermittent suction primarily to help prevent
○ 1. stimulating the client's cough reflex.
○ 2. depriving the client of sufficient oxygen supply.
○ 3. dislocating the tracheostomy tube.
○ 4. obstructing the suctioning catheter with secretions.

86. When suctioning a tracheostomy or laryngectomy tube, it is recommended that the nurse use a
○ 1. sterile catheter with each suctioning and then discard it.
○ 2. sterile catheter for all suctioning during an 8-hour period.
○ 3. sterile catheter for all suctioning during a 24-hour period.
○ 4. clean catheter with each suctioning and disinfect it between uses.

87. Outcome criteria following airway suctioning would include which of the following?
○ 1. Respirations unlabored.
○ 2. Hollow sound on chest percussion.
○ 3. Decreased mucus production.
○ 4. Breath sounds clear on auscultation.

88. Which of the following should the nurse include in a postoperative teaching plan for a client with a laryngectomy?
○ 1. Instructing the client to avoid coughing until the sutures are removed.

- ○ 2. Telling the client to speak by covering the stoma with a sterile gauze pad.
- ○ 3. Reassuring the client that normal eating will be possible after healing has occurred.
- ○ 4. Instructing the client to control oral secretions by swabbing them with tissues or by expectorating into an emesis basin.

89. A client with a new laryngectomy decides to learn about esophageal speech. The speech therapist would explain that this communication technique involves

- ○ 1. holding an electronic instrument against the esophagus.
- ○ 2. providing an access route from the trachea to the esophagus.
- ○ 3. filling the esophagus with air.
- ○ 4. replacing the larynx with scar tissue.

90. Which of the following health-promoting activities should the nurse teach the client with a new laryngectomy?

- ○ 1. Cleanse the mouth three times a day.
- ○ 2. Avoid taking tub baths.
- ○ 3. Develop an aggressive program of exercise to increase airway functioning.
- ○ 4. Dehumidify the air for comfort.

The Client With Burns

A 25-year-old male is admitted to the hospital after sustaining burns to the chest, abdomen, right arm, and right leg. The accident occurred when gasoline ignited while he was cleaning the engine of his motorcycle.

91. The client tells the emergency room nurse that when he realized his clothes were on fire, he ran into his house to telephone for help. Of the following courses of action that had been available to the client, it would have been best for him to

- ○ 1. fall to the ground and roll.
- ○ 2. take off his clothing immediately.
- ○ 3. stand still and call for help.
- ○ 4. spray his clothing with fire extinguisher liquid.

92. The shaded areas in the diagram above indicate the burned areas on the client's body. Using the "rule of nines," the nurse would determine that approximately what percentage of the client's body surface has been burned?

- ○ 1. 18%
- ○ 2. 27%
- ○ 3. 45%
- ○ 4. 64%

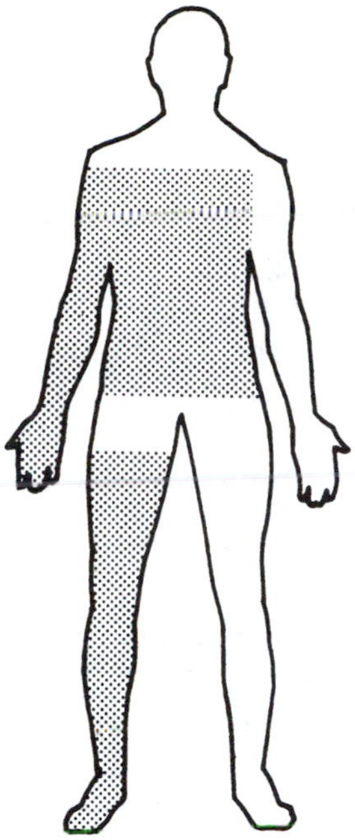

93. The nurse assesses the client for fluid shifting. The best definition of fluid shifts that are expected to occur during the emergent phase of a burn injury is that they are due to fluid moving from the

- ○ 1. vascular to interstitial space.
- ○ 2. extracellular to intracellular space.
- ○ 3. intracellular to extracellular space.
- ○ 4. interstitial to vascular space.

94. The nurse should recognize that the fluid derangement is due to a fluid shift that results from an increase in the

- ○ 1. permeability of capillary walls.
- ○ 2. total volume of intravascular plasma.
- ○ 3. total volume of circulating whole blood.
- ○ 4. permeability of the kidney tubules.

95. When bandaging the client's hand, the nurse should make certain that

- ○ 1. the hand and finger surfaces do not touch.
- ○ 2. the bandage is free of elastic.
- ○ 3. the hand and fingers are not elevated above the level of the heart.
- ○ 4. the bandage material is moistened with sterile normal saline solution.

96. A priority nursing diagnosis category for this client during the emergent period would be

- ○ 1. Fluid Volume Excess.
- ○ 2. Altered Nutrition: Less than Body Requirements
- ○ 3. High Risk for Injury Falls.
- ○ 4. High Risk for Infection.

97. Which of the following would provide the best emergency care for a burn victim at the accident site?

- ○ 1. Pouring cool water over the burned area.
- ○ 2. Applying clean, dry dressings to the area.
- ○ 3. Rinsing the area with a warm, mild soap solution.

○ 4. Applying a mild antiseptic ointment to the area.

98. During the first 48 to 72 hours of fluid resuscitation therapy following a major burn injury, the nurse would anticipate that the IV infusion rate will be adjusted by evaluating the client's
- ○ 1. daily body weight.
- ○ 2. hourly body temperature.
- ○ 3. hourly urine output.
- ○ 4. hourly urine specific gravity.

99. When the open method is used for treating burns, which of the following actions should the nurse take to help prevent discomfort caused by air currents over the client's burned skin surfaces?
- ○ 1. Keep the client well-sedated.
- ○ 2. Add humidity to the room air.
- ○ 3. Support the bed linens on a cradle.
- ○ 4. Keep the door and windows closed in the room.

100. The client is to take whirlpool baths with dressing changes. Which of the following activities should the nurse include on the client's care plan to be carried out about 1/2 hour before his daily whirlpool bath and dressing change?
- ○ 1. Soak the dressing.
- ○ 2. Remove the dressing.
- ○ 3. Administer an analgesic.
- ○ 4. Slit the dressing with blunt scissors.

101. The client with a major burn injury receives total parenteral nutrition (TPN). The primary reason for this therapy for this client is to help
- ○ 1. correct water and electrolyte imbalances.
- ○ 2. allow the gastrointestinal tract to rest.
- ○ 3. provide supplemental vitamins and minerals.
- ○ 4. ensure adequate caloric and protein intake.

102. The client hears physicians using the term "eschar" when speaking about the burn wounds; he asks the nurse what the word means. Which of the following descriptions by the nurse best defines eschar?
- ○ 1. Scar tissue in a developmental stage.
- ○ 2. Crust formation without a blood supply.
- ○ 3. Burned tissue that has become infected.
- ○ 4. Visible living tissue with a rich blood supply.

103. An advantage of using biologic burn grafts, such as porcine (pigskin) grafts, is that they appear to help
- ○ 1. encourage formation of tough skin.
- ○ 2. promote the growth of epithelial tissue.
- ○ 3. provide for permanent wound closure.
- ○ 4. facilitate development of subcutaneous tissue.

104. Which of the following factors would have the least influence on the survival and effectiveness of a burn victim's porcine (pigskin) grafts?
- ○ 1. Absence of infection in the wounds.
- ○ 2. Adequate vascularization in the grafted area.
- ○ 3. Immobilization of the area being grafted.
- ○ 4. Use of analgesics as necessary for pain relief.

105. While caring for the client with a burn injury, the nurse should observe for signs and symptoms of which complication believed to be due primarily to stress?
- ○ 1. Infection.
- ○ 2. Gastric dilatation.
- ○ 3. Nitrogen imbalance.
- ○ 4. Gastrointestinal ulceration.

106. When instructing the client about proper nutrition, the nurse would encourage him to eat which of the following meals?
- ○ 1. Chicken breast, salad, iced tea.
- ○ 2. Roast beef sandwich, milkshake, french fries.
- ○ 3. Hamburger, orange, coffee.
- ○ 4. Pasta salad, carrots, iced tea.

CORRECT ANSWERS AND RATIONALE

The letters in parentheses following the rationale identify the step of the nursing process (A, D, P, I, E); cognitive level (K, C, T, N); and client need (S, G, L, H). See the Answer Grid for the key.

The Client With Cataracts

1. 2. The most common cause of cataracts is aging, followed by eye injury. Other causes include ingestion of injurious substances, such as naphthalene, and systemic diseases, such as diabetes. (I, T, G)

2. 3. The lens focuses light rays onto the retina. The process of bringing light rays into focus from both near and far objects is called accommodation. The ciliary bodies secrete aqueous humor. The retina houses the rods and cones. The iris regulates the amount of light entering the eye. (I, T, G)

3. 2. The nurse should give a client who seems fearful of surgery an opportunity to express her feelings. Only after identifying the client's concerns can the nurse intervene appropriately. Premature explanations and cliches do not provide needed assessment data and ignore the client's feelings. (I, T, L)

4. 1. Reality orientation means frequently orienting the client to person, place, and time. Respect for the client dictates addressing her by name. Frequent visits by friends may be helpful but should not be the primary strategy for reorienting the client. Keeping the environment dim and very quiet is likely to increase the client's confusion. (I, T, G)

5. 4. Promoting safety is a priority goal for this client. Her vision will not be clear, and she may need to wear an eye patch following surgery. Orienting the client to the physical environment, assisting her during ambulation, and following other safety precautions to reduce the risk of injury are required. (P, T, S)

6. 4. After cataract surgery, a client must relearn to judge distances accurately to walk safely. The client will need glasses or contact lenses to restore vision, and cataract glasses do correct vision by magnifying objects; however, these points are not as important in discharge planning as is relearning to judge distance accurately. (I, T, H)

7. 3. A client with a cataract usually complains of blurred and hazy vision. This vision distortion is due to opacity of the lens, which blocks light rays from reaching the retina. (A, T, G)

8. 1. The accepted abbreviation for the right eye is OD, which stands for "oculis dexter." OS ("oculis sinister") refers to the left eye. OU ("Oculis uterique") refers to both eyes. RE is not an accepted abbreviation for the right eye. (I, T, S)

9. 2. Instilled in the eye, phenylephrine hydrochloride (Neo-Synephrine) acts as a mydriatic causing the pupil to dilate. It also constricts small blood vessels in the eye. (I, T, G)

10. 1. Applying pressure against the nose at the inner angle of the closed eye after administering eyedrops prevents the medication from entering the lacrimal (tear) duct. If the medication enters the tear duct, it can enter the nose and pharynx, where it may be absorbed and cause toxic symptoms. Eyedrops should be placed in the eye's lower conjunctival sac. (I, T, G)

11. 4. A prescribed antiemetic should be administered as soon as the client who has undergone cataract extraction complains of nausea. Vomiting can increase intraocular pressure, which should be avoided after eye surgery because it can cause complications. (I, T, G)

12. 2. Coughing is contraindicated after cataract extraction because it increases intraocular pressure. Other activities that are contraindicated because they increase intraocular pressure include turning to the operative side, sneezing, crying, and straining. Lying supine, ambulating, and deep breathing do not affect intraocular pressure. (I, T, G)

13. 4. Bending from the hips to pick up slippers is contraindicated after cataract surgery because it increases intraocular pressure. The client should be taught to flex her knees when picking up something from the floor. Activities such as walking, lying in bed on the nonoperative side, and performing isometric exercises are not contraindicated. (I, T, G)

14. 4. Pain and restlessness following eye surgery should suggest to the nurse that the client may be experiencing intraocular hemorrhage. The physician should be notified promptly. (A, T, G)

15. 3. Decreasing intraocular pressure is the primary concern following cataract removal. Vision will remain unclear temporarily after surgery. Infection, although it may occur, is not anticipated. IV infusion of pain medication at home is not required. (E, N, G)

16. 3. The retina is especially susceptible to damage in a client with chronic hypertension. The arterioles supplying the retina are damaged. (I, T, H)

The Client With a Retinal Detachment

17. 2. The spots, or "floaters," commonly reported by clients with retinal detachment are blood cells released into the vitreous humor by the detachment. (A, T, G)

18. 3. In retinal detachment, the two layers of the retina separate as a result of a small hole or tear, trauma, or degeneration. Vitreous humor seeps into the tear and separates the retinal layers. Vitreous humor does not leak out of the eye or cause any direct damage to the optic nerve. Increased intraocular pressure is not associated with retinal detachment. (I, T, G)

19. 1. Patching the eyes helps decrease random eye movements that could enlarge and worsen retinal detachment. (I, T, G)

20. 4. Untreated retinal detachment results in increasing detachment and eventual blindness, but 70% to 90% of clients can be successfully treated with surgery. If necessary, the surgical procedure can be repeated about 10 to 14 days after the first procedure. Many more services are available for newly blind persons, but ideally this client will not need them. (I, T, L)

21. 3. Pressure dressings are not applied to the eyes following the surgery, although general eye patching may temporarily be used. Elderly clients in particular need planned meaningful stimuli to prevent disorientation. Routine care includes range-of-motion exercises and deep breathing. Coughing should be avoided. (I, T, G)

22. 1. The scarring of the retinal tear needs time to heal completely. Therefore, resumption of activity should be gradual; the client may resume his usual activities in 5 to 6 weeks. Successful healing should allow the client to return to his previous level of functioning. (P, T, H)

23. 4. A client with retinal detachment frequently reports flashing lights in the affected eye followed by a loss of vision commonly described as like a curtain being slowly drawn across the eye. The detachment is painless, does not involve the eye muscles, and does not cause lacrimation. (A, K, G)

24. 1. Following surgery to correct a detached retina, the client requires analgesics for pain management. Decreasing intraocular pressure is another priority goal. Low-sodium diets and normothermia are not priority goals for this client. (I, N, G)

25. 4. The client's position is determined by the location of the retinal tear. The rationale for rest is the hope that the retina will fall back into place as much as possible before surgery, which will facilitate adherence of the retina to the choroid. Increased intraocular pressure is not a problem in retinal detachment. There should be no external drainage from the eye. (I, T, G)

26. 2. Using light, heat, and cold are all strategies that stimulate an inflammatory response in the area of the detachment. The eventual scarring reattaches the separated retinal layers. (P, T, G)

27. 4. A choroidal scar will form a permanent seal to close the hole or tear in the retina. A scleral buckle serves as a splint to hold the retina and choroid together until this scar can form. Loss of a portion of or the whole retina would interfere with sight. Retinal transplants are not performed. The retina is never stitched to the optic nerve. (P, T, S)

28. 2. Although restful, reading involves too much jerky eye movement and should be avoided during recovery. Watching television, walking outdoors, and visiting with friends are all appropriate activities and can be encouraged. (D, N, G)

29. 1. During recovery, the client should be instructed to avoid abrupt or jarring head movements. Such activities as shampooing or brushing the hair may be restricted. No specific eye exercises are prescribed, and depth perception is not specially affected by this surgery. (E, T, G)

The Client With Glaucoma

30. 2. In chronic open-angle glaucoma there is an obstruction to the outflow of aqueous humor, leading to increased intraocular pressure. The increased intraocular pressure eventually causes destruction of the retina's nerve fibers. This nerve destruction causes painless vision loss. The exact cause of glaucoma is unknown. (P, C, G)

31. 4. Although chronic open-angle glaucoma is usually asymptomatic in the early stages, peripheral vision gradually decreases as the disorder progresses. (A, C, G)

32. 3. Proper technique for instilling eyedrops includes maintaining sterile asepsis of the applicator tip, placing the client in a supine position, and instilling the eyedrops in the conjunctival sac. There is no need for the client to blow his nose after eyedrop administration. (E, T, S)

33. 3. A miotic agent constricts the pupil and contracts ciliary musculature. These effects widen the filtration angle and permit increased outflow of aqueous humor. Miotics also cause vasodilation of the intraocular vessels, where intraocular fluids leave the eye, also increasing aqueous humor outflow. Mydriatics cause cyclopegia, or paralysis of the ciliary muscle. (A, K, G)

34. 1. Pilocarpine hydrochloride is a commonly prescribed miotic that produces negligible systemic effects. Atropine sulfate and scopolamine hydrobromide have mydriatic effects. Acetazolamide (Diamox), a carbonic anhydrase inhibitor, decreases secretion of aqueous humor in the eye, thus lowering intraocular pressure. (P, C, G)

35. 3. The most effective health-promotion measure for a client with glaucoma is annual intraocular pressure measurements after age 40. Glaucoma is insidious and basically asymptomatic, and must be diagnosed before the client becomes aware of any vision changes. (I, T, H)

36. 2. Tonometry, which measures intraocular pressure, is a simple and painless procedure that requires no particular preparation or postprocedure care and carries no side effects. (I, C, S)

37. 3. Timolol maleate (Timoptic) is commonly administered to control glaucoma. The drug's action is not completely understood, but it is believed to reduce aqueous humor formation, thereby reducing intraocular pressure. (P, C, G)

38. 2. The cornea is very sensitive and can be injured by eyedrops falling onto it. Thus, eyedrops should be instilled into the lower conjunctival sac of the eye to avoid the risk of corneal damage. (I, T, H)

39. 4. Miotic agents may compromise a client's ability to adjust safely to night vision. For safety, extra lighting should be added to the home. The client does not need to curtail fluid intake. Bright lights are not harmful to the eyes, and exercise is permitted (although excessive exertion should be avoided). (I, N, H)

40. 4. Acute narrow-angle glaucoma produces abrupt changes in the angle of the iris. Clinical manifestations include severe eye pain, colored halos around lights, and rapid vision loss. (A, C, G)

41. 2. Atropine sulfate causes pupil dilation. This action is contraindicated for the client with glaucoma because it increases intraocular pressure. The drug does not have this effect on intraocular pressure in persons who do not have glaucoma. (P, T, G)

42. 4. To control his increased intraocular pressure, the client will need to continue taking his eye medications the rest of his life. Any loss of vision that the client has suffered will be permanent. Vision loss can occur gradually without any symptoms. (P, T, G)

43. 4. The nurse should use such nursing measures as giving a back rub, offering a bedpan, and changing the client's position in bed to promote sleep before resorting to sedative administration. But when nursing measures fail, the nurse may judge that a sedative is necessary to promote rest and sleep. Indiscriminate sedative use is indefensible. (I, N, G)

44. 3. Acute narrow-angle glaucoma is a medical emergency that rapidly leads to blindness if left untreated. Treatment typically involves miotic drugs and surgery, usually iridectomy or laser therapy. Both procedures create a hole in the periphery of the iris, which allows the aqueous humor to flow into the anterior chamber. (P, T, G)

45. 3. There are no rigid guidelines for normal periodicity and duration of sleep. What is important is that each person follow a rest pattern that maintains his well-being. (E, N, G)

The Client Undergoing Nasal Surgery

46. 2. Postoperative nursing assessment of the client after nasal surgery focuses on early detection of complications. Two common complications are airway obstruction and hemorrhage. The nasal packing can slip out of position and occlude the client's airway. Therefore, assessing the client for airway obstruction is a priority assessment. (A, N, S)

47. 4. The best way for the nurse to detect posterior nasal bleeding is to use a penlight to observe the back of the pharynx. The nasal drip pad will remain dry with posterior nasal bleeding. Nausea can occur postoperatively for several reasons, with bleeding being just one of them. Checking the client's hemoglobin and hematocrit every 8 hours will not help detect bleeding in its earliest stages. (A, N, S)

48. 3. To assist in breathing, promote comfort, and decrease edema formation after surgery, the client is most appropriately placed in a semi-Fowler's position. (P, T, S)

49. 4. The most effective way to decrease discomfort is to decrease local edema. Cold application, such as an ice compress or ice bag, is very effective. Heat dilates local vessels and increases local congestion. A semi-Fowler's position helps decrease edema and prevent aspiration. Nose blowing should be avoided for at least 48 hours after the nasal packing is removed, as it can disrupt the surgical site and lead to bleeding. (I, N, G)

50. 2. Because of the dense packing, it is relatively unusual for bleeding to be apparent through the nasal drip pad. Instead, the blood runs down the throat, causing the client to swallow frequently. The back of the throat can be assessed with a flashlight. An accumulation of blood in the stomach may cause vomiting. Increased respiratory rate occurs in shock, but is not an early sign of bleeding in the post-nasal surgery client. (I, N, G)

51. 2. The packing helps maintain hemostasis and prevent bleeding. Removing the packing is uncomfortable and must be done carefully. The surgeon generally removes the packing the day after surgery. The physician needs to assess the client before removing the packing and must be present in case bleeding occurs. (I, C, G)

52. 1. Mouth-breathing dries the oral mucous membranes. Frequent mouth care is necessary for comfort and to combat the anorexia associated with the taste of blood and loss of the sense of smell. The other interventions listed are not targeted at the effects of the packing. (I, T, G)

53. 1. Although foods as tolerated are encouraged, the nurse should encourage the client with nasal packing to increase fluid intake, because fluids are best tolerated at this time. Nasal packing makes eating very difficult and uncomfortable. The packing blocks the passage of air through the nose, creasing a partial vacuum during swallowing. A sucking action may occur when the client attempts to drink with a straw. Antiemetics are needed only if the client experiences nausea or vomiting. (I, T, G)

54. 3. A water-soluble lubricant offsets dryness and enhances comfort while healing occurs. The lubricant also prevents secretions from drying and crusting in the nose. The client should be cautioned not to disturb clots either with her fingers or applicators, as bleeding may occur. (I, N, H)

55. 1. Nasal bleeding gives stools a tarry appearance for several days; the client should be informed of this effect. Epistaxis and nausea are not expected outcomes, and some discomfort can be expected to persist after discharge. (I, T, H)

56. 1. The client should be instructed to avoid any activities that cause Valsalva's maneuver (e.g., constipation, vigorous coughing, exercise) to reduce bleeding and stress on suture lines. The client should not take aspirin because of its antiplatelet properties, which may cause bleeding. Oral hygiene is important to rid the mouth of old dried blood and to enhance the client's appetite. Cool compresses, not heat, should be applied to decrease swelling and control discoloration of the area. (I, N, H)

57. 2. The client should avoid blowing her nose for 48 hours after the packing is removed. Thereafter, she should blow her nose very gently using the open-mouth technique to minimize bleeding in the surgical area. She should also take measures to prevent coughing and avoid the use of aspirin. Constipation can cause straining during defecation, which can induce bleeding. (I, T, H)

58. 4. For the initial management of nosebleed, the client should sit up and lean forward with the head tipped downward. The soft tissues of the nose should be compressed against the septum with the fingers. The traditional head-back position allows blood to flow down the throat and can trigger vomiting. (I, T, H)

The Client With a Hearing Disorder

59. 3. Standing close to and directly in front of the client will greatly facilitate communication. Yelling at the client distorts the voice and further hinders understanding. The nurse should make sure that the client can see the nurse's mouth at all times to help facilitate lip-reading. It is best to speak slowly and clearly and to minimize distractions in the environment. The nurse should have the client validate his understanding of the conversation by repeating what was said. (I, T, S)

60. 2. Numerous drugs may cause ototoxicity; furosemide (Lasix) is one of these. Other ototoxic drugs include aminoglycoside antibiotics, antineoplastic drugs, and some thiazide diuretics. When teaching the client about ototoxic drugs, the nurse should emphasize the importance of promptly reporting any hearing loss, dizziness, or tinnitus, to help prevent permanent ear damage. (I, N, H)

61. 1. Ear irrigation is considered to be a clean procedure unless the integrity of the tympanic membrane has been damaged. The solution should be at body temperature and when instilled, should be allowed to run down the side of the ear canal. It should not be allowed to drop directly on the tympanic membrane, as this may cause discomfort or damage. Cotton pledgets should be placed loosely in the ear canal so as not to exert pressure on the tympanic membrane. (I, T, S)

62. 3. Hearing aids have limited use for clients with sensorineural hearing loss, because these clients experience problems with sound discrimination as well as volume. A hearing aid can make sound louder but not necessarily clearer. (A, C, G)

The Client With Ménière's Disease

63. 2. Ménière's disease involves the inner ear and is characterized by episodes of acute vertigo and tinnitus. It can result in progressive and irreversible hearing loss. The severe vertigo can lead to nausea and vomiting. Double vision and headache are not characteristic features of Ménière's disease. (A, C, G)

64. 3. Sensorineural hearing loss involves the inner ear and is a common degenerative problem for elderly people. The ability to hear high-pitched sounds is decreased, as is the ability to discriminate and understand sounds, especially in a noisy environment. Misinterpretation of voice levels causes these clients to speak in a louder-than-normal voice. (A, C, G)

65. 1. Vertigo is a form of hallucination in which the person perceives the environment to be moving around him or himself to be moving within the environment. Clients with Ménière's disease are not light-headed and do not faint or black out. (A, C, G)

66. 4. Many clients are able to identify an incipient attack of Ménière's disease by a feeling of fullness in the ear that reflects the evolving congestion. Ménière's disease does not affect vision. Nausea may result once the classic symptoms occur. (A, C, G)

67. 1. A low-sodium diet is frequently an effective mechanism for reducing the frequency and severity of the disease episodes. Approximately three-quarters of clients with Ménière's disease respond to treatment with a low-salt diet. A diuretic may also be ordered. (P, C, G)

68. 2. There currently is no cure for Ménière's disease, but the wide range of medical and surgical treatments allows for adequate control in many clients. The disease often worsens, but there is no indication that it spreads to the eyes. The hearing loss is usually unilateral. (E, C, G)

69. 4. The client needs to be placed in a safe and comfortable position during the attacks in Ménière's disease, which may last several hours. The client's location when the attack occurs may dictate the most reasonable position. Ideally, he should lie down immediately in a reclining or flat position to control the vertigo. The danger of a serious fall is very real. (I, T, H)

70. 1. A client with Ménière's disease may curtail social activities out of fear of embarrassment from having a dizzy spell in public. This seems likely in this situation, based on the wife's information, but would need to be validated by the client. However, the wife may be a more reliable source of information about social isolation than the client. The other three diagnoses are appropriate in Ménière's disease but are less directly related to social activity. (D, N, L)

71. 4. A wide variety of medications may be used in an attempt to control Ménière's disease, including antihistamines, anticholinergics, and diuretics. Glucocorticoids play no significant role in disease treatment. (P, T, G)

72. 2. The chronic tinnitus associated with Ménière's disease can be extremely intrusive and frustrating for clients. Quiet environments appear to worsen the client's perception of the problem. Attempting to mask tinnitus with a low-level competing sound, such as music, is often recommended. (I, T, G)

73. 1. Uncontrolled Ménière's disease can lead to irreversible hearing loss. Preventing this is the primary goal of medical treatment. The other options are important goals for both physicians and nurses during the client's care. (P, C, G)

The Client With Cancer of the Larynx

74. 2. Hoarseness occurs early in the course of most intrinsic laryngeal cancers, because the tumor prevents accurate approximation of the vocal cords during phonation. Foul breath and expectoration of blood are late symptoms. Large extrinsic tumors eventually produce difficulty and pain in swallowing. A nagging cough has no direct relationship to laryngeal cancer. (A, K, G)

75. 2. Postoperative pain is minimal, because the sensory nerves that convey pain are no longer present. The client may have a temporary laryngectomy tube, which remains in place until the wound is healed and a permanent stoma has formed, usually in 2 or 3 weeks. Speech therapy is delayed until healing occurs. Surgery permanently alters the airway and necessitates breathing through the permanent tracheal opening. (I, T, S)

76. 2. Following the client's laryngectomy, the nurse needs to establish an alternate communication pattern, since the client can no longer speak. The client needs to be able to make his needs known and express himself with dignity. The nurse should encourage him to communicate by writing or using a communication board with letters, words, or pictures, as desired. (D, N, L)

77. 1. Maintaining a patent airway is *the* priority nursing goal in the immediate postoperative period. The client's ability to cough and deep breathe is impaired, because the glottis has been removed. Promoting comfort, reducing strain on suture lines, preventing hemorrhage, and providing nutrition are important nursing goals, but maintaining a patent airway is the priority. (P, N, G)

78. 4. A nasogastric tube is usually inserted during surgery to instill food and fluids postoperatively. The tube allows the suture line to heal adequately, minimizes contamination of the pharyngeal and esophageal suture lines, and prevents fluid from leaking through the wound into the trachea before healing occurs. Normal oral feedings are resumed as soon as the nasogastric tube is removed, usually within 10 days after surgery. A tracheoesophageal fistula is a rare potential complication of total laryngectomy and may occur if radiation therapy has compromised wound healing. (P, T, G)

79. 4. The client has undergone body changes and permanent loss of verbal communication. He may feel isolated and insecure. The nurse can encourage him to express his feelings and use this information to develop an appropriate care plan. Discussing the client's behavior with his wife may not reveal his feelings. Exploring future plans is not appropriate at this time, because more information about the client's behavior is needed before proceeding to this level. The nurse can respect the client's need for privacy while also encouraging him to express his feelings. (I, T, L)

80. 2. Predisposing factors for laryngeal cancer include chronic irritants such as alcohol, cigarette smoke, and other noxious fumes. About 75% of persons who develop laryngeal cancer are smokers. The combination of smoking and heavy alcohol intake is even more strongly implicated as a causative agent in the laryngeal cancer. Epidemiologic studies indicate that a high-fat diet may be a major factor in the development of cancer of the breast, prostate, and colon. Low socioeconomic status is a predisposing factor in cervical cancer but not for laryngeal cancer. Artificial sweeteners have been related to the incidence of bladder cancer. (A, K, G)

81. 4. Clients are hyperoxygenated before suctioning to prevent hypoxia. Suction is never applied while inserting the catheter into the airway. The suction catheter should be about half the diameter of the tube; a larger-diameter suction catheter would interfere with air flow during the procedure. Laryngectomy tubes are not changed after suctioning. (I, T, S)

82. 2. Sterile normal saline is the solution of choice for instillation into a tracheostomy tube cannula to help liquefy sticky secretions. Normal saline solution is less irritating to mucous membranes than plain water, dilute hydrogen peroxide, and bacteriostatic water. The nurse may cleanse the area around a laryngectomy stoma with an applicator moistened with diluted hydrogen peroxide, but should be careful that none enters the stoma because of its irritating effects on respiratory mucosa. Furthermore, it is important to prevent aspiration. (I, T, S)

83. 3. The proper suctioning technique is to insert the suction catheter until resistance is met, withdraw the catheter 1 to 2 cm, and then begin applying intermittent suction while withdrawing the catheter. The suction catheter is inserted more than 1″ to 2″. Coughing by a client does not necessarily indicate when to begin or stop suctioning. (I, T, S)

84. 1. A client should be suctioned for no longer than 10 seconds at a time. Suctioning for longer than 10 seconds may reduce the client's oxygen level so much that he may become hypoxic. (I, T, S)

85. 2. After suctioning, the client should rest 3 minutes before suctioning is repeated, unless secretions interfere with breathing. Intermittent suctioning prevents oxygen deprivation. Hypoxia can lead to cardiac dysrhythmias and cardiac arrest. The client should receive 100% oxygen between suctionings. (I, T, S)

86. 1. The recommended technique is to use a sterile catheter for each suctioning in a client with a laryngectomy or tracheostomy tube. There is a danger of introducing organisms into the respiratory tract when strict aseptic technique, including a catheter change for each suctioning, is not used. (I, T, S)

87. 4. Auscultating for clear breath sounds is the most accurate way to evaluate the effectiveness of tracheobronchial suctioning. Auscultation should also be done to determine whether the client needs suctioning. Assessing for labored respirations, observing for cough productive of mucus, and percussing the chest for a hollow sound are not as accurate in evaluating the effectiveness of tracheobronchial suctioning. (E, T, G)

88. 3. Normal eating is possible once the suture line has healed. Coughing is essential to keep the airway patent. Since the larynx has been removed, the ability to speak is lost. Swallowing is usually not affected, nor is the ability to control oral secretions. (I, T, G)

89. 3. Esophageal speech requires filling the esophagus with air and allowing it to vibrate out. An artificial larynx (electrolarynx) is a hand-held speech aid placed against the neck. An access route from the trachea to the esophagus is required for tracheoesophageal shunting. This provides pulmonary power to the pharyngeal sphincter, which provides vibrations for a pseudo-voice. Replacing the larynx with scar tissue would not facilitate speech. (P, T, G)

90. 1. Oral hygiene is an important aspect of self-care for the laryngectomy client, who is less able to detect mouth odor. Additionally, the mouth harbors bacteria, and good mouth care reduces the risk of infection. The client is able to take tub baths with careful instruction on ways to avoid slipping, the need to make sure the water is no more than 6″ deep, and other safety measures. Air should be humidified to enhance comfort. Moderate exercise may be beneficial, but an aggressive exercise program is not usually part of the plan of care. (I, T, H)

The Client With Burns

91. 1. The priority action is to stop the burning. If the victim's clothing is on fire, he should drop to the ground and roll to extinguish the flames. Running is a natural response, but it only fans the flames. Standing still causes the flames and smoke to engulf the face, possibly igniting the hair and causing an inhalation injury. Falling to the ground and rolling would usually take less time than trying to find and use a fire extinguisher. (I, T, S)

92. 3. According to the "rule of nines," this client has sustained burns on approximately 45% of his body surface. His right arm is calculated as being 9%; his right leg is 18%; and his anterior trunk is 18%, for a total of 45%. (A, T, G)

93. 1. In a burn injury, the injured capillaries dilate and there is increased capillary permeability at the site of the burn. Plasma seeps out into the burned tissue, moving from the vascular space into the interstitial space. (A, C, G)

94. 1. When a burn occurs, the capillaries and small vessels dilate, and cell damage causes a release of a histaminelike substance. This substance causes the capillary walls to become more permeable, and significant quantities of fluid are lost. The initial fluid derangement following a burn is a plasma-to-interstitial fluid shift. (A, T, G)

95. 1. When bandaging the client's fingers and hands, the nurse must ensure that skin surfaces do not touch. Allowing skin surfaces to touch interferes with normal healing and is likely to be irritating. Bandages for burns may be elasticized and often are used to form an occlusive pressure dressing. The bandages may be impregnated with antimicrobial agents but are not ordinarily kept moist with water or normal saline solution. A bandaged hand is ordinarily elevated to prevent edema. (I, T, G)

96. 4. Infection is a priority problem for the burned victim. Fluid volume deficit and altered nutrition are not priorities during the emergent period. A high risk for falling is not a priority for this client, since the client would be on bedrest and most likely in a critical care unit. (D, N, G)

97. 1. The recommended emergency treatment for a heat burn is immersion in cool water or application of clean, cool wet packs. This treatment helps relieve pain and diminishes tissue damage by cooling the tissue. Ice is not recommended, because it may cause the victim to become hypothermic and may further damage burn lesions. Clothing should not be removed, nor should ointments be applied. Antiseptics or ointments are contraindicated, because they may lead to further tissue damage. (I, T, G)

98. 3. During the first 48 to 72 hours of fluid resuscitation therapy, hourly urine output is the most accessible and generally reliable indicator of adequate fluid replacement. Fluid volume is also assessed by monitoring mental status, vital signs, peripheral perfusion, and body weight. Pulmonary artery end-diastolic pressure (PAEDP) and even central venous pressure (CVP) are preferred guides to fluid administration, but urine output is best when PAEDP or CVP is not used. After the first 48 to 72 hours, urine output is a a less-reliable guide to fluid needs. The victim enters the diuretic phase as edema reabsorption occurs, and urine output increases dramatically. (E, T, G)

99. 3. Bed linens should be kept off a burn wound when the open method of wound care is used. To prevent drafts over the burned areas, it is best to place a cradle on the bed and drape bed linens over the cradle. Adding humidity to inspired air, keeping the client well sedated, and keeping doors and windows closed do not help prevent discomfort due to air currents passing over burned areas. (I, T, G)

100. 3. Removing dressings from severe burns will expose sensitive nerve endings to the air, which is very painful. The client should be given a prescribed analgesic about ½-hour before the dressing change to promote comfort. (P, T, G)

101. 4. Nutritional support with sufficient calories and protein is extremely important following severe burns because of the loss of plasma protein through injured capillaries and an increased metabolic rate. Gastric dilation and paralytic ileus commonly occur in severe burns, making oral fluids and foods contraindicated. TPN is also administered if the client is unable to take sufficient nourishment orally or by gastric gavage. It then becomes an effective method for supplying the body with nutrients—especially protein, which the burn victim needs in larger-than-average amounts. (I, T, G)

102. 2. Eschar is dead tissue, heavily contaminated with bacteria and without a blood supply. It is tissue that sloughs. Eschar has also been defined as devitalized skin. When eschar sloughs, an open wound that is almost always infected results. (I, T, G)

103. 2. Biologic dressings, such as porcine grafts, serve many purposes for a client with severe burns. They enhance the growth of epithelial tissues and minimize the overgrowth of granulation tissue, prevent loss of water and protein, decrease pain, increase mobility, and help prevent infection. (P, T, G)

104. 4. Analgesic administration to keep a burn victim comfortable is very important, but is unlikely to influence graft survival and effectiveness. Such factors as the absence of infection, adequate vascularization, and immobilization of the grafted area promote an effective graft. (E, T, G)

105. 4. Gastrointestinal ulceration, also known as Curling's ulcer or stress ulcer in the burn victim, occurs in about 50% of clients suffering from severe burns. The incidence of ulceration seems proportional to the extent of the burns. Such complications as infection, gastric dilation, and nitrogen imbalance may occur following burns, but they are not attributed to stress. (A, T, G)

106. 2. A roast beef sandwich, milkshake, and french fries would provide the burn victim with the extra protein and calories needed for healing. The other meals provide less calories or protein and would not be as good choices for the client with severe burns. (I, T, G)

THE NURSING CARE OF ADULTS WITH MEDICAL/SURGICAL HEALTH PROBLEMS

TEST 10: The Client With Sensory Health Problems

Directions: Use this answer grid to determine areas of strength or need for further study.

Nursing Process

A = Assessment
D = Analysis, nursing diagnosis
P = Planning
I = Implementation
E = Evaluation

Cognitive Level

K = Knowledge
C = Comprehension
T = Application
N = Analysis

Client Needs

S = Safe, effective care environment
G = Physiological integrity
L = Psychosocial integrity
H = Health promotion/maintenance

		Nursing Process					Cognitive Level				Client Needs			
Question #	Answer #	A	D	P	I	E	K	C	T	N	S	G	L	H
1	2				I				T			G		
2	3				I				T			G		
3	2				I				T				L	
4	1				I				T			G		
5	4			P					T		S			
6	4				I				T					H
7	3	A							T			G		
8	1				I				T		S			
9	2				I				T			G		
10	1				I				T			G		
11	4				I				T			G		
12	2				I				T			G		
13	4				I				T			G		
14	4	A							T			G		
15	3					E				N		G		
16	3				I				T					H
17	2	A							T			G		
18	3				I				T			G		
19	1				I				T			G		
20	4				I				T				L	
21	3				I				T			G		
22	1			P					T					H
23	4	A					K					G		

Answer Grid: 1

Nursing Process

A = Assessment
D = Analysis, nursing diagnosis
P = Planning
I = Implementation
E = Evaluation

Cognitive Level

K = Knowledge
C = Comprehension
T = Application
N = Analysis

Client Needs

S = Safe, effective care environment
G = Physiological integrity
L = Psychosocial integrity
H = Health promotion/maintenance

		Nursing Process					Cognitive Level				Client Needs			
Question #	Answer #	A	D	P	I	E	K	C	T	N	S	G	L	H
24	1				I					N		G		
25	4				I				T			G		
26	2			P					T			G		
27	4			P					T		S			
28	2		D							N		G		
29	1					E			T			G		
30	2			P				C				G		
31	4	A						C				G		
32	3					E			T		S			
33	3	A					K					G		
34	1			P				C				G		
35	3				I				T					H
36	2				I			C			S			
37	3			P				C				G		
38	2				I				T					H
39	4				I					N				H
40	4	A						C				G		
41	2			P					T			G		
42	4			P					T			G		
43	4				I					N		G		
44	3			P					T			G		
45	3					E				N		G		
46	2	A								N	S			
47	4	A								N	S			
48	3			P					T		S			
49	4				I					N		G		
50	2				I					N		G		
51	2				I			C				G		
52	1				I				T			G		

Answer Grid: 2

NURSING PROCESS

A = Assessment
D = Analysis, nursing diagnosis
P = Planning
I = Implementation
E = Evaluation

COGNITIVE LEVEL

K = Knowledge
C = Comprehension
T = Application
N = Analysis

CLIENT NEEDS

S = Safe, effective care environment
G = Physiological integrity
L = Psychosocial integrity
H = Health promotion/maintenance

		Nursing Process					Cognitive Level				Client Needs			
Question #	Answer #	A	D	P	I	E	K	C	T	N	S	G	L	H
53	1				I				T			G		
54	3				I					N				H
55	1				I				T					H
56	1				I					N				H
57	2				I				T					H
58	4				I				T					H
59	3				I				T		S			
60	2				I					N				H
61	1				I				T		S			
62	3	A						C				G		
63	2	A						C				G		
64	3	A						C				G		
65	1	A						C				G		
66	4	A						C				G		
67	1			P				C				G		
68	2					E		C				G		
69	4				I				T					H
70	1		D							N			L	
71	4			P					T			G		
72	2				I				T			G		
73	1			P				C				G		
74	2	A					K					G		
75	2				I				T		S			
76	2		D							N			L	
77	1			P						N		G		
78	4			P					T			G		
79	4				I				T				L	
80	2	A					K					G		
81	4				I				T		S			

ANSWER GRID: 3

NURSING PROCESS

A = Assessment
D = Analysis, nursing diagnosis
P = Planning
I = Implementation
E = Evaluation

COGNITIVE LEVEL

K = Knowledge
C = Comprehension
T = Application
N = Analysis

CLIENT NEEDS

S = Safe, effective care environment
G = Physiological integrity
L = Psychosocial integrity
H = Health promotion/maintenance

		Nursing Process					Cognitive Level				Client Needs			
Question #	Answer #	A	D	P	I	E	K	C	T	N	S	G	L	H
82	2				I				T		S			
83	3				I				T		S			
84	1				I				T		S			
85	2				I				T		S			
86	1				I				T		S			
87	4					E			T			G		
88	3				I				T			G		
89	3			P					T			G		
90	1				I				T					H
91	1				I				T		S			
92	3	A							T			G		
93	1			P				C				G		
94	1	A							T			G		
95	1				I				T			G		
96	4		D							N		G		
97	1				I				T			G		
98	3					E			T			G		
99	3				I				T			G		
100	3			P					T			G		
101	4				I				T			G		
102	2				I				T			G		

ANSWER GRID: 4

NURSING PROCESS

A = Assessment
D = Analysis, nursing diagnosis
P = Planning
I = Implementation
E = Evaluation

COGNITIVE LEVEL

K = Knowledge
C = Comprehension
T = Application
N = Analysis

CLIENT NEEDS

S = Safe, effective care environment
G = Physiological integrity
L = Psychosocial integrity
H = Health promotion/maintenance

		Nursing Process					Cognitive Level				Client Needs			
Question #	Answer #	A	D	P	I	E	K	C	T	N	S	G	L	H
103	2			P					T			G		
104	4					E			T			G		
105	4	A							T			G		
106	2				I				T			G		
Number Correct														
Number Possible	106	19	4	20	55	8	4	16	69	17	18	69	5	14
Percentage Correct														

Score Calculation:

To determine your **Percentage Correct**, divide the **Number Correct** by the **Number Possible.**

BIBLIOGRAPHY

Bates, B. (1991). *A guide to physical examination and history taking* (5th ed.). Philadelphia: J.B. Lippincott.

Beare, C., & Myers, J. (1990). *Principles and practice of adult health nursing.* St. Louis: C.V. Mosby.

Beckingham, A.C. (1993). *Promoting health aging: A nursing and community perspective.* St. Louis: Mosby Yearbook.

Belcher, A. (1992). *Mosby's clinical nursing series: Cancer nursing.* St. Louis: Mosby Yearbook.

Bellack, J.P., & Edlund, B.J. (1992). *Nursing assessment and diagnosis* (2nd ed.). Boston: Jones and Bartlett.

Birchenall, J.M., & Streight, M.E. (1992). *Geriatric nursing: Care of the older adult* (3rd ed.). Philadelphia: J.B. Lippincott.

Black, J.M., & Matassarin-Jacobs, E. (1993). *Luckmann & Sorensen's medical-surgical nursing: A psychophysiologic approach* (4th ed.). Philadelphia: W.B. Saunders.

Bowers, A.C., & Thompson, J.M. (1992). *Clinical manual of health assessment* (4th ed.). St. Louis: Mosby Yearbook.

Brunner, L.S., & Suddarth, D.S. (1989). *Textbook of medical-surgical nursing* (5th ed.). Philadelphia: J.B. Lippincott.

Brunner, L.S., & Suddarth, D.S. (1991). *The Lippincott manual of nursing practice* (5th ed.). Philadelphia: J.B. Lippincott.

Bullock, B., & Rosendahl, P.H. (1992). *Pathophysiology: Adaptations and alterations in function* (3rd ed.). Philadelphia: J.B. Lippincott.

Carpenito, L.J. (1993). *Handbook of nursing diagnosis* (5th ed.). Philadelphia: J.B. Lippincott.

Carpenito, L.J. (1993). *Nursing diagnosis: Application to clinical practice* (5th ed.). Philadelphia: J.B. Lippincott.

Chernecky, C.C., Berger, B.J., & Krech, R.L. (1993). *Laboratory tests and diagnostic procedures.* Philadelphia: W.B. Saunders.

Christensen, P.J., & Kenney, J.W. (1990). *Nursing process: Application of theories, frameworks, and models* (3rd ed.). St. Louis: Mosby Yearbook.

Clark, J.B., Queener, S.F., & Karb, V.B. (1992). *Pharmacologic basis of nursing practice.* (4th ed.). St. Louis: Mosby Yearbook.

Clochesy, J.M., Breu, C., Cardin, S., Rudy, E.B., & Whittaker, A. (1992). *Critical care nursing.* Philadelphia: W.B. Saunders.

Craven, R.F., & Hirnle, C.J. (1992). *Fundamentals of nursing: Human health & function.* Philadelphia: J.B. Lippincott.

Creighton, H. (1986). *Law every nurse should know* (5th ed.). Philadelphia: W.B. Saunders.

Davis, J., & Sherer, K. (1993). *Applied nutrition and diet therapy for nurses* (2nd ed.). Philadelphia: W.B. Saunders.

Davies, J.L., & Janosik, E.H. (1991). *Mental health and psychiatric nursing: A caring approach.* Boston: Jones and Bartlett.

Dittmar, S.S. (1989). *Rehabilitation nursing: Process and application.* St. Louis: Mosby Yearbook.

Dossey, B.M., Guzzetta, C.E., & Kenner, C.V. (1992). *Critical care nursing: Body-mind-spirit* (3rd ed.). Philadelphia: J.B. Lippincott.

Dossey, B.M., Keegan, L., Guzzetta, C.E., & Kolkmeier, L.G. (1988). *Holistic nursing: A handbook for practice.* Gaithersburg, MD: Aspen.

Earnest, V.V. (1993). *Clinical skills in nursing practice* (2nd ed.). Philadelphia: J.B. Lippincott.

Ebersole, P., & Hess, P. (1990). *Toward healthy aging: Human needs and nursing response* (3rd ed.). St. Louis: Mosby Yearbook.

Edelman, C.L., & Mandle, C.L. (1990). *Health promotion throughout the lifespan* (2nd ed.). St. Louis: Mosby Yearbook.

Eliopoulos, C. (1993). *Gerontological nursing* (3rd ed.). Philadelphia: J.B. Lippincott.

Ferri, R.S. (1992). *Care planning for the older adult: Nursing diagnosis in long-term care.* Philadelphia: W.B. Saunders.

Fischbach, F. (1992). *A manual of laboratory and diagnostic tests* (4th ed.). Philadelphia: J.B. Lippincott.

Flaskerud, J.H., & Ungvarski, P.J. (1992). *HIV/AIDS: A guide to nursing care* (2nd ed.). Philadelphia: W.B. Saunders.

Fogel, C.I., & Lauver, D. (1990). *Sexual health promotion.* Philadelphia: W.B. Saunders.

Fuller, J., & Schaller-Ayres, J.M. (1990). *Health assessment: A nursing approach.* Philadelphia: J.B. Lippincott.

Giger, J., & Davidhizar, R. (1991). *Transcultural nursing: Assessment and intervention.* St. Louis: Mosby Yearbook.

Gordon, M. (1991). *Manual of nursing diagnosis: 1991–1992.* St. Louis: Mosby Yearbook.

Grimes, D.E. (1991). *Mosby's clinical nursing series: Infectious diseases.* St. Louis: Mosby Yearbook.

Grimes, J., & Burns, E. (1992). *Health assessment in nursing practice* (3rd ed.). Boston: Jones and Bartlett.

Groenwald, S.L., Frogge, M.H., Goodman, M., & Yarbro, C.H. (1993). *Cancer nursing principles and practice* (3rd ed.). Boston: Jones and Bartlett.

Groer, M.W., Shekleton, M.E.: *Basic pathophysiology: A holistic approach* (3rd ed.). St. Louis: Mosby Yearbook.

Gruendemann, B.J., & Fernsebner, B. (1993). *Textbook of perioperative nursing.* Boston: Jones and Bartlett.

Haggard, A. (1989). *Handbook of patient education.* Gaithersburg, MD: Aspen.

Hartshorn, J.C., Lamborn, M., & Noll, M.L. (1993). *Introduction to critical care nursing.* Philadelphia: W.B. Saunders.

Horne, M., Heitz, U.E., & Swearingen, P.L. (1991). *Fluid, electrolyte, and acid-base balance: A case study approach.* St. Louis: Mosby Yearbook.

Huang, S.H., Kessler, A., McCulloch, C.D., & Dasher, L.A. (1989). *Coronary care nursing* (2nd ed.). Philadelphia: W.B. Saunders.

Hubbard, S.M., Green, P.E., & Knobf, M.T. (1993). *Current issues in cancer nursing practice.* Philadelphia: J.B. Lippincott.

Hudak, C.M., Gallo, B.M., & Benz, J.J. (1990). *Critical care nursing: A holistic approach* (5th ed.). Philadelphia: J.B. Lippincott.

Ignatavicius, D.D., & Bayne, M.V. (1991). *Medical-surgical nursing: A nursing process approach.* Philadelphia: W.B. Saunders.

Iyer, P.W., Taptich, B.J., & Bernocchi-Losey, D. (1991). *Nursing process and nursing diagnosis* (2nd ed.). Philadelphia: W.B. Saunders.

Jarvis, C. (1992). *Physical examination and health assessment.* Philadelphia: W.B. Saunders.

Karch, A.M. (1992). *Handbook of drugs and the nursing process* (2nd ed.). Philadelphia: J.B. Lippincott.

Kart, C.S., Metress, E.K., & Metress, S.P. (1992). *Human aging and chronic disease.* Boston: Jones and Bartlett.

Kim, M.J., McFarland, G.K., & McLane, A.M. (1992). *Pocket guide to nursing diagnosis* (5th ed.). St. Louis: Mosby Yearbook.

Kniesl, C., & Ames, S. (1990). *Adult health nursing: A biopsychosocial approach.* Menlo Park, CA: Addison-Wesley.

Kozier, B., & Erb, G. (1987). *Fundamentals of nursing: Concepts and procedures.* Menlo Park, CA: Addison-Wesley.

Lewis, S., & Collier, I. (1992). *Medical-surgical nursing.* St. Louis: C.V. Mosby.

Lewis, S., & Collier, I. (1992). *Medical-surgical nursing: Assessment and management of clinical problems* (3rd ed.). St. Louis: Mosby Yearbook.

Lewis, S., Grainger, R.D., McDowell, W.A., Gregory, R.J., & Messner, R.L. (1989). *Manual of psychosocial nursing interventions: Promoting mental health in medical-surgical settings.* Philadelphia: W.B. Saunders.

Lubkin, I.M. (1990). *Chronic illness: Impact and interventions* (2nd ed.). Boston: Jones and Bartlett.

Malasanos, L., Barkauskas, V., & Stoltenberg-Allen, K. (1990). *Health Assessment* (4th ed.). St. Louis: Mosby Yearbook.

Matteson, M.A., & McConnell, E.S. (1988). *Gerontological nursing: Concepts and practice.* Philadelphia: W.B. Saunders.

McCaffery, M., & Beebe, A. (1989). *Pain: Clinical manual for nursing practice.* St. Louis: Mosby Yearbook.

Meltzer, M., & Palau, S.M. (1993). *Reading and study strategies for nursing students.* Philadelphia: W.B. Saunders.

Metheny, N.M. (1992). *Fluid and electrolyte balance: Nursing considerations* (2nd ed.). Philadelphia: J.B. Lippincott.

Nentwich, P.F. (1990). *Intravenous therapy: A comprehensive application of intravenous therapy and medication administration.* Boston: Jones and Bartlett.

Pagana, K.D., & Pagana, T.J. (1992). *Mosby's diagnostic and laboratory test reference.* St. Louis: Mosby Yearbook.

Palmer, M.B. (1984). *Infection control: A policy and procedure manual.* Philadelphia: W.B. Saunders.

Perry, A.G., & Potter, P.A. (1990). *Clinical nursing skills and techniques* (2nd ed.). St. Louis: Mosby Yearbook.

Phipps, W., Long, B., & Woods, N. (1987). *Medical-surgical nursing: Concepts and clinical practices.* St. Louis: C.V. Mosby.

Pojman, L.P. (1992). *Life and death: Grappling with the moral dilemmas of our time.* Boston: Jones and Bartlett.

Porth, C.M. (1990). *Pathophysiology: Concepts of altered health states* (3rd ed.). Philadelphia: J.B. Lippincott.

Potter, P., & Perry, A. (1987). *Basic nursing theory and practice.* St. Louis: C.V. Mosby.

Potter, P., & Perry, A.G. (1992). *Fundamentals of nursing: Concepts, process, and practice* (3rd ed.). St. Louis: Mosby Yearbook.

Rorden, J.W., & Taft, E. (1990). *Discharge planning guide for nurses.* Philadelphia: W.B. Saunders.

Smeltzer, S.C., & Bare, B.G. (1992). *Brunner and Suddarth's textbook of medical-surgical nursing* (7th ed.). Philadelphia: J.B. Lippincott.

Swearingen, P.L. (1990). *Manual of nursing therapeutics: Applying nursing diagnoses to medical disorders.* (2nd ed.). St. Louis: Mosby Yearbook.

Swearingen, P.L., & Keen, J.H. (1991). *Manual of critical care: Applying nursing diagnoses to adult critical illness* (2nd ed.). St. Louis: Mosby Yearbook.

Taylor, C., Lillis, C.A., & LeMone, P. (1993). *Fundamentals of nursing: The art and science of nursing care* (2nd ed.). Philadelphia: J.B. Lippincott.

Thelan, L.A., Davie, J.K., & Urden, L.D. (1990). *Textbook of critical care nursing: Diagnosis and management.* St. Louis: Mosby Yearbook.

Tilkian, A.G., & Conover, M.B. (1993). *Understanding heart sounds and murmurs: With an introduction to lung sounds* (3rd ed.). Philadelphia: W.B. Saunders.

Underhill, S.L., Woods, S., Froelicher, E.S., & Halpenny, C.J. (1989). *Cardiac nursing* (2nd ed.). Philadelphia: L.B. Lippincott.

Williams, S.R. (1990). *Essentials of nutrition and diet therapy.* (5th ed.). St. Louis: Mosby Yearbook.

Workman, M.L., Ellerhorst-Ryan, J., & Hargrave-Koertge, V. (1992). *Nursing care of the immunocompromised patient.* Philadelphia: W.B. Saunders.

Section TWO

Postreview Tests

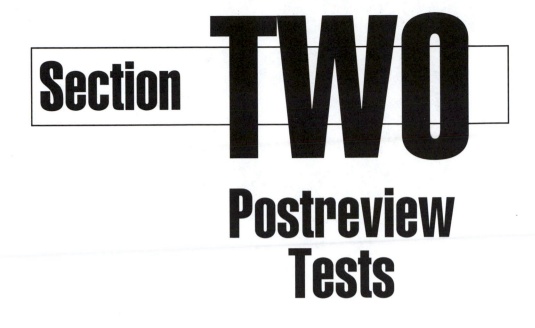

Part V

Postreview Comprehensive Tests

These four tests resemble the National Council Examination for Registered Nurses (NCLEX-RN). Just as the examination is comprehensive, so are these tests. After you have completed the four comprehensive tests, refer to the sections entitled "Correct Answers and Rationale" to reinforce or increase your knowledge and to evaluate your success. Study the rationale for each item carefully. Reading the rationale for items that you answered correctly reinforces your knowledge, while reading the rationale for items that you answered incorrectly clarifies misconceptions and expands your knowledge.

To evaluate your success on a comprehensive test, make a check mark next to the items you answered incorrectly and then determine the percentage of items you answered correctly. To do so, divide the number of your correct responses by the total number of questions in the test and multiply by 100. For example, if you answered 80 of 90 questions correctly, divide 80 by 90 and multiply by 100. The result is 89%. If you answered more than 75% of the items correctly, you are most likely prepared to take the NCLEX-RN. If, however, you answered less than 75% of the items correctly, carefully examine the items that you answered incorrectly. Did you answer incorrectly because of lack of content knowledge or because you did not read carefully? Errors attributable to not reading the question carefully indicate the need to revise your test-taking strategies (see the introduction to this book). Lack of knowledge indicates the need for further review in that content area. If you identify areas in which you need more concentrated review, you can complete the questions in the section of this book devoted to that clinical area. More information about NCLEX-RN and the format and use of this review is presented in the introduction to this book.

Select the one best answer and indicate your choice by filling in the circle in front of the option.

Comprehensive Test 1

1. Which of the following positions would permit the best assessment of a client's inguinal hernia?
- ○ 1. Standing.
- ○ 2. Sitting.
- ○ 3. Left side-lying.
- ○ 4. Right side-lying.

2. About 6 months after stabilization, a client begins to skip her prescribed doses of haloperidol (Haldol) and her counseling sessions. She tells the nurse that "I just forget to take the medication when things are going well." Which of the following interventions would the nurse include in the plan to help the client continue to take her medication?
- ○ 1. Explain the negative effects that skipping the medication will have on her condition.
- ○ 2. Consult with the staff psychiatrist about changing the medication to haloperidol decanoate (Haldol Decanoate) injections administered by the nurse.
- ○ 3. Have the client's family begin long-term commitment procedures so that her medication regimen can be supervised more closely.
- ○ 4. Refer the client to a partial hospitalization program so that she can participate regularly in group therapy sessions.

3. The nurse is caring for a primigravid client in the first trimester of pregnancy. When the client complains of morning sickness, the nurse would suggest that to help relieve the discomfort, she should eat a diet low in
- ○ 1. fat.
- ○ 2. protein.
- ○ 3. roughage.
- ○ 4. carbohydrates.

4. A client with bulimia binges twice a day. These binges would most likely involve
- ○ 1. feelings of euphoria, excitement, and gratification.
- ○ 2. feeling out of control, frightened, and disgusted with self.
- ○ 3. leaving traces of food around to attract attention.
- ○ 4. eating increasing amounts of food, resulting in substantial weight gain.

5. A client uses the telephone as often as several times an hour. This behavior is judged to be inappropriate but in keeping with his hyperactive behavior. In a nursing team conference, the team considers various ways to handle the problem and decides that the best course of action would be to
- ○ 1. take the client back to his room each time he goes to the telephone.
- ○ 2. explain to the client that because he abused his telephone privileges, he can no longer use the telephone.
- ○ 3. work out a plan with the client about the number of telephone calls he can make each day.
- ○ 4. allow the client to use the telephone when he likes until he begins to show improvement from therapy.

6. A client is scheduled for a ureterolithotomy via a flank incision. Given the specific surgical procedure, the nurse would plan to monitor the client postoperatively for signs and symptoms of
- ○ 1. parotitis.
- ○ 2. infection.
- ○ 3. deep vein thrombosis.
- ○ 4. respiratory alkalosis.

7. The nurse is caring for a primigravida in active labor. Immediately after the client's membranes rupture, the nurse assesses the fetal heart rate. The nurse would explain to the client that fetal distress due to pressure on the cord is associated with
- ○ 1. an increasingly arrhythmic fetal heartbeat before contractions.
- ○ 2. a persistently slow fetal heartbeat after contractions.
- ○ 3. a steadily increasing heartbeat during contractions.
- ○ 4. an intermittently rapid and slow fetal heartbeat between contractions.

8. A child, age 2, has just returned to the unit after a ventral-peritoneal shunt insertion. The nurse notes that the child's fontanel is slightly depressed, pupils are equal and reactive, heart rate is 100 beats/minute, respiratory rate is 24 breaths/minute, and blood pressure is 100/60 mm Hg. The nurse should
- ○ 1. elevate the head of the bed slightly, place the child on the side opposite the shunt with the head midline, and check the abdominal dressing.
- ○ 2. further assess the child by asking the child to state the date, time of day, and his age.

○ 3. notify the physician of the abnormal vital signs, then turn the child to the shunt side to increase drainage.
○ 4. repeat vital sign assessment in 15 minutes to verify their accuracy, then notify the physician.

9. During the client's final counseling session with the nurse regarding the death of his spouse, he makes the following comments. Which comment is least reflective of successful counseling outcomes?
○ 1. "I'm beginning to think I enjoy sack time (sleep) too much."
○ 2. "Did I tell you that I met a lady and we enjoy watching TV together?"
○ 3. "I would like to go on with these sessions. They are most interesting."
○ 4. "It has become a fun game to see how many different things I can do to feel better."

10. A nurse is caring for a term neonate that was delivered vaginally. Immediately after birth, the first action that the nurse plans is to assist with
○ 1. cutting the umbilical cord to prevent blood loss.
○ 2. wrapping the neonate in a warm blanket to prevent hypothermia.
○ 3. instilling erythromycin prophylaxis to protect the neonate's eyes from ophthalmia neonatorum.
○ 4. ensuring an open airway to promote pulmonary function.

11. The nurse is caring for a primigravida in active labor. The cervix is completely dilated, the fetal head is presenting, and delivery is imminent. The nurse would explain to the client that the best time to deliver the fetal head is
○ 1. midway between contractions.
○ 2. as soon as a contraction begins.
○ 3. during the last part of a contraction.
○ 4. immediately before a contraction.

12. A 23-year-old primigravida is admitted to the hospital in active labor. The client has had no complications during the pregnancy, is at 38 weeks gestation, and has attended childbirth classes. After delivering a viable neonate, the client tells the nurse, "It was really a wonderful experience to participate in my labor and delivery while wide awake." The nurse's best response would be to explain that the client's feelings of satisfaction are most likely due to the fact that she
○ 1. is at an ideal age for childbirth.
○ 2. has attended prepared childbirth classes.
○ 3. has had no complications during pregnancy.
○ 4. has delivered a neonate of lower-than-average birth weight.

13. A client referred to a psychiatric clinic for counseling describes anxiety attacks that usually occur shortly after work when he is preparing his evening meal. Which of the following questions would be most appropriate for the admitting nurse to ask the client first in an effort to learn how he can be helped?
○ 1. "When during the day do you most often think of your wife?"
○ 2. "Where do you feel most uncomfortable when you're anxious?"
○ 3. "Why do you think you feel anxious when returning from work?"
○ 4. "What do you do when you're anxious to help yourself feel better?"

14. For a client with a sucking stab wound in the chest wall, the nurse should first
○ 1. start administering oxygen.
○ 2. prepare to do a tracheostomy.
○ 3. prepare for endotracheal intubation.
○ 4. cover the wound with a petroleum-impregnated dressing.

15. The nurse would evaluate that a client is experiencing a normal side effect of an upper gastrointestinal x-ray series (upper GI) if the client experiences which of the following after the test?
○ 1. Development of diarrhea within 12 hours of the procedure.
○ 2. Elevated white blood cell count.
○ 3. Acute abdominal pain.
○ 4. Passage of white stools 24 hours after the procedure.

16. According to Erikson's theory of development, a 13-year-old client dying of cancer normally would be expected to be resolving which of the following psychosocial issues?
○ 1. Lifetime vocation.
○ 2. Social conscience.
○ 3. Personal and sexual identity.
○ 4. Sense of initiative and industry.

17. A child is brought to the clinic for a well-infant checkup and the DPT (diphtheria-pertussis-tetanus) and OPV (oral polio vaccine) immunizations. The child is recovering from a cold and is afebrile. The child's sibling has cancer and is receiving chemotherapy. Nursing considerations would include
○ 1. giving only the DPT and withholding the OPV.
○ 2. giving both the DPT and OPV.
○ 3. scheduling both immunizations for a later date.
○ 4. withholding both immunizations until the child recovers from the cold.

18. A client who is no longer delusional is being considered for discharge soon. Determining her readiness for discharge must include an assessment of her
○ 1. medication knowledge.
○ 2. activity level.
○ 3. ability to be employed.
○ 4. understanding of her disease.

19. A multigravida who delivered a 7 lb., 8 oz. (3,200g) infant at term is a candidate for early postpartal discharge 12 hours after delivery. An essential nursing assessment finding before this client is discharged is
- ○ 1. establishment of lactation.
- ○ 2. return of normal bowel function.
- ○ 3. development of lochia serosa.
- ○ 4. firmness of the fundus.

20. When performing a physical assessment on an 18-month-old child, the nurse should
- ○ 1. ask the child's mother to leave the room.
- ○ 2. assess the respiratory and cardiac systems first.
- ○ 3. carry out the assessment from head to toe.
- ○ 4. assess motor function by having the child run and walk.

21. A primary underlying problem in adult respiratory distress syndrome (ARDS) is
- ○ 1. chronic $PaCO_2$ retention.
- ○ 2. embolism causing alveolar collapse.
- ○ 3. altered alveolar-capillary membrane permeability.
- ○ 4. inadequate coronary artery perfusion.

22. The nurse is caring for a 20-year-old primigravida classified as a class II cardiac client due to a history of childhood rheumatic heart disease. The physician advises the client to have a continuous epidural anesthesia for the labor and delivery. After teaching the client about the anesthesia, the nurse would determine that she needs further instructions when she says
- ○ 1. "I may need to be catheterized if I can't empty my bladder."
- ○ 2. "I may get a 'spot' of suprapubic pain."
- ○ 3. "I could start shivering."
- ○ 4. "I could get a headache if I don't lie flat after delivery."

23. A nurse has noticed an increase in school-age children injured in automobile accidents. Most injuries are attributed to the fact that the children were not wearing seat belts. In planning an attempt to decrease these injuries, the nurse's best strategy would be to
- ○ 1. give classes on seat belt safety to the parents of the injured children.
- ○ 2. help start a seat belt safety program in local schools.
- ○ 3. lobby the legislature for stiffer fines for nonuse of seat belts.
- ○ 4. write a letter to the local newspaper outlining the problem.

24. A client dies quietly one morning. Which nursing intervention to assist the client's family would be least important at this time?
- ○ 1. Providing an unobtrusive place for family members to gather.
- ○ 2. Encouraging family members to express their feelings.
- ○ 3. Supporting the defense mechanisms in use by family members.
- ○ 4. Staying with family members while they make the funeral arrangements.

25. During a counseling session, a client says, "I could hate God for that flood." The nurse responds, "Oh, don't feel that way. We're making progress in these sessions." The nurse's statement demonstrates a failure to
- ○ 1. look for meaning in what the client says.
- ○ 2. explain to the client why he may think as he does.
- ○ 3. add to the strength of the client's support system.
- ○ 4. give the client credit for being able to solve his own problems.

26. A primipara who is breast-feeding asks the nurse if she should clean her nipples before nursing. The nurse should recommend that the client clean her nipples with
- ○ 1. alcohol.
- ○ 2. plain water.
- ○ 3. soap and water.
- ○ 4. dilute antiseptic solution.

27. A 64-year-old man is admitted to the emergency room with palpitations, a choking sensation, and tightness in the chest. He is hyperventilating. During the initial interview, the client says, "My wife left me with all the chores, and I don't know what to do. Now this. Not until she died about 6 months ago did I realize how much I need her." Physical examination and laboratory results are essentially negative. The nurse analyzes the results of arterial blood gas (ABG) studies. In this situation, the ABG studies would likely reveal excessive loss of
- ○ 1. sodium.
- ○ 2. oxygen.
- ○ 3. potassium.
- ○ 4. carbon dioxide.

28. Sodium bicarbonate is prescribed for a preterm neonate when laboratory studies reveal hyponatremia. The nurse would judge that too much sodium bicarbonate is being administered if the neonate exhibits
- ○ 1. diarrhea.
- ○ 2. fluid retention.
- ○ 3. increased irritability.
- ○ 4. spasm of the feet and hands.

29. A primigravida in the first trimester of pregnancy tells the nurse that she read a magazine article about nutrition in which trace minerals were mentioned but not defined. She asks the nurse what trace minerals are. The nurse should explain that trace minerals are important for health but are so named because they are

- ○ 1. needed by the body only during childhood.
- ○ 2. needed by the body in relatively small amounts.
- ○ 3. easily obtained by the body when milk intake is adequate.
- ○ 4. easily obtained by the body when major mineral intake is adequate.

30. A clinic's nursing staff is planning to give prenatal and parenting classes. Child care will be provided for the children of the parents attending the classes, who range in age from 12 months to 6 years. The clinic has a playroom. The staff should plan which of the following activities for the children?

- ○ 1. Free play with adult supervision.
- ○ 2. A group sing-a-long.
- ○ 3. A story hour.
- ○ 4. Viewing of cartoon videos.

31. After hearing a client with bulimia talk about her bizarre eating binges of raw pancake batter and bowls of whipped cream, the nurse feels disgusted and feels like telling her to "snap out of it." At this point, it would be best for the nurse to

- ○ 1. share her or his feelings with the client and point out that her behavior alienates people.
- ○ 2. ask the client to talk more about her eating habits, and try harder to understand her underlying problem.
- ○ 3. suggest that another nurse work with the client, because this relationship is no longer therapeutic.
- ○ 4. discuss her or his feelings with another nurse and try to resolve them.

32. During a health history, a 59-year-old male client with non-insulin-dependent diabetes mellitus says he is "not feeling right." Which of the following client statements is most probably unrelated to diabetes mellitus?

- ○ 1. "I have this cut on my hand that doesn't want to heal."
- ○ 2. "No matter how much I drink, I'm still thirsty all the time."
- ○ 3. "I seem to be unable to get an erection. I've never been impotent before."
- ○ 4. "In the past couple of weeks, I've been having a lot of trouble urinating."

33. A mother brings her 2-year-old adopted Korean child to the clinic for an initial check-up. The child has been living with the adopted family for several weeks. The nurse notes an irregular area of deep blue pigment on the child's buttocks extending into the sacral area. The nurse should

- ○ 1. ask the child in private how the bruise occurred.
- ○ 2. do nothing concerning this finding.
- ○ 3. notify social services of a case of possible child abuse.
- ○ 4. question the mother about the family's discipline style.

34. A primigravida in active labor remains 8 cm dilated for 2 hours; the physician decides to perform a cesarean section delivery due to cephalopelvic disproportion. In planning care for the neonate following cesarean section delivery, the nurse should take into consideration the neonate's

- ○ 1. increased muscle tone.
- ○ 2. high-pitched cry.
- ○ 3. increased nasopharyngeal secretions.
- ○ 4. difficulty with nipple grasping.

35. A child newly diagnosed with rheumatic fever is to receive penicillin therapy. Which of the following statements by the parents would lead the nurse to judge that they need more teaching on the reason why their child is receiving penicillin?

- ○ 1. "How long will it take for the penicillin to help relieve the joint discomfort?"
- ○ 2. "Our child should take the medication until the physician discontinues it."
- ○ 3. "We need to keep these pills out of the reach of our other children."
- ○ 4. "We should give our child the medication on a full stomach."

36. A school-age-child newly diagnosed with leukemia is admitted to the hospital. The nurse should make sure to assess which of the following on admission?

- ○ 1. Chest excursion.
- ○ 2. Mucous membrane and skin condition.
- ○ 3. Rectal temperature.
- ○ 4. Oxygen saturation of the blood.

37. After mumbling with some uncertainty when asked how she cut her finger, an elderly client says, "While cutting flowers in our garden." The client's husband later tells the nurse that they do not have a flower garden. Filling in gaps of memory, as the client has done, is called

- ○ 1. displacement.
- ○ 2. confabulation.
- ○ 3. disorientation.
- ○ 4. flight of ideas.

38. A primipara who delivered a term neonate 24 hours ago has a midline episiotomy. After teaching the client methods to alleviate perineal discomfort, the nurse would determine that the client needs further instructions when she says

- ○ 1. "I should tighten my buttocks before sitting down."
- ○ 2. "I should sit directly on my buttocks while I relax my perineal muscles."
- ○ 3. "Sometimes a lateral or side-lying position is more comfortable."
- ○ 4. "Topical application of anesthetic ointments or sprays can help alleviate the discomfort."

39. Initial nursing interventions for a child admitted to the hospital with a diagnosis of meningitis should include
- ○ 1. keeping the child well hydrated.
- ○ 2. carefully assessing the child's alertness.
- ○ 3. keeping the child positioned head down.
- ○ 4. placing the child in enteric isolation.

40. Which of the following adjustments in the average adult dosage of preoperative medications should the nurse expect for an elderly client, and why?
- ○ 1. A larger-than-average dosage; elderly clients tend to have a decreased ability to absorb drugs.
- ○ 2. A larger-than-average dosage; elderly clients tend to have a decreased ability to maintain adequate blood levels of most drugs.
- ○ 3. A smaller-than-average dosage; elderly clients tend to have an increased sensitivity to most drugs.
- ○ 4. A smaller-than-average dosage; elderly clients tend to have an increased susceptibility to allergic reactions to most drugs.

41. A 6-month-old child has been admitted to the hospital with a temperature of 103°F. The mother tells the nurse that the child is scheduled to receive the diphtheria-pertussis-tetanus (DPT) and oral polio vaccine (OPV) immunizations tomorrow, and asks the nurse to see that the child gets the immunizations as scheduled. The nurse should reply that
- ○ 1. the child should receive only the diptheria and tetanus.
- ○ 2. the immunizations must be delayed.
- ○ 3. the child should receive the OPV only, since the child is 6 months old.
- ○ 4. hold the OPV.

42. The nurse teaches a client scheduled for an intravenous pyelogram (IVP) what to expect when the dye is injected. The nurse would know that the client has correctly understood the teaching when he states that when the dye is injected, he may experience
- ○ 1. a metallic taste.
- ○ 2. flushing of the face.
- ○ 3. cold chills.
- ○ 4. chest pain.

43. The primary purpose of administering aminophylline to a client with emphysema is to
- ○ 1. relieve diaphragm spasms.
- ○ 2. relax smooth muscles in the bronchioles.
- ○ 3. promote efficient pulmonary circulation.
- ○ 4. stimulate chemoreceptors in the medullary respiratory center.

44. The nurse plans to assess the contraction pattern of a primigravida in the first stage of labor. When timing the frequency of contractions, the nurse should time the interval between the
- ○ 1. beginning and end of one contraction.
- ○ 2. end of one contraction and the beginning of the next contraction.
- ○ 3. end of one contraction and the end of the next contraction.
- ○ 4. beginning of one contraction and the beginning of the next contraction.

45. The nurse plans dietary modifications to help prevent hypokalemia in a client receiving diuretic therapy. Which of the following foods is the poorest source of potassium?
- ○ 1. Rice.
- ○ 2. Cantaloupe.
- ○ 3. Dried prunes.
- ○ 4. Grapefruit juice.

46. When teaching a sexuality class at a community center, the nurse should instruct class participants that human immunodeficiency virus (HIV) transmission can be greatly reduced, if not altogether prevented, by which of the following behaviors?
- ○ 1. Avoiding inhalant drugs.
- ○ 2. Avoiding kissing for longer than 30 minutes at a time.
- ○ 3. Using condoms during sexual intercourse.
- ○ 4. Douching after sexual intercourse.

47. What would be the priority nursing intervention for a client admitted to the emergency room with estimated 27% burns?
- ○ 1. Inserting a large-caliber intravenous line.
- ○ 2. Administering an intramuscular morphine injection.
- ○ 3. Initiating endotracheal intubation.
- ○ 4. Administering tetanus toxoid.

48. A 21-year-old gravida 1, TPAL 000, is admitted to the labor and delivery suite of the hospital. On admission, she is 4 cm dilated, 95% effaced, and at station −1, with a vertex presentation. The physician orders 1 mg butorphanol tartrate (Stadol) IV push. In planning care for the client, the nurse would plan to administer the medication
- ○ 1. between two contractions.
- ○ 2. during a period of three to five contractions.
- ○ 3. in a bolus during one contraction.
- ○ 4. in 100 ml of normal saline solution.

49. To help prevent hip flexion deformities associated with rheumatoid arthritis, several times a day the nurse should help the client assume which of the following positions in bed?
- ○ 1. Prone.
- ○ 2. Very low Fowler's.
- ○ 3. A modified Trendelenburg.
- ○ 4. Side-lying.

50. The nurse uses the concept of the wellness-illness continuum while planning care for a client with rheumatoid arthritis. This continuum will best serve to

guide the nurse when used to teach the client how to
- ○ 1. avoid the crippling effects of the disease.
- ○ 2. delay disease progression.
- ○ 3. control pain through medication management, to enhance sleep.
- ○ 4. use health strengths to function as effectively as possible.

51. A mother calls the clinic nurse and asks about home treatments for mild attacks of croup. The nurse should advise the mother to
- ○ 1. give the child an over-the-counter decongestant.
- ○ 2. run a steam vaporizer next to the child's bed at night.
- ○ 3. run the shower with hot water to fill the bathroom with steam, then sit in the room with the child.
- ○ 4. warm all foods and fluids given to the child.

52. When assessing a healthy adolescent client, the nurse should
- ○ 1. obtain a detailed prenatal and early developmental history.
- ○ 2. discuss sexual preferences and behaviors, with the parents present for legal reasons.
- ○ 3. obtain most of the information from the parents and gather any other necessary information from an interview with the adolescent.
- ○ 4. interact primarily with the adolescent, and gather any other necessary information from an interview with the parents.

53. A 77-year-old male client has been admitted to the hospital with a diagnosis of chronic peripheral arterial vascular disease. Which of the following symptoms would the nurse recognize as indicative of arterial vascular disease in the lower extremities?
- ○ 1. Distended leg veins.
- ○ 2. Ankle edema.
- ○ 3. Coolness and pallor of the feet.
- ○ 4. Peripheral pulses of 3+.

54. The nurse should plan to include which of the following interventions in the plan for care for a child with a medical diagnosis of febrile seizure?
- ○ 1. Elevate the head of the bed and keep the child supine.
- ○ 2. Keep the room temperature low and bedclothes to a minimum.
- ○ 3. Place the child in respiratory isolation and restrict visitors.
- ○ 4. Monitor intake and output and restrict fluids.

55. Which of the following disorders is a major health problem for many women, particularly elderly women?
- ○ 1. Cardiomyopathy.
- ○ 2. Crohn's disease.
- ○ 3. Vaginal bleeding.
- ○ 4. Osteoporosis.

56. The treatment team at a psychiatric hospital persuades a client to sign herself in as a voluntary client. After therapy with haloperidol (Haldol), the client is no longer considered dangerous to herself or others but remains delusional. One morning, she refuses to take the haloperidol. Which of the following interventions should the nurse take?
- ○ 1. Summon another nurse to help ensure that the client takes her medication.
- ○ 2. Tell the client that she can take the medication either orally or via injection.
- ○ 3. Withhold the medication until it is determined why the client is refusing to take it.
- ○ 4. Tell the client that she needs to take her "vitamin" to stay healthy.

57. The nurse preparing to give a child an intramuscular injection chooses to give the injection into the gluteal muscle. This site is acceptable because the child
- ○ 1. has been walking for a year.
- ○ 2. has small deltoid muscles.
- ○ 3. is older than 2 years.
- ○ 4. weighs more than 20 pounds.

58. During an early counseling session, a client says, "I guess I can't make it without my wife. I can't even sleep without her." Of the following possible responses the nurse could make, which would be the most therapeutic?
- ○ 1. "Things always look worse before they get better."
- ○ 2. "I'd say that you're not giving yourself a fair chance."
- ○ 3. "I'd bet on you to make it, given a little more time. Don't hurry yourself."
- ○ 4. "I'm interested in knowing more about what you mean when you say that you can't make it without your wife."

59. A primigravida was in labor for 14 hours in the first stage of labor, 2 hours in the second stage, and 8 minutes in the third stage. Following delivery of a viable male infant, the client tells the nurse she is "very tired, but happy." Which of the following would be the most appropriate nursing diagnosis for this client?
- ○ 1. Potential Fluid Volume Deficit related to potential for hemorrhage due to a lengthy labor.
- ○ 2. Fatigue related to lengthy second stage of labor.
- ○ 3. Potential for Altered Parenting related to ineffective bonding due to the lengthy first stage of labor.
- ○ 4. Urinary retention related to lengthy third stage of labor.

60. The nurse would judge that a client may be developing Wernicke-Korsakoff syndrome when the client exhibits
- ○ 1. fear and paranoia.
- ○ 2. aggression and hostility.

○ 3. memory loss and disorientation.
○ 4. depression and suicidal tendencies.

61. A client's husband is notified of her admission to the emergency room for acute alcohol intoxication. Which of the following statements by the man about his wife would be least typical of a person who abuses alcohol?
○ 1. "She uses alcohol and tranquilizers to steady her nerves."
○ 2. "Whenever she has a problem, she seems to hit the bottle."
○ 3. "Her drinking certainly hasn't interfered with her eating."
○ 4. "She has stopped drinking several times; sometimes for as long as 4 months."

62. The nurse teaches a client how to self-administer NPH insulin injections. Which of the following techniques for self-administering insulin is incorrect?
○ 1. Shaking the insulin vial before withdrawing the insulin.
○ 2. Introducing the needle into subcutaneous tissue with a dartlike action.
○ 3. Pulling back on the syringe plunger as soon as the needle is in place in subcutaneous tissue.
○ 4. Holding an antiseptic sponge against the needle when removing it from subcutaneous tissue.

63. A client with an obsessive-compulsive disorder washes his feet frequently. Which of the following nursing diagnoses is specifically related to this behavior?
○ 1. Self-Care Deficit.
○ 2. High Risk for Impaired Skin Integrity.
○ 3. Ineffective Individual Coping.
○ 4. Anxiety (panic).

64. Which of the following nursing diagnoses would be most appropriate for a client newly diagnosed with non-insulin-dependent diabetes mellitus?
○ 1. High Risk for Infection related to diabetes.
○ 2. Altered Nutrition: more than body requirements related to overproduction of insulin in the pancreas.
○ 3. Pain related to elevated blood glucose levels.
○ 4. Altered Health Maintenance related to lack of knowledge of proper foot care.

65. The nurse would evaluate interventions targeted at promoting comfort in an infant as successful when the
○ 1. infant is less restless and irritable.
○ 2. infant's pulse and respiratory rates increase.
○ 3. mother refuses to allow the nurse to medicate the infant.
○ 4. mother reports that the infant has been very quiet.

66. A nurse working in a community center counsels a husband and wife referred to the center because of suspected abuse of their 3-year-old daughter. The couple also has three older daughters at home. During counseling, the nurse should recognize that the parents give a typical description of an abused child when they say that their daughter
○ 1. tends to lie and cheat frequently.
○ 2. always keeps running away from home.
○ 3. does not show respect for authority.
○ 4. has always been different from her sisters.

67. A young child is admitted to the emergency room with severe dehydration. The physician orders a solution of dextrose 5% with 0.2% normal saline and 20 mEq of potassium chloride per 1,000 cc of fluid. Before administering this solution to the child, the nurse should assess
○ 1. depth and rate of respirations.
○ 2. urine output and frequency.
○ 3. apical pulse rate and regularity.
○ 4. blood pressure and temperature.

68. A 67-year-old man is admitted to the hospital for a partial gastrectomy to treat recurrent peptic ulcers. While preparing the client for surgery, the nurse assesses for psychosocial problems that may cause preoperative anxiety. It is believed that the most devastating fear a preoperative client is likely to experience is a fear of
○ 1. the unknown.
○ 2. changes in body image.
○ 3. the effects of anesthesia.
○ 4. being separated from family members.

69. The nurse is caring for a primigravida in active labor who is receiving a continuous epidural anesthetic and a continuous IV fluid infusion. The client complains of nausea, and the nurse notes that the client's blood pressure has dropped 30 mm Hg. After instructing another nurse to notify the physician, the nurse should
○ 1. place the client in Trendelenburg's position.
○ 2. decrease the IV fluid infusion rate.
○ 3. turn the client onto her left side.
○ 4. check the epidural catheter placement.

70. The nurse plans to administer an injection of heparin to a client. Which of the following techniques for heparin administration is appropriate? The nurse
○ 1. selects a 1-½", 21-gauge needle for the injection.
○ 2. makes the injection into the deltoid muscle.
○ 3. applies gentle pressure to the site for 5 to 10 seconds following the injection.
○ 4. aspirates with the plunger to check for entry into the blood vessel before injecting the heparin.

71. Treatment of diverticulitis is important to prevent the development of peritonitis from a perforated diverticulum. Nursing interventions for a client with diverticulitis should include assessing for which sign of peritonitis?

○ 1. Hyperactive bowel sounds.
○ 2. Rigid abdominal wall.
○ 3. Explosive diarrhea.
○ 4. Excessive flatulence.

72. The nurse makes a home visit to a primipara on her fourth postpartal day. In assessing the client's light-skinned neonate for jaundice, the nurse should inspect the
○ 1. skin over the forehead.
○ 2. color of the gums.
○ 3. color of the stool.
○ 4. color of the urine.

73. The nurse in a crisis center is helping clients who have suffered from the effects of a severe flood. The nurse interviews a client whose pregnant wife is missing and whose home has been destroyed. The client keeps talking rapidly about his experience and says, "I can't see how I can ever rebuild my life." Which of the following responses by the nurse would be best?
○ 1. "If you start organizing your life now, I'm sure all will be fine."
○ 2. "This has been a bad experience. Tell me more about how you feel."
○ 3. "Let me note a few of the things you said before you continue with your story."
○ 4. "Think some more of what happened tonight, so that we can continue with this tomorrow. For now, let's discuss how you might rebuild your life."

74. After 2 weeks of radiotherapy, a client with Hodgkin's disease becomes discouraged. He tells the nurse that he is so tired that he can barely keep up with his studies. What information related to the nursing diagnosis of Fatigue should the nurse use in planning a response?
○ 1. Fatigue is one of the most common problems associated with radiotherapy and will persist throughout therapy.
○ 2. Fatigue is a transient problem that will resolve as radiotherapy continues.
○ 3. Fatigue is unrelated to the radiotherapy, and another possible cause should be sought.
○ 4. Fatigue indicates that the disease is eradicated and that radiotherapy is not needed.

75. How can the emergency room nurse quickly estimate the extent of an adult client's burns?
○ 1. By correlating the percentage of the burned area with the client's admission weight.
○ 2. By dividing the body into areas equal to multiples of nine, with the calculation based on areas affected.
○ 3. By calculating the circumference of the body, then measuring and subtracting unburned areas from the total.
○ 4. By measuring the burned area in square inches, then multiplying that total by a factor of 0.862.

76. Which of the following goals would be appropriate for a client with aplastic anemia? The client will
○ 1. perform activities of daily living without fatigue or dyspnea.
○ 2. learn how to administer weekly vitamin B12 injections.
○ 3. describe how to correctly take prescribed anticoagulant drug therapy.
○ 4. describe self-care behaviors that will prevent spread of the disease to family members.

77. A client comes to the emergency department with multiple bruises on her face and arms, a black eye, and a broken nose. She says that these injuries occurred when she "fell down the stairs." The nurse suspects that the client may have been physically assaulted. During the admission interview, it would be best for the nurse to
○ 1. ask the client specifically about the possibility of physical abuse.
○ 2. tell the client that it is difficult to believe that such injuries resulted from a fall.
○ 3. tell the client that social services must be notified of the situation.
○ 4. use sensitive questioning to ask the client if she has been battered.

78. A client is admitted to the emergency room with complaints of palpitations, a choking sensation, and chest tightness. The nurse notes that he is hyperventilating. During the initial interview he states, "My wife left me with all the chores and I don't know what to do. Not until she died about 6 months ago did I realize how much I need her." The client's medical diagnosis is acute anxiety attack. Of the following nursing diagnoses, which would most accurately reflect the client's behavior?
○ 1. Anxiety (panic) related to hopelessness.
○ 2. Anxiety (panic) related to loss of wife.
○ 3. Sleep Pattern Disturbance related to anxiety.
○ 4. Powerlessness related to wife's death.

79. The nurse caring for a 21-year-old primipara following delivery of a viable neonate can promote maternal-infant bonding by allowing the client to
○ 1. nurse the neonate.
○ 2. hear the neonate cry.
○ 3. wrap the neonate in a receiving blanket.
○ 4. experience eye-to-eye contact with the neonate.

80. An infant is admitted to the hospital with a diagnosis of possible pyloric stenosis. The nurse would expect that the infant would have a history of
○ 1. abdominal distention after feedings.
○ 2. a weak suck.
○ 3. inability to burp.
○ 4. projectile vomiting after feedings.

81. A client with arthritis has been taking prescribed aspirin in large doses prior to her admission to the hospital. She complains of stomach irritation, sometimes with vomiting. Of the following foods and beverages, the one most likely contributing to her gastrointestinal irritation would be
- ○ 1. dry toast several times a day.
- ○ 2. a hard-boiled egg at least once a day.
- ○ 3. sweetened tea with each meal.
- ○ 4. several ounces of wine before her evening meal.

82. A young woman with a malignant growth on the larynx is admitted to the hospital for a laryngectomy. The client would most likely state that the earliest symptom of her health problem was
- ○ 1. a sore throat.
- ○ 2. chronic hoarseness.
- ○ 3. pain radiating to the ear.
- ○ 4. difficulty swallowing.

83. While the nurse irrigates a client's colostomy, the client complains of abdominal cramping. What would be the nurse's best course of action?
- ○ 1. Help the client turn onto her side.
- ○ 2. Remove the irrigating cone from the stoma.
- ○ 3. Have the client take several deep breaths.
- ○ 4. Slow the flow of irrigating solution temporarily.

84. A hospitalized child has a fluid restriction of 1,500 ml/day. The mother is staying with the child in the room. The nurse should plan to
- ○ 1. discuss the fluid restriction with the mother and allow her to decide how to allocate the fluids over the 24 hours.
- ○ 2. explain to the mother that only the nurses will be able to provide fluids.
- ○ 3. let the child drink until the limit is reached and then allow no more fluids.
- ○ 4. tell the mother exactly how much fluid the child can have each hour.

85. Which of the following signs and symptoms would indicate that a client with human immunodeficiency virus (HIV) infection has developed acquired immune deficiency syndrome (AIDS)?
- ○ 1. Severe fatigue at night.
- ○ 2. Pain on standing and walking.
- ○ 3. Weight loss of 10 pounds over 3 months.
- ○ 4. Herpes simplex ulcer persisting for 2 months.

86. A client tells the nurse, "Everybody smiles at me because they know that I was chosen by God for this mission." This statement reflects
- ○ 1. an idea of reference.
- ○ 2. a thought insertion.
- ○ 3. a visual hallucination.
- ○ 4. a neologism.

87. A man and woman bring their 4-year-old daughter to the emergency room with an acute ear infection. During the admission history, the nurse learns that the family lives in a rural area where the drinking water is not fluoridated. Health teaching for the family should include informing them that a significant amount of fluoride can be obtained in
- ○ 1. tea.
- ○ 2. yogurt.
- ○ 3. citrus juices.
- ○ 4. natural cheeses.

88. A 24-year-old primigravida at approximately 7 months gestation tells the nurse that she has been experiencing low backaches. The nurse instructs the client that low backaches can be decreased if she avoids wearing
- ○ 1. pull-on slacks.
- ○ 2. knee-high stockings.
- ○ 3. an elasticized girdle.
- ○ 4. sandals with flat heels.

89. Several hours after delivering a viable neonate, a client begins to cry. She tells the nurse, "I don't know why I feel this way." The nurse's best response would be
- ○ 1. "You have a lovely baby. There's no need to cry."
- ○ 2. "You're saying that you don't know why you're crying?"
- ○ 3. "Shall I call your doctor for a medication to help you?"
- ○ 4. "Many mothers cry after the birth of a baby. You'll soon feel better."

90. While examining a 12-month-old child, the nurse notes that the child can stand independently but cannot walk without support. The nurse should
- ○ 1. ask the mother if the child uses a walker at home.
- ○ 2. do nothing; this is a normal finding in a child this age.
- ○ 3. initiate a consultation with a physical therapist.
- ○ 4. tell the mother that the child may have a developmental delay.

91. The nurse is caring for a small-for-gestational age neonate in the newborn nursery after the neonate's mother has been discharged. The nurse's observation of which behavior indicates that the parents are ready to learn about caring for the neonate at home?
- ○ 1. The increasing frequency of the parent's visits to the neonate.
- ○ 2. a decline in the parents' expressions of fear about taking the neonate home.
- ○ 3. the parents' increasing involvement in the neonate's care.
- ○ 4. A decreasing number of questions that the parents ask about the neonate's condition.

CORRECT ANSWERS AND RATIONALE

The letters in parentheses following the rationale identify the step of the nursing process (A, D, P, I, E); cognitive level (K, C, T, N); client need (S, G, L, H); and nursing care area (O, X, Y, M). See the Answer Grid for the key.

1. 1. For the best assessment of an inguinal hernia, the client should be in a standing position. The sitting and side-lying positions do not help the examiner palpate for the inguinal ring. The client may be asked to lie down after being examined in the standing position to determine whether the hernia can be reduced and its sac contents returned to the abdominal cavity. (A, T, G, M)

2. 2. The nurse can most effectively monitor the client's compliance with medication therapy by administering the medication herself. Education may or may not affect the client's compliance with medication therapy. Long-term commitment is unnecessarily restrictive and would entail legal difficulties. Participation in a partial hospitalization program may be a desirable referral but would affect the client's compliance with medication therapy only indirectly. (I, T, L, X)

3. 1. Small, frequent, low-fat meals are recommended to help relieve morning sickness. Other remedies include eating a dry, starchy food, such as crackers or melba toast, before arising in the morning; limiting fluid intake with meals; eating high-protein or high-carbohydrate meals; and eating small meals five or six times a day. (I, N, H, O)

4. 2. Contrary to popular myth, binges are not enjoyable for the person with bulimia; they are frightening experiences that result in thoughts of self-deprecation. Binges are done secretively, and the person has no desire to attract attention. Because of the purging, substantial weight gain usually does not occur, although weight may fluctuate. (D, C, L, X)

5. 3. A hyperactive client needs help in setting limits on behavior. The best course of action when this client abuses telephone privileges is to work out a plan with him about the number of calls he can make each day. The agreed-upon plan should then be followed. (P, T, L, X)

6. 2. This client is at risk for infection. The flank incision, which makes it difficult to take deep breaths, predisposes the client to atelectasis and respiratory acidosis. Urinary tubes predispose him to urinary tract infection. Parotitis may occur as a secondary staphylococcal infection that develops in the parotid glands due to debilitation and poor oral hygiene. The lithotomy position—not the lateral position in which the client will be positioned intraoperatively—is associated with deep vein thrombosis. (P, N, G, M)

7. 2. It is imperative to assess the fetal heartbeat after the membranes rupture, and then again after a few minutes, to determine whether the fetus is applying pressure on the cord. A sign of fetal distress is a persistently slow fetal heartbeat after a contraction, as well as early during a contraction. The physician or other health care provider should be notified immediately of bradycardia. (I, N, G, O)

8. 1. The vital signs listed are normal for a child age 2 years. The child should be placed on the side opposite the shunt, with the head elevated and positioned midline to decrease intracranial pressure. The abdominal dressing should be assessed. A 2-year-old may or may not be able to relate the time of day, the date, and his age. (A, N, G, Y)

9. 3. Interventions can be judged to be effective when the client shows that he has learned various ways to help himself feel and sleep better and is finding interests outside himself and his own activities of daily living. The client is expressing uncertainty and continued dependence on the nurse when he says he would like to continue with the sessions. The nurse should explore these feelings of dependence to determine whether the client's strengths in handling and preventing anxiety are sufficiently strong to enable him to cope with problems effectively on his own. (E, N, L, X)

10. 4. The initial intervention after delivery is to ensure that the neonate's airway is clear. Clearing the airway begins immediately after delivery of the infant's head, when debris is cleared from the nose and mouth. The neonate is often kept in the face-down position immediately after delivery to promote drainage from the respiratory passages. Suctioning the respiratory passages is also done sometimes. After the neonate's respiratory system is functioning satisfactorily, other procedures, such as wrapping the neonate and instilling prophylactic eye drops, can be done. (P, N, G, O)

11. 1. The fetal head should be delivered slowly, about midway between contractions. Ritgen's technique is often used. In this technique, when the fetal head causes distention of the perineum as it delivers, downward pressure is placed on the occiput while forward pressure is placed on the neonate's chin. This technique allows control of the head and facilitates extension of the head to prevent perineal lacerations. (I, N, G, O)

12. 2. It is believed that prepared childbirth classes are critically important in helping a client cope and find satisfaction with the birth experience. The goal of these classes is to help a client help herself during and delivery. Although every client responds differently to the birthing process and requires individualized care, proper parental education appears to help lead to a satisfying outcome. Prepared childbirth classes typically include fathers; this also has been found to enhance the birth experience for both parents. (I, N, L, O)

13. 4. The nurse should first assess the client who is subject to anxiety attacks by determining what behavior usually relieves his anxiety. But, nursing care of an anxious client must ultimately take into account all aspects of the client's anxiety, including what leads to attacks and what happens during an attack. Only then can the nurse help the client understand his anxiety, what personal needs may be unmet, and how to cope with his problem with behavior that is more satisfactory than having an anxiety attack. (I, T, L, X)

14. 4. The first course of action for a client with a sucking chest wound is to stop air from entering the chest cavity, which will cause the lung to collapse. This is best done in an emergency situation by applying an air-occlusive dressing over the wound. Such measures as starting oxygen therapy, preparing for a tracheostomy, and preparing for endotracheal intubation may be necessary later, but do not have the same priority on admission as closing the wound. (I, N, S, M)

15. 4. The client should be instructed that for 1 to 3 days after an upper GI her stools will be whitish in color as the barium is eliminated from her system. The other side effects would not be expected and should be reported to the physician. (A, T, S, M)

16. 3. According to Erikson, a child of age 13 is normally seeking to meet his needs for developing personal identity. (D, C, L, X)

17. 1. At this time, the child should be given the DPT only. The fact that the child's sibling is immunosuppressed due to chemotherapy should alert the nurse not to give a live vaccine like the OPV. The virus can be shed in the stool of the vaccinated child and infect the immunosuppressed child. The fact that the child has a cold is not grounds for delaying the immunizations. If the child had a fever, the immunizations would be delayed. (I, N, G, Y)

18. 1. When determining the client's readiness for discharge, the nurse should give priority to assessing the client's knowledge of her medication regimen. Assessing her activity level, her ability to be employed, and her understanding of her disease are important, but not as important as assessing her medication knowledge. (A, T, L, X)

19. 4. The client with an uncomplicated labor and delivery may be discharged as soon as 6 hours after a vaginal delivery. The major criterion for early discharge is a firm uterine fundus. Lactation is not expected within the first 24 hours after delivery. Lochia will be rubra for 2 to 3 days, and the client will not be expected to have a bowel movement until the second or third day after delivery. (A, N, G, O)

20. 2. The best strategy for assessing a toddler is to start with noninvasive assessments first. Having a toddler run and be active may be tempting, but the nurse may find it difficult to settle the child down once he has been very active. A child this age needs his mother for emotional support. Starting with the head and working down is a good way to assess an older child who can tolerate invasive procedures such as ear exams. (I, N, G, Y)

21. 3. The primary pathophysiological alteration in ARDS is altered alveolar-capillary membrane permeability leading to fluid-filled alveoli and eventual alveolar collapse. Additionally, surfactant production is reduced, increasing surface tension and further contributing to the atelectasis. Massive atelectasis causes severe hypoxia, and treatment frequently requires mechanical ventilation. (A, T, G, M)

22. 4. Headache is not a side effect of epidural anesthesia, because the dura mater is not entered. Epidural anesthesia is associated with problems of bladder emptying due to a decreased urge to void. Shivering can occur due to heat loss caused by increased peripheral blood flow. A "spot" of suprapubic pain occasionally occurs with epidural anesthesia for reasons not clearly understood. (E, N, G, O)

23. 2. Although each of these strategies are acceptable, the nurse will make the most impact by targeting the children directly. School-age children can understand the reasons why certain actions are beneficial to their well-being and act on this knowledge. Parents of children who have suffered injuries know all too well why seat belt use is important in decreasing injury. Increased penalty for not using seat belts targets the parents, not the children, and often is not successful in increasing compliance. (P, N, H, Y)

24. 4. The least important intervention for the family of a client who has died is to stay with the family members while they make funeral arrangements. It is more important to provide privacy for family members, encourage them to express their feelings, and support the defense mechanisms that they may be using to ease their sorrow. (I, T, L, X)

25. 1. Individuals handle problems and situations in terms of what they consider important to them, not necessarily in terms of what others may think is important. Such cliches as "don't feel that way" are rarely helpful because they ignore the client's feelings and his interpretation of the situation in which he finds himself. They fail to focus on the client and what he feels. (E, N, L, X)

26. 2. Before breast-feeding, the client should cleanse her nipples with plain water. Water will not wash off the nipples' normal antiseptic lubricant, lysozyme. Soap, antiseptics, and alcohol tend to dry the nipples and predispose them to cracking. (I, N, H, O)

27. 4. Hyperventilation causes the excessive loss of carbon dioxide through respirations. This results in a decreased carbonic acid content of the blood. The kidneys will try to compensate by eliminating bicarbonate to maintain a normal carbonic acid-bicarbonate ratio, but this takes several days. If compensatory efforts are insufficient, the client will develop respiratory alkalosis. (E, N, G, M)

28. 2. Premature neonates' immature kidneys often cause excessive sodium loss from the urinary tract. Sodium bicarbonate is administered to correct the sodium imbalance. However, if too much is administered, fluid retention, with edema, water intoxication, and hemorrhage, may result. (D, N, G, O)

29. 2. Trace minerals, also sometimes called micronutrients, are so named because the body needs relatively small amounts of them for health. They include iron, iodine, fluorine, zinc, copper, and chromium. They are usually obtained in adequate amounts from a well-balanced, nutritious diet. Milk is very low in iron and copper, two trace minerals required by the body for health. Micronutrients are required throughout life. They do not derive from major minerals. (I, N, H, O)

30. 1. Planning any single activity that will appeal to children from age 12 months to 6 years is next to impossible. Toddlers have very short attention spans and probably will not cooperate in a group play situation for long. It would be best to allow these children to participate in free play with adult supervision. (P, N, H, Y)

31. 4. This is a countertransference reaction that can only be resolved by self-reflection and discussion with other professionals. It is inappropriate for the nurse to tell the client about her feelings; it might perpetuate the client's low self-esteem. Continuing to struggle with the problem without analyzing his or her own reactions is counterproductive for the nurse. Asking another nurse to work with the client may solve the problem momentarily, but the nurse will encounter similar problems and clients, and the client may feel rejected. (I, T, L, X)

32. 4. It is unlikely that trouble urinating is related to diabetes mellitus. Common signs and symptoms of diabetes mellitus include poor wound healing, impotence, thirst, hunger, and frequent voiding. Additional signs and symptoms may include fatigue, itching, blurred vision, irritability, and muscle cramps, especially in the legs. (A, T, G, M)

33. 2. This lesion is a mongolian spot, which is common in children of Oriental or Black heritage. The key word in the description is "pigment." A bruise results from bleeding into subcutaneous or muscle tissue; it is not a pigment change in the skin. (D, T, G, Y)

34. 3. Nasopharyngeal secretions are increased with a cesarean delivery because the neonate has not had the benefit of the squeezing action of a vaginal birth, which helps remove secretions from the nasopharynx. The neonate may have decreased muscle tone from analgesia or anesthesia. Difficulty with nipple grasping has been reported after forceps deliveries due to compression of the face, resulting in edema, but this phenomenon does not occur with cesarean section deliveries. High-pitched cry is a symptom of neurologic involvement or drug withdrawal and does not directly relate to a cesarean delivery. (P, N, G, O)

35. 1. Penicillin is given to children with rheumatic fever to eradicate the hemolytic streptococci that has triggered the autoimmune response that causes the disease. It does not decrease joint pain. Although penicillin should be given on an empty stomach, this statement does not tell the nurse what the parents know about why the drug is being given. Prevention of accidental poisoning by siblings and how long the medication must be taken also are not issues pertaining to why the drug is given to treat this disease. (E, N, G, Y)

36. 2. The child should be assessed for the condition of the skin and mucous membranes. The leukemic cells compete with other cells formed in the bone marrow. The nurse would assess for signs of infection due to a depressed white blood cell count and also for any bleeding that may be related to depressed platelet production. Rectal temperature measurement should be avoided in clients with leukemia because of possible injury and bleeding. Even though a child may be severely anemic, the oxygen saturation level may be high, because the available red blood cells are saturated to capacity with oxygen. Assessing for chest excursion is not important at this time. Unequal chest excursion would indicate an inability of one area of the lung to expand. (A, N, G, Y)

37. 2. Making up stories to fill in memory gaps is called confabulation. Displacement is a defense mechanism that refers ideas and feelings to something or someone not responsible for them. Disorientation is a loss of understanding in relation to place, time, or identity. Flight of ideas is a rapid shift of thoughts from one subject to another before any idea has been finished. (D, T, L, X)

38. 2. Relaxing the perineal muscles and sitting directly on the buttocks tends to increase discomfort. Tightening the buttocks before sitting down, assuming a lateral or side-lying position, and applying topical sprays or ointments can all help alleviate perineal discomfort. (E, N, H, O)

39. 2. The child with meningitis should be assessed for any indication of increased intracranial pressure in the acute phase. Any fluid deficit should be corrected, and then the child should be kept on low fluid maintenance to prevent cerebral edema. To decrease intracranial pressure, the child should be positioned with the head of the bed elevated and her head midline to facilitate venous return. A child with meningitis does not need to be in enteric isolation, but should be in respiratory isolation until the causative agent is identified and treated. (I, N, G, Y)

40. 3. A nurse can expect a smaller-than-average drug dosage for an elderly client because elderly clients tend to have an increased sensitivity to most drugs. Smaller-than-average doses of pharmaceutical agents are not prescribed for elderly clients because of increased susceptibility to allergic reactions—although, like younger adults, elderly clients also may be allergic to certain medications. (P, C, G, M)

41. 2. The normal immunizations given to a 6-month-old are diphtheria, pertussis and tetanus (DPT), oral polio vaccine (OPV), and haemophilus influenzae type b conjugate vaccine (HbOC). A general contraindication to all immunizations is severe febrile illness, to avoid adding the risk of adverse side effects from the vaccine in an already ill child or mistakenly identifying a symptom of the disease as having been caused by the vaccine. A minor illness such as the common cold is not a contraindication. (I, N, H, Y)

42. 2. As the dye is injected, the client may experience a feeling of warmth, flushing of the face, and a salty taste in the mouth. The client should not experience chest pain. (E, T, S, M)

43. 2. Aminophylline, a bronchodilator that relaxes smooth muscles in the bronchioles, is used in treatment of emphysema to improve ventilation by dilating the bronchioles. (I, T, G, M)

44. 4. The frequency of contractions refers to the interval between the beginning of one contraction and the beginning of the next. The duration of a contraction is the interval between the beginning and the end of one contraction. The intensity of the contractions is estimated and classified as mild when uterine muscles are somewhat tense, moderate when uterine muscles become moderately strong, and strong when the uterine muscles are so firm that the uterus cannot be indented. (P, N, H, O)

45. 1. Virtually all foods contain at least some potassium. However, rice is very low in potassium. Bananas, grapefruit and orange juice, cantaloupe, nectarines, dried prunes and figs, potatoes, and tomato juice are examples of foods especially rich in potassium. (I, T, G, M)

46. 3. Using a condom during sexual intercourse greatly reduces the risk of HIV transmission. Because HIV is most concentrated in blood and vaginal and seminal fluids, protective measures during intercourse are necessary to prevent transmission. Sharing unsterile needles for drug injections is another major mode of HIV transmission. (I, T, H, M)

47. 3. Establishing a patent airway is the priority intervention in burn trauma cases. Prophylactic intubation is initiated if heat has been inhaled or if the neck, head, or face is involved. Swelling of the upper airways can progress to obstruction. After the airway has been established, circulatory support is the next priority. Fluid replaced is best done via two large-caliber peripheral catheters. However, one peripheral line and one central line are preferable if the burn is large or complicated by inhalation injuries. Partial-thickness burns are painful, but morphine sulfate, the analgesic of choice, would not be administered until the client was stable; furthermore, the IV route would be used. Tetanus prophylaxis is begun in the emergency room, but is not the priority intervention. (I, N, G, M)

48. 2. IV analgesics should be given over a period of three to five contractions. The contractions restrict blood flow to the fetus, possibly resulting in increased maternal tissue uptake of the drug and decreased fetal uptake. Theoretically, there is more fetal uptake of IV analgesics given between contractions and in a bolus. Furthermore, a bolus of some analgesics may cause maternal vomiting. Giving the analgesic butorphanol tartrate (Stadol) via piggyback solution is not recommended. (P, N, G, O)

49. 1. To help prevent flexion deformities, a client with rheumatoid arthritis should lie in a prone position in bed for about ½ hour several times a day. This positioning helps keep the hips and knees in an extended position and prevents joint flexion. (I, T, H, M)

50. 4. The nurse should plan care for a client with rheumatoid arthritis that emphasizes how the client can avoid the crippling effects of the disease, delay disease progression, and manage pain to promote rest. But the concept of the wellness-illness continuum emphasizes teaching how a client can use remaining health strengths so that despite limitations due to a disease, the client can still function as effectively as possible. (P, N, S, M)

51. 3. The best home treatment for an attack of croup is to fill the bathroom with steam and then have the child inhale the steam. This decreases tissue edema in the tracheal and laryngeal areas, which causes the symptoms of croup. Steam vaporizers are no longer recommended, because they are a safety hazard. The nurse could recommend using a cool mist vaporizer, but the parents must be sure to carefully follow the manufacturer's instructions on cleaning. Although warm fluids and foods may not increase tracheal and laryngeal edema, they will not help decrease it either. Unless nasal secretions are a problem, a decongestant will not help this child breathe easier. (I, N, G, Y)

52. 4. When assessing an adolescent, it is appropriate to first obtain the information from the adolescent and then interview the parents for additional information. No legal reason would prohibit the nurse from discussing sexuality with the adolescent without the parents present. Obtaining prenatal and early developmental history information is usually not important for a healthy adolescent. (A, N, H, Y)

53. 3. Chronic peripheral arterial vascular disease is typically manifested by loss of hair on the lower calf and below; dry, scaly skin, delayed capillary filling, and pallor and coolness of the extremities. Pulses below the level of obstruction may be decreased or absent. (A, T, G, M)

54. 2. One nursing goal for clients with febrile seizures is to maintain temperature at a low enough level to prevent recurrence of seizures. Decreasing the environmental temperature and removing excess clothing and blankets will help decrease the client's temperature. Respiratory isolation is not necessary unless the child has a condition that warrants such an isolation. There is no reason to elevate the head of the bed and keep the child supine. This action will help decrease intracranial pressure, but a febrile seizure results from abnormal electrical activity in the brain due to elevated body temperature. The child with a fever should have an increased fluid and caloric intake. Strict intake and output monitoring is not necessary at this time. (P, N, G, Y)

55. 4. Osteoporosis is a major health problem for women, particularly after menopause. Estimates of disease incidence range from 15 to 20 million Americans. By age 75, 90% of women will have osteoporosis. The disorder, defined as a reduction in bone mass, contributes to decreased functional ability and increased susceptibility to injury in elderly women. (P, T, G, M)

56. 3. When a client refuses medication, the nurse must explore the reason for the refusal; the desire to avoid unwanted side effects is a common reason. Legally, a client cannot be forcibly medicated unless he is a danger to himself or others. Lying to a client about a medication is neither appropriate nor ethical. (I, T, L, X)

57. 1. Muscle mass determines whether or not a muscle can be safely used as an injection site. The gluteal muscle enlarges in response to use in walking. After the child has been walking for a year, it should be safe to use the gluteus maximus for injections. Weight on age have only a minor influence on muscle mass. If the deltoid is small, other injection sites, such as the ventrogluteal or vastus lateralis, are available. (I, T, S, Y)

58. 4. Here, the nurse is using a technique of communication to help the client explore his feelings by expressing interest in knowing more about his problem. Cliches and statements that make unwarranted judgments about the client are rarely, if ever, helpful. (I, T, L, X)

59. 2. The most appropriate nursing diagnosis for this client is Fatigue related to lengthy second stage of labor. The average duration of the second stage of labor for a primigravida is about 1 hour. This client had a second stage of 2 hours, which means that the client is probably very tired. The client did not have an excessively long total labor, so potential for fluid volume deficit from hemorrhage is not a priority nursing diagnosis. There are no data to suggest ineffective bonding. The third stage of labor was not excessively long, so potential for urinary retention is not a priority nursing diagnosis. (D, N, H, O)

60. 3. Memory loss, disorientation, and confabulation are typical signs of Wernicke-Korsakoff syndrome. The syndrome is believed to be due to a vitamin B deficiency and usually occurs in clients with longstanding alcoholism who have poor diets. (D, N, L, X)

61. 3. There is no precise profile of a person suffering from alcoholism, but common behavioral traits include a history of refraining from drinking for periods only to return to excessive drinking, using alcohol as a solution for personal problems, and demonstrating multiple substance abuse. An inadequate diet is common, and many chronic alcoholics suffer from malnutrition. A magnesium deficit is often noted, and Wernicke-Korsakoff syndrome, caused by a vitamin B deficiency, occurs in some alcoholics. Poor digestion and absorption of food constituents due to the damaging effect of alcohol on the stomach and small intestine, and subsequently on the liver and pancreas, also seriously compromise nutritional status in the alcoholic. (E, N, L, X)

62. 1. The client should be instructed to mix the sediment that accumulates in a vial of NPH insulin by rolling the vial gently between the palms or by turning the vial upside down several times. Shaking the vial is not recommended because it produces bubbles, which make it difficult to withdraw accurate doses of insulin. Proper techniques for self-administering insulin include introducing the needle with a dartlike action, pulling back on the plunger as soon as the needle is in place to determine whether the needle is in a vein, and holding an antiseptic sponge against the needle when removing it from tissue to prevent the discomfort of the needle pulling on the skin. (I, T, H, M)

63. 2. The nursing diagnosis High Risk for Impaired Skin Integrity related to frequent foot washing is indicated. The skin of the feet can become red and raw, providing an entry for infection. The ritualistic behavior provides relief for the client's anxiety and keeps it in check. Panic could result if the client is not allowed to perform his ritualistic behavior. (D, T, L, X)

64. 4. Knowledge of foot care is essential for the client with diabetes mellitus; improper care may lead to serious debilitating complications. Pain is not typically a problem. Overproduction of insulin would cause hypoglycemia; moreover, it would be treated by a physician. Using a medical diagnosis, such as diabetes, as an etiology in a nursing diagnosis is not appropriate, because a medical diagnosis requires treatment by the physician. (D, N, G, M)

65. 1. To assess an infant's response to interventions designed to decrease discomfort, the nurse should assess the infant's behavior. Decreased restlessness and irritability indicates that the infant is more comfortable. Physiologic indications of pain relief include decreased pulse and respiratory rates. However, such physiologic responses to the stress of pain are short-lived and are not reliable indicators of discomfort. A mother may refuse pain medications for her child for various reasons. An infant may respond to pain by becoming withdrawn and unnaturally quiet. (E, K, G, Y)

66. 4. A very typical finding when interviewing the parents of abused children is their description of the abused child as being different from other children, including siblings. They frequently say that the child whines a lot, cries, and is sullen. The nurse often will find other crisis or near-crisis situations in the home of an abused child, such as unemployment, financial strains, alcoholism, and the like. If one child in a family is being abused, siblings are also at risk for abuse. (A, N, L, X)

67. 2. Before administering an IV solution containing potassium, the nurse needs to assess the client's renal function. Severe dehydration can decrease perfusion to the kidneys due to a severe decrease in intravascular fluid. If the kidneys are damaged and cannot rid the body of excess potassium, adding this electrolyte to the child's IV fluid could result in serious, possibly even fatal, cardiac arrhythmias. (I, N, S, Y)

68. 1. Anxiety in a preoperative client may be caused by many different fears, such as fear of the effects of anesthesia, the effects of surgery on body image, being separated from family and friends, job loss, disability, pain, and death. But the fear of the unknown most likely looms as the greatest, because the client feels helpless. Therefore, an important part of preoperative nursing care is to assess the client for anxieties and explore possible causes. Interventions can then be used to help the client and to offer him emotional support so that he is in the best possible psychological condition for surgery. (A, T, L, M)

69. 3. Hypotension is a common side effect of epidural anesthesia because of its sympathetic blocking action. Nausea is an early symptom of hypotension. Placing the client on the left side may increase blood return to the heart by alleviating pressure of the uterus and fetus on the vena cava. The physician may decide to increase the IV fluid infusion rate. It is the anesthesiologist's responsibility to determine the correct placement of the epidural catheter. The client is not placed in Trendelenburg's position, because the level of anesthesia could ascend and suppress respirations. Furthermore, the vena cava would still be compressed with the client in Trendelenburg's position. (I, N, G, O)

70. 3. Heparin is administered subcutaneously, never intramuscularly. A 25- or 26-gauge, ½ to ⅝″ needle is most appropriate for heparin administration. The fatty layer of the abdomen is the preferred injection site. The nurse should select a site 1 to 2″ away from the umbilicus, scar tissue, or any bruises. To decrease the risk of hematoma formation and tissue damage, aspiration of the plunger should be avoided. Gentle pressure should be applied after the injection, but the area must not be massaged. (E, T, S, M)

71. 2. Diverticular rupture causes peritonitis from the release of intestinal contents (chemicals and bacteria) into the peritoneal cavity. The inflammatory response of the peritoneal tissue produces severe abdominal rigidity and pain, diminished intestinal motility, and retention of intestinal contents (air, fluid, and stool). (A, C, G, M)

72. 1. Neonates are routinely assessed for evidence of jaundice. Applying pressure to the skin, especially over bony prominences such as the nose and sternum, causes blanching and makes the yellowed skin more noticeable. In dark-skinned neonates, the color of the gingivae is the most reliable indicator of jaundice. (A, N, G, O)

73. 2. At the time of a major crisis, such as the flood described in this item, the client suffering a great loss is best helped by being encouraged to talk about his experience and describe his feelings. Telling the client to think more about what happened for further discussion the next day and suggesting that he start to rebuild his life are nurse-centered rather than client-centered and are unlikely to help the client. Asking the client to stop talking so that the nurse can write notes places more emphasis on the nurse's needs than on the client's needs. Cliches such as "everything will be fine" are not helpful. (I, T, L, X)

74. 1. Fatigue is one of the most common problems associated with radiotherapy. It persists during therapy and for varying periods after therapy ends. Extra rest and a reduction in normal activity are often necessary to maintain a reasonable energy level. Informing the client about the fatigue before treatment enables him to schedule his activities accordingly. (P, N, G, M)

75. 2. The rule of nines is used to quickly determine the extent of burns. A chart with the body areas divided into areas equal to multiples of nine is used. Affected areas are shaded, and the total shaded areas are calculated. Other, more detailed charts can be used later for more specific calculation. It is impractical to measure the body when critical care is indicated. Weight is not a reliable parameter to use when measuring the extent of burns. (A, C, G, M)

76. 1. An appropriate goal for the client with aplastic anemia would be to strive to perform activities of daily living without excessive fatigue or dyspnea. It is important for the client to learn to schedule rest periods throughout the day to conserve energy and reduce oxygen requirements. The client needs adequate vitamin B12 in the diet, but typically do not require vitamin B12 injections. Anticoagulants are contraindicated in clients with low platelet counts, as often occurs in aplastic anemia. Aplastic anemia is not contagious. (P, T, G, M)

77. 4. It is important to determine whether abuse is occurring to provide appropriate nursing care and support for the client. Many clients are hesitant to talk about abuse and need help to do so. The nurse should ask directly about abuse when it is suspected; however, a challenging confrontation may alienate the client and make her less willing to talk about her situation. The nurse is not legally required to report abuse of adults to social services, unless they are considered vulnerable adults. (A, T, L, X)

78. 2. The appropriate nursing diagnosis is Anxiety (panic) related to loss of wife. The symptoms of hyperventilation, palpitations, choking sensation, and chest tightness relate to a panic level of anxiety or a panic attack. The client stated that his wife died 6 months ago and he realizes that he needs her. (D, N, L, X)

79. 4. Maternal-infant bonding is best initiated when the mother has eye-to-eye contact with the neonate as soon after birth as possible. This is best accomplished by allowing the mother to assume a position so that she is face-to-face with the neonate when holding the neonate. Typically, the mother then touches the baby in an exploratory manner. (I, N, H, O)

80. 4. An infant with pyloric stenosis typically vomits after feedings. Vomiting may be projectile and may or may not immediately follow the feeding. However, the usual picture is a child who has projectile vomiting immediately after feeding. The child is usually very hungry, has a strong suck, and is willing to nipple immediately after a feeding. The child does not have a distended abdomen, because the contents of the stomach are forcibly ejected. The child usually burps well. Other signs are an olive-size mass over the pyloric sphincter and reverse peristaltic waves in the abdominal area after feedings. (A, T, G, Y)

81. 4. Gastrointestinal irritation is a common side effect of aspirin, especially when taken in large doses. Such signs and symptoms as anorexia, nausea, vomiting, diarrhea, and constipation are also common. The combination of aspirin and alcohol is especially likely to cause gastrointestinal irritation, sometimes to the point of doing direct damage to gastric mucosa. (A, T, G, M)

82. 2. Hoarseness that fails to subside with conservative care is an early sign of cancer of the larynx. Difficulty swallowing is a later symptom and occurs as the tumor enlarges to the point that it obstructs swallowing. Sore throat is not an early symptom of laryngeal cancer. Pain radiating to the ear may indicate that the tumor is metastasizing. (A, T, G, M)

83. 4. The amount of irrigating solution and the pressure at which it is given distend the bowel and promote peristalsis. Feces are then excreted through the stoma. If the client complains of cramping during irrigation, the nurse should continue with the irrigation but slow the flow rate temporarily. If cramping continues and becomes severe, it is best to halt the flow of solution for a minute or two. Deep breathing or lying on the side will not help relieve cramping during a colostomy irrigation. Cramping will usually subside when proper measures are used without removing the irrigating cone from the stoma. (I, N, S, M)

84. 1. The nurse should plan the child's fluid restriction with the mother for two reasons. First, the mother would best know her child's usual pattern of fluid intake. Second, the mother also needs to feel in control of her child's situation, and this is an area where the nurse can allow the mother some control. It is not advisable to allow a client on fluid restriction to drink all the allotted fluid at once; this may result in many thirsty hours for the client. Also, the nurse should remind the mother to count fluids used when the child takes any medications. (P, N, G, Y)

85. 4. Herpes simplex with skin ulcerations persisting longer than 1 month is categorized as an AIDS-defining illness. The Centers for Disease Control (CDC) lists opportunistic diseases that, when found in persons with laboratory evidence of HIV infection, are diagnostic of AIDS. (A, C, G, M)

86. 1. An idea of reference is a person's view that other people recognize that he or she has an important characteristic or power. Thought insertion is a person's belief that others, or a specific other, can put thoughts into his or her mind. Visual hallucinations involve seeing objects or persons not based in reality. A neologism is a word or phrase that has meaning only to the person using it. (A, T, L, X)

87. 1. Tea contains a significant amount of fluoride. Most foods contain very limited amounts. In most communities water is fluoridated, an effective and safe practice that helps prevent dental caries. Fluoride drops or tablets may also be given to provide fluorine; however, the nurse should observe careful safety measures, because children may accidentally take them in sufficient quantities to cause serious toxicity. (I, T, H, M)

88. 4. Shoes with little or no arch support are likely to contribute to backaches, leg pain, poor posture, and general fatigue for the pregnant client. Flat or low-heeled shoes with a good arch support are recommended. Knee-high stockings are not recommended, because the elastic at the top is likely to constrict circulation in the legs. However, they do not necessarily cause low back pain. A loosely elastic girdle helps support the abdomen and may relieve backaches. Pull-on slacks are satisfactory if they are comfortable. (I, N, H, O)

89. 2. When a mother cries soon after delivery and says she does not know why she is crying, the nurse should encourage her to talk about her feelings. By validating the client's statements, the nurse provides an open channel of communication. Various emotional reactions shortly after delivery are not uncommon and help relieve tension. The nurse ignores the client's feelings by telling her that there is no need to cry, asking if she needs medication, or explaining that her reactions are normal. (I, N, L, O)

90. 2. A child age 12 months is expected to cruise, but not necessarily to walk without support. Even if the child's development in walking is slow, this fact is not sufficient data on which to make a diagnosis of developmental delay. A physical therapy consult is not necessary. Using or not using a walker does not significantly affect independent walking. (D, N, H, Y)

91. 3. The parents' increased involvement in caretaking responsibilities for the sick neonate indicates their readiness for teaching. Parents will still verbalize feelings of grief and insecurity and concern for the neonate's health. However, they will demonstrate attachment behaviors as well. (D, N, H, O)

NURSING CARE COMPREHENSIVE TEST

TEST 1

Directions: Use this answer grid to determine areas of strength or need for further study.

Nursing Process

A = Assessment
D = Analysis, nursing diagnosis
P = Planning
I = Implementation
E = Evaluation

Cognitive Level

K = Knowledge
C = Comprehension
T = Application
N = Analysis

Client Needs

S = Safe, effective care environment
G = Physiological integrity
L = Psychosocial integrity
H = Health promotion/maintenance

Nursing Care Area

O = Maternity and newborn care
X = Psychosocial health problems
Y = Nursing care of children
M = Medical-surgical health problems

		Nursing Process					Cognitive Level				Client Needs				Care Area			
Question #	Answer #	A	D	P	I	E	K	C	T	N	S	G	L	H	O	X	Y	M
1	1	A							T			G						M
2	2				I				T				L			X		
3	1				I					N				H	O			
4	2		D					C					L			X		
5	3			P					T				L			X		
6	2			P						N		G						M
7	2				I					N		G			O			
8	1	A								N		G					Y	
9	3					E				N			L			X		
10	4			P						N		G			O			
11	1				I					N		G			O			
12	2				I					N			L		O			
13	4				I				T				L			X		
14	4				I					N	S							M
15	4	A							T		S							M
16	3		D					C					L			X		
17	1				I					N		G					Y	
18	1	A							T				L			X		

ANSWER GRID: 1

Nursing Process

A = Assessment
D = Analysis, nursing diagnosis
P = Planning
I = Implementation
E = Evaluation

Cognitive Level

K = Knowledge
C = Comprehension
T = Application
N = Analysis

Client Needs

S = Safe, effective care environment
G = Physiological integrity
L = Psychosocial integrity
H = Health promotion/maintenance

Nursing Care Area

O = Maternity and newborn care
X = Psychosocial health problems
Y = Nursing care of children
M = Medical-surgical health problems

		Nursing Process					Cognitive Level				Client Needs				Care Area			
Question #	Answer #	A	D	P	I	E	K	C	T	N	S	G	L	H	O	X	Y	M
19	4	A								N		G			O			
20	2				I					N		G					Y	
21	3	A							T			G						M
22	4					E				N		G			O			
23	2			P						N				H			Y	
24	4				I				T				L			X		
25	1					E				N			L			X		
26	2				I					N				H	O			
27	4					E				N		G						M
28	2		D							N		G			O			
29	2				I					N				H	O			
30	1			P						N				H			Y	
31	4				I				T				L			X		
32	4	A							T			G						M
33	2		D						T			G					Y	
34	3			P						N		G			O			
35	1					E				N		G					Y	
36	2	A								N		G					Y	
37	2		D						T				L			X		
38	2					E				N				H	O			
39	2				I					N		G					Y	
40	3			P				C				G						M
41	2				I					N				H			Y	
42	2					E			T		S							M

Answer Grid: 2

NURSING PROCESS

A = Assessment
D = Analysis, nursing diagnosis
P = Planning
I = Implementation
E = Evaluation

COGNITIVE LEVEL

K = Knowledge
C = Comprehension
T = Application
N = Analysis

CLIENT NEEDS

S = Safe, effective care environment
G = Physiological integrity
L = Psychosocial integrity
H = Health promotion/maintenance

NURSING CARE AREA

O = Maternity and newborn care
X = Psychosocial health problems
Y = Nursing care of children
M = Medical-surgical health problems

		Nursing Process					Cognitive Level				Client Needs				Care Area			
Question #	Answer #	A	D	P	I	E	K	C	T	N	S	G	L	H	O	X	Y	M
43	2				I				T			G						M
44	4			P						N				H	O			
45	1				I				T			G						M
46	3				I				T					H				M
47	3				I				T			G						M
48	2			P						N		G			O			
49	1				I				T					H				M
50	4			P						N	S							M
51	3				I					N		G					Y	
52	4	A								N				H			Y	
53	3	A							T			G						M
54	2			P						N		G					Y	
55	4			P					T			G						M
56	3				I				T				L			X		
57	1				I				T		S						Y	
58	4				I				T				L			X		
59	2		D							N				H	O			
60	3		D							N			L			X		
61	3					E				N			L			X		
62	1				I				T					H				M
63	2		D						T				L			X		
64	4		D							N		G						M
65	1					E	K					G					Y	
66	4	A								N			L			X		

ANSWER GRID: 3

Nursing Process

A = Assessment
D = Analysis, nursing diagnosis
P = Planning
I = Implementation
E = Evaluation

Cognitive Level

K = Knowledge
C = Comprehension
T = Application
N = Analysis

Client Needs

S = Safe, effective care environment
G = Physiological integrity
L = Psychosocial integrity
H = Health promotion/maintenance

Nursing Care Area

O = Maternity and newborn care
X = Psychosocial health problems
Y = Nursing care of children
M = Medical-surgical health problems

		Nursing Process					Cognitive Level				Client Needs				Care Area			
Question #	Answer #	A	D	P	I	E	K	C	T	N	S	G	L	H	O	X	Y	M
67	2				I					N	S						Y	
68	1	A							T				L					M
69	3				I					N		G			O			
70	3					E			T		S							M
71	2	A						C				G						M
72	1	A								N		G			O			
73	2				I				T				L			X		
74	1			P						N		G						M
75	2	A						C				G						M
76	1			P					T			G						M
77	4	A							T				L			X		
78	2		D							N			L			X		
79	4				I					N				H	O			
80	4	A							T			G					Y	
81	4	A							T			G						M
82	2	A							T			G						M
83	4				I					N	S							M
84	1			P						N		G					Y	
85	4	A						C				G						M
86	1	A							T				L			X		
87	1				I				T					H				M
88	4				I					N				H	O			
89	2				I					N			L		O			
90	2		D							N				H			Y	

Answer Grid: 4

Nursing Process

A = Assessment
D = Analysis, nursing diagnosis
P = Planning
I = Implementation
E = Evaluation

Cognitive Level

K = Knowledge
C = Comprehension
T = Application
N = Analysis

Client Needs

S = Safe, effective care environment
G = Physiological integrity
L = Psychosocial integrity
H = Health promotion/maintenance

Nursing Care Area

O = Maternity and newborn care
X = Psychosocial health problems
Y = Nursing care of children
M = Medical-surgical health problems

		Nursing Process					Cognitive Level				Client Needs				Care Area			
Question #	Answer #	A	D	P	I	E	K	C	T	N	S	G	L	H	O	X	Y	M
91	3		D							N				H	O			
Number Correct																		
Number Possible	91	21	12	15	33	10	1	6	35	49	8	41	24	18	21	21	19	30
Percentage Correct																		

Score Calculation:
To determine your **Percentage Correct**, divide the **Number Correct** by the **Number Possible**.

Select the one best answer and indicate your choice by filling in the circle in front of the option.

Comprehensive Test 2

1. When assessing a black client for cyanosis, the nurse should examine the client's
- ○ 1. retinas.
- ○ 2. nail beds.
- ○ 3. oral mucous membranes.
- ○ 4. skin on the inner aspects of the wrists.

2. Two adolescent clients who do not have smoking privileges are discovered smoking cigarettes in another client's room. Of the following courses of action the nurse could take in this situation, it would be best to plan to restate the limits about cigarette smoking clearly to these clients and
- ○ 1. restrict their television privileges.
- ○ 2. send them to separate rooms.
- ○ 3. discuss their behavior with them.
- ○ 4. report the incident to their physician.

3. A 30-year-old primigravida at 28 weeks gestation is admitted to the hospital with preterm labor. The client tells the nurse, "I think my water broke." After observing a cord prolapse when the client's membranes ruptured, the nurse should help the client assume which of the following positions?
- ○ 1. Supine.
- ○ 2. Knee-chest.
- ○ 3. Low Fowler's.
- ○ 4. Flat in bed on either side.

4. A client who has undergone a laryngectomy begins oral feedings 9 days postoperatively. After oral feedings start, it is important for the nurse to help the client develop the ability to
- ○ 1. cough.
- ○ 2. belch.
- ○ 3. hiccup.
- ○ 4. sneeze.

5. A 25-year-old gravida 2, TPAL 1001, who had a previous cesarean section delivery for breech presentation visits the prenatal clinic for a routine visit. The nurse instructs the client about laboratory tests that may be performed during the second trimester, including alpha-fetoprotein (AFP) testing. The nurse would determine that the client understands the instructions when the client says
- ○ 1. "My abdomen will be shaved, and a sample of amnionic fluid will be withdrawn."
- ○ 2. "I'll have to drink six glasses of water, and an ultrasonic examination will be performed."
- ○ 3. "A sample of my blood will be sent to the laboratory for analysis."
- ○ 4. "An electronic fetal monitor will be attached, and the baby's activity will be assessed."

6. Following delivery of a viable infant, the nurse plans to administer oxytocin following delivery of the placenta. The nurse would determine that the placenta is about to be delivered after noting that
- ○ 1. the uterus begins to feel soft.
- ○ 2. vaginal bleeding temporarily stops.
- ○ 3. the client begins to bear down of her own accord.
- ○ 4. the umbilical cord lengthens outside the vagina.

7. The nurse teaches the parents of a 3-year-old child who has undergone cleft palate repair how to use elbow restraints. The nurse would evaluate the teaching as successful when the parents state
- ○ 1. "The restraints should never be removed until the doctor says it's okay."
- ○ 2. "The child should wear the restraints at night, but can have them off during the day."
- ○ 3. "The restraints should be taped right to the arms so they will stay in place."
- ○ 4. "We'll take the restraints off at least three times a day to look for any redness or swelling, and then put them right back on."

8. When caring for a client receiving haloperidol (Haldol), the nurse should plan to assess for
- ○ 1. hypertensive episodes.
- ○ 2. extrapyramidal symptoms.
- ○ 3. euphoria.
- ○ 4. lithium toxicity.

9. While sitting on her mother's lap, an 18-month-old child pulls a full cup of hot coffee off the table onto her legs. The child's aunt, who is a nurse, should immediately
- ○ 1. apply an antiseptic spray to the burn.
- ○ 2. apply a topical ointment to the burn.
- ○ 3. cover the child's legs with a clean, dry dish towel.
- ○ 4. immerse the burned areas in cool water.

10. A nurse assessing a term neonate delivered vaginally should test the neonate's rooting reflex by
- ○ 1. stroking the neonate's cheek.

○ 2. placing a finger in the neonate's hand.
○ 3. pulling the neonate to a sitting position.
○ 4. supporting the neonate's head and then allowing it to drop back a short distance.

11. A client is admitted to an inpatient psychiatric unit because of an obsessive-compulsive disorder. He washes his feet endlessly because he thinks they "are so dirty that I can't put on my socks and shoes." The nurse would recognize that the client is using ritualistic behavior because of his obsessive-compulsive disorder primarily to relieve discomfort associated with feelings of
○ 1. depression.
○ 2. ambivalence.
○ 3. irrational fear.
○ 4. intolerable anxiety.

12. After noting that a 2-year-old child's anterior fontanel is slightly open, the nurse should
○ 1. check the child's head circumference.
○ 2. consider this a normal finding.
○ 3. question the mother about her delivery of this child.
○ 4. schedule a radiologic exam of the child's head.

13. A nurse at a crisis center helps a client obtain psychological counseling with another nurse, who makes plans to begin a one-to-one relationship with the client. The nurse's care plan for this client should indicate that the nurse will begin the relationship by
○ 1. having the client confirm his or her nursing diagnosis.
○ 2. setting goals that the nurse hopes to attain in the relationship.
○ 3. defining the relationship to be developed between the nurse and the client.
○ 4. planning a meeting schedule that is mutually convenient for the nurse and the client.

14. The nurse caring for a primigravida in early labor plans to perform a vaginal examination on the client. In addition to a lubricating agent, which of the following should the nurse plan to have ready?
○ 1. A speculum.
○ 2. Waterproof gloves.
○ 3. Nitrazine paper.
○ 4. A bedpan.

15. The physician orders IV aminophylline in a 1:1 drip to run at a rate of 12 cc per hour. The nurse would calculate that the client will receive how much aminophylline over 24 hours?
○ 1. 144 mgs.
○ 2. 288 mgs.
○ 3. 1.4 gms.
○ 4. 2.8 gms.

16. Mechanical ventilation is associated with which of the following complications?
○ 1. Gastrointestinal hemorrhage.
○ 2. Immunosuppression.
○ 3. Increased cardiac output.
○ 4. Pulmonary emboli.

17. After teaching the parents of a toddler about appropriate snack foods for toddlers, the nurse would judge that the instructions about not giving the child peanuts for snacks are effective when the father states, "Peanuts
○ 1. are low in nutritive value."
○ 2. are very high in sodium."
○ 3. can be easy aspirated."
○ 4. cannot be entirely digested."

18. An infant who has undergone surgery for bilateral clubfoot returns from the operating room with bilateral casts. After noting that the infant's toes are slightly cool and edematous, the nurse should first
○ 1. cut the casts.
○ 2. elevate the legs on pillows.
○ 3. notify the surgeon.
○ 4. reassess in about 15 minutes.

19. A 16-year-old primigravida tells the nurse, "My grandmother says I'll lose a tooth because I'm pregnant. Is that true?" The nurse should instruct the client that preventing tooth loss can best be accomplished through a proper diet and adequate intake of which mineral?
○ 1. Iron.
○ 2. Zinc.
○ 3. Calcium.
○ 4. Potassium.

20. As the nurse is administering a tap water enema, the client begins to complain of abdominal cramping. Which of the following actions should the nurse implement first?
○ 1. Stop infusing the enema and allow the client to evacuate the fluid.
○ 2. Temporarily stop the infusion until the cramping subsides.
○ 3. Tell the client to hold his breath and continue infusing the enema.
○ 4. Turn the client onto his back and continue infusing the enema.

21. While visiting a client with multiple sclerosis, the community health nurse observes that the client looks unkempt and sad. The client suddenly says, "I can't even find the strength to comb my hair" and bursts into tears. Which of the following responses by the nurse would be best?
○ 1. "It must be frustrating not to be able to care for yourself."
○ 2. "How many days have you been unable to comb your hair?"
○ 3. "Why hasn't your husband been helping you?"
○ 4. "Tell me more about how you're feeling."

22. During the first hour postpartum, a client who just

gave birth receives lactated Ringer's solution with 10 units of oxytocin (Pitocin) intravenously. The nurse would explain to the client that the primary purpose of the Pitocin is to

- ○ 1. replace fluids lost during labor.
- ○ 2. provide pain relief during the recovery period.
- ○ 3. lower blood pressure.
- ○ 4. contract the uterus.

23. A client with Hodgkin's disease explains to the nurse the monitoring he will be doing at home between radiation treatments. Which of the following statements would indicate that he knows how to detect a major complication?

- ○ 1. "I'll measure my neck circumference every day."
- ○ 2. "I'll take my temperature every day."
- ○ 3. "I'll monitor the loss of body hair every week."
- ○ 4. "I'll check the circulation in my arms every day."

24. Which of the following nursing measures would most help to prevent pressure ulcer formation in an at-risk client?

- ○ 1. Reposition every hour.
- ○ 2. Provide a low-protein diet.
- ○ 3. Ensure generous fluid intake.
- ○ 4. Massage any reddened areas on the sacral area.

25. The nurse is performing a gestational age assessment on a preterm neonate. After teaching the neonate's mother about gestational age assessment, the nurse would determine that the mother needs further instructions when she states that the neonate's prematurity can be validated by the

- ○ 1. birth weight.
- ○ 2. estimated date of delivery.
- ○ 3. muscle tone.
- ○ 4. pupillary reaction to light.

26. For a client with a demand pacemaker, the nurse should explain that this pacemaker functions by providing

- ○ 1. stimuli to the heart muscle only when the heart begins to beat irregularly.
- ○ 2. continuous stimuli to the heart muscle, resulting in a predetermined heart rate.
- ○ 3. stimuli to the heart muscle only when the heart rate falls below a specified level.
- ○ 4. continuous stimuli to the heart muscle whenever ventricular fibrillation occurs.

27. In the event of evisceration of an abdominal wound, which of the following actions should the nurse implement first?

- ○ 1. Call the physician immediately.
- ○ 2. Reinsert the protruding viscera into the abdominal cavity.
- ○ 3. Place the client in reverse Trendelenburg's position.
- ○ 4. Cover the wound with a sterile dressing moistened with sterile normal saline solution.

28. When assessing a 2-month-old infant, the nurse feels a "click" when abducting the infant's left hip. The nurse should then

- ○ 1. chart the finding; it is normal for a 2-month-old.
- ○ 2. check the lengths of the femurs to see if they are equal.
- ○ 3. instruct the mother to keep the leg in an adducted position.
- ○ 4. reschedule the child for a follow-up assessment of the hip problem in 1 month.

29. When admitting a 2-month-old infant with a ventral septal defect and congestive heart failure the nurse should first obtain information on

- ○ 1. labor and delivery history.
- ○ 2. feeding behavior.
- ○ 3. the presence of a smoker in the home.
- ○ 4. financial concerns of the family.

30. A 25-year-old male construction worker comes to the emergency department complaining of back and left flank pain. Initially the pain was dull and constant, but now the client is experiencing periods of complete comfort alternating with periods of excruciating pain. A tentative diagnosis of renal calculi is made. The priority nursing diagnosis category for this client would be

- ○ 1. Fluid Volume Excess.
- ○ 2. Pain.
- ○ 3. Fluid Volume Deficit.
- ○ 4. Impaired Skin Integrity.

31. An adolescent is admitted to the emergency room with dyspnea related to bronchospasms. The nurse should place the client in which of the following positions?

- ○ 1. High Fowler's.
- ○ 2. Side-lying.
- ○ 3. Prone.
- ○ 4. Supine.

32. Which of the following statements is the most accurate description of enteric precautions?

- ○ 1. A client on enteric precautions must have a private room.
- ○ 2. Health care workers may not enter the client's room without donning a gown, gloves, and a mask.
- ○ 3. The use of enteric precautions is not advocated by the Centers for Disease Control (CDC).
- ○ 4. Enteric precautions are designed to prevent the spread of infections transmitted by contact with feces.

33. A client, with bipolar disorder, manic phase, has a nursing diagnosis of Altered Nutrition: Less than Body Requirements. To help the client meet recommended daily allowances of nutrients, which of the following nursing interventions would be best?

- ○ 1. Give the client half of a meat and cheese sandwich between meals.

- ○ 2. Inform the client that snacks are available only if he eats properly at mealtime.
- ○ 3. Tell the client to sit alone at mealtime so he won't be distracted by others.
- ○ 4. Teach the client about proper nutrition.

34. An 8-year-old child with severe cerebral palsy is underweight and undersized for his age. He is currently being fed a diet of pureed foods and liquids via a syringe. An appropriate nursing diagnosis for this child would be Altered Nutrition: Less than Body Requirements related to

- ○ 1. impaired oral motor control.
- ○ 2. inability to absorb nutrients.
- ○ 3. inability to metabolize fats.
- ○ 4. increased intracranial pressure.

35. A client's husband telephones the nurse to ask for information about his wife's condition. Which of the following responses by the husband would show that he has understood the nurse's explanation about her ability to provide such information? "I'll

- ○ 1. meet you in the conference room so that we can discuss her progress."
- ○ 2. ask her doctor for permission to read her medical record."
- ○ 3. ask my wife to give you permission to discuss her care with me."
- ○ 4. try to attend my wife's next team treatment case conference."

36. A client in the third trimester of pregnancy tells the nurse that she tries to control her weight by skipping breakfast. The nurse should caution the client against this practice because of the risk of developing

- ○ 1. uremia.
- ○ 2. ketosis.
- ○ 3. hypertension.
- ○ 4. hyperglycemia.

37. A client agrees to undergo disulfiram (Antabuse) therapy. The nurse would suspect that the client most probably has drunk alcohol while taking disulfiram when the client experiences

- ○ 1. vertigo.
- ○ 2. hallucinations.
- ○ 3. diarrhea and fever.
- ○ 4. nausea and vomiting.

38. When the nurse documents the initial care of a suspected abuse victim, which of the following statements would be least helpful for others caring for the client?

- ○ 1. "Requests that her bruises not be described to a doctor."
- ○ 2. "Seems fearful to discuss how bruises on her body had been caused."
- ○ 3. "Asks that her husband not be called at work, because she says she knows he is very busy."
- ○ 4. "Refuses a follow-up appointment because she states that she has a child at home who needs her care."

39. Which of the following is an early symptom of glaucoma?

- ○ 1. Hazy vision.
- ○ 2. Loss of central vision.
- ○ 3. Impaired peripheral vision.
- ○ 4. Blurred or "sooty" vision.

40. A client with a 4-year history of severe bulimia is admitted to a psychiatric unit. The nurse would anticipate that the client's current signs and symptoms most likely will include

- ○ 1. amenorrhea, binge-eating episodes, vomiting, and high serum potassium level.
- ○ 2. normal weight, binge-eating episodes, vomiting, and low serum potassium level.
- ○ 3. severe weight loss, vomiting, compulsive exercising, and tachycardia.
- ○ 4. amenorrhea, laxative abuse, diet pill abuse, and vomiting.

41. Which one of the following would the nurse evaluate as an expected outcome for a client who has undergone surgical repair of an inguinal hernia?

- ○ 1. The client will verbalize understanding of instructions to avoid lifting for 2 to 6 weeks after surgery.
- ○ 2. The client's voiding patterns will return to normal within 6 months after surgery.
- ○ 3. The client will use a cane for assistance with ambulation for 2 to 6 weeks after surgery.
- ○ 4. The client will remain on a soft diet until the wound is healed.

42. A school-age child being treated for leukemia with chemotherapy begins to experience nausea and vomiting as a side effect of chemotherapy. The nurse should plan to administer an antiemetic

- ○ 1. as needed during therapy.
- ○ 2. as soon as the child says he is nauseated.
- ○ 3. concurrently with the chemotherapeutic agent after the child is NPO for 6 hours.
- ○ 4. 1 hour before chemotherapy starts and then every 2 to 6 hours for the next 24 hours.

43. The nurse tells a rape victim that even if she was protected against pregnancy by a contraceptive and has no intention of taking any legal action against her assailant, she should still be checked by a physician. This post-rape physical examination is recommended for early detection of

- ○ 1. veneral disease.
- ○ 2. anxiety reaction.
- ○ 3. periurethral tears.
- ○ 4. menstrual difficulties.

44. To help promote independence in the area of feeding for a child in skeletal traction, the nurse would help the child choose which of the following meals?

○ 1. Carrot sticks, celery with peanut butter, roast beef and gravy, peas, jello, and milk in a cup.
○ 2. Chicken noodle soup with crackers, grilled cheese sandwich, cottage cheese with pineapple, and chocolate milk in a cup.
○ 3. Chicken nuggets with sauce, carrot sticks, french-fried potatoes, ice cream sandwich, and milk in a carton.
○ 4. Chili, hot dog, cherry cobbler, and apple juice in a can.

45. The primary nursing goals for a client with myasthenia gravis are to conserve the client's energy and to
○ 1. ensure a safe environment.
○ 2. maintain respiratory function.
○ 3. provide psychological support and reassurance.
○ 4. promote comfort and relieve pain.

46. A nurse caring for a term newborn delivered vaginally includes an eye assessment in the nursing care plan. To facilitate this assessment, the nurse would plan to position the neonate on the
○ 1. abdomen.
○ 2. side.
○ 3. back with the head lowered.
○ 4. back with the head elevated.

47. A client develops an abscess in his abdominal incision. A debridement is done, and a small drain is left in the wound. The nurse would judge that the drain is accomplishing its intended purpose when it
○ 1. is used to irrigate the wound.
○ 2. permits the escape of wound drainage.
○ 3. decreases the discomfort in the surrounding tissues.
○ 4. allows for the introduction of antibiotics into the wound.

48. The nurse is assisting the physician in cardioversion of a client admitted with ventricular tachycardia. Cardioversion differs from defibrillation in that during cardioversion, the shock is
○ 1. unsynchronized with the R wave.
○ 2. synchronized with the R wave.
○ 3. delivered at a higher wattage.
○ 4. delivered with a different machine.

49. The physician has ordered alpha-fetoprotein studies for a pregnant client. In planning instruction for the client about the purposes of the test, the nurse should include the fact that alpha-fetoprotein studies can
○ 1. determine the sex of the fetus.
○ 2. detect open neural tube defects.
○ 3. evaluate Rh sensitization.
○ 4. identify Down syndrome.

50. A client admits to using cocaine and says, "When I stop using, I feel bad." Which of the following effects is the client most likely to describe as occurring after he stops using cocaine?
○ 1. Depression.
○ 2. Palpitations.
○ 3. Flashbacks.
○ 4. Double vision.

51. A client with peptic ulcers tells the nurse that she uses the following medications at home. Which one should the nurse teach her to avoid because of her peptic ulcers?
○ 1. Aspirin for occasional headaches.
○ 2. Scopolamine to prevent seasickness when boating.
○ 3. Psyllium hydrophilic mucilloid (Metamucil) for occasional constipation.
○ 4. Phenylephrine (Neo-Synephrine) for an upper respiratory infection.

52. Before being helped to ambulate, a client is first prepared for dangling over the side of the bed. Which of the following measures should the nurse plan to carry out before helping the client dangle?
○ 1. Administer a prescribed analgesic.
○ 2. Encourage the client to take a short nap.
○ 3. Have the client carry out leg exercises for a few minutes.
○ 4. Help the client assume a high Fowler's position for a few minutes.

53. The priority need for a client using marijuana would be
○ 1. physical activity.
○ 2. large amounts of fluid.
○ 3. reassurance in a calm environment.
○ 4. close contact with his friends.

54. At an emergency shelter, an earthquake victim tells the nurse that he is going to spend the night in his own bed at home. The nurse is not surprised by this comment and recognizes it as a self-protective mechanism. Which defense mechanism is the client exhibiting?
○ 1. Intellectualization.
○ 2. Denial.
○ 3. Rationalization.
○ 4. Undoing.

55. The nurse is caring for a primigravida in active labor at 39 weeks gestation. The client delivers a 4 lb., 4 oz. viable female neonate who is assessed to be term and small for gestational age. The client asks the nurse what problems her daughter may have. The nurse's best response would be that small-for-gestational age neonates are subject to problems with
○ 1. respirations.
○ 2. meconium staining.
○ 3. heat loss.
○ 4. sucking.

56. If a nursing goal is to increase a child's protein intake, the nurse would encourage the child to eat which of the following foods that the child likes?

○ 1. A bacon, lettuce, and tomato sandwich.
○ 2. Fruit-flavored yogurt.
○ 3. Nacho chips and salsa.
○ 4. Toast with butter and jelly.

57. After undergoing gastrectomy surgery, a client returns to his room from the postanesthesia recovery room. He is alert and oriented to person, place, and time. To minimize tension on his abdominal incision and to allow his cardiovascular and respiratory systems to function optimally, the nurse should position the client in bed in which position?
○ 1. Prone.
○ 2. Supine.
○ 3. Low Fowler's.
○ 4. Right or left Sims'.

58. A client with emphysema is receiving continuous oxygen therapy. Depressed ventilation is likely to occur unless the nurse ensures that the oxygen is administered
○ 1. warmed.
○ 2. humidified.
○ 3. at a low flow rate.
○ 4. through a nasal cannula.

59. When dressing the wounds of a child who has sustained serious burns, the nurse would likely note which characteristic of full-thickness burns?
○ 1. Blanching to the touch.
○ 2. Excessive bleeding.
○ 3. Little pain.
○ 4. Many blisters.

60. After teaching a client about myasthenia gravis, the nurse would judge that the client has formed a realistic concept of her condition when she says that by taking her medication and pacing her activities,
○ 1. she will live longer, but ultimately the disease will cause her death.
○ 2. her symptoms will be controlled, and eventually the disease will be cured.
○ 3. she should be able to control the disease and enjoy a healthy life-style.
○ 4. her fatigue will be relieved, but she should expect occasional periods of muscle weakness.

61. A client is admitted to an inpatient psychiatric unit accompanied by his wife, who reports that he has been "on a spending spree; he sent roses to everyone we know. He's playing a seductive game with women he meets, telling them that he's next in line for the throne in some country in Europe." During the admission process, the client becomes very active, moves about, and then puts his arm around the nurse in a show of affection and says to her, "I sure like you a lot, honey. I can do a lot for you in the real world out there." In this situation, what would be the nurse's best response?
○ 1. "Let's get some popcorn and a soda."
○ 2. "I'll have to tell my supervisor if you don't stop this minute."
○ 3. "You know you shouldn't do this. It's against the rules of the hospital."
○ 4. "Please stop. I'm very uncomfortable with your display of affection."

62. Arterial blood (ABG) gas values of a client with emphysema are monitored closely during hospitalization. Which of the following $PaCO_2$ values would indicate the need for immediate intervention in this client?
○ 1. 35 mm Hg.
○ 2. 45 mm Hg.
○ 3. 60 mm Hg.
○ 4. 80 mm Hg.

63. When caring for a primipara who has delivered in a lithotomy position with stirrups, the nurse would instruct the client that both legs will be removed slowly and simultaneously from the stirrups to prevent
○ 1. inverting the uterus.
○ 2. cramping in the leg muscles.
○ 3. damaging nerves in the popliteal spaces.
○ 4. overstretching blood vessels in the legs.

64. A pregnant client attending preparation for parenthood classes taught by a registered nurse asks the nurse how blood reaches the fetus and why neonates sometimes need heart surgery. The nurse would explain fetal circulation and include a description of the functioning of the foramen ovale, which allows blood in the fetal circulatory system to pass directly from the right atrium to the
○ 1. aorta.
○ 2. left atrium.
○ 3. left ventricle.
○ 4. right ventricle.

65. The nurse assesses a client for euphoria, looking for which of the following characteristic clinical manifestations?
○ 1. Inappropriate laughter and giddiness.
○ 2. Mood elevation with an exaggerated sense of well-being.
○ 3. Slurring of words when excited.
○ 4. Visual hallucinations and giddiness.

66. A 16-year-old is admitted to the hospital with an opportunistic infectious disease and is later diagnosed as having AIDS. The family insists that the diagnosis be withheld from the adolescent. The nurse should
○ 1. accept the family's wishes.
○ 2. insist that the family tell the adolescent of the diagnosis.
○ 3. plan a team meeting with the family to discuss their fears and concerns.
○ 4. tell the adolescent of the diagnosis with or without the family's support.

67. Which of the following assessments would be important for the nurse to make to determine whether a client is recovering as expected from spinal anesthesia?
- ○ 1. Level of consciousness.
- ○ 2. Rate and depth of respirations.
- ○ 3. Rate of capillary refill in the toes.
- ○ 4. Degree of response to pinpricks in the legs and toes.

68. After explaining the external fetal monitor to a primigravida in active labor, the nurse would determine that the client understands the instructions when she says
- ○ 1. "You'll apply a metal plate to my thigh."
- ○ 2. "You'll attach a small catheter to a pressure device."
- ○ 3. "You'll place an ultrasonic device across my abdomen."
- ○ 4. "You'll connect small wires to an electrocardiogram pad."

69. One goal the nurse should strive to achieve for a client with osteoarthritis is to
- ○ 1. relieve discomfort.
- ○ 2. prevent dehydration.
- ○ 3. prevent fluid volume excess.
- ○ 4. increase vitamin C intake.

70. A client is admitted to the emergency room with a cut finger that is bleeding profusely. She says, "Just let me alone. I'll be fine just as soon as you fix my finger." She displays signs of alcohol intoxication, and a blood test confirms this. After the client's wound is sutured but before she leaves the emergency room, it would be best for the nurse to ensure that the client
- ○ 1. takes a nap.
- ○ 2. does some exercising.
- ○ 3. restricts fluid intake.
- ○ 4. drinks generous amounts of black coffee.

71. While caring for a primigravida in early labor, the nurse would encourage her to assume which position for early labor?
- ○ 1. Sitting.
- ○ 2. Low Fowler's.
- ○ 3. Lying on either side.
- ○ 4. Any position of comfort.

72. A client is admitted to the inpatient psychiatric unit. The nurse observes that he is unshaven, has an odor about him, has spots on his shirt and pants, moves slowly, gazes at the floor, and has a flat affect. Which observation would point to psychomotor retardation?
- ○ 1. Slow movements.
- ○ 2. Flat affect.
- ○ 3. Unkempt appearance.
- ○ 4. Avoidance of eye contact.

73. When some clients fail to clean the hospital's recreation room after using it, a client-government meeting is held to discuss the problem. In this situation, it is best for staff members to assume a role of
- ○ 1. offering their view but agreeing to the group's decision.
- ○ 2. co-leading the meeting with assistance from any one of the clients.
- ○ 3. remaining silent while observing the group's process of decision making.
- ○ 4. allowing a client the leadership role but requiring staff approval of the group's decision.

74. A client being taught deep-breathing exercises preoperatively should be taught to take a deep inhalation and then
- ○ 1. close the glottis tightly.
- ○ 2. make a short, hacking cough.
- ○ 3. exhale slowly but thoroughly.
- ○ 4. hold the breath for a few seconds.

75. The nurse working with young parents on parenting skills and understanding their 2-year-old's development would judge her teaching as effective when the parents state, "We
- ○ 1. expect him to obey without hesitation."
- ○ 2. expect him to dress without help."
- ○ 3. try to give him some choices."
- ○ 4. want him to brush his own teeth."

76. A nurse planning a program aimed at decreasing the primary cause of disability, disease, and death in children should plan to
- ○ 1. focus on early cancer detection.
- ○ 2. promote prenatal care for mothers.
- ○ 3. teach safety practices to parents and children.
- ○ 4. encourage parents to have their children immunized.

77. To decrease anxiety in a young child admitted overnight for observation, the nurse should do which of the following when caring for him?
- ○ 1. Move quickly around the child.
- ○ 2. Keep the child away from the center of activity.
- ○ 3. Avoid using a night light.
- ○ 4. Avoid making loud noises.

78. A primigravida is scheduled for a cesarean section delivery after 12 hours of labor and a diagnosis of cephalopelvic disproportion. Even though the client's husband remained with his wife during labor, he decides not to stay with her during the cesarean section. Following delivery of a viable term neonate, the nurse would promote the father's attachment to the neonate by
- ○ 1. telling the father to meet the nurse at the nursery.
- ○ 2. asking the father if he had a preference for a boy or girl.
- ○ 3. encouraging the father to tell other relatives of the birth.

○ 4. allowing the father to carry the neonate to the nursery.

79. The nurse caring for a primigravida in the prenatal clinic plans to instruct her about methods to confirm the gestational age of the fetus. Which of the following should be included in the teaching plan?

○ 1. Increased fetal movement after meals.
○ 2. Date of quickening.
○ 3. Appearance of abdominal striae.
○ 4. Decrease in urinary frequency.

80. A primigravida at approximately 7 months gestation tells the nurse, "At times, I don't want intercourse. I don't know why. I try to remain distant from my husband at those times." In response to the client's statement, the nurse should explain that

○ 1. the sexual drive normally tends to fluctuate during pregnancy.
○ 2. a low sexual drive is often a sign of impending labor.
○ 3. a low sexual drive serves as nature's signal to discontinue sexual intimacies and intercourse until after delivery.
○ 4. the sexual drive normally is stronger during pregnancy, and the problem should be discussed with the physician.

81. The nurse is taking a nursing history on a preoperative client. Which of the following pieces of information would most likely have a significant impact on the client's recovery postoperatively? The client

○ 1. had a cold 6 weeks ago.
○ 2. has smoked 1 pack of cigarettes a day for 12 years.
○ 3. drinks about two beers a week on a regular basis.
○ 4. is 10 lbs. overweight.

82. A 70-year-old client says, "It's harder every day to be someone. Everyone is in such a hurry to get things done, and their way." After analyzing the client's comment, the nurse would judge that the client has described a common problem experienced by elderly clients whose life-style threatens the need for

○ 1. self-esteem.
○ 2. communicating effectively.
○ 3. expressing hostility openly.
○ 4. feeling secure about having adequate health care.

83. Radiation therapy is instituted for a client with Hodgkin's disease; after 1 week, the radiation site becomes red and irritated. Which of the following statements would indicate that the client treated the area appropriately at home? "I applied

○ 1. aloe vera lotion to the area."
○ 2. moist cool soaks to the area."
○ 3. nothing to the area; I just kept it dry."
○ 4. a hot-water bottle to the area."

84. About 2 weeks after receiving care in the emergency room, a client admits to her husband that she has a drinking problem and that she has "decided to do something about it." Of critical importance for her successful rehabilitation is

○ 1. her emotional support system.
○ 2. her motivation to change her behavior.
○ 3. the presence of self-help groups in the community.
○ 4. the presence of local health centers for alcoholics.

85. The nurse would plan to observe a child receiving IV aminophylline for which of the following symptoms of toxicity?

○ 1. Bradycardia, fatigue, and increased blood pressure.
○ 2. Fluid retention, ataxia, decreased blood pressure.
○ 3. Tachycardia, agitation, and decreased blood pressure.
○ 4. Tachypnea, drowsiness, and increased blood pressure.

86. The nurse answers a call on a telephone hotline from a man who was at the crisis center once in the past when he made a suicide threat. The client says, "Don't try to help me anymore. This is it. I've had enough and I have a gun in front of me now." He then hangs up the telephone. The nurse's first action in this situation would be to call

○ 1. the client back to try to calm him.
○ 2. the police to request their intervention.
○ 3. his wife at work to suggest that she hurry home.
○ 4. a neighbor to ask him to go to the client's home immediately.

87. A nurse caring for a primigravida in active labor plans to be supportive of the client throughout labor, especially when discomfort is likely to be intense. In planning the client's care, during which stage of labor should the nurse anticipate that the client will require the most encouragement and support because of the intensity of discomfort?

○ 1. Early part of stage 1.
○ 2. Transition part of stage 1.
○ 3. Stage 2.
○ 4. Stage 3.

88. After feedings are resumed in an infant who has undergone a pyloroplasty, the nurse should

○ 1. keep the head of the bed flat and the infant supine.
○ 2. offer several ounces of an oral electrolyte solution as an initial feeding.
○ 3. place the infant prone after feedings.
○ 4. start with small feedings (5 to 10 cc) and slowly increase the amounts as tolerated.

89. A client comes to the emergency room after being stung by a bee. The nurse observes the bee sting for initial signs and symptoms of acute inflammation, one of which typically is

○ 1. numbness.

○ 2. swelling.
○ 3. blanching of the skin.
○ 4. the presence of exudate.

90. A client receiving digoxin for congestive heart failure undergoes cardiac catheterization to further evaluate his condition. The procedure reveals a cardiac output of 2.2 L/min. The nurse would evaluate this cardiac output as

○ 1. high, due to the effects of digoxin.
○ 2. within normal limits, dogoxin is effective.
○ 3. within normal limits, but not adequate to support strenuous activity.
○ 4. low, requiring further medical intervention.

CORRECT ANSWERS AND RATIONALE

The letters in parentheses following the rationale identify the step of the nursing process (A, D, P, I, E); cognitive level (K, C, T, N); client need (S, G, L, H); and nursing care area (O, X, Y, M). See the Answer Grid for the key.

1. 3. In black clients, cyanosis can best be detected by examining the conjunctiva, lips, and oral mucous membranes. (A, N, G, M)

2. 3. Adolescents tend to test the limits of their surroundings as an expression of inner conflicts. The nurse needs to explore the relationship between limit setting and inner conflicts through discussion to increase the adolescents' self-awareness. Sending the clients to separate rooms or reporting the situation to their physician may be done if necessary after discussion has occurred. Restricting television privileges has no relationship to the abused privilege. (I, T, L, X)

3. 2. To help the presenting part of the fetus move off a prolapsed cord, the client should be helped into the knee-chest position. If this is impossible, the head of the bed should be lowered. The nurse can push the presenting part up off of the cord with a sterile gloved hand. Oxygen should be administered. This is a dire emergency, because the life of the fetus is at risk due to possible asphyxiation. An emergency cesarean section is usually performed. (I, N, G, O)

4. 2. A client with a total laryngectomy can eventually learn to produce sounds by ejecting air under pressure from the esophagus. At first, the client must do this by using the air of a belch. Therefore, a client should begin learning how to belch when starting to take oral feedings following a total laryngectomy. Coughing, sneezing, and hiccuping will not help the client during speech rehabilitation. (I, T, G, M)

5. 3. Maternal serum is assessed for alpha-fetoprotein (AFP) between 15 and 20 weeks gestation. If the value is elevated, a second sample is drawn. If follow-up is needed, an amniocentesis is performed and a small amount of amnionic fluid removed for analysis. A sonogram may detect serious fetal defects but does not provide AFP levels. An electronic fetal monitor is used antepartally for stress and nonstress testing. (E, N, H, O)

6. 4. Common signs of placental separation include a lengthening of the umbilical cord outside of the vagina, firming of the uterus, sudden vaginal bleeding (usually a spurt or a trickel), elevation of the uterus into the abdomen, and a change in the shape of the uterus from a disklike to a globular shape. The client is asked to gently bear down to help expel the placenta, because the urge to do so does not ordinarily occur spontaneously. (I, N, G, O)

7. 4. Elbow restraints help keep the child from placing fingers or any other object in the mouth that would cause injury to the operative site. The restraints are worn at all times, except when they are removed to check the skin. It is best to advise parents to remove only one restraint at a time and to keep hold of the child's hand on the unrestrained side. Toddlers are very quick and usually want to explore the area in the mouth that the surgery has made feel different. Taping the restraints directly to the skin is not advised, because of the skin breakdown that can occur when tape is reapplied to the same area over several weeks. The restraints can be fastened to clothing to keep them from slipping. (E, T, S, Y)

8. 2. Extrapyramidal symptoms frequently result from administration of antipsychotic medications; haloperidol (Haldol) is associated with a high incidence of severe extrapyramidal reactions. Other side effects of haloperidol include blurred vision, dry mouth, urine retention, and skin rash. Haloperidol is associated with a low incidence of sedation and a low incidence of cardiovascular effects at therapeutic dosages. Euphoria is not associated with haloperidol. Clients taking lithium should be monitored for lithium toxicity. (P, T, L, X)

9. 4. The emergency treatment of both minor and major burns includes stopping the burning process by immersing the burned area in cool (not warm) water. The burn is covered with a clean cloth to prevent contamination and alleviate pain by avoiding air contact. No ointments or sprays should be applied to the burn. (I, T, S, Y)

10. 1. The rooting reflex is best tested by stroking the neonate's cheek or the corner of the mouth. The normal neonate will turn to the stimulus and open the mouth. The grasp reflex is tested by placing a finger in the neonate's hand; the neonate will normally grasp the finger securely. The Moro reflex is best tested by supporting the neonate's head, then allowing it to drop back a short distance. Normally, the neonate will extend the arms laterally and open the hands, then flex the arms and bring them together as though embracing. Pulling the neonate to a sitting position tests head lag. (I, N, H, O)

11. 4. The client with an obsessive-compulsive disorder has an uncontrollable and persistent need to perform behavior that helps relieve intolerable anxiety. An irrational fear is called a phobia. Ambivalence refers to two simultaneous opposing feelings. In depression, the client feels extreme sadness. (D, C, L, X)

12. 1. The anterior fontanel usually closes by age 18 months. The nurse should measure the head circumference to identify if the child's head is larger than the established norms, because hydrocephalus can cause separation of the sutures of the cranium. Another factor that can cause lack of fontanel closure is slow bone growth, which may be related to hypothyroidism. Because the child is 2 years old, the delivery history probably would not be a significant factor. A radiologic exam is not necessary until other data are collected. (D, N, G, Y)

13. 3. After determining that a nurse and a client will collaborate in a one-to-one relationship, the nurse and client should define the relationship so that they become committed to a relationship that each can maintain. After the relationship is defined, other actions, such as scheduling meetings, setting goals, and developing nursing diagnoses, can be performed. Defining the relationship is described as the first phase of a working relationship, the orientation phase. This phase is followed by the working phase and finally by the resolution phase. (P, T, L, X)

14. 2. Vaginal examinations are performed to evaluate cervical dilatation and effacement and fetal position. A lubricating agent and waterproof gloves are necessary for these examinations. The gloves and agent should be sterile for the vaginal examination. A speculum is used to examine the vagina. Nitrazine test paper is used to determine whether vaginal secretions contain amnionic fluid. A bedpan is not necessary for a vaginal examination. (P, N, G, O)

15. 2. A 1:1 dilution contains 1 mg of drug per 1 cc of solution. Thus, 12 cc would contain 12 mg; 12 mg/hour times 24 hours equals 288 mg. (I, K, S, Y)

16. 1. Gastrointestinal hemorrhage occurs in approximately 25% of clients receiving prolonged mechanical ventilation. Other possible complications include incorrect ventilation, oxygen toxicity, fluid imbalance, decreased cardiac output, pneumothorax, infection, and atelectasis. (A, C, G, M)

17. 3. Peanuts are hard, smooth, and small enough to be aspirated by a child who is still learning to eat solids proficiently. Peanuts are not high in sodium unless they are salted. Peanuts are high in protein, and they are easily digestible if chewed completely. (E, N, H, Y)

18. 2. The nurse's first action here is to elevate the part that is edematous. Decreasing the edema by promoting venous return may help improve circulation and warm the toes. The nurse should follow up after a very short time to evaluate whether the intervention is effective. The toes may also be cool because plaster casts are wet and cool. There is no reason to notify the surgeon at this time, nor should the casts be cut. (I, N, G, Y)

19. 3. Adequate calcium intake will help prevent tooth loss in the pregnant client. When maternal calcium intake is low, the fetus receives calcium from the maternal body stores, often indirectly from her teeth and bones. (I, N, H, O)

20. 2. When the client initially begins complaining of abdominal cramping during an enema, it is usually most appropriate to temporarily stop the infusion until the cramping subsides. If on resuming the flow of enema fluid the client continues to complain of cramping or inability to retain further fluid, the nurse should then discontinue the enema. (I, T, S, M)

21. 4. By asking the client to tell her more about how she is feeling, the nurse is not making any assumptions about what is troubling the client. The nurse should acknowledge the client's feelings and encourage her to discuss them. (I, N, L, M)

22. 4. The primary purpose of oxytocin (Pitocin) administration during the first hour postpartum is to contract the uterus and prevent postpartum hemorrhage. Pitocin does not replace fluids lost during labor, provide pain relief, or lower blood pressure. (I, N, G, O)

23. 2. Clients with Hodgkin's disease are extremely vulnerable to infection because of the defective immune responses caused by the tumor, as well as the bone-marrow depression and low white blood cell count caused by the radiation therapy. Fever is the most sensitive indicator of infection and should be reported immediately so that treatment can be initiated. Loss of hair is unusual in radiation therapy to the neck. Neck circumference and upper extremity circulation are not related to major complications. (E, N, G, M)

24. 1. Because pressure ulcers (decubitus ulcers) are caused by pressure to the tissues, the most important measure to prevent them is relieving pressure by repositioning the client every 1 to 2 hours. Adequate caloric and protein intake is also essential. High fluid intake will not prevent ulcer formation. Massaging reddened areas and bony prominences, once thought to reduce risk of pressure ulcer formation, is now known to increase the risk of pressure ulcer formation. The Agency for Health Care Policy Research (AHCPR) has recently published guidelines for pressure ulcer prevention, which all nurses should incorporate into their practice. (I, T, G, M)

25. 4. A neonate weighing 2,500 g or less at birth is called a low-birth-weight neonate. A premature neonate is one whose birth weight is low and whose gestational age, estimated by gestational age examination and the mother's last menstrual period, is less than 37 weeks. Various criteria are used to help confirm gestational age, including a study of the status of the neonate's muscle tone. The ability of a neonate's pupils to react to light is not used to help establish prematurity. (E, N, H, O)

26. 3. In contrast to a fixed-rate pacemaker, a demand pacemaker functions only when the heart rate falls below a certain level. A fixed-rate pacemaker stimulates heart contractions at a constant rate independent of the client's heart rate. This type is much less common than the demand pacemaker. (I, T, G, M)

27. 4. In the event of wound evisceration, the nurse should first cover the wound with a sterile towel or dressing that has been moistened with sterile normal saline solution. The client is placed supine with knees flexed. Vital signs are monitored for possible signs of shock. The nurse should not attempt to reinsert any protruding viscera. The physician should be notified and the client prepared for surgery. (I, N, S, M)

28. 2. The "click" the nurse feels when abducting the femur is the head of the femur slipping into the acetabulum. This finding, referred to as Ortolani's sign, indicates a dislocated hip. Usual medical treatment involves keeping the hip joint in an abducted position; this can be achieved through diapering with three or more cloth diapers, using a Pavlik harness, and casting. The goal of all of these treatments is to keep the head of the femur centered in the acetabulum. Another sign of hip dislocation is unequal leg length, so the nurse should check for this, as well as asymmetry of the gluteal and thigh folds. (A, T, G, Y)

29. 2. A history of feeding behaviors gives the nurse information on how the infant adjusts to expending energy. Nursing requires sufficient energy and oxygen. An infant who is a poor eater may be suffering from hypoxia during feedings. The issue of a smoker in the home, although important in terms of preventing future health problems, is not an issue at this time. The infant's heart defect would not be affected by the labor and delivery process. Financial concerns, although important, can wait until after the initial assessment is complete. (A, N, G, Y)

30. 2. Pain is a priority problem for the client with renal calculi. The pain is typically described as excruciating and intermittent, occurring as the stone moves. Analgesics are a major part of therapy. (D, N, G, M)

31. 1. A dyspneic client is almost always most comfortable in a high Fowler's position or leaning over an overbed table. These positions maximize the lung's capacity to ventilate. (I, T, G, Y)

32. 4. Enteric precautions are designed to prevent the spread of organisms transmitted by contact with feces. A private room is not required unless the client has poor personal hygiene practices. Health care workers need to wear a gown and gloves only when contact with feces is likely. Enteric precautions are advocated by the CDC. (P, T, S, M)

33. 1. Here, the best nursing intervention is giving the client finger-foods high in protein and calories that he can eat while he paces or walks. Informing the client that snacks are available if he eats properly at mealtime is inappropriate, because the client is too busy and distracted to sit and eat an entire meal. Telling the client to sit alone at mealtime to decrease distractions will not help him. Teaching the client about proper nutrition ignores his need for adequate intake. The client would be unable to focus on the nurse's teaching. (I, T, L, X)

34. 1. A child with severe cerebral palsy often has a lack of oral motor control that interferes with tongue control, chewing, and swallowing. This is the reason that this child is being fed pureed foods and fluids. Lack of tongue control often causes the child to push the food back out of the mouth while trying to chew and swallow. This child should be able to absorb and metabolize ingested nutrients. A child with cerebral palsy has a nonprogressive central nervous insult. Ongoing increased intracranial pressure is not related to cerebral palsy. (D, N, G, Y)

35. 3. Only the client has the power and authority to allow persons not directly involved in his or her care to view his or her medical records. Only a client has the right to provide information to support persons. (E, N, L, X)

36. 2. A condition sometimes called accelerated starvation may occur if a pregnant woman does not eat for 12 hours or more. Blood glucose and alanine levels tend to fall below normal, and plasma-free fatty acid levels increase. The resulting condition—ketosis—threatens normal fetal intellectual development. Everyone, especially pregnant clients, should eat regularly and control their weight, if it becomes necessary, by means other than skipping meals. (I, N, G, O)

37. 4. When a client drinks alcohol while taking disulfiram (Antabuse) adverse effects that result include flushing of the face, neck, and upper trunk; hyperventilation; and rapid pulse rate. Nausea and severe vomiting then typically follow. These symptoms are often accompanied by pallor, hypotension, headaches, palpitations, dyspnea, and faintness. (A, N, L, X)

38. 2. Information documented on a client's record should be as objective as possible so that other health personnel can verify findings as necessary. Stating that a client seems fearful to discuss how bruises on her body had been caused is a subjective statement that expresses the nurse's opinion. Rather than stating an opinion, the nurse should state exactly what the client said. (E, N, L, X)

39. 3. In glaucoma, peripheral vision is impaired long before central vision is impaired. Hazy, blurred, or distorted vision is consistent with a diagnosis of cataracts. Loss of central vision is consistent with senile macular degeneration but occurs late in glaucoma. Blurred or "sooty" vision is consistent with a diagnosis of detached retina. (A, K, G, M)

40. 2. Manifestations of bulimia always include eating binges, usually include vomiting, and often include low serum potassium level secondary to the vomiting. Amenorrhea, severe weight loss, and compulsive exercise are signs of anorexia. Laxative abuse and diet pill abuse are sometimes seen in clients with bulimia. (A, C, L, X)

41. 1. The client should be instructed to avoid straining and lifting for 2 to 6 weeks after surgery. The client should be able to void without difficulty after the immediate postoperative phase. The client typically can ambulate without assistance and should not require assistive devices, unless such devices were used before surgery. The client returns to a regular diet as tolerated after surgery. Increased dietary fiber intake is suggested to avoid constipation, but the client does not need to remain on a soft diet until the wound heals. (E, T, G, M)

42. 4. Administering an antiemetic before beginning chemotherapy and then routinely around the clock helps prevent nausea. Evidence suggests that giving chemotherapy at bedtime together with a sedative reduces nausea and vomiting. Keeping the child NPO does not reduce nausea. (P, T, G, Y)

43. 1. Venereal diseases can be spread through rape. If the victim or the rapist was not using a contraceptive, postcoital contraceptive methods should be discussed. (P, T, L, X)

44. 3. To promote self-feeding, the nurse should provide the child with foods that can be eaten with the fingers or that do not spill easily. Soups, cottage cheese or puddings, gravies, and small round vegetables can easily spill from a spoon or fork when the child is eating in an unfamiliar position. Fluids should be provided in containers with straws to prevent spillage. (I, T, S, Y)

45. 2. In myasthenia gravis, major respiratory complications can result from weakness in the muscles of breathing and swallowing. The client is at risk for aspiration, respiratory infection, and respiratory failure. Providing a safe environment and emotional support are secondary goals. Pain is not a problem with myasthenia gravis. (P, T, G, M)

46. 4. A neonate's eyes are closed most of the time. To facilitate eye examination, the neonate's head should be lifted. The neonate will then tend to open the eyes spontaneously. The neonate is also likely to open the eyes when rocked. (P, T, H, O)

47. 2. A drain in a client's wound allows drainage of blood, lymph, and other debris from the wound. Most drains are not used to introduce antibiotics into a wound or to irrigate a wound. When wound drainage occurs, some discomfort may be relieved; but a drain is not used primarily to relieve discomfort. (E, C, G, M)

48. 2. In cardioversion, the shock is synchronous, which means that it is not delivered during the R wave. Cardioversion is used in ventricular tachycardia to prevent the shock from occurring during the R wave and thereby causing ventricular fibrillation. Typically, cardioversion is done at a lower wattage than defibrillation. The same machine is used for cardioversion and defibrillation; the caregiver sets the mode to synchronous or asynchronous. When set on synchronous, the machine then automatically synchronizes the shock with the R wave of the client's rhythm. (I, T, G, M)

49. 2. Alpha-fetoprotein (AFP) is a fetal serum produced in the yolk sac for the first 6 weeks and then by the fetal liver and gastrointestinal tract during the second trimester. AFP level peaks between 10 and 13 weeks gestation and then declines. Elevated levels are associated with fetal open neural tube defects. Maternal serum is assessed between 15 and 18 weeks gestation. AFP studies do not detect the sex of the fetus, Rh sensitization, or Down syndrome. (P, N, G, O)

50. 1. Depression typically occurs after a person stops using cocaine. Some people experience "cocaine bugs" and describe bugs crawling under the skin. Flashbacks, double vision, and palpitations are not associated with cocaine withdrawal. (A, C, L, X)

51. 1. Clients with peptic ulcers should be taught to avoid aspirin because it irritates the gastrointestinal mucosa. A nonaspirin analgesic should be used. Phenylephrine (Neo-Synephrine) for relieving cold symptoms, psyllium hydrophilic mucilloid (Metamucil) for occasional constipation, and scopolamine for seasickness are not necessarily contraindicated for clients with peptic ulcers. (I, T, H, M)

52. 4. Many clients feel faint and weak when helped to ambulate for the first time postoperatively. The nurse can help prevent these feelings by giving the circulatory system time to adjust before helping the client assume a standing position. This is best done by helping the client into a high Fowler's position in bed for a few minutes. After becoming accustomed to a sitting position, the client can then be helped to dangle at the edge of the bed before ambulating. Such preparations for ambulating help give the client's circulatory system time to adjust to the upright position. (I, N, S, M)

53. 3. A person suffering from the ill effects of chemical abuse needs reassurance, acceptance, and a calm, quiet environment. Various stimuli, physical activities, and fluids are less likely to provide the kind of environment the client needs at this time. (P, T, L, X)

54. 2. Denial is an unconscious refusal to admit an unacceptable idea or behavior. It protects the client in this crisis situation by blocking out the earthquake from conscious awareness. Intellectualization is the use of logical explanations without feelings. Rationalization is the attempt to prove that one's feelings are justifiable. Undoing is doing something to make up for a wrongdoing. (D, T, L, X)

55. 3. A small-for-gestational age neonate or one with intrauterine growth retardation has problems with heat loss because the small size implies a high surface-area-to-volume ratio, with attendant excessive heat loss. Diminished subcutaneous fat deposits because of defective maternal transfer of nutrients, defective placental transfer of nutrients, or defective use of nutrients by the fetus are indirect causes, but in themselves do not influence thermoregulation. Sucking difficulties and respiratory distress syndrome due to immature lungs are problems of the preterm neonate. The term, small-for-gestational age neonate has mature organs of diminished size. (I, N, G, O)

56. 2. Yogurt is high in protein because it is made from milk. The other choices are much higher in carbohydrates than protein except for bacon, which is higher in fat. (I, T, G, Y)

57. 3. A client who has had abdominal surgery is best placed in a low Fowler's position postoperatively. This positioning relaxes abdominal muscles and provides for maximum respiratory and cardiovascular function. (I, T, G, M)

58. 3. The client with emphysema has chronic retention of excessive carbon dioxide; as a result, the normal stimulus for respirations in the medulla becomes ineffective. Instead, peripheral pressoreceptors in the aortic arch and carotid arteries, which are sensitive to oxygen blood levels, stimulate respirations in response to low oxygen levels that have developed over time. If the client then receives high concentrations of oxygen, the blood level of oxygen will rise excessively, the stimulus for respiration will decrease, and respiratory failure may result. (I, N, G, M)

59. 3. Full-thickness burns are serious injuries in which all the skin layers are destroyed. Lack of pain is characteristic of full-thickness burns. Because blood supply is destroyed, blanching and bleeding are absent. Blisters characterize partial-thickness burns and do not occur in full-thickness burns. (A, T, G, Y)

60. 3. With a well-managed regimen, a client with myasthenia gravis should be able to control symptoms, maintain a normal life-style, and achieve a normal life expectancy. Myasthenia gravis can be controlled, not cured. Episodes of increased muscle weakness should not occur if treatment is well-managed. (E, T, H, M)

61. 4. The overactive client needs limits set on behavior, especially when his behavior is demanding or seductive. The nurse should tell the client to stop his behavior and explain her intolerance for it. Telling a seductive client that it is against the rules for clients and nurses to display affection toward each other does not tell the client that his behavior is unacceptable; nor will it help to threaten him by saying the supervisor will be notified. It may become appropriate to divert the client's attention (for example, by suggesting something to eat and drink), but first the nurse should set limits and explain them to the client. (I, T, L, X)

62. 4. Normal $PaCO_2$ values range from 35 to 45 mm Hg. The client with longstanding emphysema has chronic carbon dioxide retention, leading to elevated $PaCO_2$ levels. The client with emphysema and a $PaCO_2$ level of 60 mm Hg may not be in immediate danger, but the nurse would want to further evaluate the client with a level of 60 mm Hg. A $PaCO_2$ level of 80 mm Hg is life-threatening and always requires immediate intervention, possibly mechanical ventilation, to reduce the $PaCO_2$ level. (E, N, G, M)

63. 2. Muscle strain may result from the use of stirrups. Cramping and an uncomfortable twitching of leg muscles are prevented by removing the client's legs from the stirrups slowly and simultaneously. The technique is not used to prevent stretching of the blood vessels, damage to nerves in the popliteal spaces, or inversion of the uterus. (I, N, H, O)

64. 2. The blood enters the fetal heart from the inferior vena cava and empties into the right atrium. From there, most blood goes directly into the left atrium through the foramen ovale. Blood then flows to the left ventricle and from there to the aorta. The foramen ovale is a special fetal structure that helps much blood to bypass pulmonary circulation. Normally, the foramen ovale closes at birth. (I, N, H, O)

65. 2. A client with multiple sclerosis may have a sense of optimism and euphoria, particularly during remissions. Euphoria is characterized by mood elevation with an exaggerated sense of well-being. Inappropriate laughter and giddiness, slurring of words when excited, and visual hallucinations and giddiness are uncharacteristic of euphoria. (A, C, L, M)

66. 3. The client's family needs support at this time. They may be projecting their own fears and concerns about the diagnosis onto the child. When these problems are resolved, the family should be able to discuss the diagnosis with the child. The family will also need to be able to support the child when the diagnosis is revealed. The nurse needs to maintain good relations with the family to provide support to the family and child. (I, N, L, Y)

67. 4. Sensations in the toes and legs mark recovery from spinal anesthesia. The anesthesia should not alter skin color. Because the client receiving spinal anesthesia is conscious, he will not ordinarily be disoriented, nor will his respiratory rate be affected unless a complication is present. (A, C, S, M)

68. 3. In external electronic fetal monitoring, the ultrasonic device is placed across the client's abdomen at the point where the fetal heart rate signal is loudest. In internal fetal monitoring, after the catheter is properly placed it is taped securely to the client's inner thigh. A pressure catheter is used with internal uterine contraction monitoring, and the device is attached to a pressure transducer on the monitor. Electrocardiogram pads are not used with fetal monitoring. (E, N, H, O)

69. 1. The most common symptom of degenerative joint disease (osteoarthritis) is pain. A client's discomfort generally decreases with rest. In contrast, a client with rheumatoid arthritis usually feels more comfortable when active. The pain associated with osteoarthritis is related to joint degeneration and muscle spasms. Analgesics are almost always required to control pain and discomfort. (P, N, G, M)

70. 1. It is best to overcome the effects of excessive alcohol intake by "sleeping it off." Alcohol is not used directly by muscle cells; therefore, physical activity does not affect the rate at which alcohol is removed from the bloodstream. Restricting fluids or drinking black coffee does not hasten removal of alcohol from the body. (I, T, L, X)

71. 4. The client who is not being monitored, should be encouraged to assume any position of comfort. There is no need to keep the client in one position. However, the client should be encouraged not to lie on her back without a wedge under her side, as this can result in vena cava syndrome and hypotension. (I, N, H, O)

72. 1. Psychomotor retardation refers to a general slowdown of motor activity commonly seen in a depressed client. Movements appear lethargic, energy is absent or lacking, and performance of activity is slow and very difficult. (A, T, L, X)

73. 1. The milieu should foster relationship development and decision making abilities among clients. Staff members need to encourage client discussion and decision making by offering their view but agreeing to abide by the group's decision concerning unit (but not hospital) policies and issues. Co-leading a client-government meeting, remaining silent during a meeting, and requiring staff approval of the group's decision are not the most therapeutic roles for staff members in the milieu setting and may hinder effective client government. (I, T, L, X)

74. 4. The client should be instructed to take a deep breath while inhaling slowly, then hold the breath for 3 to 5 seconds before exhaling. This technique of holding the breath after inhalation allows for maximum oxygen absorption. Teaching a client how to cough properly ordinarily is done preoperatively only if a client has accumulated secretions in the airway. The client should be relaxed while deep breathing and should not be told to close the glottis tightly, because this defeats relaxation. (I, T, S, M)

75. 3. A 2-year-old needs some choices to develop a feeling of autonomy. Being responsible for brushing teeth and dressing independently is beyond the developmental level of a 2-year-old and would be more typical behavior of a 3- to 5-year-old. Obeying one's parents is an important concept for any child to master; however, a 2-year-old's favorite word is often "no." Expectation that a child of any age will always obey without hesitation could cause frustration and anger in the parents. (E, N, H, Y)

76. 3. The primary cause of disability, disease, and death in children is injury from accidents. Teaching safety measures is a way to decrease injury and accidents. (P, T, H, Y)

77. 4. Caregiver behaviors that decrease a child's fears and anxieties include moving slowly around the child, keeping the child near the center of activity, using night lights, and avoiding loud noises. (I, T, L, X)

78. 4. When a father cannot or chooses not to be present at a cesarean birth, the nurse can facilitate his involvement in the birthing and attachment process by allowing him to carry the neonate to the nursery. Other methods to promote attachment include having the father hear the neonate's first cry or having him accompany the nurse to the newborn nursery. Telling the father to meet the nurse at the nursery, asking if he had a preference for a boy or a girl, or telling him to notify other relatives of the birth do not promote attachment. (I, N, H, O)

79. 2. Quickening, or the first maternal perception of fetal movement, occurs between 18 and 20 weeks gestation. Adding 20 weeks to the date of quickening can help determine the estimated date of delivery. Sonography is also used to validate the date of delivery. Fetal movement normally increases after meals. Maternal striae appear as the abdomen stretches, but they do not occur in all clients and do not appear at any certain gestational age. Urinary frequency, which usually disappears as the fetus rises in the pelvis and reappears after the fetus has dropped into the pelvis, is an unreliable indicator of gestational age. (P, N, H, O)

80. 1. Sexual drives during pregnancy tend to fluctuate. A pregnant woman may not wish to have sexual intercourse, for no specific reason. Communication between the expectant parents is essential, and both should understand that sexual drives normally fluctuate during pregnancy. The male may also experience varying emotions from time to time during the partner's pregnancy, which can influence sexual drives. (I, N, H, O)

81. 2. A client who smokes is at increased risk for atelectasis postoperatively; thus, smoking is the most significant risk factor listed in this item. If the client has completely recovered from the cold he had 6 weeks ago, it would be irrelevant to his postoperative recovery. Although an obese client faces increased surgical risks, an excess of 10 pounds is not significant enough to pose a greater risk than the smoking. (A, N, G, M)

82. 1. A developmental task of the elderly client is to build and maintain self-esteem and feelings of worth. The client who says he finds it difficult "to be someone" displays problems with the task of developing self-esteem. His statement less clearly demonstrates that he finds it difficult to communicate effectively, feels insecure about having inadequate health care, or finds it difficult to express hostility (although these problems may also arise in the elderly client). (D, N, L, M)

83. 3. Lotions, creams, and powders may increase skin irritation and should be avoided. The area should be kept dry and open to the air. Radiated skin is temperature-sensitive, and a hot-water bottle could cause a burn. (E, N, G, M)

84. 2. The client with an alcohol problem must be motivated to change her behavior before rehabilitation can be successful. Such other factors as a support system in the home, a community health center for alcoholics, and self-help groups can play an important role, but they cannot be expected to help unless the client wants to solve her alcohol abuse problem. (P, N, L, X)

85. 3. Signs of aminophylline toxicity include tachycardia, agitation, decreased blood pressure, and vomiting. (A, T, G, Y)

86. 2. The nurse's first responsibility when a client threatens suicide is to do whatever can be done most quickly to protect the client from himself. When the nurse is in a crisis center and the client is at home, it is best to call the police to intervene. They will be able to reach the client quickly and are experienced in handling such situations. Outsiders, such as a neighbor or even the client's wife, may be hurt, especially when the client has a weapon. It is appropriate to err on the side of safety rather than to assume that the client is not serious about a suicide threat. (I, T, L, X)

87. 2. The transition part of stage 1 is ordinarily the most difficult period of labor. It is the time when clients are most likely to lose control. The client also usually suffers from fatigue during transition, may be nauseated, and has very intense and forceful contractions. (P, N, H, O)

88. 4. In a pyloroplasty, performed to treat pyloric stenosis, the pyloric sphincter is incised to allow food to pass into the small intestine. The child will have a small abdominal incision and probably will not be comfortable in a prone position. An infant who has just been fed should never be placed flat in the bed unless prone or side-lying. The infant usually will respond best if fed very small amounts, which are increased gradually. An oral electrolyte solution is acceptable as an initial feeding, but several ounces is too much in this instance. (I, N, G, Y)

89. 2. Cardinal signs of acute inflammation include swelling, warmth, pain (not numbness), redness (not blanching), and a loss of function in the part involved. Exudate is not typical of an acute inflammation but often occurs when an inflammation becomes infected or chronic. (A, T, G, M)

90. 4. Normal cardiac output is 4 to 8 L/min. The value does vary with body size, but 2.2 L/min is very low and can be life-threatening. For the client with a cardiac output of 2.2 L/min, the nurse should anticipate that the physician will adjust the medication regimen. The client may experience symptoms of dyspnea and fatigue, requiring nursing intervention. (E, T, G, M)

NURSING CARE COMPREHENSIVE TEST

TEST 2

Directions: Use this answer grid to determine areas of strength or need for further study.

Nursing Process

A = Assessment
D = Analysis, nursing diagnosis
P = Planning
I = Implementation
E = Evaluation

Cognitive Level

K = Knowledge
C = Comprehension
T = Application
N = Analysis

Client Needs

S = Safe, effective care environment
G = Physiological integrity
L = Psychosocial integrity
H = Health promotion/maintenance

Nursing Care Area

O = Maternity and newborn care
X = Psychosocial health problems
Y = Nursing care of children
M = Medical-surgical health problems

		Nursing Process					Cognitive Level				Client Needs				Care Area			
Question #	Answer #	A	D	P	I	E	K	C	T	N	S	G	L	H	O	X	Y	M
1	3	A								N		G						M
2	3				I				T				L			X		
3	2				I					N		G			O			
4	2				I				T			G						M
5	3					E				N				H	O			
6	4				I					N		G			O			
7	4					E			T		S						Y	
8	2			P					T				L			X		
9	4				I				T		S						Y	
10	1				I					N				H	O			
11	4		D					C					L			X		
12	1		D							N		G					Y	
13	3			P					T				L			X		
14	2			P						N		G			O			
15	2				I		K				S						Y	
16	1	A						C				G						M
17	3					E				N				H			Y	
18	2				I					N		G					Y	

ANSWER GRID: 1

Nursing Process

A = Assessment
D = Analysis, nursing diagnosis
P = Planning
I = Implementation
E = Evaluation

Cognitive Level

K = Knowledge
C = Comprehension
T = Application
N = Analysis

Client Needs

S = Safe, effective care environment
G = Physiological integrity
L = Psychosocial integrity
H = Health promotion/maintenance

Nursing Care Area

O = Maternity and newborn care
X = Psychosocial health problems
Y = Nursing care of children
M = Medical-surgical health problems

		Nursing Process					Cognitive Level				Client Needs				Care Area			
Question #	Answer #	A	D	P	I	E	K	C	T	N	S	G	L	H	O	X	Y	M
19	3				I					N				H	O			
20	2				I				T		S							M
21	4				I					N			L					M
22	4				I					N		G			O			
23	2					E				N		G						M
24	1				I				T			G						M
25	4					E				N				H	O			
26	3				I				T			G						M
27	4				I					N	S							M
28	2	A							T			G					Y	
29	2	A								N		G					Y	
30	2		D							N		G						M
31	1				I				T			G					Y	
32	4			P					T		S							M
33	1				I				T				L			X		
34	1		D							N		G					Y	
35	3					E				N			L			X		
36	2				I					N		G			O			
37	4	A								N			L			X		
38	2					E				N			L			X		
39	3	A					K					G						M
40	2	A						C					L			X		
41	1					E			T			G						M
42	4			P					T			G					Y	

Answer Grid: 2

Nursing Process

A = Assessment
D = Analysis, nursing diagnosis
P = Planning
I = Implementation
E = Evaluation

Cognitive Level

K = Knowledge
C = Comprehension
T = Application
N = Analysis

Client Needs

S = Safe, effective care environment
G = Physiological integrity
L = Psychosocial integrity
H = Health promotion/maintenance

Nursing Care Area

O = Maternity and newborn care
X = Psychosocial health problems
Y = Nursing care of children
M = Medical-surgical health problems

		Nursing Process					Cognitive Level				Client Needs				Care Area			
Question #	Answer #	A	D	P	I	E	K	C	T	N	S	G	L	H	O	X	Y	M
43	1			P					T				L			X		
44	3				I				T		S						Y	
45	2			P					T			G						M
46	4			P					T					H	O			
47	2					E		C				G						M
48	2				I				T			G						M
49	2			P						N		G			O			
50	1	A						C					L			X		
51	1				I				T					H				M
52	4				I					N	S							M
53	3			P					T				L			X		
54	2		D						T				L			X		
55	3				I					N		G			O			
56	2				I				T			G					Y	
57	3				I				T			G						M
58	3				I					N		G						M
59	3	A							T			G					Y	
60	3					E			T					H				M
61	4				I				T				L			X		
62	4					E				N		G						M
63	2				I					N				H	O			
64	2				I					N				H	O			
65	2	A						C					L					M
66	3				I					N			L				Y	

Answer Grid: 3

Nursing Process

A = Assessment
D = Analysis, nursing diagnosis
P = Planning
I = Implementation
E = Evaluation

Cognitive Level

K = Knowledge
C = Comprehension
T = Application
N = Analysis

Client Needs

S = Safe, effective care environment
G = Physiological integrity
L = Psychosocial integrity
H = Health promotion/maintenance

Nursing Care Area

O = Maternity and newborn care
X = Psychosocial health problems
Y = Nursing care of children
M = Medical-surgical health problems

		Nursing Process					Cognitive Level				Client Needs				Care Area			
Question #	Answer #	A	D	P	I	E	K	C	T	N	S	G	L	H	O	X	Y	M
67	4	A						C			S							M
68	3					E				N				H	O			
69	1			P						N		G						M
70	1				I				T				L			X		
71	4				I					N				H	O			
72	1	A							T				L			X		
73	1				I				T				L			X		
74	4				I				T		S							M
75	3					E				N				H			Y	
76	3			P					T					H			Y	
77	4				I				T				L			X		
78	4				I					N				H	O			
79	2			P						N				H	O			
80	1				I					N				H	O			
81	2	A								N		G						M
82	1		D							N			L					M
83	3					E				N		G						M
84	2			P						N			L			X		
85	3	A							T			G					Y	
86	2				I				T				L			X		
87	2			P						N				H	O			
88	4				I					N		G					Y	
89	2	A							T			G						M
90	4					E			T			G						M

Answer Grid: 4

Nursing Process

A = Assessment
D = Analysis, nursing diagnosis
P = Planning
I = Implementation
E = Evaluation

Cognitive Level

K = Knowledge
C = Comprehension
T = Application
N = Analysis

Client Needs

S = Safe, effective care environment
G = Physiological integrity
L = Psychosocial integrity
H = Health promotion/maintenance

Nursing Care Area

O = Maternity and newborn care
X = Psychosocial health problems
Y = Nursing care of children
M = Medical-surgical health problems

		Nursing Process					Cognitive Level				Client Needs				Care Area			
Question #	Answer #	A	D	P	I	E	K	C	T	N	S	G	L	H	O	X	Y	M
Number Correct																		
Number Possible	90	15	6	15	39	15	2	7	38	43	10	38	24	18	20	20	19	31
Percentage Correct																		

Score Calculation:
To determine your **Percentage Correct**, divide the **Number Correct** by the **Number Possible**.

Comprehensive Test 3

Select the one best answer and indicate your choice by filling in the circle in front of the option.

1. A client has been admitted to the hospital with acute osteomyelitis in the left leg. He complains of acute pain in the left leg that intensifies when he moves it. The nurse notes a temperature of 101°F and a reddened, warm area in the mid-calf region over the shaft of the tibia. Based on this information, which of the following nursing diagnoses would be most appropriate for this client?

- ○ 1. Anticipatory Grieving related to possible left lower leg amputation.
- ○ 2. Activity Intolerance related to severe left leg pain.
- ○ 3. Body Image Disturbance related to left leg swelling and inflammation.
- ○ 4. Fluid Volume Deficit related to elevated temperature of 101°F.

2. A primipara in the second trimester of pregnancy asks the nurse, "I have several beers or highballs every day. Is that okay?" After teaching the client about alcohol use during pregnancy, the nurse would determine that she understands the instructions when she says

- ○ 1. "There is probably no safe level of daily alcohol intake during pregnancy."
- ○ 2. "Drinking alcohol is probably safe during pregnancy if limited to several beers per day."
- ○ 3. "Drinking alcohol is probably safe during pregnancy if limited to several servings of wine per day."
- ○ 4. "Drinking alcohol is probably safe during pregnancy if limited to several ounces of liquor per day."

3. When preparing a client for a scheduled colonoscopy, the nurse would include

- ○ 1. inserting a nasogastric tube 12 hours before the procedure.
- ○ 2. cleansing the bowel with laxatives and/or enemas.
- ○ 3. administering an antibiotic to decrease the risk of infection.
- ○ 4. spraying a local anesthetic into the client's throat to calm the gag reflex.

4. After noting that a client's skin is dry and flaky and feels warm to the touch and that her oral mucous membrane is cracked, the nurse judges that the client is dehydrated. To most accurately validate this observation, the nurse should check the client's

- ○ 1. skin turgor.
- ○ 2. eye grounds.
- ○ 3. respiratory rate.
- ○ 4. urine specific gravity.

5. A mother of an ill child is concerned because the child "isn't eating well." Of the following strategies devised to help increase the child's intake, the nurse should advise the mother not to

- ○ 1. allow the child to choose his meals from an acceptable list of foods.
- ○ 2. allow the child to substitute items on his tray for other nutritious foods.
- ○ 3. ask the child why he is not eating.
- ○ 4. tell the child he must eat or he will not get better.

6. A child is admitted to the hospital with a diagnosis of congenital aganglionic megacolon. The nurse should

- ○ 1. ask the mother how much time elapses between feedings and subsequent emesis.
- ○ 2. accurately measure the amount and pH of any emesis.
- ○ 3. gather a complete diet history for the last 2 weeks.
- ○ 4. ask for a history of the child's bowel movements.

7. Outcome criteria for the client with osteoarthritis should include

- ○ 1. joint degeneration arrested.
- ○ 2. joint range of motion improved.
- ○ 3. able to self-administer gold compound safely.
- ○ 4. feels better than on hospital admission.

8. A mother asks the nurse if the lesions around her child's mouth could be impetigo. To verify the mother's suspicions, the nurse would look for

- ○ 1. erythema and formation of pus around hair follicles.
- ○ 2. honey-colored crusts, vesicles, and reddish macules on the skin.
- ○ 3. intense redness, swelling, and firmness of the skin.
- ○ 4. macular erythema with a "sandpaper" texture of the skin.

9. A female client comes to the emergency room complaining of vertigo and tinnitus. During physical assessment, the nurse will need to be particularly alert to identify supporting signs involving the

- ○ 1. eyes.
- ○ 2. ears.
- ○ 3. nose.
- ○ 4. throat.

10. A female client comes to the emergency room complaining of a fever and a sore throat. While examining the client, the nurse notes that she has many bruises in various stages of healing. The nurse suspects that she may be an abuse victim. When the client notes that the nurse observes her bruises, she says that her fever caused her to become confused and clumsy and that she fell several times and bruised herself. If the client is being abused and denying it, this behavior is most probably due to

- ○ 1. gaining pleasure from being abused.
- ○ 2. fearing that she will be blamed for her plight.
- ○ 3. believing that because she is ill, the abuse will now end.
- ○ 4. thinking that she can handle the problem as soon as she is well.

11. A 2-year-old child is brought to the emergency room with a broken arm. Which of the following findings would lead the nurse to suspect child abuse?

- ○ 1. The child has bruises on his shins.
- ○ 2. The child's clothes are dirty and torn.
- ○ 3. The child's father alters the story of the injury each time he tells it.
- ○ 4. The child's mother did not come to the hospital with the child.

12. A client with chronic schizophrenia is admitted for the third time to a state mental institution under a 72-hour involuntary commitment for evaluation. On admission the client tells the nurse, "I didn't do anything wrong. I was just carrying out the orders God gave me to paint an "X" on the door of all sinners." Several hours after being admitted, the client wants to leave the hospital. Besides explaining that the staff is concerned about her health and safety, the nurse would also tell the client that

- ○ 1. it will take about 3 days to complete the evaluation.
- ○ 2. she must stay at least 2 days but then may be able to leave.
- ○ 3. the court has mandated a 72-hour evaluation.
- ○ 4. the court has mandated that she stay until she is well.

13. A 24-year-old primigravida at approximately 7 months gestation has received permission from her physician to make an 8-hour automobile trip to visit relatives. After teaching the client about precautions she should take while traveling, the nurse would determine that she understands the instructions when she says that she plans to

- ○ 1. drink fluids every 1 to 2 hours.
- ○ 2. have a snack approximately every 2 hours.
- ○ 3. sleep for about 1 hour at the halfway point.
- ○ 4. take a 10- to 15-minute rest period every few hours.

14. Because a mother recently lost a friend, the mother can be expected to react to the impending loss of her child even more intensely than is usually expected. Which of the following concepts best explains this expected grief experience? Losses

- ○ 1. are cumulative in effect.
- ○ 2. taken time to resolve.
- ○ 3. affect one's emotional reserves.
- ○ 4. involve objects or people that are significant to oneself.

15. Two days after a client's wife was found dead in a flood, the client returns to the crisis center and says he thinks it would be better to "end it all right now and join my wife and kid, wherever they are." The nurse has already determined that the client has no history of major psychological problems. In terms of the seriousness of the client's suicide threat, his risk should be considered as

- ○ 1. very low; as long as the client speaks of suicide, he is unlikely to carry out the act.
- ○ 2. low; a person who has not had psychological problems in the past rarely carries out a first suicide threat.
- ○ 3. moderate; the client appears to be making an effort to gain attention and extra support.
- ○ 4. high; the client's suicide threat can be considered a call for help and should be taken seriously.

16. Health promotion activities to reduce the incidence of osteoporosis include

- ○ 1. teaching women to maintain a regular exercise program.
- ○ 2. teaching women how to safely administer pain medication.
- ○ 3. teaching women to increase caffeine intake as a preventive measure.
- ○ 4. increasing periods of bedrest for the elderly client.

17. A nurse has taught a mother about her child's sickle cell disease. No one else in the immediate family has sickle cell disease. The nurse would determine that the mother may need more teaching when she states

- ○ 1. "I need to make sure my child gets plenty of extra fluids in hot weather."
- ○ 2. "My child got this disease from both myself and my husband."
- ○ 3. "There is a one in four chance that my next child will have the same problem."
- ○ 4. "When my child complains of pain, I try to ignore it; it's just psychosomatic."

18. A female client is experiencing bladder control problems. She and the nurse identify several interventions to promote urinary continence, such as keeping the bedpan within easy reach and developing a drinking and voiding schedule. Which of the following client outcomes would indicate the success of these interventions? The client

○ 1. is continent 24 hours a day.
○ 2. states that her bladder control is improved.
○ 3. monitors herself for urine retention.
○ 4. complies with the drinking and voiding schedule.

19. Following abdominal surgery, the nurse should use which of the following measures to determine if a school-age child is ready to drink oral fluids?

○ 1. Asking if the child is thirsty.
○ 2. Auscultating the child's abdomen for bowel sounds.
○ 3. Determining that the child is fully conscious.
○ 4. Palpating the epigastric area for discomfort.

20. A nurse prepares to present a community program about women who are victims of physical abuse. Which of the following facts could the nurse stress about the incidence of battering? Battering

○ 1. rarely results in death.
○ 2. is a major cause of injury to women.
○ 3. occurs primarily in lower socioeconomic groups.
○ 4. rarely occurs in pregnant women.

21. An infant admitted to the hospital with acute rotovirus is having frequent diarrheal stools; on assessment, the nurse notes increased bowel sounds. The nurse would make a nursing diagnosis of Fluid Volume Deficit related to

○ 1. decreased gastric motility.
○ 2. insufficient antidiuretic hormone.
○ 3. inability to metabolize nutrients.
○ 4. increased gastrointestinal motility.

22. After a male client with diabetes mellitus has been on insulin therapy for some time, laboratory findings demonstrate high fasting blood sugars each morning. He is believed to be suffering from the Somogyi, or dawn, phenomenon. The nurse should understand that this condition has most often been found to be due to

○ 1. dietary noncompliance.
○ 2. excessive insulin dosages.
○ 3. early atherosclerotic changes in large arteries.
○ 4. pathologic changes in the autonomic nervous system.

23. The nurse explains to a new mother that her neonate requires a vitamin K injection shortly after birth. The nurse would instruct the mother that this injection will be given into which muscle?

○ 1. Biceps brachii.
○ 2. Biceps femoris.
○ 3. Rectus femoris.
○ 4. Gluteus maximus.

24. In burn clients, fluid resuscitation is quickly initiated with lactated Ringer's solution. Which of the following assessment findings would indicate adequate fluid resuscitation?

○ 1. Urine output greater than 30 ml/hr.
○ 2. Pulse rate above 120 beats/min.
○ 3. Systolic blood pressure above 130 mm Hg.
○ 4. A 5% weight gain in the first 72 hours.

25. A client with non-insulin dependent diabetes mellitus being taught dietary management says, "I'm Italian—how will I ever live without my pasta!" Which of the following responses by the nurse would be best in this situation?

○ 1. "After you are well regulated on insulin, maybe you can eat some pasta."
○ 2. "Many people have given up pasta, and I'm sure you'll be able to, also."
○ 3. "I think this is something to discuss with your doctor. He may allow you to eat pasta."
○ 4. "You don't need to give up pasta, but the amount you eat will need to be regulated."

26. The nurse caring for a preterm neonate with an elevated PaO_2 level who is receiving supplemental oxygen should assess frequently for signs of

○ 1. deafness.
○ 2. blindness.
○ 3. mental retardation.
○ 4. respiratory distress syndrome.

27. During a follow-up session, the nurse judges that an elderly client is beginning to accomplish a developmental task of elderly persons when observing evidence of

○ 1. trust.
○ 2. generativity.
○ 3. self-identity.
○ 4. personal integrity.

28. Which of the following nursing measures should be of highest priority when preparing a client with cancer of the larynx for total laryngectomy surgery? Ensuring that she has

○ 1. adequate nourishment.
○ 2. thorough oral hygiene.
○ 3. proper bowel elimination.
○ 4. a high fluid intake.

29. The nurse would anticipate that a client with chronic peripheral vascular disease would most likely be placed on which of the following medications for long-term drug therapy?

○ 1. Sedative.
○ 2. Antiplatelet agent.
○ 3. Heparin.
○ 4. Vasoconstrictive agent.

30. In teaching a client about Alcoholics Anonymous (AA), the nurse states that AA has helped in the rehabilitation of many alcoholics, most probably because many persons find it easier to change their behavior when they

- ○ 1. have the support of rehabilitated alcoholics.
- ○ 2. know that rehabilitated alcoholics will sympathize with them.
- ○ 3. can depend on rehabilitated alcoholics to help them identify personal problems related to alcoholism.
- ○ 4. realize that rehabilitated alcoholics will help them develop mechanisms to cope with their alcoholism.

31. Which of the following behaviors displayed by a 13-year-old male dying of leukemia would most clearly indicate his need for emotional support?

- ○ 1. Teasing his sister about her new boyfriend.
- ○ 2. Wanting to have someone with him at all times.
- ○ 3. Having the nurse wait with his bath while he makes a phone call.
- ○ 4. Complaining about the limited number of choices on the dietary list.

32. The nurse is preparing to feed a preterm neonate by gastric gavage with a tube that enters the neonate's nostril. Before inserting the gavage tube, the nurse would measure the length of tube needed to reach the neonate's stomach by measuring the distance from the

- ○ 1. neonate's mouth to the bottom of the stomach.
- ○ 2. bridge of the neonate's nose to the xiphoid process.
- ○ 3. tip of the neonate's nose to an earlobe, and then to the xiphoid process.
- ○ 4. middle of the neonate's forehead to an earlobe, and then to the bottom of the rib cage.

33. A child admitted to the hospital with a serum sodium level of 160 mmol/L is receiving dextrose 5% with 0.45 normal saline solution. The mother, who is a nurse, asks the child's nurse why the child is receiving sodium. The nurse's best reply would be, "Your child's sodium is

- ○ 1. high; I'll stop the infusion and check with the physician."
- ○ 2. high; but if serum sodium level is decreased too rapidly, it may cause seizures."
- ○ 3. low; we need to give some intravenously."
- ○ 4. normal; the solution will maintain the level."

34. Diuretic therapy with furosemide (Lasix) is started for a client with congestive heart failure. The nurse would judge that drug therapy is effective after observing that, compared to 3 days earlier, the client now

- ○ 1. eats better.
- ○ 2. weighs less.
- ○ 3. is less thirsty.
- ○ 4. has clearer urine.

35. A client is admitted to the emergency room in acute respiratory distress. When managing an acute respiratory emergency, the nurse should first

- ○ 1. start oxygen therapy.
- ○ 2. provide an open airway.
- ○ 3. give mouth-to-mouth resuscitation.
- ○ 4. start giving sodium bicarbonate intravenously.

36. A nurse must be able to distinguish cholinergic crisis (too much medication) from myasthenic crisis (too little medication) in a client receiving anticholinesterase drug therapy. Which of the following symptoms are present in cholinergic crisis?

- ○ 1. improved muscle strength after IV edrophonium chloride (Tensilon) administration.
- ○ 2. increased strength of skeletal muscles.
- ○ 3. respiratory embarrassment.
- ○ 4. decreased salivation.

37. After considering the most common cause of death in children with leukemia, the nurse caring for a child with leukemia should place priority on

- ○ 1. locating suitable blood donors.
- ○ 2. monitoring the child's temperature.
- ○ 3. monitoring the child's platelet count.
- ○ 4. encouraging increased fluid intake.

38. The nurse instructs a client to use an incentive spirometer postoperatively primarily to help

- ○ 1. promote gastric drainage.
- ○ 2. decrease cardiac irritation.
- ○ 3. promote lung expansion.
- ○ 4. prevent metabolic alkalosis.

39. During hospitalization, a client with bulimia stops vomiting but becomes fearful that she will gain weight. She tells the nurse, "I can't gain weight. I'm fat enough as it is. I'll be really disgusting if I get fatter." When responding to this client, it would be most therapeutic for the nurse to

- ○ 1. explain that the calories in her prescribed diet are not enough to cause weight gain.
- ○ 2. tell her that she is not fat and encourage her to negotiate a calorie change with the nutritionist.
- ○ 3. validate her feelings and help her identify positive aspects of herself other than appearance.
- ○ 4. reassure her that the staff will take complete control of her eating and will prevent her from gaining weight in the hospital.

40. Digoxin (Lanoxin) is prescribed for a client with congestive heart failure. While observing the client for evidence of digoxin toxicity, the nurse should be especially careful to monitor the client's

- ○ 1. pulse rate.
- ○ 2. fluid intake.
- ○ 3. blood pressure.
- ○ 4. respiratory rate.

41. A primigravida is seen in the prenatal clinic at 30 weeks gestation. When the client complains of a common discomfort of pregnancy, the nurse instructs

the client to use the "tailor-sitting" position. On the next visit, the nurse would determine that the position has been effective when the client says that she is less bothered by
○ 1. hemorrhoids.
○ 2. leaking urine.
○ 3. low backaches.
○ 4. leg varicosities.

42. The nurse is caring for a 22-year-old gravida 3, TPAL 2002, who had her last baby by cesarean section for a breech presentation. After discussing vaginal birth after cesarean section (VBAC), the nurse would determine that the client needs further instruction when she says
○ 1. "I can have only minimal if any analgesia or anesthesia if I have VBAC."
○ 2. "I may need to have another cesarean section if this baby is in a breech presentation."
○ 3. "I can use the birthing suite during labor."
○ 4. "I might need continuous electronic monitoring during labor."

43. An adolescent client immobilized in a spica cast complains of having trouble breathing after meals. The nurse should
○ 1. encourage the client to drink more between meals.
○ 2. have the client do breathing exercises each shift.
○ 3. give the client a laxative after meals.
○ 4. offer the client small feedings several times a day.

44. A client's scrotum is swollen and painful 2 days after undergoing a herniorrhaphy. The nursing measure most likely to promote comfort for this client would be to
○ 1. apply a snug binder on his abdomen.
○ 2. have him wear a truss to support the scrotum.
○ 3. elevate the scrotum and place ice bags on the area intermittently.
○ 4. have him lie on his side and place a pillow between his legs.

45. In keeping with the gate-control theory for pain relief, the nurse suggests to a client that she use effleurage when she feels discomfort. The nurse instructs the client that an anatomic characteristic believed to be important for closing the gating mechanism and halting the transmission of pain impulses is that the skin
○ 1. is well supplied with blood vessels.
○ 2. is normally well lubricated with oily sebum.
○ 3. has many large-diameter sensory nerve fibers.
○ 4. has many receptors that are responsive to pressure changes.

46. Which of the following statements best reflects a 50-year-old client's developmental concerns at this time in his life?
○ 1. It is time to reevaluate life's goals.
○ 2. The selection of a career is important.
○ 3. Leisure-time activities are a center of focus.
○ 4. Stress associated with illness precipitates a need to "settle down."

47. A 20-year-old client is admitted to the emergency room hyperventilating. A physical examination is essentially negative. The client's medical diagnosis is acute anxiety attack. While planning nursing care for this client, the nurse's behavior should reflect
○ 1. calmness.
○ 2. sympathy.
○ 3. cheerfulness.
○ 4. friendliness.

48. A 21-year-old gravida 1, TPAL 000, is admitted to a hospital's labor and delivery suite. On admission she is 4 cm dilated, 95% effaced, and at station −1, with a vertex presentation. After 4 hours, the physician ruptures the client's membranes and applies an internal scalp electrode to the fetal head. After observing that the monitor tracing is exhibiting moderate variable decelerations, the nurse's first action should be to
○ 1. turn the client onto her side.
○ 2. administer oxygen at 6 L/min. per protocol.
○ 3. chart this observation on the labor record.
○ 4. notify the physician of the decelerations.

49. Which of the following abilities that the nurse may possess is best suited to helping provide a therapeutic milieu for clients? The ability to
○ 1. display leadership and persuasiveness.
○ 2. set goals for the clients' final recovery.
○ 3. accept behavior as meaningful and motivated.
○ 4. meet the nurse's own needs while helping clients meet their needs.

50. A 10-month-old child with bronchitis is taken out of the 30% oxygen tent for breakfast because he refuses to eat unless in a high chair. During the feeding, the nurse notes that the child's respiratory rate has increased, he is becoming more irritable, and he is using accessory muscles to breathe. The nurse should
○ 1. assess the pulse rate and notify the physician.
○ 2. discontinue the feeding and place the child back in the tent.
○ 3. perform postural drainage and then complete the feeding.
○ 4. suction the child's nose with a bulb syringe.

51. Which type of chair is most suitable for the client with rheumatoid arthritis?
○ 1. A rocking chair.
○ 2. An upholstered chair.
○ 3. A straight-back chair.
○ 4. A stool with low back support.

52. When planning to monitor a preterm neonate's pulse rate, the nurse would plan to auscultate over

○ 1. a femoral artery.
○ 2. a carotid artery.
○ 3. the ascending aorta.
○ 4. the apex of the heart.

53. A nurse is reviewing a care plan that includes interventions aimed at preventing complications in a child with a low platelet count. The nurse would eliminate which of the following interventions because it is inappropriate in relation to preventing complications of a low platelet count?
○ 1. Consult with the physician about using a stool softener.
○ 2. Place the child in protective isolation.
○ 3. Use normal saline solution instead of heparin to flush intermittent IV access devices.
○ 4. Work to help the child understand the need for some activity restrictions.

54. Two boys in their early teens come to the crisis center. One says, "Can you help? Our friend is sick in the car. We don't know what's wrong but he uses lots of stuff to feel better." After bringing the client into the center, the nurse judges that the client has most probably been using marijuana, because his eyes
○ 1. are bloodshot.
○ 2. have dilated pupils.
○ 3. have pinpoint pupils.
○ 4. show rapid movement.

55. A 16-year-old primigravida delivered a viable neonate after 15 hours of labor. The nurse would plan to administer vitamin K to the neonate shortly after birth to help
○ 1. stimulate respirations.
○ 2. improve blood clotting.
○ 3. increase calcium absorption.
○ 4. start peristaltic movements.

56. The neonate of a primigravida is receiving phototherapy for physiologic jaundice. When the mother visits the neonate in the nursery, she becomes alarmed and says, "My baby is changing color!" The nurse can best allay the mother's anxiety by telling her that the
○ 1. tanning should disappear in about 3 weeks.
○ 2. darkened skin color will gradually lighten to normal during the school-age years.
○ 3. alternative to the permanent tanning is brain damage from an accumulation of bilirubin in the blood.
○ 4. apparent color change is due to the type of room lights used in the nursery.

57. A nurse is caring for a primigravida in active labor. The fetal head is presenting. The nurse instructs the client that during delivery of the fetal head, the practitioner will check for a cord around the neck. The nurse would determine that the client understands the instructions when she states that a primary danger of allowing pressure to persist on the cord is that the
○ 1. umbilical cord is likely to tear.
○ 2. placenta is likely to separate prematurely.
○ 3. fetus will fail to move through the normal delivery process.
○ 4. fetus will not receive adequate oxygen.

58. Typically, parents who abuse children
○ 1. were also abused as children.
○ 2. married at a very early age.
○ 3. did not want more than two children.
○ 4. were disappointed when all the children were of the same sex.

59. It is especially important that a client with major burns receive a diet high in protein and
○ 1. fats.
○ 2. amino acids.
○ 3. potassium.
○ 4. calorie intake.

60. A 24-year-old engineering student with a diagnosis of stage I Hodgkin's disease is discharged from the hospital and started on an outpatient chemotherapy and radiation therapy regimen. The client spends a lot of time talking with the nurse about his fate. Which of the following statements would indicate that he understands his prognosis?
○ 1. "I'm going to pack a lot of living into the 4 or 5 years that I have left."
○ 2. "I hate never having the chance to use all the education I've received."
○ 3. "If I had caught this in an early stage, it might have been better."
○ 4. "I'm very fortunate to have a cancer that has such a good chance for a cure."

61. Which of the following techniques would be least appropriate for the nurse to implement in crisis intervention?
○ 1. Encouraging the client to ventilate feelings.
○ 2. Including the client in an effort to find solutions to the problem.
○ 3. Using active and flexible approaches.
○ 4. Attacking the client's maladaptive defenses.

62. A school-age child is admitted to the hospital with newly diagnosed insulin-dependent diabetes mellitus. On admission at 10:00, his blood sugar is 180 mg/dl. His urine tests negative for ketones. He receives 10 units of regular humulin insulin subcutaneously at 10:30. The nurse should plan to
○ 1. assess the child beginning at 11:30 for shakiness, feelings of anxiety, or decreased level of consciousness.
○ 2. carefully regulate an IV solution of dextrose 5% in water and lente insulin.
○ 3. encourage the child to drink large amounts of clear liquids.
○ 4. enforce strict bedrest with bathroom privileges.

63. A client is separated from her husband and receives Supplemental Security Income. She lives with her mother and older sister and manages her own medication. The client's mother is in poor health and receives Social Security benefits; the client's sister works outside the home. The client's father is dead. Which of the following issues should the nurse address first in this client's care?
○ 1. Family.
○ 2. Marital.
○ 3. Financial.
○ 4. Medication.

64. A 2-day-old term neonate is diagnosed with physiologic jaundice and is to receive phototherapy. While the neonate is receiving phototherapy, the nurse should
○ 1. cover the neonate with a blanket.
○ 2. keep the neonate under the lights continuously.
○ 3. apply eye patches during therapy.
○ 4. cover the neonate's head with a stockinette cap.

65. An 8-year-old child is sent home by the school nurse with pediculosis. The child's mother speaks with the nurse and is obviously upset and embarrassed. Which of the following statements by the mother would indicate to the nurse that she understands how her child got pediculosis?
○ 1. "I wash her hair every other day."
○ 2. "I am very careful not to let my children get dirty."
○ 3. "Could this result from sharing batting helmets at T-ball practice?"
○ 4. "We always use a dandruff control shampoo."

66. A priority nursing problem for a client with AIDS would be
○ 1. fluid volume excess.
○ 2. fluid volume deficit.
○ 3. constipation.
○ 4. immobility.

67. The nurse is caring for a multipara on the second postpartum day when the client complains of "afterpains." The nurse would instruct the client that afterpains are most common when she
○ 1. is nursing the neonate.
○ 2. is experiencing urine retention.
○ 3. received inhalation anesthesia during labor.
○ 4. had an episiotomy during delivery.

68. The nurse should plan which of the following activities to meet the diversional and developmental needs of a school-age child on bed rest?
○ 1. Playing a board game with a friend.
○ 2. Putting together a puzzle with the nurse.
○ 3. Watching television with her mother.
○ 4. Reading a book to her father.

69. After a period of depression and preoccupation with his son's impending death, a father has started to adjust to the idea of life without his son. This phenomenon of emotionally reacting to a person's death before it actually occurs is known as
○ 1. neurotic depression.
○ 2. acute grief reaction.
○ 3. pathological mourning.
○ 4. anticipatory mourning.

70. Client government is often an important component in a therapeutic milieu. The most important advantage of this activity is that it
○ 1. saves time for the nursing and auxiliary staff.
○ 2. fosters better planning and implementation of social activities.
○ 3. bridges the gap between the hospital and community environments.
○ 4. promotes better organization for changing hospital unit policies and rules.

71. While performing a gestational age assessment on a neonate, the nurse would elicit the scarf sign by
○ 1. pulling the neonate to a sitting position and observing the head.
○ 2. holding the neonate prone on the table and measuring body length.
○ 3. flexing the neonate's thigh onto the abdomen.
○ 4. drawing the neonate's arm across the chest toward the opposite shoulder.

72. The nurse teaches the client with a pacemaker what to expect when the pacemaker begins to fail or function improperly. Which of the following statements is correct? "You will have
○ 1. nausea."
○ 2. tremors."
○ 3. headaches."
○ 4. dizziness."

73. A 21-year-old gravida 1, TPAL 000, is admitted to the hospital's labor and delivery suite at 4 cm dilated, 95% effaced, and station −1, with a vertex presentation. Over the next 3 hours, the client dilates 1 cm more. The nurse would document the client's progress on the Friedman labor pattern as
○ 1. prolonged latent phase.
○ 2. protracted active phase.
○ 3. prolonged deceleration phase.
○ 4. secondary arrest of dilation.

74. The nurse assessing a multigravida for early symptoms of pregnancy-induced hypertension would first assess for
○ 1. vaginal bleeding.
○ 2. dizziness with tinnitus.
○ 3. sudden rise in blood pressure.
○ 4. pain in the abdominal area.

75. A 4-year-old child with hemophilia is brought to the pediatrician's office with spontaneous soft tissue bleeding of the right knee. Immediately on the child's arrival, the nurse would plan to
○ 1. apply a tourniquet to the right thigh and administer aspirin for discomfort.

○ 2. elevate the right knee and apply ice to the area.
○ 3. immobilize the knee in a dependent position, then apply warm soaks to the involved knee.
○ 4. do a type and cross-match for platelets, then assess vital signs.

76. The nurse planning interventions for the victim of physical abuse would base the plan on knowledge that
○ 1. a woman in crisis is unlikely to be receptive to professional help.
○ 2. the client generally can control the batterer.
○ 3. assessing the client's level of danger is a prerequisite to intervention.
○ 4. success is least likely with a multidisciplinary approach.

77. The sign or symptom that most probably caused a client with pernicious anemia to seek health care is
○ 1. dark stools.
○ 2. a tendency to bleed.
○ 3. sudden weight loss.
○ 4. unusual fatigue.

78. For a child receiving steroids in therapeutic doses over a long period, the nurse should
○ 1. increase the child's ingestion of sodium chloride.
○ 2. give the child the drug on an empty stomach.
○ 3. monitor the child's serum glucose level.
○ 4. monitor the child's temperature to assess for infection.

79. A 16-year-old primipara is being cared for by a nurse in a maternity clinic. An admission interview indicates that the client's life-style is typical of a low socioeconomic status. The nurse should further assess the client's
○ 1. activity level.
○ 2. nutritional status.
○ 3. rest and sleep patterns.
○ 4. personal cleanliness.

80. A school-age child is in the emergency room with an acute asthma attack. The child's respiratory rate is 44 breaths/min., and his pulse rate is 134 beats/min. The child has severe intercostal and supraclavicular retractions. Which of the following findings would cause the most concern for the nurse at this time?
○ 1. Absence of wheezing.
○ 2. Prolonged expiratory phase.
○ 3. Capillary refill time under 3 seconds.
○ 4. Shortness of breath on exertion.

81. To prevent osteomyelitis in a child who has a fracture and is in skeletal traction, the nurse should plan to
○ 1. encourage good nutrition.
○ 2. administer antibiotics as ordered.
○ 3. keep the child in protective isolation.
○ 4. protect the child from visitors with colds.

82. A male client with an obsessive-compulsive disorder frequently washes his feet, which often makes him late for meals, group activities, therapy sessions, and other occasions. It probably would be best for the nurse to help the client overcome this habitual tardiness by planning to
○ 1. explain how his tardiness for scheduled activities interferes with his getting well.
○ 2. help him stop his ritualistic behavior when it is time for him to leave for scheduled activities.
○ 3. allow him to decide whether he wishes to attend scheduled activities or do his ritualistic behavior.
○ 4. remind him early enough that he can carry out his ritualistic behavior in time to arrive for scheduled activities.

83. A multigravida is admitted to the labor and delivery unit of the hospital with symptoms of pregnancy-induced hypertension. Four hours after admission, her condition worsens. The nurse would document the client's eclampsia when she
○ 1. develops anuria.
○ 2. has a convulsion.
○ 3. goes into premature labor.
○ 4. suddenly becomes hypotensive.

84. A 48-year-old male client is admitted to the hospital with a diagnosis of congestive heart failure. He presents with signs of dyspnea and fatigue. When planning care for this client, the nurse should keep in mind that the primary pathophysiology underlying the client's disease process is failure of the heart muscles to
○ 1. contract effectively.
○ 2. maintain a regular rhythm.
○ 3. experience full refractory periods.
○ 4. properly initiate electrical currents.

85. After teaching the mother of a 6-month-old child about immunization schedules and the reason why certain immunizations are given at different times, the nurse would evaluate the teaching as successful when the mother says, "My child will have to wait for the MMR (measles, mumps, and rubella) because
○ 1. oral polio vaccine and MMR cannot be given at the same time."
○ 2. research has shown that complete immunity is not achieved if the child receives the MMR before 12 months."
○ 3. since the MMR and DPT are both injections, it would be too traumatic to give them at the same time."
○ 4. there must be at least a 6-month waiting period between MMR and DPT."

86. A client tells the nurse that she has been using bicarbonate of soda frequently to relieve the heartburn and indigestion caused by her peptic ulcer. The nurse should explain that by so doing, the client increases her risk of developing

○ 1. constipation.
○ 2. dehydration.
○ 3. metabolic alkalosis.
○ 4. iron-deficiency anemia.

87. The nurse is instructing a client with chronic peripheral arterial disease (PAD) on how to improve the flow of arterial blood to his extremities. Which of the following instructions should the nurse include in the teaching?
○ 1. Rest with the legs elevated above heart level.
○ 2. Wear socks or insulated bedroom slippers at all times.
○ 3. Apply a heating pad to the lower extremities at night while sleeping.
○ 4. Avoid walking whenever possible.

88. The nurse is gathering data on a pregnant Asian-American client who has only been in the United States 2 months and speaks very little English. When assessing the client's diet, the nurse should further assess for a possible
○ 1. lactose intolerance.
○ 2. protein deficiency.
○ 3. magnesium deficiency.
○ 4. carbohydrate excess.

89. The nurse should teach a client with glaucoma to avoid activities that increase intraocular pressure, such as
○ 1. watching television.
○ 2. knitting with fine yarn.
○ 3. eating a high-fat diet.
○ 4. shoveling snow.

90. Which of the following comments by an elderly client best illustrates that the client is failing to come to terms with his life?
○ 1. "Life ends for all."
○ 2. "Life has little meaning any more."
○ 3. "Life on earth is short, but I did a lot in my time."
○ 4. "Life has not always been easy, but we learn from hardships."

91. The nurse would judge correctly that a male client with bipolar disorder, manic phase, is nearing readiness for discharge when
○ 1. he sleeps 4 hours per night.
○ 2. he is able to differentiate between reality and unrealistic situations.
○ 3. he telephones his wife and asks for a divorce.
○ 4. his affect is labile.

92. A client's belief in her "mission from God" can be referred to as a religious delusion of grandeur. A primary purpose of such a delusion is to provide
○ 1. a sexual outlet.
○ 2. comfort.
○ 3. safety.
○ 4. self-esteem.

CORRECT ANSWERS AND RATIONALE

The letters in parentheses following the rationale identify the step of the nursing process (A, D, P, I, E); cognitive level (K, C, T, N); client need (S, G, L, H); and nursing care area (O, X, Y, M). See the Answer Grid for the key.

1. 2. Based on the data given, the most appropriate nursing diagnosis is Activity Intolerance related to severe left leg pain. The other diagnoses are not supported by the data presented. (D, N, G, M)

2. 1. There is no safe level of alcohol consumption during pregnancy. It has been demonstrated that alcohol crosses the placenta, although it is not known whether it is the ethanol or the product of alcohol breakdown (acetaldehyde) that causes problems. Outright alcoholism is not required to place a fetus at risk. Using alcohol during pregnancy involves these risks: changes in fetal development and growth, low birth weight, short stature, small head, various joint and heart defects, mental retardation, motor dysfunction, and spontaneous abortion. Smoking or using other recreational ("street") drugs in addition to alcohol puts the fetus at even greater risk. (E, N, H, O)

3. 2. A colonoscopy is the visual examination of the large bowel. Typically, the client will be placed on a liquid diet 24 hours before the procedure and kept NPO after midnight the night before the procedure. The bowel is cleansed through the use of laxatives and enemas. Introducing a nasogastric tube is not part of the preparation for a colonoscopy. The client does not usually receive antibiotics before the procedure. (I, T, G, M)

4. 4. A high urine specific gravity is often the result of dehydration. Skin turgor does not accurately indicate an elderly client's hydrational status, because skin normally becomes dry and inelastic with aging. In a younger client, skin turgor accurately reflects dehydration. When a client is dehydrated, skin loses its elasticity, remaining puckered when the nurse compresses a fold of skin between the fingers. Assessing eye grounds and respiratory rate will not help the nurse validate dehydration in a client. (E, T, G, M)

5. 4. Although nutrition plays a large part in the healing process, it is not advisable to tell a child that he or she will not get better if he or she does or does not do a particular activity. Not only is this dishonest, but it also makes the child believe that his or her own actions are causing the illness. Allowing children choices often helps them feel in control. They also will be more likely to eat foods they have chosen. It is also important to find out the reason the child is not eating. Clients refuse to eat for multiple reasons, and interventions should be devised taking into consideration the reason for the child's refusal. (P, N, L, Y)

6. 4. Children with congenital aganglionic megacolon usually have constipation due to the accumulation of fecal material proximal to the defect. The defect is the absence of autonomic parasympathetic ganglion cells of the colon. The defect can also affect the internal rectal sphincter, which fails to relax and prevents evacuation of fecal material. The lack of innervation varies from child to child, so a careful history centering on bowel habits is important in planning treatment. Some children can be regulated with enemas and digital stimulation; others require temporary or permanent colostomies. (A, N, G, Y)

7. 2. One outcome criteria for the client with osteoarthritis is improved joint mobility. It is probably not possible to arrest the disease. Gold compound is administered to clients with rheumatoid arthritis, not osteoarthritis. Outcome criteria should be specific; feeling better is too general to be useful. (E, T, G, M)

8. 2. Impetigo presents as reddish macules, which turn to vesicles and then erupt and form honey-colored crusts. The lesions can be in any stage. Redness and formation of pus around a follicle describes folliculitis. Cellulitis is described as being intensely red, edematous, and firm. Macular eruption with a "sandpaper" texture describes staphylococcal scalded skin syndrome. (A, T, G, Y)

9. 2. Vertigo (dizziness) and tinnitus (ringing in the ears) are abnormal findings ordinarily associated with a disturbance in proper ear function. (A, T, G, M)

10. 2. Battered women commonly deny being abused because they are afraid that they will be blamed for their plight. It is mostly a myth that battered women are masochistic and gain pleasure from abuse. Most abused women realize that the abuse is unlikely to stop, and they suffer from fear, shame, hopelessness, and helplessness. (D, N, L, X)

11. 3. The nurse should suspect child abuse when the child's caregiver changes the story of the injury each time it is told. A child who is still learning to walk and run often will have bruises on the shins; bruises on the upper arms and thighs are suspicious. Children often become dirty and tear clothes when they play. A parent may not be able to come to the hospital with the child for many reasons, such as care of other children, illness, or lack of transportation. (D, N, G, Y)

12. 3. Clients admitted on involuntary commitment must remain hospitalized for the time allotted for the evaluation. If the treatment team completes the evaluation in less than the allotted time, they may decide to discharge the client or may institute further commitment procedures. Clients cannot sign themselves out of the hospital during this period, nor can family members release them. (I, T, L, X)

13. 4. There are few travel restrictions for a pregnant client who is free of complications and avoids undue fatigue. The client should plan to take 10- to 15-minute rest periods every few hours when traveling by car. This schedule helps prevent fatigue and, when the breaks include walking and stretching, improves circulation. Pregnant women should use shoulder and seat belts, worn below the level of the abdomen. Although drinking fluids, eating a snack, and sleeping for 1 hour may make the client more comfortable, the primary problem with long automobile trips is the potential for venous stasis from prolonged sitting. (E, N, H, O)

14. 1. Losses tend to be cumulative. Old losses are relived or reexperienced with each new loss and add to the intensity of the present grief experience. (D, T, L, X)

15. 4. The client who threatens suicide should be considered at high risk, and his threat should be taken seriously as a call for help. It is untrue that a suicide threat is only a bid for attention, that people who talk about suicide will not do it, and that a person without a history of psychological problems will be very unlikely to carry out a first threat. (D, N, L, X)

16. 1. Many factors may contribute to the development of osteoporosis. A regular program of exercise is one activity thought to reduce disease incidence. Weight-bearing exercises may be recommended as a preventive or treatment measure. Proper diet instruction would be another health promotion activity. Pain management by medication is not a health promotion activity. Bedrest and caffeine intake are considered contributing factors to osteoporosis. (I, T, H, M)

17. 4. Hemodilution is an important aspect of sickle cell crisis prevention. Keeping a child with the disease well hydrated is part of home management. Increasing fluid intake in the summer is especially important, because the child can become dehydrated from excess perspiration, increasing the risk of sickling. The disease is caused by an autosomal recessive gene that must be transferred to the child by both parents. Any subsequent children of these parents have a one in four chance of having the disease and a one in two chance of carrying the defective gene. A child in sickle cell crisis is in severe pain from tissue anoxia. (E, N, G, Y)

18. 1. The goal is to promote urinary continence; an indication that this goal has been met is that the client is continent 24 hours a day. A client's report that her bladder control is improved may indicate that the goal has been attained, but 24-hour-a-day continence is a more definite indication that the goal has been met. Monitoring for urine rentention and complying with the drinking and voiding schedule are important but do not reflect achievement of the stated goal. (E, N, G, M)

19. 2. After an uncomplicated appendectomy, fluid intake is resumed early in the postoperative period. But before providing fluids, the nurse should auscultate the child's abdomen for bowel sounds; fluids should be withheld until bowel sounds are heard. Asking the child if he is thirsty, making sure he is fully conscious, and palpating the abdomen for pain will not help determine whether he has bowel sounds and is ready to take oral fluids. (A, T, G, Y)

20. 2. Battering is a major cause of injury to women. Although battering occurs in all socioeconomic groups, it may seem more common in members of lower socioeconomic groups because they are more likely to use emergency room services. Pregnant women are frequent victims of battering. (P, C, L, X)

21. 4. Rotovirus is a type of viral infection that affects the gastrointestinal tract. It causes diarrhea, which results in fluid loss. This type of infection can be very serious in infants, who cannot adjust to fluid loss as readily as adults because of their immature kidneys. Treatment is supportive. (D, N, G, Y)

22. 2. The Somogyi, or dawn, phenomenon is due to excessive insulin administration. The client has high fasting blood glucose level each morning when dietary noncompliance is not a factor. Some clients describe middle-of-the-night symptoms resembling symptoms of hypoglycemia. It is believed that when hypoglycemia occurs, the body demonstrates a rebound hyperglycemic action that causes the high fasting blood glucose level in the morning. Usually, insulin dosages are reduced for clients suffering from the Somogyi phenomenon. (A, C, G, M)

23. 3. For a neonate, intramuscular injections should be given in the rectus femoris muscle on the anterior of the thigh. This is a relatively large muscle, convenient to use, and free of nerves that could be injured. Gluteus muscles should not be used, because of the danger of injuring the sciatic nerve. The biceps brachii muscle, located in the arm, and the biceps femoris muscle, located in the back of the leg, also are unsuitable sites. (I, N, G, O)

24. 1. Hourly urine output is the most accessible and generally reliable index of adequate fluid replacement, because of the kidneys' sensitivity to circulating volume. A pulse rate of 120 beats/min. or less indicates successful resuscitation; a higher rate indicates stress on the cardiovascular system. Systolic blood pressure above 130 mm Hg is unrealistic, because the loss of skin integrity causes severe fluid loss; systolic blood pressure around 100 mm Hg is more realistic. A weight gain of 15% to 20% is expected during the first 72 hours of fluid resuscitation. (E, N, G, M)

25. 4. When teaching a client with diabetes mellitus about dietary alterations, the nurse should take into account the client's food preferences and cultural background. Neglecting to do so often results in dietary noncompliance. In exchange lists, which most persons with diabetes mellitus are taught to use, pastas are classified as cereals. (I, T, G, M)

26. 2. Careful monitoring of PaO_2 levels is essential during oxygen administration in a premature neonate. Too-high levels can cause vasoconstriction of vessels in the neonate's retinas, a condition likely to result in retinopathy of prematurity (retrolental fibroplasia) and irreversible blindness. Although causes of retinopathy of prematurity tend to be multifactorial, high oxygen levels are one contributing factor. Respiratory distress syndrome in premature neonates is caused by a deficiency of surfactant. (A, N, G, O)

27. 4. Erik Erikson is credited with a theory that describes typical developmental tasks during various ages. The elderly person experiences positive resolution of a central task by developing integrity rather than falling into a state of despair. Typical signs of personal integrity include finding meaningfulness in life and finding new interests and relationships. Developing trust rather than suffering with mistrust typically occurs during infancy; self-identity is an important developmental task of adolescents; and generativity is a typical task of middle adulthood. (D, T, L, X)

28. 2. Preparing a client for surgery involves attending to oral hygiene, giving adequate nourishment and fluid, and providing for proper bowel elimination. However, before a laryngectomy, the highest priority is ensuring thorough and regular oral hygiene. This measure is especially significant in helping prevent postoperative infection. An antibiotic may be prescribed preoperatively, also with the intent of reducing the risk of postoperative infection. Oral hygiene is also important postoperatively to help prevent infection. In addition, because the client's exhaled air does not pass through the mouth following a total laryngectomy, the client may be unaware of halitosis. The nurse can help prevent it by ensuring good oral hygiene. (P, T, G, M)

29. 2. The client with peripheral vascular disease would most likely be placed on vasodilators, antiplatelet agents, and defibrination agents for drug therapy. Neither sedatives nor heparin would be administered for long-term therapy. Aspirin is a commonly used antiplatelet agent. (P, C, G, M)

30. 1. Membership in Alcoholics Anonymous (AA) is voluntary. Its rehabilitated members are available to support alcoholics, and the understanding and influence of these rehabilitated members often enable alcoholics to change their own behavior. The role of rehabilitated members does not include helping others abusing alcohol to identify personal problems, sympathizing with them, or helping them develop defense mechanisms to cope with alcoholism. AA is not entirely unlike other groups who organize to help persons with disorders similar to their own. For example, ostomy clubs have helped many persons with new ostomies learn to adjust to a change in their bodies and to live useful and fulfilling lives. (I, T, L, X)

31. 2. A client who wants to have someone with him at all times is displaying dependency; and for the client described in this item, who is 13 years old, the behavior illustrates regression. It would be considered normal for a 13-year-old boy to tease a sister, make the nurse wait while he uses the telephone, and complain about his dietary choices. (A, T, L, X)

32. 3. A tube used for gastric gavage in a neonate should be inserted a distance equivalent to the distance from the tip of the neonate's nose to an earlobe, and then to the xiphoid process. If the tube is inserted through the mouth, tube length should be equivalent to the distance from the bridge of the nose to the xiphoid process. These lengths ensure that the tube reaches the neonate's stomach. (I, N, G, O)

33. 2. The normal serum sodium level for a child is 138 to 146 mmol/L. The value given is high. However, a rapid decrease in serum sodium level can cause fluid shifts that will result in a rapid increase in intracranial pressure, increasing the risk of seizures. Therefore, the child's sodium level is monitored carefully and decreased slowly. A solution of 0.2% normal saline in 5% dextrose is most commonly used as a maintenance fluid. (I, K, G, Y)

34. 2. The primary purpose of a diuretic in a client with congestive heart failure is to promote sodium and water excretion through the kidneys. As a result, the excessive body water that tends to accumulate in a client with congestive heart failure is eliminated, which will cause the client to lose weight. Monitoring the client's weight daily helps evaluate the effectiveness of diuretic therapy. (E, T, G, M)

35. 2. Unless the airway is open for the entry of air or oxygen, such measures as starting oxygen therapy, giving mouth-to-mouth resuscitation, and giving sodium bicarbonate will not be of value. Ensuring that a client's airway is open is the first step in emergency care. (I, N, S, M)

36. 3. Extreme muscle weakness is present in both cholinergic and myasthenic crisis. In cholinergic crisis, IV edrophonium chloride (Tensilon), a cholinergic agent, does not improve muscle weakness; in myasthenic crisis, it does. The muscarinic effects of pyridostigmine bromide (Mestinon) overdosage cause respiratory embarrassment, abdominal cramps, and excessive salivation in cholinergic crisis. (E, C, G, M)

37. 2. The most common cause of death in children with leukemia is infection. The child should be monitored for any signs of infection, including temperature. Bleeding, although a common problem, is not the most common cause of death. (A, N, G, Y)

38. 3. Incentive spirometry is used postoperatively to promote lung expansion. The machine is set at a preselected target, and the client is taught proper breathing techniques preoperatively so that the targeted setting is reached postoperatively. Incentive spirometry most effectively enhances the inspiratory phase of respiration. (P, T, S, M)

39. 3. Bulimia involves low self-esteem and a belief that one's appearance is the only attractive aspect of oneself. Thus, this client needs to change her self-concept and challenge her negative self-perceptions. Reassurance about weight gain misses the point and probably will be rejected. Changing calories perpetuates the need to focus on eating and weight. Emphasizing the staff's control detracts from the client's sense of responsibility and capability to heal herself. (I, T, L, X)

40. 1. Common signs and symptoms of digitalis toxicity include bradycardia or tachycardia (with dysrhythmias), anorexia, nausea, vomiting, headache, and general malaise. Urine output should also be carefully monitored in a client taking digitalis preparations who has poor renal function and electrolyte depletion. (A, T, G, M)

41. 3. "Tailor-sitting" is often recommended for pregnant clients with low backaches. The knee-chest position also sometimes helps relieve backaches. Exercises that help relieve backaches include pelvic tilts and knee-chest twists. The knee-chest position often helps relieve discomfort associated with hemorrhoids. Leg elevation is recommended for leg varicosities. Pelvic floor contractions (Kegel's exercises) are recommended when leaking urine is a problem. (E, N, H, O)

42. 1. Analgesia or anesthesia is allowed in vaginal birth after cesarean section. VBAC may be considered if no contraindications exist for vaginal delivery. Electronic monitoring should be used, and facilities should be ready in the event a cesarean section becomes necessary. A cesarean section should take no longer than 30 minutes. Breech presentation may be an indication for a repeat cesarean section. A VBAC client can use the birthing suite if she meets the criteria for good labor assessment. (E, N, H, O)

43. 4. A spica cast extends up over the abdomen. When a child eats large meals the abdomen distends; since the abdomen is in a fixed space, the distention pushes the abdominal contents against the diaphragm. This results in decreased chest expansion, and the client may experience some respiratory distress. The best way to prevent the distress is to decrease abdominal distention. Since the client's complaints are associated with meals, it may be assumed that decreasing the amount of food consumed at any one time may help decrease the distress. By offering small, frequent meals, the nurse can provide nutritional support while minimizing distention. (I, N, G, Y)

44. 3. A swollen, painful scrotum following herniorrhaphy is relatively common. Elevating the scrotum, as on a rolled towel, and placing ice bags on the area intermittently are helpful. Applying a binder or a truss and having the client lie on his side with a pillow between his legs are unlikely to promote comfort when the scrotum is swollen. (I, N, S, M)

45. 3. According to the gate-control theory, stimulation of large-diameter sensory nerve fibers closes the gating mechanism to prevent pain impulses from reaching the brain. The skin has many large-diameter nerve fibers; therefore, cutaneous stimulation is a common method for relieving discomfort. (I, N, H, O)

46. 1. During middle adulthood (age 45 to 55), most persons go through a process of taking stock of their lives and become very aware of the time left to live. This appears to be especially true of men. Death now becomes more of a reality instead of something that happens only to others. Selecting career goals and leisure-time activities and settling down are more typical concerns of younger adults. (E, N, L, M)

47. 1. A nurse caring for a very anxious client should be calm and sufficiently authoritative to help the client understand that she or he can provide controls for the client when he cannot do so on his own. If possible, the client should be kept in a quiet, relatively small room, because he is already overwhelmed by external stimuli. (P, T, L, X)

48. 1. Variable decelerations occur in 50% of labors; they are due to some type of cord involvement, the most common being cord compression between the fetus and the maternal pelvis. This often can be alleviated by a maternal position change. If the condition worsens, oxygen may be administered according to protocol. It is essential to notify the physician and document the observations. (I, N, G, O)

49. 3. The milieu should provide an atmosphere that fosters growth, change, and self-responsibility. The staff needs to accept behavior as meaningful and motivated. Staff interventions should also be flexible and open and should encourage clients to achieve their own potential. Displaying leadership and persuasiveness, setting goals for clients, and meeting one's own needs while helping clients meet their needs are not well-suited for a therapeutic milieu. (E, N, L, X)

50. 2. The child with increasing respiratory difficulty after being removed from an increased oxygen environment should be placed back in the environment. The child's pulse rate will most likely be increased. The nurse does not need to notify the physician of the child's status unless no improvement occurs after the child is back in the oxygen tent. It is best to wait until a later time to feed the child, since the act of eating takes up energy and oxygen that the child does not have in sufficient supply at the moment. Unless the child has blocked nasal passages, there is no reason to suction the nares. (D, N, G, Y)

51. 3. To help prevent flexion deformities, a straight-back chair with a seat that allows the feet to rest flat on the floor is recommended. Upholstered chairs, rocking chairs, and stools with back supports do not support the body in proper alignment as well as a straight-back chair does. (P, T, H, M)

52. 4. The most frequently recommended procedure for assessing a neonate's pulse rate is to auscultate over the apex of the heart. This technique gives the most accurate data. (P, N, G, O)

53. 2. An unnecessary intervention would be to place the child in protective isolation. This intervention would be appropriate if the child had a depressed immune response. Platelets are partially responsible for the clotting process, and the child should be protected against tissue injury. The child is usually encouraged not to participate in any activity that can cause injury. Stool softeners are recommended to prevent tissue damage in the rectal area due to hard stool. Since the child is at risk for bleeding, heparin should be avoided. (E, N, G, Y)

54. 1. Marijuana causes dilation of arterioles, and this causes a marked redness of the eyes; they become bloodshot. Heroin characteristically causes pinpoint pupils; cocaine causes dilation of the pupils; and phencyclidine (PCP) causes rapid eye movements. (A, C, L, X)

55. 2. The neonate's lower gastrointestinal tract does not contain the bacteria necessary to produce vitamin K. As a result, poor blood clotting occurs. This deficiency is overcome by giving the neonate vitamin K shortly after birth. (P, N, G, O)

56. 1. Neonates receiving phototherapy sometimes tan or become "bronze." This is not a permanent condition and disappears in about 3 weeks. Explaining the process involved in phototherapy can help alleviate the mother's anxiety. (I, N, H, O)

57. 4. If the umbilical cord encircles the fetal neck, the pressure of the fetus on the cord will interfere with the oxygen supply. If the cord is too tightly encircled to be slipped over the head, it ordinarily is clamped and cut, and the neonate is delivered quickly before asphyxiation occurs. (E, N, G, O)

58. 1. Child abuse can be a vicious cycle, because abused children very often become abusive parents. Marrying at an early age, being disappointed at the child's sex, and having unwanted children are not necessarily associated with child abuse. (A, C, L, X)

59. 4. A burn client's metabolic needs can frequently double or even triple the caloric requirements needed to promote healing and prevent body wasting. A high-protein, high-calorie diet is essential. If the client cannot meet his metabolic needs through oral intake, hyperalimentation or enteral feedings may be necessary. (I, C, G, M)

60. 4. Clients with stage I Hodgkin's disease treated with chemotherapy and radiotherapy currently have a 5-year survival rate of 95% and are considered cured. In stage I, the earliest stage, the disease is limited to a single node and contiguous structure or a single extralymphatic organ or site. (E, N, S, M)

61. 4. The nurse should carefully encourage adaptive defenses and discourage maladaptive defenses. Attacking the client's defenses decreases his ability to maintain his self-esteem and ego-integrity. In crisis intervention, the time limit does not allow replacing maladaptive defenses with healthier ones. Encouraging the client to ventilate feelings increases his awareness of his feelings and reduces tension. Including the client in finding solutions to problems helps the client regain his self-worth and communicates confidence and respect. Using active and flexible approaches helps the nurse use interventions specific to each crisis situation for a healthy resolution of the crisis. (I, T, L, X)

62. 1. The peak action of regular insulin occurs from 1 to 5 hours. Since this is the first dose of insulin the child has received, the nurse should be especially careful to watch for signs of hypoglycemia. These signs include shakiness, irritability, loss of consciousness, anxiety, and hunger. The hyperglycemic child will not need to be encouraged to drink, because one of the cardinal signs of diabetes is polydipsia (excessive, prolonged thirst). The child who is not ketoacidotic will not require an insulin drip. The insulin would not initially be mixed with dextrose, but should be mixed with normal saline solution. Strict bedrest is not indicated for this child. (P, N, G, Y)

63. 4. Medication noncompliance is a primary cause of exacerbation in chronic mental illnesses. Of the issues listed in this item, noncompliance should be addressed first; other issues can be addressed as client stabilization is maintained. (P, N, L, X)

64. 3. During phototherapy, the neonate's eyes are covered to prevent exposure to the lights. Phototherapy can damage the photoreceptors in the retina. At least once each nursing shift, the neonate is removed from the lights and the eyes assessed for discharge. The neonate is placed under the fluorescent lights nude, except for minimal covering over the genitals, and is turned frequently. For phototherapy to be effective, the lights must come in contact with the skin surface. Light in the blue range is believed to decompose bilirubin through the process of photo-oxidation. Input and output should be carefully monitored, and vital signs taken frequently. A stockinette cap may be used to cover the head of a preterm neonate at 37 gestational weeks or younger; this neonate is not preterm. (I, N, G, O)

65. 3. Pediculosis, or head lice, is commonly spread by the sharing of headwear, combs, and brushes. The adult lice can also travel from one person to another if contact is close. The adult lice lay eggs, or nits. These nits are "glued" to the hair and cannot be removed unless treated with special shampoo that is formulated for just this purpose. The hair is then combed with a fine-toothed comb to remove the nits. Cleanliness does not prevent the acquisition of pediculosis. Because head lice spread so easily, a child is usually kept out of school until he or she is treated and found to be free of nits. (E, N, H, Y)

66. 2. Fluid volume deficit related to severe diarrhea, nausea, and anorexia are common problems for persons with AIDS. The fluid volume deficit is often severe and requires aggressive management, possibly including IV nutritional support at home. (D, N, G, M)

67. 1. Afterpains are common when a mother breastfeeds her neonate. Sucking releases oxytocin from the mother's pituitary gland, causing the uterus to contract. Other factors that contribute to afterpains are retention of material in the uterus and a greatly distended uterus during pregnancy. (I, N, H, O)

68. 1. Any of the listed activities would meet the child's diversional needs. However, school-age children have a need to interact with their peers and generally enjoy competition. (I, N, H, Y)

69. 4. A person who starts to adjust to life without a family member before the member actually dies is experiencing anticipatory grief or mourning. This represents an early "giving up" of the loved one and accomplishes some of the grieving for the loved one before he dies. (D, T, L, X)

70. 3. Clients are helped to bridge the gap between the hospital and community environments when they learn to function in leadership, membership, and decision-making positions in an activity that increases their awareness of the democratic process. Saving staff time, planning better social activities, and promoting better organization for changing policies and rules describe possible outcomes of client government, but none of these is the main advantage of the activity described in this item. (D, N, L, X)

71. 4. The scarf sign is elicited by placing the neonate in a supine position and drawing the arm across the chest toward the opposite shoulder until resistance is met. Pulling the neonate to a sitting position and observing the head measures head lag. Holding the neonate prone on the table and measuring length only assesses the neonate's length. Flexing the neonate's thigh onto the abdomen determines the flexibility of the joint. (I, N, H, O)

72. 4. Symptoms of a failing pacemaker result from poor perfusion of blood to the brain, heart, and skeletal muscles. The client will report such symptoms as dizziness, faintness, chest pains, palpitations, shortness of breath, and fatigue. Fluid retention also may occur, causing the client to report symptoms of peripheral edema such as swollen ankles and fingers. (E, T, G, M)

73. 2. According to Emmanuel Friedman, protracted active phase labor in a primigravida is one in which the cervix fails to dilate at least 1.2 cm per hour for 2 hours. This client was in the active stage of labor (4 cm) on admission. To detect dysfunctional labor, the nurse should first identify the client's phase of labor, then determine whether the client meets the Friedman criteria for progress. Prolonged latent phase labor occurs in the latent phase, from about 1 to 4 cm of dilation, and lasts longer than 20 hours in a primigravida. Prolonged deceleration phase labor lasts longer than 3 hours in the primigravida when the client is dilated 8 to 10 cm. Secondary arrest of dilation means that cervical dilation has ceased for an hour in the active phase of labor. Multiparas have different criteria for progress. (I, N, G, O)

74. 3. The three classic signs of pregnancy-induced hypertension are sudden hypertension (usually the earliest sign), albuminuria, and edema. Visual disturbances and pain in the epigastric area are late symptoms and may indicate an impending convulsion. Because pregnancy-induced hypertension is a serious complication of pregnancy, every pregnant client should have her blood pressure checked regularly and frequently during pregnancy, to ensure that the complication can be discovered and treated early. Vaginal bleeding, dizziness with tinnitus, and abdominal pain are not early symptoms of pregnancy-induced hypertension. (A, N, G, O)

75. 2. The goal is to decrease the bleeding. This can be aided by decreasing circulation to the area. Elevating the part and applying cold decreases circulation to the area. The child will also receive cryoprecipitate. Lack of platelets is not the problem in children with hemophilia. A tourniquet should not be used, because it can cause damage to vessels and result in additional bleeding. Aspirin is contraindicated for clients who have bleeding disorders, because it increases capillary fragility. (P, N, G, Y)

76. 3. Assessing the client's level of danger is a prerequisite to intervention, which usually requires a multidisciplinary approach. A woman is more open to change and more receptive to professional intervention during a crisis. At other times, it is easier for her to deny the problems and maintain usual patterns of interaction. The client cannot control the batterer, only her responses to the batterer and to her situation. (P, C, L, X)

77. 4. A client with pernicious anemia characteristically seeks health care because of unusual fatigue and listlessness. Energy is poor because the drop in red blood cells causes poor tissue oxygenation. The onset of pernicious anemia is usually rapid. Pernicious anemia is sometimes referred to as a vitamin B12 deficiency when there is an absence of the intrinsic factor secreted by the cells of the stomach. (A, C, G, M)

78. 3. Steroid use tends to elevate blood glucose levels, and the child should be monitored for increases. Potassium intake should be increased; sodium intake, decreased. The drug should be taken with food or milk to reduce gastrointestinal upset and ulceration. Because steroids suppress the inflammatory response, temperature measurement is no longer an effective assessment tool in identifying infections. (I, N, S, Y)

79. 2. All the factors in this item influence a client's pregnancy. However, probably the most common and important problem associated with low socioeconomic status is inadequate or poor nutrition. Especially common problems include iron-deficiency anemia and inadequate intake of vitamins A, C, and riboflavin. (A, N, H, O)

80. 1. Absence of wheezing in a child who is having an asthma attack and also exhibits symptoms of respiratory distress (e.g., increased respiratory rate, chest retractions, and increased pulse rate) would be an indication that the child's bronchioles are totally obstructed as a result of edema and bronchospasms. Wheezing, a musical sound made by the air passing through narrowed lower airways, at least indicates that some air is getting to the alveoli. The nurse would expect the child to have a prolonged expiratory phase and be short of breath on exertion. Capillary refill time is normally less than 3 seconds. (D, N, G, Y)

81. 1. The best strategy for preventing osteomyelitis is to maintain skin integrity and promote good nutrition. Protective isolation is not necessary for this child, and it may lead to social isolation. Antibiotics are not administered prophylactically when pins are inserted for traction, unless the child already has a bacterial infection. Osteomyelitis is caused by bacteria invading bone tissue. Colds are caused by a virus. (P, N, G, Y)

82. 4. Coping with compulsive behavior can be very frustrating. Interfering with the client's behavior is not helpful and may cause him to become negative and more firmly committed to the behavior. Nor does it help to explain how his behavior may interfere with getting well. Allowing the client to decide whether he will carry out his behavior or attend meals, group activities, therapy sessions, and the like usually means that he will favor his abnormal behavior over activities that he requires for healthful living. Therefore, in this situation, it would be best for the nurse to remind the client in sufficient time so that he can carry out his ritualistic behavior and arrive on time for scheduled activities. (P, T, L, X)

83. 2. A client is considered to have eclampsia when she has a convulsion. Eclampsia is almost always preceded by preeclampsia, or pregnancy-induced hypertension. (I, N, G, O)

84. 1. The primary pathophysiologic process underlying congestive heart failure involves impaired contractile properties of the heart muscle. Various causes can impair heart muscle function, including atherosclerosis, hypertension, and inflammatory or degenerative muscle disease. The heart muscle would be in a state of sustained contraction if periods of refraction did not occur. This is not part of the pathophysiology of congestive heart failure. The heartbeat is initiated in the SA node, which consists of specialized cells controlled by the autonomic nervous system. These cells initiate an impulse that travels through the heart's conduction system, allowing for contraction of the heart muscle. (P, T, G, M)

85. 2. The MMR is not given until age 12 months; if given earlier, immunity is not completely achieved. The MMR can be given with the DPT and OPV to an older child, if the child has not been immunized in early infancy and it is considered likely that the child will not return for further immunizations. Otherwise, the MMR is given 1 month after the DPT and OPV. (E, N, H, Y)

86. 3. The indiscriminate use of bicarbonate of soda may result in metabolic alkalosis. The product is emptied from the stomach very quickly. Using bicarbonate of soda is unrelated to the development of constipation, dehydration, and iron-deficiency anemia. Renal calculi, hypernatremia, and hyperkalemia can occur with excessive bicarbonate of soda use. (A, C, G, M)

87. 2. This client should wear socks or insulated bedroom slippers at all times. A client with PAD should never use a heating pad on the extremities, as sensitivity in the affected limbs is decreased. The client also should not elevate the legs above heart level, as this will further decrease arterial flow. Exercise improves arterial flow; the client should be encouraged to walk as much as possible to help increase collateral circulation. (I, N, H, M)

88. 1. Asian-American clients often experience lactose intolerance, as do Black, Hispanic, and Native American clients. Symptoms include abdominal distention, discomfort, nausea, vomiting, and diarrhea. This client needs adequate amounts of calcium, so the nurse should determine which high-calcium foods the client can tolerate. Milk in cooked form (such as custards and puddings), and sometimes cultured or fermented products, are better tolerated. In some situations, the enzyme lactase can be given to alleviate the problem. (A, N, H, O)

89. 4. Excessive exertion increases intraocular pressure, as does any activity that causes a person to perform the Valsalva maneuver. Watching television and knitting do not increase intraocular pressure. Dietary fat does not affect intraocular pressure. (I, T, H, M)

90. 2. An elderly client often has problems finding meaning and value in what remains of his or her life. Failing to find meaning and value often leads to bitterness and depression. For successful development in old age, the elderly client needs to accept his or her finiteness and come to terms with the knowledge that life ends for all. Such comments as "Life has not always been easy but we learn from hardships" and "Life on earth is short, but I did a lot in my time" suggest that the client has come to terms with the past, present, and most likely the future and has maintained integrity and self-worth. (E, N, L, M)

91. 2. The client is approaching discharge when he is able to differentiate between reality and unrealistic situations. Sleeping 4 hours per night and exhibiting a labile affect are indications that the client is still acutely ill. Asking for a divorce could indicate the client's poor judgment and inability to perceive his situation realistically. (E, N, L, X)

92. 4. Delusions of grandeur provide the client with an exaggerated sense of self-esteem that is unrelated to the client's actual achievements. Other, less grandiose, religious delusions may provide comfort or meaning for the client. Delusions of persecution are frequently related to safety issues. Delusions may also be related to sexual issues. (D, C, L, X)

NURSING CARE COMPREHENSIVE TEST

TEST 3

Directions: Use this answer grid to determine areas of strength or need for further study.

NURSING PROCESS

A = Assessment
D = Analysis, nursing diagnosis
P = Planning
I = Implementation
E = Evaluation

COGNITIVE LEVEL

K = Knowledge
C = Comprehension
T = Application
N = Analysis

CLIENT NEEDS

S = Safe, effective care environment
G = Physiological integrity
L = Psychosocial integrity
H = Health promotion/maintenance

NURSING CARE AREA

O = Maternity and newborn care
X = Psychosocial health problems
Y = Nursing care of children
M = Medical-surgical health problems

		Nursing Process					Cognitive Level				Client Needs				Care Area			
Question #	Answer #	A	D	P	I	E	K	C	T	N	S	G	L	H	O	X	Y	M
1	2		D							N		G						M
2	1					E				N				H	O			
3	3				I				T			G						M
4	4					E			T			G						M
5	4			P						N			L				Y	
6	4	A								N		G					Y	
7	2					E			T			G						M
8	2	A							T			G					Y	
9	2	A							T			G						M
10	2		D							N			L			X		
11	3		D							N		G					Y	
12	3				I				T				L			X		
13	4					E				N				H	O			
14	1		D						T				L			X		
15	4		D							N			L			X		
16	1				I				T					H				M
17	4					E				N		G					Y	
18	1					E				N		G						M

ANSWER GRID: 1

Nursing Process

A = Assessment
D = Analysis, nursing diagnosis
P = Planning
I = Implementation
E = Evaluation

Cognitive Level

K = Knowledge
C = Comprehension
T = Application
N = Analysis

Client Needs

S = Safe, effective care environment
G = Physiological integrity
L = Psychosocial integrity
H = Health promotion/maintenance

Nursing Care Area

O = Maternity and newborn care
X = Psychosocial health problems
Y = Nursing care of children
M = Medical-surgical health problems

		Nursing Process					Cognitive Level				Client Needs				Care Area			
Question #	Answer #	A	D	P	I	E	K	C	T	N	S	G	L	H	O	X	Y	M
19	2	A							T			G					Y	
20	2			P				C					L			X		
21	4		D							N		G					Y	
22	2	A						C				G						M
23	3				I					N		G			O			
24	1					E				N		G						M
25	4				I				T			G						M
26	2	A								N		G			O			
27	4		D						T				L			X		
28	2			P					T			G						M
29	2			P				C				G						M
30	1				I				T				L			X		
31	2	A							T				L			X		
32	3				I					N		G			O			
33	2				I		K					G					Y	
34	2					E			T			G						M
35	2				I					N	S							M
36	3					E		C				G						M
37	2	A								N		G					Y	
38	3			P					T		S							M
39	3				I					N			L			X		
40	1	A							T			G						M
41	3					E				N				H	O			
42	1					E				N				H	O			

Answer Grid: 2

NURSING PROCESS

A = Assessment
D = Analysis, nursing diagnosis
P = Planning
I = Implementation
E = Evaluation

COGNITIVE LEVEL

K = Knowledge
C = Comprehension
T = Application
N = Analysis

CLIENT NEEDS

S = Safe, effective care environment
G = Physiological integrity
L = Psychosocial integrity
H = Health promotion/maintenance

NURSING CARE AREA

O = Maternity and newborn care
X = Psychosocial health problems
Y = Nursing care of children
M = Medical-surgical health problems

		Nursing Process					Cognitive Level				Client Needs				Care Area			
Question #	Answer #	A	D	P	I	E	K	C	T	N	S	G	L	H	O	X	Y	M
43	4				I					N		G					Y	
44	3				I					N	S							M
45	3				I					N				H	O			
46	1					E				N			L					M
47	1			P					T				L			X		
48	1				I					N		G			O			
49	3					E				N			L			X		
50	2		D							N		G					Y	
51	3			P					T					H				M
52	4			P						N		G			O			
53	2					E				N		G					Y	
54	1	A						C					L			X		
55	2			P						N		G			O			
56	1				I					N				H	O			
57	4					E				N		G			O			
58	1	A						C					L			X		
59	4				I			C				G						M
60	4					E				N	S							M
61	4				I				T				L			X		
62	1			P						N		G					Y	
63	4			P						N			L			X		
64	3				I					N		G			O			
65	3					E				N				H			Y	
66	2		D							N		G						M

ANSWER GRID: 3

Nursing Process

A = Assessment
D = Analysis, nursing diagnosis
P = Planning
I = Implementation
E = Evaluation

Cognitive Level

K = Knowledge
C = Comprehension
T = Application
N = Analysis

Client Needs

S = Safe, effective care environment
G = Physiological integrity
L = Psychosocial integrity
H = Health promotion/maintenance

Nursing Care Area

O = Maternity and newborn care
X = Psychosocial health problems
Y = Nursing care of children
M = Medical-surgical health problems

		Nursing Process					Cognitive Level				Client Needs				Care Area			
Question #	Answer #	A	D	P	I	E	K	C	T	N	S	G	L	H	O	X	Y	M
67	1				I					N				H	O			
68	1				I					N				H			Y	
69	4		D						T				L			X		
70	3		D							N			L			X		
71	4				I					N				H	O			
72	4					E			T			G						M
73	2				I					N		G			O			
74	3	A								N		G			O			
75	2			P						N		G					Y	
76	3			P				C					L			X		
77	4	A						C				G						M
78	3				I					N	S						Y	
79	2	A								N				H	O			
80	1		D							N		G					Y	
81	1			P						N		G					Y	
82	4			P					T				L			X		
83	2				I					N		G			O			
84	1			P					T			G						M
85	2					E				N				H			Y	
86	3	A						C				G						M
87	2				I					N				H				M
88	1	A								N				H	O			
89	4				I				T					H				M
90	2					E				N			L					M

Answer Grid: 4

NURSING PROCESS

A = Assessment
D = Analysis, nursing diagnosis
P = Planning
I = Implementation
E = Evaluation

COGNITIVE LEVEL

K = Knowledge
C = Comprehension
T = Application
N = Analysis

CLIENT NEEDS

S = Safe, effective care environment
G = Physiological integrity
L = Psychosocial integrity
H = Health promotion/maintenance

NURSING CARE AREA

O = Maternity and newborn care
X = Psychosocial health problems
Y = Nursing care of children
M = Medical-surgical health problems

		Nursing Process					Cognitive Level				Client Needs				Care Area			
Question #	Answer #	A	D	P	I	E	K	C	T	N	S	G	L	H	O	X	Y	M
91	2					E				N			L			X		
92	4		D					C					L			X		
Number Correct																		
Number Possible	92	16	13	16	26	21	1	11	25	55	5	46	24	17	21	21	20	30
Percentage Correct																		

Score Calculation:
To determine your **Percentage Correct**, divide the **Number Correct** by the **Number Possible**.

ANSWER GRID: 5

Comprehensive Test 4

Select the one best answer and indicate your choice by filling in the circle in front of the option.

1. The nurse should focus on all of the following issues with a battered client except
- ○ 1. helping the client displace her feelings.
- ○ 2. giving her information on and telephone numbers of a safe home and a crisis help line.
- ○ 3. teaching the client about the cycle of violence.
- ○ 4. discussing the client's legal and personal rights.

2. A client who fell and suffered a laceration of her lower leg has profuse arterial bleeding at the wound site. After exposing the leg, the nurse should next
- ○ 1. apply a tourniquet to the leg.
- ○ 2. place a pressure dressing over the wound.
- ○ 3. place the client in modified Trendelenburg's position.
- ○ 4. apply pressure by hand on the femoral artery.

3. A client in an inpatient psychiatric unit tells the nurse, "I'm gonna divorce my no-good husband. I hope he rots in hell. But I miss him so bad. I love him. When's he gonna come get me out of here?" The client is displaying
- ○ 1. ambivalence.
- ○ 2. autistic thinking.
- ○ 3. associative looseness.
- ○ 4. auditory hallucinations.

4. The nurse is caring for a multigravida in active labor. While assessing the client during labor, the nurse notes on the fetal heart monitor that decelerations are occurring, beginning early in the contracting phase with the onset of the contraction and recovering at the end of the contraction. The nurse would document this labor pattern as
- ○ 1. early decelerations.
- ○ 2. late decelerations.
- ○ 3. mild variable decelerations.
- ○ 4. severe variable decelerations.

5. A client suspected of being an abuse victim returns to the emergency room and, sobbing, tells the nurse, "I guess you really know that my husband beats me and that's why I have bruises all over my body. I don't know what to do. I'm afraid he'll kill me one of these times." Which of the following responses would best show that the nurse recognizes the client's needs at this time?
- ○ 1. "The fear that your husband will kill you is unfounded."
- ○ 2. "We can begin by discussing various options open to you."
- ○ 3. "You can legally leave your husband, because he has no right to hurt you."
- ○ 4. "We can begin by listing ways to avoid making your husband angry with you."

6. A client is admitted to the inpatient psychiatric unit. He is unshaven, has an odor about him, and has spots on his shirt and pants. He moves slowly, gazes at the floor, and has a flat affect. The nurse's highest priority in assessing the client on admission would be to ask him
- ○ 1. how he sleeps at night.
- ○ 2. if he is thinking about hurting himself.
- ○ 3. about recent stresses.
- ○ 4. how he feels about himself.

7. The nurse is caring for a primigravida in the first trimester of pregnancy. The client's last menstrual period began April 10. Using Naegele's rule, the nurse would document the client's estimated date of delivery as
- ○ 1. December 17.
- ○ 2. January 10.
- ○ 3. January 17.
- ○ 4. February 10.

8. The nurse should assess for pediculosis capitis (head lice) in a child who
- ○ 1. has spotty baldness.
- ○ 2. has wheals with blistering on the scalp.
- ○ 3. scratches the scalp frequently.
- ○ 4. twirls strands of hair frequently.

9. A primigravida admitted to the labor and delivery unit in early active labor has suspected mild pregnancy-induced hypertension. The nurse assesses the client's blood pressure reading. Which of the following data would confirm the diagnosis of mild pregnancy-induced hypertension?
- ○ 1. Systolic blood pressure reading of at least 140 mm Hg.
- ○ 2. Diastolic blood pressure reading above 90 mm Hg.
- ○ 3. An increase in systolic and diastolic blood pressure readings of at least 20 mm Hg.
- ○ 4. An increase in systolic and diastolic blood pressure readings of at least 40 mm Hg.

10. The nurse is assessing a primigravida in the prenatal clinic. While auscultating the client's abdomen, the nurse hears funic souffles. The nurse would instruct the client that this is considered

○ 1. abnormal, as it is the sound of blood passing through a defective placenta.
○ 2. abnormal, as it is the sound of blood passing through a defective valve in the fetal heart.
○ 3. normal, as it is the sound of blood passing through uterine vessels.
○ 4. normal, as it is the sound of blood passing through the umbilical cord.

11. A multigravida is admitted to the labor and delivery unit of the hospital with symptoms of pregnancy-induced hypertension. After explaining the plan of care to the client, the nurse would determine that she needs further instructions when she says that she will

○ 1. be weighed once a week.
○ 2. have her intake and output monitored.
○ 3. be monitored for contractions.
○ 4. have her urine checked frequently for protein.

12. A client admits herself to a rehabilitation program for alcoholics. Plans are made to care for her if she begins to have delirium tremens (DTs). An appropriate intervention for the nurse to take when DTs occur is to

○ 1. help the client remain awake.
○ 2. place the client in restraints.
○ 3. keep the client's room well lighted.
○ 4. reinforce the client's visual misinterpretations.

13. A 61-year-old man is admitted to the hospital in acute respiratory distress. He has been suffering from emphysema for about 5 years. The physician orders a loading dose of 400 mg of aminophylline IV, diluted in 250 ml of dextrose. Each ampule of aminophylline contains 250 mg of the drug in 10 ml of solution. How many milliliters of the aminophylline should the nurse add to the 250 ml solution?

○ 1. 12 ml.
○ 2. 15 ml.
○ 3. 16 ml.
○ 4. 18 ml.

14. The nurse is caring for a client who has been admitted with a suspected abdominal aortic aneurysm. Late on the evening shift, the client calls the nurse to his room complaining of a sudden onset of severe, sharp abdominal pain. The nurse's initial response would be to

○ 1. obtain a Doppler probe to check dorsalis pedis pulses.
○ 2. call the physician.
○ 3. assess the client's blood pressure, pulse, and respirations.
○ 4. slow the infusion rate of IV fluids.

15. A 20-year-old single parent brings her 3-year-old son into the emergency department because "he fell." The child has bruises on his face, arms, and legs; his mother says that she did not witness the fall. Because the reported cause of injury is vague, the nurse suspects child abuse. While the nurse is examining the client, the mother says, "Sometimes I guess I'm pretty rough with him. He's so demanding! I'm alone and I try to do my best, but I just don't know how to manage him." Referral to which type of program would be most appropriate for the mother at this time?

○ 1. An assertiveness training program.
○ 2. A program for single parents.
○ 3. A parenting education program.
○ 4. A women's support group.

16. A child is being treated for tinea (ringworm) with the drug griseofulvin (Fulvicin). The nurse teaches the mother a technique to increase absorption of the drug. The nurse would evaluate the teaching as successful when the mother gives the drug

○ 1. when the child's stomach is empty.
○ 2. with a glass of water.
○ 3. with a high-fat meal.
○ 4. with a high-roughage meal.

17. Clients who abuse chemicals generally have feelings of

○ 1. depression.
○ 2. superiority.
○ 3. low self-esteem.
○ 4. exaggerated well-being.

18. A multigravida is admitted to the hospital's labor and delivery unit with symptoms of pregnancy-induced hypertension. The physician prescribes magnesium sulfate. In planning the client's care, which of the following medications should the nurse plan to have available in case the client develops magnesium toxicity?

○ 1. Atropine sulfate.
○ 2. Protamine sulfate.
○ 3. Naloxone (Narcan).
○ 4. Calcium gluconate.

19. The mother of an infant with a cyanotic heart defect tells the nurse that her child has not been gaining weight even with an increased caloric intake. The mother states that the infant starts out with a good suck but tires and quits after about 2 ounces. The infant is receiving oxygen via nasal cannula as necessary, and is on digoxin therapy. The nurse should suggest that the mother

○ 1. cut a large hole in the nipple.
○ 2. feed the infant every 2 hours.
○ 3. have the infant tested for digoxin toxicity.
○ 4. increase the oxygen for feedings.

20. A 34-year-old woman is hospitalized with rheumatoid arthritis. The nurse assesses the client's musculoskeletal system and notes crepitation, which refers to

○ 1. swelling in an affected joint.
○ 2. irregularity in the shape of an affected joint.
○ 3. elevated skin temperature over an affected joint.
○ 4. grating sounds when an affected joint is moved.

21. Which of the following statements that the nurse could make to a client suspected of being abused would most likely encourage her to admit and describe her abuse?

○ 1. "How did you hurt yourself?"
○ 2. "When were you in an accident?"
○ 3. "Is someone doing this to you?"
○ 4. "How long have you had these bruises?"

22. A primigravida in the first trimester of pregnancy tells the nurse that she has been using Alka-Seltzer and baking soda to relieve heartburn. The nurse should instruct the client to avoid these products and assess her for

○ 1. diarrhea.
○ 2. flatulence.
○ 3. fluid retention.
○ 4. urinary frequency.

23. A mother of a child with strabismus brings the child to the clinic. The physician has prescribed patching. Which of the following actions or statements by the mother would lead the nurse to judge that further teaching concerning this treatment is necessary?

○ 1. The abnormal eye is patched.
○ 2. The mother keeps the patch on even when the child fusses.
○ 3. The mother states, "I have to watch him when he walks; he's still a little clumsy."
○ 4. The mother tells the nurse that she removes the patch at night.

24. During the conversation with the nurse, a victim of physical abuse says, "Let me try to explain why I stay with my husband." Which of the following reasons would the client be least likely to mention?

○ 1. "I'm responsible for keeping my family together."
○ 2. "When it's not too bad, the abuse adds spice to our relationship."
○ 3. "I have only a sixth-grade education."
○ 4. "I'm not sure I could get a job that pays even minimum wage."

25. In which of the following instances would the nurse anticipate that a client who has been sexually assaulted will have future adjustment problems and the need for additional counseling?

○ 1. When she becomes upset when talking about the rape to anyone.
○ 2. When she seeks support from formerly ignored relatives and friends.
○ 3. When her parents show shame and suspicion about her part in the rape.
○ 4. When her life becomes focused on helping other rape victims like herself.

26. A 24-year-old primigravida at approximately 38 weeks gestation is admitted to the hospital for evaluation of labor. The client tells the nurse that she thinks she is in false labor. When assessing the client to determine whether she is in true labor, the nurse would evaluate the client's contraction pattern and whether or not the

○ 1. cervix is dilating.
○ 2. fetus is in the pelvis.
○ 3. membranes have ruptured.
○ 4. mucus plug has been expelled.

27. A client's care plan specifies that he is to be up in a chair for 1 hour three times daily. The primary purpose of this order is to help

○ 1. strengthen the heart muscle.
○ 2. improve arterial blood pressure.
○ 3. limit the volume of circulating blood.
○ 4. decrease the return of venous blood to the heart.

28. A 21-year-old gravida 1, TPAL 000, is admitted to the hospital's labor and delivery suite. On admission, she is 4 cm dilated, 95% effaced, and at station −1, with a vertex presentation. Soon after the client is admitted, the nurse applies an external electronic monitor, or tocodynamometer. The nurse should explain to the client that the external electronic monitor enables the nurse to assess

○ 1. contraction compensation.
○ 2. contraction quality.
○ 3. periodic changes in fetal heart rate.
○ 4. fetal heart baseline variability.

29. A primigravida in labor has been pushing for 90 minutes. The fetus is in ROA position, and the fetal heart rate remains between 120 and 126 beats/min. The physician makes a diagnosis of outlet dystocia due to a narrow pubic arch. The nurse would explain to the client that the neonate will most likely be delivered

○ 1. with forceps assistance.
○ 2. via cesarean section.
○ 3. in a squatting position.
○ 4. under general anesthesia.

30. The nurse planning a screening clinic for scoliosis would target

○ 1. adolescents, during periods of rapid growth.
○ 2. infants whose mothers have had no prenatal care.
○ 3. preschoolers, on entering kindergarten.
○ 4. toddlers who have diets low in calcium and vitamin D.

31. After talking with the nurse, the client admits to being physically abused by her husband. She says that she has never called the police, because her husband has threatened to kill her if she does. She says, "I don't want to get him into trouble, because he's the father of my children. I don't know what to

do!" Which of the following nursing interventions would be most therapeutic at this time?
- ○ 1. Express concern for the client's safety.
- ○ 2. Help the client identify the behaviors that provoke the abuse.
- ○ 3. Teach the client ways to reduce stress within her family.
- ○ 4. Tell the client that she should leave her husband.

32. Clients at greatest risk for adult respiratory distress syndrome (ARDS) are those who have experienced
- ○ 1. myocardial infarction.
- ○ 2. hypovolemic shock.
- ○ 3. emphysema.
- ○ 4. surgery.

33. A school-age child has her broken arm in a cast. The nurse teaches the parents about conditions that necessitate immediate medical attention in relation to the fracture and cast. The nurse would evaluate this teaching as effective when the parents state, "We will return our child to the emergency room if
- ○ 1. her fingers are cool, pale, or bluish in color."
- ○ 2. she is irritable and says the cast seems too heavy."
- ○ 3. the plaster cast is not dry in 6 hours."
- ○ 4. she has any discomfort."

34. The nurse is caring for a 16-year-old primigravida in a maternity clinic. When the nurse inquires about the client's marital status, she appears uneasy and says, "Do I have to discuss that with you?" What would be the nurse's best response?
- ○ 1. "Yes, if you want me to care for you."
- ○ 2. "Yes, because I need to know so I can complete your records."
- ○ 3. "No, but it would be helpful in planning your care."
- ○ 4. "No, but I want you to know that I'm sorry for you."

35. A preschool-age child who is hospitalized with gastroenteritis has been NPO. The physician has written an order to advance the diet as tolerated. The first feeding the nurse should offer the child is
- ○ 1. creamed cereal and milk.
- ○ 2. ice cream shake and cream soup.
- ○ 3. clear lemon carbonated beverage and popsicle.
- ○ 4. orange juice and toast.

36. The nurse and parents of a child with juvenile rheumatoid arthritis are planning interventions to reduce joint pain in the morning after arising. The plans should include
- ○ 1. having the child sleep in a sleeping bag.
- ○ 2. increasing the pain medications at bedtime.
- ○ 3. instituting an exercise regimen just after the child arises.
- ○ 4. limiting the child's nighttime sleep to no more than 5 hours.

37. When assessing a client receiving long-term lithium carbonate (Lithane) therapy, the nurse would judge that the client is exhibiting a typical sign of lithium toxicity when he demonstrates
- ○ 1. insomnia.
- ○ 2. disorientation.
- ○ 3. excessive perspiration.
- ○ 4. poor muscle coordination.

38. About 6 hours after a client delivered of a term infant, the nurse helps her to ambulate. The nurse would explain to the client that the primary purpose of walking is to prevent
- ○ 1. afterpains.
- ○ 2. endometritis.
- ○ 3. vulvar edema.
- ○ 4. thrombophlebitis.

39. The nurse planning care for a child in vaso-occlusive crisis because of sickle cell disease would include increasing fluid intake in the list of interventions, because
- ○ 1. decreased blood viscosity prevents the sickling process.
- ○ 2. decreased blood viscosity will reverse the sickling process.
- ○ 3. hemodilution increases normal red blood cell life span.
- ○ 4. increasing fluid intake increases hemolysis.

40. The nurse is teaching a client with osteomyelitis in the left leg how to ambulate with crutches. The client cannot bear any weight on his affected leg. Which of the following crutch gaits would be most appropriate for this client?
- ○ 1. Four-point gait.
- ○ 2. Two-point gait.
- ○ 3. Three-point gait.
- ○ 4. Modified three-point gait.

41. Which of the following would be an appropriate nursing diagnosis for a child who has aganglionic megacolon?
- ○ 1. Impaired Skin Integrity related to caustic excrement.
- ○ 2. Constipation related to lack of innervation in the large intestine.
- ○ 3. Altered Nutrition: Less than Body Requirements related to an alteration in feeding patterns.
- ○ 4. Altered Nutrition: Less than Body Requirements related to inability to digest nutrients.

42. A client who suffered cardiac arrest is receiving cardiopulmonary resuscitation in the emergency room after being brought in by the rescue squad. On assessment, the nurse notes that the client's pupils constrict when exposed to light. This finding would indicate an adequate oxygen supply to the client's
- ○ 1. lungs.
- ○ 2. heart.
- ○ 3. brain.

○ 4. kidneys.

43. Before discharge, the nurse teaches a client with emphysema to use pursed-lip breathing. The primary purpose of this type of breathing is to help

○ 1. increase intrapulmonic pressure.
○ 2. promote a regular breathing pattern.
○ 3. prevent collapse of alveoli.
○ 4. sensitize central chemoreceptors in the medulla.

44. The nurse is caring for a 20-year-old primigravida who, due to a history of rheumatic heart disease as a child, is classified as a class II cardiac client during the pregnancy. After teaching the client about her activities during pregnancy, the nurse would determine that she has understood the teaching when she says

○ 1. "I won't perform any physical activity during the third trimester."
○ 2. "I'll continue my usual daily activities and rest for 30 minutes each day."
○ 3. "I'll remain on bedrest throughout my pregnancy."
○ 4. "I'll walk more to increase circulation to the growing fetus."

45. A client has been hospitalized with a diagnosis of diverticulitis. After treatment with antibiotics, the client has recovered and is ready for discharge. When planning the client's discharge teaching, which of the following instructions should the nurse include in the teaching plan?

○ 1. Avoid taking hot showers.
○ 2. Maintain a sitting position for 30 minutes after meals.
○ 3. Avoid using laxatives and enemas.
○ 4. Limit intake of milk products.

46. When caring for a client with pernicious anemia, the nurse would most likely note which of the following signs and symptoms?

○ 1. Clubbing of the fingernails.
○ 2. Paresthesias in the feet and hands.
○ 3. Cyanosis of the lips.
○ 4. Urinary incontinence.

47. After assessing an obese woman with rheumatoid arthritis, the nurse establishes four broad goals of nursing care. Which should have the highest priority at this time for the client? To teach the client how to

○ 1. use correct body mechanics.
○ 2. avoid rushing through activities of daily living.
○ 3. reduce her daily food intake for weight control.
○ 4. arrange her kitchen so that utensils are easy to reach.

48. A small-for-gestational age neonate is being cared for in the newborn nursery after the neonate's mother has been discharged. When the nurse makes a home visit, the client is crying and tells the nurse, "I'm a failure. I can't even have a healthy baby." Which of the following statements by the client would indicate that the nurse's interventions were successful?

○ 1. "I appreciate your listening to me talk about my feelings."
○ 2. "I know my baby is normal, just a little small."
○ 3. "I understand that all mothers go through a period of the 'blues' after childbirth."
○ 4. "I'll go to the nursery to see how my daughter is really doing."

49. Timolol maleate (Timoptic), a beta-adrenergic receptor blocking agent, is ordered for the client with glaucoma because it does not interfere with vision. The nurse should tell the client to be aware of which common side effect?

○ 1. Slight bradycardia at rest.
○ 2. Nausea and vomiting.
○ 3. Vivid dreams.
○ 4. Migraine headaches.

50. A client with major burn injury is friendly and cooperates with the nurses, but changes the subject whenever the nurse discusses her burn injury. She repeatedly says that she is "fine" and seems almost euphoric. The client's behavior is most indicative of

○ 1. regression.
○ 2. denial.
○ 3. depression.
○ 4. flood reaction.

51. On noting that a 1-month-old infant is using the abdominal muscles to breathe, the nurse should

○ 1. chart the findings.
○ 2. check oxygen saturation level with a pulse oximeter.
○ 3. elevate the head of the bed.
○ 4. notify the physician of the findings.

52. A mother calls the emergency room and tells the nurse that she is fairly sure that her 3-year-old has eaten 10 to 12 chewable acetaminophen tablets. The nurse should tell the mother to bring the child to the emergency room, but to first

○ 1. give the child 6 to 8 ounces of milk and keep the child awake.
○ 2. give the child 6 to 8 ounces of water followed by 3 teaspoons of ipecac.
○ 3. give the child 1 teaspoon of baking soda in 4 ounces of water, followed by burnt toast.
○ 4. withhold fluids and position the child on the side.

53. An adolescent male was hurt while diving into shallow water; a spinal cord injury is suspected. The nurse would evaluate that the client's friends transported him to the hospital correctly when they moved him by placing him

○ 1. on his back on a board.
○ 2. in a sitting position on a straight-back chair.

○ 3. on their chests while using a three-carrier lift.
○ 4. on a stretcher made with a blanket and poles.

54. A young child who has undergone a tonsillectomy refuses to let the nurse look at the tonsilar beds to check for bleeding. To assess whether or not the child is bleeding from the tonsilar beds, the nurse should
○ 1. assess peripheral circulation by timing capillary refill.
○ 2. force the child to open the mouth with a tongue blade.
○ 3. monitor for decreased blood pressure.
○ 4. observe for frequent swallowing.

55. An older adult is admitted to the hospital for a permanent pacemaker insertion. Which of the following appliances in his home most likely would present a hazard, even when the pacemaker and the item are in good working order?
○ 1. Dehumidifier.
○ 2. Electric razor.
○ 3. Microwave oven.
○ 4. High-fidelity record player.

56. A client is admitted to the inpatient chemical dependency unit for alcohol detoxification. To provide the client with safe medical withdrawal from alcohol, the nurse would include all of the following nursing measures except
○ 1. monitoring vital signs.
○ 2. observing for convulsions.
○ 3. administering lorazepam (Ativan), as ordered.
○ 4. explaining the outpatient alcohol rehabilitation program.

57. The nurse caring for a client with insulin-dependent diabetes mellitus would use which of the following assessment tools to determine how well the child's insulin, diet, and exercise are balanced?
○ 1. Fasting serum glucose level.
○ 2. Interview with the child about compliance.
○ 3. Glycosylated hemoglobin level.
○ 4. 1-week diet recall.

58. A client is admitted to the inpatient psychiatric unit accompanied by his wife, who reports that he has been "on a spending spree; he sent roses to everyone we know." While being admitted to the hospital, the client becomes very active, moves about, and then puts his arm around the nurse and says to her, "I sure like you a lot, honey. I can do a lot for you in the real world out there." An important goal of nursing care for this client would be to help him
○ 1. join in group activities.
○ 2. get enough rest.
○ 3. select leisure-time activities.
○ 4. find ways to promote cardiopulmonary stimulation.

59. The nurse is caring for a neonate in the newborn intensive care nursery. When the mother visits the neonate, she tells the nurse that she has not yet chosen a name for the baby. The most appropriate nursing diagnosis for this family would be
○ 1. Grieving related to having a less-than-perfect baby.
○ 2. Ineffective Family Coping related to hospitalization of the neonate.
○ 3. Altered Family Processes related to preterm delivery.
○ 4. Powerlessness related to inability to care for the neonate.

60. The nurse who has conducted classes about substance abuse evaluates the success of the classes. Data indicate that the class to help decrease marijuana use has not been successful. The nurse would attribute this to the fact that there is
○ 1. no evidence that marijuana is harmful.
○ 2. no known cure at present for marijuana addiction.
○ 3. little social stigma attached to the use of marijuana.
○ 4. very little known about the active ingredient in marijuana.

61. An extremely angry client walks into the outpatient mental health center and tells the nurse he wants "to kill my boss" for cheating him out of his pension and forcing him into early retirement. What would be the nurse's most appropriate action?
○ 1. Talk in depth with the client about his feelings.
○ 2. Ask the client to explain more about his feelings since he lost his job.
○ 3. Help the client think through the consequences of his act if he should carry it out.
○ 4. Help the client become aware of possible resources to obtain employment.

62. A 65-year-old female is admitted to the hospital with peptic (duodenal) ulcers. The discomfort that most probably led this client to seek health care is pain that is relieved by
○ 1. eating.
○ 2. resting.
○ 3. physical activity.
○ 4. voiding.

63. While using an otoscope to examine the tympanic membrane of a 2-year-old child, the nurse should pull the pinna
○ 1. down and back.
○ 2. down and slightly forward.
○ 3. up and back.
○ 4. up and slightly forward.

64. The sputum of a client with emphysema is very thick and tenacious. In addition to a high fluid intake, which of the following measures should be included in the client's plan of care to help reduce the tenacity of respiratory secretions?

○ 1. Having the client use postural drainage.
○ 2. Humidifying the air that the client inspires.
○ 3. Giving the client low concentrations of oxygen.
○ 4. Instructing the client to use diaphragmatic breathing.

65. A 6-year-old child is scheduled for surgery to remove the appendix. It would be most appropriate for the nurse to tell the child
○ 1. that it will "hurt pretty bad" after the surgery.
○ 2. that the child will have a tube in the nose after surgery.
○ 3. that the doctor sometimes orders a "shot" before the surgery.
○ 4. where the incision will be with the use of a human figure drawing.

66. Which of the following statements that a dying client makes about himself would indicate that he has most probably come to healthy terms with his death?
○ 1. "Why did I have to get cancer?"
○ 2. "I don't want to talk about it anymore. I'm going to die anyway."
○ 3. "I'd like you to sit with me. I feel as though it's OK now."
○ 4. "I think that a cancer cure will be discovered very soon."

67. While caring for a preschool-age child with chickenpox, the nurse asks her how she got the chickenpox. The child replies, "I got it because I went too near my sister and the poxes jumped onto me!" The nurse would evaluate this as
○ 1. an understanding of the relationship of germs and illness.
○ 2. concrete logical thinking.
○ 3. magical prelogical thinking.
○ 4. repeating an explanation from her older sister.

68. A cream containing mafenide acetate (Sulfamylon Acetate) is ordered to be applied over an area of a burn victim's body. Before applying the cream, the nurse should plan to prepare the client by explaining that the cream is likely to cause
○ 1. nausea.
○ 2. a strange taste in the mouth.
○ 3. a burning sensation on the body.
○ 4. a stain on the skin surrounding the burn area.

69. Iron supplements are prescribed for a primigravida in the first trimester of pregnancy. When planning to instruct the client about the iron supplements, the nurse would include the fact that absorption of iron is improved if taken with
○ 1. milk.
○ 2. yogurt.
○ 3. orange juice.
○ 4. cranberry juice.

70. Tolbutamide (Orinase) is prescribed for a client with non-insulin-dependent diabetes mellitus. The nurse would explain that this drug functions by
○ 1. decreasing gluconeogenesis in the liver.
○ 2. potentiating the action of insulin in body cells.
○ 3. promoting the excretion of excess glucose through the kidneys.
○ 4. stimulating the beta cells in the pancreas to release insulin.

71. A client says that he is "afraid" of his pacemaker. Which of the following responses by the nurse would be most appropriate?
○ 1. "All clients are scared at first, but you have nothing to fear."
○ 2. "Tell me more about what frightens you about your pacemaker."
○ 3. "There is no need to worry if you see your doctor as scheduled."
○ 4. "Here's a manual for you to read before I begin to teach you about your pacemaker."

72. A 22-year-old female visits the prenatal clinic because she thinks she is pregnant Of the following information about the client, which would the nurse interpret as a probable sign of pregnancy?
○ 1. Morning sickness.
○ 2. Positive pregnancy test.
○ 3. Amenorrhea.
○ 4. Urinary frequency.

73. For a client admitted with a diagnosis of appendicitis, the nurse would most likely note which of the following assessment findings?
○ 1. Diarrhea alternating with constipation.
○ 2. Right lower quadrant abdominal pain.
○ 3. Hematemesis.
○ 4. Ascites.

74. A client with a ventricular demand pacemaker asks the nurse, "Where did they put the tip of my pacemaker? Is it in my heart?" The nurse should base the response on the knowledge that with this type of pacemaker, the tip of the catheter is placed in the
○ 1. left atrium.
○ 2. right atrium.
○ 3. left ventricle.
○ 4. right ventricle.

75. A client is admitted to the hospital with a possible diagnosis of myasthenia gravis. Which of the following symptoms would the nurse most likely expect to elicit from the client during the nursing history?
○ 1. Anorexia and weight loss.
○ 2. Spasticity of the leg muscles.
○ 3. Bilateral peripheral edema.
○ 4. History of ptosis or diplopia.

76. After teaching a primigravida in active labor about the need to keep the bladder empty, the nurse would determine that the client understands the instructions when she says that a full bladder during labor

○ 1. increases the risk of urinary incontinence.
○ 2. predisposes to umbilical cord prolapse.
○ 3. causes a decreased frequency of uterine contractions.
○ 4. interferes with fetal descent in the birth canal.

77. The client states he is "a worthless worm, lower than low." To convey acceptance of the client, the nurse would first
○ 1. spend time with the client by sitting with him.
○ 2. ask the client what he would like to change about himself.
○ 3. tell the client he is a worthwhile person.
○ 4. remind the client that his family cares about him.

78. As a client with an obsessive-compulsive disorder busily scrubs his feet, he tells the nurse, "Never mind if I look silly to you. I must finish before I can put on my socks and shoes and go to lunch." When analyzing the client's statement, the nurse should be guided by knowledge that clients with obsessive-compulsive disorders tend to
○ 1. be unaware of the disruptive nature of their ritualistic behavior.
○ 2. be aware of the unreasonableness of their ritualistic behavior.
○ 3. expect health professionals to stop them from performing their ritualistic behavior.
○ 4. make frequent attempts to test the skill of those helping them overcome their ritualistic behavior.

79. A multipara has just had a subdermal implant (Norplant) inserted as a contraceptive. After teaching the client about the implant, the nurse would determine that the client understands the instructions when she says
○ 1. "If I get pregnant while the device is in place, then the fetus can have congenital defects."
○ 2. "There are no side effects associated with this form of contraception."
○ 3. "This form of contraception is effective for up to 5 years."
○ 4. "This device can interrupt spermatogenesis."

80. A toddler with croup is given an epinephrine hydrochloride (Vaponephrine) updraft because of increasing restlessness and stridor. The nurse would assess the treatment effect as being successful when the child's
○ 1. color is normal.
○ 2. appetite improves.
○ 3. heart rate is 90.
○ 4. retractions are less severe.

81. A client with a large-area body burn is judged to have a negative nitrogen balance. Because of this, it is particularly important that the client receive a generous intake of which of the following nutrients?
○ 1. Fats.
○ 2. Proteins.
○ 3. Minerals.
○ 4. Carbohydrates.

82. The client asks the nurse about the effect of multiple sclerosis on sexual function, and the nurse teaches her how to combat problems that interfere with sexual activity. Which of the following statements by the client would indicate that she has understood the teaching?
○ 1. "I'll use lubricants and stimulants."
○ 2. "I'll do perineal tightening exercises every day."
○ 3. "I'll take a hot bath before having intercourse."
○ 4. "I'll rest before having intercourse."

83. A client with pernicious anemia is to receive intramuscular vitamin B12 therapy. The client asks when she can stop taking the injections. Which of the following statements should guide the nurse's response? Injections will be necessary
○ 1. for the rest of the client's life.
○ 2. between episodes of disease remission.
○ 3. until the disease process has been successfully controlled.
○ 4. until the dietary regimen has been successfully established.

84. Which of the following sequences of a child's gross motor development would the nurse consider to be normal?
○ 1. Roll over, creep, sit, stand.
○ 2. Roll over, sit, creep, stand.
○ 3. Sit, roll over, stand, creep.
○ 4. Sit, roll over, creep, stand.

85. Preoperatively, the nurse is preparing the client's skin for surgery. The primary goal of preoperative skin preparation is to
○ 1. render the operative area free of organisms.
○ 2. improve the field of vision for the physician.
○ 3. decrease the number of organisms on the skin surface.
○ 4. enhance the skin's natural defenses against organisms.

86. When a rape victim arrives at an emergency room for treatment, which of the following measures should the nursing staff be especially sure to carry out for its own and the client's legal protection?
○ 1. Keep prying, insensitive personnel away from the victim.
○ 2. Record the victim's account of the assault in her own words.
○ 3. Arrange for the victim to be escorted home by a trustworthy person.
○ 4. Hand-carry any evidence from the victim's person to the pathology laboratory.

87. The nurse instructs a 45-year-old female client on health measures to reduce the risk of osteoporosis. Which of the following statements would indicate that the client has understood the teaching?

○ 1. "I'll increase the amount of milk and dairy products in my diet."
○ 2. "I'll need to decrease the amount of tennis I play."
○ 3. "Wearing a firm girdle will help prevent osteoporosis."
○ 4. "I don't need to worry about developing osteoporosis until I'm in my sixties."

88. A nurse is caring for a primigravida in active labor. It is determined that the fetal head is presenting. About midway between the client's contractions, the nurse notes that the fetal heart rate is between 140 and 150 beats/min. with good variability. The nurse would document this finding in the client's record as a fetal heart rate
○ 1. within normal range.
○ 2. below normal range.
○ 3. slightly above normal range.
○ 4. markedly above normal range.

89. On a visit to the prenatal clinic, a primigravida says that she is "feeling life." The nurse would document which of the following in the client's record?
○ 1. Quickening.
○ 2. Lightening.
○ 3. Ballottement.
○ 4. Chadwick's sign.

90. A child with rheumatic fever has polyarthritis and chorea. An echocardiogram shows fragmentation and swelling of the cardiac tissue. The nurse would plan which of the following interventions for this child?
○ 1. Explaining to the child and family that the chorea will disappear over time.
○ 2. Keeping the child in a warm environment.
○ 3. Performing neurological checks every 4 hours until the chorea subsides.
○ 4. Promoting ambulation by giving aspirin every 4 hours.

91. A client has had a long-leg plaster cast applied to his right leg. Which of the following nursing measures would be appropriate while the cast is still wet?
○ 1. Apply a heat lamp to help dry the cast.
○ 2. Use the palms of the hands when handling the wet cast.
○ 3. Avoid turning the client until the cast is dry.
○ 4. Protect the wet cast by covering it with a blanket.

CORRECT ANSWERS AND RATIONALE

The letters in parentheses following the rationale identify the step of the nursing process (A, D, P, I, E); cognitive level (K, C, T, N); client need (S, G, L, H); and nursing care area (O, X, Y, M). See the Answer Grid for the key.

1. 1. When working with a battered woman, the nurse should help her share and discuss her feelings of anger, frustration, guilt, shame, and other feelings. Displacing or placing feelings unto another person or object is not helpful to the client and is not a healthy way for her to handle her feelings. Informing the client of safe homes and crisis lines, teaching her about the cycle of violence, and informing her about legal and personal rights are some of the issues the nurse should address with the battered client. (I, T, L, X)

2. 4. Initial emergency care for profuse bleeding involves applying pressure over the involved artery—in this situation, the femoral artery. A pressure dressing should then be applied. A tourniquet should be used only as a last resort to control bleeding. Modified Trendelenburg's position may be used later, if the client develops signs of shock due to excessive bleeding. (I, N, S, M)

3. 1. Ambivalence refers to strong, conflicting attitudes or feelings toward an object, person, goal, or situation. Autistic thinking involves attributing personal and private meanings to words and situations. Associative looseness is characterized by simultaneous expression of unrelated, or only slightly related, ideas or thoughts. Auditory hallucinations are sounds, words, or voices not heard by others. (A, T, L, X)

4. 1. Early decelerations are the mirror image of a contraction, beginning with the contraction, dipping to a nadir at the peak of the contraction, and ending with the contraction. Late decelerations begin at least 15 seconds after the beginning of the contraction, reach a nadir near the end of the contraction, and return to baseline at least 15 seconds after the end of the contraction. All types of variable decelerations are jagged at the onset, dropping abruptly from the baseline. Variable decelerations may or may not be related to the contraction. Early decelerations are due to head compression; late decelerations, to uteroplacental insufficiency; and variable decelerations, to cord compression. (I, N, G, O)

5. 2. This client is asking for help when she says that she does not know what to do about being abused by her husband. The nurse's best course of action is to explain the various options available to her. This helps the client make decisions based on appropriate knowledge. (I, T, L, X)

6. 2. The nurse's highest priority is to ask the client if he is thinking about hurting himself or to assess for suicide. Questioning the client about his sleep pattern, recent stresses, and feelings about himself are important areas of assessment for the depressed client but not as immediate a priority as assessing for suicide. (I, T, L, X)

7. 3. According to Naegele's rule, the estimated date of delivery is determined as follows: Determine the first day of the client's last menstrual period minus 3 calendar months plus 7 days plus 1 year. This client's last menstrual period began on April 10. So, April 10 minus 3 calendar months is January 10; then, adding 7 days makes the delivery date January 17 of the following year. (I, N, H, O)

8. 3. A typical sign of pediculosis capitis (head lice) is frequent scratching of the scalp, because the condition causes severe itching. Scratch marks are usually easily visible. Because head lice are easily transmitted to others, the child's family members and peers also should be examined for infestation. Spotty baldness often occurs when the client has tinea capitis (scalp ringworm). Wheals, smooth elevated areas that often itch, are common in various allergic reactions. (D, T, G, Y)

9. 4. The best description of the blood pressure changes occurring in pregnancy-induced hypertension and on which the diagnosis of mild pregnancy-induced hypertension is based on an increase of 30 mm Hg or more in systolic pressure and 15 mm Hg or more in diastolic pressure. Between 120/80 and 140/90 mm Hg is usually considered the general range of blood pressure readings in mild pregnancy-induced hypertension. Both systolic and diastolic pressures increase in pregnancy-induced hypertension. (D, N, G, O)

10. 4. Funic and uterine souffles are normal sounds heard over a pregnant uterus. Funic souffle—the soft, murmuring sound of blood passing through the umbilical cord—is a positive sign of pregnancy because it can be heard at approximately the same rate as the fetal heartbeat. Uterine souffle—the sound of blood passing through the uterine vessels—is caused by maternal blood flow and is heard at approximately the same rate as the mother's heartbeat. (I, N, H, O)

11. 1. Because the client with pregnancy-induced hypertension should be observed carefully for fluid retention and edema, she should be weighed daily. Other typical orders for a client with pregnancy-induced hypertension include monitoring intake and output, monitoring for contractions, and monitoring for proteinuria. In addition, administration of medications such as magnesium sulfate requires frequent assessment of respirations and deep tendon reflexes. Oxygen and suction equipment should be kept available at all times. (E, N, G, O)

12. 3. Delirium tremens often occurs after the client who has been abusing alcohol does not drink alcohol for about 24 to 72 hours. It is a serious, possibly even life-threatening, complication. The client should be kept in a private room, which should be well lighted to reduce shadows and visual hallucinations. A calm, nonstressful environment is recommended; the client should be given prescribed sedation. Restraints are used only as a last resort; it is preferable that the nurse stay with and calm the client with touch, reassurance, and a constant presence. The nurse's attitude of acceptance and support is important. One way to help strengthen the client's link with reality is to explain her visual misinterpretations rather than to reinforce them. (I, T, L, X)

13. 3. One formula that can be used to determine dosage is proportion:

$$250 \text{ mg}:10 \text{ ml}::400 \text{ mg}:x$$
$$250x = 4{,}000$$
$$4{,}000 \div 250 = 16 \text{ ml.}$$

Another method is as follows:

$$\frac{\text{dose desired}}{\text{dose on hand}} \times \text{quantity} = x$$

$$\frac{400 \text{ mg}}{250 \text{ mg}} \times 10 \text{ ml} = x$$

$$4{,}000 \div 250 = 16 \text{ ml}$$

(I, T, S, M)

14. 3. Abdominal aortic aneurysm rupture is usually accompanied by a sudden onset of severe abdominal pain. The client will go into immediate shock. The nurse should first assess vital signs to ascertain the client's condition. The IV fluid infusion should not be slowed, as the client will most likely require large volumes of fluid to maintain tissue perfusion. Emergency care must be implemented immediately; the likelihood of survival for a client with a ruptured abdominal aneurysm who receives prompt surgical intervention is approximately 50%. (I, N, S, M)

15. 3. Referral to a parenting education program is the most appropriate measure at this time, since this client is expressing problems with parenting. (I, T, L, X)

16. 3. Although absorption of most drugs is decreased when the drug is given with food, griseofulvin is absorbed more quickly when taken with a high-fat meal. (E, T, G, Y)

17. 3. Clients who abuse chemicals most often reveal feelings of failure, poor self-esteem, dependency, and passivity. They tend to be seeking experiences that will alter these feelings and often turn to chemicals to accomplish their goal. These feelings often make substance abuse a difficult problem, because the chemicals meet an important need in the mind of the abuser. (D, T, L, X)

18. 4. The antidote for magnesium sulfate is calcium gluconate. The antidote should be kept ready whenever a client receives magnesium sulfate. Symptoms of magnesium toxicity include lethargy, impaired respirations, absent deep tendon reflexes, and coma. Protamine sulfate is an antidote for heparin. Naloxone (Narcan) is an antidote for opiates. (P, N, G, O)

19. 4. All children use energy to ingest and digest nutrients. The body needs oxygen to utilize the calories taken in to provide energy. Usually, the caloric intake outweighs the energy needed to obtain them. A child with a heart defect that circulates unoxygenated blood to the tissues may need extra oxygen support during times of high energy consumption, such as when feeding. Without this extra support, the child may fatigue. If the child's suck is good, then enlarging the hole in the nipple will give the child too much volume with each suck and may cause the child to choke. Tiring during feedings is not a symptom of digitoxin toxicity, although lack of appetite may be. (I, N, G, Y)

20. 4. Crepitation, or crepitus, is a term used to describe various abnormal sounds or noises. In clients with rheumatoid arthritis, a characteristic grating sound is heard when an affected joint is moved. The sound is caused by the rubbing together of dry synovial surfaces in the joint. Clients with rheumatoid arthritis also may have such typical signs as joint tenderness, warmth of the skin, and irrigularities in the shape of joints. (A, T, G, M)

21. 3. A question from the nurse that helps the client describe her health problem is most helpful when abuse is suspected. Statements that help the client avoid the issue are least helpful. Even if the client does not want to discuss the cause of her bruises, helping her to express her thoughts in a supportive atmosphere often helps open channels of communication. (I, T, L, X)

22. 3. Baking soda and many over-the-counter preparations, including Alka-Seltzer, contain sodium, which tends to cause fluid retention. Better products for relieving heartburn include antacids that contain calcium or have a magnesium or aluminum base. Alternately, heartburn may be relieved by drinking milk or carbonated beverages or sipping water. Sitting up, trying to relax, or deep breathing are also often helpful. Suggestions for helping to prevent heartburn include eating small, frequent meals; wearing clothes loose at the waist; and staying in an upright position after meals. (A, N, G, O)

23. 1. When an eye patch is used to correct strabismus, the normal eye is patched. This forces the child to use the abnormal, or "lazy," eye and increases muscle strength in that eye. The patch can be removed at night while the child sleeps. Patching one eye interferes with depth perception and can cause the child to be clumsy at first. (E, N, G, Y)

24. 2. Violence is never acceptable to a victim; this myth condones the use of violence. Often an episode of battering is followed by a period of pleasant relations between the partners, during which the woman may hope that the violence will never happen again. She may stay in the relationship for that reason. Women are conditioned to be responsible for the family's well-being, and this is often a motivation for a battered woman to stay in an abusive relationship. A woman's lack of job skills and financial resources also may cause her to stay. Many women are injured or killed when they try to leave a violent relationship. (E, N, L, X)

25. 3. The potential for problems in adjusting after a rape will be increased when those around the victim treat her as though she is to blame for the rape, especially when she already may feel some guilt and shame about it. A rape victim is very likely showing adjustment to her experience when she is upset about her experience, when she seeks out formerly ignored relatives and friends for support, or when she attempts to help other rape victims. (D, N, L, X)

26. 1. A sign of true labor is gradual cervical dilation with regular contractions. In false labor, no change in the cervix is noted and contractions are usually irregular. The client's membranes may rupture before true labor starts. The presence of the fetus in the pelvis is not a sign of true labor. The mucus plug in the cervical canal and the presence of show are signs of impending labor. (A, T, G, O)

27. 4. Having the client sit in a chair and elevating the head of the bed while the client is in bed help decrease the return of venous blood to the heart and lungs. Decreased venous return reduces myocardial workload and gives the diaphragm maximum space to function. Sitting in a chair does not limit the volume of circulating blood, improve arterial blood pressure, or increase the strength of the heart muscle. (I, T, G, M)

28. 3. The external fetal monitor works by ultrasound. It monitors the fetal heart rate and periodic changes, but not the true R–R interval of the fetal heart rate, which is the baseline variability. The baseline variability can be assessed only through internal monitoring with a fetal scalp electrode. The external contraction monitor works via a pressure transducer placed across the mother's abdomen. It displays the frequency and duration of the contractions but not the true intensity or quality. Measuring the true intensity or quality requires an internal pressure device, because maternal tissues lie between the pressure transducer and the uterus. (I, N, H, O)

29. 1. A client diagnosed with outlet dystocia due to a narrow pubic arch will most likely need a forceps-assisted delivery. There is no immediate need for a cesarean section. A squatting position will not alleviate the outlet dystocia in this situation. This client does not need general anesthesia. (I, N, G, O)

30. 1. Adolescents are at greatest risk for scoliosis. Incidence is higher in females than in males. Incidence also increases during periods of rapid growth. A toddler with a diet low in vitamin D is prone to develop rickets. There is no relationship between poor prenatal care and scoliosis. (P, T, G, Y)

31. 1. The nurse's expression of concern for the client's safety may help the client validate her fears and choose to take action. Telling her to leave her husband is inappropriate advice. The idea of leaving the marriage may be so overwhelming that it may push the client away from the nurse as a support person. Talking to the client about changing her behavior or reducing family stress are forms of victim blaming. They reinforce the message that the client is responsible for the abuse—the same message that she is likely getting from the abuser and others. (I, T, L, X)

32. 2. A client who has experienced episodes of hypovolemic shock is at increased risk for adult respiratory distress syndrome (ARDS). Other risk factors include any type of shock, massive trauma, sepsis, aspiration or infectious pneumonia, near drowning, and inhalation of toxic substances. (A, C, G, M)

33. 1. The child should return to the emergency facility or receive prompt medical assessment if any signs of circulatory or neurological impairment is noted. Changes in temperature and loss of color indicate circulatory compromise, which may result from a tourniquet effect caused by the cast. If circulation is not restored, the result could be tissue loss due to anoxia. Cast drying takes more than 6 hours (possibly up to 24 hours). The child will experience some discomfort due to the fracture, and the cast will seem heavy. (E, N, S, Y)

34. 3. Because of the problems particular to pregnant unmarried adolescents, it is important for the nurse to learn about psychosocial factors in the client's life. When psychosocial problems exist, as they often do for these young women, the nurse can plan in cooperation with other health team members, whatever actions possible to make the client's pregnancy a healthful experience. To help a reluctant client, the nurse should convey a nonjudgmental and accepting attitude and keep channels of communication open. Threatening to withhold care if certain information is not given, saying that information is necessary for the record, and offering sympathy are unlikely to gain the client's trust and cooperation. (I, T, H, O)

35. 3. A child with gastroenteritis should receive clear liquids first. When the child can tolerate the clear liquids, a BRAT diet (bananas, rice cereal, applesauce, and toast) may be instituted. Milk-based foods are not recommended, because a child with gastroenteritis may become lactose-intolerant for a period following the acute illness. (I, N, G, Y)

36. 1. Keeping the child in a warm sleep environment will help decrease joint pain in the morning. Other good methods of keeping the child warm include using a heated water bed or an electric blanket. Having the child take a warm bath upon arising can also help. Any stress, such as lack of sleep, can exacerbate the joint stiffness and pain. Increasing pain medications at bedtime might help the child sleep more soundly, but blood levels would not last for the 8 to 10 hours that the child sleeps. Exercise prevents stiffness, but does not decrease the pain felt on arising. (P, N, G, Y)

37. 4. Poor muscle coordination and weakness are typical signs of lithium toxicity; so also are drowsiness and dehydration, marked by dry skin and mucous membranes. Additional untoward reactions to the drug may affect the central nervous system, cardiovascular system, gastrointestinal system, genitourinary system, and autonomic nervous system. (D, C, L, X)

38. 4. Early ambulation is credited with helping to prevent thrombophlebitis and pulmonary embolus. Early ambulation also helps prevent subinvolution of the uterus and complications related to urinary and intestinal elimination. Most clients feel less weak and psychologically better with early activity after delivery. Early ambulation does not prevent afterpains, endometritis, or vulvar edema. (I, N, H, O)

39. 1. Treatment of a child in vaso-occlusive crisis from sickle cell disease includes measures to prevent further sickling. Sickling occurs in the presence of decreased oxygen tension and alterations in pH. The hard sickle-shaped cells catch on each other and can eventually occlude vessels, which decreases oxygenation of the area and increases the sickling process. Increasing fluids will increase hemodilution and prevent the "clumps" of sickled cells from occluding vessels. Once a red blood cell has "sickled," it cannot be returned to the normal shape. The life span of a normal red blood cell is 120 days; there is no way to increase this life span. Hemolysis refers to the breakdown of red blood cells, something to be avoided in a child with sickle cell disease. (P, N, G, Y)

40. 3. The three-point gait, in which the client does not touch his affected leg to the ground, is the appropriate gait for this client to use. The other gaits require that the client be able to touch both feet to the ground. (P, C, S, M)

41. 2. Congenital aganglionic megacolon (Hirschsprung's disease) results in constipation due to lack of motility in a portion of the large intestine, which can include the rectal sphincter and may reach as far as the small intestine. The lack of motility is due to a congenital absence of the autonomic parasympathetic ganglion cells of the colon. Fecal material accumulates distal to the defect, resulting in constipation. Failure of the rectal sphincter to relax prevents evacuation of solids, liquids, and gas. Feeding methods are not altered, nor does the child have difficulty digesting nutrients. (D, N, G, Y)

42. 3. Pupil constriction in the presence of light during cardiopulmonary resuscitation generally indicates that the brain is receiving an adequate flow of oxygenated blood. A sufficient flow of oxygen to the brain is vital to sustain life. (E, T, G, M)

43. 3. Pursed-lip breathing helps prevent the collapse of alveoli in the lungs. In the presence of emphysema, a chronic state of hyperinflation results because of obstruction of bronchioles and a loss of elasticity in the lower pulmonary system, causing alveoli to collapse. Hyperinflation can be relieved somewhat by forcefully exhaling accumulated air through pursed-lip breathing to reduce intrapulmonary pressure. When alveoli function effectively, gas exchange in the lungs occurs properly. Pursed-lip breathing is not used primarily to promote a regular breathing pattern, although more regular breathing may result, nor is it used to sensitize central chemoreceptors in the medulla. (I, T, G, M)

44. 2. This client has class II cardiac disease. According to the New York Heart Association, the class II cardiac client has no symptoms at rest and has only minor activity restrictions. The client should get adequate rest and limit strenuous activity. The class III cardiac client is comfortable at rest but experiences excessive fatigue, palpitations, or dyspnea with less than ordinary physical activity. This client should have moderate to marked physical activity limitations. The class IV cardiac client has symptoms of cardiac insufficiency or of the anginal syndrome at rest and with any physical activity. This client may need to be maintained on bedrest for all or part of the pregnancy. (E, N, H, O)

45. 3. A client with diverticular disease should be instructed to avoid laxatives and enemas. These can lead to bowel perforation, especially during an acute episode of diverticulitis. Bulk-forming laxatives are acceptable. There is no need to avoid hot showers or milk products or to maintain a sitting position for 30 minutes after meals. (P, N, H, M)

46. 2. Vitamin B12 is essential for normal nervous system function. A client with pernicious anemia has a Vitamin B12 deficiency and is likely to develop neurological abnormalities if this deficiency is not corrected. (A, C, G, M)

47. 3. All of these goals are typical and appropriate for a client with rheumatoid arthritis. However, for an overweight client with rheumatoid arthritis, weight loss is especially important, because obesity increases stress on weight-bearing joints, increasing the risk of further damage. (P, T, G, M)

48. 1. This client is expressing the need to discuss her feelings. By encouraging her to do so, the nurse does not make any assumptions about what is bothering her. (E, N, H, O)

49. 1. Timolol maleate (Timoptic) eye drops reduce elevated, as well as normal, intraocular pressure and help prevent visual field loss. As with other topical ophthalmic drugs, this drug is absorbed systemically; its major side effects are slight bradycardia at rest, anorexia, and headache. Nausea and vomiting and vivid dreams are side effects of oral timolol maleate (Blocadren), an antihypertensive agent. (I, T, G, M)

50. 2. Denial is a coping mechanism used when a client is unable to accept his or her present condition. It buffers the client from the impact of overwhelming crisis. The behavior indicates a distorted comprehension of the burn. Regression produces infantile, demanding behavior. Depression results in lethargic, apathetic behavior. Flood reaction refers to an urgent attempt to settle family and financial problems. (D, T, L, M)

51. 1. Small infants often breathe using the abdominal muscles. A respiratory rate of 30 breaths/min. is normal for a 1-month-old infant. No intervention is necessary, and the assessment finding can be documented with no further action. (D, N, G, Y)

52. 2. When a child ingests a nonprescribed medication, the initial emergency treatment is to empty the stomach. This can be achieved by giving syrup of ipecac with fluids. If the child does not vomit within ½ hour, the dose can be repeated. Because medications are often rapidly absorbed, it is important that the parents attempt to empty the child's stomach before or during transport to the emergency room. Vomiting should not be induced in the child who has ingested a caustic material or a volatile liquid. (I, N, S, Y)

53. 1. A client with a possible spinal cord injury should be transported in such a way as to minimize movement, twisting, turning, and bending of the spine. Injury to the cord may be increased if the spine is not held straight. The best way to transport a client with possible spinal cord injury is to place him flat on his back on a flat board. (E, N, S, M)

54. 4. By observing for frequent swallowing, the nurse can evaluate whether or not the child is bleeding. Using a tongue blade to force open the mouth can result in broken teeth or tissue damage from a splintered tongue blade. Although a drop in blood pressure is a sign of blood loss, it is a very late sign in children. Decreased peripheral perfusion may also be a sign of blood loss; however, it is also a late sign. (A, N, G, Y)

55. 3. A microwave oven may interfere with proper pacemaker function. Microwave ovens have a particular frequency and wavelength of electromagnetic energy that may be picked up by the pacemaker and cause pacemaker stimulation. Some microwave ovens are advertised as safe for persons with pacemakers, and they probably are. The client should be taught that there appear to be few if any electrical hazards with the pacemakers and ovens now being manufactured, but that he should check to be sure. (I, T, S, M)

56. 4. Monitoring the client's vital signs, observing for convulsions, and administering lorazepam (Ativan) as ordered are important nursing actions for the client withdrawing from alcohol. Explaining the outpatient alcohol program to the client is inappropriate at this time. Explanations about rehabilitation programs should be provided when the client is physically more stable and able to comprehend the nurse's explanation. (I, T, L, X)

57. 3. Assessment tools that yield objective data are always preferable to those that yield subjective data. A fasting serum glucose level gives only a picture of the child's control in the immediate past. A glycosylated hemoglobin level gives the nurse data about the average blood glucose level over a 120-day span. It is an excellent tool for assessing control, detecting incorrect testing techniques by the child or family, monitoring the effectiveness of treatment changes, defining client goals, and detecting nonadherence. (A, N, G, Y)

58. 2. A client displaying manic behavior is commonly "on the go" almost constantly, often to the point of jeopardizing his or her health from a lack of rest and sleep. Therefore, the nurse should make concerted efforts to ensure that this client gets sufficient rest. Most often, a manic client does not need assistance in joining groups, finding things to do, and promoting cardiopulmonary activity; in fact, almost the opposite is true. (P, T, L, X)

59. 1. Parents of what they perceive as a less-than-perfect neonate may spend much time working through their grief. This process requires them to come to terms with the loss of the conceptualized ideal neonate and the reality of the less-than-perfect real neonate. One manifestation of nonacceptance of the neonate, or premature grieving of the death of a neonate, is the parents' failure to name the baby. There are no data to indicate ineffective coping, altered family functioning, or powerlessness related to inability to care for the neonate. (D, N, H, O)

60. 3. It is estimated that millions of Americans use marijuana regularly, and many people believe it should be legalized. Punitive measures and educational efforts to decrease its use have not fared well, most probably because little social stigma is attached to its use. Marijuana is not generally considered addictive, but it may cause psychological dependency. The active ingredient in marijuana has been well studied and its effects have been documented. Marijuana is not without harmful effects. (E, N, L, X)

61. 3. The nurse should discourage the client from focusing on his feelings of anger, because the feelings are out of control in this situation. Helping the client focus on thinking about the consequences of his actions would be safer and more productive for the client. Focusing on feelings in this situation would not be helpful to the client and may serve to escalate his anger. Helping the client find resources to obtain employment would come later in the process of crisis intervention; it ignores the client's immediate needs. (I, T, L, X)

62. 1. The pain of a duodenal peptic ulcer is ordinarily relieved by eating or by taking an alkali substance. The food and alkali help neutralize the excess acids that irritate gastrointestinal mucosa. The pain will gradually go away when secretion of stomach acid eventually stops. (A, C, G, M)

63. 1. When examining the tympanic membrane of a child under age 3, the nurse should pull the pinna down and back. For a child over age 3, the nurse should pull the pinna up and back to view the tympanic membrane. (A, T, G, Y)

64. 2. Measures to reduce the tenacity of respiratory secretions include humidifying inspired air and encouraging increased fluid intake. In postural drainage, the force of gravity is used to help promote drainage of secretions. Diaphragmatic breathing helps strengthen and increase the use of the diaphragm in breathing but does not reduce the tenacity of sputum. Oxygen does not reduce the tenacity of respiratory secretions. (P, T, G, M)

65. 4. The nurse should inform the child of events that will definitely happen. The physician may not order a "shot" or a nasogastric tube. If the nurse learns that these measures are ordered, then the child can be informed. The nurse should be honest about pain, but telling the child that it will "hurt really bad" may be frightening and may be untrue. The use of a human figure drawing gives the child concrete information about where the surgery will occur. (I, N, G, Y)

66. 3. When the child indicates that "it's OK now," he is indicating acceptance of his impending death. If the child says that he does not want to talk about his illness, he is probably showing denial, or maybe anger. When the child says that he does not want to talk because he is going to die anyway, he reveals bitterness and anger. The belief that a cure for his illness may be found suggests that the child is probably bargaining or denying his illness. (E, N, L, X)

67. 3. Preschool-age children engage in prelogical thinking. They also attribute occurrences to "magical" causes. At first glance, this child seems to understand that she is the victim of a contagious disease. However, the "jumping" of the "pox" when a person is close to another child is magical and not logical. If it were logical, everyone who came close to the ill child would automatically get the "pox." The "pox" takes on magical qualities; it is invisible when it jumps and can make you sick. (A, N, H, Y)

68. 3. Mafenide acetate (Sulfmylon Acetate) causes a burning pain when applied to a burn area. The discomfort is sometimes so severe that the nurse should consider administering a prescribed analgesic before applying the cream. (P, C, G, M)

69. 3. Taking iron supplements with citrus fruit juice, such as orange juice, improves iron absorption. Ferric iron is poorly absorbed, which means it has a low bioavailability within the intestinal tract. However, absorption is improved in the presence of an acid medium. Vitamin C (ascorbic acid) has been found to be particularly helpful in reducing Fe^{+++} to Fe^{++} for better absorption of supplemental iron and of dietary iron. (P, N, H, O)

70. 4. The primary action of oral hypoglycemic agents is to stimulate insulin release by the beta cells in the islets of Langerhans in the pancreas. The sulfonylureas may also alter cell-receptor sensitivity to insulin. Oral hypoglycemics can be used only when some function of the beta cells remains; they cannot be used when beta cells no longer function. The sulfonylureas do not influence urinary excretion of glucose, gluconeogenesis in the liver, or the action of insulin in body cells. (P, C, G, M)

71. 2. The nurse should give the frightened client an opportunity to express his fears rather than suggesting that there is no need for concern or handing him a manual to read. Listening to the client's fears gives the nurse a chance to select appropriate nursing interventions that may help alleviate these fears. (I, N, L, M)

72. 2. Probable signs of pregnancy include a positive pregnancy test, an enlarged uterus, Hegar's sign, and Braxton–Hicks contractions. A fetal outline can be distinguished. Presumptive signs of pregnancy include amenorrhea, morning sickness, frequency of voiding, breast tenderness, pigmentation of the skin, and quickening. Positive signs of pregnancy include fetal heart sounds, fetal movements, and a fetal outline visible on an x-ray examination or ultrasonography. (D, N, H, O)

73. 2. Although the physical manifestations of appendicitis may vary, it is common for the client to report tenderness or pain in the right lower quadrant of the abdomen (McBurney's point). Nausea, vomiting, and anorexia may also be present. The client may be mildly febrile (99–100.6°F). White blood cell count is frequently elevated. The client may feel the urge to defecate, but episodes of diarrhea alternating with constipation are not characteristic. Hematemesis (bloody emesis) and the presence of ascites are not typical of appendicitis. (A, C, G, M)

74. 4. The tip of the ventricular demand pacemaker is placed in the apex of the right ventricle, which is more muscular and thicker than the atrial wall. There is less tendency for the lead to become dislodged or rupture through the wall in this location. There are also atrial-ventricular pacemakers, in which the right atrium and right ventricle are paced and atrial output is maintained. (I, T, G, M)

75. 4. Myasthenia gravis is a chronic neuromuscular disease caused by a decrease in the number or effectiveness of acetylcholine receptors at the neuromuscular junction. Common symptoms include ptosis of the eyelids, diplopia, fatigue, and muscle weakness that increases with activity. The client also may experience respiratory difficulty, choking, and difficulty swallowing and chewing. (A, C, G, M)

76. 4. A full bladder during labor may impede labor primarily by interfering with the descent of the fetus in the birth canal. A full bladder also adds to the client's discomfort and predisposes to urine retention after delivery. It also may increase the intensity of the uterine contractions. If the client is unable to void, consideration may need to be given to catheterizing the client. However, the nurse should first attempt to promote normal voiding. (E, N, H, O)

77. 1. To show acceptance of the client, the nurse would first spend time with the client. Asking the client what he would like to change about himself ignores the client's needs and feelings at this time and would be more appropriate later during the client's hospitalization. Telling the client that he is a worthwhile person and that his family loves him are platitudes that will not help the client and ignores his feelings. (I, T, L, X)

78. 2. A common characteristic of the client with an obsessive-compulsive disorder is that he recognizes that his behavior is irrational but cannot change it. (D, C, L, X)

79. 3. Norplant acts by preventing ovulation in most women. Six silastic capsules containing the progestin levonorgestral are implanted surgically into the client's arm. These implants are effective for up to 5 years. Possible side effects include amenorrhea, irregular bleeding, spotting, weight gain, headaches, and depression. The implants are not known to cause congenital defects. The device does not interrupt spermatogenesis. (E, N, H, O)

80. 4. Croup results in inflammation in the trachea and larynx. The air being pulled through the narrowed upper airway causes stridor. The child must also use accessory muscles of respiration to pull the air past the obstruction, resulting in retractions. The harder the child works to breathe, the more severe the retractions. A child with croup often is able to maintain normal color and oxygen saturation. A low oxygen concentration and cyanosis indicate that the airway is becoming totally occluded. Vaponephrine is used to decrease the swelling of the tracheal and laryngeal tissue; it also tends to cause an increase in heart rate. (E, N, G, Y)

81. 2. Nutritionists often speak of protein nutrition in terms of nitrogen balance, because nitrogen is the element that makes proteins different from carbohydrates and fats. Large amounts of protein are lost with the exudate from burn wounds; therefore, a client in a state of negative nitrogen balance needs increased protein intake to return to nitrogen balance. (I, T, G, M)

82. 4. Fatigue, emotional lability, and loss of self-esteem and self-worth are some problems that may interfere with sexual activity for a client with multiple sclerosis. Resting before intercourse will help relieve some fatigue. Spasms of the adductor thigh muscles in women can make intercourse difficult, and these spasms do not respond to treatment with lubricants or stimulants. Perineal tightening exercises do not relieve any problem that interferes with sexual activity in a client with multiple sclerosis. Hot baths should be avoided, because they can increase weakness. (E, T, H, M)

83. 1. Vitamin B12 therapy for pernicious anemia must continue for life to prevent recurrence of symptoms, because the intrinsic factor does not return to gastric secretions, even with therapy. (P, C, G, M)

84. 2. Neuromuscular development follows a cephalocaudal direction. Head control is achieved first, followed by use of the arms and trunk, and then the legs. A child usually rolls over from the stomach to the back first, because as the head is raised to a 90-

degree angle, the weight of the head pulls the body over. Sitting requires trunk and arm control. Creeping and standing use leg muscles. (A, T, H, Y)

85. 3. Preoperative skin preparation is done primarily to reduce the number of organisms in the operative area. The skin cannot be rendered free of organisms. Skin preparation does not improve the field of vision for the physician. The skin's defenses are not necessarily improved, but reducing the number of organisms does decrease the likelihood of postoperative infection. (P, K, G, M)

86. 2. It is most important to obtain the rape victim's description of the assault. It may be desirable, but is not necessarily a legal requirement, to hand-carry evidence to a pathology laboratory, keep prying persons away from the victim, and have the victim escorted home. (I, T, S, X)

87. 1. An increased calcium intake is essential to help prevent osteoporosis. Postmenopausal women are at increased risk for osteoporosis, as are Caucasians and thin, petite women. Osteoporosis can and does develop before age 60. Middle-aged women are encouraged to increase their calcium intake and to decrease their consumption of alcohol, caffeine, and tobacco. Weight-bearing exercise is important to stimulate bone formation. (E, T, H, M)

88. 1. The normal range for the fetal heart rate about midway between contractions is 120 to 160 beats/min. During and immediately after a contraction, this range may be slightly lower. (I, T, G, O)

89. 1. The term "quickening" is synonymous with "feeling life." It is a probable sign of pregnancy, rather than a positive sign, because the sensation of feeling life can be confused with the movement of flatus in the intestines. Chadwick's sign, a dark discoloration of the vaginal tissues, is a presumptive sign of pregnancy. Ballottement is present when the fetus can be moved about in the uterus; it is a probable sign of pregnancy. Lightening occurs when the uterus descends into the pelvis, usually about 2 or 3 weeks before labor in primiparas and at or near the onset of labor in multiparas. (I, N, H, O)

90. 1. It is important for the child and family to understand that chorea associated with rheumatic fever is not permanent. The clumsiness and uncontrolled actions can be very upsetting to both the child and family. It is not necessary to assess the child's neurologic status or to keep the child warm. Since the child has cardiac involvement, ambulation is contraindicated. Aspirin is used primarily as an anti-inflammatory drug, and secondarily for pain relief. (P, N, G, Y)

91. 2. The nurse should handle a wet cast with the palms to prevent indentations in the cast. The cast should not be covered, as this will inhibit drying. A heat lamp should not be used to dry a cast, as this can cause the cast to crack and crumble. The client should be turned every 1 to 2 hours to promote cast drying. (I, T, S, M)

NURSING CARE COMPREHENSIVE TEST

TEST 4

Directions: Use this answer grid to determine areas of strength or need for further study.

NURSING PROCESS

A = Assessment
D = Analysis, nursing diagnosis
P = Planning
I = Implementation
E = Evaluation

COGNITIVE LEVEL

K = Knowledge
C = Comprehension
T = Application
N = Analysis

CLIENT NEEDS

S = Safe, effective care environment
G = Physiological integrity
L = Psychosocial integrity
H = Health promotion/maintenance

NURSING CARE AREA

O = Maternity and newborn care
X = Psychosocial health problems
Y = Nursing care of children
M = Medical-surgical health problems

		Nursing Process					Cognitive Level				Client Needs				Care Area			
Question #	Answer #	A	D	P	I	E	K	C	T	N	S	G	L	H	O	X	Y	M
1	1				I				T				L			X		
2	4				I					N	S							M
3	1	A							T				L			X		
4	1				I					N		G			O			
5	2				I				T				L			X		
6	2				I				T				L			X		
7	3				I					N				H	O			
8	3		D						T			G					Y	
9	4		D							N		G			O			
10	4				I					N				H	O			
11	1					E				N		G			O			
12	3				I				T				L			X		
13	3				I				T		S							M
14	3				I					N	S							M
15	3				I				T				L			X		
16	3					E			T			G					Y	
17	3		D						T				L			X		
18	4			P						N		G			O			

NURSING PROCESS

A = Assessment
D = Analysis, nursing diagnosis
P = Planning
I = Implementation
E = Evaluation

COGNITIVE LEVEL

K = Knowledge
C = Comprehension
T = Application
N = Analysis

CLIENT NEEDS

S = Safe, effective care environment
G = Physiological integrity
L = Psychosocial integrity
H = Health promotion/maintenance

NURSING CARE AREA

O = Maternity and newborn care
X = Psychosocial health problems
Y = Nursing care of children
M = Medical-surgical health problems

		Nursing Process					Cognitive Level				Client Needs				Care Area			
Question #	Answer #	A	D	P	I	E	K	C	T	N	S	G	L	H	O	X	Y	M
19	4				I					N		G					Y	
20	4	A							T			G						M
21	3				I				T				L			X		
22	3	A								N		G			O			
23	1					E				N		G					Y	
24	2					E				N			L			X		
25	3		D							N			L			X		
26	1	A							T			G			O			
27	4				I				T			G						M
28	3				I					N				H	O			
29	1				I					N		G			O			
30	1			P					T			G					Y	
31	1				I				T				L			X		
32	2	A						C				G						M
33	1					E				N	S						Y	
34	3				I				T					H	O			
35	3				I					N		G					Y	
36	1			P						N		G					Y	
37	4		D					C					L			X		
38	4				I					N				H	O			
39	1			P						N		G					Y	
40	3			P				C			S							M
41	2		D							N		G					Y	
42	3					E			T			G						M

ANSWER GRID: 2

Nursing Process

A = Assessment
D = Analysis, nursing diagnosis
P = Planning
I = Implementation
E = Evaluation

Cognitive Level

K = Knowledge
C = Comprehension
T = Application
N = Analysis

Client Needs

S = Safe, effective care environment
G = Physiological integrity
L = Psychosocial integrity
H = Health promotion/maintenance

Nursing Care Area

O = Maternity and newborn care
X = Psychosocial health problems
Y = Nursing care of children
M = Medical-surgical health problems

		Nursing Process					Cognitive Level				Client Needs				Care Area			
Question #	Answer #	A	D	P	I	E	K	C	T	N	S	G	L	H	O	X	Y	M
43	3				I				T			G						M
44	2					E				N				H	O			
45	3			P						N				H				M
46	2	A						C				G						M
47	3			P					T			G						M
48	1					E				N				H	O			
49	1				I				T			G						M
50	2		D						T				L					M
51	1		D							N		G					Y	
52	2				I					N	S						Y	
53	1					E				N	S							M
54	4	A								N		G					Y	
55	3				I				T		S							M
56	4				I				T				L			X		
57	3	A								N		G					Y	
58	2			P					T				L			X		
59	1		D							N				H	O			
60	3					E				N			L			X		
61	3				I				T				L			X		
62	1	A						C				G						M
63	1	A							T			G					Y	
64	2			P					T			G						M
65	4				I					N		G					Y	
66	3					E				N			L			X		

ANSWER GRID: 3

Nursing Process

A = Assessment
D = Analysis, nursing diagnosis
P = Planning
I = Implementation
E = Evaluation

Cognitive Level

K = Knowledge
C = Comprehension
T = Application
N = Analysis

Client Needs

S = Safe, effective care environment
G = Physiological integrity
L = Psychosocial integrity
H = Health promotion/maintenance

Nursing Care Area

O = Maternity and newborn care
X = Psychosocial health problems
Y = Nursing care of children
M = Medical-surgical health problems

		Nursing Process					Cognitive Level				Client Needs				Care Area			
Question #	Answer #	A	D	P	I	E	K	C	T	N	S	G	L	H	O	X	Y	M
67	3	A								N				H			Y	
68	3			P				C				G						M
69	3			P						N				H	O			
70	4			P				C				G						M
71	2				I					N			L					M
72	2		D							N				H	O			
73	2	A						C				G						M
74	4				I				T			G						M
75	4	A						C				G						M
76	4					E				N				H	O			
77	1				I				T				L			X		
78	2		D					C					L			X		
79	3					E				N				H	O			
80	4					E				N		G					Y	
81	2				I				T			G						M
82	4					E			T					H				M
83	1			P				C				G						M
84	2	A							T					H			Y	
85	3			P			K					G						M
86	2				I				T		S					X		
87	1					E			T					H				M
88	1				I				T			G			O			
89	1				I					N				H	O			
90	1			P						N		G					Y	

Answer Grid: 4

NURSING PROCESS

A = Assessment
D = Analysis, nursing diagnosis
P = Planning
I = Implementation
E = Evaluation

COGNITIVE LEVEL

K = Knowledge
C = Comprehension
T = Application
N = Analysis

CLIENT NEEDS

S = Safe, effective care environment
G = Physiological integrity
L = Psychosocial integrity
H = Health promotion/maintenance

NURSING CARE AREA

O = Maternity and newborn care
X = Psychosocial health problems
Y = Nursing care of children
M = Medical-surgical health problems

		Nursing Process					Cognitive Level				Client Needs				Care Area			
Question #	Answer #	A	D	P	I	E	K	C	T	N	S	G	L	H	O	X	Y	M
91	2				I				T		S							M
Number Correct																		
Number Possible	91	14	11	15	35	16	1	11	37	42	10	42	21	18	21	20	20	30
Percentage Correct																		

Score Calculation:
To determine your **Percentage Correct**, divide the **Number Correct** by the **Number Possible**.

ANSWER GRID: 5

State Boards of Nursing

Appendix

For further information about NCLEX-RN, write to the National Council of State Boards of Nursing, Inc.:

National Council of State Boards of Nursing, Inc.
676 North St. Clair Street
Suite 550
Chicago, Illinois 60611
(312) 787-6555

For information about the dates, requirements, and specifics of writing the examination in your state, contact the appropriate state board of nursing. The address and telephone number for each state board of nursing are provided below.

ALABAMA
Board of Nursing
RSA Plaza
Suite 250, 770 Washington Avenue
Montgomery, Alabama 36130
(205) 242-4060

ALASKA
Board of Nursing
Dept. of Commerce and Economic Development
Div. of Occupational Licensing
3601 C Street, Suite 722
Anchorage, Alaska 99503
(907) 561-2878

For Examination, License Verifications and Information:
Alaska Board of Nursing
P.O. Box 110806
Juneau, Alaska 99811-0806
(907) 465-2544

AMERICAN SAMOA
Health Service Regulatory Board
LBJ Tropical Medical Center
Pago Pago, American Samoa 96799
(684) 633-1222 Ext. 206

ARIZONA
Board of Nursing
2001 W. Camelback Road
Suite 350
Phoenix, Arizona 85015
(602) 255-5092

ARKANSAS
Arkansas State Board of Nursing
Univ. Tower Bldg.
Suite 800, 1123 South University
Little Rock, Arkansas 72204
(501) 686-2700

CALIFORNIA—RN
Board of Registered Nursing
P.O. Box 944210
Sacramento, California 94244-2100
(916) 322-3350

CALIFORNIA—VN
Board of Vocational Nurse and Psychiatric Technician Examiners
1414 K. Street, Suite 103
Sacramento, California 95814
(916) 445-0793

COLORADO
Board of Nursing
1560 Broadway, Suite 670
Denver, Colorado 80202
(303) 894-2430

CONNECTICUT
Board of Examiners for Nursing
150 Washington Street
Hartford, Connecticut 06106
(203) 566-1041

For Exam Information:
Examinations and Licensure Div. of Medical Quality Assurance
Dept. of Health Services
150 Washington Street
Hartford, Connecticut 06106
(203) 566-1032

DELAWARE
Board of Nursing
Margaret O'Neill Building
P.O. Box 1401
Dover, Delaware 19903
(302) 739-4522

DISTRICT OF COLUMBIA
Board of Nursing
614 H. Street, N.W.
Washington, District of Columbia 20001
(202) 727-7468

For Exam Information:
(202) 727-7454

FLORIDA
Board of Nursing
111 Coastline Drive, East, Suite 516
Jacksonville, Florida 32202
(904) 359-6331

For Exam Information:
Dept of Professional Regulation
1940 N. Monroe Street
Tallahassee, Florida 32399-0750
(904) 488-5952

GEORGIA—PN
Board of Licensed Practical Nurses
166 Pryor Street, S.W.
Atlanta, Georgia 30303
(404) 656-3921

For Exam Information:
Exam Development & Testing Unit
(404) 656-3903

GEORGIA—RN
Board of Nursing
166 Pryor Street, S.W.
Atlanta, Georgia 30303
(404) 656-3943

GUAM
Board of Nurse Examiners
P.O. Box 2816
Agana, Guam 96910
011-(671) 734-7295(6)
011-(671) 734-7304

HAWAII
Board of Nursing
P.O. Box 3469
Honolulu, Hawaii 96801
(808) 586-2695

IDAHO
Board of Nursing
280 North 8th Street, Suite 210
Boise, Idaho 83720
(208) 334-3110

ILLINOIS
Dept. of Professional Regulation
320 West Washington Street
3rd Floor
Springfield, Illinois 62786
(217) 785-9465
(217) 785-0800

For Exam Information:
Application Requests
Licensure Information
Asst. Nursing/Act Coordinator
(217) 782-0458
(217) 782-8556
(217) 785-9465

INDIANA
Board of Nursing
Health Professions Bureau
402 West Washington Street
Room #041
Indianapolis, Indiana 46204
(317) 232-2960

IOWA
Board of Nursing
State Capitol Complex
1223 East Court Avenue
Des Moines, Iowa 50319
(515) 281-3255

KANSAS
Board of Nursing
Landon State Office Building
900 S.W. Jackson, Suite 551-S
Topeka, Kansas 66612-1256
(913) 296-4929

KENTUCKY
Board of Nursing
312 Wittington Parkway, Suite 300
Louisville, Kentucky 40222-5172
(502) 329-7000

LOUISIANA—RN
Board of Nursing
912 Pere Marquette Building
150 Baronne Street
New Orleans, Louisiana 70112
(504) 568-5464

LOUISIANA—PN
Board of Practical Nurse Examiners
Tidewater Place
1440 Canal Street, Suite 1722
New Orleans, Louisiana 70112
(504) 568-6480

MAINE
Board of Nursing
State House Station #158
Augusta, Maine 04333-0158
(207) 624-5275

MARYLAND
Board of Nursing
4201 Patterson Avenue
Baltimore, Maryland 21215-2299
(301) 764-4741

MASSACHUSETTS
Board of Registration in Nursing
Leverett Saltonstall Building
100 Cambridge Street, Room 1519
Boston, Massachusetts 02202
(617) 727-9962

MICHIGAN
Bureau of Occupational and
Professional Regulation
Dept. of Commerce
Ottawa Towers North
611 West Ottawa
Lansing, Michigan 48933
(517) 373-1600

For Exam Information:
Office of Testing Services
Department of Commerce
P.O. Box 30018
Lansing, Michigan 48909
(517) 373-3877

MINNESOTA
Board of Nursing
2700 University Avenue, West #108
St. Paul, Minnesota 55114
(612) 642-0567

MISSISSIPPI
Board of Nursing
239 N. Lamar Street, Suite 401
Jackson, Mississippi 39201-1311
(601) 359-6170

MISSOURI
Board of Nursing
P.O. Box 656
Jefferson City, Missouri 65102
(314) 751-0681

MONTANA
Board of Nursing
Dept. of Commerce
Arcade Building, Lower Level
111 North Jackson
Helena, Montana 59620-0407
(406) 444-4279

NEBRASKA
Bureau of Examining Boards
Dept. of Health
P.O. Box 95007
Lincoln, Nebraska 68509
(402) 471-2115

NEVADA
Board of Nursing
1281 Terminal Way, Suite 116
Reno, Nevada 89502
(702) 786-2778

NEW HAMPSHIRE
Board of Nursing
Health & Welfare Building
6 Hazen Drive
Concord, New Hampshire 03301-6527
(603) 271-2323

NEW JERSEY
Board of Nursing
P.O. Box 45010
Newark, New Jersey 07101
(201) 504-6493

NEW MEXICO
Board of Nursing
4253 Montgomery Blvd., Suite 130
Albuquerque, New Mexico 87109
(505) 841-8340

NEW YORK
Board of Nursing
State Education Department
Cultural Education Center,
Room 3023
Albany, New York 12230
(518) 474-3843/3845

For Exam Information:
Div. of Professional Licensing
Services
State Education Department
Cultural Education Center
Albany, New York 12230
(518) 474-6591

NORTH CAROLINA
Board of Nursing
P.O. Box 2129
Raleigh, North Carolina 27602
(919) 782-3211

NORTH DAKOTA
Board of Nursing
919 South 7th Street, Suite 504
Bismarck, North Dakota 58504-5881
(701) 224-2974

NORTHERN MARIANA ISLANDS
Commonwealth Board of Nurse
Examiners
Public Health Center
P.O. Box 1458
Saipan, MP 96950
011-670-234-8950

OHIO
Board of Nursing
77 South High Street, 17th Floor
Columbus, Ohio 43266-0316
(614) 466-3947

OKLAHOMA
Board of Nurse Registration
& Nursing Education
2915 North Classen Blvd., Suite 524
Oklahoma City, Oklahoma 73106
(405) 525-2076

OREGON
Board of Nursing STE 465
800 NE Oregon St. #25
Portland, Oregon 97232
(503) 731-4745

PENNSYLVANIA
Board of Nursing
P.O. Box 2649
Harrisburg, Pennsylvania 17105
(717) 783-7142

PUERTO RICO
Commonwealth of Puerto Rico
Board of Nurse Examiners
Call Box 10200
Santurce, Puerto Rico 00908
(809) 725-8161

RHODE ISLAND
Board of Nurse Registration
& Nursing Education
Cannon Health Building
Three Capitol Hill, Room 104
Providence, Rhode Island 02908-5097
(401) 277-2827

SOUTH CAROLINA
Board of Nursing
220 Executive Center Drive, Suite 220
Columbia, South Carolina 29210
(803) 731-1648

SOUTH DAKOTA
Board of Nursing
3307 South Lincoln Avenue
Sioux Falls, South Dakota 57105-5224
(605) 335-4973

TENNESSEE
Board of Nursing
283 Plus Park Blvd.
Nashville, Tennessee 37247-1010
(615) 367-6232

TEXAS—RN
Board of Nurse Examiners
P.O. Box 140466
Austin, Texas 78714
(512) 835-4880

TEXAS—VN
Board of Vocational Nurse Examiners
9101 Burnet Road, Suite 105
Austin, Texas 78758
(512) 835-2071

UTAH
Board of Nursing
Div. of Occupational & Prof. Licensing
P.O. Box 45805
Salt Lake City, Utah 84145-0805
(801) 530-6628

VERMONT
Board of Nursing
Redstone Building
26 Terrace Street
Montpelier, Vermont 05602-1106
(802) 828-2396

VIRGIN ISLANDS
Board of Nurse Licensure
P.O. Box 4247, Veterans Drive Station
St. Thomas, U.S. Virgin Islands 00803
(809) 776-7397

VIRGINIA
Board of Nursing
1601 Rolling Hills Drive
Richmond, Virginia 23229-5005
(804) 662-9909

WASHINGTON—RN
Board of Nursing
Dept. of Health
P.O. Box 47864
Olympia, Washington 98504-7864
(206) 753-2686

WASHINGTON—PN
Board of Practical Nursing
1300 S.E. Quince Street
P.O. Box 47865
Olympia, Washington 98504-7865
(206) 753-2807

WEST VIRGINIA—RN
Board of Examiners for Registered
Professional Nurses
101 Dee Drive
Charleston, West Virginia 25311-1688
(304) 558-3596

WEST VIRGINIA—PN
Board of Examiners for Practical
Nurses
101 Dee Drive
Charleston, West Virginia 25311-1688
(304) 558-3572

WISCONSIN
Bureau of Health Service Professions
1400 East Washington Avenue
P.O. Box 8935
Madison, Wisconsin 53708-8935
(608) 266-0257

WYOMING
Board of Nursing
Barrett Building, 2nd Floor
2301 Central Avenue
Cheyenne, Wyoming 82002
(307) 777-7601

NCLEX Practice Test Program Instructions

This software program has been designed to be used with an IBM or IBM compatible computer. To start the program, insert the diskette in the floppy drive and set the default to the floppy drive (e.g., Drive A or Drive B). At the prompt (A:\> or B:\>), type GO and press the Enter key.

This program enables you to answer 100 questions on the computer similar to the way in which you will take the NCLEX Examination after the NCLEX-CAT is implemented.

As in the NCLEX Examination, all questions on this program are multiple choice. To answer questions, you will need only three computer keys—the up and down Arrows and the Enter key. Use the Arrow keys to highlight the answer you want to select. To enter the highlighted answer as your choice, simply press the Enter key. (The actual NCLEX Examination will require you to use the Space Bar to move the cursor among the answer choices and to press the Enter key twice to select the answer choice.)

This practice test allows you two testing options and an option to see your test results. Each computer screen has prompts at the bottom of the screen that will provide any needed instructions. The program menu will look like this.

1. Instructions
2. Take the Test
3. Try Again
4. Review Your Results
5. Quit

The "Take the Test" option will allow you to answer all 100 questions and will store your answers in memory. To do this, select number two (2) from the menu. You can choose to have the test timed, to have the program show you the time remaining, and to have the program show you the number of questions you have completed. When you have completed the test, you can choose to see the "Review Your Results" screen. You can also choose the "Review Your Results" option, (4) from the menu, which will show you a chart that indicates the following (the chart will look like the Answer Grids that appear after each review test in the book):

- question number
- whether you answered the questions correctly (a checkmark indicates that you answered the question correctly, an "X" indicates that you answered the question incorrectly, and no mark indicates that you did not answer the question)
- the Attributes for each question
  —Nursing Process Step
  —Client Need
  —Nursing Care Area

This way, you can see how well you did on this sample test.

The "Try Again" option, (3) from the menu, will give you all 100 questions again with a check mark next to each question you answered correctly. All questions without a check mark were either answered incorrectly or not answered. The "Try Again" option allows you to work on those questions that you got wrong or did not answer. This way, you can practice questions that were a problem. This option will give you three tries to answer the question (the screen will say "NO, try again"). If your third answer choice is also incorrect, the program will show you the correct answer. If your second (or third) answer choice is correct, the screen will say "That's right." (As the Preface of this book describes, the NCLEX Examination will not allow you to try a question a second time and will, of course, not provide you with test results.)

Good luck and enjoy practicing on this disk before you take the real examination!